Molecular Biomethods Handbook

Second Edition

Molecular Biomethods Handbook

Second Edition

Edited by

John M. Walker

Professor Emeritus
School of Life Sciences
University of Hertfordshire
Hatfield, Hertfordshire, UK

Ralph Rapley

School of Life Sciences
University of Hertfordshire
Hatfield, Hertfordshire, UK

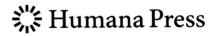 Humana Press

Editors
John M. Walker
Professor Emeritus School of Life Sciences
University of Hertfordshire
Hatfield, Hertfordshire, UK

Ralph Rapley
School of Life Sciences
University of Hertfordshire
Hatfield, Hertfordshire, UK

ISBN (hardcover): 978-1-60327-370-1   e-ISBN: 978-1-60327-375-6
ISBN (softcover): 978-1-60327-374-9
DOI: 10.1007/978-1-60327-375-6

Library of Congress Control Number: 2008923167

Cover illustration: Fig. 55.3(B), "Confocal Microscopy," by Guy Cox

Printed on acid-free paper

9 8 7 6 5 4 3 2 1

springer.com

Preface

There have been numerous advances made in many fields of the biosciences in recent years, and perhaps the most dramatic advances have been in our ability to investigate and define cellular processes at the molecular level. These insights have been largely owing to the development and application of powerful new techniques in molecular biology—nucleic acid, protein, and cell-based methodologies, in particular.

In the first edition of the *Molecular Biomethods Handbook*, we introduced the reader to a selection of analytical and preparative techniques that we considered to be frequently used by research workers in the field of molecular biology. Clearly, within the constraints of a single volume we had to be selective in the techniques we described. Since the first edition was published, science has continued to move on apace. For example, the use of microarray technology is now commonplace, nanotechnology has entered the scientific literature, microfluidic technology has been developed, the tremendous potential of stem cells has been recognized, single-cell analysis is becoming routine, the human genome has been sequenced, and new techniques for mapping and RNA expression have been introduced. The second edition is consequently significantly expanded, with over 1100 pages compared to the 720 pages of the first edition.

As with the first edition, we have aimed to describe the theory, outline practical procedures, and provide the applications of the techniques described. For those who require detailed laboratory protocols, these can be found in the references cited in each chapter and in the laboratory protocol series *Methods in Molecular Biology*™ published by Humana Press.

This book should prove useful to undergraduate students (especially project students), Masters students, postgraduate research students, and research scientists and technicians who wish to understand and use new techniques, but who do not have the necessary background for setting up such techniques. In addition, this book will be useful for those wishing to update their knowledge of particular techniques. All the chapters have been written by well-established research scientists who run their own research programs and who use the methods on a regular basis. We hope that this edition will prove to be a useful source of information in the molecular biosciences and a valuable text for those engaged in or entering the field of molecular biology.

John M. Walker
Ralph Rapley

Contents

Part B Protein and Cell Methods

Contributors

Marie-Isabel Aguilar, BSc, PhD
Department of Biochemistry and Molecular Biology, Monash University, Clayton, Victoria, Australia

Rob Aitken, BSc, PhD
Division of Infection and Immunity, Institute of Biomedical and Life Sciences, Glasgow Biomedical Research Centre, University of Glasgow, Glasgow, Scotland, UK

Maher Albitar, BSc, PhD
Department of Hematopathology, Nichols Institute, Quest Diagnostics, San Juan Capistrano, CA

Marilena Aquino de Muro, BSc, PhD
University of Caxias of the South, Francisco Getulio Vargas, Petropolis, Caxias of the South, RS, Brazil

Katja M. Arndt, BSc, PhD
Institute of Biology III, Albert-Ludwigs-University of Freiburg, Freiburg, Germany

Jane Bayani, BSc, MHSc
Department of Applied Molecular Oncology, Princess Margaret Hospital, University Health Network, Toronto, Ontario, Canada

Erica E. Benson, BSc, PhD
Environmental Science and Biotechnology, Cupar Muir, Cupar, Fife, Scotland, UK

Terry D. Butters, BSc, PhD
Glycobiology Institute, Department of Biochemistry, Oxford University, Oxford, Oxfordshire, UK

Adam Charlton, BSc, PhD
Industrial Biotechnology, CSIRO Molecular and Health Technology, Clayton, Victoria, Australia

Yann-Jang Chen, MD, PhD
Faculty of life Sciences, National Yang-Ming University, Taipei, Taiwan; and
Department of Pediatrics, Taipei Veterans General Hospital, Taipei, Taiwan

Quan Jason Cheng, BSc, PhD
Department of Chemistry, University of California, Riverside, CA

Chellu S. Chetty, BSc, PhD
Department of Natural Sciences and Mathematics, Savannah State University,
Savannah, GA

Charlotte H. Clarke, BSc, PhD
Ciphergen, Fremont, CA

Lisa Montoya Cockrell, BSc, PhD
Graduate Program of Molecular and Systems Pharmacology, Emory
University School of Medicine, Atlanta, GA

Gayle Corkill, BSc, PhD
Cyprotex, Macclesfield, Cheshire, UK

Guy Cox, BSc, PhD
Electron Microscope Unit, University of Sydney, Sydney, New South Wales,
Australia

John Crowther, BSc, PhD
International Atomic Energy Agency, Vienna, Austria

Mare Cudic, BSc, PhD
Department of Chemistry and Biochemistry, Florida Atlantic University,
Boca Raton, FL

Paul Cutler, BSc, PhD
GlaxoSmithKline, Stevenage, Hertfordshire, UK

Ian A. Darby, BSc, PhD
Microvascular Biology Lab, School of Medical Sciences, RMIT University,
Bundoora, Victoria, Australia

Ian Davidson, BSc, PhD
School of Medical Sciences, University of Medical Sciences, IMS Building,
Foresterhill, Aberdeen, Scotland, UK

John G. Day, BSc, PhD
Curator CCAP, Culture Collection of Algae and Protozoa, Scottish
Association for Marine Science, Dunstaffnage Marine Laboratory, Dunbeg,
Argyll, Scotland, UK

C. De-la-Peña, BSc, PhD
Department of Horticulture and Landscape Architecture, Colorado State
University, Fort Collins, CO

Patricia de Winter, BSc, PhD
Cardiovascular Division, School of Medicine, King's College London,
London Bridge, London, UK

Arnis Druka, BSc, PhD
Department of Genetics, SCRI Invergowrie, Dundee, Scotland, UK

Yuhong Du, BSc, PhD
Department of Pharmacology, Emory University School of Medicine,
Atlanta, GA

Phillip G. Febbo, MD
Duke Institute for Genome Science and Policy, Departments of Medicine
and Molecular Genetics and Microbiology, Duke University, Durham, NC

Gregg B. Fields, BSc, PhD
Department of Chemistry and Biochemistry, Florida Atlantic University,
Boca Raton, FL

Haian Fu, BSc, PhD
Department of Pharmacology, Emory University School of Medicine,
Atlanta, GA

Birte Fuchs, BSc, PhD
Institut fur Molekularbiologie and Biochemi, Freie Universitat Berlin,
Berlin, Germany

Eric T. Fung, BSc, PhD
Ciphergen, Fremont, CA

Annette Gaida, BSc, PhD
Institute for Biology III, Albert-Ludwigs University of Freiburg,
Freiburg, Germany

R. M. Galaz-Ávalos, BSc, PhD
Centro de Investigacion Cientificia de Yucatan, Yucatan, Mexico

Lúcia Maria da Cunha Galvão, BSc, PhD
Departamento de Parasitologia, Instituto de Ciências Biológicas (ICB),
Universidade Federal de Minas Gerais (UFMG), Belo Horizonte, Minas
Gerais, Brazil

Patricia Gravel, BSc, PhD
V.P. Medicinal Product and Regultory Affairs, Triskel Integrated Services,
Geneva, Switzerland

Simon G. Gregory, BSc, PhD
Center for Human Genetics, Durham, NC

Urs B. Hagemann, BSc, PhD
Institute of Biology III, Albert-Ludwigs-University of Freiburg,
Freiburg, Germany

Keith C. Harding, BSc, PhD
Environmental Science and Biotechnology, Cuparmuir, Cupar, Fife,
Scotland, UK

Bronwen M. Harvey, BSc, PhD
GE Healthcare, Medical Diagnostics, Group Centre, Amersham,
Buckinghamshire, UK

Jonathan Havel, BSc, PhD
Graduate Program of Molecular and Systems Pharmacology, Emory
University School of Medicine, Atlanta, GA

Pete Hedley, BSc, PhD
Department of Genetics, SCRI Invergowrie, Dundee, Scotland, UK

Tim D. Hewitson, BSc, PhD
Department of Medicine, University of Melbourne, Melbourne,
Victoria, Australia

Charles Z. Hotz, BSc, PhD
True Materials Inc., San Francisco, CA

William P. Janzen, BSc, PhD
Amphora Discovery Sciences "(retired)," Chapel Hill, NC

Gareth J. S. Jenkins, BSc, PhD
School of Medicine, Swansea University, Singleton Park, Swansea,
Wales, UK

Eva M. Jouaux, BSc, PhD
Institute of Biology III, Albert-Ludwigs-University of Freiburg,
Freiburg, Germany

Christoph Kannicht, BSc, PhD
Institut fur Molekularbiologie and Biochemi, Freie Universitat Berlin,
Berlin, Germany

Katherine A. Kantardjieff, BSc, PhD
Department of Chemistry and Biochemistry, California State University,
Fullerton, CA

Andrea Kasinki, BSc, PhD
Graduate Program of Genetics and Molecular Biology, Emory University
School of Medicine, Atlanta, GA

Anna C. Kinsella, BSc, PhD
Department of Chemistry, Saint Louis University, St. Louis, MO

Ludmila Kousoulidou, BSc, PhD
Department of Cytogenetics, The Cyprus Institute of Neurology and
Genetics, Nicosia, Cyprus

John Kuo, BSc, PhD
Centre for Microscopy and Microanalysis, The University of Western
Australia, Crawley, Western Australia, Australia

Eliane Lages-Silva, BSc, PhD
Departamento de Ciências Biológicas, Universidade Federal do Triângulo
Mineiro, Uberaba, Minas Gerais, Brazil

Simon P. Langdon, BSc, PhD
Cancer Research Centre, University of Edinburgh, Edinburgh, Scotland, UK

Tzong-Hsien Lee, BSc, PhD
Department of Biochemistry and Molecular Biology, Monash University,
Clayton, Victoria, Australia

Kim Hung Leung, BSc, PhD
Department of Health Technology and Informatics, The Hong Kong
Polytechnic University, Hung Hom, Kowloon, Hong Kong SAR, China

Chi-Hung Lin, MD, PhD
Institute of Microbiology and Immunology/Institute of Biophotonics
Engineering, Yang-Ming Genome Research Center, National Yang-Ming
University, Taipei, Taiwan

Victor M. Loyola-Vargas, BSc, PhD
Centro de Investigacion Cientificia de Yucatan, Yucatan, Mexico

Jody M. Mason, BSc, PhD
Institute of Biology III, Albert-Ludwigs-University of Freiburg,
Freiburg, Germany

Shelley D. Minteer, BSc, PhD
Department of Chemistry, Saint Louis University, St. Louis, MO

Glenn E. Morris, BSc, PhD
Centre for Inherited Neuromuscular Disease (CIND), Leopold Muller ARC
Building, Robert Jones and Agnes Hunt Orthopopaedic Hospital, Oswestry,
Shropshire, UK

Kristian M. Müller, BSc, PhD
Institute of Biology III, Albert-Ludwigs-University of Freiburg,
Freiburg, Germany

Graeme I. Murray, BSc, PhD
Department of Pathology, University Medical Buildings, University of
Aberdeen, Foresterhill, Aberdeen, Scotland, UK

Jayanthi Nadarajan, BSc, PhD
Millennium Seed Bank, Royal Botanic Gardens, Ardingly, Haywards Heath,
W. Sussex, UK

David C. A. Neville, BSc, PhD
Glycobiology Institute, Department of Biochemistry, Oxford University,
Oxford, Oxfordshire, UK

Paula O'Connor, BSc, PhD
School of Medical Sciences, University of Medical Sciences, IMS Building,
Foresterhill, Aberdeen, Scotland, UK

Paul A. O'Farrell, BSc, PhD
Senior Lecturer in Biochemistry, Royal College of Surgeons in Ireland-
Medical University of Bahrain, Adliya, Kingdom of Bahrain

Siobhan O'Sullivan, BSc, PhD
Department of Biochemistry, University College Cork,
Lee Maltings, Mardyke, Cork, Ireland

Constance Oliver, BSc, PhD
Departamento Biologia Celular e Molecular e Bioagentes Patogênicos,
Faculdade de Medicina de Ribeirão Preto – USP, Ribeirão Preto, SP, Brasil

Hae Ryoun Park, BSc, PhD
Pusan University, Namgu, Busan, Korea

Philippos C. Patsalis, PhD
Department of Cytogenetics, The Cyprus Institute of Neurology and
Genetics, Nicosia, Cyprus

Dorien J. M. Peters, BSc, PhD
Center for Human and Clinical Genetics, LUMC, Sylvius Laboratory,
Leiden, The Netherlands

K. Scott Phillips, BSc, PhD
Department of Physiology and Biophysics, University of California, Irvine, CA

Pottumarthi V. Prasad, BSc, PhD
Department of Radiology, MRI, Evanston Northwestern Healthcare,
Evanston, IL

F. R. Quiroz-Figueroa, BSc, PhD
Department of Molecular Biology of Plants, Istituto de Biotechnologia,
Universidad Nacional Autonoma de Mexico (UNAM), Cuernavaca, Morelos,
Mexico

Ralph Rapley, BSc, PhD
School of Life Sciences, University of Hertfordshire, Hatfield,
Hertfordshire, UK

Bernd H. A. Rehm, BSc, PhD
Institute of Molecular BioSciences, Massey University, Palmerston North,
New Zealand

Frank Reinecke, PhD
Institut für Medizinische Physik und Biophysik, Elektronenmikroskopie und
Analytik, Universitätsklinikum Münster, Westfälische Wilhelms-Universität,
Münster, Germany

Jeroen H. Roelfsema, BSc, PhD
Center for Human and Clinical Genetics, LUMC, Sylvius Laboratory,
Leiden, The Netherlands

Bernhard Rupp, BSc, PhD
q.e.d. Life Science Discoveries, Livermore, CA

Beatriz Sanchez-Vega, BSc, PhD
Head of the Genomics Laboratory, Hospital General Universitario Reina
Sofia, Murcia, Spain

David Sheehan, BSc, PhD
Department of Biochemistry, University College Cork, Lee Maltings,
Mardyke, Cork, Ireland

Nameeta Shah, BSc, PhD
Institute for Data Analysis and Visualization (IDAV), Department of
Computer Science, University of California, Davis, CA

Carolina Sismani, BSc, PhD
Department of Cytogenetics, The Cyprus Institute of Neurology and
Genetics, Nicosia, Cyprus

Jonathan D. Smith, PhD
Department of Cell Biology, Cleveland Clinic Foundation, Cleveland, OH

Pirkko Soundy, BSc, PhD
GE Healthcare, The Grove Centre, Amersham, Buckinghamshire, UK

Jeremy A. Squire, BSc, PhD
Division of Applied Molecular Oncology, Ontario Cancer Institute,
Princess Margaret Hospital, University Health Network, Toronto,
Ontario; and University of Toronto, Toronto, Ontario, Canada

Kenneth G. Standing, BSc, PhD
Department of Physics and Astronomy, University of Manitoba, Winnipeg,
Manitoba, Canada

Sabine C. Stebel, BSc, PhD
Institute of Biology III, Albert-Ludwigs-University of Freiburg,
Freiburg, Germany

Maryalice Stetler-Stevenson, BSc, PhD
Laboratory of Pathology, NCI, NIH, Bethesda, MD

Pippa Storey, BSc, PhD
Department of Radiology, MRI, Evanston Northwestern Healthcare,
Evanston, IL

Mark Strege, BSc, PhD
Lilly Research Laboratories, Eli Lilly and Co., Lilly Corporate Center,
Indianapolis, IN

David Sugden, BSc, PhD
Reader in Cellular Endocrinology, Division of Reproduction and
Endocrinology, School of Biomedical and Health Sciences, King's College
London, London Bridge, London, UK

Anu Suomalainen, BSc, PhD
Research Program of Molecular Neurology, Biomedicum-Helsinki,
University of Helsinki, Helsinki, Finland

Ann-Christine Syvänen, PhD
Department of Medical Sciences, Uppsala University,
Research Department 2, University Hospital, Uppsala, Sweden

Bimal D. M. Theophilus, BSc, PhD
Department of Haematology, Birmingham Children's Hospital, NHS Trust,
Birmingham, West Midlands, UK

Francisca Reyes-Turcu, BSc, PhD
Department of Biochemistry, Emory University School of Medicine,
Atlanta, GA

Mohan C. Vemuri, BSc, PhD
Invitrogen Corporation, Grand Island, NY

John M. Walker, BSc, PhD
Professor Emeritus, School of Life Sciences, University of Hertfordshire,
Hatfield, Hertfordshire, UK

Peng-Hui Wang, MD
Department of Obstetrics and Gynecology, Taipei Veterans General Hospital;
National Yang-Ming University School of Medicine, Taipei, Taiwan

Robbie Waugh
Department of Genetics, SCRI Invergowie, Dundee, Scotland, UK

James L. Weaver, BSc, PhD
Department of Applied Pharmacology Research, CDER, White Oak, MD

Keith D. Wilkinson, BSc, PhD
Department of Biochemistry, Emory University School of Medicine,
Atlanta, GA

Thomas Willemsen, BSc, PhD
Institute of Biology III, Albert-Ludwigs-University of Freiburg,
Freiburg, Germany

Craig Winstanley, BSc, PhD
Division of Medical Microbiology and Genitourinary Medicine, University
of Liverpool, Liverpool, UK

Shea Ping Yip, BSc, PhD
Department of Health Technology and Informatics, The Hong Kong
Polytechnic University, Hung Hom, Kowloon, Hong Kong SAR, China

Michael Zachariou, PhD
Director Project Management, Technical Operations, Bio Marin
Pharmaceutical Inc., Novato, CA

Zhong J. Zhang, BSc, PhD
Hematopathology, Nichols Institute, Quest Diagnostics, San Juan
Capistrano, CA

Jing Zhao, BSc, PhD
Department of Pharmacology, Emory University School of Medicine,
Atlanta, GA

Part A
Nucleic Acid Methods

1

The Manipulation of Nucleic Acids
Basic Tools and Techniques

Gayle Corkill and Ralph Rapley

1. Introduction

There have been many developments over the past three decades that have led to the efficient manipulation and analysis of nucleic acids and proteins. Many of these have resulted from the isolation and characterization of numerous DNA-manipulating enzymes, such as DNA polymerase, DNA ligase, and reverse transcriptase. However, perhaps the most important was the isolation and application of a number of enzymes that enabled the reproducible digestion of DNA. These enzymes, termed *restriction endonucleases* or *restriction enzymes*, provided a turning point for not only the analysis of DNA but also the development of recombinant DNA technology and provided a means for the detection and identification of disease and disease markers.

1.1. Enzymes Used in Molecular Biology

Restriction endonucleases recognize specific DNA target sequences, mainly 4–6 bp in length, and cut them, reproducibly, in a defined manner. The nucleotide sequences recognized are of an inverted repeat nature (typically termed *palindromic*), reading the same in both directions on each strand *(1)*. When cut or cleaved, they produce a flush or blunt-ended, or a staggered, cohesive-ended fragment depending on the particular enzyme as indicated in **Fig. 1.1**. An important property of cohesive ends is that DNA from different sources (e.g., different organisms) digested by the same restriction endonuclease will be complementary (termed "sticky") and so will join or anneal to each other. The annealed strands are held together only by hydrogen-bonding between complementary bases on opposite strands. Covalent joining of nucleotide ends on each of the two strands may be brought about by the introduction of the enzyme DNA ligase. This process, termed *ligation*, is widely exploited in molecular biology to enable the construction of recombinant DNA molecules (i.e., the joining of DNA fragments from different sources). Approximately 500 restriction enzymes have been characterized to date that recognize over 100 different target sequences. A number of these, termed *isoschizomers*,

From: *Molecular Biomethods Handbook, 2nd Edition.*
Edited by: J. M. Walker and R. Rapley © Humana Press, Totowa, NJ

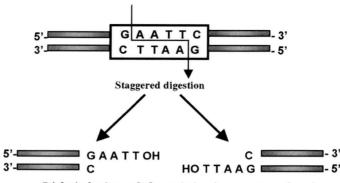

Fig. 1.1. The cleavage of a DNA strand with a target site for the restriction enzyme EcoR1 indicating the ends of the DNA formed following digestion.

recognize different target sequences but produce the same staggered ends or overhangs. With the vast number of restriction endonucleases it can be difficult and laborious to determine the number of restriction sites present within a given DNA sequence. There are many instances where it would be beneficial to attain this information quickly and easily; design of plasmids, site-directed mutagenesis investigations, PCR primer design etc. Programs are available free of charge on the Internet that identify restriction sites according to criteria defined by the user within the Input DNA sequence (e.g., Webcutter).

In addition to restriction enzymes a number of other enzymes have proved to be of value in the manipulation of DNA and are indicated at appropriate points within this chapter.

2. Extraction and Separation of Nucleic Acids

2.1. DNA Extraction Techniques

The use of DNA for medical analysis or for research-driven manipulation usually requires that it be isolated and purified to a certain degree. DNA is usually recovered from cells by methods that include cell rupture but that prevent the DNA from fragmenting by mechanical shearing. This is generally undertaken in the presence of EDTA, which chelates the magnesium ions needed as cofactors for enzymes that degrade DNA, termed *DNase*. Ideally, cell walls, if present, should be digested enzymatically (e.g., lysozyme in the bacteria or bacterial cell). In addition the cell membrane should be solubilized using detergent. Indeed, if physical disruption is necessary, it should be kept to a minimum and should involve cutting or squashing of cells, rather than the use of shear forces. Cell disruption and most of the subsequent steps should be performed at 4°C, using glassware and solutions that have been autoclaved to destroy DNase activity. After release of nucleic acids from the cells, RNA can be removed by treatment with ribonuclease (RNase) that has been heat treated to inactivate any DNase contaminants; RNase is relatively stable to heat as a result of its disulfide bonds, which ensure rapid renaturation of the molecule on cooling. The other major contaminant, protein, is removed by shaking the solution gently with water-saturated phenol, or with a phenol/chloroform mixture, either of which will denature proteins but not nucleic acids. Centrifugation of the emulsion formed by this mixing produces a lower, organic phase, separated from the upper, aqueous phase by an interface of denatured protein. The aqueous solution is recovered and deproteinized repeatedly, until no more material is seen at the interface. Finally, the deproteinized DNA preparation is mixed with two volumes of absolute ethanol, and the DNA is allowed to precipitate out of solution in a freezer. After centrifugation, the DNA pellet is redissolved in a buffer containing EDTA to inactivate any DNases present. This solution can be stored at 4°C for at least a month. DNA solutions can be stored frozen, although repeated freezing and thawing tends to damage long DNA molecules by shearing. A flow diagram summarizing the extraction of DNA is given in **Fig. 1.2**. The above-described procedure is suitable for total cellular DNA. If the DNA from a specific organelle or viral particle is needed, it is best to isolate the organelle or virus before extracting its DNA, because the recovery of a particular type of DNA from a mixture is usually rather difficult. Where a high degree of purity is required, DNA may be subjected to density gradient ultracentrifugation through cesium chloride, which is particularly useful for the preparation plasmid DNA. It is possible to check the integrity of the DNA by agarose gel electrophoresis and determine the concentration of the DNA by using the fact that 1 absorbance unit equates to 50 μg/mL of DNA:$50A_{260}$ = Concentration of DNA sample (μg/mL). The identification of contaminants may also be undertaken by scanning ultraviolet (UV)-spectrophotometry from 200–300 nm. A ratio of 260:280 nm of approx 1.8 indicates that the sample is free of protein contamination, which absorbs strongly at 280 nm.

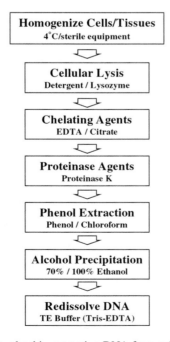

Fig. 1.2. General steps involved in extracting DNA from cells or tissues.

2.2. RNA Extraction Techniques

The methods used for RNA isolation are very similar to those described above for DNA; however, RNA molecules are relatively short and, therefore, less easily damaged by shearing, so cell disruption can be rather more vigorous *(2)*. RNA is, however, very vulnerable to digestion by RNases, which are present endogenously in various concentrations in certain cell types and exogenously on fingers. Gloves should therefore be worn, and a strong detergent should be included in the isolation medium to immediately denature any RNases. Subsequent deproteinization should be particularly rigorous, because RNA is often tightly associated with proteins. DNase treatment can be used to remove DNA, and RNA can be precipitated by ethanol. One reagent in particular that is commonly used in RNA extraction is guanadinium thiocyanate, which is both a strong inhibitor of RNase and a protein denaturant. It is possible to check the integrity of an RNA extract by analyzing it by agarose gel electrophoresis. The most abundant RNA species, the rRNA molecules, are 23S and 16S for prokaryotes and 18S and 28S for eukaryotes. These appear as discrete bands on the agarose gel and indicate that the other RNA components are likely to be intact. This is usually carried out under denaturing conditions to prevent secondary structure formation in the RNA. The concentration of the RNA may be estimated by using UV spectrophotometry in a similar manner to that used for DNA. However in the case of RNA at 260 nm, 1 absorbance unit equates to 40 µg/mL of RNA. Contaminants may also be identified in the same way by scanning UV spectrophotometry; however, in the case of RNA, a 260:280 nm ratio of approx 2 would be expected for a sample containing little or no contaminating protein *(3)*.

In many cases, it is desirable to isolate eukaryotic mRNA, which constitutes only 2–5% of cellular RNA from a mixture of total RNA molecules. This may be carried out by affinity chromatography on oligo(dT)-cellulose columns. At high salt concentrations, the mRNA containing poly(A) tails binds to the complementary oligo(dT) molecules of the affinity column, and so mRNA will be retained; all other RNA molecules can be washed through the column by further high-salt solution. Finally, the bound mRNA can be eluted using a low concentration of salt *(4)*. Nucleic acid species may also be subfractionated by more physical means such as electrophoretic or chromatographic separations based on differences in nucleic acid fragment sizes or physicochemical characteristics.

2.3. Electrophoresis of Nucleic Acids

To analyze nucleic acids by size, the process of electrophoresis in an agarose or polyacrylamide support gel is usually undertaken. Electrophoresis may be used analytically or preparatively and can be qualitative or quantitative. Large fragments of DNA such as chromosomes may also be separated by a modification of electrophoresis termed *pulsed field gel electrophoresis* (PFGE), which uses alternating directions of DNA migration *(5)*. The easiest and most widely applicable method is electrophoresis in horizontal agarose gels as indicated in **Fig. 1.3**. To visualize the DNA, staining has to be undertaken, usually with a dye such as ethidium bromide. This dye binds to DNA by insertion between stacked base-pairs, termed *intercalation*, and exhibits a strong orange/red fluorescence when illuminated with UV light. Alternative

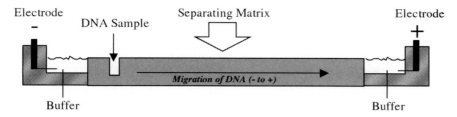

Fig. 1.3. Schematic illustration of a typical horizontal gel electrophoresis setup for the separation of nucleic acids.

stains such as SYBRGreen or Gelstar, which have similar sensitivities, are also available and are less hazardous to use. In general, electrophoresis is used to check the purity and intactness of a DNA preparation or to assess the extent of an enzymatic reaction during, for example, the steps involved in the cloning of DNA. For such checks "mini-gels" are particularly convenient, because they need little preparation, use small samples, and provide results quickly. Agarose gels can be used to separate molecules larger than about 100 base pairs (bp). For higher resolution or for the effective separation of shorter DNA molecules, polyacrylamide gels are the preferred method. In recent years, a number of acrylic gels have been developed that may be used as an alternative to agarose and polyacrylamide.

When electrophoresis is used preparatively, the fragment of gel containing the desired DNA molecule is physically removed with a scalpel. The DNA is then recovered from the gel fragment in various ways. This may include crushing with a glass rod in a small volume of buffer, using agarase to digest the agrose leaving the DNA, or by the process of electroelution. In this method, the piece of gel is sealed in a length of dialysis tubing containing buffer and is then placed between two electrodes in a tank containing more buffer. Passage of an electrical current between the electrodes causes DNA to migrate out of the gel piece, but it remains trapped within the dialysis tubing and can, therefore, be recovered easily.

3. Nucleic Acid Blotting and Gene Probe Hybridization

3.1. Nucleic Acid Blotting

Electrophoresis of DNA restriction fragments allows separation based on size to be conducted; however, it provides no indication as to the presence of a specific, desired fragment among the complex sample. This can be achieved by transferring the DNA from the intact gel onto a piece of nitrocellulose or Nylon membrane placed in contact with it. This provides a more permanent record of the sample because DNA begins to diffuse out of a gel that is left for a few hours. First the gel is soaked in alkali to render the DNA single stranded. It is then transferred to the membrane so that the DNA becomes bound to it in exactly the same pattern as that originally on the gel (*6*). This transfer, named a Southern blot after its inventor Ed Southern, is usually performed by drawing large volumes of buffer by capillary action through both gel and membrane, thus transferring DNA from the gel to the membrane. Alternative methods are also available for this operation such as electrotransfer or vacuum assisted transfer. Both are claimed to give a more even transfer and are much more rapid, although they do require more expensive equipment than the capillary transfer system. Transfer of the DNA from the gel to the membrane allows the membrane to be treated with a labeled DNA gene probe. This single-stranded DNA probe will hybridize under the right conditions to complementary single-stranded DNA fragments immobilized onto the membrane.

3.2. Hybridization and Stringency

The conditions of hybridization are critical for this process to take place effectively. This is usually referred to as the stringency of the hybridization and it is particular for each individual gene probe and for each sample of DNA. Two of the most important components are the temperature and the salt concentration. Higher temperatures and low salt concentrations, termed *high stringency*, provide a favorable environment for perfectly matched probe and template sequences, whereas reduced temperatures and high salt concentrations, termed *low stringency*, allow the stabilization of mismatches in the duplex. In addition, inclusions of denaturants such as formamide allow the hybridization temperatures to be reduced without affecting the stringency. A series of posthybridization washing steps with a salt solution such as SSC, containing sodium citrate and sodium chloride, is then carried out to remove any unbound probe and control the binding of the duplex. The membrane is developed using either autoradiography if the probe is radiolabeled or by a number of nonradioactive methods.

The precise location of the probe and its target may be then visualized. The steps involved in Southern blotting are indicated in **Fig. 1.4**. It is also possible to analyze DNA from different species or organisms by blotting the DNA and then using a gene probe representing a protein or enzyme from one of the organisms. In this way, it is possible to search for related genes in different species. This technique is generally termed Zoo blotting. A similar process of nucleic acid blotting can be used to transfer RNA separated by gel electrophoresis onto membranes similar to that used in Southern blotting. This process, termed *Northern blotting*, allows the identification of specific mRNA sequences of a defined length by hybridization to a labeled gene probe *(7)*. It is possible with this technique to not only detect specific mRNA molecules, but it may also be used to quantify the relative amounts of the specific mRNA present in a tissue or sample. It is usual to separate the mRNA transcripts by gel electrophoresis under denaturing conditions because this improves resolution and allows a more accurate estimation of the sizes of the transcripts. The format of the blotting may be altered from transfer from a gel to direct application to slots on a specific blotting apparatus containing the Nylon membrane. This is termed *slot* or *dot blotting* and provides a convenient means of measuring the abundance of specific mRNA transcripts without the need for gel electrophoresis, it does not, however, provide information regarding the size of the fragments. Hybridization techniques are essential to many molecular biology experiments; however, the format of the hybridization may be altered to improve speed sensitivity and throughput.

One interesting alternative is termed *surface plasmon resonance* (SPR). This is an optical system based on difference between incident and reflected

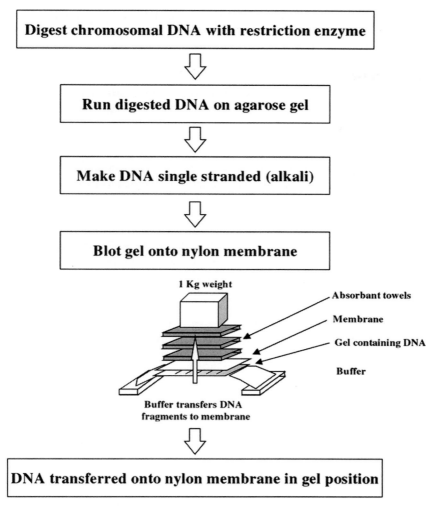

Fig. 1.4. The procedure involved in a typical Southern blot indicating the construction of a simple capillary transfer setup.

light in the presence or absence of hybridization. Its main advantage is that the kinetics of hybridization can be undertaken in real time and without a DNA label. A further exciting method for hybridization is also in use, which uses arrays of single-stranded DNA molecules tethered to small hybridization chips. Hybridization to a DNA sample is detected by computer, allowing DNA mutations to be quickly and easily identified.

3.3. Production of Gene Probes

The availability of a gene probe is essential in many molecular biology techniques; yet, in many cases, it is one of the most difficult steps. The information needed to produce a gene probe may come from many sources, but with the development and sophistication of genetic databases, this is usually one of the first stages *(8)*. There are a number of genetic databases such as those at Genbank and EMBL and it is possible to search these over the Internet and identify particular sequences relating to a specific gene or protein. In some cases, it is possible to use related proteins from the same gene family to gain information on the most useful DNA sequence. Similar proteins or DNA sequences but from different species may also provide a starting point with which to produce a so-called heterologous gene probe. Although, in some cases, probes are already produced and cloned, it is possible, armed with a DNA sequence from a DNA database, to chemically synthesize a single-stranded oligonucleotide probe. This is usually undertaken by computer-controlled gene synthesizers, which link dNTPs together based on a desired sequence. It is essential to carry out certain checks before probe production to determine that the probe is unique, is not able to self-anneal, or is self complementary, all of which may compromise its use. Where little DNA information is available to prepare a gene probe, it is possible in some cases to use the knowledge gained from analysis of the corresponding protein. Thus, it is possible to isolate and purify proteins and sequence part of the N-terminal end of the protein. From our knowledge of the genetic code, it is possible to predict the various DNA sequences that could code for the protein and then synthesize appropriate oligonucleotide sequences chemically. Because of the degeneracy of the genetic code, most amino acids are coded for by more than one codon; therefore, there will be more than one possible nucleotide sequence that could code for a given polypeptide. The longer the polypeptide, the larger the number of possible oligonucleotides that must be synthesized. Fortunately, there is no need to synthesize a sequence longer than about 20 bases, as this should hybridize efficiently with any complementary sequences and should be specific for one gene. Ideally, a section of the protein should be chosen that contains as many tryptophan and methionine residues as possible, because these have unique codons and there will therefore be fewer possible base sequences that could code for that part of the protein. The synthetic oligonucleotides can then be used as probes in a number of molecular biology methods.

3.4. DNA Gene Probe Labeling

An essential feature of a gene probe is that it can be visualized by some means. In this way, a gene probe that hybridizes to a complementary sequence may be detected and identify that desired sequence from a complex mixture. There are two main ways of labeling gene probes, traditionally this has been carried out using radioactive labels, but gaining in popularity are nonradioactive labels. Perhaps the most used radioactive label is phosphorous-32 (^{32}P), although for certain techniques sulfur-35 (^{35}S) and tritium (^{3}H) are used. These may be detected by the process of autoradiography where the labeled probe molecule, bound to sample DNA, located, for example, on a Nylon membrane, is placed in contact with an X-ray-sensitive film. Following exposure, the film is developed and fixed just as a black-and-white negative and reveals the precise location of the labeled probe and, therefore, the DNA to which it has hybridized.

3.5. Nonradioactive DNA Labeling

Nonradioactive labels are increasingly being used to label DNA gene probes. Until recently, radioactive labels were more sensitive than their nonradioactive counterparts. However, recent developments have led to similar sensitivities, which, when combined with their improved safety, have led to their greater acceptance. The labeling systems are either termed direct or indirect. Direct labeling allows an enzyme reporter such as alkaline phosphatase to be coupled directly to the DNA. Although this may alter the characteristics of the DNA gene probe, it offers the advantage of rapid analysis because no intermediate steps are needed. However indirect labeling is, at present, more popular. This relies on the incorporation of a nucleotide that has a label attached. At present, three of the main labels in use are biotin, fluorescein, and digoxigenin. These molecules are covalently linked to nucleotides using a carbon spacer arm of 7, 14, or 21 atoms. Specific binding proteins may then be used as a bridge between the nucleotide and a reporter protein such as an enzyme. For example, biotin incorporated into a DNA fragment is recognized with a very high affinity by the protein streptavidin. This may either be coupled or conjugated to a reporter enzyme molecule such as alkaline phosphatase or horseradish peroxidase (HRP). This is usually used to convert a colorless substrate into a colored insoluble compound and also offers a means of signal amplification. Alternatively, labels such as digoxigenin incorporated into DNA sequences may be detected by monoclonal antibodies, again conjugated to reporter molecules, including alkaline phosphatase. Thus, rather than the detection system relying on autoradiography, which is necessary for radiolabels, a series of reactions resulting in either a color or a light or a chemiluminescence reaction takes place. This has important practical implications because autoradiography may take 1–3 d, whereas color and chemiluminescent reactions take minutes. In addition, no radiolabeling and detection minimize the potential health and safety hazards encountered when using radiolabels.

3.6. End Labeling of DNA

The simplest form of labeling DNA is by 5'- or 3'-end labeling. 5'-End labeling involves a phosphate transfer or exchange reaction, where the 5' phosphate of the DNA to be used as the probe is removed and in its place a labeled phosphate, usually ^{32}P, is added. This is usually carried out by using two enzymes, the first, alkaline phosphatase, is used to remove the existing phosphate group from the DNA. Following removal of the released phosphate from the DNA, a second enzyme polynucleotide kinase is added that catalyzes the transfer of a phosphate group (^{32}P labeled) to the 5' end of the DNA (see **Fig. 1.5**). The newly labeled probe is then purified, usually by chromatography through a Sephadex column and may be used directly. Using the other end of the DNA molecule, the 3' end, is slightly less complex. Here, a new dNTP, which is labeled (e.g., $^{32}PadATP$ or biotin-labeled dNTP), is added to the 3' end of the DNA by the enzyme terminal transferase as indicated in **Fig. 1.6**. Although this is a simpler reaction, a potential problem exists because a new nucleotide is added to the existing sequence and so the complete sequence of the DNA is altered, which may affect its hybridization to its target sequence. End labeling methods also suffer from the fact that only one label is added to the DNA, so these methods are of a lower activity in comparison to methods that incorporate labels along the length of the DNA.

3.7. Random Primer Labeling of DNA

The DNA to be labeled is first denatured and then placed under renaturing conditions in the presence of a mixture of many different random sequences of

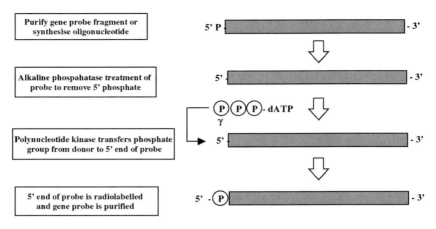

Fig. 1.5. End labeling of a gene probe at the 5' end with alkaline phosphatase and polynucleotide kinase.

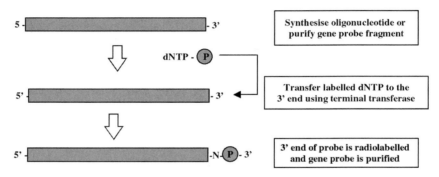

Fig. 1.6. End labeling of a gene probe at the 3' end using terminal transferase. Note that the addition of a labeled dNTP at the 3' end alters the sequence of the gene probe.

hexamers or hexanucleotides. These hexamers will, by chance, bind to the DNA sample wherever they encounter a complementary sequence and, thus, the DNA will rapidly acquire an approximately random sprinkling of hexanucleotides annealed to it. Each of the hexamers can act as a primer for the synthesis of a fresh strand of DNA catalyzed by DNA polymerase because it has an exposed 3' hydroxyl group, as seen in **Fig. 1.7**. The Klenow fragment of DNA polymerase is used for random primer labeling because it lacks a 5'–3' exonuclease activity. This is prepared by cleavage of DNA polymerase with subtilisin, giving a large enzyme fragment that has no 5' to 3' exonuclease activity, but which still acts as a 5' to 3' polymerase. Thus, when the Klenow enzyme is mixed with the annealed DNA sample in the presence of dNTPs, including at least one that is labeled, many short stretches of labeled DNA will be generated. In a similar way to random primer labeling, polymerase chain reaction (PCR) may also be used to incorporate radioactive or nonradioactive labels.

3.8. Nick Translation Labeling of DNA

A traditional method of labeling DNA is by the process of nick translation. Low concentrations of DNase I are used to make occasional single-strand nicks in the double-stranded DNA that is to be used as the gene probe. DNA polymerase then fills in the nicks, using an appropriate deoxyribonucleoside

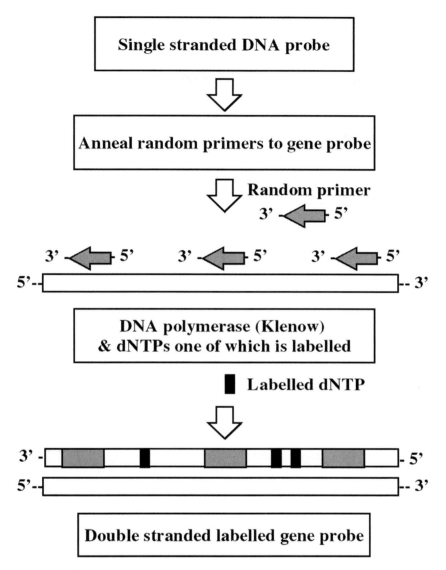

Fig. 1.7. Random primer gene probe labeling. Random primers are incorporated and used as a start point for Klenow DNA polymerase to synthesize a complementary strand of DNA while incorporating a labeled dNTP at complementary sites.

triphosphate (dNTP), at the same time making a new nick to the 3' side of the previous one. In this way, the nick is translated along the DNA. If labeled dNTPs are added to the reaction mixture, they will be used to fill in the nicks, as indicated in **Fig. 1.8**. In this way, the DNA can be labeled to a very high specific activity.

4. RNA Interference

Another of the important developments of recent times was the discovery of RNA interference (RNAi), which has been extensively used as a tool in the identification of the function of specific genes and the effect of gene silencing.

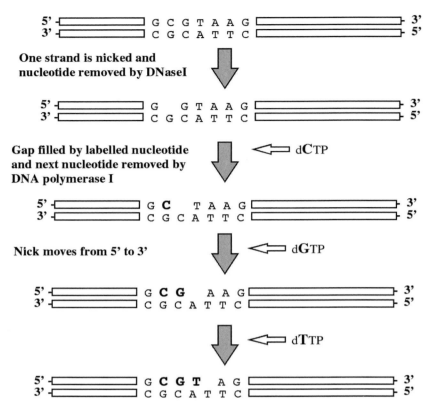

Fig. 1.8. Nick translation. The removal of nucleotides and their subsequent replacement with labeled nucleotides by DNA polymerase I makes the gene probe more labeled as nick translation proceeds.

RNAi is a process in which double-stranded RNA (dsRNA) triggers the degradation of a homologous messenger RNA (mRNA). Once in the cell, the dsRNA (>30 bp) is recognized and cleaved by the enzyme Dicer (member of the RNAse III family) to form small interfering RNA (siRNA, 21–25 bp) each with 2-nucleotide overhangs at the 3' end. The siRNA is unwound and the guide strand (usually antisense strand) *(9)* incorporated into the protein complex, RNA-induced silencing complex (RISC) where it guides the RISC to its complementary mRNA *(10)*. The complementary mRNA is then cleaved by the enzyme Argonaute 2, at a single site at the center of the duplex region between the siRNA and the target mRNA, resulting in the inhibition of protein synthesis and gene expression. This is also known as *gene silencing*. The siRNA strand is protected from degradation and can direct the cleavage of many mRNA molecules.

In addition to this natural process of RNAi, synthetic dsDNA and siRNAs may be introduced directly into the cytoplasm or vector-mediated using plasmids or viral vectors.

The high specificity and potency of RNAi on gene expression has made this not only a valuable research tool in the laboratory, being well studied in model organisms such as *Caenorhabditis elegans* (nematode worm) and *Drosophila melanogaster* (fruit fly), but has potential as a therapeutic approach. RNAi has the capability to reduce the expression of pathological proteins and has been demonstrated in a number of animal models by local administration of siRNAs or short hairpin RNAs (shRNAs). Efficacy has been demonstrated in rodent and monkey model of viral infections *(11)*, ocular neovascularization, diseases of the nervous system *(12,13)* and cancer *(14)*. See Bumcrot *et al* for a review *(15)*. One obstacle in using siRNAs as a therapeutic is the lack of drug-like properties impeding delivery and stability. Chemical modifications and conjugations have been made to the sugar, backbone and bases, improving the stability, potency, and cellular uptake *(15)*.

References

1. Smith HO, Wilcox KW (1970) A restriction enzyme from Haemophilus influenzae: purification and general characterization. J Mol Biol 51:379
2. Jones P, Qiu J, Rickwood D (1994) RNA isolation and analysis. Bios Scientific. Oxford
3. Heptinstall J (2000) Spectrophotometric analysis of nucleic acids. In: Rapley R (ed) The nucleic acid protocols handbook. Humana, Totowa, NJ
4. Bryant S, Manning DL (2000) Isolation of mRNA by affinity chromatography. In: Rapley R (ed) The nucleic acid protocols handbook. Humana, Totowa, NJ
5. Maule J (2000) Pulsed-field gel electrophoresis. In: Rapley R (ed) The nucleic acid protocols handbook. Humana, Totowa, NJ
6. Southern EM (1975) Detection of specific sequences among DNA fragments separated by gel electrophoresis. J Mol Biol 98:503
7. Alwine JC, Kemp DJ, Stark GR (1977) Method for the detection of specific RNAs in agarose gels by transfer to diazobenzyloxymethyl paper and hybridization with DNA probes. Proc Natl Acad Sci *USA* 74:5350
8. Aquino de Muro M, Rapley R (2002) Gene probes: principles and protocols. Humana, Totowa, NJ
9. Zamore PD, Tuschi T, Sharp PA, Bartel DP (2000) RNAi: double-stranded RNA directs the ATP-dependent cleavage of mRMA at 21 to 23 nucleotide intervals. Cell 101 (1):25–33
10. Nykanen A, Haley B, Zamore PD (2001) ATP requirements and small interfering RNA structure in the RNA interference pathway. Cell 107 (3):309–321
11. Bitko V, Musiyenko A, Shulyayera O, Barik S (2005) Inhibition of respiratory viruses by nasally administered siRNA. Nat Med 11:50–55
12. Gonzalez-Alegre P (2007) Therapeutic RNA interference for neurodegenrative diseases: from promise to progress. Pharmacol Therap Epub ahead of print
13. Andersen ND, Monahan TS, Malek JY, Jain M, Daniel S, Caron LD, Pradhan L, Ferran C, LoGerto FW (2007) Comparison of gene silencing in human vascular cells using small interfering RNAs. J Am Col Surg 204:399–408
14. Masiero M, Nardo G, Indraccolo S, Favaro, E (2007) RNA interference: implications for cancer treatment. Mol Aspects Med 28:143–166
15. Bumcrot D, Manoharan M, Koteliansky V, Sah DWY (2006) RNAi therapeutics: a potential new class of pharmacological drugs. Nat Chem Biol 2 (12):711–719

2

Restriction Enzymes

Tools in Clinical Research

Gareth J. S. Jenkins

1. Restriction Enzymes

Restriction enzymes (or restriction endonucleases) are bacterial enzymes capable of cleaving double-stranded DNA. Even though the enzymes are bacterial in origin, because of the universal nature of DNA they can digest DNA from any species, including humans. Importantly, restriction enzymes (REs) carry out this cleavage at specific sites in DNA governed by the sequence context (so-called recognition sequences). Hence, REs are known to be extremely sequence-specific; subtle alterations in the recognition sequence render the sites indigestible. This fact is the basis of their usefulness in clinical research and diagnostics. **Table 2.1** is a list of a few of the common REs showing their sequence specificities. **Figure 2.1** shows the interaction of a RE with DNA. The RE interacts with DNA via multiple hydrogen bonds (typically 10–15) plus numerous van der Waals interactions. Only when the RE–DNA complex is tightly bound does the catalytic domain cause DNA cleavage *(2)*.

Restriction enzymes were first discovered in the 1950s and their subsequent isolation in the 1970s paved the way for modern recombinant DNA technologies *(3)*. In fact, without REs, gene cloning technologies (e.g., the construction of genetically modified organisms) would not have become as ubiquitous as they currently are. Therefore, REs have a central place in current DNA manipulation methodologies, but as will be seen here, they are also being used to answer questions about the integrity of DNA in clinical specimens. The clinical use of REs relies on their extreme sequence specificity.

Restriction enzymes can be grouped into three main groups, known as type I, type II, and type III. This chapter focuses on the role of the type II REs, which are the most commonly used REs in DNA manipulation. Type II REs cleave DNA within the same sequences that are recognized by the enzyme, hence an internal digestion. The other two types of RE are more complex (e.g., type I REs cleave DNA outside of this recognition sequence). There are currently well over 1,000 type II REs characterized, with over 200 commercially available. A searchable database exists online (rebase.neb.com) containing the specific details of a large number of available REs and the companies that sell them *(4)*.

From: *Molecular Biomethods Handbook, 2nd Edition.*
Edited by: J. M. Walker and R. Rapley © Humana Press, Totowa, NJ

Table 2.1. List of six commonly used restriction enzymes.

Name	Host bacteria	Recognition sequence	Digestion temperature
*Hae*III	*Haemophilis parainfluenzae*	GGCC	37°C
*Pvu*II	*Proteus vulgaris*	CAGCTG	37°C
*Eco*RI	*Escherichia coli*	GGATCC	37°C
*Hha*I	*Haemophilus haemolyticus*	GCGC	37°C
*Msp*I	*Moraxella species*	CCGG	37°C
*Taq*I	*Thermus aquaticus*	TCGA	65°C

Note: Included are details of the bacteria from which they were isolated and some of their reaction characteristics, including their recognition sequences.

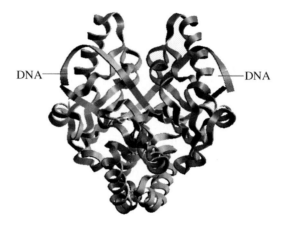

Fig. 2.1. Restriction enzyme (*Pvu*II) interaction with DNA (Taken from the nucleic acid database [http://ndbserver.rutgers.edu/] deposited by the authors of **ref.** *1*.)

2. Function of REs

Restriction enzymes were first identified in bacterial strains that were shown to be resistant to certain bacteriophages (virus equivalents in bacteria). This phenomenon was termed "hostcontrolled restriction" and was later shown to be caused by the presence of specific REs within these bacteria, which destroyed the bacteriophage DNA before it could insert itself into the bacterial genome. Obviously, the bacteria's own DNA would normally be susceptible to similar digestion, but for the presence of DNA-modifying enzymes, which modify the bacterial genome and protect it. Hence, particular species of bacteria produce REs and modifying enzymes (actually DNA methylases) that recognize the same DNA sequences. The bacterial DNA is methylated by the methylase enzyme, protecting it from RE-mediated digestion while incoming unmethylated bacteriophage DNA is destroyed.

3. Sequence Specificity of REs

Restriction enzymes usually recognize four to six basepair sequences, often in the form of palindromes (read same sequence in the 5′ to 3′ direction on both strands). Each species of bacteria produces a different RE recognizing a different DNA sequence. In fact, REs are named after the bacterial species from which they were isolated (see **Table 2.1**). Where bacteria produce more than one RE, they are known as *Pvu*I, *Pvu*II, and so forth. REs produced by different bacteria but with the same recognition sequence are known as isoschizomers.

If one assumes that the human genome contains a random sequence of the A, C, G, and T bases and that all four bases are present at the same frequency, it can be estimated that REs cut human DNA every 256–4096 bp (4-bp cutters, 6-bp cutters, respectively). Hence, in the 3 billion bases of the human genome, there would be, on average, 10 million sites for a 4-base cutting RE and on average 700,000 sites for a 6-base cutting RE. Given the availability of over 200 different REs, it is easy to see how frequent RE sites are in human DNA; in fact, RE sites are estimated to cover 50% of the genome *(5)*.

4. Role of REs in Clinical Research and Diagnostics

It is the sequence specificity of REs that is exploited in clinical research. Alteration of a single base within a RE site removes the ability of the RE to digest that particular stretch of DNA. Hence, DNA sequence changes can be inferred by the loss of corresponding RE sites. Given that up to 50% of the genome is covered by one or another of the 200 available REs, it is relatively straightforward to monitor the integrity of these RE sites for the presence of clinically related DNA alterations (mutation, deletion). The alteration of known RE sites can be readily examined in large numbers of clinical specimens simultaneously, allowing the study of DNA alterations linked to a particular clinical condition. For example, if mutation of a single base leads to loss of a particular RE site and this is linked to the occurrence of a disease as a result of the altered protein produced by this gene, then RE analysis is able to rapidly screen large numbers of samples for this particular sequence change. In the following subsections are listed several molecular approaches involving REs currently used for the analysis of clinical specimens.

4.1. Restriction Fragment Length Polymorphism

Restriction fragment length polymorphism (RFLP) analysis is widely used to examine the sequences of large numbers of samples simultaneously. RFLP involves the digestion of individual DNA samples with a particular RE, followed by separation of the daughter products by electrophoresis. This allows the study of the integrity of the recognition sites of one particular RE at a time and, thereby, the integrity of the DNA sequence contained within the RE site. Hence, alterations in the distribution of the RE sites for each RE in turn can be assessed in large numbers of samples. This process has been particularly useful in studying population differences in individuals of many species, not just humans.

In the past, RFLP analysis was carried out as follows: Genomic DNA was initially digested with each RE in turn; the DNA was then electrophoresed and probed for specific sequences by Southern blotting. However, more recently, with the advent of polymerase chain reaction (PCR), a simpler approach has become available. Currently, the gene of interest (or gene region) is initially PCR-amplified from the genomic DNA; this PCR product is then digested with the RE and the RE fragments are separated and visualized by electrophoresis. **Figure 2.2** shows the result of this process. In **Fig. 2.2**, the digested PCR products from two different individuals are shown. It should be borne in mind that every human somatic cell contains two copies of every gene. Hence, analysis of the integrity of a particular gene sequence is actually carried out in duplicate each time. In **Fig. 2.2** the right-hand digested PCR product is from an individual who is homozygous for the RE site sequence (both DNA sequences digest, hence both RE sites intact), whereas the left-hand digested PCR product is from an individual who is heterozygous for the sequence of this particular RE site (one copy digests, one copy does not). RFLP patterns can be easily produced for many RE sites (up to 50% of genome) within a gene of interest and these patterns of digestion can be compared among large numbers of clinical samples for differences. By this method, mutations at particular RE sites that lead to loss of RE sites and are important in clinical conditions have been identified.

Such RFLP analysis can actually detect two separate molecular events in the clinical samples, namely, mutations and deletions. Point mutations within the particular RE site under study will be detected by the loss of digestion at one site leading to loss of two daughter strands post electrophoresis. As was seen above, this process is monitored in both copies of each gene simultaneously (heterozygous versus homozygous changes). Conversely, the development of a new RE site within a particular PCR product by mutation can lead to an extra pair of daughter fragments on the gel. These new RE sites are identified by the presence of smaller than expected digestion fragments. Furthermore, deletions of DNA tracts will be detected by the loss of specific RE sites. These deletions can also sometimes be seen by the size of the amplified PCR product changing. RE analysis can also be used to study specific deletions in heterozygous individuals. This is particularly useful in cancer research, where tumor suppressor genes are often deleted during tumor evolution. Where heterozygosity (one cut band, one uncut band) is present in the normal tissue but is lost in the tumor (either cut band or uncut band alone), this indicates that one copy of the particular sequence has been deleted. Therefore, choosing RE sites in tumor suppressor genes for which the individual is heterozygous is the key for this type of analysis.

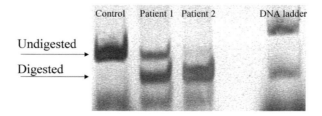

Fig. 2.2. RFLP analysis. PCR-amplified DNA is digested with a RE. Left lane shows undigested PCR product. Right lane shows DNA size ladder. Patient 1 shows a heterozygous individual (one sequence digests, one sequence does not digest). Patient 2 shows individual homozygous for the RE site sequence (both sequences digest)

In both cases (mutation and deletion), RFLP analysis is used as an initial screen for alterations in large numbers of samples. The alterations are always confirmed by DNA sequencing.

The use of DNA sequencing provides important information on the type of mutation (G to A, A to G, etc.) present in the DNA and the position of such mutations (base and codon preference). In the case of deletion events, sequencing can identify the size of the deleted region and the points at which the deletion occurred. In terms of mutations, much can be gained from studying the actual mutation types in clinical tissues as a result of the fact that chemical mutagens that lead to the mutation being induced produce a characteristic pattern of mutations (types and position). Therefore, causative mutagens can be retrospectively identified from the pattern of mutations seen in clinical tissues. This can provide important information on mutagen exposures, potentially leading to a reduction in such exposures in the future.

The advantage of RFLP analysis lies in its simplicity, high-throughput nature, and low cost. Sequencing the gene of interest from a large number of individuals would be the ideal way of looking for sequence changes that might be clinically important. However, this would be an extremely time consuming and expensive process. Hence, we use alternative screening methods like RFLP to reduce the amount of sequencing necessary.

There are two research areas in which RFLP analysis can be particularly useful in clinical research. These are the study of DNA polymorphisms and the study of tumor mutations.

4.1.1. DNA Polymorphisms

Polymorphisms are natural sequence variations that can lead to interindividual phenotypic differences. These polymorphisms (p/ms) occur on average once in every 1,000 bp. Most p/ms do not produce profound phenotypic differences, as selection has acted during evolution to rid our gene pool of these disadvantageous changes. However, many p/ms do modulate an individual's risk of developing certain diseases, hence the current focus on mapping large numbers of p/ms in large numbers of individuals to study their effect on disease etiology. For example, cytochrome P450 enzymes (P450s) metabolize exogenous chemicals that enter the body in an effort to detoxify them, occasionally, this metabolism increases the toxicity or carcinogenicity of the parent compound. Hence, overactivity or underactivity of particular P450s can be linked to cancer risk if the metabolic product or the parent compound is carcinogenic, respectively. Therefore, p/ms that affect P450 activity can modulate cancer risks in individuals (see **Table 2.2**). RFLP analysis is a very suitable methodology for scanning a large number of p/ms in cancer-modulating genes in large numbers of individuals. Examples of gene p/ms important in increasing cancer risks are shown in **Table 2.2**.

4.1.2. Tumor Mutations

Tumors result from genetic damage accumulated in normal tissue during an individual's life-span. This genetic damage often occurs in genes involved in the control of cell division, such that mutant clones are produced that divide uncontrollably. The cell division genes targeted are known as oncogenes (promote division) and tumor suppressor genes (suppress division). The genetic damage inflicted in these genes includes point mutations and deletions and often occurs early in tumor development such that mature tumor tissue

Table 2.2. Some of the polymorphisms present in cancer-related genes that have been studied by RE analysis.

Gene	Cancer type	Region	RE	References
DCC gene	Colon	Codon 201	SalI	*(6)*
p53 gene	All	Intron 7	ApaI	*(7)*
CYP1A1	All	3′ UTR	MspI	*(8)*
H-ras	Bladder	Intron 4	BstEII	*(9)*
CYP17	Breast	5′ Promoter	MspI	*(10)*

Note: UTR = untranslated region.

contains cells in which the genetic damage (e.g., mutation) is ubiquitous. This means that the mutations are readily detectable in tumor tissue by methods such as RFLP and DNA sequencing. Indeed, REs have been widely used to study the activation of oncogenes such as the *K-ras* oncogene, which is activated through mutation at codon 12 *(11,12)*. Furthermore, the *p53* gene, commonly mutated in tumor development, has been shown to acquire mutations most frequently at codon 248 (www.iarc.fr/p53), which contains a *Msp*I site (CCGG), hence allowing RE-based analysis to provide information on tumor-specific *p53* mutations. Rarer mutations (present in <10% of the cells) such as those present in precancerous tissue would not be detectable by RFLP or sequencing. This is a consequence of the limited sensitivity of the detection step in RFLP analysis (i.e., the identification of a band on a gel). For these rare mutations, more sensitive mutation detection methods are needed.

4.2. Restriction Site Mutation

Restriction site mutation (RSM) employs REs to detect mutations, particularly those involved in tumor formation. RSM has been developed to detect mutations when they occur very infrequently, when RFLP is not suitable (for a review, see **ref**. *(13)*. RSM is capable of detecting point mutations when they are present in a 10,000-fold excess of nonmutated DNA *(14,15)*. Therefore, RSM is highly suited to detecting cancer-causing mutations early in tumor evolution (i.e., in premalignant tissue). RSM is able to detect such rare mutations because of a reversal of the digestion and PCR steps compared to RFLP (see **Fig. 2.3**). With RSM, the DNA is digested first in order to destroy nonmutated sequences, mutations arising in target RE sites render those particular RE sites resistant to digestion. Subsequent PCR amplification of digested DNA ensures that only undigested (i.e., mutated) sequences are amplified. This arrangement is the basis of the sensitivity of RSM.

We developed RSM in our laboratory over 10 years ago *(16)* and have since been continually validating and optimizing the methodology *(13,15)*. We have used RSM to detect the action of mutagenic chemicals through the analysis of induced mutations in tissues and cells exposed to putative mutagens. In addition, we have recently studied a range of early premalignant tissues for the presence of initiating mutations (e.g., of the *p53* tumor suppressor gene). **Table 2.3** is a summary of some of the recent research carried out by ourselves

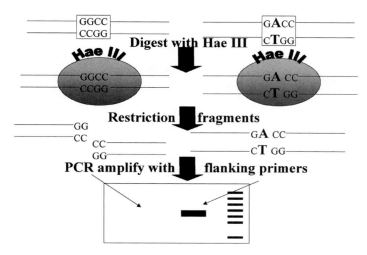

Fig. 2.3. The principle of RSM. DNA is initially digested with the RE whose site is under mutation analysis (*Hae*III in this case). This digestion cleaves the unmutated DNA copies (as seen on the left), but leaves the mutated copies intact (as seen on the right). Subsequent PCR amplifies the mutated DNA, producing a band after electrophoresis, digested DNA will not PCR, hence no band on the gel. A second digestion step is often included to remove any amplified un-mutated DNA after PCR

Table 2.3. A summary of published RSM data showing the detection of mutations in both clinical samples and in vitro mutagen experiments.

Subject analyzed	Gene	Codon	Mutation types identified	References
Fibroblasts treated with oxidizing agent 4-NQO	*p53*	248	GC to AT	*(17)*
Fibroblasts treated with reactive oxygen species generator	*p53*	248	GC to TA, GC to AT	*(18)*
Fibroblasts treated with reactive oxygen species generator	*p53*	248	GC to AT	*(14)*
Premalignant esophageal tissue	*p53*	248	GC to AT	*(15)*
Premalignant gastric tissue	*p53*	248	GC to AT	*(19)*

Note: These data show the similarity between the mutation induced in vitro by oxidative agents and the mutations identified in upper gastrointestinal (GI) tract tissues, suggesting a role of oxygen free radicals in upper GI tract cancer.

and others, using RSM to detect DNA mutations in chemically exposed cells or in premalignant tissue. **Figure 2.4** illustrates the potential of RSM to detect *p53* mutations in premalignant clinical samples. This RSM approach has also been used by other groups looking at the presence of early cancer-causing mutations in clinical tissue *(20)*. Our aims in these clinical studies have been threefold. First, how early are *p53* mutations in these tumor types? Second, by comparison to in vitro studies on putative mutagens, can we identify

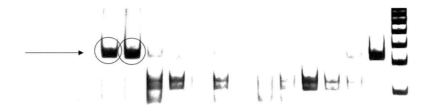

Fig. 2.4. RSM analysis of premalignant esophageal tissue from 12 individuals for *p53* mutations at codon 248 (*Msp*I restriction site). On the right of the gel is a DNA size ladder and next to this is a positive control for the PCR amplification, showing the expected band size. Lanes 1 and 2 show an undigested PCR product of the correct size as a result the presence of a *p53* mutation at codon 248 in the *Msp*I restriction site. These two samples are actually from the same individual

causative mutagens based on the mutation patterns? For example, as shown in **Table 2.3**, we have recently identified a similarity between the premalignant mutations present in esophageal and gastric tissue and those mutations induced experimentally by reactive oxygen species (ROS), suggesting a role for ROS in gastrointestinal (GI) tract carcinogenesis *(14,17,19)*. Finally, as *p53* is a key tumor suppressor in humans whose loss coincides with tumor development, can early *p53* mutations predict cancer progression in individual cases? We have found early *p53* mutations in a subset of premalignant clinical tissue samples by use of RSM (esophageal, gastric, colon, and bladder). We are now following up these patients closely in order to determine if the presence of an early *p53* mutation predicts which patients progress to cancer fastest. If this proves to be the case, then RSM analysis of early mutations in genes such as *p53* may be useful in assessing cancer risk on an individual basis.

4.3. DNA Methylation Analysis

DNA methylation is a frequent modification in the DNA of genomes *(21)*. It is widely accepted that methylation (which occurs at 5′ CG 3′ sequences in mammals) is responsible for the silencing of unwanted genes in specific cell types. The loss of this methylation pattern will, therefore, switch on genes that should be silent, whereas *de novo* methylation will switch off genes that should be switched on. The involvement of DNA methylation abnormalities in cancer development is now well established, often seen as the silencing of tumor suppressor genes by *de novo* methylation *(22)*. Therefore, methods to study DNA methylation are being developed *(23)*. REs are particularly useful in studying DNA methylation *(24)*. This is the result of the fortuitous existence of pairs of REs (isoschizomers) that are differentially sensitive to DNA methylation. For example, *Hpa*II and *Msp*I both recognize the CCGG sequence, but *Hpa*II will not digest this sequence if the internal C is methylated. *Msp*I will digest both methylated and unmethylated sequences. This feature of pairs of REs can be exploited to monitor the methylation status of tumor suppressor genes in clinical samples. Because CG sites are methylated in mammals, RE sites containing CG sequences such as *Hpa*II are particularly useful. **Figure 2.5** is the outline of how RE analysis can measure DNA methylation.

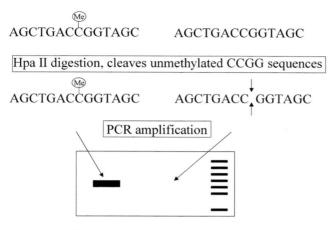

Fig. 2.5. Mammalian DNA is methylated at the five carbon position of the cytosine base in a CG sequence context, as shown. To detect this methylation, DNA is initially digested with a methylation sensitive RE (*Hpa*II in this case). This RE cuts unmethylated DNA, but fails to cut methylated DNA (marked Me). Subsequent PCR amplification allows the methylated (undigested) DNA to be amplified. Hence, methylation is ultimately detected by the presence of a PCR band on a gel.

5. Concluding Remarks

In conclusion, REs are remarkable enzymes that have been exploited in molecular biology for over 30 yr. In that time, REs have played a paramount role in genetic manipulation (cloning, etc.) as well as in clinical research. The basis of the usefulness of REs is their sequence specificity. The fact that each RE stringently digests only its own recognition sequence and fails to recognize this sequence even if only 1-bp changes has led to their widespread use with clinical samples. In fact, the sequence specificity of REs is such that they can also recognize chemical modifications of normal DNA bases (so-called DNA adducts). Hence, REs can be employed to detect modified DNA after exposure to DNA-damaging chemicals resulting from the failure of REs to digest these modified sequences *(25,26)*.

As has been seen here, the use of REs in clinical research is widespread. REs are regularly used to analyze the DNA of clinical samples for the presence of mutations, deletions, and methylation abnormalities. RFLP analysis of human pathogens (bacteria, viruses, and other micro-organisms) has also been important in the study of human disease, through the identification, at the DNA level, of virulent strains and strains resistant to drug therapy.

Importantly, hundreds of REs are now available with different sequence combinations, thus allowing their application to many different DNA sequences. Furthermore, in an effort to increase the application of REs in mutational analysis, PCR-based methods have been developed that artificially create RE sites at specific sequences. These methods employ mismatched primers during the PCR step, hence producing PCR products containing unique RE sites for mutation analysis *(11,12)*. It is hoped that future research involving REs will benefit from new RE's being discovered, with new recognition sequences. Importantly, advances in protein engineering can also, in the near future, allow the design of new REs with tailor made recognition sequences not currently available.

References

1. Horton JR, Nastri HG, Riggs PD, Cheng X (1998) Asp34 of PvuII endonuclease is directly involved in DNA minor groove recognition and indirectly involved in catalysis. J Mol Biol 284:1491–1504
2. Pingoud A, Jeltsch A (2001) Structure and function of type II restriction endonucleases. Nucleic Acids Res 29:3705–3727
3. Brown TA (1990) Gene Cloning, 2nd edn. Chapman & Hall, London
4. Roberts RJ, Macelis D (2001) REBASE: restriction enzymes and methylases. Nucleic Acids Res 29:268–269
5. Cotton GH (1989) Detection of single base changes in nucleic acids. Biochem J 263:1–10
6. Minami R, Aoyama N, Honsako Y, Kasuga, M, Fujimura T, Maeda S (1997) Codon 201 (arg/gly) polymorphism of DCC (deleted in colorectal cancer) gene in flat and polypoid type colorectal tumours. Dig Dis Sci 42:2446–2452
7. Prosser J, Condie A (1991) Biallelic Apa I polymorphism of the human p53 gene (TP53). Nucleic Acids Res 19:4799
8. Garte S (1998) The role of ethnicity in cancer susceptibility gene polymorphisms: example of CYP1A1. Carcinogenesis 19:1329–1332
9. Cohen JB, Levinson AD (1988) A point mutation in the last intron responsible for increased expression and transforming activity of the c-Ha-ras oncogene. Nature 334:119–124
10. Ye Z, Parry JM (2002) The CYP17 MspA1 polymorphism and breast cancer risk: a meta-analysis. Mutagenesis 17:119–126
11. Levi S, Urbano-Ispizua Gill R et al (1991) Multiple K-ras codon 12 mutations in cholangiocarcinomas demonstrating a sensitive polymerase chain reaction technique. Cancer Res 51:3497–3502
12. Ward R, Hawkins N, O'Grady R et al (1998) Restriction endonuclease mediated selective polymerase chain reaction. Am J Pathol 153:373–379
13. Jenkins GJS, Suzen HS, Sueiro RA, Parry JM (1999) The restriction site mutation (RSM) assay. A review of the methodology development and the current status of the technique. Mutagenesis 14:439–448
14. Jenkins GJS, Morgan C, Parry EM, Baxter JN, Parry JM (2001) The detection of mutations induced *in vitro* in the human p53 gene by a model reactive oxygen species (ROS) employing the restriction site mutation (RSM) assay. Mutat Res 498:135–144
15. Jenkins GJS, Doak SH, Griffiths AP, Baxter JN, Parry JM (2003) Early p53 mutations in non-dysplastic Barrett's tissues detected by the restriction site mutation (RSM) methodology. Br J Cancer 88:1271–1276
16. Parry JM, Shamsheer M, Skibinski D (1990) Restriction site mutation analysis, a proposed methodology for the detection and study of DNA base changes following mutagen exposure. Mutagenesis, 5:209–212
17. Jenkins GJS, Chalestori MH, Song H, Parry JM (1998) Mutation analysis using the restriction site mutation (RSM) assay. Mutat Res 405:209–220
18. Perwez Hussain SP, Aguilar F, Amstad P, Cerutti P (1994) Oxyradical induced mutagenesis of hotspot codons 248 and 249 of the human p53 gene. Oncogene 9:2277–2281
19. Morgan C, Jenkins GJS, Ashton T, et al (2003) The detection of p53 mutations in pre-cancerous gastric tissue using the RSM assay. Br J Cancer 89:1314–1319
20. Perwez Hussain S, Amstad P, Raja K, et al (2000) Increased p53 mutation load in noncancerous colon tissue from ulcerative colitis: a cancer prone chronic inflammatory disease. Cancer Res 60:3333–3337
21. Ehrlich M, Wang RHY (1981) 5-Methylcytosine in eukaryotic DNA. Science 212:1350–1357

22. Toyota M, Issa JPJ (2000) The role of DNA hypermethylation in human neoplasia. Electrophoresis 21:329–333
23. Fraga ME, Esteller M (2002) DNA methylation: a profile of methods and applications. Biotechniques 33:632
24. Oakeley EJ (1999) DNA methylation analysis: a review of current methodologies. Pharmacol Ther 84:389–400
25. Puvvada MS, Hartley JA, Jenkins TC, Thurston DE (1993) A quantitative assay to measure the relative DNA-binding affinity of pyrrolo[2,1-c][1,4]benzodiazepine (pbd) antitumor antibiotics based on the inhibition of restriction-endonuclease BamHI. Nucleic Acids Res 21:3671–3675
26. Denissenko MF, Venkatachalam S, Ma YH, Wani AA (1996) Site-specific induction and repair of benzo[a]pyrene diol epoxide DNA damage in human H-ras protooncogene as revealed by restriction cleavage inhibition. Mutation Res 36:27–42

3

Principles and Medical Applications of the Polymerase Chain Reaction

Bimal D. M. Theophilus

1. Introduction

The polymerase chain reaction (PCR) is currently one of the mainstays of medical molecular biology. One of the reasons for the wide adoption of PCR is the elegant simplicity of the way in which the reaction proceeds and the relative ease of the practical manipulation steps. Indeed, combined with the relevant bioinformatics resources for the practical design and for the determination of the required experimental conditions, it provides a rapid means for DNA diagnostic identification and analysis. It has also opened up the investigation of cellular and molecular processes to those outside the field of molecular biology and also contributed in part to the successful sequencing of the human genome project. Polymerase chain reaction is an in vitro amplification method able to generate a relatively large quantity (about 10^5 copies, or approx 0.25–0.5 µg) of a specific DNA sequence from a small amount of a heterogeneous DNA target, often comprising the total cellular genome. The sensitivity of PCR is such that successful amplification can be achieved from a single cell, as in single-sperm typing and preimplantation diagnosis, or from a minority DNA population that is present among an excess of background DNA (e.g., from viruses infecting only a few cells, or from low levels of "leaky" RNA transcription from nonexpressing tissues). The PCR process consists of incubating a reaction sample containing the DNA substrate and required reactants repeatedly between three different temperature incubations: denaturation, annealing, and extension. Many current investigators, the author included, recall their initial introduction to PCR as comprising the laborious transfer of sample tubes between three water baths heated to different temperatures representing the three incubations. Fortunately and no doubt instrumental to the wide implementation of PCR in numerous areas of fundamental research and applications is the automation of the process. This was the result of the development of programmable thermal cylcers that were developed only a few years subsequent to the invention of PCR by Mullis in 1983. Today, the technology has advanced to modern thermal cyclers that use Peltier heating and cooling elements to produce fast temperature changes or ramp rates of

From: *Molecular Biomethods Handbook, 2nd Edition.*
Edited by: J. M. Walker and R. Rapley © Humana Press, Totowa, NJ

around 3°C/s and that maintain accurate temperature control across the entire sample block. In addition PCR undertaken in 96-well microtiter plate systems is now possible, which is useful for high-throughput analysis of clinical samples.

2. Elements of PCR

2.1. PCR Practical Procedures

Polymerase chain reaction achieves near-exponential amplification of a DNA sequence, the length of which is defined by a pair of oligonucleotide primers, complementary to 20–25 bp of sequences at the 5' and 3' ends of the target molecule, respectively. It is relatively straightforward for the PCR to amplify up to approx 2 kb of sequences, but special modifications such as the use of a cocktail of enzymes are required to amplify larger sequences of up to 40 kb in a process termed "long-range PCR." Typical sources of target DNA include blood, mouthwashes or buccal scrapes, chorionic villus (for antenatal diagnosis), one to two cells from an eight-cell embryo (for preimplantation diagnosis), hair, and Guthrie spots. Extracted DNA does not need to be particularly pure and could even be partially fragmented, as in the case of archival material such as that derived from paraffin-embedded tissues. In the case of blood samples, simple boiling releases enough DNA for successful amplification. A PCR reaction mix is usually 5–50 µl in volume and is set up in 0.2-ml or 0.5-ml thin-walled reaction tubes or, as indicated, in 96-well microtiter plates. It comprises reaction buffer (optimized for magnesium chloride), deoxynucleotide triphospates (dNTPs), the oligonucleotide primers, a thermostable DNA polymerase (usually *Taq* DNA polymerase), which synthesizes DNA by incorporating dNTPs and extending the annealed primers, and, finally, the template to be amplified.

2.2. Steps Involved in a PCR Cycle

The initial step of PCR involves incubation of around 94°C for 5 min to denature the target genomic DNA into single strands. This step is not usually necessary when using cDNA derived from RNA as the template. The subsequent and main part of the process comprises the sequential incubation of the sample at three different temperatures, which together constitute one PCR cycle (see **Fig. 3.1**). The first step in a cycle involves incubation at 94–96°C for 10 s to 1 min to denature newly synthesized template DNA. Subsequent incubation is at a temperature determined by the melting properties of the primers, ideally around 56°C, optimized to allow them to anneal only to their specific target sequences. The third incubation is usually 72°C for 20 s to 2 min, during which *Taq* DNA polymerase extends the primers mediating the synthesis of DNA using the target sequence as the template. Normally, 30–35 such cycles are performed to comprise a PCR reaction, which typically takes about 3 h to complete. In the first cycle of PCR, primers can only anneal to the original target DNA. In this case, the primer defines the 5' end of each newly synthesized strand, but the 3' end is undefined and variable. However, in subsequent cycles, as newly synthesized DNA from one cycle becomes a template in the next cycle, the synthesized DNA will be defined at both ends by each primer. Because the synthesis of the latter species increases exponentially while DNA

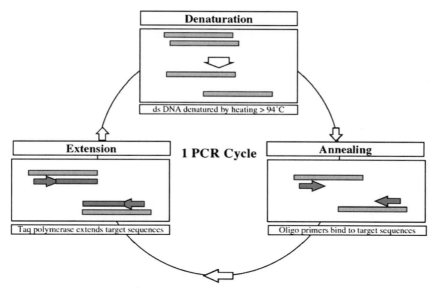

Fig. 3.1. Simplified scheme of one PCR cycle that involves denaturation, annealing and extension

synthesized from the original target only increases linearly, the predominant product (termed *amplicon*) resulting from PCR will be defined by the location of the forward and reverse primers (see **Fig. 3.2**). Whereas amplification is exponential in the earlier cycles, it plateaus out in later cycles because of the exhaustion of reaction components. For this reason, quantitative comparisons or estimates of PCR products should be based on the exponential phase of the reaction using "real time PCR". It is safe to leave the finished reaction in the thermal cycler at room temperature for several hours or overnight, although, typically, a final incubation "hold" temperature of 4–12°C is programmed after the final PCR cycle.

2.3. Primer Design and PCR

The specificity of PCR lies in the design of the two oligonucleotide primers. These not only have to be complementary to sequences flanking the target DNA but must not be self-complementary or bind each other to form dimers because both prevent DNA amplification (see **Fig. 3.3**). They also have to be matched in their GC content and have similar annealing temperatures. The increasing use of bioinformatics resources such as Oligo, Generunner, and Genefisher in the design of primers makes the design and the selection of reaction conditions much more straightforward. These resources allow the sequences to be amplified and the primer length, product size, GC content, and so forth, to be input, and, following analysis, they provide a choice of matched primer sequences. Indeed, the initial selection and design of primers without the aid of bioinformatics would now be unnecessarily time-consuming. With careful consideration of primer sequences and reaction conditions, it is possible to amplify more than one region in a single PCR. This process is termed *multiplex PCR* and is used extensively in molecular-based diagnostics, although it does require a degree of optimization.

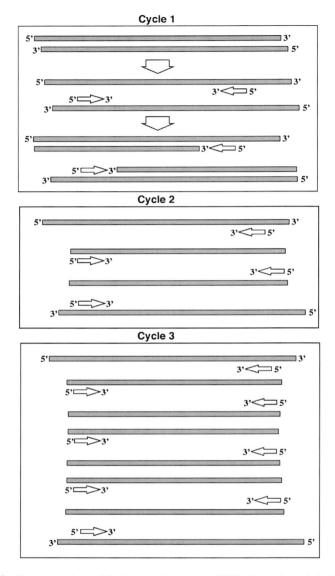

Fig. 3.2. Representation of further cycles in the PCR. Note the original template strands can also be copied, whereas newly synthesised PCR products are amplified exponentially

2.4. Sensitivity and Contamination in PCR

The enormous sensitivity of the PCR is also one of its main drawbacks because the very large degree of amplification makes the reaction vulnerable to contamination. Even a trace of foreign DNA, such as that contained in dust particles, may be amplified to significant levels and may give false-positive results. Hence, cleanliness is paramount when carrying out PCR, and dedicated equipment and, in some cases, laboratory areas and even laboratories are used. It is possible that previously amplified products may also contaminate PCR. However, this may be overcome by a number of methods including

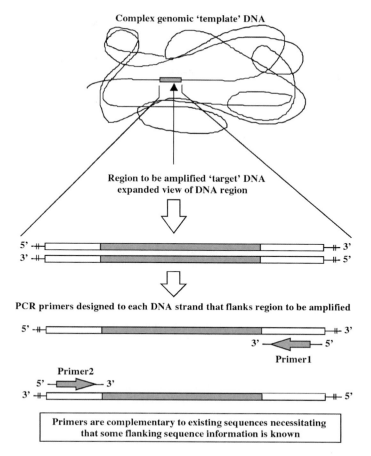

Fig. 3.3. The location of PCR primers. PCR primers designed to sequences adjacent to the region to be amplified, allowing a region of DNA (e.g., a gene) to be amplified from a complex starting material of genomic template DNA

ultraviolet (UV) irradiation to damage the already amplified products so that they cannot be used as templates. A further interesting solution is to incorporate uracil into PCR and then treat the products with the enzyme uracil-N-glycosylase (UNG), which degrades any PCR amplicons with incorporated uracil, rendering them useless as templates. In addition, most PCRs are now undertaken using hotstart. Here, the reaction mixture is physically separated from the template or the enzyme. When the reaction begins, mixing occurs and thus avoids any mispriming that might have arisen.

3. Medical Applications and PCR

The main areas of medical diagnosis to which PCR is applied are the detection of infectious pathogens (e.g., associated with sexually transmitted diseases or respiratory tract infections) and the identification of mutations in genes that are either responsible or constitute risk factors for human disease. In some tests, the result is simply found in the presence, size, or color of the PCR product, whereas in other situations, PCR is used to generate sufficient specific starting material on which to perform a number of post-PCR manipulations to obtain the result.

3.1. Polymorphism Detection: RFLPs, VNTRs, and STRs

Before specific genes and associated mutations were fully characterized, genetic diagnosis was often carried out using restriction fragment length polymorphisms (RFLPs). RFLPs are variations in the length of restriction fragments between alleles arising from the presence or absence of specific restriction enzyme sites. RFLPs within or closely linked to an affected gene were therefore used as markers to track inheritance of a faulty gene through a family pedigree. VNTRs (variable number of tandem repeat sequences) and STRs (short tandem repeats) are polymorphic sequences applied in a manner similar to RFLPs, but arise from variations in the number of tandem repeat sequences at a given locus between different alleles. They are performed by PCR using primers flanking the polymorphic region, incubation with a restriction enzyme (in the case of RFLPs), and analysis of the fragment sizes following gel electrophoresis. Subsequent research and the completion of the human genome project means that the underlying basis of most common single-gene disorders is now understood and so these methodologies are less widely used. However, they are still of use where the causative mutation in a particular family or disease remains elusive or where limited facilities or expertise prevents complete screening of a gene to identify a mutation.

3.2. PCR-Based Mutation Screening

One of the major clinical applications of PCR that has spawned numerous diagnostic laboratories is the screening of multiexon genes, without clearly defined founder mutations, and where, therefore, a significant number of heterogeneous mutations may be responsible for the disease phenotype in different families or populations (e.g., hemophilia, Gaucher disease, certain breast and ovarian cancers [which arise from mutations in the *BRCA1* and *BRCA2* genes], and colon cancer. Unfortunately, there is no single, quick, inexpensive, and reliable mutation screening method of universal application. The majority of techniques can only analyze 200–500 nucleotides at a time for maximum sensitivity, which corresponds to the size of most exons. Individual exons and their intron/exon boundaries (which may be the site of exon splice site mutations) are amplified using PCR primers complementary to flanking intronic sequence. Large exons are usually amplified as several overlapping segments.

3.2.1. Reverse Transcriptase PCR

A number of screening methods are able to analyze 1 kb or more at a time, in which case, PCR-amplified complementary or cDNA may be used. This is DNA synthesized using messenger RNA (mRNA) as a template mediated by the enzyme reverse transcriptase (see **Fig. 3.4**). This procedure, referred to as RT-PCR, enables the screening of multiple contiguous exons in a single analysis, which enables the identification of gene rearrangements and splicing

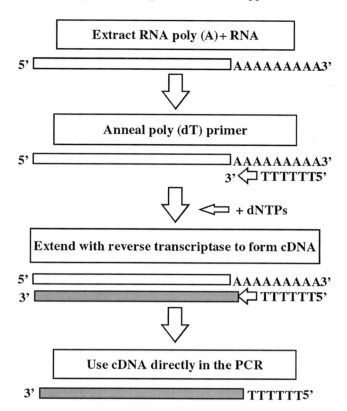

Fig. 3.4. Reverse-transcriptase PCR (RT-PCR). In RT-PCR, mRNA is converted to complementary DNA (cDNA) using the enzyme reverse transcriptase. The cDNA is then used directly in PCR

defects that may remain undetected by analysis of the genomic DNA coding sequence. However, RNA has a short half-life and is easily degraded; therefore, great care must be exercised in handling it. In addition, there is evidence that mutation-containing RNA may be less stable than normal RNA, therefore, the mutant allele may be underrepresented, or absent, in the RT-PCR product from a heterozygous sample. Finally, the gene under analysis may not be expressed in tissues that are readily accessible for analysis (e.g., blood), although sufficient "ectopic" RNA may be expressed by the so-called "leaky" transcription for successful PCR and analysis. Although mutation screening and detection methods are able to identify sequence differences between a normal and a patient sample, they do not indicate whether the change is pathogenic or simply a sequence polymorphism. This distinction usually depends on the nature of the change, the location of the change with regard to functional domains of the encoded protein, conservation of the affected amino acid residue among homologous proteins, and whether the change has been observed previously (by reference to mutation databases). Many mutation-detection methods depend on differences in the melting properties of DNA during gel electrophoresis. Single-strand conformation polymorphism (SSCP) analysis *(1)* is based on differences in the electrophoretic mobility of single-stranded DNA conformers in a nondenaturing gel system. It is a popular choice because it is simple to perform, but it is only able to analyze PCR products up to about 200 bp and it has limited sensitivity. Conformation-sensitive gel electrophoresis (CSGE) *(2)* is based on the electrophoretic mobility of DNA heteroduplexes under mildly denaturing conditions. It is only slightly more demanding to perform than SSCP, but has close to 100% detection efficiency. Denaturing gradient gel electrophoresis (DGGE) *(3)* identifies mismatch-containing heteroduplexes based on an abnormal denaturing profile on electrophoresis through a gradient of increasing denaturant concentration. Denaturing high-performance liquid chromatography (dHPLC) is a recently introduced method that is rapidly gaining in popularity. dHPLC distinguishes heteroduplexes from homoduplexes by ion-pair reverse-phase liquid chromatography according to differences in their melting behavior *(4)*. Positive ions in a buffer coat DNA in a hydrophobic layer, which interacts with a hydrophobic polystyrene matrix in a length- and sequence-specific manner. DNA is eluted from the matrix by a linear acetonitrile gradient. Although preliminary work is required to optimize the conditions for each PCR product, once established it is a rapid, highly automated, and sensitive technique able to detect close to 100% of mutations.

3.2.2. PCR-Based Mismatch Detection

Some other methods are based on chemical or enzymatic cleavage of mismatches in DNA heteroduplexes *(5,6)*. The protein truncation test (PTT) *(7)* identifies frame shift, splice site, and nonsense mutations by virtue of their ability to result in premature protein truncation, and it is applied to diseases where these types of mutation predominate, such as adenomatous polyposis coli (APC). Mutation-screening methods merely indicate that a mutation is present, which must then be characterized by DNA sequencing. With the development of automated fluorescent sequencers, many laboratories now sequence the complete coding sequence of a gene to identify mutations without the prior application of a mutation-screening method. Although the most laborious part of this process is often visual analysis of the sequence generated, there has been significant progress in the development of sequence analysis software, which is able to highlight sequence differences between two aligned sequences. However, these programs are not perfect, and it is often necessary to check sequences manually, especially in the case of heterozygous mutations. Also, although often considered the gold standard method of mutation detection, sequencing technology itself is not 100% accurate and may miss mutations or produce artifacts that must be investigated further.

3.3. PCR-Based Mutation Detection

Some conditions arise from one or a few clearly defined mutations. In these cases, one of a number of methods can be applied that detect the presence or absence of a defined sequence change. These are generally technically simpler and more rapid tests than those used for mutation screening described in Section 3.2.

3.3.1. Restriction Enzyme Analysis

If, fortuitously, a mutation creates or destroys a restriction site, then it may be identified simply by restriction enzyme analysis as described for RFLPs. For example, PCR followed by digestion with the restriction enzyme *Mnl*I is used to detect factor V Leiden, which arises from a point mutation in exon 13 of the factor V gene and constitutes the most frequent genetic risk factor for venous thrombosis. Alternatively, for mutations that do not alter a site for a restriction enzyme, a diagnostic site may be "engineered" into a PCR product using mutagenic primers.

3.3.2. Deletion Analysis

The most common cystic fibrosis (CFTR) allele is a three-nucleotide deletion, F508del. Simply amplifying the region by PCR using flanking primers and distinguishing the normal and mutant alleles by size on gel electrophoresis can identify this allele. Similarly, 60–65% of mutations causing Duchenne muscular dystrophy (DMD) are deletions of one or more exons within the dystrophin gene, 98% of which can be identified by two multiplex PCR reactions.

3.3.3. Analysis of Gene Rearrangements

Gene rearrangements are a feature of hematological malignancies, as well as certain nonmalignant diseases, such as the intron 1 and intron 22 inversion mutations responsible for approx 50% of severe hemophilia A. In the case of hematological malignancies, the novel chimeric transcripts arising from rearrangements are identified by RT-PCR (8). In hemophilia A, the intron 1 inversion mutation is detected by a standard PCR reaction, whereas the intron 22 inversion requires long-range PCR or Southern blotting for identification.

3.3.4. Allele-Specific PCR

Allele-specific oligo PCR (ASO-PCR, also known as the amplification refractory mutation system, ARMS) involves the hybridization of three primers in a single reaction. These comprise normal and mutant forward primers in which the final (3') base of the primer is homologous to either the normal or mutant sequences, respectively, together with a common reverse primer. The primer annealing temperature is optimized to ensure that primers only anneal to a perfectly matched template sequence, which is a requirement for subsequent extension by *Taq* DNA polymerase. Separate PCR reactions may be performed with the normal and mutant primers, respectively or a single reaction may be performed if the normal and mutant primers are distinguishable (e.g., with diffe rent fluorescent labels). Clearly, in order to design specific primers, the nature of the mutation to be detected must be known. An example of its use is to screen for a G to A transition at position 20210 in the 3' untranslated region of the prothrombin gene (9). The A allele is associated with elevated plasma prothrombin levels and carriers have a 2.8-fold increased risk of venous thrombosis. In addition, a multiplex ARMS test has been designed and marketed in kit form to test for a panel of common cystic fibrosis mutations.

3.3.5. 5' Nuclease/TaqMan™ Assay

The 5' Nuclease or TaqMan™ assay also involves the use of three primers: two allele-specific forward primers and a common reverse primer, which in this case is labeled with a "reporter" fluorophore at its 5' end and a "quencher" fluorophore at its 3' end. As with the allele-specific PCR, only the perfectly matched primer is extended by *Taq* DNA polymerase. On encountering the labeled reverse primer, the latter will be degraded by the 5' $\rightarrow$ 3' exonuclease activity of *Taq* DNA polymerase. This will result in the separation of the reporter and quencher fluorophores and a consequent increase in fluorescence. TaqMan is used for mutation detection and for screening specific subtypes of microbial pathogens. It is also used for association studies, which involve the correlation of single-nucleotide polymorphisms (SNPs) with complex disorders such as diabetes, heart disease, cancer, and mental disorders *(10)* SNPs are also of interest in the rapidly emerging field of pharmacogenetics, where they are analyzed for their role in determining variations between individuals in their responses to specific drugs or drug toxicity (e.g., in the cytochrome P450 genes) *(11)*. It is anticipated that this will lead to the identification of novel drug targets and aid in the production of individually tailored "designer" drugs.

3.3.6. Quantitative and Real-Time PCR

Real-Time PCR requires the use of special DNA cyclers such as the Roche Lightcycler that couples PCR with fluorescent detection, thereby enabling the detection of PCR product as it is synthesized. In its simplist form, a DNA-binding dye such as SYBR green is included in the reaction. As amplicons accumulate, SYBR green binds the dsDNA. This binding is proportional although nonspecific and fluorescence emission is detected following excitation. Diagnostically, real-time PCR enables the determination of a viral load in infectious diseases by comparing the amount of virus-specific product to a standard curve generated from samples containing known concentrations of DNA. Real-time PCR also has many research applications such as comparisons of gene expression between different tissues or at different stages of development. Although relatively expensive in comparison to other methods for determining expression levels, it is simple, rapid, and reliable. In addition to the quantitative nature, real-time PCR systems may also be used for genotyping and for accurate determination of the amplicon melting temperature using a so-called melting curve analysis. PCR has also been extended to further developments such as sequencing by minisequencing or pyrosequencing *(12,13)*. In addition, the new technology of microarrays uses, in some cases, PCR-derived material *(14)*. It is this area that may form the future of rapid nucleic acid diagnostic; however, PCR is still and no doubt will continue to be a mainstay of genetic-based diagnostics.

References

1. Orita M, Iwahana H, Kanazawa H, Hayashi K, Sekiya T (1989) Detection of polymorphisms of human DNA by gel electrophoresis as single-strand conformation polymorphisms. Proc Natl Acad Sci USA 86:2766–2770
2. Williams IJ, Goodeve AC (2002) Conformation-sensitive gel electrophoresis. In Theophilus BDM, Rapley R (eds) PCR mutation detection protocols. Humana, Totowa, NJ
3. Fischer SG, Lerman LS (1983) DNA fragments differing by a single base-pair substitution are separated in denaturing gradient gels: correspondence with melting theory. Proc Natl Acad Sci USA 80:1579–1583
4. Huber CG, Oefner PJ, Bonn GK (1995) Rapid and accurate sizing of DNA fragments by ion-pair chromatography on alkylated nonporous poly(styrenedivinylbenzene) particles. Anal Chem 67:578–585
5. Cotton RGH, Rodrigues NR, Campbell RD (1988) Reactivity of cytosine and thymine in single base-pair mismatches with hydroxylamine and osmium tetroxide

and its application to the study of mutations. Proc Natl Acad Sci USA 85: 4397–4401

6. Heisler L, Lee C-H (2002) Cleavase® fragment length polymorphism analysis for genotyping and mutation detection. In Theophilus BDM, Rapley R (eds) PCR mutation detection protocols. Humana, Totowa, NJ

7. Roest PAM, Roberts RG, Sugino S, van Ommen G-JB, den Dunnen JT (1993) Protein truncation test (PTT) for rapid detection of translation-terminating mutations. Hum Mol Genet 2:1719–1721

8. Cotter FE (1996) Molecular diagnosis of cancer. Humana, Totowa, NJ

9. Poort SR, Bertina RM, Vos HL (1997) Rapid detection of the prothrombin 20210 variation by allele specific PCR. Thromb Haemost 78:11,157–11,163

10. Chakravarti A (1999) Population genetics–making sense out of sequence. Nat Genet 21:56–60

11. McCarthy JJ, Hilfiker R (2000) The use of single-nucleotide polymorphism maps in pharmacogenomics. Nat Biotechnol 18:505–508

12. Hacia JG (1999) Resequencing and mutational analysis using oligonucleotide microarrays. Nat Genet 21:42–47

13. Syvanen AC (1999) From gels to chips: "minisequencing" primer extension for analysis of point mutations and single nucleotide polymorphisms. Hum Mutat 13: 1–10

14. Ronaghi M, Uhlen M, Nyren P (1998) A sequencing method based on real-time pyrophosphate. Science 281:363–365

4

Probe Design, Production, and Applications

Marilena Aquino de Muro

1. Introduction

A probe is a nucleic acid molecule (single-stranded DNA or RNA) with a strong affinity with a specific target (DNA or RNA sequence). Probe and target base sequences must be complementary to each other, but depending on conditions, they do not necessarily have to be exactly complementary. The hybrid (probe–target combination) can be revealed when appropriate labeling and detection systems are used. Gene probes are used in various blotting and in situ techniques for the detection of nucleic acid sequences. In medicine, they can help in the identification of microorganisms and the diagnosis of infectious, inherited, and other diseases.

2. Probe Design

The probe design depends on whether a gene probe or an oligonucleotide probe is desired.

2.1. Gene Probes

Gene probes are generally longer than 500 bases and comprise all or most of a target gene. They can be generated in two ways. Cloned probes are normally used when a specific clone is available or when the DNA sequence is unknown and must be cloned first in order to be mapped and sequenced. It is usual to cut the gene with restriction enzymes and excise it from an agarose gel, although if the vector has no homology, this might not be necessary.

Polymerase chain reaction (PCR) is a powerful procedure for making gene probes because it is possible to amplify and label, at the same time, long stretches of DNA using chromosomal or plasmid DNA as template and labeled nucleotides included in the extension step (see Sections 2.2. and 3.2.3.). Having the whole sequence of a gene, which can easily be obtained from databases (GenBank, EMBL, DDBJ), primers can be designed to amplify the whole gene or gene fragments. A considerable amount of time

From: *Molecular Biomethods Handbook, 2nd Edition.*
Edited by: J. M. Walker and R. Rapley © Humana Press, Totowa, NJ

can be saved when the gene of interest is PCR amplified, for there is no need for restriction enzyme digestion, electrophoresis, and elution of DNA fragments from vectors. However, if the PCR amplification gives nonspecific bands, it is recommended to gel purify the specific band that will be used as a probe.

Gene probes generally provide greater specificity than oligonucleotides because of their longer sequence and because more detectable groups per probe molecule can be incorporated into them than into oligonucleotide probes (1).

2.2. Oligonucleotide Probes

Oligonucleotide probes are generally targeted to specific sequences within genes. The most common oligonucleotide probes contain 18–30 bases, but current synthesizers allow efficient synthesis of probes containing at least 100 bases. An oligonucleotide probe can match perfectly its target sequence and is sufficiently long to allow the use of hybridization conditions that will prevent the hybridization to other closely related sequences, making it possible to identify and detect DNA with slight differences in sequence within a highly conserved gene, for example.

The selection of oligonucleotide probe sequences can be done manually from a known gene sequence using the following guidelines (1).

- The probe length should be between 18 and 50 bases. Longer probes will result in longer hybridization times and low synthesis yields, shorter probes will lack specificity.
- The base composition should be 40–60% G-C. Nonspecific hybridization may increase for G-C ratios outside of this range.
- Be certain that no complementary regions within the probe are present. These may result in the formation of "hairpin" structures that will inhibit hybridisation to target.
- Avoid sequences containing long stretches (more than four) of a single base.
- Once a sequence meeting the above criteria has been identified, computerized sequence analysis is highly recommended. The probe sequence should be compared with the sequence region or genome from which it was derived, as well as to the reverse complement of the region. If homologies to nontarget regions greater than 70% or eight or more bases in a row are found, that probe sequence should not be used.

However, to determine the optimal hybridization conditions, the synthesized probe should be hybridized to specific and nonspecific target nucleic acids over a range of hybridization conditions.

These same guidelines are applicable to design forward and reverse primers for amplification of a particular gene of interest to make a gene probe. It is important to bear in mind that, in this case, it is essential that the 3' end of both forward and reverse primers have no homology with other stretches of the template DNA other than the region you want to amplify. There are numerous software packages available (LaserDNA™, GeneJockey II™, etc.) that can be used to design a primer for a particular sequence or even just to check if the pair of primers designed manually will perform as expected.

3. Labeling and Detection

3.1. Types of Label

3.1.1. Radioactive Labels

Nucleic acid probes can be labeled using radioactive isotopes (e.g., ^{32}P, ^{35}S, ^{125}I, and ^{3}H). Detection is by autoradiography or Geiger–Muller counters. Radiolabeled probes used to be the most common type but are less popular today because of safety considerations as well as cost and disposal of radioactive waste products. However, radiolabeled probes are the most sensitive, as they provide the highest degree of resolution currently available in hybridization assays *(1,2)*. High sensitivity means that low concentrations of a probe–target hybrid can be detected; for example, ^{32}P-labeled probes can detect single-copy genes in only 0.5 µg of DNA and Keller and Manak *(1)* list a few reasons:

- ^{32}P has the highest specific activity.
- ^{32}P emits β-particles of high energy.
- ^{32}P-Labeled nucleotides do not inhibit the activity of DNA-modifying enzymes, because the structure is essentially identical to that of the nonradioactive counterpart.

Although ^{32}P-labeled probes can detect minute quantities of immobilized target DNA (<1 pg), their disadvantages is the inability to be used for high-resolution imaging and their relatively short half-life (14.3 d); ^{32}P-labeled probes should be used within a week after preparation.

The lower energy of ^{35}S plus its longer half-life (87.4 d) make this radioisotope more useful than ^{32}P for the preparation of more stable, less specific probes. These ^{35}S-labeled probes, although less sensitive, provide higher resolution in autoradiography and are especially suitable for *in situ* hybridization procedures. Another advantage of ^{35}S over ^{32}P is that the ^{35}S-labeled nucleotides present little external hazard to the user. The low-energy β-particles barely penetrate the upper dead layer of skin and are easily contained by laboratory tubes and vials.

Similarly, ^{3}H-labeled probes have traditionally been used for *in situ* hybridization because the low-energy β-particle emissions result in maximum resolution with low background. It has the longest half-life (12.3 yr).

The use of ^{125}I and ^{131}I has declined since the 1970s with the availability of ^{125}I-labeled nucleoside triphosphates of high specific activity. ^{125}I has lower energies of emission and a longer half-life (60 d) than ^{131}I, and are frequently used for in situ hybridization.

3.1.2. Nonradioactive Labels

Compared to radioactive labels, the use of nonradioactive labels have several advantages:

- Safety.
- Higher stability of probe.
- Efficiency of the labeling reaction.
- Detection in situ.
- Less time taken to detect the signal.

Concern over laboratory safety and the economic and environmental aspects of radioactive waste disposal have been key factors in their development and use. Some examples are as follows:

- Biotin: This label can be detected using avidin or streptavidin which have high affinities for biotin. Because the reporter enzyme is not conjugated directly to the probe but is linked to it through a bridge (e.g., streptavidin–biotin), this type of nonradioactive detection is known as an indirect system. Usually, biotinylated probes work very well, but because biotin (vitamin H) is a ubiquitous constitutent of mammalian tissues and because biotinylated probes tend to stick to certain types of Nylon membrane, high levels of background can occur during hybridizations. These difficulties can be avoided by using nucleotide derivatives, including digoxigenen-11-UTP, -11-dUTP, and -11-ddUTP, and biotin-11-dUTP or biotin-14-dATP. After hybridization, these are detected by an antibody or avidin, respectively, followed by a color or chemiluminescent reaction catalysed by alkaline phosphatase or peroxidase linked to the antibody or avidin *(1,2)*.
- Enzymes. The enzyme is attached to the probe and its presence usually detected by reaction with a substrate that changes color. Used in this way, the enzyme is sometimes referred to as a "reporter group," Examples of enzymes used include alkaline phosphatase and horseradish peroxidase (HRP). In the presence of peroxide and peroxidase, chloronaphtol, a chromogenic substrate for HRP, forms a purple insoluble product. HRP also catalyzes the oxidation of luminol, a chemiluminogenic substrate for HRP *(2,3)*.
- Chemiluminescence. In this method, chemiluminescent chemicals attached to the probe are detected by their light emission using a luminometer. Chemiluminescent probes (including the above enzyme labels) can be easily stripped from membranes, allowing the membranes to be reprobed many times without significant loss of resolution.
- Fluorescence chemicals attached to probe fluoresce under ultraviolet (UV) light. This type of label is especially useful for the direct examination of microbiological or cytological specimens under the microscope–a technique known as fluorescent in situ hybridization (FISH). Hugenholts et al have some useful considerations on probe design for FISH *(4)*.
- Antibodies. An antigenic group is coupled to the probe and its presence detected using specific antibodies. Also, monoclonal antibodies have been developed that will recognize DNA–RNA hybrids. The antibodies themselves have to be labeled, using an enzyme, for example.
- DIG system. It is the most comprehensive, convenient, and effective system for labeling and detection of DNA, RNA, and oligonucleotides. Digoxigenin (DIG), like biotin, can be chemically coupled to linkers, and nucleotides and DIG-substituted nucleotides can be incorporated into nucleic acid probes by any of the standard enzymatic methods. These probes generally yield significantly lower backgrounds than those labeled with biotin. An antidigoxigenin antibody–alkaline phosphatase conjugate is allowed to bind to the hybridized DIG-labeled probe. The signal is then detected with colorimetric or chemiluminescent alkaline phosphatase substrates. If a colorimetric substrate is used, the signal develops directly on the membrane. The signal is detected on an X-ray film (as with ^{32}P- or ^{35}S-labeled probes) when a chemiluminescent substrate is used. Roche Biochemicals has a series of kits for DIG labeling and detection, as well as comprehensive detailed guides *(5,6)* with protocols for single-copy gene detection of human genome on Southern blots, detection of unique mRNA species on Northern blots, colony and plaque screening, slot/dot blots, and *in situ* hybridization.

The one area in which nonradioactive probes have a clear advantage is in situ hybridization. When the probe is detected by fluorescence or color reaction, the signal is at the exact location of the annealed probe, whereas radioactive probes can only be visualized as silver grains in a photographic emulsion some distance away from the actual annealed probe (7).

3.2. Labeling Methods

The majority of radioactive labeling procedures rely upon enzymatic incorporation of a nucleotide labeled into the DNA, RNA, or oligonucleotide.

Table 4.1 summarizes the various types of label (2).

3.2.1. Nick Translation

Nick translation is one method of labeling DNA, which uses the enzymes pancreatic Dnase I and *Escherichia coli* DNA polymerase I. The nick translation reaction results from the process by which *E. coli* DNA polymerase I adds nucleotides to the 3'-OH created by the nicking activity of Dnase I, while the 5' to 3' exonuclease activity simultaneously removes nucleotides from the 5' side of the nick. If labeled precursor nucleotides are present in the reaction, the pre-existing nucleotides are replaced with labeled nucleotides. For radioactive labeling of DNA, the precursor nucleotide is an $[\alpha\text{-}^{32}P]dNTP$. For nonradioactive labeling procedures, a digoxigenin or a biotin moiety attached to a dNTP analog is used (2).

3.2.2. Random-Primed Labeling (or Primer Extension)

Gene probes, cloned or PCR-amplified, and oligonucleotide probes can be random-primed labeled with radioactive isotopes and nonradioactive labels (e.g., DIG). Random-primed labeling of DNA fragments (double- or single-stranded DNA) was developed by Feinberg and Volgestein (8,9) as an alternative to nick translation to produce uniformly labeled probes. Double-stranded DNA is denatured and annealed with random oligonucleotide primers (6-mers). The oligonucleotides serve as primers for the 5' to 3' polymerase (the Klenow fragment of *E. coli* DNA polymerase I), which synthesizes labeled probes in the presence of a labeled nucleotide precursor. **Figure 4.1A** shows the steps involved in random-primed DIG labeling as an example.

Table 4.1. Types of label.

Radioactive labels

^{32}P
^{35}S
^{125}I
^{131}I
^{3}H

Nonradioactive labels

Biotin
Chemiluminescent enzyme labels (acridinium
    ester, alkaline phosphatase,
    β-D-galactosidase, horseradish peroxidase
    [HRP], isoluminol, xanthine oxidase)
Fluorescence chemicals (fluorochromes)
Antibodies
Digoxigenin system

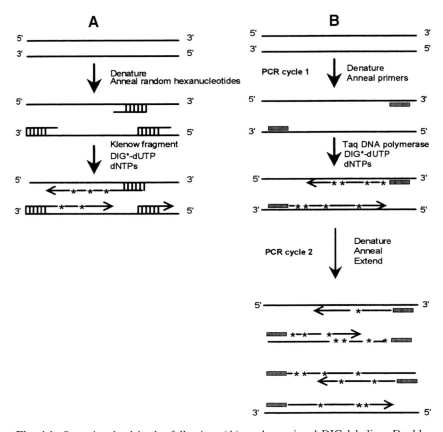

Fig. 4.1. Steps involved in the following: **(A)** random-primed DIG labeling: Double-stranded DNA is denatured and annealed with random oligonucleotide primers (6-mers); the oligonucleotides serve as primers for the 5' to 3' Klenow fragment of *E. coli* DNA polymerase I, which synthesizes labeled probes in the presence of DIG–dUTP. **(B)** PCR–DIG labelling: DIG–dUTP is incorporated during PCR cycles into the DNA strands amplified from the DNA target. The asterisk represents the digoxigenin molecule incorporated along the DNA strands

3.2.3. DIG–PCR Labeling

A very robust method for labeling a gene probe with DIG uses PCR. The probe is PCR-amplified using the appropriate set of primers and thermocycling parameters, however, the dNTP mixture has less dTTP because the labeled DIG–dUTP will also be added to the reaction. (Similarly, when this method is used with $[\alpha\text{-}^{32}P]dCTP$, the dNTP mixture will not have dCTP.) The advantage of PCR–DIG labeling, over random-primed DIG labeling, is the incorporation of a higher number of DIG moieties along the amplified DNA strands during the PCR cycles. It is worth noting that the random incorporation of large molecules of DIG–dUTP along the DNA strands during the PCR cycles makes the amplified fragment run slower on an agarose gel. A control PCR reaction, without DIG–dUTP, should also be prepared at the same time to verify whether the size of the amplified fragment with incorporated DIG (labeled probe) corresponds to the desired gene fragment. **Figure 4.1B** shows the steps involved in PCR–DIG labeling, and Refs. *(10–12)* describe successful examples of use of PCR–DIG labeling.

3.2.4. Photobiotin Labeling

Photobiotin labeling is a chemical reaction, not an enzymatic one. Biotin and DIG can be linked to a nitrophenyl azido group that is converted by irradiation with UV or strong visible light to a highly reactive nitrene that can form stable covalent linkages to DNA and RNA *(2)*. The materials for photobiotin labeling are more stable than the enzymes needed in nick translation or oligonucleotide labeling and are less expensive, and it is a method of choice when large quantities of probe but not very high sensitivities *(3,13)*.

3.2.5. End Labeling

End labeling of probes for hybridization is mainly used to label oligonucleotide probes (for a review, see **ref. *14***).

Roche Biochemicals *(6)* has developed three methods for labeling oligonucleotides with digoxigenin:

- The 3'-end labeling of an oligonucleotide 14–100 nucleotides in length with 1 residue of DIG-11-ddUTP per molecule
- The 3' tailing reaction, where terminal transferase adds a mixture of unlabeled nucleotides and DIG-11-dUTP, producing a tail containing multiple digoxigenin residues
- The 5' end labeling in a two-step synthesis with first an aminolinker residue on the 5' end of the oligonucleotide, and then after purification, a digoxigenin-*N*-hydroxy-succinimide ester is co-valently linked to the free 5'-amino residue.

Oligonucleotides can also be labeled with radioisotopes by transferring the γ-^{32}P from [γ-^{32}P]ATP to the 5' end using the enzyme bacteriophage T4 polynucleotide kinase. If the reaction is carried out efficiently, the specific activity of such probes can be as high as the specific activity of [γ-^{32}P]ATP itself *(2)*.

Promega has a detailed guide *(15)* with protocols on radioactive and nonradioactive labeling of DNA. The choice of probe labeling method will depend on the following:

- Target format: Southern, Northern, slot/dot, or colony blot (see Section 4.)
- Type of probe: gene or oligonucleotide probe
- Sensitivity required for detection: single-copy gene or detection of PCR-amplified DNA fragments

For example, 3'- and 5'-end labeling of oligonucleotides give good results on slot and colony hybridization in contrast with poor sensitivity when using Southern blotting.

4. Target Format

4.1. Solid Support

A convenient format for the hybridization of DNA to gene probes or oligonucleotide probes is immobilization of the target nucleic acid (DNA or RNA) onto a solid support while the probe is free in solution. The solid support can be a nitrocellulose or Nylon membrane, Latex or magnetic beads, or microtiter plates. Nitrocellulose membranes are very commonly used and produce low background signals; however, they can only be used when colorimetric detection will be performed and no probe stripping and reprobing is planned. For these purposes, positively charged Nylon membranes are recommended, and they also ensure an optimal signal-to-noise ratio when the DIG system is used. Although nitrocellulose membranes are able to bind large quantities of DNA, they become brittle and gradually release DNA during the hybridization step. Activated cellulose membranes, on the other hand, are more difficult to prepare, but they can be reused many times because the DNA is irreversibly bound [2].

After size fractionation of nucleic acids by electrophoresis, they are transferred to a filter membrane, which is then probed. The presence of target is confirmed by the detection of a probe on the filter membrane, for example, radiolabeled probe can be detected by autoradiography and the location of the target sequence in the bands in the original gel determined.

The different immobilization techniques include the following: Southern blots, when whole or digested chromosomal DNA is electrophoresed in an agarose gel, denatured, and blotted onto a membrane; Northern blots, when the same procedure is used for RNA; slot blots, when whole RNA or denatured DNA is loaded under vacuum into slots onto membranes (similar procedure for dot blots); colony blots, when colonies are treated with lysozyme on plates and further treatment with protease, and denaturation and neutralization solutions are applied and the procedure adjusted according the microorganism's peculiarities. The great advantage of colony blotting over slot blotting is that strains with a specific sequence can be rapidly detected from plates and the DNA preparation procedure can then be done only for the strains of interest. In a similar way, the slot blotting procedure has the advantage of quickly highlighting which DNA sample has the gene sequence of interest when a gene probe is hybridized to whole-DNA samples. The Southern blotting procedure, which involves the digest of DNA with restriction enzymes and gel electrophoresis, takes a longer preparation time than slot blotting but can provide information on the size and position of the gene as well as grouping the samples based on the similar patterns when different restriction enzymes are used to digest the samples. Schleicher and Schuell has a detailed manual on solid supports and DNA transfer (16).

4.2. In Solution

Both the probe and the target are in solution. Because both are free to move, the chances of reaction are maximized and, therefore, this format generally gives faster results than others.

4.3. *In Situ*

In this format, the probe solution is added to fixed tissues, sections, or smears, which are then usually examined under the microscope. The probe label (e.g., a fluorescent marker) produces a visible change in the specimen if the target sequence is present and hybridization has occurred. However, the sensitivity might be low if the amount of target nucleic acid present in the specimen is low. This can be used for the gene mapping of chromosomes and for the detection of microorganisms in specimens.

5. Hybridization Conditions

Many methods are available to hybridize probes in solution to DNA or RNA immobilized on nitrocellulose membranes. These methods can differ in the solvent and temperature used, the volume of solvent and the length of time of hybridization, the method of agitation, when required, and the concentration of the labeled probe and its specificity, the stringency of the washes after the hybridization. However, basically, target nucleic acid immobilized on membranes by the Southern blot, Northern blot, slot or dot blot, or colony blot procedures are hybridized in the same way. The membranes are first prehybridized with hybridization buffer minus the probe. Nonspecific DNA binding sites on the membrane are saturated with carrier DNA and synthetic polymers. The prehybridization buffer is replaced with the hybridization buffer containing the probe and incubated to allow hybridization of the labeled probe to the target nucleic acid. The optimum hybridization temperature is experimentally determined, starting with temperatures 5°C below the melting temperature (T_m). The T_m is defined as the temperature corresponding to the midpoint in transition from helix to random coil and depends on length, nucleotide composition and ionic strength for long stretches of nucleic acids. G-C pairs are more stable than A-T pairs because G and C form three H bonds as opposed to two between A and T. Therefore, double-stranded DNA rich in G and C has a higher T_m (more energy required to separate the strands) than A-T rich DNA. For oligonucleotide probes bound to immobilized DNA, the dissociation temperature, T_d, is concentration dependent. Stahl and Amman *(17)* discussed in detail the empirical formulas used to estimate T_m and T_d.

Following the hybridization, the unhybridized probe is removed by a series of washes. The stringency of the washes must be adjusted for the specific probe used. Low-stringency washing conditions (higher salt and lower temperature) increases sensitivity; however, these conditions can give nonspecific hybridization signals and high background. High-stringency washing conditions (lower salt and higher temperature, closer to the hybridization temperature) can reduce background and only the specific signal will remain. The hybridization signal and background can also be affected by probe length, purity, concentration, sequence, and target contamination *(1)*.

In aqueous solution, RNA–RNA hybrids are more stable than RNA–DNA hybrids, which are, in turn, more stable than DNA–DNA ones. This results in a difference in T_m of approx 10°C between RNA–RNA and DNA–DNA hybrids. Consequently, more stringent conditions should be used with RNA probes *(8)*.

In general, the hybridization rate increases with probe concentration. Also, within narrow limits, sensitivity increases with increasing probe concentration. The concentration limit is not determined by any inherent physical property of nucleic acid probes, but by the type of label and nonspecific binding properties of the immobilization medium involved.

6.   Applications in Medical Research

At least three basic applications of nucleic acid probes in medical research can be mentioned: (1) detection of pathogenic microorganisms, (2) detection of changes to nucleic acid sequences, and (3) detection of tandem repeat sequences. **Table 4.2** presents only a few examples of recently published literature on applications of nucleic acid probes in medical research.

6.1. Detection of Pathogenic Microorganisms

The application of nucleic acid probes has particularly been evident in microbial ecology, where probes can be used to detect unculturable microorganisms

Table 4.2. Examples of the applications of nucleic acid probes in medical research.

Application	Ref.
Detection of tumor suppressor genes in human bladder tumors	*21*
Identification of *Leishmania* parasites	*22*
Detection of malignant plasma cells of patients with multiple myeloma	*23*
Diagnosis of human papillomavirus	*24*
Visual gene diagnosis of HBV and HCV	*25*
Detection and identification of pathogenic *Vibrio parahaemolyticus*	*26*
Detection of *Vibrio cholerae*	*27–29*
Molecular analysis of tetracycline resistance in *Salmonella enterica*	*30*
Identification of fimbrial adhesins in necrotoxigenic *E. coli*	*31*
Epidemiological analysis of *Campylobacter jejuni* infections	*32*
Molecular analysis of NSP4 gene from human rotavirus strains	*33*
Physical mapping of human parasite *Trypanosoma cruzi*	*34*
Detection and identification of African trypanosomes	*35*
Changes related to neurological diseases (Alzheimer's, Huntington's)	*36*
Detection and identification of pathogenic *Candida* spp.	*37, 38*
Identification of *Mycobacterium* spp.	*39*
Detection of rifampin resistance in *Mycobacterium tuberculosis*	*40*
Identification of *Staphylococcus aureus* directly from blood cultures	*41*
Detection of rabies virus genome in brain tissues from mice	*42*

and pathogens in the environment or simply provide rapid identification of species and group levels. Through the development of DNA–DNA and RNA–DNA hybridization procedures and recombinant DNA methodology, the isolation of species-specific gene sequences is readily achieved *(18,19)*. Oligonucleotide hybridization probes complementing either small ribosomal subunits, large ribosomal subunits, or internal transcribed spacer regions have now been developed for a wide variety of microorganisms *(20)*, such as *Actinomyces, Bacteriodes, Borrelia, Clostridium, Campylobacter, Candida, Haemophilus, Helicobacter, Lactococcus, Mycoplasma, Neisseria, Proteus, Rickettsia, Vibrio, Streptococcus, Plasmodium, Pneumocystis, Trichomonas, Desulfovibrio, Streptomyces*, including some uncultivated species such as marine proteobacteria and thermophilic cyanobacterium, and *Chlamydia* species, *Rickettsia* species, *Trypanosoma* species, *Treponema pallidum, Pneumocystis carinii*, and *Mycobacterium* species to mention only a few examples with medical relevance. Detection of a nucleic acid sequence unique to a particular microorganism would demonstrate its presence in a specimen and, perhaps, confirm an infectious disease.

6.2. Detection of Changes to Nucleic Acid Sequences

A change to the DNA sequence is a mutation, which could involve deletion, insertion, or substitution. Changes in certain gene sequences can cause inherited diseases such as cystic fibrosis, muscular dystrophies, phenylketonuria, apoli-poprotein variants, and sickle cell anemia, and they can be diagnosed by probe detection. Nucleic acid probes have successfully been used to detect those mutations. With some inherited diseases, more than one type of mutation can cause the disease, in which case, a probe might have to be used under low stringency (to allow hybridization to a range of sequences) or several probes might be used to ensure hybridization to all target sequences.

6.3. Detection of Tandem Repeat Sequences

Tandem repeat sequences are usually 30–50 bp in length. Their size and dis-tribution are distinctive for an individual. They can be detected using nucleic acid probes and PCR. They are the basis of so-called "DNA fingerprinting," which can be used in forensic science to confirm the identity of a suspect from specimens (any body fluid, skin, and hair) left at the scene of a crime. This technique can also be used for paternity tests, sibling confirmation, and tissue typing.

References

1. Keller GH, Manak MM (1989) DNA probes, Stockton, NY
2. Sambrook J, Russell DW (2001) Molecular cloning:a laboratory manual, 3rd edn. Cold Spring Harbor Laboratory Press, Cold Spring Harbor, NY
3. Karcher SJ (1995) Molecular biology:a project approach. Academic, San Diego, CA
4. Hugenholtz P, Tyson GW, Blackall LL (2002) Design and evaluation of 16S rRNA-targeted oligonucleotide probes for fluorescence in situ hybridization. In: Aquino de Muro, Rapley R (eds) Gene probes:principles and protocols. Humana, Totowa, NJ, pp. 29–42
5. Boehringer Mannheim GmbH (1995) The DIG system user's guide for filter hybridisation. Boehringer Mannheim, Mannheim, Germany
6. Boehringer Mannheim GmbH (1996) Nonradioactive in situ hybridisation man-ual:application manual, 2nd edn. Boehringher Mannheim GmbH, Mannheim, Germany
7. Alphey L, Parry HD (1995) Making nucleic acid probes. In: Glover DM, Hames BD (eds) DNA cloning 1:core techniques, IRL, Oxford, pp. 121–141
8. Feinberg AP, Vogelstein B (1983) A technique for radiolabeling DNA restriction endonuclease fragments to high specific activity. Analy Biochem 132:6–13
9. Feinberg AP, Vogelstein B (1984) Addendum. Analy Biochem 137:266–267
10. Aquino de Muro M, Priest FG (1994) A colony hybridization procedure for the identification of mosquitocidal strains of *Bacillus sphaericus* on isolation plates. J Invertebr Pathol 63:310–313
11. Aquino de Muro M, Priest FG (2000) Construction of chromosomal integrants of Bacillus sphaericus 2362 by conjugation with Escherichia coli. Res. Microbiol. 151:547–555
12. Garratt LC, McCabe MS, Power JB, Davey MR (2002) Detection of single-copy genes in DNA from transgenic plants. In: Aquino de Muro M, Rapley R (eds) Gene probes: principles and protocols Humana, Totowa, NJ, pp. 211–222
13. Hilario E (2002) Photobiotin labeling. In Aquino de Muro M, Rapley R (eds) Gene probes:principles and protocols. Humana, Totowa, NJ, pp. 19–22
14. Hilario E (2002) End labeling procedures. In: Aquino de Muro M, Rapley R (eds) Gene probes:principles and protocols. Humana, Totowa, NJ, pp. 13–18
15. Promega Corp (1996) Protocols and applications guide, 3rd edn. Promega Corp., Madison, WI

16. Schleicher & Schuell Inc (1995) Blotting, hybridization and detection: an S&S laboratory manual, 6th edn. Schleicher & Schuell, Inc., Keene, NH

17. Stahl DA, Amman R (1991) Development and application of nucleic acid probes. In: Stackebrandt E, Goodfellow M (eds) Nucleic acid techniques in bacterial systematics. Wiley, Chichester, pp. 205–244

18. Brooker JD, Lockington RA, Attwood GT, Miller S (1990) The use of gene and antibody probes in identification and enumeration of rumen bacterial species. In: Macario AJL, Conway de Macario E (eds) Gene probes for bacteria Academic, San Diego, CA, pp. 390–416

19. Stahl DA, Kane MD (1992) Methods in microbial identification, tracking and monitoring of function. Curr Opin Biotechnol 3:244–252

20. Ward DM, Bateson MM, Weller R, Ruff- Roberts AL (1992) Ribosomal RNA analysis of micro-organisms as they occur in nature. Adv Microb Ecol 12:219–286

21. Orlow I, Cordon-Cardo C (2002) Evaluation of alterations in the tumor suppressor genes INK4A and INK4B in human bladder tumors. In: Aquino de Muro M, Rapley R (eds) Gene probes:principles and protocols. Humana, Totowa, NJ, pp. 43–59

22. Mendoza-Leon A, Luis L, Martinez C (2002) The β-tubulin gene region as a molecular marker to distinguish Leishmania parasites. In: Aquino de Muro M, Rapley R (eds) Gene probes:principles and protocols. Humana, Totowa, NJ, pp. 61–83

23. Brown RD, Joy Ho P (2002) Detection of malignant plasma cells in the bone marrow and peripherical blood of patients with multiple myeloma. In: Aquino de Muro M, Rapley R (eds) Gene probes:principles and protocols. Humana, Totowa, NJ, pp. 85–91

24. Nuovo G J (2002) Diagnosis of human papillomavirus using in situ hybridization and in situ polymerase chain reaction. In: Aquino de Muro M, Rapley R (eds) Gene probes:principles and protocols Humana, Totowa, NJ, pp. 113–136

25. Wang Y, Pang D, Zhang Z, Zheng H, Cao J, Shen J (2003) Visual gene diagnosis of HBV and HCV based on nanoparticle probe amplification and silver staining enhancement. J Med Virol 70(2):205–211

26. Cook DW, Bowers JC, DePaola A (2002) Density of total and pathogenic (tdh+) *Vibrio parahaemolyticus* in Atlantic and Gulf Coast molluscan shellfish at harvest. J Food Protect 65(12):1873–1880

27. Dalsgaard A, Serichantalergs O, Forslund A et al (2001) Clinical and environmental isolates of *Vibrio cholerae* serogroup 0141 carry the CTX phage and the genes enconding the toxin-coregulated pili. J Clin Microbiol 39(11):4086–4092

28. Kondo S, Kongmuang U, Kalnauwakul S, Matsumoto C, Chen CH, Nishibuchi M (2001) Molecular epidemiologic analysis of *Vibrio cholerae* O1 isolated during the 1997–8 cholera epidemic in southern Thailand. Epidemiol Infect 127(1):7–16

29. Nair GB, Bag PK, Shimada T et al (1995) Evaluation of DNA probes for specific detection of *Vibrio cholerae* O139 Bengal. J Clin Microbiol 33(8):2186–2187

30. Frech G, Schwarz S (2000) Molecular analysis of tetracycline resistance in *Salmonella enterica* subsp. *enterica* serovars Typhimurium, Enteritidis, Dublin Choleraesuis, Hadar and Sàintpaul:construction and application of specific gene probes. J Appl Microbiol 89(4):633–641

31. Mainil JG, Gerardin J, Jacquemin E (2000) Identification of the F17 fimbrial subunit- and adhesin-enconding (f17A and f17G) gene variants in necrotoxigenic *Escherichia coli* from cattle, pigs and humans. Vet Microbiol 73(4):327–335

32. Fujimoto S, Umene K, Saito M, Horikawa K, Blaser MJ (2000) Restriction fragment length polymorphism analysis using random chromosomal gene probes for epidemiological analysis of *Campylobacter* jejuni infections. J Clin Microbiol 38(4):1664–1667

33. Kirkwood CD, Gentsch JR, Glass RI (1999) Sequence analysis of the NSP4 gene from human rotavirus strains isolated in the United States. Virus Genes 19(2): 113–122

34. Santos MRM, Lorenzi H, Porcile P et al (1999) Physical mapping of a 670-kb region of chromosomes XVI and XVII from the human protozoan parasite Trypanosoma cruzi encompassing the genes for two immunodominant antigens. Genome Res 9(12):1268–1276

35. Radwanska M, Magez S, Perry-O'Keefe H et al (2002) Direct detection and identification of African trypanosomes by fluorescence in situ hybridization with peptide nucleic acid probes. J Clin Microbiol 40(11):4295–4297

36. Higgins GA, Mah VH (1989) In situ hybridisation approaches to human neurological disease. In: Conn PM (ed) Gene probes. Academic, San Diego, CA, pp. 183–196

37. Rigby S, Procop GW, Haase G, et al (2002) Fluorescence in situ hybridization with peptide nucleic acid probes for rapid identification of *Candida albicans* directly from blood culture bottles. J Clin Microbiol 40(6):2182–2186

38. Oliveira K, Haase G, Kurtzman C, Hyldig- Nielsen JJ, Stender H (2001) Differentiation of *Candida albicans* and *Candida dubliniensis* by fluorescent in situ hybridization with peptide nucleic acid probes. J Clin Microbiol 39(11): 4138–4141

39. Cloud JL, Neal H, Rosenberry R et al (2002) Identification of *Mycobacterium* spp. by using a commercial 16S ribosomal DNA sequencing kit and additional sequencing libraries. J Clin Microbiol 40(2):400–406

40. El Hajj HH, Marras SAE, Tyagi S, Kramer FR, Alland D (2001) Detection of rifampin resistance in *Mycobacterium tuberculosis* in a single tube with molecular beacons. J Clin Microbiol 39(11):4131–4137

41. Oliveira K, Procop GW, Wilson D, Coull J, Stender H (2002) Rapid identification of *Staphylococcus aureus* directly from blood cultures by fluorescence in situ hybridization with peptide nucleic acid probes. J Clin Microbiol 40(1):247–251

42. Reddy CC, Jayakumar R, Kumanan K, Nainar AM (2002) Detection of rabies virus genome in brain tissues by using in situ hybridization. Indian J Anim Sci 72(1):3–5

5

Southern Blotting as a Diagnostic Method

Bronwen M. Harvey and Pirkko Soundy

1. Introduction

Nucleic acid hybridization is a process in which complementary single strands of nucleic acids combine to achieve a stable double-stranded nucleic acid molecule. This action has been used to establish a molecular or genetic relatedness among organisms and to characterize their genomes. Furthermore, this technique is one of several diagnostic tools useful for detecting a wide variety of conditions. Since the determination of the basic principles of duplex formation and stability in the 1950s, many variations of the hybridization techniques have been developed. Southern first transferred DNA fragments from agarose, after electrophoretic separation, onto nitrocellulose *(1)*. The technique is known as Southern blotting. Alwine et al *(2)* described shortly afterward a similar Northern blotting technique in which separated RNA strands are transferred from an agarose gel to a suitable solid support. A logical extension of these blotting techniques has been the dot or slot blot in which the sample is applied directly to the solid support without prior size separation *(3)*. Over the years, these techniques have been further developed and modified extensively by many researchers across the world. The application of these methods is as varied as the procedures used (e.g., to determine the changes in the nutritional state of an environment, to establish taxa genetically, to distinguish pathogenic from nonpathogenic viruses, to analyze gene structure).

This chapter restricts itself to the application of Southern blotting to provide information relating to genetic diseases. The DNA sample, which can include blood, tissue biopsies, buccal scraps, amniotic fluid, cultured cells, and so forth, is generally digested using a restriction endonuclease and then subjected to electrophoresis in a horizontal agarose gel. After sufficient time has elapsed to achieve adequate separation of the required fragments, the gel is soaked in an alkali solution to achieve denaturation of the double-stranded nucleic acid, then neutralized and prepared for transfer. Transfer to a nitrocellulose, polyvinylidene (PVDF), or Nylon membrane is achieved by a process of blotting in which buffer is drawn through the gel and the membrane. The fragments carried

From: *Molecular Biomethods Handbook, 2nd Edition.*
Edited by: J. M. Walker and R. Rapley © Humana Press, Totowa, NJ

with the buffer are retained on the surface of the membrane. The retention is made more permanent through a fixation process. The blot can then be used in a hybridization with labeled probes to identify the fragments of interest.

There are many variations on this basic theme (*4,5*). Those procedures requiring the identification of fragments in excess of 10,000 bases advocate the use of a depurination step to improve the efficiency of large-fragment transfer. Methodologies using positively charged nylon membranes often omit the neutralization step and advocate the use of alkaline transfer buffer, which can also serve as a fixative. There are many ways to achieve the transfer of DNA from the gel to the solid support. Southern's original method (*1*) describes the use of a capillary transfer procedure, and this remains the most widely used technique by far because of its low cost and convenience, transfer is often an overnight step (see **Fig. 5.1.**). If speed is a requirement, the transfer process can be shortened by using specialized vacuum blotting apparatus or electroblotting devices. Such techniques allow transfer in 30–60 min compared to several hours for capillary transfer.

The membrane of choice is determined by the sensitivity required and the detection method to be used. The quantity of sample has a significant effect on both of these. The use of nitrocellulose usually results in low backgrounds and is recommended when the level of target is high. Nitrocellulose membrane is available in supported and unsupported forms, depending on the manufacturing method employed; however, the handling characteristics of the latter can be poor. Unsupported membranes are produced when the active substrate is cast as a pure sheet. Because of their fragile nature, unsupported membranes should be handled with care. Supported membranes are those for which the active substrate is cast onto an inert "web" or support.

Nitrocellulose membrane can bind 80–125 µg nucleic acid/cm^2, which is significantly less than the binding capacity of 400–600 µg/cm^2 for a nylon

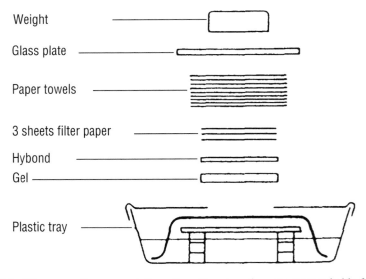

Fig. 5.1. Diagrammatic representation of capillary transfer apparatus; suitable for the transfer of DNA or RNA fragments separated by gel electrophoresis to a suitable Nylon or nitrocellulose membrane for example. Hybond is available from GE Healthcare Bio-Sciences

membrane. Its ability to bind small molecules (<400 nts) is also poor, and transfer buffers must contain high salt concentrations to ensure efficient nucleic acid binding. Nylon membranes are available in uncharged and positively charged supported forms. Charged nylon has a higher binding capacity and is particularly useful when working with low-molecular-weight nucleic acid. Binding to a nylon membrane is independent of the ionic strength of the transfer buffer. However, backgrounds can be elevated. Where repeated use of a membrane in hybridization assays is needed, the use of nylon membranes is strongly advised. Nylon is also recommended for use with medium- or low-abundance targets and is, in general, the membrane of choice when working with nucleic acids. PVDF membranes behave similarly to uncharged nylon, but because of its hydrophobic nature, use in nucleic acid blotting is limited.

Fixation bonds the target nucleic acid to the membrane. Suboptimal fixation will lower sensitivity by reducing target concentration and is particularly harmful if the blot is to be used more than once. The principal fixation methods of heat and ultraviolet (UV) light can be used with all types of membrane. Heat fixation is very reproducible but requires a vacuum oven for nitrocellulose. UV crosslinking, performed using an UV crosslinker (constant energy setting), is faster than heat. Alkali provides a third alternative method when charged Nylon membranes are used.

Original methods describe the use of a DNA probe radioactively labelled by random priming or nick translation with (^{32}P)dCTP to detect specific nucleic acid fragments immobilized on nitrocellulose membrane. Since then, many different methods for labeling nucleic acid probes ranging from short oligonucleotides to longer DNA or RNA fragments have been developed *(6,7)*. Nonradioactive labeling kits and reagents are also available, finding favor in a number of niche areas *(8)*. The role of the hybridization buffer is to provide conditions that promote hybridization between the labeled probe molecules and its complementary sequence immobilized on the membrane, and to simultaneously limit hybridization between sequences that are not perfectly matched *(6)* **Table 5.1** lists factors affecting the hybridization rate and stringency *(4–6)*. Many different formulations of hybridization buffers have been developed, containing inorganic salts and blocking agents such as Denhardt's solution (mixture of bovine serum albumin (BSA), Ficoll 400, and polyvinyl pyrrolidone), denatured DNA from salmon sperm (or other

Table 5.1. Factors affecting hybridization rate and stringency.

Factor	How hybridization is affected
Temperature	High temperature increases hybridization stringency; temperatures below T_m are recommended (for RNA long probe, 10–15°C below T_m; for DNA long probe, approx 25°C below T_m)
Ionic strength	Optimal hybridization in the presence of 1.5 M Na$^+$; lowering ionic strength increases stringency.
Destabilizing agents (or T_m modifiers)	For example, formamide and urea; used to lower the effective hybridization temperature
Mismatched basepairs	Mismatches lower hybridization rate
Duplex length	Hybridization rate increases with increased probe length
Viscosity	Increases rate of filter hybridization

species), and heparin *(4–6)*. A short prehybridization step in hybridization buffer is usually carried out to reduce nonspecific background hybridization before adding the labeled probe. This is especially important in genomic Southern blots that contain all genomic sequences on the membrane. Hybridization with the probe is usually carried out for several hours to allow hybridization between low-abundance sequences. Although various rapid-hybridization buffers containing volume excluders are available to speed up this step. After hybridization, the blot is washed to remove unhybridized probe. The stringency of washing is usually controlled by stepwise reductions in the ionic strength of wash buffer and/or by temperature *(4–6)*. The replacement of the old plastic bag technology with specialized temperature-controlled rotisserie devices for performing hybridization and washes has resulted in more consistent results and safer handing of radioactivity. After washing, the blot is subjected to autoradiography with X-ray film to visualize the bound probe *(9)*.

2. Southern Blotting in the Diagnosis of Human Disease

Southern blotting has been applied to the diagnosis of many human diseases at the molecular level. These genetic diseases are caused by point mutations, gene rearrangements, or the amplification of genes or specific sequences within the genome. These methods have in common that restriction-digested genomic DNA is size-separated in agarose gel electrophoresis, transferred onto the membrane, and hybridized with gene-specific probes.

Restriction fragment length polymorphism (RFLP) analysis was one of the early methods to diagnose point mutations implicated in genetic diseases. This method was based on the observation that if a point mutation changes a restriction fragment recognition sequence, it is possible to detect this change by Southern blotting analysis in which the affected restriction enzyme is used to cut genomic DNA before analysis. The change in the size of detected fragments with a gene-specific probe signals the presence of mutation in the analyzed gene. For example, this method has been applied to the diagnosis of hemophilia A, which is the most common inherited bleeding disorder, affecting approx 1 in 5,000 males worldwide. Hemophilia A is an X-linked, recessively inherited bleeding disorder that results from a deficiency of procoagulant factor VIII (FVIII). Affected males suffer from joint and muscle bleeds and easy bruising, the severity of which is closely correlated with the level of activity of coagulation factor VIII (FVIII:C) in their blood. Gitschier et al. demonstrated using Southern blotting that it was possible to diagnose the disease in 42% of affected families *(10)*. Having identified the *Bcl*I polymorphism, X-linked inheritance was demonstrated in three generations of a Utah family. DNA from a family member was restricted with *Bcl*I, electrophoresed on a 0.8% agarose gel, and blotted on to nylon membrane and probe with a complementary sequence within the factor VIII gene labeled with radioactivity. Twelve bands were observed by autoradiography. Eleven hybridizing bands remained constant, and one varied in position at either approx 0.9 or 1.1 kb in size.

The presence of gene point mutations has also been diagnosed with Southern blotting using allele-specific probes. These are usually short oligonucleotides in which the mismatched sequence is situated in the middle. By carefully controlling the hybridization and wash conditions (temperature and ionic strength of wash buffers), it is possible to distinguish between the binding of oligonucleotides differing by only one nucleotide. This method has been applied, for example, to distinguish between the normal human β-globin gene and the sickle cell β-globin gene *(11,12)*. Sickle cell anemia is caused by a single base change, resulting in the replacement of glutamic acid residue at position 6 of the protein (hemoglobin) by a valine residue.

Gene rearrangements can be diagnosed with Southern blotting if a probe hybridizing to the affected areas is used. Rearrangement is detected by observing change in the size and pattern of hybridized genomic restriction fragments. This type of analysis has been applied to the diagnosis of acute promyelocytic leukemia (APL), a subtype of acute myeloid leukemia. The disease is characterized by abnormal, heavily granulated promyelocytes, a form of white blood cells. APL results in the accumulation of these atypical promyelocytes in the bone marrow and peripheral blood, and they replace normal blood cells. At the molecular level, the disease involves translocation between the retinoic acid receptor-α (*RAR*-α) on chromosome 17 and the promyelocytic leukemia locus *(PML)* on chromosome 15. This results in the transcription of novel fusion messenger RNAs. By separating restriction-digested genomic DNA in pulse field gel electrophoresis followed by hybridization with probes derived from *PML* and *RAR*-α genes, it was possible to detect translocation events that correlated with disease progression *(13)*.

Gene amplifications are implicated in many diseases. Charcot–Marie–Tooth (CMT) syndrome is a common autosomal-dominant neuromuscular disorder. The disease is characterized by a slowly progressive degeneration of the muscles in the foot, lower leg, hand, and forearm and a mild loss of sensation in the limbs, fingers, and toes. The first sign of CMT is generally a high arched foot or gait disturbances. Other symptoms of the disorder may include foot bone abnormalities such as high arches and hammer toes, problems with hand function and balance, occasional lower leg and forearm muscle cramping, loss of some normal reflexes, occasional partial sight and/or hearing loss, and, in some patients, scoliosis (curvature of the spine). Genetically, the disorder is usually characterized by duplication of a region on chromosome 17 through unequal crossover. As a result, affected patients carry three copies of this region. One diagnostic approach to CMT, type 1A exploits Southern blot hybridization and the relative intensity for three polymorphic *Msp*I RFLP bands within the duplicated area to judge whether patients have two or three copies of this region using a region-specific probe. To normalize the observed intensity of the signal resulting from the CMT gene probe, another probe derived from unconnected sequences is used *(14)*.

The most significant changes in the use of Southern blotting in diagnosis have been seen since the introduction of primer-specific polymerase chain reaction (PCR) and automated nonradioactive sequencing techniques. Mutation and gene deletions once detected via Southern blot analysis are now routinely analyzed with these rapid and inexpensive methods, which are often fully automated. Cystic fibrosis, Duchenne muscular dystrophy, sickle cell anemia, and thalassaemia, to name a few, are now diagnosed by PCR. PCR methods can be completed in as little as 4 h, whereas Southern blotting can take up to 5 d to achieve the same result. More important, the amount of DNA required for analysis is significantly less with PCR amplification methods. The Southern blotting diagnosis method generally requires 5–10 µg of genomic DNA. The introduction of a PCR-based method is generally only achieved once the gene defect has been characterized at the molecular level. Hence research into disorders where the defect is unknown or further information is required still uses Southern blot analysis as an important research tool. In the routine laboratory, the use of Southern blotting is restricted to those diseases that require additional information the Southern blot can provide. One such disease is Fragile X; however prescreening using PCR analysis is common.

2.1. Fragile X Syndrome

Fragile X syndrome is a common genetic disease. This inherited form of mental retardation affects 1 in 4,000 males and 1 in 8,000 females *(15)*. Males with fragile X often exhibit characteristic physical features and accompanying autistic and attention-deficit behaviors. Individual IQs are in the range 35–70 *(16–18)*. Approximately 30% of females with full mutations are mentally retarded, and their level of retardation is, on average, less severe than that seen in males.

In 1943, Martin and Bell *(19)* were able to link the cognitive disorder to an unidentified mode of X-linked inheritance. In 1967, Lubs *(20)* discovered excessive genetic material extending beyond the low arm of the X chromosome in affected males. Diagnosis was originally based on cytogenetic analysis of metaphase spreads, but less than 60% of the affected cells in affected individuals showed a positive result. With this variability in the test, the carrier status of individuals could not be determined. Interpretation of the result is further complicated by the presence of other fragile sites in the same region of the X chromosome.

The fragile X gene (*FMR1*) is located in chromosomal band Xq27.3 and encodes an RNA-binding protein, which was initially characterized in 1991 *(21–23)* and contains a tandemly repeated trinucleotide sequence (CGG) end at its 5' end. The disease is caused by the absence of a functional *FMR1* gene product *(24)*. A small number of individuals classified as fragile X cytogentically have expansion at the nearby *FRAXE* locus, which also contains an unstable CGG repeat *(25–28)*. The normal distribution of the repeat in the unaffected population varies from 6 to 50. Affected individuals are classified into one of two major groups; premutations of approx 50–200 repeats and full mutations with more than 200 repeats. Some alleles with approx 45–55 copies of the repeat are unstable and expand from generation to generation; others are stably inherited *(29–31)*. The larger the size of the female premutation, the greater the risk of expansion during meiosis *(32)*. Individual male or females carrying a premutation are unaffected *(20,29,30)*. Males pass on the mutation relatively unchanged to all their daughters, all of whom are unaffected.

In some cases of premutation, an accurate estimate of the size of the expansion is required, most especially in family studies. This increase in resolution is achieved by Southern blot assay, using *Pst*I digestion of genomic DNA and detection with a probe close to the repeat array. Characteristic of the full mutation is methylation of the promotor region of the gene (CpG island) *(33)*; this correlates directly to gene inactivation. This is an important event in the disease pathogenesis, its effect on clinical severity is, however, unpredictable, especially in females.

Today, two main approaches are used in diagnosis of fragile X syndrome: PCR (36–39) and Southern blot analysis (40). The use of flanking primers allows the amplification of the region of DNA containing the repeats. The size of the PCR product is therefore indicative of the number of repeats present. However, the efficiency of the PCR reactions inversely relates to the number of repeats; hence, large mutations are more difficult to amplify and can fail to yield a PCR product. False negatives by PCR can also be an issue caused by the presence of normal and full mutations in some male patients (41). No information as to the extent of methylation can be determined by a PCR-based assay. Southern blotting allows both the size of the repeat segment and methylation status to be assayed simultaneously. Methylation- sensitive restriction enzymes such as *Eag*I or *Nru*I can be used to distinguish between methylated and unmethylated alleles. When combined with *Eco*RI, these enzymes give fragment sizes of 2.6 kb from normal unmethylated *FMR-1* genes. Methylated normal genes are not cut by these enzymes and yield 5.1-kb *Eco*RI fragments. Methylated and unmethylated expansions are indicated by the presence of bands or smears above the 5.1-kb and 2.6-kb fragments, respectively.

It is common practice in diagnosis laboratories to use PCR for prescreening and only to proceed to Southern blotting for those samples that fail to amplify (males) or show a single normal allele (females). If the etiology of mental impairment is unknown, DNA analysis for fragile X syndrome should be performed as part of a comprehensive genetic evaluation, which includes routine cytogenetic analysis. Cytogenetic studies are critical because constitutional chromosome abnormalities have been identified as frequent or more frequently than fragile X mutations in mentally retarded individuals referred for fragile X testing. For individuals who are at risk because of an established family history of fragile X syndrome, DNA testing alone is sufficient. If the diagnosis of the affected relative was based on previous cytogenetic testing for fragile X syndrome, then it is advised that at least one affected relative should be included in the DNA testing profile. Prenatal testing (42) of a fetus is indicated following a positive carrier test in the mother. When the mother is a known carrier, DNA testing can be offered to determine whether the fetus inherited the normal or mutant *FMR1* gene. Results must be interpreted with caution because the methylation status of the *FMR1* gene is often not yet established in chorionic villi at the time of sampling. Follow-up amniocentesis might be necessary to resolve an ambiguous result. In a very small number of patients, deletions or point mutations (43–48) rather than trinucleotide expansion are responsible for the syndrome. In these cases, linkage (31,49,50) or rare mutation studies are more useful.

References

1. Southern EM (1975) Detection of specific sequences among DNA fragments separated by gel electrophoresis. J Mol Biol 98:503–517
2. Alwine JC, Kemp DJ, Stark GR (1977) Method for detection of specific RNAs in agarose gels by transfer to diazobenzyloxymethyl-paper and hybridization with DNA probes. Proc Natl Acad Sci USA 74:5350–5354
3. Kafatos FC, Jones CW, Efstratiadis A (1979) Determination of nucleic acid sequence homologies and relative concentrations by a dot hybridization procedure. Nucleic Acid Res 7(6):1541–1552
4. Rapley R (ed) (2000) The nucleic acid protocols handbook. Humana, Totowa, NJ

5. Sambook J, Russel DW, Sambrook J (2000) Molecular cloning: A laboratory manual. Cold Spring Harbor Laboratory Press, Cold Spring Harbor, NY

6. Hames BD, Higgins SJ (1985) Nucleic acid hybridisation: A practical approach. IRL, Oxford, UK

7. Cunningham MW, Harris DW, Mundy C (1990) In vitro labelling: nucleic acids. In Salter RJ (ed) Radioisotopes in Biology IRL, Oxford, UK pp. 137–189

8. Isaac PG (1994) Protocols for nucleic acid anaylsis by nonradioactive probes. Humana, Totowa, NJ

9. Laskey RA (1990) Radioisotope detection using X ray film. In Salter RJ (ed) Radioisotopes in Biology: IRL, Oxford, UK

10. Gitschier J, Drayna D, Tuddenham EG, White RL, Lawn RM (1985) Genetic mapping and diagnosis of haemophilia A achieved through a BclI polymorphism in the factor VIII gene. Nature 314:738–740

11. Conner BJ, Reyes AA, Morin C, Itakura K, Teplitz RL, Wallace RB (1983) Detection of sickle cell beta S-globin allele by hybridization with synthetic oligonucleotides. Proc Natl Acad Sci USA 80:278–82

12. Feldenzer J, Mears JG, Burns AL, Natta C, Bank A (1979) Heterogeneity of DNA fragments associated with the sickle-globin gene. J Clin Invest 64:751–755

13. Xiao YH, Miller WH, Jr, Warrell RP, Dmitrovsky E, Zelenetz AD (1983) Pulsed-field gel electrophoresis analysis of retinoic acid receptor-alpha and promyelocytic leukemia rearrangements. Detection of the t(15;17) translocation in the diagnosis of acute promyelocytic leukemia. Am J Pathol 143:1301–1311

14. Chen KL, Wang YL, Dodson LA, et al (1996) Normalized Southern hybridization to enhance testing for Charcot–Marie–Tooth disease, Type 1A. Mol Diagn 1:65–71

15. Murray J, Cuckle H, Taylor G, Hewison J (1997). Screening for fragile X syndrome. Health Technol Assess 1:1–71

16. de Vries BBA, Halley DJJ, Oostra BA, Niermeijer MF (1998) The Fragile X syndrome. J Med Genet 35(7):579–589

17. Hagerman RJ, Silverman AC (1991) Fragile X syndrome: Diagnosis treatment, and research, Johns Hopkins University Press, Baltimore, MD

18. Warren ST, Nelson DL (1994) Advances in molecular analysis of fragile X syndrome. JAMA 271:536–542

19. Martin JP, Bell J (1943) A pedigree of mental defect showing sex-linkage. J. Neurol. Psychiatry 6:154–157

20. Lubs H (1969) A marker X chromosome. Am. Hum. Genet. 21:231

21. Heitz D, Rousseau F, Devys D, et al (1991) Isolation of sequences that span the fragile-X and identification of a fragile-X related CpG island. Science 251:1236–1239

22. Kremer EJ, Pritchard M, Lynch M, et al (1991) Mapping of DNA instability at the Fragile-X to a trinucleotide repeat sequence P(CCG)N. Science 252:1711–1714

23. Verkerk A, Pierelt M, Sutcliff JS, et al (1991) Identification of a gene (FMR-1) containing a CGG repeat coincident with a breakpoint cluster region exhibiting length variation in fragile-X syndrome. Cell 65:905–914

24. Hagerman RJ, Hull CE, Safanda JF, et al (1994) High functioning fragile-X males—demonstration of an unmethylated fully expanded Fmr-1 mutation associated with protein expression. Am J Med Genet 51:298–308

25. Gu YH, Shen Y, Gibbs RA, Nelson DJ (1996) Identification of FMR2, a novel gene associated with the FRAXE CCG repeat and CpG island. Nature Genet 13:109–113

26. Gecz J, Gedeon AK, Sutherland GR, Mulley JC (1996) Identification of the gene FMR2, associated with FRAXE mental-retardation. Nature Genet 13:105–108

27. Knight SJL, Flannery A, Hirst MC, et al (1993) Trinucleotide repeat amplification and hypermethylation of a CpG island in FRAXE mental-retardation. Cell 74:127–134

28. Knight SJL, Voelckel MA, Hirst MC, et al (1994) Triplet repeat expansion at the FRAXE locus and X- linked mild mental handicap. Am J Hum Genet. 55:81–86

29. Abramowicz MJ, Parma J, Cochaux P (1996) Slight instability of a FMR-1 allele over 3 generations in a family from the general-population. Am J Med Genet 64:268–269

30. Mornet E, Chateau C, Hirst MC, et al (1996) Analysis of germline variation at the FMR1 CFF repeat shows variation in the normal-premutated borderline range. Hum Mol Genet 5:821–825

31. Zhong N, Ju W, Pietrofesa J, Wang D, Dobkin C, Brown WT (1996) Fragile-X "gray zone" alleles—AGG patterns, expansion risks, and associated haplotypes. Am J Med Genet 64:261–265

32. Fu YH, Kuhl DP, Pizzuti A, et al (1991) Variation of the CGG repeat at the fragile-X site results in genetic instability—resolution of the Sherman paradox. Cell 67:1047–1058

33. Fisch GS, Snow K, Thibodeaa SN, et al (1995) The fragile-X premutation in carriers and its effect on mutation size in offspring. Am J Hum Genet 56:1147–1155

34. Heitz D, Rousseau F, Devys D, et al (1991) Isolation of sequences that span the fragile-X and identification of a fragile-X related CpG island. Science 251: 1236–1239

35. Haddad LA, Mingroninetto RC, Viannamorgante AM, Pena SDJ (1996) A PCR-based test suitable for screening for fragile-X syndrome among mentally-retarded males. Hum Genet 97:808–812

36. Brown WT, Nolin S, Houck G, Jr, et al (1996) Prenatal-diagnosis and carrier screening for fragile-X by PCR. Am J Med Genet 64:191–195

37. Goonewardena P, Zhang JA (1995) Single tube nonradioactive PCR assay for the detection of the full spectrum or FMR1 CGG repeats seen in the normal, carrier and fragile-X syndrome individuals. Am J Hum Genet 57:1914–1914

38. Wang Q, Green EP, Mathew CG, Bobrow M (1994) Nonradioactive PCR based screening for fragile-X syndrome. J Med Genet 31:173–173

39. Brown WT, Houck GE, Jr, Jeziorowska A, et al (1993) Rapid fragile-X carrier screening and prenatal- diagnosis using a nonradioactive PCR test. JAMA 270: 1569–1575

40. Gold B, Radu D, Balanko A, Chiang CS (2000) Diagnosis of fragile X syndrome by Southern blot hybridization using a chemiluminescent probe: a laboratory protocol Mol Diagn 5:169–178

41. Bullock S, et al (1995) Molecular DNA testing of a family manifesting fragile-X syndrome in both the fragile X—a full mutation and mosaic forms. J Med Genet 32:153

42. Yamauchi M, Nagata S, Seki N, et al (1993) Prenatal diagnosis of fragile X syndrome by direct detection of the dynamic mutation due to an unstable DNA sequence. Clin Genet 44:169–172

43. Mannermaa A, Pulkkinen L, Kajanoja E, Ryynanen M, Saarikoski S (1996) Deletion in the FMR1 Gene in a Fragile-X Male. Am J Med Genet 64:293–295

44. Deboulle K, et al (1993) A point mutation in the FMR-1 gene associated with fragile-X mental-retardation. Nature Genet 3:31–35

45. Hart PS, Olson SM, Crandall K, Tarleton J (1995) Fragile-X syndrome resulting from a 400 basepair deletion within the FMR1 gene. Am J Hum Genet 57:1395–1395

46. Hirst M, Grewal P, Flannery A, et al (1995) Two new cases of FMR1 deletion associated with mental impairment. Am J Hum Genet 56:67–74

47. Dreyfuss JC (1992) Clinical fragile-X syndrome due to total or partial gene deletion. Med Sci 8:878–878

48. Hammond LS, Macia MM, Tarleton JC, and Shashidhar Pai G (1997) Fragile X syndrome and deletions in FMR1: new case and review of the literature. Am J Med Genet 72:430–434

49. Hirst MC, Grewal PK, Davies KE (1994) Precursor Arrays For Triplet Repeat Expansion At the Fragile-X Locus. Hum Mol Genet 3:1553–1560

50. Eichler EE, Macpherson JN, Murray A, Jacobs PA, Chakravarti A, Nelson DL (1996) Haplotype and interspersion analysis of the FMR1 CGG repeat identifies 2 different mutational pathways for the origin of the fragile-X syndrome. Hum Mol Genet 5:319–330

6

Capillary Electrophoresis of DNA

Biomedical Applications

Beatriz Sanchez-Vega

1. Principles of Capillary Electrophoresis

Capillary electrophoresis (CE) separations are carried out inside a capillary tube, which usually has a diameter of 50 µm to facilitate temperature control. The length of the capillary differs in different applications, but it is typically in the region of 20–50 cm. The capillaries most widely used are fused silica covered with an external protective coating. A small portion of this coating is removed to form a window for detection purposes. The ends of the capillary are dipped into reservoirs filled with the electrolyte. Electrodes made of an inert material such as platinum are also inserted into the electrolyte reservoirs to complete the electrical circuit. The capillary is filled with running buffer, one end is dipped into the sample, and an electric field (electrokinetic injection) or pressure is applied to introduce the sample inside the capillary. Migration through the capillary is driven by application of a high-voltage current (10–30 kV).

The molecules are detected as they pass through the window at the opposite end of the capillary. The most frequently used detector is laser-induced fluorescence (LIF), which detects fluorochromes attached to the DNA molecules; alternative detectors include ultraviolet (UV) absorbance and fluorescence. Given the short path, detection requires monitoring by sensitive equipment such as charge-coupled device (CCD) cameras. The detectors are interfaced with computers responsible not only for collecting and displaying the data but also for maintaining the timing between filter wheels and controling timing exposures, readouts of the CCD cameras, and run-time processing of the CCD images and spectral data. The molecules are detected as fluorescent peaks as they pass through the detector. An electropherogram, which is a plot of the detector response with time, is generated. Because the area of each peak is proportional to the concentration of the DNA molecule, integrated peak areas are routinely used for semiquantification due to their greater dynamic range than peak heights (see **Fig. 6.1**).

Analysis times are in the range of 3–30 min, depending on the complexity of the separation. Modern instruments are relatively sophisticated and may contain fiber-optical detection systems, high-capacity autosamplers, and temperature-control devices.

From: *Molecular Biomethods Handbook, 2nd Edition.*
Edited by: J. M. Walker and R. Rapley © Humana Press, Totowa, NJ

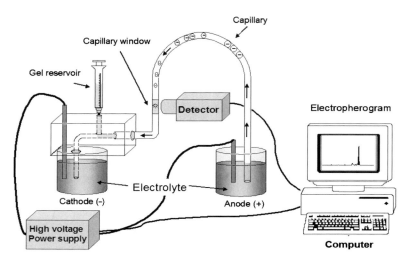

Fig. 6.1. Schematic diagram of a capillary electrophoresis system

Separation of DNA fragments by CE has advantages over the classical slab gel–based separations in terms of speed and resolution, especially now that instruments that can run more than one sample at a time are available. The principle behind DNA sequencing by an instrument with many capillaries is identical to that of using a single capillary, although the design of the sheath flow cuvet and the fluorescence detection systems is considerably more complicated. At present, 8-, 16-, 48-, 96-, and 384-capillary instruments are commercially available for DNA analysis.

1.1. Capillary Gel Electrophoresis

There is a special situation for biopolymers such as RNA, DNA, or sodium dodecyl sulfate (SDS)–loaded proteins, which have a constant charge-to-size ratio, that is, the increase in the charge is directly related to the increase in size of the molecule. Molecules with a constant charge-to-size ratio may have very similar electrophoretic mobilities, so no electrophoretic separation occurs in free solution. In these cases, separations are performed in capillaries filled with a gel solution. In capillary gel electrophoresis (CGE), a sieving effect occurs as solutes of various sizes migrate through the gel-filled capillary toward the detector. Smaller ions are able to migrate quickly through the gel, whereas larger ions become entangled in the gel matrix, reducing their migration rate.

Initially, the gels used in CGE were polyacrylamide covalently bonded to the capillary wall. These fixed gels suffered, however, from problems of shrinkage and blockage and could have relatively short lifetimes. In addition, if sample components contaminated the gel, it could not be reused and would have to be discarded. There has been a recent tendency, therefore, to use pumpable gel solutions, which can be used to fill the capillary with a non-cross-linked liquid gel matrix in which pores are created by the tangling of long linear polymers. These have the advantage of being introduced into the capillary under low pressure, extending the life of the capillary. The use of liquid gels also allows replacement of the gel between injections, reducing the contamination problems encountered with fixed gels.

1.2. Resolution

Good resolution in CE data means achieving sharp peaks and optimal separations between peaks. Peak spacing is the separation distance multiplied by the intrinsic velocity difference between two distinct molecules. This intrinsic velocity difference, in turn, is dependent on the physical properties of the molecule itself and on the separation medium (e.g., composition, concentration, and ionic strength). Diffusion, thermal gradient, and initial peak width are the major contributors to the peak width. Electric field strength, capillary dimensions, and polymer concentration, in turn, mainly influence these three factors. Each of these factors is considered in detail in this chapter.

An increase in electric field strength should lead to a decrease in diffusion due to shorter run times. It should, however, also lead to an increase in peak dispersion as a result of an increase in the heat generated when the electric current is applied through the capillary (Joule heat). Thus, the electric field strength should be 150 V/cm or lower for long sequencing reads. On the other hand, the diameter of the capillary influences the efficiency in dissipating the Joule heat. The narrower the capillary, the smaller the thermal gradient and, therefore, the peak width. A reduction of capillary diameter to less than 50 µm does not improve resolution, indicating that effects other than the thermal gradient determine the peak width in narrower capillaries.

The small cross-sectional area of the capillary creates the phenomenon of electroendosmosis. Because CE is normally carried out in capillaries made from fused silica, the negatively charged silanol groups on the surface of the capillary result in a high proportion of unbound, hydrated positive ions. Although some of these cations are tightly bound to the immobilized negative charges, the application of an electric field results in movement of the remainder toward the cathode. Since they are hydrated, the consequence is a bulk flow of liquid in the same direction, termed *electroendosmotic flow* (EOF). Many of the CE techniques rely on EOF to pump the solutes toward the detector. The EOF is produced along the entire length of the capillary, generating a constant flow rate at all distances along the capillary. The consequence is that the solutes are being swept along at the same rate throughout their transport along the capillary, minimizing sample diffusion.

Separation is improved with increasing polymer concentration, but at the cost of lower mobility and, therefore, increased run times. Low polymer concentrations are useful for fast screenings at low resolution, whereas higher concentrations produce higher resolutions. Whereas in cross-linked gels the concentration can be lowered easily, in the absence of cross-linking a decrease in the concentration results in a dilute solution. To compensate for this effect, an increase in the polymer length will keep the solution well entangled, allowing for low viscosity at the same time. To cover a large range of separation sizes, it is better to use low polymer concentrations; therefore, the polymer length must be increased to ensure sufficient entanglement. This leads to a more uniform resolution in function of the DNA size and is especially important for DNA sequencing, in which long reads are required *(1)*.

When analyzing the same DNA sample with the same parameters under native and denaturing conditions, the resolution is better in the environment that denatures the DNA molecules. If high resolution is necessary, denaturing conditions (such us the use of formamide in the sample preparation) should be used.

2.   Applications of CE to Biomedicine

Small alterations in DNA sequences of genes lead to many human diseases, such as cancer, diabetes, heart disease, myocardial infarction, atherosclerosis, cystic fibrosis, and Alzheimer's disease. These alterations in DNA sequence include many types of mutations and polymorphisms, such as nucleotide substitutions, deletion or insertion of some sequence, differences in a variable number of tandem repeat (VNTR) locus, and instability of microsatellite repeat sequences. CGE is a particularly suitable method for carrying out analysis of DNA fragments for diagnostic purposes. Currently available methods for analysis of mutations and polymorphisms include some modified polymerase chain reaction (PCR) techniques, restriction fragment length polymorphism (RFLP), single-strand conformation polymorphism (SSCP), VNTR, and short tandem repeats (STRs) analysis, and hybridization techniques, as well as PCR analysis itself (see **Fig. 6.2**).

Labeled DNA fragments to be analyzed by CE are obtained by the incorporation of fluorescent-dye-labeled nucleotides or fluorescent dye-labeled primers during the PCR reaction. The range of available dyes and the reduction

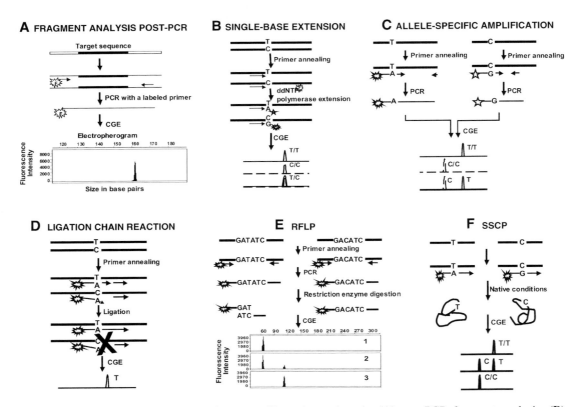

Fig. 6.2. Scheme of the methods applied to capillary electrophoresis: (**A**) post-PCR fragment analysis; (**B**) single-base extension; (**C**) allele-specific amplification; (**D**) ligation chain reaction; (**E**) RFLP and an example of its application to detect the D835 mutation on the *FLT3* gene in patients with acute leukemia: wild type (*1*), heterozygote (*2*), and homozygote (*3*) for the D835 mutation; (**F**) SSCP; (**G**) analysis of repetitive sequences; (**H**) hybridization technique; (**I**) detection of DNA damage; (**J**) analysis of methylation levels; and (**K**) sequencing

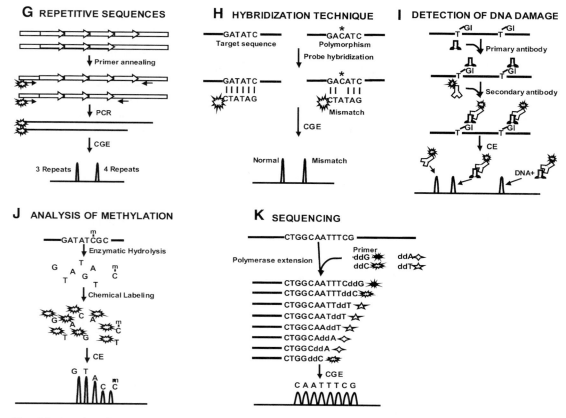

Fig. 6.2. (continued)

in costs over recent years have allowed modification of existing tests to take advantage of the four/five-color detection system and the degree of automation offered by commercially available CE electrophoresis systems. Four-color, highresolution analysis is particularly useful for the rapid mapping of genetic traits, leading to gene discovery and eventual diagnostic testing. Automation is essential for rapid gene-based mutation analysis in clinical laboratories to screen a large number of DNA samples.

2.1. Post-PCR Fragment Analysis

DNA amplification by PCR has been applied to clinical diagnosis of infectious diseases, genetic disorders, and cancer. After amplification of the DNA region of interest, the sensitivity and speed of the method of analysis is crucial in clinical diagnosis. The use of CGE with LIF detection has been proved to yield better performance than conventional slab gel electrophoresis in the clinical laboratory *(2)* (see **Fig. 6.2A**).

2.1.1. Detection of Viral Sequences

The PCR technique is a powerful tool for detecting the presence of a virus earlier than any discernible antibody response in a person infected with a virus. Detection of specific DNA or RNA regions of a certain virus genome by multiplex PCR using CE has been applied to the detection of human immuno-deficiency virus (HIV) *(3–5)* polio virus *(6)* and hepatitis C virus *(7,8)*.

2.1.2. Detection of Intragene Deletion and Duplication Sequences

Capillary gel electrophoresis has been applied to the analysis of PCR products in the detection of small gene deletions in several genetic diseases. Examples of this application include the detection of over 98% of deletions occurring on the dystrophin gene for the diagnosis of Duchenne muscular dystrophy *(9,10)*,; an 8-bp deletion in exon 3 of the *P450c21B* gene in individuals affected by 21-hydroxylase deficiency, a recessively inherited disease *(11)*, and the ΔF508 mutation, a 3-bp deletion in the gene *CFTR* that is the most frequently muta-tion found in individuals affected with cystic fibrosis *(12)*. Another example is detection of the internal tandem duplication (ITD) in the juxtamembrane domain-coding sequence of the *FLT3* gene in acute leukemias. The mutation of this receptor is important in acute myelogenous and lympho blastic leuke-mias because patients with this mutation generally have a poorer prognosis for survival than patients without it *(13)* (*see* **Fig. 6.3**).

2.1.3. Detection of Gene Rearrangements

Fluorescent PCR combined with CE analysis has been used to identify mono-clonal rearrangements in the T-cell receptor (*TCR*) *(14)* and immunoglobulin heavy-chain (*IgH*) *(15)* genes in order to detect residual disease in lymphoprolif-erative disorders. Normal lymphocytes rearrange the *TCR* and *IgH* genes ran-domly during normal development, thus, a normal polyclonal population shows many different rearrangements. Neoplastic cells exhibit a single rearrangement of the *TCR* or *IgH* gene. These rearrangements can be detected by PCR if the ampli-fication is conducted across the sequence where the gene rearranges. Polyclonal samples show a gaussian-like distribution of the peaks, whereas monoclonal or neoplastic cases display a single predominant peak. Four or five separate peaks are consistent with oligoclonal populations and almost always are the result of immunological reactive processes to unknown antigens (see **Fig. 6.4**).

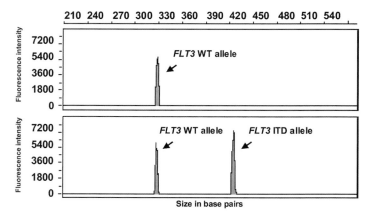

Fig. 6.3. Example of post-PCR detection showing the results of amplifying the ITD region of the *FLT3* wild-type (WT) allele in a healthy individual (upper panel) and in a patient with acute leukemia (lower panel)

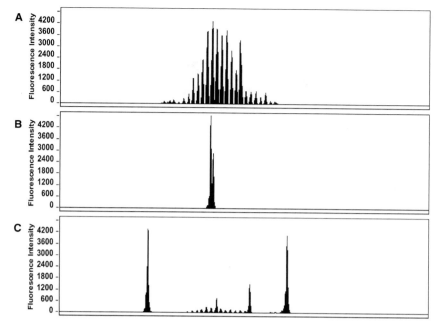

Fig. 6.4. *IgH* gene rearrangement results. The electropherograms show (**A**) a normal polyclonal B-cell population, (**B**) a monoclonal peak from a lymphoma patient, and (**C**) an oligoclonal population from an immunological reactive process

2.1.4. Detection of Chromosomal Reorganizations

Chromosomal translocations and inversions are often detected in many types of cancer. Chromosomal translocations result in juxtaposition of segments from two different genes, giving rise to a fusion gene that encodes chimeric proteins with transforming activity. In general, both genes involved in the fusion contribute to the transforming potential of the chimeric oncoprotein *(16)*. CE has been applied to the detection of many fusion transcripts, such as the bcr/abl transcript in chronic myeloid leukemia *(17)*.

On the other hand, gene activation often results from chromosomal reorganizations that relocate a proto-oncogene close to the regulatory elements of the *IgH* or *TCR* locus. This event causes deregulation of the proto-oncogene expression, which can then lead to neoplastic transformation of the cell. One of these proto-oncogenes is the *BCL-2* gene, which is translocated close to the regulatory element of the *IgH* gene in persons with follicular lymphoma. The different PCR products can be resolved by CGE *(18)*.

2.2. Single-Base Extension or Single Nucleotide Primer Extension

Single-base extension (SBE) is a method used for the accurate detection of single-nucleotide polymorphism variants in transcripts. Standard labeled Sanger dideoxynucleotide terminators (ddNTP), which lack the 3' hydroxyl group needed for chain elongation, are used in the extension reaction; as a result, the primer is extended by a single nucleotide. The reaction mixture is subsequently separated by CGE *(19)* (**Fig. 6.2B**).

For example, Leber's hereditary optic neuropathy was detected by annealing a primer immediately 5' to the mutation on the template and extending the primer by one fluorescently labeled ddNTP complementary to the mutation. By using two or more differently labeled terminators, both the mutant and wild-type sequences could be detected simultaneously *(20)*. In addition, multiplexed SBE genotyping has been applied to the detection of known point mutations on the *p53* gene using three unique primers that probe for mutations of clinical importance on this gene *(21)* and to the diagnosis of multiple endocrine neoplasia type 2 by the analysis of codons 634 and 918 on the *RET* proto-oncogene *(22)*.

A different field of application is the determination of ovine prion protein allelic variants at codons 136, 154, and 171, where the four mutations responsible for amino acid changes are typed simultaneously *(23)*.

2.3. Allele-Specific Amplification

Allele-specific amplification (ASA) allows simultaneous analysis of multiple specific alleles, known point mutations, or known polymorphisms at the same locus. Specificity is achieved in a single PCR reaction by designing one or both PCR primers so that they overlap the site of sequence difference between the amplified alleles. This results in simultaneous amplification of numerous DNA fragments differing in size, which are subsequently separated by CGE (see **Fig. 6.2C**).

This technique was applied to the detection of K329E, the most prevalent mutation in medium-chain acyl-coenzyme A dehydrogenase deficiency. The mutant allele produces a DNA fragment that differs in size from the DNA fragment generated by the normal allele *(24)*. ASA also can be used to detect multiple mutations in a locus. For example, several point mutations on the 21-hydroxylase gene of a patient with congenital adrenal hyperplasia were analyzed simultaneously by this method *(25)*.

Familial defective apolipoprotein B-100 (FDB) is a dominantly inherited disorder characterized by a decreased affinity of low-density lipoprotein (LDL) for the LDL receptor. This phenotype is a consequence of a substitution of adenine by guanine in exon 26 of the *FDB* gene in the region coding for the putative LDL receptor-binding domain of the mature protein. Mutation screening for *FDB* is performed by ASA followed by CGE *(26)*.

Another mutation that can be detected by ASA and CGE is the G1691A point mutation in the coagulation factor V gene, the most common genetic cause of thrombophilia. This mutation has been shown to cause resistance to cleavage by activated protein C and is associated with an increased thrombotic risk *(27)*.

2.4. Ligase Chain Reaction

In this method, a thermostable ligase is used to specifically bond two adjacent oligonucleotides, which hybridize to a complementary target with perfect base pairing at the junction. This approach enables single base pair differences to be detected at the ligation junction (see **Fig. 6.2D**). The design of primers with distinct labels for different base substitutions allows for simultaneous detection of several changes. This technique has been applied to the screening of the 31 most frequent mutations in the cystic fibrosis gene in a multiplex oligonucleotide ligation assay *(28)*.

Sickle cell disease refers to a collection of autosomal recessive genetic disorders characterized by a hemoglobin variant (Hb S) which differs from hemoglobin A in having a single amino acid substitution on the β-chain. Individuals who are affected with other types of sickle cell disease are compound heterozygotes, possessing one copy of the Hb S variant and one copy of a different β-globin gene variant such as Hb C or Hb β-thalassemia. CE has been applied to the detection of both hemoglobin forms Hb S and Hb C in prenatal diagnoses of sickle cell diseases *(29)*.

2.5. Restriction Fragment-Length Polymorphism Analysis

Restriction fragment-length polymorphism (RFLP) analysis is a powerful tool for the detection of known mutations and polymorphisms, which result in the loss or creation of a recognition site at which a particular restriction enzyme cuts. RFLPs are usually caused by mutation at a cutting site. DNA carrying the different allelic form will give different sizes of DNA fragments when digested with the appropriate restriction enzyme (see **Fig. 6.2E**).

The E4 allele on the *APOE* gene has been proven to be a major risk factor for late-onset familial and sporadic Alzheimer's disease. DNA samples for *APOE* genotyping are prepared by PCR amplification and subsequent digestion with that *Hha*I restriction enzyme to yield constant fragments of 16, 18, and 35 base pairs and four typical polymorphic fragments of 48, 72, 83, and 91 base pairs, corresponding to alleles E1, E2, E3, and E4, respectively *(30)*. The risk of developing Alzheimer's disease for the individual having the E4/E4 genotype is about 90%, for the individual having the E3/E3 genotype, 20%; and for the individual having the E3/E4 genotype, 47%.

Capillary gel electrophoresis has also been applied to resolve DNA fragments digested with *Bst*NI endonuclease to detect mutations in codon 12 of *K-RAS* *(31)* and to detect the D385 mutation in the *FLT3* gene, in which amplification of the sequence of interest is followed by *Eco*RV digestion.

A different application of the RFLP method is mitochondrial DNA typing. The polymorphic control region of mitochondrial DNA (mtDNA) is being used more and more commonly in forensic applications to differentiate among individuals in a population. Two hypervariable regions (HV1 and HV2) are often sequenced following amplification of the mtDNA by PCR. A methodology has been developed that uses restriction endonuclease digestion of the PCR-amplified mtDNA by *Rsa*I and *Mnl*I and CGE to separate and size the RFLP fragments *(32)*.

2.6. Single-Strand Conformation Polymorphism

The SSCP method is based on the principle that the electrophoretic mobility of single-stranded DNA in a nondenaturing condition depends not only on its size but also on its sequence. Single-stranded DNA has a folded structure that is determined by intramolecular interactions. This sequence-based secondary structure affects the mobility of the DNA during electrophoresis under nondenaturing conditions. A DNA molecule containing a mutation, even a single-base substitution, will have a different secondary structure than the wild type, resulting in a different mobility shift during electrophoresis than that of the wild type (see **Fig. 6.2F**). The technological aspects of CE-SSCP as well as the potential of CE-SSCP for routine genetic analysis were reviewed by Kourkine et al. in 2002 *(33)*.

Some examples of applications of SSCP by CGE include analysis of the *p53* tumor suppressor gene for DNA diagnosis of cancer *(34)*, detection of mutations on the *K-RAS* oncogene *(35)*, detection of a *Mycobacterium tuberculosis*–specific amplified DNA fragment *(36)*, detection of mutations in the β-*globin* gene promoter *(37)* and the lipoprotein lipase and breast cancer 2 (*BRCA2*) genes *(38)*, and identification of multiple mycobacterial species in a sample *(39)*.

CE-SSCP also has been used for the separation of fully supercoiled molecules, single topoisomers, and relaxed and open circular DNA forms in research on novel anticancer molecules targeting the activity of topoisomerase I *(40)*.

One approach that combines restriction enzyme digestion of fluorescence-labeled PCR products with SSCP by CE has been developed to screen exon 11 mutations of the breast cancer 1 (*BRCA1*) gene *(41)*. The large size of the *BRCA1* gene and the many mutations found throughout its entire coding sequence make screening for mutations in this gene particularly challenging. Capillary RFLP-SSCP electrophoresis appeared as a technically convenient technique to test mutations in this gene, requiring amplification of fewer PCR fragments than traditional SSCP.

2.7. Analysis of Repetitive DNA Sequences

The human genome contains large numbers of repetitive DNA sequences, some of which are arrayed as tandem repeat units. Polymorphic tandem repeats occur in two general families: VNTRs and STRs. VNTR or minisatellite DNA consists of variable numbers of a repeating unit from 15 to 100 nucleotides long. The repeated unit in STR or microsatellite DNA ranges from two to six bases.

Products of different lengths can be amplified by using primers complementary to conserved sequences flanking the tandem repeat regions; the length of each amplification product is directly proportional to the number of repeats. These amplification products can be resolved to individual alleles by CGE. Thus, a person can have at most two different alleles, one from each chromosome (see **Fig. 6.2G**).

Laser-induced fluorescence detection of fluorescence-labeled PCR products and multicolor analysis enable the rapid generation of multilocus DNA profiles.

2.7.1. VNTR

Capillary gel electrophoresis has been applied to the analysis of the human apolipoprotein B gene (*APOB*). This gene maps to the short arm of chromosome 2, and a VNTR is located immediately downstream. The *APOB* VNTR alleles generally contain 25–52 repeats of a basic 16-bp unit. Larger alleles containing more than 38 repeat units are more common in people who have myocardial infarction and show a significant association with coronary disease *(42)*.

Capillary gel electrophoresis also has been used to determine the lung cancer risk associated with rare *HRAS1* VNTR alleles *(43)*.

2.7.2. STR

The number of tandem repeats for a STR is highly variable from individual to individual and can be as many as 15 different alleles in a certain locus. These sequences also show high levels of heterozygosity, which make them very useful as genetic markers.

2.7.2.1. Highly Polymorphic Markers

1. *Genetic Mapping.* The almost random distribution of microsatellites and their high level of polymorphism greatly facilitated the construction of genetic maps and enabled subsequent positional cloning of several genes. A comprehensive genetic map of the human genome based on 5264 microsatellites (*44*) and a genetic map of the mouse genome based on 4006 simple sequence length polymorphisms (*45*) were constructed with these markers. When a trait or disease is inherited through a family and all of the affected members in the family also share a STR that is inherited together, it can be concluded that the disease and marker must be close to each other on a chromosome. This linkage is the first step in the isolation of disease-causing genes and their localization to an area of DNA. Linkage disequilibrium scanning of the human genome with many thousands of genetic markers has been used to map complex diseases such as schizophrenia (*46*) and autistic disorder (*47*).

2. *Trisomies.* The D21S11 locus, a highly polymorphic (90% heterozygosity) microsatellite marker, was amplified and analyzed by CGE for prenatal DNA diagnosis of Down's syndrome (*48*). In the analysis of this microsatellite marker, trisomic individuals are expected to fall into two major groups: those with three bands of similar intensities or those with two bands with a ratio of 2:1.

3. *Duplication in Chromosomes.* The Charcot–Marie–Tooth 1A disease is the result of a 1.5-Mb duplication in chromosome subband 17p11.2-p12. Suitable dinucleotide repeat markers within this region are amplified by using fluorescence-labeled primers and separated by CGE. The results are two peaks corresponding to two alleles with a dosage difference (*49*).

4. *Forensic DNA Typing.* In forensic work, DNA from a biological sample and from a known reference material (most often, buccal swabs or blood) are amplified by multiplex PCR with fluorescence-labeled primers and separated by CGE. As a result, unique DNA profiles are generated from both the evidence and the known reference sample and compared to determine whether the patterns are similar. If the DNA profiles match, then the suspect cannot be excluded as a source of the questioned sample. Likewise, if the DNA profiles do not match, the suspect can be excluded as the donor of the questioned sample. The analysis of 6–10 STRs provides a random match probability of approx 1 in 5 billion.

   DNA typing is a useful tool in crime solving, not only for blood samples, sperm, or saliva but also for traces of DNA left on tools or pieces of clothing used in burglaries or thefts. On these kinds of samples, the sources of DNA are extremely small amounts of skin debris left after gripping tools. When a sensitive technique such as PCR coupled with CGE is used, it is possible to get a profile from these low amounts of DNA (*50*). CE provides efficient separation, resolution, sensitivity, and precision for a reliable genotyping of STR loci. Sizing precision of <0.16 nucleotide standard deviation is obtained with this system, thus allowing the accurate genotyping of variants that differ in length by a single nucleotide (*51*).
   Automated fluorescent detection of a 10-loci multiplex has been applied to paternity testing (*52*). DNA is extracted from blood samples of the mother,

child, and alleged father and subjected to STR analysis. By using 10–15 STRs, the calculated probability of paternity usually exceeds 99.99%.

5. *Chimerism.* Analysis of the relative amounts of donor and recipient DNA in bone marrow after bone marrow transplantation is frequently used to determine the status of the transplant. One method involves testing the patient and donor for genetic profiles before the transplant and then comparing these with the profile obtained from the patient after transplant. The analysis of chimerism in patients who have undergone allogeneic stem cell transplantation by CE systems was reviewed by Lion in 2003 *(53)* (see **Fig. 6.5**).

2.7.2.2. Microsatellite Instability: Microsatellite instability (MSI) has been shown to be relevant to various diseases, including cancers. Cells with mutations in one of the genes responsible for DNA mismatch repair (MMR) accumulate mutations at a very high rate. Because DNA mismatches are more likely to occur in DNA microsatellites, defective DNA MMR leads to the phenomenon of MSI, in which the progeny of the defective cells have varying

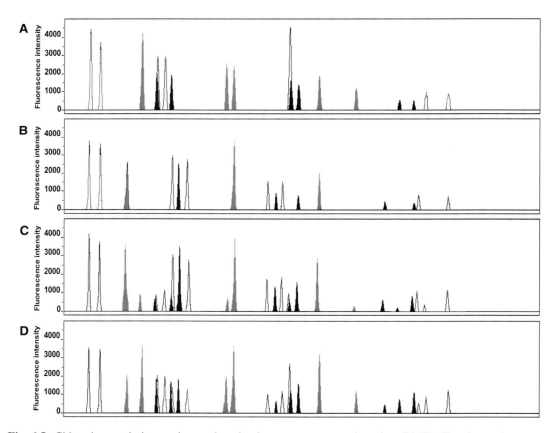

Fig. 6.5. Chimerism study in a patient undergoing bone marrow transplantation (BMT). The electropherograms show the genetic profiles of (**A**) the patient before BMT, (**B**) the donor, (**C**) the patient 1 mo after BMT, showing a mixed profile with patient and donor markers, (**D**) the patient 6 mo after BMT, showing an increase in the patient pre-BMT markers. This indicates a rejection of the transplant

lengths of a given microsatellite. The microsatellite reference panel to study MSI is BAT25, BAT26, D5S346, D2S123, and D17S250 *(54)*.

Studies of MSI are performed routinely in patients with colorectal cancer because of the defective MMR phenotype of colorectal carcinomas. The electrophoretic profile of the amplified products is compared between tumor and normal DNA from the same patient *(55)* (see **Fig. 6.6**).

2.7.2.3. Loss of Heterozygosity: Loss of heterozygosity (LOH) refers to a mutation that results in the loss of one allele at a specific locus. This phenomenon is very frequent in cancer cells. Whereas normal cells are heterozygous at many loci, tumor cells are homozygous at the same loci. LOH can be detected by CGE in bladder carcinoma *(56)*, lung cancer *(57)*, breast cancer *(58)*, renal cancer *(59)*, and other solid tumors *(60)*.

2.7.2.4. Dynamic Mutations: Some microsatellite repeats can undergo an increase in copy number by a process of dynamic mutations, typically by expansion of an unstable trinucleotide repeat. These repeat regions are polymorphic in unaffected individuals, so the number of repeated triplets varies within a certain range. In affected individuals, the number of repeats exceeds the normal range. When, in a family, the number of repeats increases in the normal range, the phenomenon is called a permutation. In such cases, there is a strong possibility of further expansion to a full mutation during inheritance

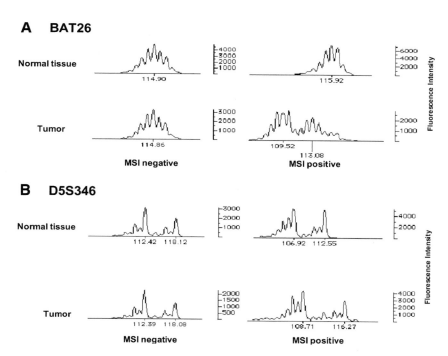

Fig. 6.6. Microsatellite instability results from BAT26 **(A)** and D5S346 **(B)** markers in two tumor samples. The left panels show MSI-negative tumor tissues and the right panels show MSI-positive tumor tissues when compared with normal tissue from the same patient

from parent to child. The high resolving power of CGE allows separation of heterozygous microsatellite bands differing by only one triplet.

Spinocerebellar ataxia type 2 results from an expansion of a stretch of polyglutamine repeats within the coding sequence of the ataxin-2 gene. The clinical phenotype arises when more than 32–35 glutamine residues are found in this region *(61)*. Other examples are fragile X syndrome *(62)*, myotonic muscular dystrophy *(63)*, Kennedy's disease *(64)* spinocerebellar ataxia type 1 *(65)*, and Huntington's disease *(66)*.

2.8. Hybridization Technique

In this technique, a probe of known sequence is capable of recognizing a specific DNA sequence in a mixture of many different DNA sequences. The probe can be a synthetic oligonucleotide, a peptide nucleic acid (PNA), a DNA sequence, an RNA sequence, or DNA-based drugs such as DNA vaccines, antisense DNA, protein-binding oligonucleotides, and ribozymes. The probe is generally labeled with a fluorochrome that can be detected after the hybridization takes place.

In a DNA hybridization assay, the sample DNA is heated to separate the two DNA strands and then exposed to the probe. The degree of DNA sequence identity is detected through a hybridization reaction between the DNA and the probe. The hybridization products are then resolved by CGE (see **Fig. 6.2H**).

This method has applications in such diverse areas as analysis of pooled genomic DNA samples, detection of mutations, screening of populations for polymorphisms, and identification of species in environmental mixtures.

2.8.1. Analysis of Heteroduplex DNA

Heteroduplex DNA is formed by pairing an unknown nucleic acid strand with a reference strand of a known sequence. Single-stranded nucleic acids with complementary sequences come together and form a double-stranded hybrid molecule in which hydrogen bonds form only between complementary base pairs. The thermal stability of DNA is related to the number of hydrogen bonds between complementary base pairs; therefore, the greater the similarity in nucleotide sequences between two samples of DNA, the more hydrogen bonds will be present in the heteroduplexes produced. Heteroduplexes generated with a mismatch in the sequence between the two strands will have a different sequence-dependent electrophoretic mobility than homoduplex DNA generated with perfectly matched sequences.

Heteroduplex analysis also can be done to detect different sequences in a mixture by using different probes labeled with different colors. Multiplex analysis has been applied to the simultaneous detection of six heterozygous mutations in *BRCA1* and *BRCA2* *(67)*, screening of the three common prothrombotic polymorphisms pl(A), factor V Leiden, and MTHFR (C677T) *(68)*, rapid genetic screening of hemochromatosis *(69)*, genetic diagnosis of factor V Leiden *(70)*, clinical diagnosis of rifampin-resistant tuberculosis strains *(71)*, and analysis of complex mutational spectra of human cells in culture *(72)*.

Heteroduplex technology is frequently combined with other screening techniques such as SSCP or ASA. Some examples of the combination of heteroduplex analysis with SSCP are detection of mutations, polymorphisms, and variants in *BRCA1* and *BRCA2* genes *(73)* and detection of mutations in the *p53* gene *(74)*. Heteroduplex analysis has been combined with ASA in order to detect specific mutations in the *BRCA1* and *BRCA2* genes *(75)*.

2.8.2. Synthetic Oligonucleotides Probes

The use of oligonucleotides as probes for hybridization has been used to determine the specificity of PCR products. One example is the use of oligonucleotides to target specific HIV-1 sequences. When these oligonucleotides are mixed with genomic DNA amplified by PCR, the presence of the HIV-1 virus within an individual can be detected *(76)*.

2.8.3. Peptide Nucleic Acid Probes

Peptide nucleic acids are molecules in which the bases are conjugated to a polyamide back-bone. The distance between bases and the complementarity are the same as in a DNA or RNA molecule. The PNA probe is hybridized to a DNA sample amplified by PCR, denatured at low ionic strength, and resolved by CE. The neutral backbone of PNA ensures an efficient CE separation of the PNA/DNA hybrids from both double-stranded and single-stranded DNA. DNA strands fully complementary to the target PNA are retarded compared to single-nucleotide mismatched strands *(77)*.

This method can be used to perform multiplex analyses on several mutations simultaneously when using different amplicon lengths and a set of mutation-specific PNAs. Each targeted mutation can be identified by the size of its corresponding amplicon. Its genotype is further characterized by its interaction with a specific PNA that can differentiate between wild-type and mutant alleles. This approach has been applied to the detection of R553X and R1162X single-base mutations in patients with cystic fibrosis *(78)* and to identification of the H63D, S65C, and C282Y mutations in the hereditary hemochromatosis gene *(79)*.

2.8.4. Analysis of DNA-Based Drugs

Antisense oligonucleotides are synthetic oligomers that bind a target mRNA or DNA, forming duplexes and thereby blocking its translation into a peptide or triggering its degradation. Among several DNA analogs proposed as antisense DNA drugs, antisense DNA in which the backbone is modified into phosphorothioate is the most promising for therapeutic application because of its resistance to nuclease degradation.

This methodology is a useful tool for synthesis control and analysis of phosphorothioate analogs *(80)* and for the determination of their subcellular distribution *(81)*, in vitro stability *(82)*, tissue half-life *(83)*, purity *(84)*, and metabolism *(85)*.

2.9. Temperature Gradient Capillary Electrophoresis

In temperature gradient CE (TGCE), a continuous, gradually decreasing temperature gradient is established during the electrophoresis. This approach can be applied to detection of DNA mutations based on thermodynamic stability and mobility shift during electrophoresis. By spanning a wide temperature range, it is possible to perform simultaneous heteroduplex analysis for various mutation types that have different melting temperatures *(86)*.

Genomic DNA also can be amplified with one fluorescence-labeled primer and one GC-clamped primer and analyzed by TGCE under denaturing temperature conditions. This tactic has been applied to the detection of mutations in exon 8 of the *p53* gene from tumor samples and controls *(87)*.

2.10. Quantification of DNA Damage

Damage to cellular DNA is implicated in the early stages of carcinogenesis and in the cytotoxicity of many anticancer agents, including ionizing radiation. CE is a sensitive technique for measuring cellular levels of DNA damage through the detection of specific DNA lesions by specific monoclonal antibodies. The detection is done by the use of a secondary antibody labeled with a fluorochrome. This method has been applied to the determination of thymine glycol residues in DNA generated by irradiation of cells during radiation therapy. The sensitivity of detection is in the range of zeptomoles *(88)* (see **Fig. 6.2I**).

Another way to detect DNA damage is the evaluation of DNA laddering during apoptosis. A key step in the onset of apoptosis is cleavage of the genomic DNA between nucleosomes, resulting in polynucleosome-sized fragments of DNA that give rise to a characteristic DNA laddering pattern. A fluorescent intercalating dye is used to label the DNA molecules that will be resolved by CGE. Also, the use of a DNA standard curve allows quantification of the apoptotic DNA. The use of CGE with LIF detection permits analysis of DNA laddering with improved automation and much greater sensitivity *(89)*.

2.11. Analysis of Methylation Status

DNA methylation refers to the addition of a methyl group to the 5-position of cytosine residues that are followed immediately by a guanine (so-called CpG dinucleotides). Small stretches of DNA known as CpG islands are rich in CpG dinucleotides. These CpG islands are frequently located within the promoter regions of human genes, and methylation within the islands has been shown to be associated with transcriptional inactivation of the corresponding gene. Changes in DNA methylation profiles are common features of development *(90)*, and DNA methylation is also involved in X-chromosome inactivation *(91)* and allele-specific silencing of imprinted genes *(92)*. Aberrant changes in methylation profiles are associated with many serious pathological consequences such as tumorigenesis *(93)*. Methylation of CpG islands has been shown to be important in transcriptional repression of numerous genes that function to prevent tumor growth or development. This phenomenon includes both genome-wide hypomethylation and gene-specific hypermethylation.

Capillary electrophoresis has been applied to the evaluation of the relative methylation degree of genomic DNA methylation. In this approach, genomic DNA is enzymatically hydrolyzed to single nucleotides. Single nucleotides are then labeled with a fluorescent marker and separated by CE to identify cytosine and 5-methyl cytosine residues *(94)* (see **Fig. 6.2J**).

This method has been applied to determine DNA methylation levels and their oncogenic potential in chronic lymphocytic leukemia *(95)* and it could be useful for the diagnosis of genetic diseases that have specific DNA methylation pattern alterations such as Angelman and Prader–Willi syndromes.

2.12. Sequencing

DNA sequencing is the determination of the order of nucleotides in a DNA molecule. The most popular method for doing this is called the Sanger sequencing method or chain-termination method. This method uses synthetic nucleotides that lack the 3′ hydroxyl group and are unable to form the 3′–5′ phosphodiester bond necessary for chain elongation. These nucleotides are called dideoxynucleotides (ddNTPs).

The sequencing reaction consists in a single-stranded template DNA to which a short complementary primer is annealed and extended by a DNA polymerase. The sequencing reaction contains a low concentration of ddNTPs, each labeled with a different fluorochrome, in addition to the normal deoxynucleotides. Once a ddNTP is incorporated in the elongating chain, it blocks further chain extension; as a result, a mixture of chains of lengths determined by the template sequence is accumulated. This mixture can then be resolved by CGE. CGE resolution allows separation of chains that differ in length by only one nucleotide (see **Fig. 6.2K**).

Sequencing by using CGE has been in constant development with steady advances in speed *(96)*, separation media *(97)*, and data collection and large-scale instruments *(98)*. DNA sequencing is considered the standard for identification of nucleic acids and detection of mutations, and CGE is routinely used in research and clinical situations in which panels of mutations or large numbers of samples are analyzed and when turnaround time is critical.

Direct sequencing of amplified fragment-length polymorphism bands also has been used as a polymorphism isolation strategy of population genetic parameters in genomic DNA of nongenomic model species *(99)*.

The combination of direct cycle sequencing of PCR products with CGE also provides a simple and rapid method convenient for routine hepatitis C virus genotyping analysis *(100)*.

2.12.1. Polymorphism Ratio Sequencing

In the polymorphism ratio sequencing (PRS) method, dideoxy-terminator extension ladders generated from a sample and a reference template are labeled with different fluorescent dyes and coinjected into a capillary for comparison of relative signal intensities. PRS allows detection and genotyping of single- nucleotide polymorphisms in the analysis of individual or multiplexed samples *(101)*.

2.12.2. Simulseq or Simultaneous Sequencing of Multiple PCR Products

This strategy allows multiple PCR products to be sequenced in a single sequencing reaction and analyzed simultaneously in a single lane or capillary. To achieve this separation, the different primers used for the sequencing reactions have long tails of nucleotides with different lengths *(102)*.

3. Microchips

Microchip analysis has become an attractive option in CE for clinical applications, not only because these kinds of analysis require usage of complex samples that are often limited in quantity but also because this system could allow clinicians to make quicker treatment and drug therapy decisions.

The use of CE in the microchip format allows high-speed separations of very small samples, and multiple channel systems have great potential for high-throughput analysis. The first report of DNA separation on a microchip device was published by Woolley and Mathies in 1994 *(103)*. Since then, great progress has been made in the design of these devices, going from single-channel to multiple-channel chips, allowing analysis of several DNA samples. The design of these systems was reviewed by Gao et al. in 2001 *(104)*.

A typical microchip device consists of one or several separation channels of 3–10 cm in length and 10–100 μm in diameter. There are also buffer, waste, and sample reservoirs. High voltages of 2–30 kV can be applied to the reservoirs by platinum electrodes because these systems disperse the heat very efficiently. The small samples used in the CE microchips require extremely sensitive detection techniques. LIF is the most commonly used detection method in CE microchips, although electrochemical, ultraviolet (UV), chemiluminiscence, and indirect fluorescence detection methods have been combined with these systems.

The applications of conventional CE can be scaled to microchip systems. Detection of mutations in hereditary hemochromatosis, STR genotyping, and rapid mitochondrial DNA sequence polymorphism analysis have all been done by these devices *(105)*.

The high-throughput capabilities of these systems were demonstrated by the simultaneous separation of multiple STR amplicons in 96 channels in 8 min *(106)*. Some other clinical applications carried out on microchip CE systems were reviewed by Wessagowit and South and Gawron et al., including DNA sequencing, genetic analysis, immunoassays, and protein and peptide analyses *(107, 108)*.

The applications and designs of microchip systems are constantly expanding. Integration of sample preparation and separation in a single microchip can be addressed in a few years, which will lead to a tremendous impact on high-throughput DNA analysis.

References

1. Heller C (2001) Principles of DNA separation with capillary electrophoresis. Electrophoresis 22:629–643
2. Liu MS, Chen FT (2000) Rapid analysis of amplified double-stranded DNA by capillary electrophoresis with laser-induced fluorescence detection. Mol Biotechnol 15:143–146
3. Gong X, Yeung ES (2000) Genetic typing and HIV-1 diagnosis by using 96 capillary array electrophoresis and ultraviolet absorption detection. J Chromatogr, B: Biomed Sci Appl 741:15–21
4. Zhang N, Yeung ES (1998) On-line coupling of polymerase chain reaction and capillary electrophoresis for automatic DNA typing and HIV-1 diagnosis. J Chromatogr B Biomed Sci Appl 714:3–11
5. Lu W, Han DS, Yuan J, Andrieu JM (1994) Multi-target PCR analysis by capillary electrophoresis and laser-induced fluorescence. Nature 368:269–271
6. Rossomando EF, White L, Ulfelder KJ (1994) Capillary electrophoresis: separation and quantitation of reverse transcriptase polymerase chain reaction products from polio virus. J Chromatogr B: Biomed Sci Appl 656:159–168
7. Li N, Tan WG, Tsang RY, Tyrrell DL, Dovichi NJ (2002) Quantitative olymerase chain reaction using capillary electrophoresis with laser-induced fluorescence detection: analysis of duck hepatitis B Anal Bioanal Chem 374:269–273
8. Tan WG, Tyrrell DL, Dovichi NJ (1999) Detection of duck hepatitis B virus DNA fragments using on-column intercalating dye labeling with capillary electrophoresis-laser-induced fluorescence. J Chromatogr A 853:309–319
9. Gelfi C, Orsi A, Leoncini F, et al (1995) Amplification of 18 dystrophin gene exons in DMD/BMD patients: simultaneous resolution by capillary electrophoresis in sieving liquid polymers. Biotechniques 19:254–258, 260–263
10. Shen Y, Xu Q, Han F, et al (1999) Application of capillary nongel sieving electrophoresis for gene analysis. Electrophoresis 20:1822–1828

11. Guttman A, Barta C, Szoke M, Sasvari-Szekely M, Kalasz H (1998) Real-time detection of allele-specific polymerase chain reaction products by automated ultra-thin-layer agarose gel electrophoresis. J Chromatogr A 828:481–487
12. Gelfi C, Righetti PG, Brancolini V, Cremonesi L, Ferrari M (1994) Capillary electrophoresis in polymer networks for analysis of PCR products: detection of delta F508 mutation in cystic fibrosis. Clin Chem 40:1603–1605
13. Kiyoi H, Naoe T (2002) FLT3 in human hematologic malignancies. Leukemia Lymphoma 43:1541–1547
14. Greiner TC, Rubocki RJ (2002) Effectiveness of capillary electrophoresis using fluorescent-labeled primers in detecting T-cell receptor gamma gene rearrangements. J Mol Diagn 4:137–143
15. Novella E, Giaretta I, Elice F, et al (2002) Fluorescent polymerase chain reaction and capillary electrophoresis for IgH rearrangement and minimal residual disease evaluation in multiple myeloma. Haematologica 87:1157–1164
16. Knudson AG (2002) Cancer genetics. Am J Med Genet 111:96–102
17. Martinelli G, Testoni N, Montefusco V, et al (1998) Detection of bcr-abl transcript in chronic myelogenous leukemia patients by reverse-transcription-polymerase chain reaction and capillary electrophoresis. Haematologica 83:593–601
18. Sanchez-Vega B, Vega F, Medeiros LJ, Lee MS, Luthra R (2002) Quantification of bcl-2/JH fusion sequences and a control gene by multiplex real-time PCR coupled with automated amplicon sizing by capillary electrophoresis. J Mol Diagn 4:223–229
19. Matyas G, Giunta C, Steinmann B, Hossle JP, Hellwig R (2002) Quantification of single nucleotide polymorphisms: a novel method that combines primer extension assay and capillary electrophoresis. Hum Mutat 19:58–68
20. Piggee CA, Muth J, Carrilho E, Karger BL (1997) Capillary electrophoresis for the detection of known point mutations by single-nucleotide primer extension and laser- induced fluorescence detection. J Chromatogr, A 781:367–375
21. Vreeland WN, Meagher RJ, Barron AE (2002) Multiplexed, high-throughput genotyping by single-base extension and end-labeled free-solution electrophoresis. Anal Chem 74:4328–4333
22. Bugalho MJ, Domingues R, Sobrinho L (2002) The minisequencing method: a simple strategy for genetic screening of MEN 2 families. BMC Genet 3:8
23. Zsolnai A, Anton I, Kuhn C, Fesus L (2003) Detection of single-nucleotide polymorphisms coding for three ovine prion protein variants by primer extension assay and capillary electrophoresis. Electrophoresis 24:634–638
24. Arakawa H, Uetanaka K, Maeda M, Tsuji A, Matsubara Y, Narisawa K (1994) Analysis of polymerase chain reaction-product by capillary electrophoresis with laser-induced fluorescence detection and its application to the diagnosis of medium-chain acyl-coenzyme A dehydrogenase deficiency. J Chromatogr A 680:517–523
25. Barta C, Sasvari-Szekely M, Guttman A (1998) Simultaneous analysis of various mutations on the 21- hydroxylase gene by multi-allele specific amplification and capillary gel electrophoresis. J Chromatogr A 817:281–286
26. Lehmann R, Koch M, Pfohl M, Voelter W, Haring HU, Liebich HM (1996) Screening and identification of familial defective apolipoprotein B-100 in clinical samples by capillary gel electrophoresis. J Chromatogr A 744:187–194
27. van de Locht LT, Kuypers AW, Verbruggen BW, Linssen PC, Novakova IR, Mensink EJ (1995) Semi-automated detection of the factor V mutation by allele specific amplification and capillary electrophoresis. Thromb Haemost 74:1276–1279
28. Gomez-Llorente MA, Suarez A, Gomez-Llorente C, et al (2001) Analysis of 31 CFTR mutations in 55 families from the South of Spain. Early Hum Dev 65(Suppl.):S161–S164
29. Day NS, Tadin M, Christiano AM, Lanzano P, Piomelli S, Brown S (2002) Rapid prenatal diagnosis of sickle cell diseases using oligonucleotide ligation assay coupled with laser-induced capillary fluorescence detection. Prenat Diagn 22: 686–691

30. Somsen GW, Welten HT, Mulder FP, Swart CW, Kema IP, de Jong, GJ (2002) Capillary electrophoresis with laser-induced fluorescence detection for fast and reliable apolipoprotein E genotyping. J Chromatogr B: Anal Technol Biomed Life Sci 775:17–26

31. Mitchell CE, Belinsky SA, Lechner JF (1995) Detection and quantitation of mutant Kras codon 12 restriction fragments by capillary electrophoresis. Anal Biochem 224:148–153

32. Butler JM, Wilson MR, Reeder DJ (1998) Rapid mitochondrial DNA typing using restriction enzyme digestion of polymerase chain reaction amplicons followed by capillary electrophoresis separation with laser-induced fluorescence detection. Electrophoresis 19:119–124

33. Kourkine IV, Hestekin CN, Barron AE (2002) Technical challenges in applying capillary electrophoresis-single strand conformation polymorphism for routine genetic analysis. Electrophoresis 23:1375–1385

34. Atha DH, Kasprzak W, O'Connell CD, Shapiro BA (2001) Prediction of DNA single-strand conformation polymorphism: analysis by capillary electrophoresis and computerized DNA modeling. Nucleic Acids Res 29:4643–4653

35. Liu MS, Rampal S, Hsiang D, Chen FT (2000) Automated DNA mutation analysis by single-strand conformation polymorphism using capillary electrophoresis with laser-induced fluorescence detection. Mol Biotechnol 15:21–27

36. Gillman LM, Gunton J, Turenne CY, Wolfe J, Kabani AM (2001) Identification of Mycobacterium species by multiple—fluorescence PCR-single-strand conformation polymorphism analysis of the 16S rRNA gene. J Clin Microbiol 39:3085–3091

37. Glavac D, Potocnik U, Podpecnik D, Zizek T, Smerkolj S, Ravnik-Glavac M (2002) Correlation of MFOLD- predicted DNA secondary structures with separation patterns obtained by capillary electrophoresis single-strand conformation polymorphism (CE-SSCP) analysis. Hum Mutat 19:384–394

38. Rozycka M, Collins N, Stratton MR, Wooster R (2000) Rapid detection of DNA sequence variants by conformation-sensitive capillary electrophoresis. Genomics 70:34–40

39. Iwamoto T, Sonobe T, Hayashi K (2002) Novel algorithm identifies species in a polymycobacterial sample by fluorescence capillary electrophoresis-based single-strand conformation polymorphism analysis. J Clin Microbiol 40:4705–4712

40. Raucci G, Maggi CA, Parente D (2000) Capillary electrophoresis of supercoiled DNA molecules: parameters governing the resolution of topoisomers and their separation from open forms. Anal Chem 72:821–826

41. Kringen P, Egedal S, Pedersen JC, et al (2002) BRCAl mutation screening using restriction endonuclease fingerprinting-single-strand conformation polymorphism in an automated capillary electrophoresis system. Electrophoresis 23:4085–4091

42. Baba Y, Tomisaki R, Sumita C, et al (1995) Rapid typing of variable number of tandem repeat locus in the human apolipoprotein B gene for DNA diagnosis of heart disease by polymerase chain reaction and capillary electrophoresis. Electrophoresis 16:1437–1440

43. Lindstedt BA, Ryberg D, Zienolddiny S, Khan H, Haugen A (1999) Hrasl VNTR alleles as susceptibility markers for lung cancer: relationship to microsatellite instability in tumors. Anticancer Res 19:5523–5527

44. Dib C, Faure S, Fizames C, et al (1996) A comprehensive genetic map of the human genome based on 5,264 microsatellites. Nature 380:152–154

45. Dietrich WF, Miller JC, Steen RG, et al (1994) A genetic map of the mouse with 4,006 simple sequence length polymorphisms. Nature Genet 7:220–245

46. Breen G, Sham P, Li T, Shaw D, Collier DA, St Clair D (1999) Accuracy and sensitivity of DNA pooling with microsatellite repeats using capillary electrophoresis. Mol Cell Probes 13:359–365

47. Cook EH, Jr, Courchesne RY, Cox NJ, et al (1998) Linkage-disequilibrium mapping of autistic disorder, with 15q11-13 markers. Am J Hum Genet 62:1077–1083

48. Gelfi C, Cossu G, Carta P, Serra M, Righetti PG (1995) Gene dosage in capillary electrophoresis: pre-natal diagnosis of Down's syndrome. J Chromatogr A 718: 405–412

49. Latour P, Boutrand L, Levy N, et al (2001) Polymorphic short tandem repeats for diagnosis of the Charcot-Marie- Tooth lA duplication. Clin Chem 47:829–37

50. Van Hoofstat DE, Deforce DL, Hubert De Pauw IP, Van den Eeckhout EG (1999) DNA typing of fingerprints using capillary electrophoresis: effect of dactyloscopic powders. Electrophoresis 20:2870–2876

51. Moretti TR, Baumstark AL, Defenbaugh DA, Keys KM, Brown AL, Budowle B (2001) Validation of STR typing by capillary electrophoresis. J Forensic Sci 46:661–676

52. Laszik A, Brinkmann B, Sotonyi P, Falus A (2000) Automated fluorescent detection of a 10 loci multiplex for paternity testing. Acta Biol Hung 51:99–105

53. Lion T (2003) Summary: reports on quantitative analysis of chimerism after allogeneic stem cell transplantation by PCR amplification of microsatellite markers and capillary electrophoresis with fluorescence detection. Leukemia 17:252–254

54. Boland CR, Thibodeau SN, Hamilton SR, et al (1998) A National Cancer Institute Workshop on Microsatellite Instability for cancer detection and familial predisposition: development of international criteria for the determination of microsatellite instability in colorectal cancer. Cancer Res 58:5248–5257

55. Berg KD, Glaser CL, Thompson RE, Hamilton SR, Griffin CA, Eshleman JR (2000) Detection of microsatellite instability by fluorescence multiplex polymerase chain reaction. J Mol Diagn 2:20–28

56. Wada T, Louhelainen J, Hemminki K, et al (2000) Bladder cancer: allelic deletions at and around the retinoblastoma tumor suppressor gene in relation to stage and grade. Clin Cancer Res 6:610–615

57. Yoshino I, Fukuyama S, Kameyama T, Shikada Y, Oda S, Maehara Y, Sugimachi K (2003) Detection of loss of heterozygosity by high-resolution fluorescent system in non-small cell lung cancer: association of loss of heterozygosity with smoking and tumor progression. Chest 123:545–550

58. Murthy SK, DiFrancesco LM, Ogilvie RT, Demetrick DJ (2002) Loss of heterozygosity associated with uniparental disomy in breast carcinoma. Mod Pathol 15:1241–1250

59. Fukunaga K, Wada T, Matsumoto H, Yoshihiro S, Matsuyama H Naito K (2002) Renal cell carcinoma: allelic loss at chromosome 9 using the fluorescent multiplex-polymerase chain reaction technique. Hum Pathol 33:910–914

60. Sell SM, Patel S, Stracner D, Meloni A (2001) Allelic loss analysis by capillary electrophoresis: an accurate, automated method for detection of deletions in solid tumors. Genet Test 5:267–268

61. Hussey J, Lockhart PJ, Seltzer W, et al (2002) Accurate determination of ataxin-2 polyglutamine expansion in patients with intermediate-range repeats. Genet Test 6:217–220

62. O'Connell CD, Atha DH, Jakupciak JP, Amos JA, Richie K (2002) Standardization of PCR amplification for fragile X trinucleotide repeat measurements. Clin Genet 61:13–20

63. Kiba Y, Baba Y (2001) Analysis of triplet-repeat DNA by capillary electrophoresis. Methods Mol Biol 163:221–229

64. Nesi M, Righetti PG, Patrosso MC, Ferlini A, Chiari M (1994) Capillary electrophoresis of polymerase chain reaction-amplified products in polymer networks: the case of Kennedy's disease. Electrophoresis 15:644–646

65. Dorschner MO, Barden D, Stephens K (2002) Diagnosis of five spinocerebellar ataxia disorders by multiplex amplification and capillary electrophoresis. J Mol Diagn 4:108–113

66. Williams LC, Hegde MR, Herrera G, Stapleton PM, Love DR (1999) Comparative semi-automated analysis of (CAG) repeats in the Huntington disease gene: use of internal standards. Mol Cell Prohes 13:283–289

67. Tian H, Brody LC, Landers JP (2000) Rapid detection of deletion, insertion, and substitution mutations via heteroduplex analysis using capillary- and microchip-based electrophoresis. Genome Res 10:1403–13

68. O'Connor F, Fitzgerald DJ, Murphy RP (2000) An automated heteroduplex assay for the Pi(A) polymorphism of glycoprotein IIb/IIIa, multiplexed with two pro-thrombotic genetic markers. Thromb Haemost 83:248–252

69. Jackson HA, Bowen DJ, Worwood M (1997) Rapid genetic screening for haemo-chromatosis using heteroduplex technology. Br J Haematol 98:856–859

70. Bowen DJ, Standen GR, Granville S, Bowley S, Wood NA, Bidwell J (1997) Genetic diagnosis of factor V Leiden using heteroduplex technology. Thromb Haemost 77:119–122

71. Thomas GA, Williams DL, Soper SA (2001) Capillary electrophoresis-based heterodu-plex analysis with a universal heteroduplex generator for detection of point mutations associated with rifampin resistance in tuberculosis. Clin Chem 47:1195–1203

72. Khrapko K, Coller HA, Hanekamp JS, Thilly WG (1998) Identification of point mutations in mixtures by capillary electrophoresis hybridization. Nucleic Acids Res 26:5738–5740

73. Kozlowski P, Krzyzosiak WJ (2001) Combined SSCP/duplex analysis by capillary electrophoresis for more efficient mutation detection. Nucleic Acids Res. 29:E71

74. Kourkine IV, Hestekin CN, Magnusdottir SO, Barron AE (2002) Optimized sample preparation for tandem capillary electrophoresis single-stranded conformational polymorphism/heteroduplex analysis. Biotechniques 33:318–320, 322, 324, 325

75. Tian H, Brody LC, Fan S, Huang Z, and Landers, JP (2001) Capillary and micro-chip electrophoresis for rapid detection of known mutations by combining allele-specific DNA amplification with heteroduplex analysis. Clin Chem 47:173–185

76. Bianchi N, Mischiati C, Feriotto G, et al (1994) Capillary electrophoresis: detec-tion of hybridization between synthetic oligonucleotides and HIV-1 genomic DNA amplified by polymerase-chain reaction. J Virol Methods 47:321–329

77. Armitage BA (2003) The impact of nucleic acid secondary structure on PNA hybridization. Drug Discoy. Today 8:222–228

78. Basile A, Giuliani A, Pirri G, and Chiari M (2002) Use of peptide nucleic acid probes for detecting DNA single-base mutations by capillary electrophoresis. Electrophoresis 23:926–929

79. Igloi GL (2001) Simultaneous identification of mutations by dual-parameter mul-tiplex hybridization in peptide nucleic acid-containing virtual arrays. Genomics. 74:402–407

80. Freudemann T, von Brocke A, Bayer E (2001) On-line coupling of capillary gel electrophoresis with electrospray mass spectrometry for oligonucleotide analysis. Anal Chem 73:2587–2593

81. McKeon J, Khaledi MG (2001) Quantitative nuclear and cytoplasmic localization of antisense oligonucleotides by capillary electrophoresis with laser-induced fluo-rescence detection. Electrophoresis 22:3765–3770

82. Gilar M, Belenky A, Budman Y, Smisek DL, Cohen AS. (1998) Study of phos-phorothioate-modified oligonucleotide resistance to 3′-exonuclease using capillary electrophoresis. J Chromatogr B: Biomed Sci Appl 714:13–20

83. Zellweger T, Miyake H, Cooper S, et al (2001) Antitumor activity of antisense clusterin oligonucleotides is improved in vitro and in vivo by incorporation of 2′-O-(2-methoxy)ethyl chemistry. J Pharmacol Exp Ther 298:934–40

84. DeDionisio LA (2001) Analysis of modified oligonucleotides with capillary gel electrophoresis. Methods Mol Biol 162:353–370

85. Lagu AL (1999) Applications of capillary electrophoresis in biotechnology. Electrophoresis 20:3145–3155

86. Zhu L, Lee HK, Lin B, Yeung ES (2001) Spatial temperature gradient capillary electrophoresis for DNA mutation detection. Electrophoresis 22:3683–3687

87. Kristensen AT, Bjorheim J, Ekstrom PO (2002) Detection of mutations in exon 8 of TP53 by temperature gradient 96-capillary array electrophoresis. Biotechniques 33:650–653

88. Weinfeld M, Xing JZ, Lee J, Leadon SA, Le XC (2002) Immunofluorescence detection of radiation-induced DNA base damage. Mil Med 167:2–4

89. Fiscus RR, Leung CP, Yuen JP, Chan HC (2001) Quantification of apoptotic DNA fragmentation in a transformed uterine epithelial cell line, HRE-H9, using capillary electrophoresis with laser-induced fluorescence detector (CE-LIF). Cell Biol Int 25:1007–1011

90. Reik, W., Dean, W., and Walter, J. (2001) Epigenetic reprogramming in mammalian development. Science 293:1089–1093

91. Panning B, Jaenisch R (1996) DNA hypomethylation can activate Xist expression and silence X-linked genes. Genes Dev 10:1991–2002

92. Li E, Beard C, Jaenisch R (1993) Role for DNA methylation in genomic imprinting. Nature 366:362–365

93. Jones PA, Baylin SB (2002) The fundamental role of epigenetic events in cancer. Nature Rev. Genet 3:415–428

94. Fraga MF, Rodriguez R, Canal MJ (2000) Rapid quantification of DNA methylation by high performance capillary electrophoresis. Electrophoresis 21: 2990–2994

95. Stach D, Schmitz OJ, Stilgenbauer S, et al (2003) Capillary electrophoretic analysis of genomic DNA methylation levels. Nucleic Acids Res 31:E2

96. Kotler L, He H, Miller AW, Karger BL (2002) DNA sequencing of close to 1000 bases in 40 minutes by capillary electrophoresis using dimethyl sulfoxide and urea as denaturants in replaceable linear polyacrylamide solutions. Electrophoresis 23:3062–3070

97. Albarghouthi MN, Barron AE (2000) Polymeric matrices for DNA sequencing by capillary electrophoresis. Electrophoresis 21:4096–40111

98. Dolnik V (1999) DNA sequencing by capillary electrophoresis. J Biochem Biophys Methods 41:103–119 (review)

99. Nicod JC, Largiader CR (2003) SNPs by AFLP (SBA): a rapid SNP isolation strategy for non-model organisms. Nucleic Acids Res 31:e19

100. Doglio A, Laffont C, Thyss S, Lefebvre JC (1998) Rapid genotyping of hepatitis C virus by direct cycle sequencing of PCR-amplified cDNAs and capillary electrophoresis analysis. Res Virol 149:219–227

101. Blazej RG, Paegel BM, Mathies RA (2003) Polymorphism ratio sequencing: a new approach for single nucleotide polymorphism discovery and genotyping. Genome Res 13:287–293

102. Murphy KM, Eshleman JR (2002) Simultaneous sequencing of multiple polymerase chain reaction products and combined polymerase chain reaction with cycle sequencing in single reactions. Am J Pathol 161:27–33

103. Woolley AT, Mathies RA (1994) Ultra-high- speed DNA fragment separations using microfabricated capillary array electrophoresis chips. Proc Natl Acad Sci USA 91:11,348–11,352

104. Gao Q, Shi Y, Liu S (2001) Multiple-channel microchips for high-throughput DNA analysis by capillary electrophoresis. Fresenius J Anal Chem 371:137–145

105. Medintz IL, Paegel BM, Blazej RG, et al (2001) High-performance genetic analysis using microfabricated capillary array electrophoresis microplates. Electrophoresis 22:3845–3856

106. Medintz IL, Berti L, Emrich CA, Tom J, Scherer JR, Mathies RA (2001) Genotyping energy-transfer-cassette-labeled short-tandem-repeat amplicons with capillary array electrophoresis microchannel plates. Clin Chem 47:1614–1621

107. Wessagowit V, South AP (2002) Dermatological applications of DNA array technology. Clin Exp Dermatol 27:485–492

108. Gawron AJ, Martin RS, Lunte SM (2001) Microchip electrophoretic separation systems for biomedical and pharmaceutical analysis. Eur J Pharm Sci 14:1–12

7

Denaturing High-Performance Liquid Chromatography (DHPLC) for Nucleic Acid Analysis

Kim Hung Leung and Shea Ping Yip

1. Introduction

1.1. DNA Sequence Variants

Since the completion of the Human Genome Project, it is clear that the human genome carries about 30,000 genes occupying less than 5% of the 3 billion base pairs (bp) of DNA sequence. Meanwhile, the human genome was also found to carry a very large number of sequence variations (*1*). On average, there are about 3 million sequence differences (0.1% of the whole genome) between any two unrelated individuals from a population. The analysis of DNA sequence variations is very important in genetic studies. Two broad types of DNA sequence variations are classified: polymorphisms and disease-causing mutations. Polymorphisms refer to those sequence variations that are found in normal individuals and do not result in diseased phenotypes. They include single nucleotide polymorphisms (SNPs), microsatellites, and minisatellites. A SNP (pronounced as sn*i*p) is a sequence variation owing to change in a single nucleotide. Microsatellites and minisatellites are caused by variations in the number of repeat units that are themselves a short stretch of DNA sequence. They are very useful in research for locating the position of genes in our chromosomes, a process known as gene mapping. On the other hand, disease-causing mutations are those sequence variations that result in diseased phenotypes because they adversely affect the functions of the proteins, either qualitatively or quantitatively. The identification of mutations is important for the diagnosis of genetic diseases in clinical medicine.

To examine DNA sequence variations in various genetic studies, both unknown and known variations can be investigated (*2*). Unknown sequence variations refer to those that are not known to exist previously and have to be detected by a group of methods called screening or scanning methods. Known sequence variations are known to exist and their genotypes can be determined by a group of methods known as diagnostic methods. Numerous techniques are available for detecting and identifying sequence variations, and vary from each other in terms of the principle of the method, cost, ease of optimization and use, requirement of special instruments, and turnaround time. Examples

From: *Molecular Biomethods Handbook, 2nd Edition.*
Edited by: J. M. Walker and R. Rapley © Humana Press, Totowa, NJ

of methods for analysis of sequence variations include DNA sequencing, single strand conformation analysis (SSCP), denaturing high-performance liquid chromatography (DHPLC), denaturing gradient gel electrophoresis (DGGE), restriction endonuclease digestion, allele-specific hybridization and allele-specific polymerase chain reaction. For DHPLC, the WAVE DNA fragment analysis system (Transgenomic) provides an automatic medium-throughput analytical tool for both screening unknown sequence variations and genotyping known sequence variations.

1.2. Denaturing High-Performance Liquid Chromatography (DHPLC)

1.2.1. The Principle of DHPLC

DHPLC is a chromatographic technique for the separation and analysis of DNA fragments with different length and/or base composition. This technique can be applied for mutation detection in DNA fragments of 200–1000 bp in length with a high sensitivity (>96%) and specificity (>99%) (3). In addition, the high resolving power of DHPLC allows the distinction of short nucleic acid fragments such as primer extension products for allelic discrimination.

DHPLC is based on a reversed phase system in which the stationary phase is nonpolar and the mobile phase polar (4,5). The hydrophobic stationary phase, *DNASep* column marketed by the company Transgenomic, is made up of alkylated nonporous poly(styrene-divinylbenzene) particles 2–3 μm in diameter. The polar mobile phase is acetonitrile (CH_3-CN). However, DNA molecules are large anions because of the negative charges on the phosphate groups in the phosphate-sugar backbones of the DNA strands. Organic cations are required to allow interaction between DNA anions and the nonpolar stationary phase. The organic cation carries a positively charged portion to interact with the negative charge of DNA molecules on the one hand, and also a hydrophobic portion to interact with the nonpolar stationary phase on the other hand.

The most commonly used organic cation is triethylammonium, $(CH_3CH_2)_3N^+$, in the form of triethylammonium acetate (TEAA). Thus, TEAA is used as an ion pairing reagent. The triethylammonium cations bind to the phosphate groups of DNA molecules and hence effectively coat the DNA molecules with a hydrophobic layer (the triethyl portion). The number of TEAA molecules coating the DNA molecules is proportional to the length of the DNA molecules and in turn determines the degree of interaction between the DNA molecules and the stationary phase. DNA molecules are eluted from the column in an increasing gradient of acetonitrile, which weakens the interaction between coated DNA molecules and the stationary phase. In other words, coated DNA molecules bind onto the stationary phase and will be released from the stationary phase when acetonitrile in the mobile phase reaches a specific concentration. Thus, shorter DNA molecules are eluted earlier from the column than and hence separated from longer DNA molecules under the same buffer condition. In summary, the separation of DNA molecules is based on the principle of ion-pair reversed phase liquid chromatography (4,5).

1.2.2. Modes of DHPLC

Three modes of operation are available for chromatographic analysis of nucleic acids, depending on the temperature of the column (4). They are nondenaturing, partially denaturing, and completely denaturing modes. Each mode of operation serves a different purpose in nucleic acid analysis. In brief, the nondenaturing condition is applied to the size-dependent separation of double strand (ds) DNA molecules. The partially denaturing condition is used for screening of putative SNPs or detection of unknown mutations. The third operation mode performed under completely denaturing condition is used for the analysis of short DNA fragments such as products of primer extensions and synthetic oligonucleotides, as well as RNA. Nucleic acid chromatography is most widely used under partially or completely denaturing conditions, and hence is frequently called denaturing HPLC (DHPLC).

1.2.2.1. Nondenaturing HPLC: Nondenaturing HPLC is used for the size-dependent separation of dsDNA molecules, which depends on the length of the molecules, but not the base composition *(4,5)*. After polymerase chain reactions (PCR), the amplified DNA fragments are directly injected into the DHPLC analysis system. The column temperature is maintained at 50°C and DNA molecules remain double-stranded. The concentration of the eluent (acetonitrile) is increased with time. The shorter DNA fragments will be eluted and detected first, followed by the longer fragments. The eluted DNA fragments are detected by the ultraviolet (UV) detector and the chromatographic peaks representing the corresponding DNA fragments are demonstrated on the computer screen (**Fig. 7.1**). Similar to conventional gel electrophoresis, nondenaturing

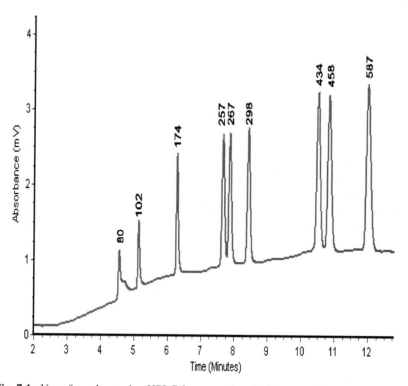

Fig. 7.1. Use of nondenaturing HPLC for separating double-stranded DNA molecules. The chromatogram shows the elution profile of DNA molecules of known size (size standards) with the size in basepairs indicated above the peaks

HPLC can accurately determine the size of the amplicons. Unlabeled products can be used for analysis even with a UV detector if the injection volumes are large *(6)*. Use of unlabeled products reduces the cost of analysis. With small injection volumes, reliable quantification can also be achieved by adding dsDNA intercalation dye such as SYBR Green I and measuring the green fluorescence with a fluorescence detector *(7)*. The dye is mixed with the DNA samples after elution from the column (postcolumn addition). The throughput of such analyses can further be increased by multiplex PCR in which several fragments of different sizes are amplified in the same tube *(6,7)*.

1.2.2.2. Partially Denaturing HPLC: The major application of DHPLC is to screen for unknown mutations and putative SNPs *(4,8)*. To achieve this, the partially denaturing HPLC mode is used and the column temperature is maintained above 50°C, but below 70°C. The column temperatures vary with different DNA fragments to be analyzed and depend on the melting domains in the fragments. Before the DHPLC analysis, the DNA fragments are amplified by PCR. The PCR product from a test sample is mixed with a homozygous reference PCR product in equal volume. The mixed DNA fragments are denatured and allowed to reanneal by gradually lowering the temperature. With this process of heteroduplex formation, two dsDNA molecules that differ by a single base pair (e.g., A-T vs G-C) will give two heteroduplexes and two homoduplexes (**Fig. 7.2**). Stability of the DNA duplexes determines the order of elution from the column: the more stable the duplexes, the longer the elution time. Heteroduplexes with mismatches are less stable than and are thus eluted before homoduplexes. The partially denaturing HPLC allows separation of homoduplexes and heteroduplexes produced as a result of even a single base difference between two otherwise identical dsDNA molecules at an optimized column temperature. With reference to a homozygous wild type control, any difference in the elution profile is indicative of the presence of a sequence variation. In fact, a 4-peak pattern is not frequently seen. The test DNA samples are then sequenced to confirm the presence and characterize the nature of the mutations. Nevertheless, false positive results can sometimes be obtained and an altered elution pattern is demonstrated for DNA fragments without sequence variations (see the following). The ideal size of PCR products is 150–450 bp for detection of unknown sequence variations although mutations have been detected in fragments as large as 1500 bp. Long DNA fragments tend to have more than 1 melting domain and hence require several column temperatures for complete screening of the fragment.

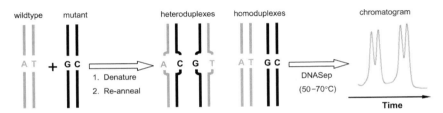

Fig. 7.2. Use of partially denaturing HPLC to separate homoduplexes and heteroduplexes. This mode of operation allows detection of sequence variations, either known or unknown

The column temperature is the most important parameter for the detection of sequence variations. Some sequence variations can be detected only at a particular temperature whereas others can be detected at several temperatures *(9)* (**Fig. 7.3**). The column temperature for the analysis of a particular PCR fragment can be automatically determined by a predictive algorithm of the software packages WAVEMAKER or NAVIGATOR (Transgenomic) as well as the freeware MELT (http://insertion.stanford.edu/melt.html). Experience has shown that optimized analysis temperature may differ from the one recommended by software packages *(8)*.

Partially denaturing HPLC is very sensitive in detecting heteroduplexes even though the heteroduplexes may be present in small amounts only. Not being error-proof, DNA polymerase can misincorporate nucleotides during PCR and

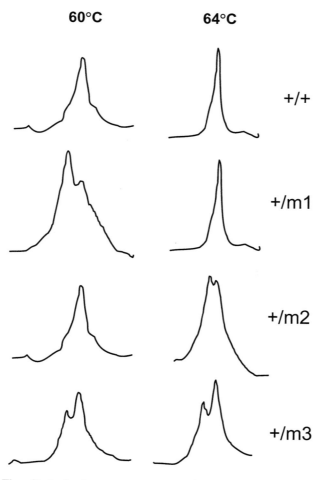

Fig. 7.3. The effect of column temperature on the detection of sequence variations. The diagram shows the elution profiles at two column temperatures (60°C and 64°C) for three different hypothetical heterozygous mutations (+/m1, +/m2 and +/m3) in comparison with the homozygous normal (+/+). The mutations are found within the same DNA fragment in different individuals. Mutation m1 is detected at 60°C only and mutation m2 at 64°C only whereas mutation m3 is detected at both temperatures

hence generate in the test mixture a small proportion of heteroduplexes, which may produce a shoulder peak or background heteroduplex peaks. Such false positive results have to be excluded by follow-up study with DNA sequencing (*8*), and are thus wastage of time and money. Use of DNA polymerase with proofreading activity or a mixture of such enzyme and *Taq* DNA polymerase can help reduce such errors (*5*).

1.2.2.3. Completely Denaturing HPLC: The mode of operation is completely denaturing if the column temperature is maintained between 70°C and 80°C (*4,5*). Under such a high temperature, DNA molecules are completely denatured and become single-stranded. Completely denaturing HPLC can differentiate single-stranded (ss) DNA (and RNA) molecules with the separation depending on both the length and the base composition of the single-stranded nucleic acid molecules. It can be used to analyze and isolate synthetic oligonucleotides and RNA molecules. More commonly, it is used to analyze the products from primer extension (PE) reactions (also known as minisequencing).

In PE reaction, an extension primer is annealed immediately upstream of the polymorphic site. In the presence of a modified DNA polymerase (e.g., Thermo Sequenase from GE Healthcare) and appropriate unlabeled dideoxynucleotides (ddNTPs), the primer is then extended in a template-dependent manner (**Fig. 7.4**). The allele-specific extension products with different sequence compositions are then detected and discriminated by completely denaturing HPLC. As such, completely denaturing HPLC provides a robust platform of medium throughput for genotyping known mutations or SNPs. The throughput can be increased by multiplexing several primer extensions in a single reaction (*10*).

1.3. The Hardware of DHPLC

The hardware of DHPLC consists of components similar to those in conventional HPLC (**Fig. 7.5**). Together with a gradient system, a pressure pump delivers buffers or solvents from buffer reservoirs in appropriate proportions to a column for the separation of DNA molecules. The buffer is the mobile phase while the column is the stationary phase. DNA samples are placed in an autosampler plate and injected into the column through an injection unit. The column is housed in a temperature-controlled oven. Under appropriate conditions, DNA molecules are separated in the column into individual components and then eluted from the column. The eluted components are monitored by a detector and the data collected in a computer system. A UV detector is

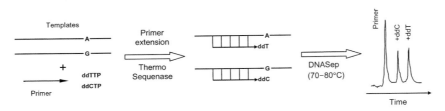

Fig. 7.4. Use of completely denaturing HPLC for analyzing primer extension products. Under this condition, genotypes can be determined for known sequence variations for individual DNA samples or DNA pools

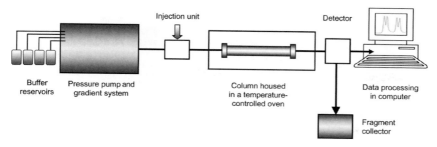

Fig. 7.5. Hardware components of HPLC for nucleic acid analysis. The heart of the system lies in the separation column housed in a temperature-controlled oven

the most common option for measuring DNA molecules at a wavelength of 260 nm although a fluorescence detector can also be installed. The results are displayed as chromatograms or elution profiles showing the amounts and elution times for various components separated by the column. An optional fragment collector can be connected to the detector to collect the separated components into vials for further analysis and processing. The heart of the system lies in the column—the stationary phase. The most widely used column is DNASep (Transgenomic). DNA separating columns (e.g., Eclipse and Helix columns) from other manufacturers use a different type of stationary phase, and are less popular when compared with DNASep *(4)*.

2. Methods

2.1. DNA Sample Preparation

Before DHPLC analysis, the target DNA fragments of interest are first amplified by PCR (**Fig. 7.6**). Three DNA polymerases are suggested for use with DHPLC analysis, including Optimase® Polymerase, Maximase™ Polymerase and T-Taq™ Polymerase (Transgenomic). The functional integrity of the column might be adversely affected if other DNA polymerases are used (http://www.transgenomic.com/lib/ug/602032.pdf). It is also important to note that under no circumstances should PCR additives such as mineral oil, dimethyl sulfoxide, and formamide be used. Otherwise, the column would be damaged.

The amplified PCR products can be injected directly into the separation column if they are to be analyzed under the nondenaturing condition (**Fig. 7.6**). Otherwise, they are further processed as described in the following sections on the basis of the purpose of the analysis.

2.1.1. Heteroduplex Formation

For mutation detection, the PCR product from a test sample is mixed with a homozygous reference PCR product in a 1:1 (v/v) ratio. The mixed DNA fragments are denatured at 95°C and then cooled slowly for reannealing of the DNA strands by gradually lowering the temperature at a rate of 1°C per 20 seconds from 95°C to 25°C (**Fig. 7.6**). A single base pair difference between the test and reference fragments will produce two heteroduplexes and two homoduplexes (**Fig. 7.2**). The mixture of DNA samples are then analyzed by DHPLC under partially denaturing conditions (**Fig. 7.6**).

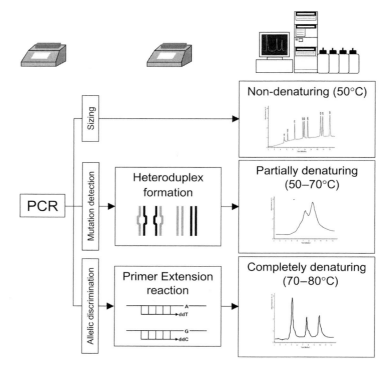

Fig. 7.6. Method outline for DHPLC analysis under three different modes of operation. The top panel shows the instruments (thermal cycler or DHPLC system) to be used in different steps shown in the bottom part

2.1.2. Primer Extension Reactions

For allelic discrimination, the amplicons containing the target polymorphic site serve as templates for PE reactions (**Fig. 7.6**). Prior to the PE reactions, the amplicons are purified by treatment at 37°C with exonuclease I and shrimp alkaline phosphatase in order to remove the unincorporated single strand oligo primers and deoxynuclotides respectively. The enzymes are then inactivated at 80°C. After purification, the PCR products are mixed with Thermo Sequenase (GE Healthcare) and appropriate ddNTPs. The PE reactions are carried out in a thermal cycler with a universal thermal cycling condition that includes denaturation at 96°C, annealing at 43°C followed by extension at 60°C (**Fig. 7.6**). The single strand extended products are analyzed by DHPLC under completely denaturing condition.

2.2. DHPLC Analysis

Regardless of the operation mode, the DNA samples are placed in the cooled 96-well autosampler compartment of the DHPLC system. It is controlled by the software from the manufacturer of the system (e.g. the WAVEMAKER software for the WAVE DNA Fragment Analysis System from Transgenomic). All the analytical parameters are entered into the program, including the sample information (sample identity and volume to be injected), application types, column temperature (mode of HPLC), and the linear gradient profile (the percentage of acetonitrile in the mobile phase). A linear gradient of 1.8–2.0%

per minute at a flow rate of 0.9 ml/min is usually used. In general, the start- and end-points of the gradient are adjusted according to the size of the DNA fragments. For the detection of unknown mutation, the optimal column temperature and the linear gradient profile are calculated by the algorithm of the software. The gradient profile for each injection includes the column regeneration and equilibrium steps prior to the next injection. The eluted DNA fragments are shown as peaks in the chromatogram (**Fig. 7.6**). The retention time and the intensity of the peaks (height or area) are determined by the software.

2.3. Data Analysis

After sample injection, the signal intensity of DHPLC profile is shown real-time on the computer screen. A DNA fragment appears as a peak in the chromatogram with the corresponding intensity and retention time. Interpretation of DHPLC data is based on the comparison between sample and reference chromatograms. For sizing of a DNA fragment, the sample peak is compared with a series of DNA fragments of known size or commercial size standards (**Fig. 7.1**). Because the retention time increases with increasing DNA fragment size, the retention time becomes a measure of DNA fragment size. Accordingly, the size of a DNA fragment is determined by comparing the retention time obtained and the retention times of the size standards.

In mutation detection, the elution profile of a test sample is compared with that of the wild type sample. Any altered elution profile such as shoulder peak and additional peak(s) implies the presence of heteroduplexes and hence mutation(s) in the DNA fragment (see, for example, **Fig. 7.3**). The DHPLC profile of a test sample showing any aberrant elution profile is then confirmed by direct sequencing.

In allelic discrimination, the alleles are distinguished by the retention times of allele-specific PE products. Different sequence compositions of PE products give different retention times, which can then be verified by DNA samples of known genotypes. The genotype of a test sample can be determined on the basis of the number of elution peaks and their corresponding retention times. In addition, the detected DNA samples can be quantified by the peak height or area. Accordingly, the amount of DNA samples and the allele frequencies of DNA pools can be estimated.

3. Applications

In the past years, DHPLC has been used for various research and diagnostic purposes. Under appropriate conditions, DHPLC can be used to size and quantify PCR products, detect unknown (and known) sequence variations, and genotype individual samples or DNA pools by analysis of primer extension products.

3.1. Mutation Detection

The most significant function of DHPLC is mutation detection. Partially denaturing HPLC is used to detect unknown sequence variations. Heteroduplexes are generated before analysis (see Section 2.1.1). This step is essential for the detection of X-linked mutations in males and homozygous mutations. The screening throughput can be increased by mixing several test samples with 1 reference sample *(8,11)*. As has been mentioned above, the ideal size of PCR products is 150–450 bp for detection of unknown sequence variations. Long DNA fragments tend to have more than 1 melting domain and require several column temperatures for complete screening of the fragment.

There are occasions in which several sequence variations are found within a small DNA region in different chromosomes (i.e., in different individuals). These are well illustrated by the diverse mutations in the *CFTR* and *HBB* genes *(9,12)*. Mutations in *CFTR* result in cystic fibrosis whereas mutations in *HBB* give rise to β-thalassemia or sickle cell disease. Distinct mutations in a PCR product usually give consistent distinct chromatograms. Therefore, partially denaturing HPLC can also be used to genotype known sequence variations (**8**), particularly known mutations, once their corresponding distinct chromatograms have been established. However, it is still possible that different mutations may share indistinguishable chromatograms.

Partially denaturing HPLC is the most widely used mode of operation for DNA chromatography. To date, over 300 genes have been analyzed by partially denaturing HPLC (http://insertion.stanford.edu/dhplc_genes1.html). For screening mutations, its sensitivity and specificity approach 100% in many published studies and compare very favorably with direct DNA sequencing, which is widely regarded as the gold standard for comparison. Partially denaturing HPLC can also detect mosaic mutations that account for only a small proportion of alleles in a PCR product and that may remain undetected even by DNA sequencing *(13,14)*. Mosaic mutations are found in tumor samples where tumor cells with mutations are surrounded by normal cells without mutations, and in minimal residual disease where malignant cells are not completely eradicated.

3.1.1. Direct Detection of Deletions and Duplications

Nondenaturing HPLC can be used to quantify PCR products. To allow for quantification of PCR products, the number of PCR cycles has to be around 25 so that the amount of product amplified is proportional to the initial gene copy number. This type of analysis is very useful for detecting gene rearrangements such as deletions and insertions.

Applications are exemplified by the detection of large deletions of the X-linked dystrophin gene in Duchene muscular dystrophy *(6)* and the demonstration of exon deletions and duplications in the *RB1* tumor suppressor gene *(7)*. With a wild type or normal chromatogram for comparison, homozygous deletion is indicated by the absence of a particular elution peak, and heterozygous deletion (or a carrier) by a peak of half height (**Fig. 7.7**).

3.2. Allelic Discrimination

3.2.1. Individual Genotyping

The PE reaction in combination with completely denaturing HPLC analysis offers a simple, robust and automatic genotyping platform because a single analytic condition can be used *(15)*. The accuracy and sensitivity can be increased by using fluorescent-labeling method. Equipped with the DNASep-High Throughput (HT) column and the High Sensitive Detector, the 4500HT-HS model of the WAVE System (Transgenomic) is developed for high-throughput genotyping.

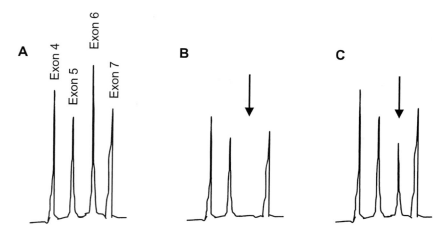

Fig. 7.7. Use of nondenaturing HPLC to detect exon deletions. The chromatograms show the elution profiles of multiplex PCR products amplified from exons 4 to 7 of a hypothetical X-linked gene. Panel A shows the profile for a normal female, panel B for an affected hemizygous male with deletion of exon 6, and panel C for a carrier female with a heterozygous deletion of exon 6. Note that the peak height for exon 6 in the carrier female is about half that of the normal female

The PE/DHPLC genotyping platform has been used in the genotyping of the mutations of the hemochromatosis gene and the β-globin gene for the diagnosis of hereditary hemochromatosis and β-thalassemia respectively. Two mutation sites (C282Y and H63D) of the hemochromatosis gene were simultaneously genotyped in a multiplex format including the PCR, PE reactions and DHPLC detection *(16,17)*. For β-thalassemia, two different studies demonstrated the successful simultaneous genotyping of five common mutations within the β-globin gene. Amplicons containing the five common mutations were amplified, and the mutations distinguished by multiplex PE reactions followed by DHPLC analysis *(10,18)*. This approach would help the development of diagnostic mutation panels for the diagnosis of β-thalassemia and other genetic diseases showing extensive allelic heterogeneity.

3.2.2. Quantitative Genotyping—Allele Frequency Estimation for DNA Pools

In completely denaturing HPLC analysis, the PE products can be quantified by their absorbance at 260 nm. If the starting test sample is a mixture prepared by pooling many DNA samples in equal amounts (a process known as DNA pooling), the relative allele frequencies of a SNP in the DNA pool can be estimated by measuring the relative signal intensities of the two extension products of the DNA pool with reference to those of a heterozygote sample *(19)*. Note that a SNP only has two alleles and their relative allele frequencies sum up to 1. This provides a very cost-effective method for estimating the relative allele frequencies of a large number of different samples. Conventionally, estimation of allele frequencies is achieved by genotyping all samples individually, and this approach is of course very expensive and time-consuming if the number of samples is very large (in the range of several hundreds, or more preferably over 1,000 in genetic association studies, see the following).

In other words, completely denaturing HPLC coupled with primer extension provides a convenient method for estimating relative allele frequencies
in DNA pools, and is very useful in mapping genes involved in complex
diseases. Many human diseases are complex in nature in that they are caused
by genetic factors, environmental factors such as lifestyle and diet, and possibly the interaction between genetic and environmental factors. Examples of
complex diseases include diabetes, hypertension, myopia, infectious diseases,
and many others. Many genes are expected to be involved in a complex
disease and the effect of each gene on the disease is usually small. Genetic
association studies are very powerful in identifying genes of small effects in
complex diseases (20). One approach of genetic association studies is called
case-control study, in which the allele frequencies of a SNP in a candidate
gene are compared between a group of patients with the same disease under
study (the "cases") and a group of control individuals without the disease (the
"controls"). Instead of genotyping all samples one by one, estimation of relative allele frequencies in DNA pools is a very attractive alternative (21). Two
DNA pools are usually constructed: 1 *case pool* prepared from all patients'
samples and 1 *control pool* from all control samples in equal amounts. Once
estimated, the allele frequencies of DNA pools can be compared by statistical
tests. If initial comparison of DNA pools shows statistically significant difference in allele frequencies, confirmatory study is carried out by genotyping
individual samples. If initial comparison does not show any significant difference, then the SNP will not be further investigated. Therefore, this approach
allows more time and effort to be spent on sequence variations that are worthy
of further investigation, and unpromising sequence variations are abandoned
after initial testing. In brief, completely denaturing HPLC plays an important
role in mapping genes involved in complex diseases.

3.3. Microbial Analysis

In addition to the applications in human genetic studies, DHPLC has been
used in the investigation of microbes because the method is cost-effective and
time-saving. One application is the characterization of drug resistance in different bacterial pathogens. DHPLC was first applied to mutation screening in
Staphylococcus aureus (22). The study showed that DHPLC provided a rapid
detection platform of identifying the quinolone resistance alleles of *gyrA*,
gyrB, *grlA,* and *grlB* genes. Similarly, mutations in the quinolone resistance-
determining regions of *Salmonella enterica* (*gyrA*, *gyrB*, *parC*, and *parE*)
(23,24) and *Yersinia pestis* (*gyrA*) *(25)* could also be detected by DHPLC.
Multiplex PCR together with DHPLC analysis has also been developed for the
detection of plasmid-mediated *ampC* β-lactamase gene mutations in Gram-
negative bacteria *(26)*. For the investigation of the drug-resistance genes of
Mycobacterium tuberculosis, mutations were detected by DHPLC in six genes
including *katG*, *rpoB*, *emB*, *gyrA*, *pncA*, and *rpsL*, which are responsible for
isoniazid, rifampicin, ethambutol, fluoroquinolone, pyrazinamide, and streptomycin resistance respectively *(27)*. Besides, the DHPLC analysis system
was also introduced to high-throughput bacterial identification *(28)*. Through
analysis of the prokaryotic 16S rRNA gene, different species could be differentiated by the corresponding distinctive DHPLC peak profiles. This application showed an overall specificity of 100% and a sensitivity of 91.7%.

An enhanced version of the WAVE DHPLC system known as the WAVE Microbial Analysis System (Transgenomic) has been developed specifically for the purpose of microbial analysis. One recent application is the high-throughput typing of *M. tuberculosis* strains based on twelve loci of variable number of tandem repeat present in mycobacteria *(29)*. Typing results based on nondenaturing HPLC showed 100% concordance with those generated by agarose gel electrophoresis. It should be noted that such applications do not fully utilize the benefits of nondenaturing HPLC because the amounts of PCR products are not measured. DHPLC can also be used for the detection and identification of fungal species in blood culture and fecal samples *(30)*. This approach provides a simpler and quicker method than the culture-based approach.

The DHPLC system also allows rapid detection and identification of bacterial species in mixed populations. By separation of PCR-amplified species-specific 16S rRNA, various bacterial species in microbial communities can be identified. A culture-independent 16S rRNA-based approach was set up to identify pathogenic bacteria in urinary tract after renal transplantation *(31)*. The rapid identification of urinary tract infections in the renal transplant recipients would facilitate immediate and appropriate antibiotic therapy to decrease the risk of graft rejection. Furthermore, the technology can be used to display the complex intestinal bacterial communities *(32)*. Because the interruption of the gut flora homeostasis would indicate gastrointestinal disorders, rapid monitoring of the changes in the intestinal microbiota from fecal samples by DHPLC would help in guiding the antimicrobial therapy. The capability of the technology in the analysis of complex microbial communities would allow and extend the investigation to different kinds of bacterial populations from different environments of interest *(33)*.

3.4. Quantification of Gene Expression

The DHPLC technology can be employed for accurate, absolute quantification of gene expression, which is estimated by the competitive reverse transcription (RT) PCR *(34,35)*. Competitive RT-PCR is based on competitive coamplification of a dilution series of known concentrations of internal standard RNA (competitor) together with a constant amount of total RNA (target) in one reaction tube. The amplified RT-PCR products are verified by restriction fragment analysis. Fragments of expected sizes are then quantified by DHPLC analysis. The use of DHPLC in the quantification process offers a rapid, accurate, and automated measurement of gene expression. It is superior to the time-consuming and labor-intensive gel electrophoresis with the use of radiolabeled or fluorescent components. In a recent breast cancer study, the quantitative method identified that nine candidate genes were over-expressed in breast tumor cells *(36)*. The method was also used for studying the differences in quantitative gene expression of α and γ sodium pump subunits of nephron segments from hypertensive rats *(37)*.

3.5. Purification and Isolation of Nucleic Acids

Conventionally, nucleic acids are analyzed by gel electrophoresis for the purposes of separation, identification, and purification. However, the process of the gel-based analysis involves labor-intensive steps such as sample and gel preparations, sample loading, gel staining, and photographic processing. The DHPLC system has high resolving power and thus allows the automatic purification and isolation of nucleic acids. It has been demonstrated that dsDNA, ssDNA, and RNA can be separated, quantified, and then recovered by the fragment collector of the DHPLC system (**Fig. 7.5**). Under nondenaturing conditions, dsDNA molecules such as PCR products and restriction fragments are separated. The isolated dsDNA fragments can then be collected for downstream applications such as sequencing and cloning (*38*). In purification and isolation of ssDNA, DHPLC can directly separate ssDNA from dsDNA under fully denaturing conditions (75°C) (*39*). The purification is facilitated by using a tagged primer, which has a hydrophobic moiety such as a biotin group or fluorescein, in PCR. The hydrophobicity of the ssDNA generated by the tagged primer is increased and leads to the increased retention time in DHPLC analysis. As a result, the two ssDNA species from the dsDNA PCR products can be separated. DHPLC is a simpler and faster method of purifying ssDNA than other techniques involving a variety of analytical molecular biology procedures. Moreover, the fully denaturing conditions can be applied to the purification and quantification of mRNA from total RNA (*40*). In DHPLC analysis, RNA degradation and spurious transcription can also be detected, and hence the quality and integrity can be determined. DHPLC greatly improves the analysis and purification of RNA as compared to the conventional methods by simplifying the lengthy experimental procedures.

3.6. DNA Methylation Analysis

DNA methylation is the modification of DNA by the addition of a methyl group to the 5-position of cytosines. The process is implicated in gene regulation, genomic imprinting, embryonic development, and cell growth and differentiation (*41*). Alteration of DNA methylation may lead to diseases including cancer. As a result, it is important to investigate patterns of DNA methylation status. Different traditional techniques have been used in methylation studies, including sequencing of bisulfite-treated DNA (*42*), methylation-sensitive restriction enzymes and Southern blotting (*43*), methylation-sensitive enzymes and PCR amplification (*44*). However, these methods are labor-intensive and time-consuming. DHPLC provides an efficient alternative for rapid and reliable methylation detection. DHPLC analyzes the methylation-specific PCR products under partially denaturing HPLC condition (*45*) or the PE products under completely denaturing HPLC condition (*46*). The DHPLC method is capable of distinguishing overall methylation profiles of differentially methylated regions of imprinted genes (*47*). The technique also allows the quantification of relative amounts of methylated and unmethylated molecules.

3.7. Forensic Applications

In forensic investigations, mitochondrial DNA (mtDNA) is used to obtain genetic information from forensic samples. The great abundance and stability of mtDNA facilitate the successful investigation of limited quantity of samples obtained from crime scenes (*48*). Hypervariable regions 1 and 2 (HV1/HV2) of the displacement loop are usually examined for mtDNA analysis. Apart from DNA sequencing, the analysis can also be done by immobilized sequence-specific oligonucleotide probes, DGGE, SSCP, microarray, and mass spectrometry. However, some limitations of these methods would influence the accuracy of the results. DHPLC has recently been used to screen the HV1 and HV2 regions of the mtDNA displacement loop (49). The screening method is used to separate mixtures of DNA molecules obtained from body fluid mixtures. The target regions of mtDNA from DNA mixtures are amplified by PCR. Under the partially denaturing HPLC conditions, the homo- and hetero-duplexes are evaluated, and hence the mtDNA species from forensic sample mixtures are resolved and separated. DHPLC provides a rapid, accurate and cost-effective platform for forensic investigations.

3.8. Concluding Remarks

The use of HPLC for nucleic acid analysis depends very much on the separation column that is capable of separating DNA molecules under different conditions (nondenaturing, partially denaturing or completely denaturing). Under appropriate conditions, "DHPLC" or, more correctly, DNA chromatography can be used to size and quantify PCR products, detect unknown (and known) sequence variations, and genotype individual samples or DNA pools by analysis of primer extension products. Such applications can be used for both research and diagnostic purposes, and in genetic, microbiological and forensic studies.

Acknowledgments: Work with DHPLC was funded by the following research grants: PolyU Big Equipment Grant (G.53.27.9027), PolyU Central Research Grants (G-YD47, G-YD74 and G-U069), Dean's Reserve (1.53.09.87AV) and RGC Competitive Earmarked Research Grant (B-Q04A).

References

1. The International SNP Map Working Group (2001) A map of human genome sequence variation containing 1.42 million single nucleotide polymorphisms. Nature 49:928–933
2. Cotton RGH (1997) Mutation Detection. Oxford University Press, Oxford
3. Xiao W, Stern D, Jain M, Huber CG, Oefner PJ (2001) Multiplex capillary denaturing high-performance liquid chromatography with laser-induced fluorescence detection. Biotechniques 30:1332–1338
4. Xiao WH, Oefner PJ (2001) Denaturing high-performance liquid chromatography: a review. Hum Mutat 17:439–474
5. Gjerde DT, Hanna CP, Hornby D (2002) DNA chromatography. Wiley-VCH, Weinheim
6. Hung CC, Su YN, Lin CY, Yang CC, Lee WT, Chien SC, Lin WL, Lee CN (2005) Denaturing HPLC coupled with multiplex PCR for rapid detection of large deletions in Duchenne muscular dystrophy carriers. Clin Chem 51:1252–1256
7. Dehainault C, Lauge A, Caux-Moncoutier V, Pages-Berhouet S, Doz F, Desjardins L, Couturier J, Gauthier-Villars M, Stoppa-Lyonnet D, Houdayer C (2004) Multiplex PCR/liquid chromatography assay for detection of gene rearrangements: application to RB1 gene. Nucleic Acids Res 32:e139
8. Han W, Yip SP, Wang J, and Yap MKH (2004) Using denaturing HPLC for SNP discovery and genotyping, and establishing the linkage disequilibrium pattern for the all-trans-retinol dehydrogenase (RDH8) gene. J Hum Genet 49:16–23
9. Ravnik-Glavac M, Atkinson A, Glavac D, Dean M (2002) DHPLC screening of cystic fibrosis gene mutations. Hum Mutat 19:374–383

10. Yip SP, Pun SF, Leung KH, Lee SY (2003) Rapid simultaneous genotyping of five common Southeast Asian β-thalassemia mutations by multiplex minisequencing and denaturing HPLC. Clin Chem 49:1656–1659

11. Chu MY (2003) Mutational analysis of the RLBP1 and CHM genes in Chinese patients with retinal degeneration. MSc Dissertation. The Hong Kong Polytechnic University, Hong Kong SAR, China

12. Colosimo A, Guida V, De Luca A, Cappabianca MP, Bianco I, Palka G, and Dallapiccola B. (2002) Reliability of DHPLC in mutational screening of beta-globin (HBB) alleles. Hum Mutat 19:287–295

13. Lilleberg SL, Durocher J, Sanders C, Walters K, Culver K (2004) High sensitivity scanning of colorectal tumors and matched plasma DNA for mutations in APC, TP53, K-RAS, and BRAF genes with a novel DHPLC fluorescence detection platform. Ann NY Acad Sci 1022:250–256

14. zur Stadt U, Rischewski J, Schneppenheim R, Kabisch H (2001) Denaturing HPLC for identification of clonal T-cell receptor gamma rearrangements in newly diagnosed acute lymphoblastic leukemia. Clin Chem 47:2003–2011

15. Hoogendoorn B, Owen MJ, Oefner PJ, Williams N, Austin J, O'Donovan MC (1999) Genotyping single nucleotide polymorphisms by primer extension and high performance liquid chromatography. Hum Genet 104:89–93

16. Liang Q, Davis PA, Thompson BH, Simpson JT (2001) High-performance liquid chromatography multiplex detection of two single nucleotide mutations associated with hereditary hemochromatosis. J Chromatogr B Biomed Sci Appl 754: 265–270

17. Devaney JM, Pettit EL, Kaler SG, Vallone PM, Butler JM, Marino MA (2001) Genotyping of two mutations in the HFE gene using single-base extension and high-performance liquid chromatography. Anal Chem 73:620–624

18. Wu G, Hua L, Zhu J, Mo QH, Xu XM (2003) Rapid, accurate genotyping of beta-thalassaemia mutations using a novel multiplex primer extension/denaturing high-performance liquid chromatography assay. Br J Haematol 122:311–316

19. Hoogendoorn B, Norton N, Kirov G, Williams N, Hamshere ML, Spurlock G, Austin J, Stephens MK, Buckland PR, Owen MJ, O'Donovan MC (2000) Cheap, accurate and rapid allele frequency estimation of single nucleotide polymorphisms by primer extension and DHPLC in DNA pools. Hum Genet 107:488–493

20. Lewis CM (2002) Genetic association studies: design, analysis and interpretation. Brief Bioinform 3:146–153

21. Norton N, Williams NM, O'Donovan MC, Owen MJ (2004) DNA pooling as a tool for large-scale association studies in complex traits. Ann Med 36:146–152

22. Hannachi-M'Zali F, Ambler JE, Taylor CF, Hawkey PM (2002) Examination of single and multiple mutations involved in resistance to quinolones in *Staphylococcus aureus* by a combination of PCR and denaturing high-performance liquid chromatography (DHPLC). J Antimicrob Chemother 50:649–655

23. Eaves DJ, Liebana E, Woodward MJ, Piddock LJ (2002) Detection of *gyrA* mutations in quinolone-resistant Salmonella enterica by denaturing high-performance liquid chromatography. J Clin Microbiol 40:4121–4125

24. Randall LP, Coldham NG, Woodward MJ (2005) Detection of mutations in Salmonella enterica gyrA, gyrB, parC and parE genes by denaturing high performance liquid chromatography (DHPLC) using standard HPLC instrumentation. J Antimicrob Chemother 56:619–623

25. Hurtle W, Lindler L, Fan W, Shoemaker D, Henchal E, Norwood D (2003) Detection and identification of ciprofloxacin-resistant Yersinia pestis by denaturing high-performance liquid chromatography. J Clin Microbiol 41:3273–3283

26. Perez-Perez FJ Hanson ND (2002) Detection of plasmid-mediated AmpC beta-lactamase genes in clinical isolates by using multiplex PCR. J Clin Microbiol 40: 2153–2162

27. Shi R, Otomo K, Yamada H, Tatsumi T, Sugawara I (2006) Temperature-mediated heteroduplex analysis for the detection of drug-resistant gene mutations in clinical isolates of Mycobacterium tuberculosis by denaturing HPLC, SURVEYOR nuclease. Microbes Infect 8:128–135

28. Hurtle W, Shoemaker D, Henchal E, Norwood D (2002) Denaturing HPLC for identifying bacteria. Biotechniques 33:386–391

29. Evans JT, Hawkey PM, Smith EG, Boese KA, Warren RE, Hong G (2004) Automated high-throughput mycobacterial interspersed repetitive unit typing of Mycobacterium tuberculosis strains by a combination of PCR and nondenaturing high-performance liquid chromatography. J Clin Microbiol 42:4175–4180

30. Goldenberg O, Herrmann S, Adam T, Marjoram G, Hong G, Gobel UB, Graf B (2005) Use of denaturing high-performance liquid chromatography for rapid detection and identification of seven Candida species. J Clin Microbiol 43:5912–5915

31. Domann E, Hong G, Imirzalioglu C, Turschner S, Kuhle J, Watzel C, Hain T, Hossain H, Chakraborty T (2003) Culture-independent identification of pathogenic bacteria and polymicrobial infections in the genitourinary tract of renal transplant recipients. J Clin Microbiol 41:5500–5510

32. Goldenberg O, Herrmann S, Marjoram G, Noyer-Weidner M, Hong G, Bereswill S, Gobel UB (2007) Molecular monitoring of the intestinal flora by denaturing high performance liquid chromatography. J Microbiol Methods (in press)

33. Barlaan EA, Sugimori M, Furukawa S, Takeuchi K (2005) Profiling and monitoring of microbial populations by denaturing high-performance liquid chromatography. J Microbiol Methods 61:399–412

34. Becker-Andre M, Hahlbrock K (1989) Absolute mRNA quantification using the polymerase chain reaction (PCR). A novel approach by a PCR aided transcript titration assay (PATTY). Nucleic Acids Res 17: 9437–9446

35. Freeman WM, Walker SJ, Vrana KE (1999) Quantitative RT-PCR: pitfalls and potential. Biotechniques 26:112–125

36. Leerkes MR, Caballero OL, Mackay A, Torloni H, O'Hare MJ, Simpson AJ, de Souza SJ (2002) In silico comparison of the transcriptome derived from purified normal breast cells and breast tumor cell lines reveals candidate upregulated genes in breast tumor cells. Genomics 79:257–265

37. Hayward AL, Hinojos CA, Nurowska B, Hewetson A, Sabatini S, Oefner PJ, Doris PA (1999) Altered sodium pump alpha and gamma subunit gene expression in nephron segments from hypertensive rats. J Hypertens 17:1081–1087

38. Hecker KH, Green SM, Kobayashi K (2000) Analysis and purification of nucleic acids by ion-pair reversed-phase high-performance liquid chromatography. J Biochem Biophys Methods 46:83–93

39. Dickman M, Hornby DP (2000) Isolation of single-stranded DNA using denaturing DNA chromatography. Anal Biochem 284:164–167

40. Azarani A, Hecker KH (2001) RNA analysis by ion-pair reversed-phase high performance liquid chromatography. Nucleic Acids Res 29:e7

41. Robertson KD, Wolffe AP (2000) DNA methylation in health and disease. Nat Rev Genet 1:11–19

42. Frommer M, McDonald LE, Millar DS, Collis CM, Watt F, Grigg GW, Molloy PL, Paul CL (1992) A genomic sequencing protocol that yields a positive display of 5-methylcytosine residues in individual DNA strands. Proc Natl Acad Sci USA 89: 1827–1831

43. Southern EM (1975) Detection of specific sequences among DNA fragments separated by gel electrophoresis. J Mol Biol 98:503–517

44. Singer-Sam J, Grant M, LeBon JM, Okuyama K, Chapman V, Monk M, Riggs AD (1990) Use of a HpaII-polymerase chain reaction assay to study DNA methylation in the Pgk-1 CpG island of mouse embryos at the time of X-chromosome inactivation. Mol Cell Biol 10:4987–4989

45. Baumer A (2002) Analysis of the methylation status of imprinted genes based on methylation-specific polymerase chain reaction combined with denaturing high-performance liquid chromatography. Methods 27:139–143

46. El-Maarri O, Herbiniaux U, Walter J, Oldenburg J (2002) A rapid, quantitative, non-radioactive bisulfite-SNuPE-IP RP HPLC assay for methylation analysis at specific CpG sites. Nucleic Acids Res 30:e25

47. Couvert P, Poirier K, Carrie A, Chalas C, Jouannet P, Beldjord C, Bienvenu T, Chelly J, Kerjean A (2003) DHPLC-based method for DNA methylation analysis of differential methylated regions from imprinted genes. Biotechniques 34: 356–362

48. Holland MM, Parsons TJ (1999) Mitochondrial DNA Sequence Analysis: validation and use for forensic casework. Forensic Sci Rev 11:21–50

49. LaBerge GS, Shelton RJ, Danielson PB (2003) Forensic utility of mitochondrial DNA analysis based on denaturing high-performance liquid chromatography. Croat Med J 44:281–288

8

Denaturing Gradient Gel Electrophoresis (DGGE)

Jeroen H. Roelfsema and Dorien J. M. Peters

1. Introduction

Denaturing gradient gel electrophoresis (DGGE) is a robust method for point mutation detection that has been widely used for many years (*1*). It is a polymerase chain reaction (PCR)-based method, the principle being the altered denaturing temperature of a PCR product with a mutation compared to the wild-type product. PCR performed on DNA of an individual with a point mutation in one of two genes will lead to a mixture of different products. PCR products from both the wild-type gene and the mutated gene will be formed. These are known as the homoduplex products. The difference in melting temperature between these two products, however, is subtle. Another type of product, heteroduplexes, consisting of a wild-type strand combined with a mutant strand of DNA, will also be formed during the last cycles of the reaction. The real strength of DGGE lies in the fact that the heteroduplex PCR products will have much lower melting temperatures compared to the homoduplex PCR products, because the heteroduplexes have a mismatch (see **Fig. 8.1**).

To visualize the different melting temperatures of these homoduplexes and heteroduplexes, the products should be run on an acrylamide gel with a gradient of denaturing agents: urea and formamide. These denaturing agents alone are not sufficient. In addition, the gel should be run at a high temperature, usually 60°C. During electrophoresis, the PCR products will run through the gel as double-stranded DNA until they reach the point where they start to denature. Once denatured, the PCR products could continue running through the gel as single-stranded DNA, but the fragments have to remain precisely where they denatured. To achieve this, a so-called GC clamp is attached, to prevent complete denaturing. This GC clamp is a string of 40–60 nucleotides composed only of guanine and cytosine and is attached to one of the PCR primers. PCR with a GC clamp results in a product with one end having a very high denaturing temperature. A PCR product running through a DGGE gel will, therefore, denature partially. The GC clamp remains double stranded. The fragment will form a Y-shaped piece of DNA that will stick firmly at its position on the gel.

From: *Molecular Biomethods Handbook, 2nd Edition.*
Edited by: J. M. Walker and R. Rapley © Humana Press, Totowa, NJ

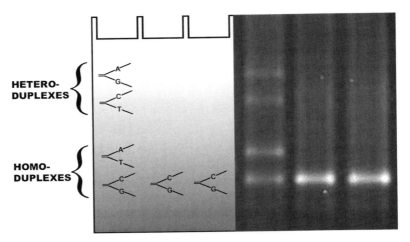

Fig. 8.1. Diagram of a DGGE gel and the actual result. During PCR, two homoduplex and two heteroduplex PCR products will be formed, as shown in the diagram. All four types of product will have different melting temperatures and will, therefore, melt at different positions in a gradient gel. The two heteroduplex products will melt earlier than the two homoduplex products because of their mismatch. On the gel, an example of a mutation resulting in four bands on a DGGE is visible. This is a *de novo* mutation in the gene coding for CREB-binding protein in a patient with Rubinstein–Taybi syndrome. The two adjacent lanes contain the wild-type products from the parents of the patient

2. Practical Steps

2.1. Designing the PCR Products

The melting characteristics of PCR products screened for point mutations are crucial for DGGE. It is important that the fragment, when it reaches the critical point in the gel, denatures immediately, instead of slowly denaturing at one end and progressing with this process as the product runs deeper in the gel. Such a slow-melting process will result in fuzzy bands or smears, rendering mutation detection impossible. Because the melting characteristics are vital for success, primers to amplify the target should be chosen with great care. With this aim, special software that analyzes the melting curves of possible PCR products is used for primer selection. A number of programs are available for various platforms, either commercially (e.g., Winmelt from Bio-Rad Laboratories and Meltingeny from Ingeny International) or for free. There are websites where a sequence can be analyzed online as well. The experimenter will usually see a rather irregular melting curve when analyzing a target sequence. Attachment of a GC clamp of 40–60 nucleotides most often flattens this curve dramatically (see **Fig. 8.2**). The curve should be flat within a range of 1°C. Of course, the melting temperature around the GC clamp is very high. If attaching a GC clamp at one side does not flatten the curve, one should try attaching it to the other side, because for DGGE, it does not matter whether the GC clamp is attached to the forward or to the reverse primer. The selection process involves trying various combinations of forward and reverse primers to find products with a good flat curve and primers that will work well together

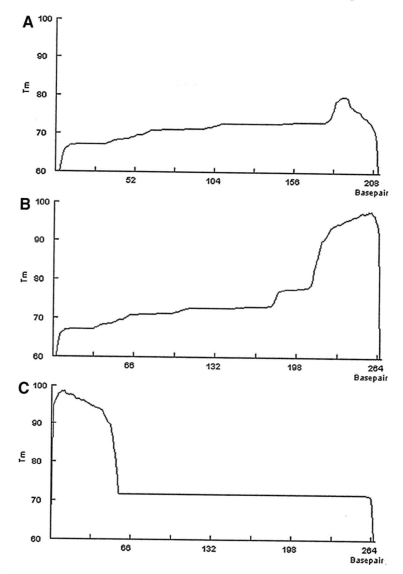

Fig. 8.2. Melt maps made with the program Meltingeny (Ingeny International): **(A)** The melt map of the PCR product without the attachment of a GC clamp. **(B)** The melt map with the GC clamp attached to the right side (cgcccgccgcgcccccgcgcccg-gcccgccgcccccgcccgcgcccccggcccggg). The curve reveals a number of different melt domains. It is unlikely that this product would be successful in DGGE analysis. **(C)** The map with the GC clamp attached at the left side of the product. Now, only two melt domains remain: the high-melt domain of the sequence of the GC clamp and the lower-melt domain of the target sequence. Note that the curve is completely flat. Obviously, the GC clamp at the left side should be chosen

in a PCR. DGGE products typically range from 200 to 400 bp. It is difficult to find the correct melting curve for products longer than 400 bp.

The length of the GC clamp also alters the melting behavior of the entire product. A GC clamp of 55 nucleotides (nt) is routinely used but sometimes 60 nt are necessary, especially with GC-rich sequences. Eventually, most target sequences will produce a good, flat curve in the computer analysis. However, there are troublesome sequences for which one has to use some tricks *(2)*. For instance, if the melting curve of a product goes down at the end without a GC clamp, one can attach a second, smaller GC clamp. This is known as bipolar clamping. Strings of 8–20 nt are used in the rare cases where this is needed. Special attention is also required for GC-rich sequences for which the melting curve does not make a sharp turn where the GC clamp starts, but climbs to a higher melting temperature as it gets closer to the GC clamp. Here, the addition of a few A's and T's between the GC clamp and the annealing part of the primer may cause a sharp turn in the curve.

As mentioned above, a GC clamp consists of 40–60 guanines and cytosines. Using a GC clamp with a sequence that has been proven to work in practice is recommended. Designing your own GC clamp may prove difficult, perhaps resulting in a GC clamp that forms a very stable hairpin structure during PCR. Several melting prediction programs offer a sequence of a GC clamp. Performing a PCR using primers with a GC-clamp does not require special arrangements. The protocol is the same as any other PCR and there are no changes in annealing or denaturing temperatures.

Denaturing gradient gel electrophoresis is a very suitable method for mutation screening on genomic DNA, because the majority of exons are shorter than 400 bp and can be analyzed as one fragment. Methods that can screen larger fragments thus offer little advantage for small exons. Over the years, mutation analysis in many genes has revealed a large number of mutations affecting the consensus splice sites *(3)*. Primers in the intronic sequences flanking the exons are, therefore, selected in such a way that the splice sites are screened as well as the exonic sequence. The remainder of the intron is much less likely to harbor deleterious mutations, but is more likely to contain harmless polymorphisms when compared to coding sequences. Therefore, it is wise not to include too much intronic sequence within the DGGE fragment.

2.2. Visualization of Mutations

To separate the homoduplexes and heteroduplexes, DGGE fragments are run on acrylamide gels. Gels with 9% acrylamide ensure sharp bands and are easy to handle. To pour these gradient gels, two types of stock solution are used: 9% 37.5:1 acrylamide/bisacrylamide in 0.5X TAE and the same stock solution with 7*M* urea and 40% formamide. The former is called 0% denaturant and the latter is called 100% denaturant.

Gradients from 100% to 0% are rarely used because, in such a broad gradient, the denaturing points of the homoduplexes and heteroduplexes would probably be very close to each other; therefore, a range of 30% for the gradients is recommended. To select a urea/formamide gradient, the predicted melting temperature (T_m) of a product as obtained from the computer analysis is used in the empirical formula $T_m \times 3.2 - 182.4 = \%$ denaturant. The melting point is positioned approximately in the center of the gel by simply adding and subtracting 15% from this calculated urea/formamide concentration to obtain the desired 30% gradient. Acrylamide gels with gradients of urea and formamide are poured using a simple gradient mixer that consists of two reservoirs that are connected at the base with a short tube. Such a system is widely used for pouring all types of gradient.

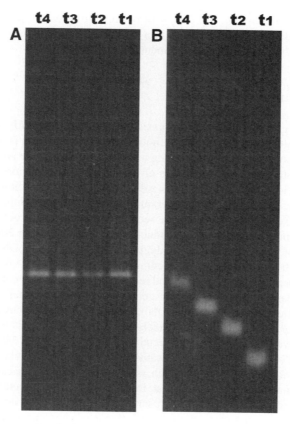

Fig. 8.3. Time travel gels for two different PCR products. In each gel, the same product is loaded at four different time-points. A good result is shown in (**A**). In (**B**), however, the bands do not stay at the same position in the gel. Note the fuzzy bands. This is a clear example of a product that denatures slowly and is, therefore, probably not suitable for DGGE analysis

The first electrophoresis run for a product is on a so-called time-travel gel on which the DGGE products are loaded at 15- to 20-min time intervals in consecutive lanes of the gel. After the electrophoresis run, the denatured products in all lanes should be at the same height in the gel, regardless of what time they were loaded. If this is not the case, then the system probably has to be redesigned (see **Fig. 8.3**). If a product does not result in sharp bands or gets stuck at a position too high or too low in the gel, the gradient used should be adjusted.

Technically, the most challenging problem with DGGE experiments is performing the electrophoresis at 60°C. There are various possible methods to achieve a temperature of 60°C, but usually the glass plates, with the acrylamide gel in between, are submerged in a tank of water that is heated to a constant temperature with the help of a thermostat. There are a number of commercially available systems with total equipment kits suitable for DGGE, in which the lower buffer chamber forms the water bath that is heated. The electrophoresis is usually performed overnight at 90 V in 0.5×TAE buffer, but shorter runs during the day with higher voltages are possible. After electrophoresis, the gels are soaked in a 0.5×TAE solution containing ethidium bromide to visualize the DNA fragments.

3. Applications of DGGE

Denaturing gradient gel electrophoresis is a method to identify small mutations (e.g., point mutations). The definition of a point mutation is the transition or transversion of one nucleotide into another. However, there are more types of small mutation such as deletions or insertions of one or more nucleotides that can be identified by DGGE as well. In fact, these mutations will cause a large difference in melting temperatures in both the homoduplexes and the heteroduplexes and can therefore be seen quite clearly on the gels.

As mentioned earlier, DGGE products typically range from 200 to 400 bp, making DGGE well suited for analyzing exons in genomic DNA, although DGGE can be applied to RNA screening as well. However, RNA is more vulnerable to degradation than DNA and requires conversion into complementary (cDNA). Scanning for mutations in genes involved in hereditary disorders is therefore often done on genomic DNA for both diagnostic purposes and for research. For instance, DGGE is widely applied in the analysis of the various genes involved in hereditary colorectal cancer such as APC, MSH2, MSH6, MLH1, and so forth *(4–6)* Presymptomatic diagnosis is particularly important with a potentially lethal disease such as colorectal cancer that can be treated. Mutation analysis has revealed that in families with colorectal cancer, the mutation is often unique. Obviously, screening a family for an unknown mutation requires a technique, such as DGGE, that is tried and proven, particularly when the stakes are very high. However, for research purposes, reliability is important as well. Investigation into types of mutation requires that the screening will reveal almost all point mutations so that an unbiased analysis of the mutation spectrum can be made.

Duchenne muscular dystrophy is caused by mutations in a huge gene, coding for dystrophin, on chromosome X. Most of these mutations are large deletions or duplications, but approx 30% of the mutations are point mutations somewhere in 1 of the more than 70 exons, or their flanking splice sites *(7)*. To increase the speed of the screening procedure, the PCR products are grouped together, ranging from three to six fragments and run in one lane. Of course, this multiplexing technique is not limited to the large genes. An example is the α-1-antitrypsin gene. The entire gene can be screened using two multiplex amplification reactions. The products of both reactions can be analyzed on the same gel, thus allowing the rapid screening of a large number of individuals *(8)*.

The primary strength of DGGE is its ability to easily detect the heteroduplexes that will be formed if a mutation is present. During the screening for mutations in genes that are involved in dominant hereditary diseases, the heteroduplexes will be formed during PCR. However, is DGGE applicable to recessive hereditary diseases? Cystic fibrosis is one of the most frequently inherited recessive diseases known. Mutation detection performed since the identification of the CFTR gene in 1989 has revealed that a few mutations are frequent, most notably the Δ508 mutation, a deletion of three nucleotides causing an in-frame deletion of amino acid phenylanaline on position 508 *(9)*. Such a frequent mutation is often analyzed by other methods, designed to screen for specific mutations that are known. For the remainder of the mutations that are rare and may never have been identified previously, DGGE is very well suited. The fact that cystic fibrosis is a recessive gene does not hamper screening for the simple reason that DNA obtained from the parents of an affected child will usually be screened. These parents are heterozygote carriers of a mutation. Nevertheless, screening patients can be done without many problems, because rare mutations are seldom found in both genes. However, one has to be aware that homozygosity of rare mutations will be found much more frequently in communities that are isolated by geographical or cultural conditions. Even then, careful analysis of DGGE gels will also reveal the homozygote mutations in the majority of cases. It is, however, possible to mix the DNA that is screened with DNA from unaffected individuals in order to create heteroduplexes. From a technical point of view, there is no difference between a recessive disorder and an X-linked disorder. Again, it is often the heterozygote mothers who are screened.

Point mutation detection is not limited to genetic disorders. It is also applied to tumor samples. Cancer is caused by a series of mutations in genes and these mutations vary from the loss of whole chromosome arms to point mutations. The amount of DNA from a surgically removed tumor may not be great and, depending on the tumor and the DNA isolation method, DNA may be degraded into relatively small fragments. In general, this will not be a problem for DGGE because the PCR fragments are usually small anyway. Another problem is the fact that tumor samples do not solely consist of tumor cells. Blood vessels and connective tissue may be present as well. Especially, malignant invasive tumors may lead to samples with a high percentage of unaffected cells. In our experience, and that of others, DGGE is sensitive enough to find mutations when present. Typical genes that are often screened in this type of research are *TP53* and *K-*, *N-*, and *H-RAS (10,11)*. Mutation detection on the *TP53* gene is often limited to exons 5–8 that are thought to harbor the majority of mutations. However, mutation analysis of the entire gene has shown that this leads to a neglect of many mutations *(12)*. Immunohistochemistry is often used to investigate the *p53* status in tumors. The researcher should be aware that immunohistochemistry cannot replace DGGE and that DGGE cannot replace immunohistochemistry. Both ways of looking at *p53* in tumors are complementary.

An entirely different application for DGGE is to assess the number and types of different bacteria species. The genes encoding for ribosomal RNA are used as a target because these genes are highly conserved among different species. Primers that anneal in the most conserved parts can be used to amplify the genes in completely different species. Sequence variations in the less conserved parts of the fragments can be revealed by DGGE and used to identify different species. This technique was developed first in microbiological ecology to investigate the number of species living in soil or water. The method is now also used to assess species of bacteria living in or on the human body *(13,14)*. One application, for instance, is monitoring patients treated with antibiotics *(15)*.

Point mutation detection is often performed using either single-strand conformation polymorphism (SSCP) analysis or DGGE *(16)*. Both methods have been around for more than a decade and are relatively inexpensive compared to new, state-of-the-art technologies that usually require very expensive equipment. Therefore, when does one decide to use SSCP or to use DGGE? DGGE is a robust method; once optimized for a product, it will work. The results are very easy to score, because a quick glance on an ultraviolet (UV) illuminator will reveal mutations immediately. The clarity of the results is a very strong advantage of DGGE. Another strong advantage is the fact that radioactive labels are not needed. SSCP needs radioactive PCR, or silver staining, and the results are less clear. On the other hand, SSCP takes less time to optimize compared to DGGE and can be done without an investment in expensive material. It is also the number of samples that determines the method of choice. For instance, screening candidate genes with a small number of samples typically calls for SSCP. DGGE is best suited for screening a large number of samples over a longer period.

After finding an aberrant band on a gel, it is only clear that there is a sequence variation present within that specific product from that specific sample. The nature or exact location of the variation is not known. For this, sequencing the PCR product is needed. Why, if sequencing is needed at the end, is mutation screening not performed using sequencing rather than DGGE? The answer is twofold. First, DGGE results are very clear. Mutations present in DGGE products can be seen immediately, whereas sequencing requires either very sophisticated software or very tedious scrutinizing behind the computer. Second, and often the deciding factor, when large numbers of samples have to be screened, DGGE is less expensive.

Primers are selected in the intronic sequences flanking the exons to screen the entire coding region and the flanking splice sites as well. Screening exons from genomic DNA with DGGE products that encompass relatively large pieces of intronic DNA can be cumbersome with some genes because of the large amount of polymorphisms found in the intronic sequences. Screening those genes by DGGE will result in samples showing aberrant bands on a gel of which the majority turns out to be polymorphisms after sequencing. Researchers working on those genes usually resort to direct sequencing of their samples as a method for point mutation detection.

Denaturing gradient gel electrophoresis is the method of choice if one wants to screen a large number of samples for unknown mutations. Because radioactive markers are not needed, it is considered a user-friendly technique. This together with the reliability and the cost-effectiveness are the strong points for DGGE.

Acknowledgment: We thank Stefan White for critically reading the manuscript.

References

1. Sheffield VC, Cox DR, Lerman LS, Meyers RM (1989) Attachment of a 40-base-pair G+C-rich sequence (GC-clamp) to genomic DNA fragments by the polymerase chain reaction results in improved detection of single-base changes. Proc Natl Acad Sci USA 86:232–236
2. Wu Y, Hayes VM, Osinga J, et al (1998) Improvement of fragment and primer selection for mutation detection by denaturing gradient gel electrophoresis. Nucleic Acids Res 26:5432–5440

3. Krawczak M, Reiss J, Cooper DN (1992) The mutational spectrum of single base-pair substitutions in mRNA splice junctions of human genes: causes and consequences Hum Genet 90:41–54

4. van der Luijt RB, Khan PM, Vasen HF, et al (1997) Molecular analysis of the APC gene in 105 Dutch kindreds with familial adenomatous polyposis: 67 germline mutations identified by DGGE, PTT, and southern analysis. Hum Mutat 9:7–16

5. Wagner A, Hendriks Y, Meijers-Heijboer EJ, et al (2001) Atypical HNPCC owing to MSH6 germline mutations: analysis of a large Dutch pedigree. J Med Genet 38:318–322

6. Wijnen J, Vasen H, Khan PM, et al (1995) Seven new mutations in hMSH2, an HNPCC gene, identified by denaturing gradient-gel electrophoresis. Am J Hum Genet 56:1060–1066

7. den Dunnen JT, Grootscholten PM, Bakker E, et al (1989) Topography of the Duchenne muscular dystrophy (DMD) gene: FIGE and cDNA analysis of 194 cases reveals 115 deletions and 13 duplications. Am J Hum Genet 45:835–847

8. Hayes VM (2003) Genetic diversity of the alpha- 1-antitrypsin gene in Africans identified using a novel genotyping assay. Hum Mutat 22:59–66

9. Kerem B, Rommens JM, Buchanan JA, et al (1989) Identification of the cystic fibrosis gene: genetic analysis. Science 245:1073–1080

10. Soussi T Beroud C (2001) Assessing TP53 status in human tumours to evaluate clinical outcome. Nature Rev Cancer 1:233–240

11. Nedergaard T, Guldberg P, Ralfkiaer E, Zeuthen J (1997) A one-step DGGE scanning method for detection of mutations in the K-, N-, and H-ras oncogenes: mutations at codons 12, 13 and 61 are rare in B-cell non-Hodgkin's lymphoma. Int J Cancer 71:364–369

12. Hartmann A, Blaszyk H, McGovern RM, et al (1995) p53 gene mutations inside and outside of exons 5-8: the patterns differ in breast and other cancers. Oncogene 10:681–688

13. Tannock GW (2002) Analysis of the intestinal microflora using molecular methods Eur J Clin Nutr 56 (Suppl. 4):S44–S49

14. Favier CF, Vaughan EE, De Vos WM, and Akkermans AD (2002) Molecular monitoring of succession of bacterial communities in human neonates. Appl Environ Microbiol 68:219–226

15. Donskey CJ, Hujer AM, Das SM, et al (2003) Use of denaturing gradient gel electrophoresis for analysis of the stool microbiota of hospitalized patients. J Microbiol Methods 54:249–256

16. Orita M, Suzuki Y, Sekiya T, Hayashi K (1989) Rapid and sensitive detection of point mutations and DNA polymorphisms using the polymerase chain reaction. Genomics 5:874–879

9

Single Strand Conformation Polymorphism (SSCP) Analysis

Kim Hung Leung and Shea Ping Yip

1. Introduction

Variations in DNA sequences underlie the differences among different members of the same species and also between different species. DNA sequence variations are usually known as polymorphisms if the commonest allele is less than 0.99 in a given population *(1)*. DNA polymorphisms are widespread in many different species, particularly in humans *(2,3)*. Examples include single nucleotide polymorphisms (SNPs), microsatellites, minisatellites, small insertions/ deletions, and large insertions/deletions. DNA polymorphisms may not have any phenotypic effect at the protein level or at the level of the whole organism. On the other hand, they are usually called disease-causing or pathogenic mutations if they cause a change in the phenotype and results in a disease status. The frequencies of individual mutations are usually not high because of selection pressure against such less favorable base changes. It is thus important to study DNA sequence variations in various branches of biological sciences.

1.1. Types of Methods for Detecting Sequence Variations

There are two broad groups of methods for identifying DNA sequence variations: screening (or scanning) methods and diagnostic methods *(4)*. From a technical point of view, sequence variations may or may not be known to exist in a stretch of DNA in a given sample before the search is begun. Screening methods are used to search *unknown* sequence variations; for example, a sample from a patient with a certain genetic disease is screened for disease-causing mutations in the different exons of a putative disease gene. Diagnostic methods are used to determine the genetic make-up (or genotype) of a sample for a *known* sequence variation at a known location; for instance, a pregnant woman is genotyped for her Rh(D) status at the *RHD* locus. Single strand conformation polymorphism (SSCP) analysis of DNA fragments amplified by polymerase chain reaction (PCR) can be used as a screening method, a diagnostic method or both in any single electrophoretic run, depending on the purpose of the experiments and the region of DNA sequences being examined.

From: *Molecular Biomethods Handbook, 2nd Edition.*
Edited by: J. M. Walker and R. Rapley © Humana Press, Totowa, NJ

On the basis of the size of the DNA sequences involved, sequence variations can be of small or large scale. Small-scale sequence variations involve a few basepairs (bp), such as base substitutions and small insertions/deletions. Large-scale sequence variations involve a large stretch of DNA sequences, and are exemplified by large insertions/deletions and gross gene arrangements. There are no definitive cut-offs between small-scale and large-scale sequence variations. However, small-scale and large-scale sequence variations, either known or unknown, do require different methods for detection. Many more

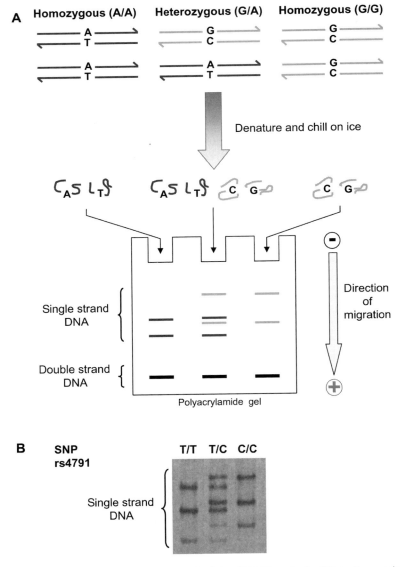

Fig. 9.1. PCR-SSCP analysis. (**A**) The principle of SSCP analysis. (**B**) A silver-stained SSCP banding pattern for a single nucleotide polymorphism (rs4791, T>C). Note that number of single strand bands is 3 for each of *the homozygotes*, and 6 for the heterozygote

methods are available for detecting small-scale than for large-scale sequence variations. SSCP analysis is used to detect small-scale sequence variations.

To detect small-scale sequence variations, it is usual to amplify by PCR the DNA region that is to be screened for unknown base changes or that contains the known base changes to be genotyped. PCR enables the target DNA region to be amplified within a few hours to such a large quantity that detection of the target DNA fragment after electrophoresis can be performed using nonisotopic methods such as silver staining or fluorescence-based protocols. As such, the method described here can be called PCR-SSCP analysis. SSCP analysis was first described in 1989 *(5)*. It is one of the most popular methods for detecting sequence variations, as is evident from the large number of results (>8,300 as of November 2006) from a keyword search in Ovid Medline.

1.2. Principle of SSCP Analysis

DNA molecules have two strands intertwined with each other in antiparallel direction with the base-pairing of A with T and C with G. The two strands are complementary to each other, but not identical. The two strands of a PCR-amplified product can be separated into single strands by heat (**Fig. 9.1A**). Each single strand can coil around itself to form a 3-dimensional structure (or conformation) through intramolecular (or intrastrand) hydrogen bonds. This conformation is dependent on the length of the strand and its base composition. The two complementary strands may form different conformers because they are not identical. If the DNA fragment contains a single base change (e.g., A-T changed to G-C basepairs, **Fig. 9.1A**), there are four different single strands on denaturation, which may form four different conformers. These conformers may have different 3-dimensional sizes and shapes, and hence migrate at different speeds in a polyacrylamide gel. Thus, different samples may give different banding patterns because of the presence of a base change in the amplified DNA region.

2. Methods

2.1. Outline of PCR-SSCP Analysis

PCR is used to amplify a DNA region to be analyzed (**Fig. 9.2**). The PCR products are diluted in a loading solution that contains formamide and indicator dyes (e.g., bromophenol blue and xylene cyanol FF). The diluted PCR products are heated to over 90°C for a few minutes to denature the products into single strands and then cooled immediately in ice water. High concentration of formamide (a chemical denaturant) in the loading solution and immediate cooling are required to keep a sizable proportion of the products in single strands.

The denatured PCR products are then loaded onto a nondenaturing polyacrylamide gel (i.e., without chemical denaturants). Samples diluted in formamide are denser than the buffer and will sink to the bottom of the wells. Separation of the single strands is achieved by electrophoresis. The duration of electrophoresis depends on the gel composition, voltage applied, buffer/gel temperature, and the size and base composition of the PCR products. After electrophoresis, the DNA bands are visualized by silver staining *(6)* or, less commonly, SYBR Green II *(7)*. Though less popular now, PCR products

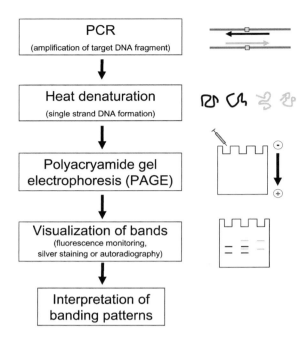

Fig. 9.2. Method outline for SSCP analysis

can also be radioactively labeled and the bands detected by autoradiography. Banding patterns of samples are compared. The presence of different banding patterns among samples indicates that sequence variations exist in the DNA sequence amplified by the two PCR primers. Silver-stained gels can be dried in a gel dryer and the dried gels kept for permanent records if so desired.

2.2. Interpretation of SSCP Results

The interpretation of SSCP results is simple. What one is looking for is a variation in the SSCP banding patterns among different samples. The variation can be a band shift or some additional bands. Depending on such factors as gel composition and electrophoresis temperature, the variation can be very conspicuous in some cases, but subtle in other cases. Subtle changes in banding patterns may be difficult to recognize if the bands are very broad as in the case of sample overloading, which should thus be avoided. Clean and specific PCR products are also a prerequisite for easy interpretation of banding patterns.

Representative samples with distinctive SSCP patterns can then be sequenced to define the underlying sequence variations. In this way, initially unknown sequence variations can be identified and defined. Alternatively, known sequence variations can be correlated with specific banding patterns if SSCP is used as a diagnostic method.

If the DNA samples are from diploid organisms like human beings, then the banding patterns are additive. In other words, if one type of homozygote (e.g., A/A) has a particular pattern and another type of homozygote (e.g., G/G) has another pattern, then the heterozygote (A/G) has a banding pattern that is the summation of these two patterns (**Fig. 9.1A**). However, this additive property is not applicable to the analysis of the X chromosome in human males, DNA from mitochondria or chloroplasts (except in heteroplasmy), and DNA from bacteria (haploid organisms).

It is very often that the two complementary single strands of a duplex DNA molecule do *not* give two SSCP bands (**Fig. 9.1B**). The number of SSCP bands can vary from one to several under a particular condition, and cannot be predicted. This indicates that any single DNA strand can exist in one or more conformers. Sometimes, broad or diffuse bands are seen with or without background smearing *(8)*. This is owing to the occurrence of numerous single strand conformers with similar, but not identical, migration rates.

2.3. Size of PCR Products

The ability of detecting sequence variations in a PCR product decreases with increasing length of the products *(9)*. It is recommended that the size of PCR products be less than 300 bp to increase the chance of picking up sequence variations in the fragments although sequence variations can sometimes be detected in fragments larger than 1,000 bp. The throughput of SSCP analysis can be increased by running in the same lane two or more small products of different sizes *(6,10–12)*, or several small products generated by restriction digestion of a long PCR product *(13,14)*. The gel must of course be large enough for the required separation.

2.4. Gel Composition, Buffer System, and Electrophoresis System

Polyacrylamide gels are defined by two parameters: %T and %C. The %T refers to the total amount in grams of acrylamide and N,N'-methylene-*bis*-acrylamide (a common crosslinker, usually abbreviated as *bis*) in 100 mL solution. The %C refers to the proportion of the total monomers (acrylamide plus *bis*) that is the crosslinker (*bis*). The %C can also be expressed in another format as the ratio of acrylamide to *bis*; for example, 2%C is equivalent to an acrylamide:*bis* ratio of 49:1. The probability of detecting sequence variations in a PCR product is higher if the %C is lower *(9)*. Low levels of crosslinking produce large pores in the gels, and thus allow efficient separation of bulky single strand conformers. We use a nondenaturing gel of 10%T/1%C as a starting point in conjunction with a conventional vertical electrophoresis system (e.g., SE600 from Hoefer) and a medium-sized gel (e.g., 16 × 14 cm). Large-sized gels of 5%T and 1–2%C are also commonly used together with conventional electrophoresis systems for manual sequencing *(9,15)*. Another commercially available gel matrix called Mutation Detection Enhancement (MDE) Gel is also widely used for SSCP analysis *(7,16)*. It is a polyacrylamide-like matrix and is claimed to be very sensitive to DNA conformational changes.

The buffer most commonly used in SSCP analysis is Tris-borate-EDTA buffer with an alkaline pH. However, low pH buffer (e.g., Tris-MES-EDTA, pH 6.3) can still maintain very high sensitivity of detecting sequence variations for PCR fragments up to 800 bp in length *(15)*.

Glycerol at 5–10% (v/v) can be incorporated in gels prepared in Tris-borate-EDTA buffer to enhance the sensitivity of detecting sequence variations. It is because of the reduction of buffer pH by the reaction between glycerol and borate ions *(15)*. Gels used in SSCP analysis are usually nondenaturing so that stable single strand conformers can be maintained. However, denaturants like formamide, urea and sodium dodecyl sulfate can selectively be added to the gels to change the conformation of single strands *(8,17,18)*. The denaturant will disrupt the intramolecular hydrogen bonds, alter the single strand conformers and hence change their mobility. Depending on base composition and sequence context, this can sometimes enhance resolution and clear up smearing background.

Temperature is one of the most critical factors affecting the conformation of single strand DNA fragments and hence the sensitivity of SSCP analysis *(9)*. A heat exchanger or cooling unit that is immersed in the buffer and connected to an external thermostatically controlled circulator can efficiently and actively control the temperature of the gel and the buffer at the desired level and hence ensure reproducible banding patterns *(6,10–12)*. Other methods of maintaining any desired temperature in the electrophoresis system can also be used as long as reproducible thermal profiles can be maintained from run to run. It is not unusual that sequence variations are detected at a particular temperature, but not at another temperature.

Thin precast gels are commercially available in several gel sizes and are to be used in conjunction with dedicated flatbed electrophoresis systems (PhastSystem and GenePhor DNA Separation System from GE Healthcare) with built-in or separate components for automated silver staining *(19,20)*. Precast gels (about 12 cm wide) for GenePhor System are about twice the size of those for PhastSystem, and thus have twice the separation distance and resolving power in addition to higher sample throughput. These flatbed electrophoresis systems have very efficient built-in temperature control units and produce highly reproducible banding patterns for SSCP analysis. The advantage of highly reproducible patterns may probably outweigh the disadvantages of higher cost incurred and limited choice of gel composition from the manufacturer, particularly in the setting of in vitro diagnostics.

2.5. SSCP Analysis Using an Automated Electrophoresis System

SSCP analysis can be performed in an automated electrophoresis system, typically an automated DNA sequencer, which monitors the mobility of the fluorescently labeled DNA fragments during electrophoresis. PCR products can be fluorescently labeled in a number of ways. Target DNA regions can be amplified by forward and reverse primers labeled with the same single fluorescent dye *(21)* or two dyes of different colors *(22)*. Post-PCR labeling can also be done easily and is more cost-effective because unlabeled primers are used *(23–25)*. Internal labeling of PCR products is another option *(26)*. The automated DNA sequencer can be gel-based *(21–23,24,26)* or, more commonly now, capillary-based *(23,25,27,28)*. Throughput can be increased by analysis in the same lane or capillary of multiple PCR fragments labeled with multiple colors *(28)*. Mobility of DNA fragments can be standardized by inclusion in the test sample of an internal mobility standard that contains DNA fragments of known size and labeled with a color different from those of the fragments being analyzed. Electrophoresis can be performed at ambient temperature or above because most automated DNA sequencers are equipped with a built-in heating device, but not a cooling unit.

One exciting development is microchip electrophoresis, i.e., performance of electrophoresis in microchannels *(29)*. Microchip SSCP analysis can be finished within a few minutes, and thus greatly reduces the analysis times by more than 100-fold when compared with conventional methods. This may revolutionize molecular genetic testing in diagnostic laboratories in the future.

3. Applications

SSCP analysis can be used to screen for unknown sequence variations, to genotype known sequence variations, or to detect both known and unknown variations. Applications of SSCP analysis are centered on these themes.

3.1. Screening for Unknown Mutations in Human Genetic Disorders

SSCP analysis is widely used to screen or detect disease-causing mutations in hereditary disorders. A keyword search in PubMed can tell its popularity in this application. This method is simple and economical, and does not require any special equipment. Any laboratory with a basic electrophoresis system can use this method without any difficulty. However, this method does not indicate the position of the sequence variation once a variant banding pattern is found. The identity and position of the sequence variation have to be determined by DNA sequencing. In addition, SSCP analysis cannot tell whether the sequence variation is disease-causing or not – a feature shared by most mutation screening methods.

In this application, one critical issue is the sensitivity of SSCP analysis – the probability of detecting mutations, usually unknown, in samples from patients with a particular genetic disease under study. It is well known that the sensitivity never reaches 100% if SSCP analysis is performed under a single condition. Therefore, it is important to note that a negative result under a single condition does not automatically signify the absence of mutations in the PCR fragment being analyzed. It is generally expected that the sensitivity is over 90% for most fragments less than 200 bp, and probably over 80% for fragments about 300–350 bp in size (*9*). It is generally accepted that the sensitivity can reach 100% if a few sets of conditions are used (*4,9,12,30–32*). The following four conditions are used in our laboratories for screening unknown mutations: 10%T/1%C gels with or without 5% glycerol incorporated in the gel, and electrophoresis using SE600 system (from GE Healthcare) at 20°C and at 4°C (in cold room) (*12*).

There are modifications to the standard SSCP method to increase the sensitivity of mutation detection. Dideoxy fingerprinting (ddF) is a hybrid method combining dideoxy terminator sequencing and SSCP, and has been shown to be 100% sensitive (*33*). A dideoxy chain terminator sequencing reaction is performed with a single primer on PCR-amplified template in the presence of normal deoxynucleotide triphosphates (dNTPs) and a *single* dideoxynucleotide triphosphate (ddNTP; say, ddCTP for the purpose of illustration) (instead of four ddNTPs as in conventional dideoxy sequencing). Here, a series of ddCTP-terminated single-stranded products are produced and then separated in a large nondenaturing gel as in SSCP analysis (**Fig. 9.3**). An additional ddCTP-terminated fragment is produced if a C base replaces another base. On the contrary, a ddCTP-terminated fragment is missing if a C base is replaced by another base. Thus, the relative position of a base change (involving a C base in this example) can be deduced from the extra or missing ddCTP-terminated

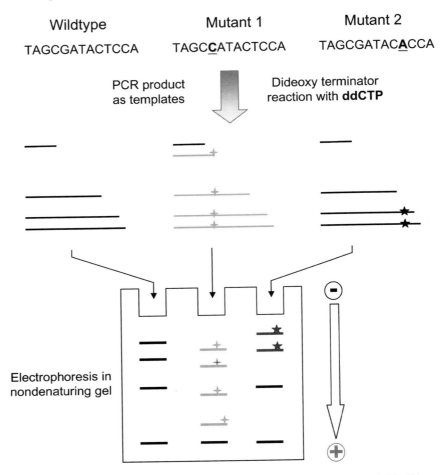

Fig. 9.3. The principle of dideoxy fingerprinting (ddF). Note that mutant 1 (G>C base change) has both an informative dideoxy component and an informative SSCP component whereas mutant 2 (T>A base change) has only an informative SSCP component. See texts for details

fragment. This part is known as the informative dideoxy component of the ddF method. In addition, a series of ddCTP-terminated single strands of different lengths are produced and hence carry a mutation in different sequence contexts. Thus, a series of single strands may show altered mobility, which in turn increases the sensitivity of the method. This part is known as the informative SSCP component of the ddF method. Mutations in larger PCR fragments of up to 600 bp can be detected with 100% sensitivity if two primers are used to perform a bi-directional chain termination reaction and hence the fragment is interrogated from two opposing ends *(34)*. This modification is known as di-directional ddF. These methods are further improved via automation by separating the fluorescently labeled single strands in an automated DNA sequencer *(35,36)*.

SSCP analysis and heteroduplex analysis (HA) are two separate methods for screening mutations, but can be combined and performed in the same

Heterozygous (G/A)

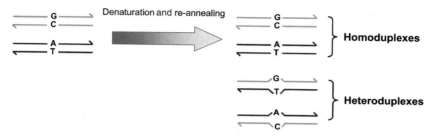

Fig. 9.4. The formation of both homoduplexes and heteroduplexes from a heterozygous DNA sample

lanes on a single gel or in the same capillary. When a DNA fragment carrying a heterozygous mutation is denatured and then cooled to allow reannealing of the strands, four types of duplex molecules are formed (**Fig. 9.4**). Half of the duplex molecules are identical to the original input duplex molecules without any mismatch (homoduplexes), and half are hybrid duplex molecules with a mismatch between the two strands at the mutation site (heteroduplexes). Heteroduplexes may have a kink or a mismatch bubble, and thus migrate through a gel with greater difficulty and hence more slowly than homoduplexes *(37)*. This is the principle underlying HA. Although SSCP analysis relies on single strand conformers and HA depends on homoduplexs and heteroduplexes, both methods can use similar electrophoresis system and gels. Both methods each do not achieve 100% sensitivity of mutation detection under a single condition, but can be combined to give 100% sensitivity *(38–40)*.

3.2. Genotyping Known Mutations and Polymorphisms in Humans

Once mutations and polymorphisms are well characterized, they can be genotyped regularly for many samples by SSCP analysis. This is best exemplified by well-known mutations underlying thalassemia *(11)* and hereditary hemochromatosis *(41)*, and polymorphisms underlying apolipoprotein E *(42)*, cytochrome P450 enzymes *(43)* and ABO blood group system *(6)*. Samples carrying known mutations or polymorphisms are used to optimize SSCP conditions so that all known sequence variations can be distinguished from each other reliably by their distinctive banding patterns. The following parameters can be varied to achieve this purpose: gel composition, electrophoresis temperature and duration, and incorporation of additives like glycerol in the gel. One modification known as snapback SSCP analysis can be used to enhance the detection of known mutations *(44)*. This requires the use of a special primer with additional bases that are attached to the 5' end of the sequence-specific portion of the primer, and that can introduce a conformational change into the single strand carrying, say, the mutation.

One advantage of SSCP analysis is that it may detect new sequence variations within the amplified fragment when known mutations or polymorphisms are being genotyped *(6,41,45)*. If there are several sequence variations simultaneously found on the same PCR fragment, specific combinations of the alleles at these several sites define the haplotypes. Different haplotypes may form distinct single strand conformers and hence give distinct haplotype-specific banding patterns under appropriate SSCP conditions. Therefore, another advantage of SSCP analysis is that it can determine haplotypes *(6,46,47)*.

3.3. Detection and Differentiation of Microorganisms

Conventionally, bacteria are cultured for detection and identification. Culturing of bacteria is a time-consuming process, particularly for fastidious or slow-growing bacteria. An alternative is to study the genetic variation of bacterial ribosomal genes amplified by PCR. The 16S rRNA gene is highly conserved and is found in all bacteria *(48)*. But it also contains variable regions that can be used to discriminate between bacteria of different genera and species. SSCP analysis of PCR-amplified 16S rRNA sequences can be used advantageously to allow rapid identification of bacteria *(49)* in clinical *(50,51)* or nonclinical *(52,53)* settings. Similar approaches can be applied to the study of rRNA gene sequences by SSCP analysis for the recognition and differentiation of fungi *(54,55)*. Identification and genotyping of viruses can also be achieved by SSCP analysis of appropriate viral sequences *(56–58)*.

Successful treatment of infectious diseases relies on appropriate use of anti-microbial drugs. Excessive use of such drugs results in the increasing occurrence of drug-resistant microbes. Drug-resistant microbes can be identified by SSCP analysis of the genes responsible for the resistance to drugs *(59–61)*.

3.4. Estimation of Relative Allele Frequencies of SNPs in DNA Pools

With the completion of the Human Genome Project, more research effects are focused on the identification of the genes involved in complex diseases. In contrast to single gene disorders, complex diseases are caused by multiple genes, multiple environmental factors and possibly their interactions. Complex diseases are common. Examples include diabetes, hypertension, coronary heart disease, myopia and even infectious diseases. One powerful method to identify such genes is genetic association study. One common approach of genetic association study is to compare the allele frequencies of single nucleotide polymorphisms between two groups of subjects, one group with the disease under study (the cases) and another group without the disease (the controls) *(62)*. This approach is also known as case-control study. In practice, genotypes have to be determined for a large number of samples (at least several hundred and preferably over a thousand) and for many SNPs from many potential candidate genes that may be involved in the complex disease under study. If the allele frequencies of a particular SNP are different between the cases and the controls, then it is said to be associated with the disease. This is the first step towards identifying a causative SNP and hence a causative gene underlying a complex disease, but only very few SNPs may turn out to be associated with the disease.

One way to cut the cost and to increase the speed of screening a large number of SNPs is by means of a DNA pooling approach *(63)*. In the simplest form, all case DNA samples are mixed in equal amounts to construct a *case pool*, and all control DNA samples also mixed in equal amounts to give a *control pool*. Then, the relative allele frequencies of the two alleles of a SNP are estimated by a quantitative genotyping method, and compared between the two DNA pools. If the two pools are found to differ significantly in the relative allele frequencies, the positive result can be confirmed by genotyping all case and control samples *individually*. In this process, a good quantitative genotyping method is important. Capillary-based SSCP analysis of fluorescently labeled PCR products can precisely estimate the allele frequencies of pooled DNA samples *(64)*. Appropriate software for this purpose is also available *(65,66)*.

3.5. Other Applications

SSCP analysis is most widely used to detect sequence variations in humans and microorganisms as discussed above. In fact, it can be applied to detect sequence variations in *any* living organism, be it an animal like roundworm *(67)*, mosquito *(68)*, lizard *(69)* and even panda *(70)*, or a plant like grape *(71)*, apple *(72)*, and wheat *(73)*. SSCP analysis is also very popular in studies of population genetics and phylogenetics *(67,74)*.

In summary, SSCP analysis is a simple and rapid method for detecting both known and unknown sequence variations in nucleic acids from any living organism. Many modifications are available to make it more sensitive and to adapt it to a variety of applications.

References

1. Harris H (1980) *Human Biochemical Genetics*, 3rd revised ed., Elsevier/North-Holland Biomedical Press, Amsterdam, The Netherlands
2. Sachidanandam R, Weissman D, Schmidt SC et al (2001) A map of human genome sequence variation containing 1.42 million single nucleotide polymorphisms. Nature 409:928–933
3. Redon R, Ishikawa S, Fitch KR et al (2006) Global variation in copy number in the human genome. Nature 444:444–454
4. Cotton RGH (1997) Mutation detection. Oxford University Press, Oxford
5. Orita M, Iwahana H, Kanazawa H, Hayashi K, Sekiya T (1989) Detection of polymorphisms of human DNA by gel electrophoresis as single-strand conformation polymorphisms. Proc Natl Acad Sci USA 86:2766–2770
6. Yip SP (2000) Single-tube multiplex PCR-SSCP analysis distinguishes seven common ABO alleles and readily identifies new alleles. Blood 95:1487–1492
7. Emanuel JR, Damico C, Ahn S, Bautista D, Costa J (1996) Highly sensitive nonradioactive single-strand conformational polymorphism. Detection of Ki-ras mutations. Diagn Mol Pathol 5:260–264
8. Yip SP, Hopkinson DA, Whitehouse DB (1999) Improvement of SSCP analysis by use of denaturants. BioTechniques 27:20–24
9. Hayashi K, Yandell DW (1993) How sensitive is PCR-SSCP? Hum Mutat 2: 338–346
10. Yip SP, Lovegrove JU, Rana NA, Hopkinson DA, Whitehouse DB (1999) Mapping recombination hotspots in human phosphoglucomutase (PGM1). Hum Mol Genet 8:1699–1706
11. Yip SP, Fung LF, Lo ST (2004) Rapid detection of common southeast Asian beta-thalassemia mutations by nonisotopic multiplex PCR-SSCP analysis. Genet Test 8: 104–108
12. Lim KP (2005) Mutational analysis of RHO, RDS and PRPF31 genes in Chinese patients with retinitis pigmentosa. MPhil thesis, The Hong Kong Polytechnic University, Hong Kong SAR, China
13. Liu Q, Sommer SS (1995) Restriction endonuclease fingerprinting (REF): a sensitive method for screening mutations in long, contiguous segments of DNA. Biotechniques 18:470–477

14. Kringen P, Egedal S, Pedersen JC, Harbitz TB, Tveit KM, Berg K, Borresen-Dale AL, Andersen TI (2002) BRCA1 mutation screening using restriction endonuclease fingerprinting-single-strand conformation polymorphism in an automated capillary electrophoresis system. Electrophoresis 23:4085–4091

15. Kukita Y, Tahira T, Sommer SS, Hayashi K (1997) SSCP analysis of long DNA fragments in low pH gel. Hum Mutat 10:400–407

16. Vidal-Puig A, Moller DE (1994) Comparative sensitivity of alternative single-strand conformation polymorphism (SSCP) methods. Biotechniques 17:490–496

17. Paccoud B, Bourguignon J, Diarra-Mehrpour M, Martin JP, Sesboüé R (1998) Transverse formamide gradients as a simple and easy way to optimize DNA singlestrand conformation polymorphism analysis. Nucleic Acids Res 26:2245–2246

18. Blancé H, Valette C, Bellanné-Chantelot C (1997) Optimization of non isotopic PCR-single-strand conformation polymorphism analysis. Clin Chem 43:2190–2192

19. Mohabeer AJ, Hiti AL, Martin WJ (1991) Non-radioactive single strand conformation polymorphism (SSCP) using the Pharmacia "Phast system." Nucleic Acids Res 19:3154

20. Campos B, Diez O, Cortes J, Domenech M, Pericay C, Alonso C, Baiget M (2001) Conditions for single-strand conformation polymorphism (SSCP) analysis of BRCA1 gene using an automated electrophoresis unit. Clin Chem Lab Med 39:401–404

21. Makino R, Yazyu H, Kishimoto Y, Sekiya T, Hayashi K (1992) F-SSCP: fluorescence-based polymerase chain reaction-single-strand conformation polymorphism (PCR-SSCP) analysis. PCR Methods Appl 2:10–13

22. Iwahana H, Yoshimoto K, Mizusawa N, Kudo E, Itakura M (1994) Multiple fluorescence-based PCR-SSCP analysis. BioTechniques 16:296–305

23. Inazuka M, Tahira T, Hayashi K (1996) One-tube post-PCR fluorescent labeling of DNA fragments. Genome Res 6:551–557

24. Iwahana H, Adzuma K, Takahashi Y, Katashima R, Yoshimoto K, Itakura M (1995) Multiple fluorescence-based PCR-SSCP analysis with postlabeling. PCR Methods Appl 4:275–282

25. Inazuka M, Wenz HM, Sakabe M, Tahira T, Hayashi K (1997) A streamlined mutation detection system: multicolor post-PCR fluorescence labeling and single-strand conformational polymorphism analysis by capillary electrophoresis. Genome Res 7:1094–1103

26. Iwahana H, Fujimura M, Takahashi Y, Iwabuchi T, Yoshimoto K, Itakura M (1996) Multiple fluorescence-based PCR-SSCP analysis using internal fluorescent labeling of PCR products. Biotechniques 21:510–519

27. Baba S, Kukita Y, Higasa K, Tahira T, Hayashi K (2003) Single-stranded conformational polymorphism analysis using automated capillary array electrophoresis apparatuses. Biotechniques 34:746–750

28. Doi K, Doi H, Noiri E, Nakao A, Fujita T, Tokunaga K (2004) High-throughput single nucleotide polymorphism typing by fluorescent single-strand conformation polymorphism analysis with capillary electrophoresis. Electrophoresis 25:833–838

29. Tian H, Jaquins-Gerstl A, Munro N, Trucco M, Brody LC, Landers JP (2000) Single-strand conformation polymorphism analysis by capillary and microchip electrophoresis: a fast, simple method for detection of common mutations in BRCA1 and BRCA2. Genomics 63:25–34

30. Leren TP, Solberg K, Rodningen OK, Ose L, Tonstad S, Berg K (1993) Evaluation of running conditions for SSCP analysis: application of SSCP for detection of point mutations in the LDL receptor gene. PCR Methods Appl 3:159–162

31. Larsen LA, Christiansen M, Vuust J, Andersen PS (1999) High-throughput single-strand conformation polymorphism analysis by automated capillary electrophoresis: robust multiplex analysis and pattern-based identification of allelic variants. Hum Mutat 13:318–327

32. Liu Q, Feng J, Buzin C, Wen C, Nozari G, Mengos A, Nguyen V, Liu J, Crawford L, Fujimura FK, Sommer SS (1999) Detection of virtually all mutations-SSCP (DOVAM-S): a rapid method for mutation scanning with virtually 100% sensitivity. Biotechniques 26:932–942

33. Sarkar G, Yoon HS, Sommer SS (1992) Dideoxy fingerprinting (ddE): a rapid and efficient screen for the presence of mutations. Genomics 13:441–443

34. Liu Q, Feng J, Sommer SS (1996) Bi-directional dideoxy fingerprinting (Bi-ddF): a rapid method for quantitative detection of mutations in genomic regions of 300–600 bp. Hum Mol Genet 5:107–114

35. Ellison J, Squires G, Crutchfield C, Goldman D (1994) Detection of mutations and polymorphisms using fluorescence-based dideoxy fingerprinting (F-ddF). Biotechniques 17:742–753

36. Shevchenko YO, Bale SJ, Compton JG (2000) Mutation screening using automated bidirectional dideoxy fingerprinting. Biotechniques 28:134–138

37. Keen J, Lester D, Inglehearn C, Curtis A, Bhattacharya S (1991) Rapid detection of single base mismatches as heteroduplexes on Hydrolink gels. Trends Genet 7:5

38. Ravnik-Glavac M, Glavac D, Dean M (1994) Sensitivity of single-strand conformation polymorphism and heteroduplex method for mutation detection in the cystic fibrosis gene. Hum Mol Genet 3:801–807

39. Axton RA, Hanson IM, Love J, Seawright A, Prosser J, van Heyningen V (1997) Combined SSCP/heteroduplex analysis in the screening for PAX6 mutations. Mol Cell Probes 11:287–292

40. Kozlowski P, Krzyzosiak WJ (2001) Combined SSCP/duplex analysis by capillary electrophoresis for more efficient mutation detection. Nucleic Acids Res 29:e71

41. Simonsen K, Dissing J, Rudbeck L, Schwartz M (1999) Rapid and simple determination of hereditary haemochromatosis mutations by multiplex PCR-SSCP: detection of a new polymorphic mutation. Ann Hum Genet 63:193–197

42. Tsai MY, Suess P, Schwichtenberg K, Eckfeldt JH, Yuan J, Tuchman M, Hunninghake D (1993) Determination of apolipoprotein E genotypes by single-strand conformational polymorphism. Clin Chem 39:2121–2124

43. Daly AK, King BP, Leathart JB (2006) Genotyping for cytochrome P450 polymorphisms. Methods Mol Biol 320:193–207

44. Wilton SD, Honeyman K, Fletcher S, Laing NG (1998) Snapback SSCP analysis: engineered conformation changes for the rapid typing of known mutations. Hum Mutat 11:252–258

45. Quaranta S, Chevalier D, Bourgarel-Rey V et al (2006) Identification by single-strand conformational polymorphism analysis of known and new mutations of the CYP3A5 gene in a French population. Toxicol Lett 164:177–184

46. Kamio K, Matsushita I, Tanaka G, Ohashi J, Hijikata M, Nakata K, Tokunaga K, Azuma A, Kudoh S, Keicho N (2004) Direct determination of MUC5B promoter haplotypes based on the method of single-strand conformation polymorphism and their statistical estimation. Genomics 84:613–622

47. Beheshti I, Hanson NQ, Copeland KR, Garg U, Tsai MY (1995) Single-strand conformational polymorphisms (SSCP): studies of the genetic polymorphisms of exon 4 of apolipoprotein C III. Clin Biochem 28:303–307

48. Clarridge JE III (2004) Impact of 16S rRNA gene sequence analysis for identification of bacteria on clinical microbiology and infectious diseases. Clin Microbiol Rev 17:840–862

49. Widjojoatmodjo MN, Fluit AC, Verhoef J (1994) Rapid identification of bacteria by PCR-single-strand conformation polymorphism. J Clin Microbiol 32:3002–3007

50. Turenne CY, Witwicki E, Hoban DJ, Karlowsky JA, Kabani AM (2000) Rapid identification of bacteria from positive blood cultures by fluorescence-based PCR-single-strand conformation polymorphism analysis of the 16S rRNA gene. J Clin Microbiol 38:513–520

51. Gillman LM, Gunton J, Turenne CY, Wolfe J, Kabani AM (2001) Identification of Mycobacterium species by multiple-fluorescence PCR-single-strand conformation polymorphism analysis of the 16S rRNA gene. J Clin Microbiol 39:3085–3091

52. Schwieger F, Tebbe CC (1998) A new approach to utilize PCR-single-strand-conformation polymorphism for 16S rRNA gene-based microbial community analysis. Appl Environ Microbiol 64:4870–4876

53. King S, McCord BR, Riefler RG (2005) Capillary electrophoresis single-strand conformation polymorphism analysis for monitoring soil bacteria. J Microbiol Methods 60:83–92

54. Walsh TJ, Francesconi A, Kasai M, Chanock SJ (1995) PCR and single-strand conformational polymorphism for recognition of medically important opportunistic fungi. J Clin Microbiol 33:3216–3220

55. Kumar M, Shukla PK (2006) Single-stranded conformation polymorphism of large subunit of ribosomal RNA is best suited to diagnosing fungal infections and differentiating fungi at species level. Diagn Microbiol Infect Dis 56:45–51

56. Soares CC, Volotao EM, Albuquerque MC, Nozawa CM, Linhares RE, Volokhov D, Chizhikov V, Lu X, Erdman D, Santos N (2004) Genotyping of enteric adenoviruses by using single-stranded conformation polymorphism analysis and heteroduplex mobility assay. J Clin Microbiol 42:1723–1726

57. Golijow CD, Perez LO, Smith JS, Abba MC (2005) Human papillomavirus DNA detection and typing in male urine samples from a high-risk population from Argentina. J Virol Methods 124:217–220

58. Mackiewicz V, Roque-Afonso AM, Marchadier E, Nicand E, Fki-Berrajah L, Dussaix E (2005) Rapid investigation of hepatitis A virus outbreak by single strand conformation polymorphism analysis. J Med Virol 76:271–278

59. Telenti A, Honore N, Cole ST (1998) Detection of mutations in mycobacteria by PCR-SSCP (single-strand conformation polymorphism). Methods Mol Biol 101:423–430

60. Kim BJ, Lee KH, Yun YJ, Park EM, Park YG, Bai GH, Cha CY, Kook YH (2004) Simultaneous identification of rifampin-resistant Mycobacterium tuberculosis and nontuberculous mycobacteria by polymerase chain reaction-single strand conformation polymorphism and sequence analysis of the RNA polymerase gene (rpoB). J Microbiol Methods 58:111–118

61. Beckmann L, Muller M, Luber P, Schrader C, Bartelt E, Klein G (2004) Analysis of gyrA mutations in quinolone-resistant and -susceptible Campylobacter jejuni isolates from retail poultry and human clinical isolates by non-radioactive single-strand conformation polymorphism analysis and DNA sequencing. J Appl Microbiol 96:1040–1047

62. Cordell HJ, Clayton DG (2005) Genetic association studies. Lancet 366:1121–1131

63. Norton N, Williams NM, O'Donovan MC, Owen MJ (2004) DNA pooling as a tool for large-scale association studies in complex traits. Ann Med 36:146–152

64. Sasaki T, Tahira T, Suzuki A, Higasa K, Kukita Y, Baba S, Hayashi K (2001) Precise estimation of allele frequencies of single-nucleotide polymorphisms by a quantitative SSCP analysis of pooled DNA. Am J Hum Genet 68:214–218

65. Higasa K, Kukita Y, Baba S, Hayashi K (2202) Software for machine-independent quantitative interpretation of SSCP in capillary array electrophoresis (QUISCA). Biotechniques 33:1342–1348

66. Tahira T, Okazaki Y, Miura K, Yoshinaga A, Masumoto K, Higasa K, Kukita Y, Hayashi K (2006) QSNPlite, a software system for quantitative analysis of SNPs based on capillary array SSCP analysis. Electrophoresis 27:3869–3878

67. Gasser RB, Chilton NB (2001) Applications of single-strand conformation polymorphism (SSCP) to taxonomy, diagnosis, population genetics and molecular evolution of parasitic nematodes. Vet Parasitol 101:201–213

68. Bosio CF, Harrington LC, Jones JW, Sithiprasasna R, Norris DE, Scott TW (2005) Genetic structure of Aedes aegypti populations in Thailand using mitochondrial DNA. Am J Trop Med Hyg 72:434–442

69. Godinho R, Domingues V, Crespo EG, Ferrand N (2006) Extensive intraspecific polymorphism detected by SSCP at the nuclear C-mos gene in the endemic Iberian lizard Lacerta schreiberi. Mol Ecol 15:731–738

70. Wan QH, Zhu L, Wu H, Fang SG (2006) Major histocompatibility complex class II variation in the giant panda (*Ailuropoda melanoleuca*). Mol Ecol 15:2441–2450

71. Di Gaspero G, Cipriani G (2003) Nucleotide binding site/leucine-rich repeats, Pto-like and receptor-like kinases related to disease resistance in grapevine. Mol Genet Genomics 269:612–623

72. Baldi P, Patocchi A, Zini E, Toller C, Velasco R, Komjanc M (2004) Cloning and linkage mapping of resistance gene homologues in apple. Theor Appl Genet 109: 231–239

73. Ohsako T, Wang GZ, Miyashita NT (1996) Polymerase chain reaction-single strand conformational polymorphism analysis of intra- and interspecific variations in organellar DNA regions of Aegilops mutica and related species. Genes Genet Syst 71:281–292

74. Sunnucks P, Wilson AC, Beheregaray LB, Zenger K, French J, Taylor AC (2000) SSCP is not so difficult: the application and utility of single-stranded conformation polymorphism in evolutionary biology and molecular ecology. Mol Ecol 9: 1699–1710

10

Randomly Amplified Polymorphic DNA (RAPD)

A Useful Tool for Genomic Characterization of Different Organisms

Lúcia Maria da Cunha Galvão and Eliane Lages-Silva

1. Introduction

Genetic variability or molecular biodiversity, besides being important for evolution, can be used as instrument of inquiry in diverse areas, for example, to verify the affinities and the limits between species, to detect forms of reproduction and familiar structure, to evaluate levels of migration and dispersion in populations and for the identification of species threatened with extinction. The basic data for these studies are the called molecular markers, which are genetic loci that present some variability, different rates of substitution/evolution between individuals, populations or species.

In the past decade, several techniques have been developed for identifying and typing prokaryotic and eukaryotic organisms at the DNA level, which differ in their taxonomic range, discriminatory power, reproducibility, interpretation, and standardization.

Molecular techniques using polymerase chain reaction (PCR)-based assays for DNA amplification have provided new insights into the systematic and evolutionary trends of different organisms. The most commonly used methods are PCR-hybridization, PCR-size polymorphism, random PCR-restriction fragment length polymorphism, and random amplified polymorphic DNA-PCR.

However, one limitation for the immediate wide scale implantation of PCR technology, for genetic analysis of diverse organisms of interest, was the requirement of prior knowledge of the genome nucleotide sequences of the organisms for the design and synthesis of the primers. To solve this limitation, a PCR-based arbitrarily primed genetic assay called random amplified polymorphic DNA (RAPD), also referred to as arbitrarily primed PCR (AP-PCR) or DNA Amplification Fingerprinting (DAF), was described simultaneously by different authors (1–3) as a rapid and sensitive PCR method that enabled the identification of a large number of independent genetic loci representative of the target genome that are not biased towards particular sequences or types of sequences.

The molecular markers of the RAPD type are now used world-wide for molecular studies, therefore they present Mendelian segregation (1) and can be used as genetic markers.

From: *Molecular Biomethods Handbook, 2nd Edition.*
Edited by: J. M. Walker and R. Rapley © Humana Press, Totowa, NJ

This technique has been developed for genetic mapping, fingerprinting, and is widely used in inter- and intraspecific population polymorphism analyses of different organisms. It has proved to be powerful tool for discriminating different species or subspecies and for genetic analysis of phylogenetic relationships among strains or populations for a variety microorganisms, plants, and mammals (1–4), hence all sorts of organisms are accessible.

The RAPD assay is based on the amplification of genomic DNA with single short primers of arbitrarily chosen sequence, which, because they are shorter and less specific, bind to complementary sequences of both DNA strands at low annealing temperatures, resulting in the amplification of intervening regions. The amplification reaction proceeds in conditions of low stringency, allowing for the occurrence of pairing between the primers and the DNA-target, even though two totally complementary sequences do not occur. As result, a set of amplified fragments are produced, which, when separated by gel electrophoresis, produce a standard of specific bands known as genomic fingerprinting. Complex banding profiles are generated, varying in size and intensity, associated with the genetic sequences of the organism under analysis. In theory, the primer annealing occurs at many regions of the genome simultaneously. However, geometric amplification only occurs in those regions in which the 3' end of the annealed primers face one another on opposite strands and are no more than 3 kilo bases apart. These conditions suggest that the primer annealing sites must be inverted repeats. Moderate and highly repetitive DNA segments in centromeric, telomeric and heterochromatic genomic regions are rich in inverted repeats, as are various classes of dispersed repetitive and mobile elements. RAPD is biased in its amplification of these repetitive regions, but amplifies unique regions as well. This technique essentially scans the genome for these small inverted repeats and amplifies intervening DNA sequences of variable length. The genotypes are evaluated by means of markers; the common bands for all individuals are interpreted as genetic similarities and the noncommon bands, as differences. The results are codified to generate a similarity (or dissimilarity) matrix that can be graphically interpreted by grouping multivariate analysis.

For the PCR reaction to work, the primers must anneal in a manner that they point towards each other and within a reasonable distance of one another. The primers are represented by arrows, where a large fragment of DNA is used as a template in a PCR reaction containing many copies of a single arbitrary primer (see following diagrams available on http://avery.rutgers.edu/WSSP/StudentsScholars/Project/archives/omnions/rapd.html):

RAPD reaction #1

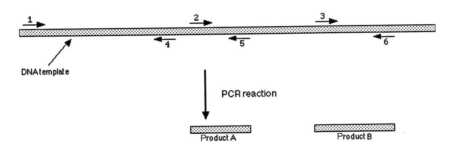

In this scheme the arrows represent multiple copies of a primer, and the direction of the arrow also indicates how the procedure of DNA synthesis occurs. The numbers are the locations on the DNA template where the primers anneal. In this example, only two RAPD PCR products are formed. Product A is generated by PCR amplification of the DNA sequence that lies in between the primers bound at positions 2 and 5. Product B is generated by PCR amplification of the DNA sequence that lies in between the primers bound at positions 3 and 6. No PCR product is formed by the primers bound at positions 1 and 4 because these primers are too far apart to permit completion of the PCR reaction. Note that no PCR products are produced by the primers bound at positions 4 and 2 and positions 5 and 3 because these primer pairs are not oriented towards each other. For eliciting differences among genomes using RAPD analysis consider the previous figure. If another DNA template (genome) was obtained from a different yet related source, some differences in the DNA sequence of the two templates would probably occur. Suppose there was a change in the sequence at primer annealing.

RAPD reaction #2

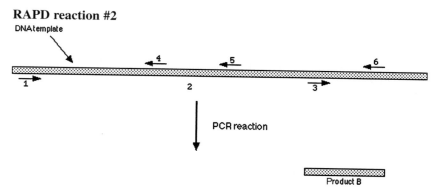

The primer is no longer able to anneal to position 2 and thus the PCR product A is not produced, only product B. If the two RAPD PCR reactions shown in the above diagrams are run on agarose gel they would be visualized as follows:

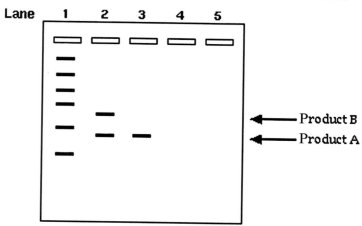

Lane 1: molecular weight markers

Lane 2: RAPD Rxn. #1

Lane 3: RAPD Rxn. #2

In comparison with others polymorphism methods, RAPD offers many advantages like: a combination of simplicity with no radioactivity; amplification of anonymous fragments of the target DNA; the requirements of minimum amounts of target DNA; the acceptance of an unlimited number of primers; no requirements of previous knowledge of the sequences to be amplified and hybridization analysis; a rapid procedure for performing and screening a large number of loci and more loci (and individuals) simultaneously, in a much shorter time than screening for other genetic assays. Therefore, RAPD profiles remain stable and present good reproducibility under rigidly controlled conditions, even when using DNA from different extractions or the same sample under different conditions (5,6) and after prolonged parasite culture up to 100 generations of a *T. cruzi* clone (6).

The RAPD protocol is simple, quick to assay a large number of samples and accessible under minimum molecular laboratory conditions, requiring a moderate investment: a thermocycler, agarose gel or polyacrylamide electrophoresis apparatus, a power supply (with outputs of at least 200 V), an ultraviolet transiluminator (light box), the laboratory set up will have to include taking photographs of agarose and/or acrylamide gels or use a digital image capture system (e.g., a CCD camera, a computer, and image analysis software), and a spectrophotometer or fluorometer for determining DNA concentration.

Different researchers have pointed out that RAPD presents problems of reproducibility, mainly between distinct laboratories, because the profiles might dependent on many variables, such as the sequence of the primer, the concentration and quality of the DNA template, the composition of the buffer and batches of the *Taq* polymerase enzyme used (7,8). An optimization step capable of fulfilling the requirements under laboratory conditions and previous acquaintance of molecular tools are necessary for initiating studies based on the types of markers required for obtaining reliable data.

The main disadvantages are that the sequences of the amplified DNA fragments are unknown, because the primers are not directed against any particular genetic locus and many of the priming events are the result of imperfect hybridization between the primer and the target site. Thus, the determination of homology between species and the possible functions of these loci is problematic owing to the reproducibility of some amplified markers (1,2,8–11).

As RAPD markers are dominant, there is no way to determine whether a single band on the gel corresponds to a homozygous or heterozygous individual. Owing to the fact that primers anneal randomly, there is little guarantee of homology between comigrating bands (12). In parentage analysis, an excess of nonparental bands has been observed (7). Regarding RAPD markers, some bands are easily determined and their interpretation is clear, whereas others are ambiguous as a consequence of the reduced power of a specific primer for discriminating distinct sites of amplification and competition between different sites. Especially because the presence of certain fragments can interfere in the amplification of others fragments, thus influencing the final phenotype bands.

Finally, the use of random primers requires extreme caution to minimize contamination and problems with reproducibility, so although it is a relatively straightforward procedure, it requires meticulous sample processing to avoid contamination with foreign DNA (13).

2. RAPD-PCR Method Optimization

Several points must be taken into account regarding RAPD optimization to maintain the reaction sensitivity conditions and reproducibility of amplified markers. A true representation of the particular organism analyzed is sensitive to a set of variables and slight changes may affect the reaction. Among these variables, the following must be considered: the quality and purity of the DNA template; the quality of all reagents and buffers used; primer size; thermal cycling conditions (especially annealing temperature); the type, activity and concentration of thermostable polymerase (*Taq* DNA polymerase enzyme); magnesium concentration; the number of reaction cycles, and the type of thermocycler. The experimental conditions must be kept constant and all steps must avoid contamination, gloves and goggles must also be worn and the reactions carried out in the most sterile environment available. These limitations can be easily overcome with the careful standardization of techniques and reagents.

On setting up these kinds of experiments for diverse species, assaying under a variety of conditions is recommended, to make the most of the RAPD technique as described below:

2.1. DNA Extraction

The most important factor regarding the reproducibility of RAPD profiles is the suitable preparation of the DNA template with a high level of purity and free from contaminating DNA *(14)*. Different procedures are used for DNA extraction with specific protocol for mammals, plants, fungi, bacteria, protozoan, helminthes, insects, and others. In specific cases, such as insects, contamination can be reduced by hypochlorite treatment before extraction to avoid contact with foreign DNA *(15)*. DNA preparation includes the digestion of samples using different lysis buffers, which contain proteinase K at several concentrations. DNA purification has been performed by the classical phenol-chloroform extraction and ethanol precipitation *(16)*. Further treatment with RNAse and a further round of extraction and precipitation has been recommended *(5,17)*. Negative controls using distilled water instead of a DNA sample can detect possible environmental or reagent contaminants. DNA sample purity and molecular weight must be controlled by agarose gel electrophoresis with 0.4–0.8% ethidium bromide stain. The DNA can be suspended in TE buffer (Tris-HCl and EDTA pH 8.0) or double-distilled water.

PCR reactions using DNA obtained by cell boiling is routine in many laboratories worldwide, seems to be very efficient, simple and may be used in the RAPD technique. The low number of steps required in this procedure is one of the positive aspects, because a higher number of samples can be processed per day, it is not necessary to change tubes during incubation, no hazardous wastes are produced, it is much less expensive, special drugs or equipment are not required, neither is additional RNAse treatment or purification required for reproducible results. This methodology has been used on bacteria, but little information exists concerning the efficiency and sensibility of this protocol using different organisms *(18)*.

2.2. DNA Quantification

Clear RAPDs profiles are obtained when the same DNA concentration is used in each sample and varies from 1 to 25 nanograms per 25 µL reaction according to the organism analyzed (5,9). RAPD amplification is no longer reproducible below a certain genomic DNA concentration and produces "smears" or results in poor resolution if the DNA concentration is high. It is important to consider that DNA amplification in this assay can be inhibited at high DNA concentrations or by the presence of inhibitory compounds (19), it also is advisable to amplify a dilution series of the template using one or two primers. DNA concentration can be determined by comparison with samples of known standards through electrophoresis in agarose gel (0.8–2%) stained with ethidium bromide or by spectrophotometry at 260–280 ηm using 10 µL of DNA template (20).

2.3. RAPD-PCR Reagents

For preparing all reagents and daily premixes, sterile double-distilled water must be used.

2.3.1. Primers

The choice of adequate set primers will determine the degree of reproducibility in genome scanning by RAPD, where only a single oligonucleotide random sequence is used at low stringency conditions and no prior knowledge of the genome submitted to analysis is required. Normally, some sets must be tried and tested individually, to determine which primers in particular differentiate one species from another and those that show reproducible banding patterns should be used for genetic studies on each organism. The primer concentration varies from 1.0 to 25 pmoles for each PCR reaction, according to proposal studies.

The use of random designed primers, each with its own optimal reaction conditions and reagents, also makes standardization of the technique difficult (21). The sequences of the RAPD primers that generate the best DNA pattern for differentiation must be determined empirically. Recently, a consensus M13 DNA sequencing primer was used in RAPD assays for bacteria, which allows for some standardization of the procedure (22). Usually, RAPD markers are detected by the use of random decamer primers (10-mers) with 50–80% GC content are preferred (23). Decamer primers are commercially available in sets of 10 to 20 from several suppliers (e.g., Operon, Genosys).

However, complex banding patterns have also been generated with primers as short as five bases (3,24,25). Few reports exist regarding the use of long primers (over 12 bases), owing to the high probability of random nonreproducible amplification patterns with long primers. Increasing the primer length may also increase its nonspecific annealing; consequently, the genomic target sites should decrease owing to the diminished chances of finding perfect or near perfect homologies (4).

Because oligonucleotides are capable of binding to any complementary DNA, the DNA template must be free from contaminating DNA, otherwise the banding pattern obtained would not be a true representation (14). For a given primer, a difference of only one band when comparing two stocks isolated from the same origin should be considered as an artifact, a mutation or a limited genomic rearrangement. However, the occurrence of artifact bands can be eliminated by checking all patterns and by the correct determination of primer and template concentrations *(26)*.

2.3.2. Taq DNA Polymerase

The quality of the thermostable DNA polymerase enzyme used in the reaction is an important variable to take into account in RAPD assays. Specific polymerases may be required, such as native polymerases or Ultratools, because different thermostable DNA polymerase activities may amplify different RAPD products *(27)*. Some batches of enzymes, although perfectly adequate for the amplification of DNA sequences using specific primers under standard conditions, may induce perfectly reproducible DNA sequences, whereas others fail to produce arbitrarily primed products or produce very limited and irreproducible profiles *(5)*. Each amplification reaction is carried out in a final volume from 10–60 µL (mean 25 µL) containing 0.8–1.0 units of *Taq* DNA polymerase.

2.3.3. PCR-Mix Reagents

The magnesium chloride ($MgCl_2$) concentrations should be optimized for RAPD technique, but may differ for each primer, *Taq* DNA polymerase type, and DNA template species studied. Different $MgCl_2$ concentrations may affect the number and intensity of bands, because low magnesium concentrations produce few RAPD bands. The optimal concentration for a particular application should be empirically determined. The standard value varies from 1.5 to 2.0 m*M*, however, different concentrations of $MgCl_2$ ranging from 1 to 5 m*M* must be tried. The presence of EDTA in TE buffer (up to 1 m*M*), sometimes used to dissolve genomic DNA, can produce complex magnesium and reduce its effective concentration. In this case, the magnesium concentration in the reaction should be increased to compensate this effect.

For each reaction, 100–200 µ*M* of DNTP, 50 m*M* of KCl, and 10 m*M* Tris-HCl buffer are used. When stored frozen, the DNA should also be thawed out and mixed gently. Assembled reactions are sealed, vortexed, centrifuged and placed in the thermocycler for DNA amplification. Add oil when recommended by the thermocycler manufacturer.

2.4. Thermal Cycling and PCR Amplification Parameters

RAPD is particularly sensitive to thermal cycling parameters and, therefore, strongly depends on the thermocycler used. PCR amplification conditions, such as temperature, time and the number of cycles should be optimized; the use of the same thermocycler is always recommended *(22)*. The standard annealing temperature for RAPD is 35°C; this choice depends on both the size and oligonucleotide sequence of the random primer. Change in the shape of the temperature profile (i.e., temperature ramp) will affect the way the primers anneal to the template DNA. Usually, the amplification program in a thermal cycler operates between 35–45 cycles. A high cycle number frequently leads to the amplification of unspecific bands in the pattern.

Different thermocyclers exhibit different rates of heating and cooling, even when programmed using identical settings. This may even occur within the same model of apparatus. Furthermore, thermocyclers that use Peltier devices for heating and cooling can exhibit decay in the ability to heat and dissipate heat as these unit work. In some units that lack internal temperature probes, a considerable difference in temperature between the block and the sample can occur and such differences can be important for the success of RAPD amplification. Whenever possible, it is advisable to use a thermocouple combined with a chart recorder to confirm temperature variation in the thermocycler unit.

Cycling conditions may be modified depending on the thermocycler used. With average speed thermocyclers (e.g., Perkin-Elmer model 480) use 40–45 cycles of 1 min at 94°C, 1 min at 36°C, 2 min at 72°C, followed by 1 cycle of 7 min at 72°C and 1 at 4°C. With faster thermocyclers (e.g., Perkin-Elmer model 9600) a shorter protocol can be used: 40–45 cycles of 15 s at 94°C, 30 s at 36°C and 1 min at 72°C. An initial denaturation step of 3 min at 94°C and/or a final 7 min extension at 72°C can be added to the amplification protocol, depending on the templates used.

2.5. PCR Controls

DNAs from known amplification profiles of previous gels are used in each PCR run as positive controls, with the aim of ensuring comparison reliability between gels and monitoring the reproducibility of the technique. Negative controls for each PCR reaction containing all components except the template DNA are recommended. Contamination with DNA seen with some brands of *Taq* polymerase may cause the appearance of bands in the "no DNA" controls.

2.6. Electrophoresis Gel

Use electrophoresis gels under standard conditions, typically 5–10 V/cm gel length. Stain gels with ethidium bromide, if not already included in the gel and buffer. Depending on the objective of the experiment, make a note of polymorphisms, segregating bands and the appearance of overall patterns within fingerprint databases. Traditionally, RAPD products are analyzed by electrophoresis at 3–10 V/cm gel length in 1.2–2.0% agarose gels containing ethidium bromide 0.5 μg/mL in both gel and TBE electrophoresis running buffer, are then examined and the gels are photographed under UV light. The electrophoresis should be complete after the bromophenol blue dye has reached three-quarters of the gel length. Alternatively, stain the gel with ethidium bromide after electrophoresis or use other dyes (SYBR-green; Molecular Probes). Normally, the agarose gel concentration used is 1.4%, though the concentration should be adjusted appropriately when analyzing lower molecular weight amplification products. Higher concentrations can also be used routinely (up to 2.5% agarose or up to 3–4% NuSieve® agarose, FMC Bioproducts). However, more information can be obtained when RAPD products are separated in 4.0–6.0% polyacrylamide gels (PAGE) and revealed by staining with 0.2% silver nitrate. Alternatively, high-resolution agarose can be used, which is capable of detecting length differences as short as 6 base pairs. Amplified DNA products should be stored at 4°C until analysis *(28)*.

2.7. Choice and Interference of Genetic Profiles

The ideal conditions having been achieved, it is important to check whether the banding patterns produced are reproducible among different preparations of DNA from the same source. For this purpose, the highest possible number of samples should be analyzed, especially those from different DNA extractions. Although some inconsistencies in products can occur, even in independent amplifications of the same DNA preparation, owing to nonspecific priming or heteroduplex formation, these should not be considered as genetic markers. RAPD amplified fragments can be assumed to be unique, because the procedure does not amplify two distinct fragments that comigrate on gels owing to a similar size; however, this fact is not always true. RAPD markers are usually scored as dominant alleles, the presence or absence of bands produced with a single primer is often assumed to be independent. In some cases, the amplification of certain bands competes to amplify other bands *(29)*. Homology between bands of apparently the same molecular weight from the same primer is another potential problem for RAPD surveys. When this occurs between comigrating bands in different individuals, it is a good assumption that these individuals are from the same population.

2.8. RAPD Data Analysis

The bands or fragments that can be identified with confidence on the basis of their intensity and separation from others products on the gels must be considered for analysis. Individual bands should be converted into binary data matrices, where 0 represent the absence of a fragment and 1 its presence. The analysis is performed by dividing each gel into horizontal regions, each of which lies between two bands of molecular weight marker.

The RAPD Distance Program, version 1.0, for analyzing RAPD bandings is available at ftp://life.anu.edu.au/pub/sofware/RAPDistance or http://life.anu.edu.au/molecular/software/rapd.html.

The genetic differences among stocks or genetic divergence are estimated by Jaccard's phenetic distances and are calculated by the formula $D = 1 - [a/(a + b + c)]$, where a = the number of bands that are common to the two compared genotypes, b = the number of bands present in the second *(30,13)*. Correlation between two sets of similarity indices (Jaccard's distance) may be conducted by the Mantel t test *(31)*.

The relationships between genotypes used to cluster organisms are analyzed by the unweighted pair group method with arithmetic averages (UPGMA) *(32)*.

Phylogenetic relationships among stocks can be visualized by the software package PHYLLIP, version 3.5 *(33)* and phylogenetic trees are drawn with the TREEVIEW program *(34)*. The genetic information is arranged in a matrix of binary data and crossed with the (UPGMA) algorithm to construct phenograms using Jaccard's dissimilarity index to compare each pair of individuals. The support of each node can be tested by bootstrap analysis *(35)*.

RAPD markers used to study the genetic diversity of parasites, for example, different *T. cruzi* populations, can be seen in **Fig. 10.1**. Each arbitrary primer directed the synthesis of several DNA segments simultaneously at different genome points, thus resulting in diverse bands on the gel. RAPD profiles using two different random primers demonstrated that the *T. cruzi* populations isolated from humans (HTC) constitute a distinct genetic group to those isolated from sylvatic reservoirs (STC), which differ completely, and also when compared with *T. rangeli* populations. A high intraspecific similarity between the RAPD profiles of these populations was observed, associated with parasite origin HTC and STC generated by each primer.

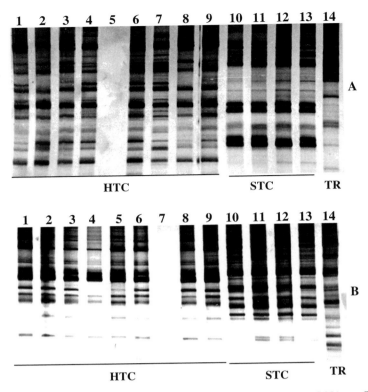

Fig. 10.1. A silver-stained 5% polyacrylamide gel showing RAPD-DNA profiles of *Trypanosoma cruzi* populations isolated from humans (HTC, lanes1–9), sylvatic reservoirs (STC, lanes 10–13, and lane 14 *Trypanosoma rangeli* (TR, obtained using the primers L15996 (**A**) and M13-40F (**B**))

3. Applications of RAPD Analysis

Molecular genetic markers have been developed into powerful tools to analyze genetic relationships and genetic diversity. The discovery that PCR random primers can be used to amplify a set of randomly distributed loci in any genome facilitated the development of genetic markers for a variety of purposes *(1,3)*. The ease and simplicity of the RAPD technique has stimulated the interest of many scientists in many fields, such as agriculture, biology, medicine and others. As already discussed, its success may be owing to the gain of a large number of genetic markers that require small amounts of DNA, without requiring cloning, sequencing or any other form of molecular characterization of the genome of the species under study and permits direct comparison of the effects on genotypes at the DNA level, hence, all sorts of organisms are accessible *(1,3,13)*.

RAPD analysis has been successfully used in genetic mapping and fingerprinting applications. Certainly, one of the most widely used applications of this method is the identification of markers linked to traits of interest, without the necessity for mapping the complete genome *(36)*. In genetic mapping, only the RAPD amplification products in coupling with the segregating trait are informative, i.e., amplification products from the parent that carries the dominant form of the gene being mapped. In these situations a suitable statistical test to confirm the segregation ratios must be used. For this and other applications, errors can result from incorrect allele assignment owing to small differences in band mobility. It is advisable to verify that homologous bands are in fact allelic *(37)*. In fingerprinting applications, the RAPD assay is not an appropriate technique when the difference (localized or dispersed) between the two genomes being compared is limited to an extremely small genomic fraction, in this case the use of more powerful techniques for analysis is recommended.

However, RAPD can efficiently identify differences that constitute a significant fraction of a genome, but tend to underestimate genetic distances between distantly related individuals, for example in interspecific comparisons. Therefore, be cautious when using RAPD for taxonomic studies above the species level.

Besides the features already described, the RAPD fragment can be excised, eluted from gel, cloned and partially sequenced. The sequence characterized amplified regions (SCARs) are PCR-based markers that represent a specific locus. The sequence of these primers is derived from a band identified as a RAPD marker linked to a gene of interest that contains a primer decamer used for RAPD at end 5' and an internal region immediately adjacent, at end 3'. These markers can be applied in the development of hybridization probes and PCR primers and can also be used as physical reference points on the genome and mapping proposal or genetic markers, which could be used in a wide variety of species. SCARs present higher reproducibility than RAPD markers and can be more advantageous in commercial breeding programs, if a quick plus/minus assay can be developed to detect the presence or absence of the product *(38)*.

The RAPD technique continues to spread through the scientific community, in the last few years it has became an important tool used in genetic diversity and variability studies of several species of plants and for improvements in vegetable breeding. The ability of the RAPD technique to reveal intraspecific variation can be used in screening for the degree of inbreeding in commercial plant and animal species to prevent further increase in the frequency of deleterious recessive alleles in certain populations *(36)*. Many studies have reported success in using RAPD assays to distinguish bacterial strains among diverse species and it has been successfully used to identify markers linked to disease resistance genes in different vegetables *(29)*.

RAPDs have shown potential for the identification of inter and intraspecific somatic hybrids in the potato and the potential identification of true nuclear hybrids from parental types at an early stage following fusion, would represent an excellent predictive tool for somatic cell genetics *(39)*. A fast and efficient method based on the amplification of random sequences from genomic DNA *(1)* to isolate DNA segments linked to certain traits and applied to a pair of tomato near-isogenic lines (NILs), succeeded in identifying three additional markers that are linked to a gene conferring resistance to the pathogen *Pseudomonas syringae* pv. tomato. Therefore, markers that show polymorphisms between these lines are probably linked to the gene of interest *(40)*. The main limitation of NILs is the availability of a pair of NILs and the long generation time for many species *(36)*. RAPD technique can be used in molecular ecology to determine taxonomic identity, to assess kinship relationships, to analyze mixed genome samples and to create specific probes *(41)*.

The RAPD method has emerged as an effective genetic marker for the analysis of parasite population variability (20), to investigate the nature of the six double-drug-resistance *T. cruzi* clones (42). Differences among the strains, their genetic diversity or variability, can be easily revealed by RAPD analysis, which has been successfully used in regard to a wide range of protozoan and metazoan parasites. Some genetic diversity has been reported for *Taenia solium* (43). This genetic variability has relevant epidemiological implications, such as the development of the parasite, its pathogenicity and drug susceptibility. The variation in populations of *Echinococcus granulosus* has contributed to the identification of different strains and helped elucidate transmission patterns (44). Up to now, many studies have been conducted with the aim of finding correlations among clinical variations of a disease and the diversity of infectious agent populations. Metronidazole resistance in *Trichomonas vaginalis*, suggested the existence of genetic markers associated with clinical features (45). Although findings of the genetic polymorphism of isolates of this parasite using RAPD technique showed a correlation with the presence of mycoplasma and its susceptibility to metronidazole, no correlation between genetic polymorphism and virulence, geographic origin and the severity of infections by *T. vaginalis* was found (46). Recently, a specific 490 base pairs marker was found be specific for symptomatic isolates, but not asymptomatic isolates; this is the first description of a possible virulence marker for *T. vaginalis* (47). RAPD also confirmed the evidence of multiple infections by different genotypes in the same patient, despite low genetic variability among *Trypanosoma brucei gambiense* stocks (28).

In relation to *T. cruzi*, RAPD has been useful at obtaining highly variable DNA markers, establishing genetic relations among the isolates and for differentiating *T. cruzi* and *T. rangeli* (5,13,19,48–52). RAPD profiling was also used to corroborate the *T. cruzi* taxon division in two major lineages (49,51–53). A complex and strain-specific banding revealed by RAPD for different *T. cruzi* populations was not related to the clinical aspects of the disease. *T. cruzi* isolates showed distinct grouping in tree topology, however no correlation between the isolates and the clinical forms of Chagas' disease was established (54).

Regarding the advantages and disadvantages of the method here described, it would pertinent to emphasize its ability for analyzing a large number of samples and the fact that an unlimited number of different primers can be used. The problems that have been reported can be solved by following suitable protocols for optimization and by confirming reproducibility. However, the best choice of the molecular method that can be used for a particular study will depend upon relevant features that will contribute to the selection, interpretation of the results, the level of ability of the researchers and resources of the laboratory in question.

References

1. Williams JG, Kubelik AR, Livak KJ, Rafalsky JA, Tingey SV (1990) DNA polymorphisms amplified by arbitrary primers are useful genetic markers. Nucleic Acids Res 18:6531–6535
2. Caetano-Anolles G, Bassam BJ, Gresshoff PM (1991) DNA amplification fingerprinting using very short arbitrary oligonucleotide primers. Bio/Technology 9: 553–557
3. Welsh J, McClelland M (1990) Fingerprinting genomes using PCR with arbitrary primers. Nucleic Acids Res 18:7213–7218

4. Rafalski JA, Tingey SV, William JGK (1991) RAPD markers – a new technology for genetic mapping and plant breeding. AgBiotech News Inform 3:645–648

5. Steindel M, Dias-Neto E, Menezes CLP, Romanha AJ, Simpson AJG (1993) Random amplified polymorphic DNA analysis of *Trypanosoma cruzi* strains. Mol Biochem Parasitol 60:71–80

6. Zingales B, Pereira MES, Almeida KA, Umezawa ES, Nehme NS, Oliveira RP, Macedo A, Souto RP (1997) Biological parameters and molecular markers of clone CL Brener – the reference organism of the *Trypanosoma cruzi* genome project. Mem Inst Oswaldo Cruz 92:811–814

7. Riedy MF, Hamilton III WJ, Aquadro CF (1992) Excess of non-parental bands in offspring from known primate pedigrees assayed using RAPD PCR. Nucleic Acids Res 20:918

8. Ellsworth DL, Rittenhouse KD, Honeycut RL (1993) Artifactual variation in randomly amplified polymorphic DNA banding patterns. BioTechniques 14: 214–217

9. Parar I, Kesseli R, Michelmore R (1991) Identification of restriction fragment length polymorphism and random amplified polymorphic DNA markers linked to downy mildew resistance genes in lettuce, using near-isogeniclines. Genome 34: 1021–1027

10. Macedo AM, Melo MN, Gomes R, Pena SDJ (1992) DNA fingerprints: a tool for identification and determination of the relationships between species and strains of *Leishmania*. Mol Biochem Parasitol 53:63–70

11. Theodorakis CW, Bickham JW (2004) Molecular characterization of contaminant-indicativ e RAPE markers. Ecotoxicology 13:303–309

12. Black WC 4TH (1993) PCR with arbitrary primers: approach with care. Insect Mol Biol 2:1–6

13. Tibayrenc M, Neubauer K, Barnabé C, Guerrini F, Skarecky D, Ayala FJ (1993) Genetic characterization of six parasitic protozoa: parity between random-primer DNA typing and multilocus enzyme electrophoresis. Proc *Natl* Acad Sci USA 90: 1335–1339

14. Singh B (1997) Molecular methods for diagnosis and epidemiological studies of parasitic infections. Int J Parasitol 27:1135–1145

15. Jaramilo C, Montana MF, Castro LR, Vallejo GA, Guhl F (2001) Differentiation and genetic analysis of *Rhodnius prolixus* and *Rhodnius colombiensis* by rDNA and RAPD amplification. Mem Inst Oswaldo Cruz 96:1043–1048

16. Sambrook J, Fritsch EF, Maniatis T (1989) Molecular cloning: a laboratory manual. Cold Spring Harbor Laboratory, Cold Spring Harbor, New York.

17. Macedo AM, Martins MS, Chiari E, Pena SDJ (1992) DNA fingerprinting of *Trypanosoma cruzi*: a new tool for characterization of strains and clones. Mol Biochem Parasitol 55:147–154

18. Araújo WL, Angelis DA, Azevedo JL (2004) Direct RAPD evaluation of bacteria without conventional DNA extraction. Braz Arch Biol Technol 47:375–380

19. Dias-Neto E, Steindel M, Passos LK, Souza CP, Rollinson D, Katz N, Romanha AJ, Pena SD, Simpson AJ (1993) The usse of RAPDs for the study of the genetic diversity of *Schistosoma mansoni* and *Trypanosoma cruzi*. EXS 67:339–345

20. Bosseno MF, Barnabé C, Magallón-Gastélum E, Kasten FL, Ramsey J, Espinoza B, Brenière SF (2002) Predominance of *Trypanosoma cruzi* lineage I in Mexico. J Clin Microbiol 40:627–632

21. Meunier JR, Grimont PAD (1993) Factors affecting reproducibility of random amplified polymorphic DNA fingerprinting. Res Microbiol 144:373–379

22. Olive DM, Bean P (1999) Principles and applications of methods for DNA-based typing of microbial organisms. J Clin Microbiol 37:1661–1669

23. Lodhi MA, Weeden NF, Reisch BI (1997) Characterization of RAPD markers in *Vitis*. Vitis 36:133–140

24. Masumi Y, Hiromi A, Michiharu N, Akira N (2002) PCR-based molecular markers in Asiatic hybrid lily. Sci Horticult 1831:1–10

25. Welsh J, McClelland M (1991) Genomic fingerprinting using arbitrarily primed PCR and a matrix of pairwise combinations of primers. Nucleic Acids Res 19: 5275–5279

26. Muralidharan K, Wakeland EK (1993) Concentration of primer and template qualitatively affects products in random-amplified polymorphic DNA PCR. BioTechniques 14:362–364

27. Schierwater B, Ender A (1993) Different thermostable DNA polymerases may amplify different RAPD products. Nucleic Acids Res 21:4647–4648

28. Oury B, Jamonneau V, Tibayrenc M, Truc P (2004) Characterization of *Trypanosoma brucei gambiense* isolated from humans by RAPD fingerprinting in Côte d'Ivoire: another evidence for multiple infections. J Biotechnol 3:94–98

29. Paran I, Kesseli R, Michelmore R (1991) Identification of restriction-fragment-length-polymorphism and random amplified polymorphic DNA markers linked to downy mildew resistance genes in lettuce, using near isogenic lines. Genome 34: 1021–1027

30. Jaccard P (1908) Nouvelles recherches sur la distribution florale. Bull Soc Vaudoise Sci Nat 44:223–270

31. Mantel N (1967) The detection of disease clustering and a generalized regression approach. Cancer Res 27:209–220

32. Barnabe C, Brisse S, Tibayrenc M (2003) Phylogenetic diversity of bat trypanosomes of subgenus *Schizotrypanum* based on multilocus enzyme eletrophoresis, random amplified polymorphic DNA, and cytochrome *b* nucleotide sequence analyses. Infect Genet Evol 2:201–208

33. Felsenstein J (1993) Phylogeny interference package (PHYLIP). 3.5c. Seattle: distributed by the author. Department of Genetics, University of Washington

34. Page RDM (1996) TREEVIEW: an application to display phylogenetic trees on personal computers. Comput Appl Biosci 12:357,358

35. Felsenstein J (1985) Confidence limitson phylogenies: an approach utilizing the bootstrap. Evolution 39: 783–791

36. Bardakci F. (2001) Random amplified polymorphic DNA (RAPD) markers. Turk J Biol 25: 185–196

37. Williams JG, Hanafey MK, Rafalski JA, Tingey SV (1993) Genetic analysis using random amplified polymorphic DNA markers. Methods Enzymol 218: 704–740

38. Paran I, Michelmore RW (1993) Development of reliable PCR-based markers linked to downy mildew resistance genes in lettuce. Theor Appl Genet 85:985–993

39. Baird E, Cooper-Bland S, Waugh R, DeMaine M, Powell W (1992) Molecular characterization of inter- and intra-specific somatic hybrids of potato using randomly amplified polymorphic DNA (RAPD) markers. Mol Gen Genet 233: 469–475

40. Martin GB, Williams JGK, Tanksley SD (1991) Rapid identification of markers linked to a Pseudomonas resistance gene in tomato by using random primers and near-isogenic lines. Proc Natl Acad Sci USA 88:2336–2340

41. Hadrys H, Balick M, Schierwater B (1992) Applications of random amplified polymorphic DNA (RAPD) in molecular ecology. Mol Ecol 1:55–63

42. Gaunt MW, Yeo M, Frame IA, Stothard JR, Carrasco HJ, Taylor MC, Mena SS, Veazey P, Miles GAJ, Acosta N, Arias AR, Miles MA (2003) Mechanism of genetic exchange in American trypanosomes. Nature 421:936–939

43. Maravilla P, Souza V, Valera A, Romerp-Valdovinos M, Lopex-Vidal Y, Dominguez-Alpizar JL, Ambrosio J, Kawa S, Flisser A (2003) Detection of genetic variation in *Taenia solium*. J Parasitol 89:1250–1254

44. Campbell G, Garcia HH, Nakao M, Ito A, Craig PS (2006) Genetic variation in *Taenia solium*. Parasitol Int 55:S121–S126

45. Snipes LJ, Gamard PM, Narcisi EM, Beard CB, Lehmann T, Secor WE (2000) Molecular epidemiology of metronidazole resistance in a population of *Trichomonas vaginalis* clinical isolates. J Clin Microbiol 38:3004–3009

46. Hampl J, Vanacova S, Kulda J, Flegr J (2001) Concordance between genetic relatedness and phenotypic similarities of *Trichomonas vaginalis*. BMC Evol Biol 48: 1–11

47. Rojas L, Fraga J, Sariego I (2004) Genetic variability between *Trichomonas vaginalis* isolates and correlation with clinical presentation. Infect Genet Evol 4: 53–58

48. Steindel M, Dias-Neto E, Pinto CJ, Grisard E, Menezes CLP, Murta SMF, Simpson AJG, Romanha AJ (1994) Random amplified polymorphic DNA (RAPD) and isoenzyme analysis of *Trypanosoma rangeli* strains. J Euk Microbiol 41:261–267

49. Souto RP, Fernandes O, Macedo AM, Campbell D, Zingales B (1996) DNA markers define two major phylogenetic lineages of *Trypanosoma cruzi*. Mol Biochem Parasitol 83:141–152

50. Fernandes CD, Murta SMF, Cerávolo IP, Krug LP, Vidigal PG, Steindel M, Nardi N, Romanha AJ (1997) Characterization of *Trypanosoma cruzi* isolated from chronic chagasic patients, triatomines and opossums naturally infected from state of Rio Grande do Sul, Brazil. Mem Inst Oswaldo Cruz 92:343–351

51. Brisse S, Barnabé C, Tibayrenc M (2000) Identification of six *Trypanosoma cruzi* phylogenetic lineages by random amplified polymorphic DNA and multilocus enzyme electrophoresis. Int J Parasitol 30:35–44

52. Murta SMF, Gazzinelli RT, Brener Z, Romanha AJ (1998) Molecular characterization of susceptible and naturally resistant strains of *Trypanosoma cruzi* to benznidazole and nifurtimox. Mol Biochem Parasitol 93:203–214

53. Tibayrenc M (1995) Population genetics of parasitic protozoa and other microorganisms. Adv Parasitol 36:48–115

54. D'Ávila DA, Gontijo ED, Lages-Silva E, Meira WSF, Chiari E, Galvão LMC (2006) Random amplified polymorphic DNA profiles of *Trypanosoma cruzi* isolates from chagasic patients with different clinical forms. Parasitol Res 98: 455–461

11

Quantification of mRNA Using Real Time RT-PCR

The SYBR Solution

David Sugden and Patricia de Winter

1. Introduction

Commonly used methods to quantify RNA and DNA include Northern and Southern blotting, RNase protection assays and in situ hybridization. Although these methods are direct in that they analyze nonamplified RNA or DNA, they are of low sensitivity and require relatively large amounts of nucleic acid. Another method, thousands of times more sensitive than these traditional techniques, combines reverse transcription (RT) and the polymerase chain reaction (PCR). Although RT-PCR is an exquisitely sensitive and specific technique, obtaining quantitative data presents a difficult challenge *(1–4)*.

The goal of all quantitative PCR methods is to determine the initial number of molecules of a given target DNA from the amount of product generated during PCR. A major obstacle to achieving this goal is the exponential nature of PCR itself. Under ideal conditions, when the reaction efficiency is 100% (i.e., $E = 1$), the amount of product generated increases exponentially, doubling with each cycle of PCR. In practice, the efficiency of amplification may be considerably less than this and can vary substantially. Reaction efficiency depends on many factors, including the primer sequences, the length of the amplicon and its GC content, and sample impurities *(5)*. These factors affect primer binding, the melting point of the target sequence and the processivity of the *Taq* polymerase. Importantly, amplification of exactly the same sequence in replicate tubes using the same PCR block can give substantial variations in efficiency values (e.g., $E = 0.8$–0.99) even when a master mix of reaction components is used *(6)*. This occurs because of small sample-to-sample differences in cycling conditions, perhaps in different regions of the block (e.g., center versus edge), which lead to small variations in reaction efficiency. Because of the exponential nature of PCR, this results in substantial differences in product yield as the reaction progresses. A difference in efficiency of as little as 5% between two samples with the same initial copy number can result in one sample having twice as much product after 26 cycles of PCR *(7)*.

A further difficulty in obtaining quantitative data is that the relationship between the number of molecules of a target present in a sample at the start and

From: *Molecular Biomethods Handbook, 2nd Edition.*
Edited by: J. M. Walker and R. Rapley © Humana Press, Totowa, NJ

at the end of the PCR reaction is linear *only* during the exponential phase of PCR. During PCR product accumulates exponentially initially, but then slows typically reaching a plateau. Various factors may contribute to this plateau effect, including the accumulation of polymerase inhibitors, the loss of *Taq* activity, and increasing reassociation of the sense and antisense strands of the amplicon (at the expense of primer binding) as the target product accumulates. Despite these difficulties, quantitative PCR methods have been devised that use equipment and techniques common to most molecular biology laboratories (a PCR block, agarose gel electrophoresis, and densitometry analysis). These methods endeavor to overcome the difficulties of tube-to-tube variation in efficiency and the limitations imposed by the need for measurement during the exponential phase of PCR. These "end-point" methods separate the amplicon from other reaction components by agarose gel electrophoresis and quantitate by staining with ethidium bromide (EtBr) *(8)*, incorporate radiolabeled nucleotides or primers followed by autoradiography or phosphoimaging, or use hybridization strategies such as Southern blotting using radiolabeled amplicon-specific probes, to measure the quantity of amplicon synthesized. However, to ensure that measurements are made during the exponential phase it is necessary to sample and analyze the product every cycle or to run multiple serial dilutions of each DNA amplified.

Another approach is competitive RT-PCR, which has the important advantage that products can be analyzed when the PCR process has reached a plateau and not only during the exponential phase *(9)*. In this method, an internal standard that shares the same primer sequences as the target is amplified in the same tube leading to competition for reagents. The internal standard product is designed to have a small difference in size to the target amplicon (or a unique restriction site) allowing the amplicon generated from the internal standard to be distinguished from the target amplicon by agarose gel electrophoresis and enabling both products to be quantified by gel densitometry. A series of PCRs are run with a fixed amount of cell or tissue cDNA and varying concentrations of competitor. A graph of the logarithm of the ratio of target amplicon intensity/competitor amplicon intensity versus concentration of competitor spiked into the reaction is linear. The concentration of target cDNA can be determined from this graph as the logarithm of the ratio of target amplicon intensity/competitor amplicon intensity is zero when the concentration of target and competitor were equal at the start of PCR *(10–12)*.

Competitive RT-PCR is an ingenious and elegant procedure that circumvents some of the substantial problems in making PCR quantitative. However, competitive PCR assays are labor-intensive, unsuited to high throughput requiring post-PCR processing for all reactions, have a limited dynamic range and are expensive to run. These substantial practical problems limit the utility of this technique for quantitating gene expression.

2. Real-Time PCR

Techniques like competitive RT-PCR, rely on "end-point" analysis of amplicon and have been largely superseded in the last few years by the development of real-time PCR instruments that combine rapid amplification with fluorescence detection and quantitation of product. Such instruments allow cycle-by-cycle quantitation of accumulating product in real-time, so that the entire course of the PCR process can be accurately defined, making possible reproducible determination of starting template concentration. Real-time PCR assays have many advantages over "end-point" assays. These include a very large dynamic range (>8 log units), high throughput, and a very high sensitivity, with a typical assay able to measure as little as 10 copies of an amplicon. Furthermore, real-time PCR assays have high precision—interassay and intra-assay coefficients of variation are <10% when measuring only 100 copies. Assays run in a closed tube system and no handling or manipulation of PCR products is required, minimizing the risk of cross-contamination between samples. A large number of fluorescence detection strategies have been developed. These include the use of "nonspecific" DNA-binding dyes such as SYBR Green I that will be the focus of this review, and a variety of probe-based methods that rely on hybridization of a specific fluorescent probe to a sequence unique to the amplicon. These probe-based methods have the potential for multiplex assays to measure two or more products in a single tube, as many real-time PCR instruments have the capability to measure signals generated from multiple fluorophores simultaneously.

The use of real-time PCR to measure levels of expression of specific mRNA requires isolation of RNA, conversion of RNA into cDNA by the enzyme reverse transcriptase (RT) and finally amplification and detection of accumulating products in real-time. The advantages of real-time PCR assays have led many users to give insufficient consideration to some of the steps in the process. Standard operating procedures have not yet been developed for real-time PCR assays, though recent detailed guidelines *(13,14)* represent an important step towards improving quality control of these quantitative assays.

2.1. RNA Extraction and Purification

When extracting RNA, a critical consideration is the quality of the purified RNA. Disruption of cellular material leads to the release of RNases, enzymes that rapidly degrade RNA. Hence a crucial step in minimizing degradation is the inhibition of RNases. This is usually achieved by the inclusion of guanidine isothiocyanate (GITC), a powerful RNase inhibitor, in the homogenization buffer. It is also necessary to use RNase-free consumables, such as tubes and pipet tips, throughout the purification procedure. Cleanliness is paramount; work surfaces and pipets should be wiped with diluted bleach or commercial RNase-inhibiting detergents. For isolation of RNA from tissues we strongly recommend placing tissue in RNA*later*® to stabilize the RNA and limit degradation. There are various means of extracting RNA from cells and tissues, both manual and automated.

Manual extraction by phenol-chloroform remains popular, but is labor-intensive and therefore suitable for only a small number of samples at any one time. Furthermore, phenol is hazardous and several phenol-free commercial kits are now available. The method is based on modifications of the original paper by Chirgwin et al. *(15)* and relies on removal of proteins by a phenol-chloroform mixture and the recovery of RNA in the aqueous phase. Commercial solutions of phenol with GITC are available from several companies. Cells are lysed or tissues are homogenized in this solution, to which chloroform is then added. The homogenate is then centrifuged separating the mixture into a lower, organic phase, containing proteins and an upper, aqueous phase containing RNA.

The white layer visible between the two phases is the interphase, containing DNA. The aqueous phase is removed, RNA is precipitated by the addition of isopropyl alcohol, pelleted by centrifugation, washed with ethanol, and finally dried and resuspended in RNase-free water or buffer.

An alternative technique uses spin-columns containing a silica-based membrane and buffers that allow the selective binding of RNA. Cells are usually lysed in an SDS-based buffer containing GITC, ethanol is added, and the lysate is transferred to a column containing a silica membrane. The column fits into a microfuge tube and samples are then centrifuged; RNA adheres to the membrane and proteins, DNA and other cellular constituents are contained in the flow-through collected in the tube and discarded. The RNA is washed and finally eluted in water.

Spin-column technology has been incorporated into high-throughput procedures in which a silica membrane in a 96-well plate format is used rather than individual columns. The advantage of this format is that it allows for automation. Several robotic liquid handing systems are available that will pipet the required solutions into the wells. The solutions can be passed through the membrane using either suction (the plate is attached to an automated or manually operated vacuum manifold) or by centrifugation. One potential drawback of these systems is that if the cell lysate is too viscous or tissue is not well homogenized, the membrane becomes clogged and both RNA yield and purity may be very low. For very confluent cell monolayers, concentrated cell suspensions or for tissue, a preliminary experiment to optimize the volume of lysis buffer is advisable before proceeding with sample processing.

A variation of spin-column technology uses silica-coated magnetic beads rather than a silica membrane. Beads are incubated with cell or tissue lysate and RNA binds to the silica coating. A robotic system handles all the pipeting and incorporates a strong magnet that allows the beads to be collected and deposited into the various buffers and solutions through the wash steps to elution of the RNA. One advantage is that clogging is not a problem as the system is membrane-free. The disadvantage is that the hardware is more expensive than that for the membrane-based systems described above. Plate-based isolation, either using a vacuum or magnetic bead system, is more convenient when extracting RNA from many cell or tissue samples. Our experience suggests that yields tend to be slightly greater with the magnetic bead system. For extracting RNA from tissues we prefer to use the aqueous phase of the phenol-chloroform method, which is then processed using a magnetic bead system or spin columns. Effective homogenization of tissues ensuring rapid inactivation of RNases is an important step. This can be achieved reliably and extremely effectively using a bead-mill homogenization method (e.g., Qiagen Tissuelyser).

It is also possible to isolate poly(A) containing mRNA directly using magnetic beads coupled to oligo(dT). This procedure is effective and allows elution of mRNA for reverse transcription in a small volume. Though the mRNA obtained in this way may be very suitable for subsequent reverse transcription and quantitative PCR, the amount of mRNA obtained is often so low that it is not easy to check its quantity and quality before downstream analysis.

2.2. RNA Quality and Concentration

The issue of assessing RNA quality has been much debated, but it is generally agreed that one should make all possible efforts to minimize degradation of RNA and to obtain RNA that is free from contamination by DNA and proteins *(14)*. Rapid cell or tissue lysis in a buffer able to inhibit RNases is critical. A greater number of cultured cells or tissue mass does not mean a higher RNA yield *unless* you can ensure that the RNases of all cells are immediately inactivated. Perhaps the commonest method to assess integrity of RNA is to run samples on a formaldehyde-agarose (denaturing) gel containing ethidium bromide and to quantify the ratio of 28S to 18S ribosomal RNA by densitometry. The intensity of the 28S band should be at least twice that of the 18S band. The Agilent Bioanalyser or Biorad Experion are rapid automated capillary electrophoresis systems for analyzing RNA integrity. Both systems return the 28S/18S ratio but the former also computes a RIN (RNA integrity number), using an algorithm that includes the 28S/18S ratio *(16)*. The drawback of both systems is the expense of the hardware and consumables compared with the conventional gel method. Recently Nolan et al. *(14)* reported a method for assessing RNA degradation by priming three regions of GAPDH: the 5' end, the middle and the 3' end and quantifying the relative amounts of each amplicon by multiplex qPCR. Intact RNA should have equal (or at least similar) amounts of each. This assay, termed the 3':5' assay, may be adapted for different RNA targets.

In practice it is not always possible to obtain intact RNA, for example, degradation is very common in samples extracted from formalin-fixed and paraffin-embedded (FFPE) tissue. Similarly, if it is not possible to dissect postmortem tissue immediately, some RNA degradation may well occur owing to the release of RNases. In all cases, it is important to ensure that RNA integrity is similar between all samples to be compared; that is, one should not use intact RNA from a control group and degraded RNA from a treated group. Indeed, very degraded RNA from FFPE samples can be used as long as all the samples exhibit a similar degree of degradation *(17,18)*.

The purity of the RNA is a further quality control consideration. Purity can be determined from the ratio of the sample absorbance at 260 and 280 nm. Pure RNA should have a ratio of around 2. Small volume spectrophotometers like the NanoDrop spectrophotometer are useful, though the 260/280 ratio can be determined in any UV-spectrophotometer. The NanoDrop requires only 1.5 µL of undiluted sample, thereby eliminating dilution errors and preserving the precious RNA sample. It is important to realize that although a low 260/280 ratio may signify protein contamination; an acceptable ratio does not preclude contamination from DNA, which will also be detected at 260 nm. Therefore, routine treatment of all RNA samples with DNase, either during the RNA purification process with an "on-column" digest or by adding a DNase step in the magnetic bead extraction protocol, or after purification is advisable to reduce the likelihood of amplification of products from contaminating genomic DNA. RNA concentration is derived from the absorbance at 260 nm, the length of the light path and the molar extinction coefficient. An absorbance reading of 1 equals 40 ng RNA. An alternative means of measuring RNA quantity is the use of the fluorescent dye RiboGreen, which shows a very large increase in fluorescence when bound to RNA *(19)*. RiboGreen assays are linear over a wide range, suitable for quantitating RNA in large numbers of samples simultaneously on a plate reader and are much more sensitive than measurement of absorbance at 260 nm.

2.3. Reverse Transcription

The polymerase chain reaction relies on a DNA polymerase to amplify the starting template, DNA. Therefore, to quantify gene expression, cell or tissue RNA and must first be converted to a DNA template before amplification can occur. Fortunately, retroviruses contain an enzyme that can do just that—convert RNA to DNA. This is because the retroviral genome is composed of RNA and genome replication depends upon conversion of the viral RNA to DNA inside a host cell. The enzyme used in reverse transcription is a retroviral reverse transcriptase, commonly from the Moloney murine leukaemia virus (MMLV) or the avian myeloblastosis virus (AMV), although some commercial kits now contain modified recombinant enzymes from other sources. Naturally occurring reverse transcriptases also have an RNase H activity, which degrades RNA hybridized to DNA. The enzymes used in the laboratory reaction do not possess the latter function.

To reverse transcribe RNA before PCR, the reverse transcriptase, requires the four deoxynucleotides, dATP, dCTP, dGTP, and dTTP (generically termed dNTPs), the appropriate buffer and salts, and a primer. Three types of primer are commonly used; random primers, oligo (dT) primers, and gene-specific primers. Random primers consist of short strands of deoxynucleotides, usually 6–10 bases long, in random sequences. As their name suggests, these bind randomly to complementary RNA sequences and therefore provide a good representation of the RNA population, including ribosomal RNA. Oligo (dT) primers consist of short strands (usually ~18 bases long) of thymine deoxynucleotides, and target the poly A tail of mRNA. They cannot, therefore, prime cDNA synthesis of ribosomal RNA. Oligo (dT) priming tends to give a biased representation of the 3'-end of mRNAs. If the target amplicon sequence is at the 5'-end of the mRNA this may make it more difficult to quantitate genes that are expressed in low abundance. We routinely use a mixture of random and oligo (dT) primers for reverse transcription to maximize the probability of representing the greater part of the RNA population within a sample. The RT-PCR reaction primed by either or both of these types of primers will produce complementary DNA (cDNA) copies of the different RNA molecules in the sample. Gene-specific primers allow reverse transcription of only the specific genes that the researcher intends to measure by qPCR. Their advantage is that very rare genes within a sample, which might not be well represented by using random or oligo (dT) primers, can be reverse transcribed. A practical disadvantage is that any genes not targeted in the initial RT reaction cannot subsequently be quantified from that sample.

The RT procedure itself usually consists of an RNA denaturation step (heating the RNA sample to 65–70°C in the presence of primer and quickly cooling on ice) followed by addition of the RT enzyme and all other reaction components (dNTPs and enzyme buffer). An RNase inhibitor is often added to protect unstable RNA from RNases. The components are heated to the ideal working temperature for the particular enzyme (37°C or 42°C usually) for 15 min to 1 h. Finally the RT enzyme is inactivated by heating at 95°C. Some RNAs have significant secondary structure and some protocols use higher reaction temperatures to increase reaction efficiency. Before quantitative PCR the reaction is diluted 5- to 100-fold with transfer RNA (tRNA, 10 μg/ml) in nuclease-free water. tRNA is added as a carrier to minimize loss of cDNA onto surfaces; tRNA itself does not generate any PCR products. cDNA is diluted before quantitative PCR as undiluted cDNA added to the PCR reaction may alter the optimum salt and pH conditions resulting in lower reaction efficiency in undiluted cDNA than in diluted cDNA. Undiluted cDNA may even fail to generate any PCR product, whereas a 10-fold dilution of cDNA amplifies with high efficiency. Often it is recommended that the cDNA makes up at most 20% of the qPCR reaction volume. Typically, we dilute cDNA 10-fold then make the cDNA 20% of the volume of the reaction to ensure a low background fluorescence and high efficiency in the amplification step (**Fig. 11.1**). When using a standard (this could be the purified PCR product or a linearized plasmid containing the target gene) it is essential to show that these standards amplify with the same efficiency as the cDNA. After all in the standard reaction tubes, the only template that is likely to be copied is the expected one so this may well be amplified very efficiently, whereas the cDNA will contain many thousands of potential templates, so that misprimed products are much more likely to occur, or even PCR inhibition resulting from inhibitors carried over from the initial RNA isolation. To ensure standards and cDNA amplify with comparable efficiency, the slope of the standard curve can be compared with the slope of a

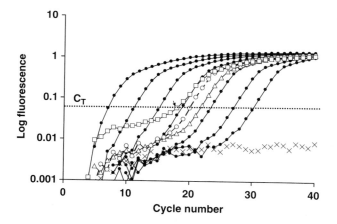

Fig. 11.1. Appropriate dilution of cDNA is required before amplification by real-time quantitative PCR. The figure illustrates the problem that high background fluorescence, because of insufficient dilution of cDNA, may cause. The standards (•) were produced from serial 10-fold dilutions of a 10^8 copies/μL of PCR product amplified from the same source as the samples, purified and then quantified. Fluorescence from the NTC (no template control, X) never exceeds that of the background (below the dotted horizontal line that represents the threshold cycle). A sample (Δ) that was diluted 50-fold following RT gives an amplification curve that is parallel to the standards and a background fluorescence equivalent to that observed in the standards. A sample that was diluted only 5-fold following RT is also shown ($\square$); the background fluorescence in this sample is high and the curve is not parallel with those of the standards. The calculated C_T for this sample (17.6) is represented by the arrow. The dotted line (○) illustrates approximately where the curve should be and its C_T value is 19.6. Thus, a difference of 2 cycles means that the copy number obtained for this sample is ~4-fold greater than its real value simply because of the high background. It is therefore important to ensure that samples are diluted sufficiently before quantitative PCR. This can be checked by making a serial dilution of sample cDNA and comparing it against the amplification plots of the standards

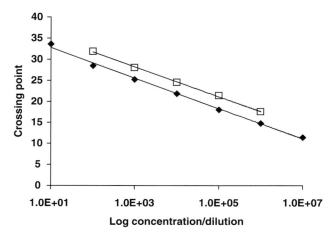

Fig. 11.2. Confirmation that the standards (i.e., a serial dilution of the purified PCR product) and a cDNA sample amplify with very similar efficiency. The experiment ran a dilution series of the standard (♦ 10^7 to 10^1 copies) and a 10-fold dilution series of a pool of cDNAs (□) obtained from 24 rat pineal glands. The amplification efficiency of the standards was 89% whereas the efficiency of cDNA amplification was 92%

dilution series of a cDNA. **Fig. 11.2** shows an example of this; the efficiency of amplification of standards is 89%, whereas cDNA amplifies with a very similar efficiency, 92%. In our experience, as long as cDNA is diluted before PCR, standard and cDNA amplify with very similar efficiencies.

Another important consideration is that reverse transcription efficiency is probably the most variable step in the whole process of quantification of gene expression. Efficiency may vary from sample to sample and for different targets within the same reaction. To minimize such potential variation, reverse transcription should be done on all RNA samples in an experiment at the same time using a common master mix using the same quantity of RNA in all reactions.

3. Real-Time Quantitative PCR

3.1. DNA Binding Dyes – SYBR Green I

SYBR Green I is a minor groove DNA binding dye *(20)*. In solution (i.e., not bound to DNA) its fluorescence is low but on binding to double-stranded DNA, fluorescence increases **(Fig. 11.3)**. Of the detection chemistries available for real-time PCR it is the least expensive, does not require the synthesis of a target specific probe, and can be used with any pair of primers to measure any gene. Many manufacturers now offer quantitative real-time PCR kits using SYBR Green I suitable for use in all of the instruments available. It is generally possible to develop a real-time quantitative assay using primers already optimized in regular block PCR. However, it is preferable to design primers specifically with real-time assays in mind.

Most kits now include a hot-start *Taq* polymerase, rendered inactive at room temperature, either by complexing with an antibody or by chemical modification. The *Taq* enzyme must be activated in a preliminary heating step

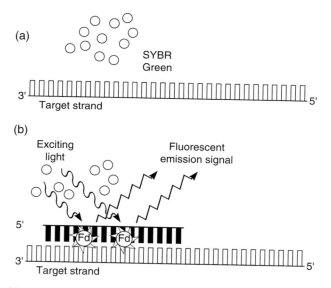

Fig. 11.3. Use of SYBR Green I to detect accumulating amplicons in real-time quantitative PCR. SYBR Green I shows a large increase in fluorescence on binding to the double-stranded amplicon. Fd, fluorescent dye

allowing reaction set-up on the bench. Most kits have an optimized reaction buffer formulation that dispenses with the need to run preliminary reactions to determine the concentration of Mg^{2+} giving the best yield and specificity. As the PCR progresses, greater amounts of SYBR Green I bind to the accumulating double-stranded amplicon, giving an increase in fluorescence that is proportional to the concentration of the product. Fluorescence is measured once each cycle at the end of each extension step. Quantitative real-time assays using SYBR Green I are as sensitive as those using any of the sequence specific fluorescence detection strategies. One potential drawback of using SYBR Green I is that it will detect not only the specific target, but also any nonspecific products that may be amplified or even primer-dimers if they are formed. However, this is not a difficulty in practice if sufficient care is taken in designing specific primers (as it should be in any PCR). In any case, it is possible to verify the identity of the product in all amplified samples by using the melting analysis function available on many real-time instruments. At the end of amplification, the temperature of the instrument is lowered to 5°C above the annealing temperature, allowing all double-stranded products to anneal and SYBR Green I to bind, giving maximum fluorescence. The instrument is then programmed to increase temperature slowly (0.1°C/s) while continuously monitoring the fluorescence signal. If a single product has been generated during PCR, the measured fluorescence will fall dramatically as all of the identical amplicon molecules denature as their melting temperature is reached. The first negative derivative (i.e., the change in fluorescence divided by the change in temperature, −dF/dT) is plotted against temperature, and a single peak is generated for a single amplicon species. If primer-dimers have been generated these will typically melt at a lower temperature, as they will be shorter than the genuine product. **Fig. 11.4** shows a comparison of the melting

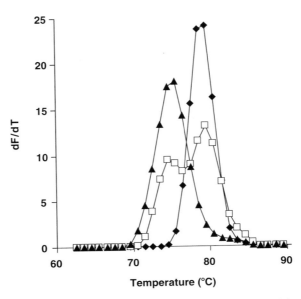

Fig. 11.4. An illustration of the generation of primer-dimers. The melting curve of the standard (◆purified PCR product) gives a single melting peak at ~79.5°C, whereas the NTC sample (△) has a peak at ~75.5°C. When cell cDNA is amplified (□) 2 peaks are apparent at ~79.5°C corresponding to genuine PCR product and ~75.5°C corresponding to primer-dimer

peaks of a standard, a cDNA sample and a NTC sample for a particular gene in which primer-dimers were a problem. In the absence of any genuine template (i.e., the standard or in cDNA samples expressing only very small amounts of the gene of interest) primer-dimers were often found (T_m ~75.5°C). The cDNA shown generated both a genuine amplicon (T_m ~79.5°C) and primer-dimers and thus fluorescence readings for this sample could not be used. Once the T_m of the genuine amplicon is established, the amplification step of each cycle of the real-time assay program can be modified to include an additional heating step to a temperature ~2–3°C below the product T_m before acquiring fluorescence. In this way, fluorescence caused by primer-dimers is eliminated, because these have melted before the acquisition temperature is reached, whereas that produced by the genuine amplicon is retained and collected.

Additional fluorescent dyes have been synthesized that offer some advantages over SYBR Green I. These include SYTO9 *(21)*, EvaGreen *(22)*, BOXTO *(23)*, LCGreen *(24)* and SYBR GreenER. Increased stability even after multiple freeze-thaw cycles, improved enhancement of fluorescence on DNA binding and reduced inhibition of PCR are some of the features of the newer dyes. In addition, as SYBR Green I has a tendency to inhibit the PCR reaction it is used in real-time PCR at a concentration that may not saturate the amplicon. This makes SYBR Green I unsuitable for high resolution melting (HRM) analysis, an emerging method useful in genotyping and SNP scanning *(25)*, as molecules of SYBR Green I released from double-stranded amplicons as they melt may redistribute, binding to un-occupied sites or other molecules of amplicon. Fluorescent dyes that can be used at a higher concentration, without compromising PCR efficiency, are more suited to HRM, and may supersede SYBR Green in time.

3.2. Probe Based Assays

An alternative, widely-used strategy for detecting the amplicon during the PCR process relies on the use of a probe containing an oligonucleotide sequence that is complementary to the target amplicon. A popular probe format is the use of hydrolysis or Taqman probes (**Fig. 11.5**). A detailed discussion of probe-strategies can be found in Wong and Medrano (**26**). Probe-based detection ensures that the only amplicon detected is the target amplicon; nonspecific products and primer-dimers cannot be detected. Thus, unlike SYBR Green I and other minor groove binding dyes, probe-based detection methods have an intrinsic additional specificity built-in. However, this does not mean that probe-based assays require less stringent assay conditions or primer design, as inefficient amplification can severely limit their sensitivity and reliability.

The probes used in quantitative PCR typically have a reporter dye whose fluorescence increases on hybridization with the specific amplicon. For most probe formats, in the absence of the target amplicon, probe fluorescence is inhibited by a quencher. A wide range of dyes and quenchers are available with different excitation and emission spectra, allowing the dyes to be distinguished from one another, and thus allowing simultaneous detection and measurement of multiple PCR products. This is referred to as multiplex

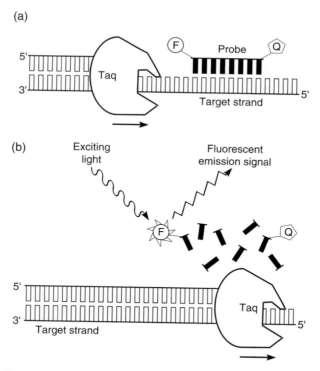

Fig. 11.5. Example of probe-based strategy for detecting accumulating product in quantitative PCR. Principle of hydrolysis or Taqman probes. A probe complementary to the specific target is synthesized with a 5'-fluophore (F) and a 3'-quencher dye (Q). The probe hybridizes to the target amplicon, but in the intact probe the quencher inhibits fluorescence emission (a). During the extension phase of PCR (b), the 5'→3' exonuclease activity of *Taq* polymerase cleaves the probe, releasing the fluophore allowing it to emit a fluorescent signal

PCR. Most quantitative PCR instruments are able to measure fluorescence at multiple wavelengths and thus are capable of multiplex PCR. Although attractive in principle, multiplex quantitative PCR is not a routine procedure as a considerable investment in time and effort may be required for optimization to ensure that each target is amplified truly independently. Of course, there are circumstances when the time taken in developing a reliable multiplex assay is worthwhile, for example, in establishing diagnostic assays or when setting up high throughput quantitative PCR assays that will be used for a prolonged period of time.

3.3. Primer and Assay Design

The "rules" for primer design apply equally to the design of quantitative PCR primers. No additional purification of primers is needed and desalted primers from reputable manufacturers work well. Well-designed primers and probes are a prerequisite of successful quantitative RT-PCR. Primers should be approximately 18–30 nucleotides long with a GC content of 40–60%. Complementarity within the primers and repeats of 3 or more G or C should be avoided, and primers with sequence complementarity should not be used to avoid primer-dimers. If possible, primers that span or flank an intron should be used to prevent, or at least identify, potential amplification of genomic DNA. Secondary structure within the amplicon should be avoided and can be checked using MFold (http://mfold.burnet.edu.au/). Fortunately, primer design software programs such as primer 3 (http://frodo.wi.mit. edu/cgi-bin/primer3/primer3_www.cgi) are freely available, and the manufacturers of a number of quantitative PCR instruments and/or consumables offer free design services. In addition, a growing library of assays exists in a public database (RTPrimerDB http://medgen.ugent. be/rtprimerdb/), which lists primer and probe sequences, submitted by researchers, which have been validated in real-time quantitative PCR assays. The database was set-up to prevent unnecessary and time-consuming primer design and experimental optimization, and to introduce a degree of uniformity and standardization among different laboratories.

For quantitative PCR we design all of our primers to have a very similar annealing temperature (59–60°C) and always choose primers that will synthesize short products between 60–140 bp. This allows a single common PCR run program for all assays so that multiple real-time PCR assays can be performed at the same time. Amplification of short products generally gives assays with very high efficiency that are more tolerant of reaction conditions. For example, the standard curves from quantitative PCR assays for 10 rat genes chosen at random from an unpublished microarray validation study are shown in **Fig. 11.6**. In these particular assays product sizes varied between 60 and 200 bp. PCR efficiency ranged from 94.8% to 100.6% and correlation coefficients (r^2) were all excellent (0.9978–1.0000). Like the quantitative PCR assays in **Fig. 11.6** nearly all assays are linear over a very large concentration range (10^8 log units).

Primer design is crucial to establishing a specific and sensitive real-time assay. When measuring gene expression, primers should be designed to anneal to separate exons. This, combined with RNase-free DNase treatment of the initial RNA sample before reverse transcription (see RNA quality and concentration above), can eliminate the risk that the product generated occurs by amplification of contaminating genomic DNA. The use of SYBR Green I detection necessarily requires that a single amplicon be generated. Although hybridization detection strategies may at first sight appear to be more forgiving of amplification of nonspecific products, in practice such mis-amplification or primer dimerization will reduce assay sensitivity and/or reliability. Time devoted to careful choice of primers and to optimising assay conditions is always time well-spent.

We have, on occasion, employed primers already in use in our laboratory for qualitative PCR, that generate specific, if rather long, products to establish workable real-time quantitative assays. The longest of these generated an amplicon of >900 bp. In such cases, assay sensitivity is reduced, typically to >100 copies rather than 10 copies usually achievable with shorter amplicons. Shorter amplicons are to be preferred even if new primers must be designed and synthesized as optimization of a poorly performing assay may be considerably more trouble than simply designing new primers and developing a quantitative PCR assay with them. Some reviewers recommend the design and testing of several primers pairs, optimization of primer concentrations and even testing amplification using several Mg^{2+} concentration to develop a quantitative PCR that is highly sensitive and specific *(14)*. In the past we have done this, but in the last two years we have adopted a simple strategy of using a fixed concentration of forward and reverse primer (500 n*M*), a common annealing temperature for all assays (57°C) and have used SYBR Green I kits from a manufacturer that contain a fixed concentration of Mg^{2+} (2.5 m*M*). In the great majority of cases this gives quantitative PCR assays that are sensitive; 10 copies of a PCR product standard can not only be detected but this point falls squarely on the standard curve of copy number against crossing point (see **Fig. 11.6**). In addition, agarose gel electrophoresis shows that a single product is produced and this is confirmed by melting curve analysis. Careful design of primers can enable assays to be set-up that can quantitate highly homologous

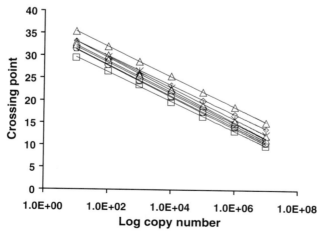

Fig. 11.6. Typical examples of standard curves obtained with SYBR Green RT-qPCR assays. Oligonucleotide primers specific for ten rat genes were synthesized and used to amplify standards (10^1 to 10^7 copies of the PCR products generated from tissue cDNA). All standard curves were linear with correlation coefficients (r^2) close to 1 (range 0.9978 to 1.000) and high amplification efficiency ($E = 94.8$ to 100.6%)

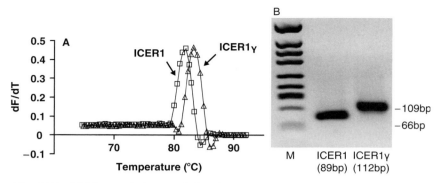

Fig. 11.7. Melting analysis can distinguish closely-related amplicons. Distinct isoforms of the transcription factor, inducible cAMP early repressor (ICER) could be amplified and quantitated from the same cDNA sample using isoform specific primers. Melting curve analysis on the LightCycler (**A**) confirms agarose gel analysis (**B**) that distinct products are formed

transcripts (for example mRNA encoding tryptophan hydroxylase 1 and 2 genes; *27*) or alternatively spliced transcripts of a gene (**Fig. 11.7**). Occasional assays, no more than 1 in 20, fail to meet these standards. In our experience of such failed assays, either the primer pair does not amplify any product (in which case redesign and synthesis of primers is the best option) or efficiency is less than ideal. In one recent example from our laboratory an assay was linear with a very good correlation coefficient ($r^2 = 0.9998$) but it had a low efficiency (~85%) so that the standard curve could measure only to ~100 copies. In practice, this was not a problem as the tissue cDNA being measured contained many tens of thousands of copies.

PCR efficiency is best measured by fitting a regression line to the graph of crossing point (C_T) versus the logarithm of the template concentration and calculating the slope of this line. The efficiency is given by the equation $10^{-1/slope}$. Ideally this calculation should give a value of 2, indicating an efficiency of 100%. The ten SYBR Green I quantitative PCR assays shown in **Fig. 11.6** had a mean efficiency of 98.4%, all were linear with correlation coefficients very close to 1 (mean $r^2 = 0.9994$).

4. Avoiding Contamination

A common problem when many quantitative PCR reactions are run in a laboratory can be the appearance of small amounts of amplicon in NTC tubes. Typically very small numbers of copies of the amplicon made during previous reactions find their way into subsequent assays. This is always irritating but if your NTC contains <10 copies whereas the cDNAs you are measuring contain many thousands of copies then such "contamination" may be of little consequence. Of course, when quantitating low abundance mRNA such contamination is much more than irritating. In our experience, the problem occurs more frequently if a particular assay is run many times, or if the particular gene being measured is very abundant (for example with some reference genes used for normalization). Colleagues who have used linearized plasmids as standards, which were prepared in very large amounts have had contamination problems more frequently. If you consider that a product (120 bp) from a single PCR that is clearly visible after staining with ethidium bromide on an agarose gel may be ~10 ng, this is equivalent to ~8 × 10¹⁰ copies, and quantitative PCR routinely can measure 10 copies, it is clear that extreme care must be taken to prevent any carry-over of products into future reactions. **Fig. 11.8** shows a dilution series of a PCR standard (10⁹ to 10¹ copies/tube) amplified for 40 cycles. In this example, amplification of the highest concentration of template (10⁹ copies) seems to be inhibited (at least during the early cycles of PCR) because tubes containing 10⁹ and 10⁸ copies increase almost in parallel. In addition, in this particular assay the NTC sample is contaminated with some copies of the PCR product carried over from earlier runs. As a result though the graph of CT versus log copy number remains linear over a wide concentration range, distinct bends occur at the each end of the concentration range.

Measures taken to avoid such contamination include sensible steps such as the use of a dedicated set of pipets with filter tips for reaction set-up, regular decontamination of pipets and frequent changes of gloves especially after handling standards. Avoid opening quantitative PCR tubes in the room where other samples will be set up and if agarose gels are run to visualize products do this in a separate laboratory. Users of our instruments are advised that it is best to set up all of their reactions in their own laboratory, then bring only their reaction tubes over to the quantitative PCR laboratory. We also suggest that they do not take their reactions tubes back to their laboratory after a run. This is not because we are unfriendly or even short of space (though we are of course!); it is simply that if the products of previous reactions never enter the area set aside for reaction set-up then the chances of this sort of contamination

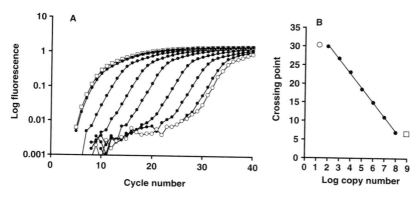

Fig. 11.8. When very high copy numbers of the target are present in either cDNA or the standard (□, 10⁹ copies of standard in this example) amplification may be inhibited (**A**). Poor amplification at high copy number is most likely owing to hybridization of complementary strands during annealing, which prevents the polymerase from copying them. If nontemplate controls (NTC) are also contaminated with a small amount of the target amplicon as was also the case in this assay (○, 10¹ copies of standard) the extremes of the standard curve (e.g., 10¹ and 10⁹ copies) can appear curved giving the standard curve a distinct S-shape. The other standards (●, 10⁸ (left) to 10² (right) copies) amplify as expected and give a linear standard curve (**B**) with good linearity ($r^2 = 0.9986$) if 10⁹ and 10¹ samples are omitted

are minimized. In addition, we clean the set-up area daily with 3% bleach, and are often tempted into covering the area with a new sheet of benchcote, especially if several reactions have been set-up during the day. You may think us paranoid, but we also prefer to work with the air conditioning off; when you have had small numbers of copies of PCR product spoil your otherwise excellent standard curve, you will understand our concern.

Routinely, we first thaw reagents (primers, water and the SYBR Green I kit containing DNA polymerase, dNTPs, reaction buffer and SYBR Green I dye) required to prepare the master mix, make this up and return these reagents to the freezer before even handling any standards or cDNA.

There is another approach to preventing this sort of contamination *(28)*. Many SYBR Green I master mix reagents contain dUTP substituting for dTTP, so that the amplicon generated contains dUMP rather than dTMP. The enzyme uracil-*N*-glycosylase (UNG) can be added to the quantitative PCR and an additional incubation step (50°C for 2 min) included in the cycling programme before activation of the *Taq* DNA polymerase. UNG removes uracil from dUMP, thus if any amplicons generated in previous runs contaminate any of the samples, the contamination will be degraded. During the *Taq* activation step (95°C for 15 min.) the UNG is inactivated and contaminating molecules are destroyed ensuring that during amplification only the target DNA is amplified.

5. Normalization and Data Analysis

The basis of quantitative PCR is the linear relationship between crossing point (C_T) and the logarithm of the initial concentration of template amplified. Defining C_T values can be accomplished manually by setting a threshold in the linear or exponential region of the amplification curve. However, many instruments have software that defines the C_T for the user automatically. It is important to have some understanding of the procedure used in this automatic analysis because an experienced user may readily notice (and thus discard) samples with high background fluorescence or anomalous samples that clearly do not amplify with the expected high efficiency. The availability of melting analysis with SYBR Green I detection also enables each and every cDNA sample to be examined to make sure that a single melting peak is observed indicating that the expected PCR product has been generated.

The methods used for analysis of real-time PCR assays give data that is either absolute or relative. Absolute quantification requires that standards of known copy number are amplified in the same run, whereas relative quantification allows the fold-change between samples to be calculated. Analysis software is provided by the manufacturers of real-time PCR instruments enabling the user to determine C_T values for each sample (i.e., the fractional cycle when the fluorescence signal reaches a threshold set by the user within the linear phase of the reaction). Absolute quantitation requires that the standards and sample unknowns amplify with equal efficiency. Recent publications have discussed the merits of relative and absolute quantitation *(29)* and described the use of new algorithms allowing automated detection and characterization of the exponential phase of amplification curves to give increased precision in the determination of C_T values *(30)*.

It is necessary to normalize quantitative PCR data to account for variations in starting material, mRNA (or DNA) extraction and differences in reverse transcription efficiency between samples. The issue of which method is most appropriate for normalization has been much discussed *(31,32)*, but not satisfactorily resolved. Normalizing gene expression data relative to the amount of RNA taken for reverse transcription has been used *(32)*. However, this method does not correct for differences in cDNA synthesis efficiency, and may give problems if comparisons between quiescent and proliferating cells are made as ribosomal RNA quantity may differ. Measurement of 18S and 28S ribosomal RNA has also been used *(33,34)*, although its suitability has been questioned *(35)*. Ribosomal RNA comprises approximately 95% of total RNA and as such suffers from similar criticisms as those given for total RNA. Furthermore ribosomal RNAs are not polyadenylated unlike mRNAs proscribing the use of oligo(dT) as a primer for reverse transcription. Most commonly, an endogenous reference gene is quantitated in the same samples as the gene of interest. Ideally, this internal reference gene should be expressed at a constant level in different tissues and should not vary with experimental treatment. Often "housekeeping" genes such as GAPDH and β-actin are used, although there is evidence that the expression of these genes can vary substantially. At present, the most widely accepted way to normalize is to use the geometric mean of several reference genes *(36)*. The underlying principle of using multiple reference genes is an important one. If mRNA in one sample has been reverse transcribed less efficiently than in another then not only will the amount of cDNA for the gene of interest be lower but also those for reference genes. This also applies if less RNA was added into the reaction in the first instance. Measuring a single reference gene and using it to normalize the amount of a gene of interest is no longer recommended as it is difficult to be sure any given reference gene is stably expressed. Comparison of multiple reference genes allows the most stable to be selected and averaged therefore reducing variability between samples. To minimize the risk of a treatment or condition affecting the reference genes it is advisable to choose genes involved in different physiological functions in the cell. Methods of selecting the most stable reference genes have been published *(36,37)* and the software can be down-loaded free of charge (for example, GeNorm, http://medgen.ugent.be/~jvdesomp/genorm/; BestKeeper, http://www.gene-quantification.info/).

6. Applications of Quantitative Real-Time PCR

The use of quantitative real-time PCR has increased enormously in the last five years. A PubMed search using the key word "real-time PCR" gave only 45 citations for 1998–1999, but more than 4,600 citations for 2005. This rapid growth in real-time quantitative PCR has been driven by a growing awareness that this is a practicable technique that can generate reliable and valuable data, given appropriate care in template preparation, assay design, use and analysis. The specificity, sensitivity, accuracy and speed of real-time quantitative PCR make it the method of choice for measurement of gene expression. A number of real-time PCR cyclers have been brought to the market by a variety of established instrument manufacturers. In addition, improvements in primer and probe design, the development of additional fluorescent dyes and detection strategies and the availability of quantitative PCR kits from many manufacturers, have made these assays more affordable. Another important factor in the rapid growth of this technique is the remarkable range of applications of the technique itself in a very wide variety of basic biological and clinical research areas and its use in diagnostics. There seems little doubt that this method will become even more widely used in the future.

References

1. Wang AM, Doyle MV, Mark DF (1989) Quantitation of mRNA by the polymerase chain reaction. Proc Natl Acad Sci USA 86:9717–9721
2. Foley KP, Leonard MW, Engel JD (1993) Quantitation of RNA using the polymerase chain reaction. Trends Genet 9:380–385
3. Eidne KA (1991) The polymerase reaction and its uses in Endocrinology. Trends Endo Med 2:69–175
4. Becker-Andre M, Hahlbrock K (1989) Absolute mRNA quantification using the polymerase chain reaction (PCR). A novel approach by a PCR aided transcript titration assay (PATTY). Nucleic Acids Res 17:9437–9446
5. McDowell DG, Burns NA, Parkes HC (1998) Localised sequence regions possessing high melting temperatures prevent the amplification of a DNA mimic in competitive PCR. Nucleic Acids Res 26:3340–3347
6. Wiesner RJ (1992) Direct quantification of picomolar concentrations of mRNAs by mathematical analysis of a reverse transcription/exponential polymerase chain reaction assay. Nucleic Acids Res 20:5863–5864
7. Freeman WM, Walker SI, Vrana KE (1999) Quantitative RT-PCR: pitfalls and potential. Biotechniques 26:112–122, 124–125
8. Ririe KM, Rasmussen RP, Wittwer CT (1997) Product differentiation by analysis of DNA melting curves during the polymerase chain reaction. Anal Biochem 245:154–160
9. Siebert PD, Larrick JW (1992) Competitive PCR. Nature 359:557–558
10. Sugden D, McArthur AJ, Ajpru S, Duniec K, Piggins H (1999) Expression of mt$_1$ melatonin receptor mRNA in the entrained rat suprachiasmatic nucleus: a quantitative study across the diurnal cycle. *Brain Res* Mol Brain Res 72:176–182
11. McArthur AJ, Coogan AN, Ajpru S, Sugden D, Biello SM, Piggins HD (2000) Gastrin-releasing peptide shifts suprachiasmatic nuclei neuronal rhythms in vitro. J Neurosci 20:5496–5502
12. Ajpru S, McArthur AJ, Piggins HD, Sugden D (2002) Identification of PAC1 receptor isoform mRNAs by real-time PCR in rat suprachiasmatic nucleus. Mol Brain Res 105:29–37
13. Bustin SA (2004) A–Z of Quantitative PCR. IUL Biotechnology Series, IUL, USA
14. Nolan T, Hands RE, Bustin SA (2006) Quantification of mRNA using real-time RCR. Nature Protocols 1:1559–1582
15. Chirgwin JM, Przybyla AE, MacDonald RJ, Rutter WJ (1979) Isolation of biologically active ribonucleic acid from sources enriched in ribonuclease. Biochemistry 18:5294–5299
16. Schroeder A, Mueller O, Stocker S, Salowsky S, Leiber M, Gassmann M, Lightfoot S., Menzel W., Granzow M., and Ragg T. (2006) The RIN: an RNA integrity number for assigning integrity values to RNA measurements. BMC Mol Biol 7:3
17. Fleige S, Walf V, Huch S, Prgomet C, Sehn J, Pfaffl MW (2006) Comparison of relative mRNA quantification models and the impact of RNA integrity in quantitative real-time RT-PCR. Biotechnol Lett 28:1601–1613
18. Fleige S, Pfaffl MW (2006) RNA integrity and the effect on the real-time qRT-PCR performance. Mol Aspects Med 27:126–139

19. Jones LJ, Yue ST, Cheung CY, Singer VL (1998) RNA quantitation by fluorescence-based solution assay: RiboGreen reagent characterization. Anal Biochem 265:368–374

20. Morrison TB, Weis JJ, Wittwer CT (1998) Quantification of low-copy transcripts by continuous SYBR Green I monitoring during amplification. Biotechniques 24: 954–958, 960, 962

21. Paul TM, Steven G, Christopher PS (2005) Comparison of SYTO9 and SYBR Green 1 for real-time polymerase chain reaction and investigation of the effect of dye concentration on amplification and DNA melting curve analysis. Anal Biochem 340:24–34

22. Wang W, Chen K, Xu C (2006) DNA quantification using EvaGreen and a real-time PCR instrument. Anal Biochem 356:303–305

23. Karlsson HJ, Bergqvist MH, Lincoln P, Westman G (2004) Syntheses and DNA-binding studies of a series of unsymmetrical cyanine dyes: structural influence on the degree of minor groove binding to natural DNA. Bioorg Med Chem 12: 2369–2384

24. Wittwer CT, Reed GH, Gundry CN, Vandersteen JG, Pryor RJ (2003) High-resolution genotyping by amplicon melting analysis using LCGreen. Clin Chem 49: 853–860

25. Herrman MG, Durtschi JD, Bromley LK, Wittwer CT, Voelkerding KV (2006) Amplicon DNA melting analysis for mutation scanning and genotyping: cross-platform comparison of instruments and dyes. Clin Chem 52:494–503

26. Wong ML, Medrano JF (2005) Real-time PCR for mRNA quantitation. Biotechniques 39:75–85

27. Sugden D (2003) Comparison of circadian expression of tryptophan hydroxylase isoform mRNAs in the rat pineal gland using real-time PCR. J Neurochem 86: 1308–1311

28. Longo MC, Berninger MS, Hartley JL (1990) Use of uracil DNA glycosylase to control carry-over contamination in polymerase chain reactions. Gene 93:125–128

29. Peirson SN, Butler JN, Foster RG (2003) Experimental validation of novel and conventional approaches to quantitative real-time PCR data analysis. Nucleic Acids Res 31:e73

30. Wilhelm J, Pingoud A, Hahn M (2003) Validation of an algorithm for automatic quantification of nucleic acid copy numbers by real-time polymerase chain reaction. Anal Biochem 317:218–225

31. Bustin SA (2000) Absolute quantification of mRNA using real-time reverse transcription polymerase chain reaction assays. J Mol Endocrinol 25:169–193

32. Bustin SA (2002) Quantification of mRNA using real-time reverse transcription PCR (RT-PCR): trends and problems. J Mol Endocrinol 29:23–39

33. Goidin D, Mamessier A, Staquet MJ, Schmitt D, Berthier-Vergnes O (2001) Ribosomal 18S RNA prevails over glyceraldehyde-3-phosphate dehydrogenase and beta-actin genes as internal standard for quantitative comparison of mRNA levels in invasive and noninvasive human melanoma cell subpopulations. Anal Biochem 295, 17–21

34. Schmittgen TD, Zakrajsek BA (2000) Effect of experimental treatment on housekeeping gene expression: validation by real-time, quantitative RT-PCR. J Biochem Biophys Methods 46:69–81

35. Solanas M, Moral R, Escrich E (2001) Unsuitability of using ribosomal RNA as loading control for Northern blot analyses related to the imbalance between messenger and ribosomal RNA content in rat mammary tumors. Anal Biochem 288: 99–102

36. Vandesompele J, De Preter K, Pattyn F, Poppe B, Van Roy N, De Paepe A, Speleman F (2002) Accurate normalization of real-time quantitative RT-PCR data by geometric averaging of multiple internal control genes. Genome Biol 3:0034

37. Pfaffl MW, Tichopad A, Prgomet C, Neuvians TP (2004) Determination of stable housekeeping genes, differentially regulated target genes and sample integrity: BestKeeper – Excel-based tool using pair-wise correlations. Biotechnol Lett 26: 509–515

12

Quantitative Analysis of DNA Sequences by PCR and Solid-Phase Minisequencing

Anu Suomalainen and Ann-Christine Syvänen

1. Introduction

The PCR technique provides a highly specific and sensitive means for analyzing nucleic acids, but it does not allow their direct quantification. This limitation is because the efficiency of PCR depends on the amount of template sequence present in the sample, and the amplification is exponential only at low template concentrations (*1*). Owing to this plateau effect of PCR, the amount of amplification product does not directly reflect the original amount of template. Moreover, subtle differences in reaction conditions, such as material from biological samples, may cause significant sample-to-sample variation in the final yield of the PCR product.

The problem of performing accurate quantitative PCR analyses has been addressed by two principal approaches. A quantitative PCR result can be obtained by "kinetic PCR," in which the amplification process is monitored at numerous times or concentration points (*2,3*). Most conveniently, the amplification process can be monitored in real time by, for example, the homogeneous TaqMan 5' nuclease assay or molecular beacon probes using a fluorescence detection instrument (*4,5*). The other approach, known as competitive PCR, utilizes an internal quantification standard sequence that is coamplified in the same reaction as the target sequence (*6–8*). The efficiency of the amplification is affected by the sequence of the PCR primers as well as the size and sequence of the template. Therefore, the internal standard should be as similar to the target sequence as possible to ensure that the ratio of the two sequences remains constant throughout the amplification. An ideal PCR quantification standard differs from the target sequence only at one nucleotide position, by which the two sequences can be identified and quantified after the amplification. Determination of the relative amounts of PCR products originating from the target and standard sequences allows calculation of the initial amount of the target sequence. If two target sequences are present as a mixture in a sample, it is easy and often sufficient to measure their relative amounts. To determine the absolute amount of a target sequence, it is necessary to add a known amount of standard sequence to the sample before amplification.

From: *Molecular Biomethods Handbook, 2nd Edition.*
Edited by: J. M. Walker and R. Rapley © Humana Press, Totowa, NJ

In this case, a measure of the amount of the analyzed sample, such as the number of cells or the total amount of DNA, RNA, or protein, is needed.

We have developed a solid-phase minisequencing method for the identification of point mutations or nucleotide variations in human genes *(9)*. This method is based on the distinct detection of two sequences that differ from each other only at a single nucleotide, making the method an ideal tool for quantitative analysis of DNA *(10)* and RNA *(11)* sequences by competitive PCR. In the solid-phase minisequencing method, a DNA fragment containing the variable nucleotide is first amplified using one biotinylated and one unbiotinylated PCR primer. The PCR product carrying a biotin residue at the 5' end of one of its strands is captured on an avidin-coated solid support and denatured. The nucleotides at the variable site in the immobilized DNA strand are then identified by two separate primer extension reactions, in which a DNA polymerase incorporates a single-labeled deoxynucleotide triphosphate (dNTP) (see **Fig. 12.1**). Our first-generation assay format utilizes [³H]dNTPs as labels and streptavidin-coated microtiter plates as a solid support *(12)*. The results of the assay are numeric counts per minute (cpm) values expressing the amount of [³H]dNTP incorporated in the minisequencing reactions. The ratio between the cpm values obtained in the minisequencing assay (R value) directly reflects the ratio between the two sequences in the original sample (see **Fig. 12.2**). The method allows quantitative determination of a sequence that represents less than 1% of a mixed sample; that is, the dynamic range for the quantitative analysis spans five orders of magnitude *(10,14)*. Furthermore, because the two sequences differ from each other by a single nucleotide, they

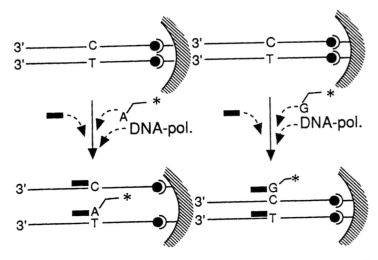

Fig. 12.1. Principle of the solid-phase minisequencing method. Analyses for two nucleotides performed in separate wells are shown on the left and right. ***Top panel***: one PCR primer is biotinylated at its 5' end, resulting in a PCR product carrying biotin at the 5'end of one of its strands (filled circle). The product is captured in a streptavidin-coated microtiter well and denatured. ***Lower panel***: A detection step primer hybridizes to the single-stranded template, 3' adjacent to the variant nucleotide. The DNA polymerase extends the primer with the [³H]-labeled dNTP if it is complementary to the nucleotide present at the variable site. After washing, the sample is denatured and the eluted radioactivity expressing the amount of incorporated label is measured

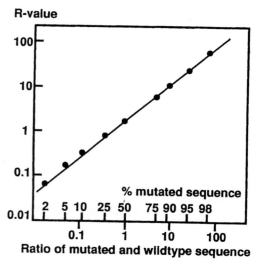

Fig. 12.2. Solid-phase minisequencing standard curve prepared by analyzing mixtures of two 63-mer oligonucleotides differing from each other at one nucleotide in the mitochondrial tRNA[Leu(UUR)] gene *(16)*. The C_{cpm}/T_{cpm} ratio obtained from the minisequencing reactions is plotted as a function of the original ratio between two oligonucleotides in the mixtures. (From **ref. *13*.**)

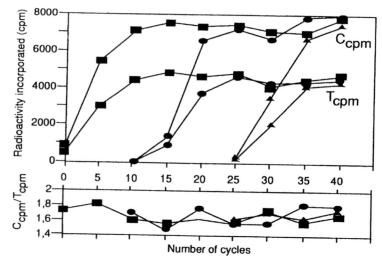

Fig. 12.3. Result of the solid-phase minisequencing assay obtained at different PCR cycles and amounts of template. Mixtures of equal amounts (10^3, 10^7, or 10^{11} molecules) of the same oligonucleotide as in **Fig. 12.2** were analyzed. The upper panel shows the cpm values obtained in the minisequencing assay at different PCR cycles, and the lower panel shows the corresponding C_{cpm}/T_{cpm} ratios

are amplified with equal efficiency during PCR, and the R value obtained is not affected by the amount of template present in the reaction (see **Fig. 12.3**). Consequently, the quantitative analysis can be performed irrespective of the phase of the PCR process. If two sequences are not present in the sample itself, quantitation by minisequencing can be done relative to a standard added to the sample, as described above.

2. Practical Steps

The basic materials and equipment needed for solid-phase minisequencing are available in most molecular genetics laboratories. Routine contamination-free PCR facilities are needed, as well as a PCR machine. In addition, microtiter plates with streptavidin-coated wells (e.g., BioBind assembly strip; Thermo-Labsystems, Finland) are required, and use of a multichannel pipet and microtiter plate washer speed up the procedure, but are optional. A shaker at 37°C and a water bath or incubator at 50°C, as well as a liquid scintillation counter are needed. Exact descriptions of the materials and methods are in given in *(14)*.

2.1. PCR Primer Design

Initially, PCR primers are designed so that one PCR primer is biotinylated at its 5' end during its synthesis, using a biotin–phosphoramidite reagent. If oligonucleotides are to be used as quantification standards (see **Section 2.2.**), the length of oligonucleotides that can be synthesized with acceptable yields sets an upper limit for the length of the PCR product at about 80–100 bp. The detection step primer for the minisequencing reaction is an oligonucleotide complementary to the biotinylated strand of the PCR product designed to hybridize with its 3' end immediately adjacent to the variant nucleotide to be detected (see **Fig. 12.1**). The detection step primer should be at least five nucleotides nested in relation to the unbiotinylated PCR primer.

2.2. Quantification Standards

To accurately quantify a sequence in a sample that contains only one sequence type, a standard should be designed to differ from the target sequence at the nucleotide to be detected in the minisequencing reaction (see **Fig. 12.1**). To construct a standard curve, a second standard identical to the target sequence is required. Oligonucleotide standards can be synthesized using a DNA synthesizer; PCR products or cloned DNA fragments also can be used. First, the molecular concentrations of the standards have to be determined. The optimal amount of the standard added to a sample depends on the abundance of the target sequence in the original sample. The ratio of the target-to-standard sequence should preferably be between 0.1 and 10. If no estimate of the target sequence is available, it might be necessary to initially titrate the optimal amount of the standard in the analysis (e.g., 10^2, 10^4, or 10^6 molecules). For accurate quantification, standards representing both sequence variants should be available, and analysis of mixtures of known amounts of the two standards should be analyzed to construct a standard curve, as demonstrated in **Figs. 12.1** and **12.2** and **Table 12.3**.

2.3. PCR

Polymerase chain reaction follows routine protocols except that the amount of biotin-labeled primer should be reduced, not to exceed the biotin-binding capacity of the microtiter well. If high binding capacity is required, avidin-coated polystyrene beads can also be used. The PCR should be optimized so that one-tenth of the PCR product produces a single visible band after agarose gel electrophoresis and staining with ethidium bromide.

2.4. Solid-Phase Minisequencing (see Fig. 12.1)

The detection of biotin-labeled PCR product starts with affinity capture: The PCR product binds from its 5' biotin to the streptavidin-coated micro-titer well. Each nucleotide to be detected at the variant site needs to be analyzed in a separate well. Thus, minimally two wells are needed per PCR product. After capture, the wells are washed carefully to remove PCR-derived dNTPs. Then, the PCR product is denatured in the wells, after which only the biotin-labeled DNA strand of the PCR product remains attached to the well wall and the complementary strand is washed off. Next, the minisequencing solution is added. This consists of a thermostable DNA polymerase, such as *Taq* polymerase, in its buffer, supplemented with [³H]-labeled dNTP specific to the mutation to be detected, as well as a detection step primer, which hybridizes its 3' end adjacent to the nucleotide to be detected. If the labeled dNTP matches the variant site, the polymerase extends the detection primer with this nucleotide, and the primer becomes [³H] labeled. After denaturation of the primer, the amount of incorporated nucleotide is measured by a liquid scintillation counter. The ratio between the cpm values for the two nucleotides detected in separate wells reflects the ratio between the two sequences in the original sample. Because the specific activities of [³H]-labeled dNTPs vary, these have to be corrected before calculating the final ratio. Alternatively, a standard curve can be used to correct for these factors.

Our standard assay format uses [³H]-labeled dNTPs because of their low radioactivity and high chemical resemblance to natural dNTPs such as polymerase substrates. However, dNTPs or dideoxy-nucleotides labeled with other isotopes or with fluorophores can also be used. Furthermore, streptavidin-coated microtiter plates made of scintillating polystyrene are available. These allow direct detection of the extended primer after the minisequencing reaction, but a scintillation counter for microtiter plates is needed *(15)*.

3. Examples of Applications

3.1. Determination of Allele Frequencies by Quantitative Analysis of Pooled DNA Samples

We have developed a system for forensic DNA typing, in which a panel of 12 single-nucleotide polymorphisms (SNPs) is analyzed by the solid-phase minisequencing method *(12)*. The statistical interpretation of forensic and paternity testing results requires information on allele frequencies of the analyzed markers in each particular population. To rapidly obtain this information in the Finnish population, we utilized the quantitative nature of the solid-phase minisequencing method to determine allele frequencies of polymorphic markers by analyzing pooled DNA samples derived from hundreds of individuals. The ratio between the two sequences at each polymorphic locus in the pooled DNA samples is equivalent to the allele frequencies in the population. **Table 12.1** shows the results from the analysis of allele frequencies of a polymorphism in the *PROS1* gene on chromosome 13. A good correlation between allele frequencies determined from the pooled samples and those determined from about 100 alleles individually were observed *(12)*. This possibility of determining the allele frequencies of common SNPs with good accuracy in pooled samples has recently been used in many association studies as an approach to increase the throughput of genotyping SNP markers. We also have determined the carrier frequency of a rare disease allele causing recessively inherited aspartylglucosaminuria in Finland by determining the frequency of the mutant allele (**Table 12.2**) by quantitative analysis of large pooled DNA samples *(10)*.

Table 12.1. Example of the determination of the allele frequencies of a polymorphism in the PROS1 gene by quantitative analysis of pooled DNA samples.

Sample[a]	[³H]dNTP incorporated (cpm)[b]		R value (A_{cpm}/G_{cpm})	Allele frequency[c]	
	A reaction	G reaction		A allele	G allele
Pool 1390	2750	1280	2.14	0.59	0.41
Pool 860	2240	1048	2.15	0.59	0.41
Pool 920	2510	1190	2.11	0.58	0.42
Control (AA)	2100	52	40	—	—
Control (GG)	96	1930	0.050	—	—
Control (AG)	2480	1660	1.49	—	—
No DNA	64	39	—	—	—

[a]The numeral gives the number of individuals in each pool. AA, GG, and AG indicate the genotype of the individual control samples.
[b]Mean values of five (pools) or two (individual controls) parallel assays. The specific activities of [³H]dATP and [³H]dGTP were 58 and 32 Ci/mmol, respectively.
[c]The allele frequencies determined from 50 individual samples were 0.61 (A) and 0.39 (G) *(12)*.

Table 12.2. Determination of the copy number of the aspartylglucosaminidase Gene.

Karyotype of sample	$C_{cpm}/(C_{cpm} + G_{cpm})$	Deduced AGA gene copy number
46,XY,−4,+der(4) t(4;12) (q31.3;p12.2)mat	0.28–0.33[a]	1
46,XX,del(4)(q33)	0.26–0.32[a]	1
46,XX,−21,+der(21) t(4;21) (q28;p13)mat	0.63–0.70[a]	3
Controls[b]	0.50–0.54	2

[a]Range of variation of five parallel assays.
[b]DNA from individuals heterozygous for the target nucleotide in the aspartylglucosaminidase gene.
Source: **ref.** *19*

3.2. Detection of Heteroplasmic Point Mutations of Mitochondrial DNA

Disease-causing point mutations of mitochondrial DNA (mtDNA) are most often heteroplasmic; that is, the tissues of patients contain both mutant and normal mtDNA. The solid-phase minisequencing method is particularly useful for detecting heteroplasmic mtDNA mutations, allowing both identification and quantification of the mutation in the same assay. Using this method, we have observed a correlation between the degree of heteroplasmy and the severity and age of disease onset in two mitochondrial disorders associated with mtDNA point mutations (13,16) (**Table 12.3**). Furthermore, a decline of a mutant mitochondrial DNA population was shown to occur during aging (17,18). The method is widely used in clinical DNA diagnosis laboratories for routine detection of point mutations.

3.3. Determination of Gene Copy Numbers

We have developed an alternative method to the widely used fluorescence in situ hybridization techniques in the determination of the copy number of human genes. The copy number of the aspartylglucosaminidase gene, located on the chromosome 4q, was determined by solid-phase minisequencing in the samples of three patients with either deletions or duplications involving the distal region of chromosome 4q. A known amount of DNA from a patient homozygous for a mutation in the marker gene was mixed with the DNA samples to be analyzed to serve as an internal standard, and the relative amount of normal sequence was determined by the solid-phase minisequencing

Table 12.3. Example of the result of a solid-phase minisequencing analysis of mixtures of two 63-Mer oligonucleotides differing from each other at one nucleotide in the mitochondrial tRNA$^{Leu(UUR)}$ gene.

Ratio of wild-type sequence to mutated sequence	T_{cpm} (wt oligo)[a]	C_{cpm} (mut oligo)[b]	R value (C_{cpm}/T_{cpm})
Wild type	3110	44	0.014
50 : 1	3640	190	0.05
20 : 1	2780	420	0.15
10 : 1	2830	730	0.26
4 : 1	2520	1690	0.67
1 : 2	1650	2810	1.7
1 : 4	790	3630	4.6
1 : 10	350	3790	10.8
1 : 20	210	4760	22.7
1 : 50	120	4800	40.0
Mutant	43	4580	106.5
H_2O	41	23	—

[a]The specific activities of the [^{3}H] dNTPs: dTTP=126 Ci/mmol; dCTP=67 Ci/mmol.
[b]In this case, two [^{3}H] dCTPs were incorporated into the mutant sequence.
Source: **ref. 13**.

method *(19)*. This application demonstrates the suitability of the method for determining monosomies, trisomies, and loss of heterozygosity, provided that a DNA standard containing a suitable polymorphism is available.

3.4. Identification of Mixed Samples

The *R* values obtained by solid-phase minisequencing, when individual genomic DNA samples are analyzed for a variable nucleotide, fall into three distinct categories that unequivocally define the genotype of the sample. *R* Values falling outside of these three categories that normally differ from each other by a factor of 10 suggest the presence of contaminating DNA in the sample *(12)*. The ability of the method to identify a mixed sample is an advantage in forensic analyses, where stain samples could contain DNA from several individuals, as well as in prenatal diagnosis, where placental biopsy samples could contain contaminating maternal DNA, and for mutation analysis in tumor samples that could contain normal DNA. Recently, we have utilized the possibility of quantitative genotyping of mixed samples to monitor the success of allogenic stem cell transplantation in leukaemia patients. In this application, the change of each patient's blood cell genotypes to that of the donor were assessed quantitatively after the transplantation *(20)*.

3.5. High-Throughput Genotyping of SNPs

Single-nucleotide polymorphisms (SNPs) are the most abundant form of genetic variation, occurring approx every 1–2 kb in the human genome *(21)*. New assay formats with low reagent costs are required for highly multiplexed SNP genotyping, which is becoming of increasing importance in association studies of complex disorders. Solid-phase minisequencing meets that challenge when adapted to a microchip format *(22)*. In this format, minisequencing primers, or tags homologous to the detection primers, are attached on a glass chip, and the detection of minisequencing reaction is based on the incorporation of a fluorescent dye. The microarray-based minisequencing allows simultaneous, quantitative analysis of up to 100 SNPs in 56 samples per microscope slide, detecting 2% of the minority alleles *(23)*.

In conclusion, solid-phase minisequencing is an accurate high-sensitivity, low-cost method applicable to a routine molecular genetic laboratory for single-nucleotide detection. It is widely used in DNA diagnostic laboratories for nuclear gene mutation detection as well as relative quantification of mitochondrial DNA mutations. It also is applicable to the microarray format for efficient screening and genotyping of SNPs.

References

1. Syvänen AC, Bengtström M, Tenhunen J, Söderlund H (1988) Quantification of polymerase chain reaction products by affinity-based hybrid collection. Nucleic Acids Res 16:11,327–11,338.
2. Murphy LD, Herzog CE, Rudick JB, Fojo AT, Bates SE (1990) Use of the polymerase chain reaction in the quantitation of mdr-1 gene expression. Biochemistry 29:10,351–10,356
3. Noonan KE, Beck C, Holzmayer TA, et al (1990) Quantitative analysis of MDR1 (multidrug resistance) gene expression in human tumors by polymerase chain reaction. Proc Natl Acad Sci USA 87:7160–7164

4. Livak KJ, Flood SJ, Marmaro J, Giusti W, Deetz K (1995) Oligonucleotides with fluorescent dyes at opposite ends provide a quenched probe system useful for detecting PCR product and nucleic acid hybridization. PCR Methods Appl 4:357–362

5. Tyagi S, Kramer FR (1996). Molecular beacons: probes that fluoresce upon hybridization. Nat Biotechnol 14:303–308

6. Chelly J, Kaplan JC, Maire P, Gautron S, Kahn A (1988) Transcription of the dystrophin gene in human muscle and non-muscle tissue. Nature 333:858–860

7. Wang AM, Doyle MV. and Mark DF (1989) Quantitation of mRNA by the polymerase chain reaction. Proc Natl Acad Sci USA 86:9717–9721.

8. Gilliland G, Perrin S, Blanchard K, and Bunn HF (1990) Analysis of cytokine mRNA and DNA: detection and quantitation by competitive polymerase chain reaction. Proc Natl Acad Sci USA 87:2725–2729.

9. Syvänen AC, Aalto-Setälä K, Harju L, Kontula K, Söderlund H (1990) A primer-guided nucleotide incorporation assay in the genotyping of apolipoprotein E. Genomics 8:684–692

10. Syvänen AC, Ikonen E, Manninen T, et al (1992) Convenient and quantitative determination of the frequency of a mutant allele using solid-phase minisequencing: application to aspartylglucosaminuria in Finland. Genomics 12:590–595

11. Ikonen E, Manninen T, Peltonen L, Syvänen AC (1992). Quantitative determination of rare mRNA species by PCR and solid-phase minisequencing. PCR Methods Appl 1:234–240

12. Syvänen AC, Sajantila A, Lukka M (1993). Identification of individuals by analysis of biallelic DNA markers, using PCR and solid-phase minisequencing. Am J Hum Genet 52:46–59.

13. Suomalainen A, Majander A, Pihko H, Peltonen L, Syvänen AC (1993) Quantification of tRNA 3243(Leu) point mutation of mitochondrial DNA in MELAS patients and its effects on mitochondrial transcription. Hum Mol Genet, 2:525–534

14. Suomalainen A, Syvänen AC (2000) Quantitative analysis of human DNA sequences by PCR and solid-phase minisequencing. Mol. Biotechnol. 15:123–131

15. Ihalainen J, Siitari H, Laine S, Syvänen AC, Palotie A (1994) Towards automatic detection of point mutations: use of scintillating microplates in solid-phase minisequencing. BioTechniques 16:938–943

16. Suomalainen A, Kollmann P, Octave JN, Söderlund H, Syvänen AC (1993) Quantification of mitochondrial DNA carrying the tRNA(8344Lys) point mutation in myoclonus epilepsy and ragged-red-fiber disease. Eur J Hum Genet 1:88–95

17. Rahman S, Poulton J, Marchington D, Suomalainen A (2001) Decrease of 3243 A→G mtDNA mutation from blood in MELAS syndrome: a longitudinal study. Am J Hum Genet 68:238–240

18. Olsson C, Johnsen E, Nilsson M, Wilander E, Syvänen AC, Lagerström-Fermer M (2001) The level of the mitochondrial mutation A3243G decreases upon ageing in epithelial cells from individuals with diabetes and deafness. Eur J Hum Genet 9:917–921.

19. Laan M, Grön-Virta K, Salo A, et al (1995) Solid-phase minisequencing confirmed by FISH analysis in determination of gene copy number. Hum Genet 96:275–280

20. Fredriksson M, Barbany G, Liljedahl U, Hermanson M, Kataja M, Syvänen AC (2004) Assessing hematopoietic chimerism after allogeneic stem cell transplantation by multiplexed SNP genotyping using microarrays and quantitative analysis of SNP alleles. Leukemia 18:1–12

21. Sachidanandam R, Weissman D, Schmidt SC, et al (2001) A map of human genome sequence variation containing 1.42 million single nucleotide polymorphisms. Nature 409:928–933

22. Syvänen AC (1999) From gels to chips: "minisequencing" primer extension for analysis of point mutations and single nucleotide polymorphisms. Hum Mutat 13:1–10.
23. Lindroos K, Sigurdsson S, Johansson K, Rönnblom L, Syvänen AC (2002) Multiplex SNP genotyping in pooled DNA samples by a four-colour microarray system. Nucleic Acids Res 30:e70

13

Multiplex Amplifiable Probe Hybridization (MAPH)

Carolina Sismani, Ludmila Kousoulidou, and Philippos C. Patsalis

1. Introduction

Changes in DNA copy number can result in a wide range of pathological conditions such as mental retardation, malformations, developmental delay, neurological disorders and congenital anomalies. These copy number changes may be large or small and they may include the entire or segments of a chromosome. Conventional chromosomal analysis (karyotyping) allows detection of chromosomal aberrations larger than 5 Mb, however smaller aberrations are not detectable with the existing G-banding analysis. Microdeletion syndromes, subtle deletions and complex rearrangements in the subtelomeric regions are typical examples of small abnormalities that cause clinical phenotypes but are not visible by routine cytogenetics. Such small imbalances, called "submicroscopic," can only be detected using other methods that provide high-resolution analysis.

Several methodologies have been developed to detect these submicroscopic genetic imbalances. The introduction of fluorescence in situ hybridization (FISH) led to the identification of cryptic chromosomal imbalances that were undetectable with high-resolution G-banding chromosomal analysis. Examples include detection of most of the known microdeletion syndromes, microduplications, interstitial segment imbalances and subtelomeric rearrangements (1–5), using locus-specific or subtelomeric specific FISH probes. Although FISH methodology provided significant improvements in the field of cytogenetics, it does not offer an alternative approach to G-banded chromosomal analysis, as it is a targeted method, which does not provide genome-wide analysis.

DNA-based methods such as quantitative PCR or real time PCR can also be applied to determine small copy number changes (6,7). These are high-resolution methods but are also targeted to specific known loci. Simultaneous analysis of multiple loci is technically challenging and it is therefore difficult to screen large genomic regions and identify new genes.

Until now, the only alternative method to chromosomal analysis, for genome wide screening was comparative genomic hybridization (CGH). Conventional CGH analysis uses metaphases and permits the detection of

From: *Molecular Biomethods Handbook, 2nd Edition.*
Edited by: J. M. Walker and R. Rapley © Humana Press, Totowa, NJ

chromosomal deletions or duplications as small as 3 Mb *(8)*. The advancement from metaphase chromosome-based CGH to microarray based-CGH using BAC and PAC clones has increased the resolution to higher than 1 Mb *(9,10)*. Microarray-based CGH has been performed successfully to screen total genome to identify subtle abnormalities in cancer samples *(11)*, mental retardation *(12)*. The sensitivity and specificity of array-CGH was further increased with recent improvements and modifications, such as tiling resolution BAC arrays covering the entire human genome with approximately one clone per 100 kb *(13)*, hybridization of genomic representations to CGH arrays *(14)*, arraying long oligonucleotide probes *(15)*, Affymetrix SNP arrays *(16,17)* and other commercial solutions with extreme resolution *(18)*. Array-CGH has been proven to be very sensitive and is rapidly becoming the method of choice for high-resolution genome-wide screening to detect known and unknown copy-number changes.

A new DNA-based method for the reliable determination of locus copy number in complex genomes is multiplex amplifiable probe hybridization (MAPH) *(19)*. This method relies on the fact that probes can be quantitatively recovered and amplified after hybridization to genomic DNA template. MAPH uses probes that can be specifically designed for any locus, telomere, chromosomal segment, whole chromosome or the total human genome at extremely high resolution, and enable the sensitive detection of loss or gain of genomic DNA sequences as small as 150 bp. However gel-based detection places a limit to the multiplicity of MAPH, as in most cases only 30–50 probes per assay are included.

The latest advancement in MAPH methodology is the introduction of microarrays, resulting in the development of microarray-based MAPH (array-MAPH) *(20,21)*. This new method combines the high specificity and sensitivity of MAPH with the high multiplicity of microarray format. Array-MAPH could be applied as a potential alternative to array-CGH, offering several advantages for the detection of copy number changes in the human genome.

2. Methods

2.1. Multiplex Amplifiable Probe Hybridization

2.1.1. Probe Preparation

MAPH and array-MAPH are illustrated in **Fig. 13.1**. Both methodologies require probe selection and preparation. Correct selection of probes is one of the key steps towards a successful MAPH experiment and it is based on a number of important criteria. Probe sequences should be: unique in the human genome, nonrepetitive, nonpolymorphic, well localized, size varying from 100 bp to 600 bp, evenly spaced over the studied genomic region and have similar GC% (around 50%) to ensure similar hybridization conditions. Each probe should represent a specific sequence of interest, which might be any locus of human genome including genes, non-coding specific loci, subtelomeric or subcentromeric regions.

There are two different strategies of probe preparation (**Fig. 13.1A**). The first is to identify the DNA sequence in the region of interest, amplify the sequence with specific primers and subclone the amplicon (probe) into a plasmid vector *(21)*. A new web interface called MAPHDesigner is now available

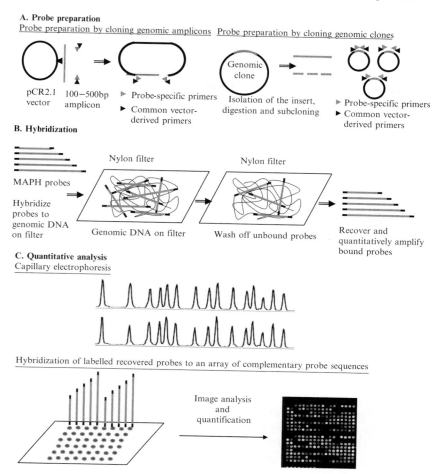

Fig. 13.1. MAPH methodology

at http://bioinfo.ebc.ee/MAPH and allows to rapidly design probes and PCR primers with the desired criteria to cover any chromosome segment, any chromosome, or the whole genome. The second strategy is to insert blunt-ended restriction fragments from genomic clones into the EcoRV site of pZero2 (*19*). In both cases all probes subcloned in the same plasmid vector are flanked by common vector-derived primer sequences and can be amplified simultaneously in a single reaction directly from bacterial cells.

A clone library is created by culturing and cryopreserving selected clones in LB medium with 10% glycerol. Clone identity is confirmed for every probe by sequencing or PCR amplification using the probe-specific primer sets (*21*). These primers have no other homologous sequences in the Human genome, or in bacterial genome. Therefore they can only bind to a specific probe sequence and give a distinct product only if a specific probe sequence is inserted.

Amplifiable probes are prepared by PCR amplification using common primers flanking the vector-cloning site. A probe mixture (set) is formed by mixing in equal quantities a number of selected probes.

2.1.2. Hybridization

The probe mixture is hybridized to denatured genomic DNA immobilized on a small nylon membrane (**Fig. 13.1B**). An excess of probe is used, to drive hybridization to completion so that all probes can fully anneal to all homologous genomic sequences. Calculations related to hybridization kinetics and probe concentrations can be found at http://www.nottingham.ac.uk/~pdzjala/ maph/maph.html. After stringent washing of filter for the removal of unbound probes, bound probes are released by denaturing at 95°C for 5 min. Released bound probes are simultaneously and quantitatively amplified with common vector-derived primers for no more than 20–25 cycles and the quantity of amplification product for each probe reflects the copy number of the corresponding locus.

2.1.3. Quantitative Analysis

Amplification products are visualized on polyacrylamide gel or capillary electrophoresis; each band (peak) is identified by its size and quantified against other probes with known copy number (**Fig. 13.1C**). Quantification procedure is described in detail in the literature (*19,22,23*) and full experimental details have been published (*19*) with regular updates and practical notes in a website (http://www.nottingham.ac.uk/~pdzjala/maph/maph.html) (*23*).

2.2. Microarray-Based Multiplex Amplifiable Probe Hybridization (array-MAPH)

A recent advancement in MAPH methodology is the introduction of microarray technology (*20,21*). Two different methodological approaches were used in two different pilot studies. In both cases the final quantification step was replaced by hybridization to an array of target sequences, complementary to individual MAPH probes. The first (*20*) is an oligonucleotide-based PamGene 3-Dimentional Flow-Through microarray platform and the second (*21*) is based on 500 bp PCR amplifiable sequences.

2.2.1. Oligo-Based PamGene 3-Dimentional Flow-Through Microarray (PamChip): Microarray Preparation

Microarray target sequences are 60mer oligonucleotides, complementary to individual MAPH probes (*20*). Three complementary oligonucleotides with CG content as close as possible to 50%, are designed for each probe. Each target oligonucleotide is synthesized and spotted in duplicate, giving a total of six arrays spots per probe.

2.2.1.1. Hybridization: MAPH filter hybridization is performed as described above (**Fig. 13.1B**). At the final step, the recovered probe mixture is labeled with either Cy3 or Cy5 by PCR amplification with labeled common primers. Reference sample and test sample are differentially labeled. Labeled reference sample is produced by amplifying a number of MAPH primary products from five normal male samples. These are purified and pooled in a homogenous reference DNA (*20*).

2.2.1.2. Quantitative Analysis: Quantitative analysis is performed by microarray hybridization (**Fig. 13.1C**). Differentially labeled reference and test probe solutions are mixed together, denatured and cohybridized to the oligonucleotide microarray. PamChips are loaded into the Olympus FD10 microarray instrument according to the manufacturer's instructions and processed with a custom hybridization protocol (20).

Images of are scanned using the software pre-installed on the FD10 and then loaded into PamChip Analyzer. Median spot intensity minus background value is calculated for each spot. Cy3/Cy5 ratios are calculated and then normalized in two levels: (a) to address differences in sample DNA concentrations, by assuming a 1:1 ratio for autosomal control probes in each sample and return all ratios for that sample to the mean of these probes, (b) to address differential PCR amplification of individual probes in reference and test samples: the ratios of individual probes are adjusted to the corresponding mean ratios among normal control samples.

The values of normalized ratios are indicative of locus copy number as in capillary MAPH (19).

2.2.2. Microarray of 500bp PCR Amplifiable Sequences

This methodology was used to develop and validate a chromosome X specific MAPH microarray (21). Several modifications of the standard MAPH protocol were made, to adjust the whole procedure to the new methodological challenges of the new microarray platform, such as high multiplicity (up to 800 loci analyzed simultaneously), two consecutive hybridization steps etc.

2.2.2.1. *Probe Preparation*: Probe mixture is prepared as described above, with two modifications: (1) The size range of probes is narrowed down to 400–600bp, instead of 100–600p, to ensure more uniform amplification and hybridization properties, achieving higher hybridization efficiency. There is no need to separate probe sequences based on size, as they are identified by their position on the microarray. (2) Unlike gel-based MAPH, where a maximum of 60 probes can be used in a mixture, array-MAPH probe mixture consists of up to 800 different probes (21).

2.2.2.2. *Microarray Preparation*: Array-MAPH target sequences are amplified for spotting onto the microarray, using specific PCR primers for every cloned probe. Each array-MAPH target sequence is spotted onto microarray slides in duplicate. All probes are arrayed in random order, to minimize the possibility that a spatial artifact during array hybridization will be incorrectly interpreted as an aberration.

2.2.2.3. *Hybridization*: MAPH filter hybridization is performed as described above (**Fig. 13.1B**), with some modifications in the protocol, such as a twofold increase in starting DNA quantity, mainly due to the large number of simultaneously amplified and hybridized probes. At the final step, the recovered probe mixture is purified and labeled by nick translation using aminoallyl-dUTP-s and later treatment with amino-reactive Cy3 or Cy5 dye.

2.2.2.4. *Quantitative Analysis*: Quantitative analysis is performed by single sample hybridization of the labeled probe mixture to the microarray (**Fig. 13.1C**). The microarrays are scanned; raw signal intensities are extracted and analyzed using MAPH-Stat software, which is specifically designed for array-MAPH.

Microarray signals are normalized with respect to the median of autosomal probe-specific signals from the given microarray (21). Raw data is adjusted to normal distribution for correct calculation of confidence intervals by taking logarithm of signal intensity values with base 2. Average and 90% tolerance interval (*TI 90%*) values are calculated for each probe using data (signal intensity values) from the control panel. The control panel is used as reference and it is a set of five separate microarray hybridizations, performed with five DNA samples of phenotypically normal individuals. A male and female control panel is created and used for analyzing male and female DNA, respectively.

Signal intensity values of at least two adjacent probes with the intensity above or below the *TI 90%* values were considered indicative for a potential copy number change in the analyzed region. However the use of one, two or three adjacent probes as an indication of a copy number change, depends on the expected rate of false-positives, based on the quality of the experiment.

3. Applications

3.1. MAPH

MAPH can be used as a diagnostic or research tool to determine deletions or duplications in the genome. Such genetic imbalances may be located in known or unknown positions and therefore MAPH can be used as a targeted approach or for screening in "unknown locations" anywhere in the genome.

Several MAPH tests have been developed to identify genetic defects of known loci, such as *DMD* (deletions or duplications cause Duchenne/Becker muscular dystrophy), *SNRPN* (deletions or duplications cause Prader-Willi/ Angelman syndrome), *TBX5* (deletions cause Holt-Oram syndrome (HOS)), *PMP22* (duplication cause Charcot-Marie-Tooth disease (CMT1A)) and deletions that cause hereditary neuropathy with liability to pressure palsies (HNPP), MBP (MBP gene encodes the second most abundant CNS myelin protein, deletions or duplications may cause leukodystrophies), sarcogly-can genes (*SGCA, SGCB, SGCG,* and *SGCD*), the candidate genes *TSGs* at 16q22.1 (deletion may cause lobular and low grade nonlobular invasive carcinoma of the breast), *BRC-ABL1* genes (fusion and amplification causes chronic myeloid leukemia (CML), *BRACA1* (deletions and duplications cause breast cancer) and *MLH1/MSH2* (deletions or duplications causes hereditary nonpolyposis colorectal cancer (HNPCC).

The establishment and validation of MAPH methodology was first illustrated for specific genomic loci, by Armour et al. (2000) *(19)*. In this initial study, the power and specificity of MAPH was demonstrated by simultaneous assessment of copy number at a set of 40 probes, including the locus for Duchenne muscular dystrophy (*DMD*), Prader-Willi/Angelman (*SNRPN*), sex determining region Y (*SRY*) and other loci from chromosomes 16, 17, 22. Microdeletions and microduplication on the above syndromes and X and Y copy number in males and females were accurately determined in 10 human DNA samples *(19)*.

Akrami et al. (2001) *(24)*, applied MAPH to search for large-scale deletions or duplications at *TBX5*. The authors used probe mixture consisting of three probes from the promoter region, 13 probes from the nine exons of the gene, two probes from downstream of exon 9 and as controls, six probes from other autosomes, two from the sex chromosomes and one from a nonhuman DNA probe. The *TBX5* MAPH assay demonstrated reproducible results in all unaffected controls, whereas in 20 unrelated HOS patients with no known mutation in *TBX5* showed that MAPH assay can be used to determine the "missing" mutations due to exonic deletions.

White et al. (2002) *(25)* adapted the MAPH assay for screening of *DMD* gene, mutations in which cause Duchenne and Becker muscular dystrophy. The authors engineered probes for each of the 79 exons of *DMD* gene and analyzed them by capillary electrophoresis-based MAPH methodology. Probe sets A and B were prepared containing 40 and 39 *DMD* exons, respectively. Nine probe control mixtures were made specifically for use with each probe set. Probes were initially tested by hybridization to control DNA from 24 healthy individuals and to DNA from a complete *DMD* gene deletion. A total of 125 patients samples were screened in a semiblind manner and a large number of novel rearrangements were detected, especially small, one- and two-exon duplications. A year later *(26)* the above method was also validated using the Bioanalyzer 2100 (Agillent) and the "Lab-on-a-chip" electrophoresis, which process quantitatively 12 samples in 30 min. The MAPH DMD approach demonstrated a reliable, inexpensive and rapid method, which takes less than 24 h for the detection of deletions or duplications, and can be easily implemented in routine practice of diagnostic laboratories. In 2005, Dent et al. *(27)*, used a combination of single condition amplification/internal primer (SCAIP) sequencing analysis with MAPH analysis to report the frequency of mutations in a large cohort of 84 unselected dystrophinopathy patients from 68 families. Forty-five proband were clinically affected with DMD, 21 with BMD, and two females were manifesting carriers. They identified disease-causing mutations in over 93% of the clinically affected individuals using the two methods. Buzin et al. (2005) *(28)* performed duplication scanning of *DMD* deletion-negative patients, using MAPH probes for all of the *DMD* gene exons. In this case, each probe contained an exon-specific region in the middle and two primer-specific regions at each end. From a total of 141 *DMD* deletion-negative patients screened, 18 duplications involving many segments of the gene were detected. Eight of them were previously found by other methodology, and 10 of them were previously undetected.

MAPH was also successfully applied for the detection of copy number at *PMP22* in CMT1A/HNPP patients *(29)*. They developed an efficient and sensitive MAPH assay with 19 probes, consisting of seven probes for *PMP22* gene, nine probes from other autosomes, two from the sex chromosomes and a nonhuman DNA probes. The overall specificity and reliability of the probes were tested in 94 unaffected controls, with one duplication and one deletion previously known. The *PMP22* MAPH assay successfully distinguished five HNPP from unaffected samples among a blind test on 10 samples, and 31 from a blind study on 62 samples collected from a previous study. Apart from minor discrepancies, all diagnoses agreed with results from other methods, showing that the *PMP22* MAPH assay is a simple, fast and accurate screening test for molecular diagnosis of CMT1A and HNPP.

White et al. (2005) *(30)* designed a MAPH probe set with 28 probes to screen for pathogenic deletions or duplications in the sarcoglycan genes (*SGCA, SGCB, SGCG,* and *SGCD*) in limb-girdle muscular dystrophy (LGMD) patients. They screened six patients five unrelated patients diagnosed as possible homozygous but segregation of the mutations could not be confirmed in the parents and one patient where a mutation was found only in one allele. Although copy number changes in sarcoglycan genes are rare, they found one paternally inherited heterozygous deletion of *SGCG* exon 7.

In a recent publication, Vaurs-Barriere et al. (2006) *(31)* used a combination of quantitative multiplex PCR short fluorescent fragments (QMPSF), and

MAPH to look for genomic copy number at the Goll*i-MBP* (myelin basic protein) locus in 195 patients with cerebral MRI suggesting a myelin defect, that do not have *PLP1* (proteolipoprotein gene) mutation. The (*MBP*) gene encodes the second most abundant CNS myelin protein after *PLP1*. In this study no abnormal gene quantification was found using MAPH and QMPSF. In addition no discrepancies were observed between the two methods. Based on their findings, the authors suggested that *Golli-MBP* deletion or duplication is rarely involved in inherited defects of myelin formation. In another study by the same group *(32)* they screened 262 hypomyelinating patients for intragenic copy number changes along the *PLP1*gene. Among these patients, 56 were known *PLP1* duplication patients, one *PLP1* triplication and 205 patients had a leukodystrophy of unknown origin. MAPH identified all the known copy number changes of *PLP1* and also identified one partial triplication and two partial deletions of *PLP1*. The above study showed that MAPH is a reliable technique for the diagnosis of *PLP1* copy number changes.

Besides the investigation on constitutional genetics, MAPH is also applied in cancer genetics. In a recent study the DNA copy-number was measured in patients with both lobular and low-grade nonlobular invasive carcinoma of the breast in the candidate genes *TSGs* (*CDH1, CDH3, CDH5, CDH16, E2F-4, CTCF AND TRF2*) at 16q22.1 using MAPH methodology *(33)*. The MAPH probe set included 27 probes, where each gene was represented by at least two probes of different sizes. Twenty-two cases out of 35 informative cases (63%) found to have deletions whereas the remaining 13 did not show copy number changes. This study shows that MAPH is a promising technique in measuring of DNA copy number alterations in malignant tissues. Any genomic loss of heterozygosity in cancer cells is possible and probe sets for scanning the whole genome for detection of deletions or duplications are planned.

Rad et al. (2001) *(34)* also established a MAPH assay for breast cancer on BRCA1 gene, using a set of 32 separate probes that cover all 23 BRCA1 exons and other control regions.

MAPH technique was adapted and successfully applied for quantification of constitutional genomic imbalances in tumor DNA samples. Reid et al. (2003) *(35)* used MAPH to investigate amplifications of *BCR-ABL1* causing chronic myeloid leukemia (CML), as well as extensive deletion of chromosomes 9 and 22 material from the der(9)t(9;22), which are found in 15% of CML patients and associated with the worse disease prognosis. Ten MAPH probes were designed for this study: six probes were designed from the 9q34 and 22q11 regions to map the der(9) deletions; two probes were designed from the *BCR* exon 1 and *ABL1* exon 11 to detect the *BCR-ABL1* amplification; and two probes were designed outside the detected region on the der(9) to be used as control probes in the MAPH data analysis. The CML MAPH assay was applied to DNA extracted from the CML cell line MC3, to a normal lymphoblastoid cell line (HRC575), as well as MC3 "tumor DNA" diluted with HRC575 "normal DNA" to concentrations of 50, 60, 70, and 90%. The der(9) deletions were not found in the normal cell line and were successfully mapped in the CML cell line (MC3). MAPH probes *ABL1*1 and *BRC*1 indicated overrepresentation of the *BCR-ABL1* fusion. Furthermore, der(9) deletions were successfully found in the samples of 90, 80, and 70% concentrations of MC3 DNA. *BCR-ABL1* amplification, revealed in the undiluted MC3 DNA sample by use of MAPH probes *ABL*11 and *BRC*1, remained detectable in all dilutions of MC3 DNA tested. These data demonstrate that MAPH reliably detects both deletions and amplification, even when present in 70% of cells only. Having shown that MAPH may be successfully applied to screen clonal cell populations, the CML MAPH assay with 10 probes was applied to DNA samples isolated from nine CML patients' bone marrow samples. The assay detected all deletions. FISH confirmed all of the above results. To assess the sensitivity of MAPH in quantifying amplifications, two patients, a normal individual and the cell lines MEG-01, SUP-B15, MC3, K562, and KCL22 with different levels of *BCR-ABL1* copy number (1, 2, 3, 5, and 38 copies), were used. In consistency with previous FISH results, MAPH accurately detected the number of copies of the *BCR-ABL1* loci in all of the above cell lines. In this study MAPH assay demonstrated the ability to (i) quantify acquired genomic copy number changes at numerous loci simultaneously with high precision and (ii) perform effectively on DNA samples extracted from fresh or methol/acetic acid-fixed clonal cell populations. Furthermore, the results of this study demonstrated that MAPH is a reproducible high-throughput method suitable for the assessment of genomic imbalances of multiple loci in tumor DNA samples with heterogeneous cell populations at a resolution of 100–300 bp.

MAPH assay was also developed for the detection of copy number changes of *MLH1/MSH2* genes in HNPCC patients (*36*). They created a single MAPH assay consisting of probes from the 19 exons of MLH1 and 16 exons of MSH2, and three control probes. They tested 50 HNPCC patients in whom no point mutations had been found, and detected 10 copy number changes. The authors proposed that since MAPH is a very cost effective method, it could be used to prescreen HNPCC samples by MAPH before screening for point mutations.

MAPH tests have been also developed to screen and identify genetic unbalances of "unknown locations," such as numerical chromosomal abnormalities, loss or gains of subtle chromosomal segments in subtelomeric region easily missed or not visible with conventional cytogenetics, as well as interstitial submicroscopic cryptic abnormalities of unknown location that could be located anywhere in the human genome and they are not easy or impossible to be detected by high-resolution G-banding.

The initial study of establishment and validation of MAPH methodology first demonstrated the identification of numerical abnormalities for 16, 17, 22, X, and Y chromosomes (*19*). Additional numerical abnormalities for chromosomes 13, 15, 18, and 21 were also accurately identified using different set of probes (*22*).

Sismani et al. (2001) (*37*) described the use of MAPH telomeric assay by developing subtelomeric specific amplifiable probes for all human chromosome ends. The MAPH assay accurately analyzed 70 patients with idiopathic mental retardation, 25 unrelated samples with normal karyotype, 20 samples with known subtelomeric chromosomal rearrangements and four samples with know numerical chromosomal abnormalities. FISH analyses confirmed in a blinded parallel study all MAPH findings, showing that the new MAPH telomeric assay can accurately detect numerical chromosomal anomalies, subtle subtelomeric unbalances of unknown locations, that can be easily missed or not be able to see with classical cytogenetics methods due to their small size or pattern similarity.

A year later, another study has established and demonstrated the MAPH subtelomeric assay by constructing a second generation set of 47 MAPH probes with each subtelomeric region represented at least once, so that one gel lane can assay the copy number at all chromosome ends in one person (23). Several positive controls with known chromosomal aberrations were used to assess the sensitivity of the probes and 83 normal controls were used to assess the frequency of polymorphic copy number with no apparent phenotypic effect. Furthermore, a cohort of 37 males with idiopathic mental retardation was used to identify unknown cryptic chromosomal defects near the telomeric regions. Six of them were found to changes in the copy number of a subtelomeric region and were further confirmed by dosage PCR.

Using the same panel of probes, Pickard et al. (2004) (38), screened a group of 69 patients comorbid for mental retardation and psychiatric illness and other positive and negative controls, using MAPH subtelomeric assay. One patient with loss of one copy of the 4q subtelomeric region was found and confirmed by FISH. Additional MAPH probes were designed and determined the extent of the 4q subtelomeric deletion. The identification of such cryptic DNA losses of "unknown locations" associated with certain conditions can identify candidate genes for further study. The above three studies showed that MAPH can be used to screen for unknown subtelomeric region imbalances in a very fast, efficient, effective, and cost effective manner.

Kriek et al. (2004) (39) used MAPH methodology to screen loci known to be involved in mental retardation, such as subtelomeric and pericentromeric regions. Those regions affected in microdeletion syndromes, as well as interstitial genes are randomly spaced throughout the genome. The authors designed several probe sets covering a total of 162 different loci, including 41 subtelomeric probes, five genes near the centromere on the q arm of the acrocentric chromosomes, pericentromeric regions for all chromosomes, 27 probes from 21 genes involved in microdeletion syndromes, 19 probes from genes on chromosome 22 with 1 Mb spacing and 68 other interstitial genes spread throughout the genome. The probe sets were validated with known normal and known abnormal patient samples. Overall, 188 developmentally delayed patients were screened for deletions and duplications at 162 loci, resulting in the detection of 19 copy number changes. From those, ~65% would have not been detected by conventional cytogenetic analysis. A significant fraction (46%) of the rearrangements found to be interstitial, despite the fact that only a limited number of these loci have so far been tested. Such high-resolution duplication/deletion screening by MAPH will help in the future identification of the specific genes that are responsible for mental retardation.

In another recent study by Kriek et al. (2006) (40), 105 patients with developmental delay and/or congenital malformations were screened for copy number changes using a specifically designed MAPH assay. The MAPH assay contained 63 exon-specific single-copy sequences from duplicon-flanked regions (selected from targeted hot spots of genomic instability including some from known disease loci). The same patients were also tested using a set of probes derived from 58 genes outside the duplicons. They identified six cases of copy number variations in the regions flanked by duplicons and two in the region outside the duplicons. In this study two previously undescribed reciprocal duplication of more Williams Beuren syndrome critical region were detected. In addition, they demonstrated that copy number imbalances were more frequent within duplicon-containing regions and provided further evidence that regions flanked by duplicons are enriched for copy number variations.

MAPH has also been demonstrated to be very useful for phenotype-genotype correlations. Aldred et al. (2004) *(41)* used MAPH to define for the first time minimal deletion intervals for all the major phenotypes associated with 2q37 monosomy. They analyzed 20 patients with 2q37.3 monosomy using a MAPH assay containing single copy sequences from 2q37 chromosomal region.

3.2. Microarray MAPH

The introduction of microarrays in MAPH methodology has been a major step towards the advancement of DNA copy-number detection. The first published pilot study on microarray MAPH is based on oligonucleotide PamGene 3-Dimentional Flow-Through microarray platform *(20)*. Gel electrophoresis was replaced by an array of 60mer oligonucleotides complementary to individual MAPH probes. The array was co hybridized with Cy3 labeled probes from test samples and Cy5 labeled probes from reference samples. In this study, the copy number of 6 different probes from *PMP22* gene was assessed and a comparison with gel-based (capillary) MAPH showed a nice correlation of the two platforms in gene dosage determination.

The second array-MAPH pilot study aimed to develop and validate a chromosome X-specific microarray containing a total of 558 target sequences, with median spacing of 238kb over the entire human chromosome X *(21)*. Gel electrophoresis was replaced by single-fluorophore hybridization to an array of PCR amplifiable 500bp target sequences, identical to MAPH probes and comparison to a control panel of normal individuals. DNA samples from normal individuals and patients with known and unknown chromosome X aberrations were analyzed. Deletions and duplications of various sizes were detected and confirmed (**Fig. 13.2**), including an unknown deletion of 23kb, which was detected based on a single probe deviation (**Fig. 13.2C**).

The above data demonstrated the specificity and sensitivity of the two new microarray-based platforms that allowed increasing multiplicity and throughput in locus copy-number assessment, providing an alternative approach, which is expected to contribute significantly to genomic analysis, along with other microarray-based methods.

The main advantages of array-MAPH are derived from probe and primer design, which is based on uniqueness, avoiding polymorphisms and repeats, optimized size (400–600bp), uniform CG% and the option to vary probe spacing on any selected genomic region *(21)*. As a result, besides the obvious gain in flexibility, specificity, sensitivity and resolution, there is also the advantage of easy confirmation: instead of ordering and culturing BAC, PAC or other clones, one can use the existing probe-specific primers to perform PCR-based confirmation for any detected copy-number alteration or, if needed, use the well-established methodology for rapid selection of additional primers from any genomic region *(21)*.

As a methodological approach, microarray MAPH provides means to amplify the quantity of studied genomic sequences, as in ROMA technology *(15)*. Consequently the signal to noise ratio is increased, which is critical for obtaining reliable data *(14,42,43)*. PamChip platform provides improved hybridization kinetics, thereby shortening the microarray hybridization step to less than an hour *(20)*. The use of a single fluorophore in combination with a control panel in amplicon-based array-MAPH *(21)*, allows saving on materials

A. Patient A-2879

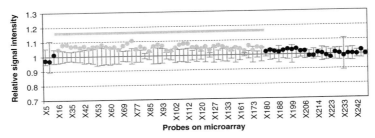

B. Patient 22467

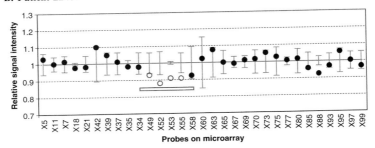

C. Patient A045

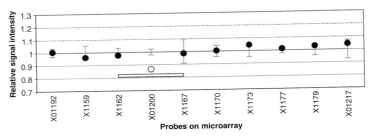

X axis: Probes arranged according to location.

Y axis: log₂(relative signal intensity).

─────── Normalized median value of the signal intensities of probes on the control panel.

○ ● ● Normalized values of fluorescence intensities in the test DNA.

⊥ Tolerance Intervals (*TI90%*) of the control panel for each probe.

─────── Duplicated region, detected by Array-MAPH and confirmed by FISH analysis.

═════ Deleted region detected by array-MAPH.

Fig. 13.2. Array-MAPH chromosome X profiles of patients **A.** A-2879, female with approximately 15 Mb duplication **B.** 22467, male with 1.5 Mb deletion and **C.** A045, male with 23 kb deletion

and analysis time and also gives the flexibility to vary the features of reference samples (control panel), depending on the aims of the project.

However there are certain limitations that at present may prevent microarray MAPH from being actively applied in clinical practice. One of these limitations is the need of two hybridization steps, adding in labor-intensiveness and adds errors to the final analysis. Another source of biases in single fluorophore array-MAPH *(21)* is the comparison of results obtained from different microarray hybridizations. Time and effort is consumed on probe development, especially when dealing with more than 700 loci *(21)*. PamGene microarray-MAPH *(20)* uses specialized equipment and software, which might not be easily accessible by a diagnostic laboratory, even if it acquires microarray facilities, related to array-CGH.

Further optimization is expected to fully reveal the power of microarray MAPH and successfully implement this new technique in a variety of research topics such as high-resolution screening of patients with abnormal phenotype and no genetic findings, detection of microdeletions, microduplications, genotype-phenotype correlations, gene identification and studying genetic variation.

References

1. Battaglia A, Carey JC (1998) Wolf-Hirschhorn syndrome and Pitt-Rogers-Danks syndrome. Am J Med Genet 75:541
2. Donnai D, Karmiloff-Smith A (2000) Williams syndrome: from genotype through to the cognitive phenotype. Am J Med Genet 97:164–171
3. Cassidy SB, Dykens E, Williams CA (2000) Prader-Willi and Angelman syndromes: sister imprinted disorders. Am J Med Genet 97:136–146
4. Knight SJ, Flint J (2000) Perfect endings: a review of subtelomeric probes and their use in clinical diagnosis. J Med Genet 37:401–409
5. Patsalis PC, Evangelidou P, Charalambous S, Sismani C (2004) Fluorescence in situ hybridization characterization of apparently balanced translocation reveals cryptic complex chromosomal rearrangements with unexpected level of complexity. Eur J Hum Genet 12:647–653
6. Kim J, Yu W, Kovalski K, Ossowski L (1998) Requirement for specific proteases in cancer cell intravasation as revealed by a novel semiquantitative PCR-based assay. Cell 94:353–362
7. Kalinina O, Lebedeva I, Brown J, Silver J (1997) Nanoliter scale PCR with TaqMan detection. Nucleic Acid Res 25:1999–2004
8. Kirchhoff M, Rose H, Lundsfeen C (2001) High resolution comparative genomic hybridisation in clinical cytogenefics. J Med Genet 38:740–744
9. Snijders AM, Nowak N, Segraves R, Blackwood S, Brown N, Conroy J, Hamilton G, Hindle AK, Huey B, Kimura K, Law S, Myambo K, Palmer J, Ylstra B, Yue JP, Gray JW, Jain AN, Pinkel D, Albertson DG (2001) Assembly of microarrays for genome-wide measurement of DNA copy number. Nat Genet 29:263–264
10. Albertson DG, Pinkel D. (2003) Genomic microarrays in human genetic disease and cancer. Hum Mol Genet 12:145–152
11. Kraus J, Pantel K, Pinkel D, Albertson DG, Speicher MR (2003) High-resolution genomic profiling of occult micrometastatic tumour cells. Genes Chromosomes Cancer 36:159–166
12. Shaw-Smith C, Redon R, Rickman L, Rio M, Willatt L, Fiegler H, Firth H, Sanlaville D, Winter R, Colleaux L, Bobrow M, Carter NP (2004) Microarray based comparative genomic hybridisation (array-CGH) detects submicroscopic chromosomal deletions and duplications in patients with learning disability/mental retardation and dysmorphic features. J Med Genet 41:241–248
13. Ishkanian AS, Malloff CA, Watson SK et al (2004) A tiling resolution DNA microarray with complete coverage of the human genome. Nat Genet 36:299–303
14. Lucito R, West J, Reiner A et al (2000) Detecting gene copy number fluctuations in tumor cells by microarray analysis of genomic representations. Genome Res 10: 1726–1736

15. Lucito R, Healy J, Alexander J et al (2003) Representational oligonucleotide microarray analysis: a high-resolution method to detect genome copy number variation. GenomeRes 13:2291–2305

16. Zhao X, Li C, Paez JG et al (2004) An integrated view of copy number and allelic alterations in the cancer genome using single nucleotide polymorphism arrays. Cancer Res 64:3060–3071

17. Huang J, Wei W, Zhang J et al (2004) Whole genome DNA copy number changes identified by high density oligonucleotide arrays. Hum Genomics 1:287–299

18. Selzer RR, Richmond TA, Pofahl NJ et al (2005) Analysis of chromosome breakpoints in neuroblastoma at sub-kilobase resolution using fine-tiling oligonucleotide array CGH. Genes Chromosomes Cancer 44:305–319

19. Armour JAL, Sismani C, Patsalis PC, Cross G (2000) Measurements of locus copy number by hybridisation with amplifiable probes. Nucl Acids Res 28:605–609

20. Gibbons B, Datta P, Wu Y, Chan A, Armour J (2006) Microarray-MAPH: accurate array-based detection of relative copy number in genomic DNA. BMC Genomics 7:163

21. Patsalis PC, Kousoulidou L, Männik K, Sismani C, Žilina O, Parkel, S, Puusepp H, Tõnisson N, Palta P, Remm M, Kurg A (2007) Detection of small genomic imbalances using microarray based Multiplex Amplifiable Probe Hybridization (array-MAPH). Eur J Hum Genet 15:162–172

22. Sismani C, Al Armour J, Flint J, Girgalli C, Regan R, Patsalis PC (2001) Screening for subtelomeric chromosomes abnormalities in children with idiopathic mental retardation using multiprobe telomeric FISH and the new MAPH telomeric assay. Eur J Hum Genet 9:527–532

23. Hollox EJ, Atia T, Cross G, Parkin T, Armour JAL (2002) High throughput screening of human subtelomeric DNA for copy number changes using multiplex amplifiable probe hybridisation (MAPH). J Med Genet 39:790–795

24. Akrami SM, Winter RM, Brook JD, Armour JAL (2001) Detection of a large TBX5 deletion in a family with Holt-Oram syndrome. J Med Genet 38:44

25. White SJ, Kalf M, Liu Q, Villerius M, Engelsma D, Kriek M, Vollebregt E, Bakker B, van Ommen GJB, Breuning MH, den Dunnen JT (2002) Comprehensive detection of genomic duplications and deletions in the dmd gene, by use of multiplex amplifiable probe hybridization. Am J Hum Genet 71:365–374

26. White SJ, Sterrenburg E, van Ommen GJB, den Dunnen JT, Breuning MH (2003) An alternative to FISH: detecting deletion and duplication carriers within 24 hours. J Med Genet 40:1–5

27. Dent KM, Dunn DM, Niederhausern AC, Aoyagi AT, Kerr L, Bromberg MB, Hart KJ, Tuohy T, White S, den Dunnen JT, Weiss RB, Flanigan KM (2005) Improved molecular diagnosis of dystrophinopathies in an unselect clinical cohort. Am J Med Genet 30:295–298

28. Buzin CH, Feng J, Yan J, Scaringe W, Liu Q, den Dunnen J, Jerry Mendel JR, Sommer SS (2005) Mutation rates in the dystrophin gene: a hotspot of mutation at a GpG dinucleotide. Hum Mutat 25:177–188

29. Akrami SM, Rowland JS, Taylor GR, Armour JAL (2003) Diagnosis of gene dosage alterations at the PMP22 gene using MAPH. J Med Genet 40:123

30. White SJ, Uitte de Willige S, Verbove D, Politano L, Ginjaar I, Breuning MH, den Dunnen JT (2005) Sarcoglycanopathies and the risk of undetected deletion alleles in diagnosis. Hum Mutat 26:59

31. Vaurs-Barriere C, Bonnet-Dupeyron MN, Combes P et al (2006) Golli-MBP copy number analysis by FISH, QMPSF and MAPH in 195 patients with hypomyelinating leukodystrophies. Ann Hum Genet 70:66–77

32. Combes P, Bonnet-Dupeyron MN, Gauther-Barichard F et al (2006) PLP1 and GPM6B intragenic copy number analysis by MAPH in 262 patients with hypomyelinating leukodystrophies: identification of one partial triplication and two partial deletions of PLP1. Neurogenetics 7:31–37

33. Rakha EA, Armour JAL, Pinder SE, Paish CE, Ellis IO (2005) High-resolution analysis of 16q22.1 in breast carcinoma using DNA amplifiable probes (multiplex amplifiable probe hybridization technique) and immunohistochemistry. Int J Cancer 114:720–729

34. Rad IA, Sharif AL, Raeburn JA, Evans G, Lalloo F, Morrison P, Armour JAL, Cross GS (2001) Detection of BRCA1 whole exon deletions andduplications in breast/ovarian cancer families from UK by Multiplex Amplifiable Probe Hybridisation (MAPH). J Med Genet 38:S22

35. Reid AG, Tarpey PS, Nacheva N (2003) High-resolution analysis of acquired genomic imbalances in bone marrow samples from chronic myeloid leukemia patients by use of multiple short DNA probes. Genes, Chromosomes Cancer 37:282–290

36. Akrami SM, Dunlop MG, Farrington SM, Frayling IM, MacDonald F, Harvey JF, Armour JAL (2005) Screening for exonic copy number mutations at MSH2 and MLH1 by MAPH. Fam Cancer 4:145–149

37. Sismani C (2003) Genetic factors in mental retardation. PhD Thesis, University of Nottingham

38. Pickard BS, Hollox EJ, Malloy MP, Porteous DJ, Blackwood DHR, Armour JAL, Muir WJ (2004) A 4q35.2 subtelomeric deletion identified in a screen of patients with co-morbid psychiatric illness and mental retardation. BMC Med Genet 5:21

39. Kriek M, White SJ, Bouma MC, Dauwerse HG, Hansson KBM, Nijhuis JV, Bakker B, van Ommen GJB, den Dunnen JT, and Breuning MH (2004) Genomic imbalances in mental retardation. J Med Genet 41:249–255

40. Kriek M, White SJ, Szuhai K, Knijnenburg J, van Ommen GJB, den Dunnen JT, Breuning MH (2006) Copy number variation in regions flanked (or unflanked) by duplicons among patients with developmental delay and/or congenital malformations: detection of reciprocal and partial Williams-Beuren duplications. Eur J Hum Genet 14:180–189

41. Aldred MA, Sanford ROC, Thomas NS, Barrow MA, Wilson LC, Brueton LA, Bonaglia MC, Hennekam RCM, Eng C, Dennis NR, Trembath RC (2004) Molecular analysis of 20 patients with 2q37.3 intervals monosomy: definition of minimum deletion intervals for key phenotypes. J Med Genet 41:433–439

42. Lucido R, Nakimura M, West JA, Han Y, Chin K, Jensen K, MacCombie R, Gray JW, Wigler M (1998) Genetic analysis using genomic representations. Proc Natl Acad Sci U S A 95:4487–4492

43. Kennedy GC, Matzuzaki H, Dong C, Liu WM et al (2003) Large-scale genotyping of complex DNA. Nat Biotechnol 21:1233–1237

14

Gene Expression Profiling

Arnis Druka, Robbie Waugh, and Pete Hedley

1. Introduction

Gene expression profiling measures the relative abundance of a large number of individual mRNA species within the context of a total mRNA population that has been isolated and purified from a target biological sample. The technology for achieving this evolved from low-throughput membrane-based probe-to-target hybridization assays (northern and Southern blotting) commonly used in molecular biology labs since the 1980s (reviewed in *1*). Scaling these assays down in size and up in number by redesigning the assay into a "target-to-probe" hybridization has enabled efficient and highly parallel genome-wide gene expression analysis. The technology platforms that emerged are generically called microarrays. A comprehensive review of microarrays, their history, application, and analysis is given by Schena *(2)*.

The goal of gene expression profiling, achieved by microarray analysis, is to aid the biologist in identifying groups of genes that are functionally associated with certain biological processes. "Guilt by association" is a classical approach that is based on correlation analysis of mRNA abundance measures taken from biological samples subjected to various experimental factors (variables or conditions) *(3)*. Typical variables are genotype (e.g., mutant vs. wild type), tissue, time, and treatment, or combinations of these. Visual representation of the results of correlation analysis are frequently dendrograms and "heat-maps" of expression values ordered (clustered) for each gene and/or each condition based on statistical measures of similarity. The underlying data provides the leads for hypothesis development and further experimentation.

In this chapter we have chosen to restrict our discussion to the two current and most commonly used microarray formats: spotted arrays and Affymetrix GeneChips. The basic principles of microarray analysis are outlined in **Fig. 14.1A, B**. As many components of a microarray experiment—e.g., sample choice, preparation and analysis—are largely similar across both of these platforms, we consider these aspects together, but discuss the different technologies separately. We conclude by considering examples and summarize the need for adequate data standards and public access.

From: *Molecular Biomethods Handbook, 2nd Edition.*
Edited by: J. M. Walker and R. Rapley © Humana Press, Totowa, NJ

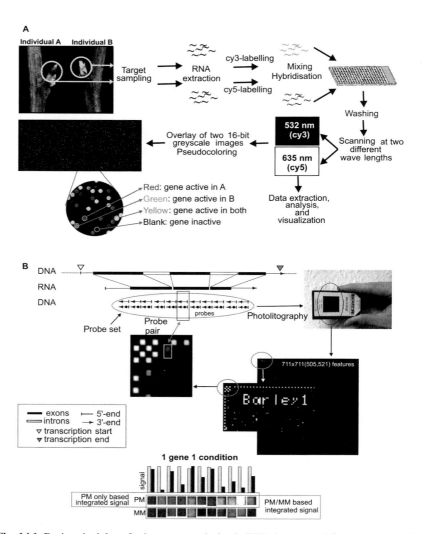

Fig. 14.1 Basic principles of microarray analysis. **A.** RNA is extracted from target samples to be compared (Individual A and B) and is subjected to independent fluorescent labeling (A, Cy5 red, B, Cy3 green). Mixing and hybridization to a pre-prepared spotted microarray followed by washing allows complementary sequences to bind. Relative levels of gene (probe) expression between targets is determined by scanning hybridized arrays at two different wavelengths and analyzing ratios of fluorescent intensities at each spot. **B.** Design principle and expression detection using Affymetrix' expression GeneChip is shown at the top where RNA and DNA sequences are used to design oligonucleotide probes. At the right hand side is a picture of an Affymetrix array. The panels below show scanned images of the 22 K GeneChip features after hybridization showing some of the design elements. They also show the markings (corners, edges and identifier) that are revealed by the Control Oligos (B2). Bottom image and graph shows the probe pairs from a single unigene. The probe pairs are randomly distributed across the microarray, but the 11 PM and 11 MM probes from a single pair are always together. Measurements of the pixel values (bar graphs) for all 22 probes representing an "average" gene, in terms of expression level are shown above the individual probe pairs. In this image the individual features have been brought together to demonstrate variability of the signal difference between PM and MM probes of different probe pairs. Only a few MM probes report a higher signal than PM probe. For genes that are very highly or lowly expressed, this variability is much higher. It was this observation that promoted the development of alternative algorithms for calculation of the expression values.

2. Methods

2.1. Key Components of Experimental Design

Key to the eventual success of a microarray experiment lies in both the selection and implementation of the variables that will yield the most informative data for a given biological question. An appropriate experimental design, which maximises reproducibility and minimises false positive and false negative associations is therefore paramount. Experimental design has been discussed extensively elsewhere *(4)*, and so only some key considerations are summarized here.

2.1.1. Sample Preparation and Replication

A microarray experiment consists of many technically complex stages, all of which have associated errors, albeit to different degrees. Although good experimental practice and application of standard operating procedures can reduce many of these, replication is essential to minimise and assess systematic errors (reviewed in *4*). Technical replication, including multiple representation of genes (probes) on the microarray and repetition of array hybridizations from identical mRNA sources (see Section 2.3), can identify sources of error within protocols. However, applying biological replication from completely independent sample preparations enables application of statistical filtering and extrapolation of biological inference. In some cases, pooling of biological material may be necessary when sample material is limited, but this masks variability, and it remains essential to replicate these pools biologically.

2.1.1.1. Time of Sampling: It is important to consider the possible effects of temporal factors, such as cell cycle, circadian rhythm, photoperiod, and physiological or developmental differences that, if neglected, can generate biases in gene expression level estimates, leading to incorrect interpretation of the results. For example, microarray experiments have shown that at least 6% of Arabidopsis genes are rhythmically expressed during the day/night cycle, with peaks of expression at all different times during the night and the day (reviewed in *5*). In some cases genes that affect a common pathway or process peak at the same time. Thus, just before sunrise, the transcript abundance of many of the genes encoding enzymes in the biochemical pathway that synthesise photoprotective pigments (i.e., the phenylpropanoid pathway) peak, possibly to guarantee the accumulation of sufficient of these pigments in advance of dawn *(6)*. So, harvesting material for a microarray experiment at various times throughout the day will sample different subsets of genes that are regulated by the circadian clock. It is therefore important to schedule sampling at the same time each day.

2.1.1.2. Tissue Complexity: Samples (targets) to be compared may be whole organisms, organs, dissected tissues, specific cells or cell types. Loss of information may be a concern when using whole organisms or organs, compared to dissected tissue or cell types. Genes that appear to be expressed at similar levels in a complex tissue sample may actually be expressed in completely different component cell types and by different degrees (**Fig. 14.2A, B**). Simple logic suggests that lower tissue complexity provides higher spatial resolution and more information. Several approaches have been adopted to sample mRNAs directly from specific cell types, including laser-capture microdissection

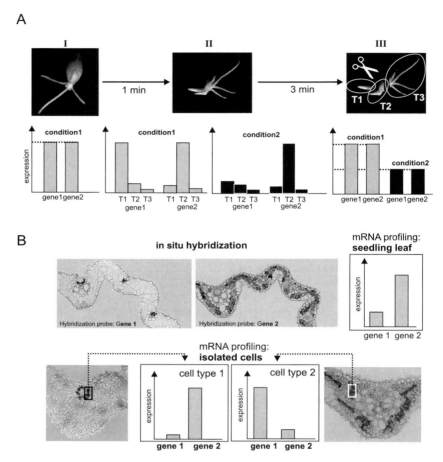

Fig. 14.2. Possible loss of information when profiling complex tissues. **A**. Different complexity levels of the tissues from germinating barley grain are shown with the time required for the dissection. I – the whole grain 4 days after imbibition, II – dissected embryo-derived tissue, III – further dissection of embryo-derived tissues, separating seminal roots, mesocotyl and coleoptile. The bar graphs below show how expression levels of two genes in two conditions can vary under these different tissue complexity situations. Selection of more informative conditions (experimental variables) may justify using simpler sampling procedures. **B**. Cell specificity effect on the detection of gene expression in rice seedling leaves. Expression of Gene1 is restricted to the phloem cells, while Gene2 is expressed in mesophyl. The expression of the two genes may appear different in a complex tissue. But in fact, it is the number of cells expressing these genes that is different. Individual cell isolation methods, such as one shown in the next figure can resolve such situations.

and microsampling *(7)*. In an elegant set of experiments, Birnbaum *(8)* used a series of *Arabidopsis* lines expressing green fluorescent protein under cell type specific promoters to characterize the transcriptomes of specific *Arabidopsis* root cell types (**Fig. 14.3**). Root tissues of transgenic plants at the defined developmental stages were used to generate protoplasts that were separated into fluorescent and nonfluorescent fractions using fluorescence assisted cell sorting. The different fractions were then subjected to expression profiling, providing an important insight into the dynamics of the transcriptomes of individual or groups of root cells.

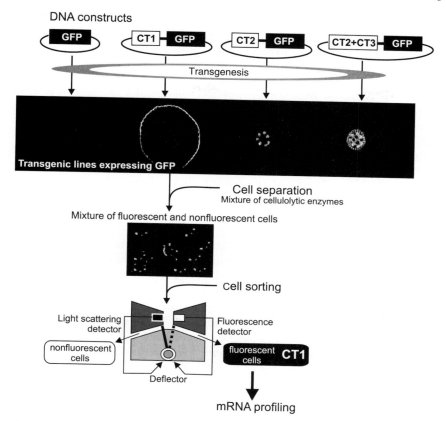

Fig. 14.3. Principle of isolation of specific root cell types as described by Birnbaum et al. (8). The key to this experiment was the transgenic *Arabidopsis* lines expressing Green Fluorescent Protein (GFP) in specific root cells. Expression specificity was achieved by using cell-specific promoters (CT1–CT3 as illustrated in the DNA constructs illustration at the top). In the histological sections the location of GFP expression is shown by the bright white areas. The root tissue cells were enzymatically separated from each other and fractionated into the fluorescent and nonfluorescent fractions using a Fluorescence Assisted Cell Sorting machine (FACS). Cross-sections of rice seedling roots are used to illustrate the principle.

2.2. mRNA Purification

After tissues have been sampled, total RNA (including mRNA) is extracted from the targets of interest, generally now using commercial RNA preparation kits to ensure the RNA is of the highest quality with respect to both integrity and purity. It is highly recommended that RNA intended for use in microarray experiments is column purified (e.g., Qiagen RNeasy, http://www1.qiagen.com/). Before labeling, RNA is quality control (QC) checked using spectrophotometry and gel electrophoresis or commonly by the Bioanalyzer Lab-on-a-Chip system (http://www.chem.agilent.com/).

2.3. Spotted Microarrays

Microarrays are informative because they are effective at measuring the abundance of individual messenger RNA (mRNA) molecules in a complex sample. These measures are then interpreted as an indirect measure of relative gene activity between samples. The primary advantage of using microarrays for this process is that many thousands of genes can be assayed simultaneously. Spotted microarrays were the first true microarrays to be developed (9).

2.3.1. Array Generation

The basic principles of spotted, or 2-color, microarrays are outlined in **Fig. 14.1A**. The first stage is the generation of high-quality arrays. Today, several commercial vendors, including Agilent (http://www.chem.agilent.com/), manufacture off-the-shelf and custom arrays in this format for many commonly studied species. Agilent uses patented Ink Jet *in situ* Synthesis (IJISS) to build oligonucleotide sequences (60 mers), or probes, which represent genes of interest, directly onto the surface of modified glass slides. This produces very high-quality arrays with extremely flexible formatting depending upon the number of genes to be studied, with up to 240,000 gene sequences represented on a single slide.

For organisms where no commercial arrays are available, custom arrays can be generated using robotic deposition. Dedicated microarray robots, from companies such as Genetix (http://www.genetix.co.uk/), can array many thousands of probes (< 20,000 per slide), which can either be specifically designed oligonucleotides or fragments of genes (usually out of EST collections) generated by the polymerase chain reaction (PCR). Glass slides, onto which the arrays are deposited, are commercially available (e.g., Schott Nexterion, http://www.schott.com/; UltraGaps, http://catalog2.corning.com/) and have different modified surface chemistries to allow binding of different probe types. Probe spot sizes are usually in the order of 1/10 mm in diameter, thereby allowing moderate to high density arrays to be produced.

2.3.2. Target Labeling, Hybridization, and Microarray Scanning

Spotted microarrays rely upon fluorescent detection of interactions between sample targets and the gene fragments (probes) immobilized on the microarray substrate. As RNA is highly susceptible to degradation, owing to its single-stranded structure, it is converted into double-stranded complementary DNA (cDNA) by reverse transcription. During this enzymatic process, fluorescent dye molecules are directly incorporated into the cDNA or indirectly via chemical linkage. Excess dye is removed using column purification and the efficiency of dye incorporation is determined spectrophotometrically. Commercial labeling kits are now available that have very high sensitivity (e.g., Array900, http://www.genisphere.com/) and therefore require small quantities of target RNA (less than 1 μg), an extremely important consideration for analyzing dissected samples.

With spotted microarrays, the relative expression profiles of two targets (samples A and B in **Fig. 14.1A**) are compared on a single array. This is achieved by labeling each target with a different dye, each of which has a specific excitation wavelength and can subsequently be detected independently (represented as red [A] and green [B]).

Following fluorescent labeling, the two targets to be compared are mixed and applied to the surface of the array. Overnight hybridization enables the labeled target molecules to specifically bind to complementary gene probe sequences. This may be performed manually, by simply applying a glass cover slip and incubating overnight at a predetermined hybridization temperature for optimal binding, or using an automated hybridization station (e.g., HS400 Pro, http://www.tecan.com/). Unbound target is removed by stringent washing procedures and the array is dried ready for scanning.

Detection of bound target is achieved using a specialised microarray scanner, such as GenePix (http://www.moleculardevices.com/), which scans the array area sequentially with a laser at each wavelength corresponding to the two dyes and at high resolution (~1/100 mm). Independent images are therefore generated, which can be false-colored (red and green), to enable visualization of relative gene expression levels of each target sample for every gene probe (**Fig. 14.1A**).

2.4. Affymetrix GeneChip Arrays

Affymetrix has for some time been one of the leading companies in microarray development and production. By the end of 2006 there were over 7,000 scientific publications that use or review this technology *(10)*. The company has invested in the development of instrumentation, standardized assays and reagents, as well as data management and analysis tools, arguably offering a complete microarray solution.

2.4.1. Array Fabrication

The basic building blocks of Affymetrix GeneChip microarrays are 25-base long oligodeoxynucleotides (probes) that are synthesized at specific locations (features) on a coated quartz surface by photolithography *(10,11)*. Over a million features per microarray are usually available for the probe synthesis, allowing multiple (typically 22) probes per gene (**Fig. 14.1B**). Eleven of these (PM probes) are perfectly complimentary to the mRNA sequence of the representative gene (often called the "exemplar"). The remaining 11 mismatch (MM) probes have a noncomplementary middle base designed to detect and eliminate any false or contaminating signal within the gene expression measurement. The assumption is that the MM probe will hybridize to nonspecific sequences (background) as effectively as the PM probe, thus allowing spurious signals to be quantified and subtracted. This logic is incorporated into the statistical algorithms that estimate a single expression value using all 22 probes from the probe set. However, there is a well-founded opinion, that MM probe signals are actually poor background estimators. This comes from the frequency of observations where MM values are higher than PM values. This has led to the development of alternative statistical algorithms, where MM signal is not used for the calculation of relative expression values *(12)*.

2.4.2. Target Labeling, Hybridization, and Microarray Scanning

For Affymetrix GeneChips, the labeling process and signal generation is different from that for the spotted arrays, the main differences being synthesis and labeling of cRNA with biotin, followed by a 2-step signal enhancement procedure. Standard Affymetrix target labeling starts with first strand cDNA synthesis, which involves annealing a $T7(dT)_{24}$ primer to the poly(A) mRNA. The $T7(dT)_{24}$ primer consists of two domains; a promoter for the phage T7 DNA-dependent RNA polymerase and an oligo dT tract to bind to the polyA tail of mRNA. Annealed mRNA is reverse transcribed into cDNA followed by second DNA strand synthesis. The next step is *in vitro*-transcription biotin labeling (IVT labeling), which involves synthesising cRNA from the double-stranded cDNA using biotin labeled ribonucleotides and T7 RNA polymerase. The resulting cRNA is cleaned up and fragmented. The hybridization cocktail contains fragmented labeled cRNA, a control oligo (B2) and "spiked in" controls. Hybridization, washing and staining is set up as an automated process using the Affymetrix GeneChip Fluidics Station 400. Staining to reveal quantitative hybridization of target to probe involves treatment with a streptavidin-R-phycoerythrin conjugate (streptavidin binds to the biotin, that is incorporated in the cRNA), followed by biotinylated antistreptavidin antibody treatment and a second round of streptavidin-R-phycoerythrin conjugate binding to amplify the signal. Scanning is again an automated process conducted using an Affymetrix GeneChip scanner.

2.5. Data Acquisition and Analysis

In both types of array the output is a scanned image. However, scanned image visualization only indicates general trends in gene expression. To obtain accurate estimates of the relative gene expression profiles of many thousands of probes, dedicated microarray software is required. The initial software used is for data acquisition (e.g., GenePix Pro (http://www.moleculardevices.com/), which identifies all of the probes on each array and extracts intensity values for both the spot/feature and the local background, for each labeled target (i.e., for two in spotted arrays). Poor quality arrays, spots and features can be flagged at this point and removed from downstream analysis.

Data from the acquisition process is then generally loaded into dedicated analysis software, such as Genespring (http://www.chem.agilent.com/). Microarray data analysis is complex and has been described in detail elsewhere *(13)*. Essentially, array data is normalized to account for technical variation in labeling between the two dyes over the dynamic range of the scanning, and to allow comparison between different microarrays in the same experiment (which could potentially be hundreds of arrays). Data from replicate samples can then be combined, which enables statistical analysis (such as Student's *t*-test, principle components analysis (PCA) and analysis of variance (ANOVA)) to be carried out. Statistically significant data can then be filtered and lists of potential candidate genes for the biological process identified. Therefore from many thousands of genes on the array, manageable numbers (10s to 100s) can be taken forward for validation assays.

2.5.1. Processing the Gene Expression Matrix

The minimal gene expression matrix consists of the expression values of every gene for every condition, gene names (probe set names) and condition names. This is sufficient for mathematical analysis, but to extract meaningful biological information more data describing genes (rows) and conditions (column) may be necessary. Such information when provided as additional rows and columns in the matrix is called an extended or annotated gene expression matrix. Depending on whether annotations are taken into account from the very beginning or not, analysis of the expression matrix is termed either supervised or unsupervised. The goal of supervised analysis may be to identify sets of genes that are diagnostic for a certain set of conditions and uses the annotation information. Here the annotations are used to define the criteria that group the conditions. In contrast, unsupervised analysis ignores annotations at the initial phase. Instead it is the analysis of the data that groups genes or conditions, commonly achieved using some sort of clustering analysis (e.g., principle coordinate analysis). Annotations subsequently determine whether the identified groups of genes are enriched in functionally related categories.

In reality, combinations of supervised and unsupervised analyzes are often used. Unsupervised analysis (clustering) is generally known as data mining or exploratory data analysis, while supervised analysis is hypothesis driven. It is however important to remember that computational analysis and information processing are only the first step towards knowledge acquisition, and follow-up lab experiments are needed to accept or reject erected hypotheses.

3. Applications

Arrays are readily regarded as the most cost-efficient means to identify putative gene targets. There are now thousands of published examples of where they have been used to identify candidate genes for a given biological process and we refer the reader to the primary literature for some excellent examples *(14,15)*. Here we summarize three types of experiment that illustrate the wide use of gene expression profiling.

3.1. Identification of Genes Involved in Dormancy Break in Raspberry

The process of dormancy and dormancy break is poorly understood in many perennial plant species, but it is known that the physiological status of buds outside the growing season determines the potential harvest of soft fruit crops, including raspberry *(16)*. Mazzitelli and colleagues used a microarray approach to help identify genes and their associated metabolic pathways, which could potentially be involved in this process *(16)*. As no commercial microarrays, or even large numbers of gene sequences, were available for raspberry, they generated libraries of cDNA clones (representing expressed RNA species) at critical dormancy stages. These formed the basis for the generation of a custom raspberry microarray. PCR was used to generate ~5,000 anonymous (unsequenced) cDNA fragments that were purified and spotted as probes onto modified glass slides using a robotic spotter. Each probe was spotted in triplicate to allow for any technical variation during processing.

An experimental design was devised that provided the most efficient use of the microarrays and optimized comparisons between samples (**Fig. 14.4**). Samples of raspberry buds were collected every week for a 15-week period over the winter and early spring, flash-frozen and stored at −80°C to preserve RNA integrity. RNA was extracted from pooled bud samples (owing to their small size), labeled, and hybridized to the custom raspberry arrays. The entire experiment was replicated to allow downstream statistical analysis. Data was extracted from each of the processed raspberry microarrays and loaded into Genespring analysis software for normalization. Statistical analysis (ANOVA and PCA) identified probes with the most significant expression profiles corresponding to transition between dormancy states (**Fig. 14.1A**). Sets of probes for each expression pattern (approx 100 of each) were subsequently sequenced and compared to public databases of known genes to assign potential biological function. Many raspberry probes were found to be closely related to genes whose products have known roles in dormancy physiology in model species, advocating the microarray approach. However, several novel genes were also identified that had no previously reported significance in this process. Thus, using this straightforward and relatively low investment approach, Mazzitelli and colleagues generated temporal gene expression profiles over the most

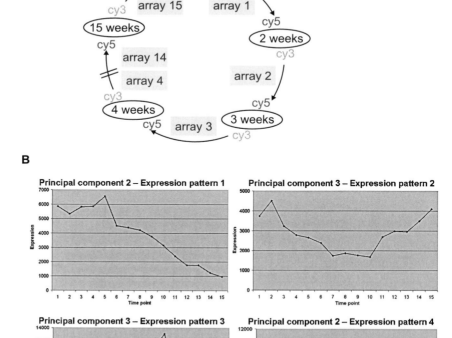

Fig. 14.4. Application of spotted microarrays to gene expression profiling during dormancy in raspberry buds. **A.** Loop-type experimental design, whereby consecutive time-points (weeks), labeled with different dyes, were compared on individual microarrays (1–15). Panel **B.** shows expression patterns (1–4), representing primary changes. These were derived from analysis of variance (ANOVA) and principle components analysis (PCA). They corresponded directly to major phases in dormancy determined through physiological characterisation (weeks 1–7 = endodormant; weeks 8–15 = paradormant), thereby directly identifying important genes in the process.

important stages of dormancy "phase change" identified by physiological studies and highlighted a group of candidate genes whose expression profiles were highly correlated with this physiological process. This list of putative candidate genes is the subject of further study.

3.2. Identification of Genes Associated with Host–Pathogen Interactions

To provide new insights in the understanding of compatibility and incompatibility in host–pathogen interactions, Caldo and colleagues designed and performed the expression profiling experiment outlined in **Fig. 14.5**. The aim of the experiment

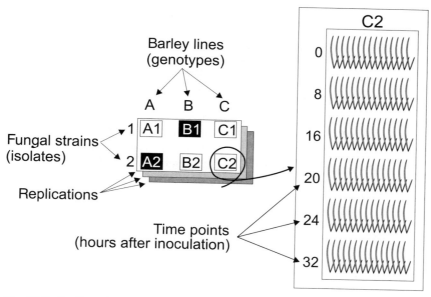

Fig. 14.5. Outline of the mRNA profiling experiment to identify genes involved in barley plant interaction with the powdery mildew fungus. Three barley cultivars (A, B and C) were challenged with two fungal isolates *(1,2)*. Compatible interactions (i.e., those where disease develops) are shown in white boxes, incompatible (i.e., no disease) in black. The interaction type is determined by the barley combination of plant resistance gene and fungal avirulence gene. In this case, combinations of barley carrying different resistance genes and different fungal avirulence genes were tested. Samples were taken at 6 time points (experiment C2; 0, 8, 16, 20, 24, 32h, 15 seedlings each), and the whole experiment was replicated 3 times. This provided a dataset consisting of 108 experimental units (GeneChips)(2 strains X 3 genotypes X 3 replications X 6 time points). Rigorous statistical analysis was applied to each of the 22,792 probe sets on the Barley1 GeneChip. The analysis included terms for the effects of genotype, isolate, time point, and all interactions between these 3 factors, as well as random effects for replications and random interactions corresponding to whole-plot, split-plot, and split-split-plot experimental units, ultimately leading to the identification of 14 genes.

was to identify genes whose average expression between compatible and incompatible interactions of the barley plant with powdery mildew fungus varied significantly across time, as well as those involved in pathways that distinguish *Mla*-specified *Rar1*-dependent from *Rar1*-independent interactions *(17)*.

Caldo and colleagues observed increased levels of defence-related transcripts, but found no difference in transcript accumulation up to 16h after infection (hai) between incompatible and compatible interactions. This was consistent with observations that fungal attachment and germination are accompanied by the release of proteins, carbohydrates, lipids, glycoproteins, and peptides from the spores that trigger general host defence responses. However, in incompatible interactions the expression of some of these genes increased or remained steady from 16 to 32hai. This suggested that one of the outcomes of recognition of a cognate avirulence effector by the host is the maintenance of increased levels of defence-related transcripts, consistent with the phenomenon of induced resistance. Delivery and recognition of mildew fungus avirulence effectors most likely occurs during membrane-to-membrane contact after penetration and during early haustorial development.

As a result, the difference between expression can only be seen after 16 hpi. In these experiments 14 genes were identified that are potentially involved in *Mla*-specified *Rar1*-dependent and -independent barley interactions; they are now being assessed using alternative functional analyses.

3.3. Combining Expression Profiling with Genetics

In 1994 J. Damerval et al. *(18)*, in their paper "Quantitative trait loci underlying gene product variation: a novel perspective for analyzing regulation of genome expression" described a method to "dissect the genetic architecture of quantitative variation of numerous gene products simultaneously." They concluded that "such a methodology might help understand the architecture of regulatory networks and the possible adaptive or phenotypic significance of polymorphism in the genes involved" (citations from *18*). About a decade later this approach, termed "the genetics of gene expression" or "genetical genomics" (GG) *(19)*, has become a standard for the dissection of genetic mechanisms underlying phenotypic variation. The development of large scale mRNA profiling platforms, high throughput genotyping and genome sequencing have been key factors in developing this approach (for the reviews see *20,21*).

The basis of GG emerges from comparisons of mRNA abundance between different genotypes of the same species. Such comparisons revealed that hundreds or even thousands of genes are differentially expressed in a genotype-dependent manner and considerable research effort is currently focussed on identifying and understanding the underlying causes. GG involves expression profiling individuals from an experimental mapping population derived from a cross between two distinct genotypes (parents). The resulting mRNA abundance measurements in each of the progeny is then considered a "phenotype" (referred to as an expression QTL or eQTL), which can be analyzed using the well established statistical tools of genetic analysis.

Several groups have recently applied this approach to plants *(22–24)*. These studies have shown that for a given proportion of genes, mRNA abundance values unambiguously fall into two easily definable classes. When this happens, these can effectively be treated the same way as DNA polymorphisms (i.e., as a binary (Mendelian or discrete) trait, **Fig. 14.6A)** *(25)*. However, for the majority

---

Fig. 14.6. (continued) all nonsignificant associations. This is usually determined by applying permutation tests. The 'best marker' for the trait is determined by bootstrap analyzes and assigned the amount of genetic variation that it contributes to the overall trait. In this case, Marker 4 is most closely associated and contributes ~60% of the observed trait variation. P1, P2, indicates parental values; cM, centiMorgan (i.e., measure of genetic distance), LRS, likelihood ratio statistic; LOD, Logarithm of the Odds statistic. **B**. Dissecting the genetic variation in mRNA abundance observed using microarray analysis of a segregating population using QTL mapping. By using a segregating population it is possible to determine whether the observed difference in mRNA abundance between two parental lines is caused by a sequence difference within the gene itself or close to it (*cis*-eQTL) or to a factor from a different location (*trans* or distal eQTL). If it is possible to map both the gene itself (a binary trait) and the variation in the abundance of mRNA expressed from that gene (a quantitative trait) onto the chromosomes (as above) then *cis*- and *trans*-regulation can be easily differentiated. If they colocalize then it is likely that variation either in, or close to the gene itself, is the cause of the observed difference (left hand diagram). However if they do not then regulation is likely caused by a trans-acting factor that controls the expression of the target gene (right hand diagram). Transcription factors are strong candidates for *trans*-acting factors.

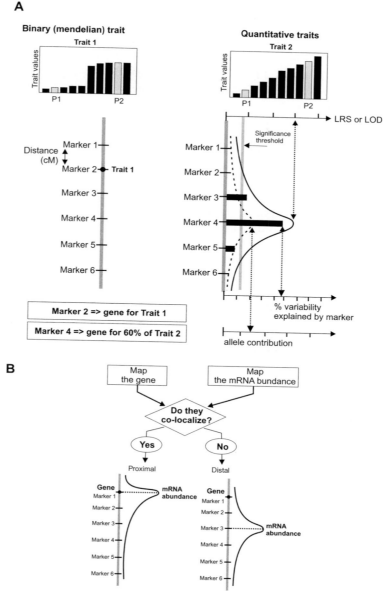

Fig. 14.6. Trait value distributions and linkage mapping parameters for binary (mendelian) and quantitative traits (**A**). The histograms show the distribution of scores for two traits, with the parents colored grey and other members of the population black. For trait 1 the population can be easily split into two groups (i.e., two classes, high and low, = binary). For trait 2 the distribution is continuous. This is the expectation for a quantitative or polygenic trait. The grey vertical lines below the histograms represent a linear chromosome of a plant, with black intersecting lines defined as gene-based markers. These can be used to follow the inheritance of the surrounding chromosome segments in a population of plants. The distance between the markers is given as a recombination measure termed a centiMorgan. For trait 1, the binary score of the trait shows exactly the same inheritance pattern in the population as Marker 2. Marker 2 could therefore be a candidate gene for trait 1 (however this is unlikely given the fairly large number of other unknown genes that will also be inherited with Marker 2). Similar logic, but with more mapping parameters, is applied when dealing with trait 2, the quantitative trait. In this case the gene controlling the trait does not map clearly to a single location along the chromosome. Instead statistical approaches are used to identify its most likely position, which is indicated here as the point in the curve with the highest statistical association with the trait (calculated as a Likelyhood ratio or LOD statistic). As statistical analyzes are used to identify the location of the trait genes, a significance threshold (grey vertical line parallel to chromosome) is applied that provides a measure for declaring

of genes, their mRNA abundance value distribution is continuous, resembling that of a quantitative phenotypic trait. By applying standard QTL mapping procedures to the mRNA abundance "phenotype," these studies revealed that many genes have eQTL peaks linked to the gene itself (which are called *cis*-eQTL) (**Fig. 14.6B**). However, for many genes eQTL are observed that are not at the same position on the genome as the underlying gene, suggesting the presence of a genetic factor that controls the mRNA abundance of the studied gene (i.e., a trans-eQTL). In general terms, *cis*-regulation reflects differences in the local sequence elements controlling the expression of the studied gene while transregulation represents regulators (or "key drivers") that control the expression of several-to-many other genes (including the studied gene).

Not unexpectedly, exploiting the potential of GG in crop plants lags behind model organisms (especially those with fully sequenced genomes). However the potential of GG was nicely demonstrated by Schadt and colleagues *(26)* who developed a model to link genetic loci, gene expression and phenotypic traits. Different sets of mRNA profiling data, extensive genotyping data, physiological trait data and the almost complete genome sequence of both of the parents used to develop the recombinant inbred mapping population, were combined to identify new causal genes controlling obesity. A similar approach is being taken in a number of plant species to unravel the underlying genetic determinants of several quantitative traits.

4. Data Standards and Sharing

Public access to microarray data will have a profound impact on the functional genomics field. The sheer amount and multifaceted nature of the data generated even from a simple profiling experiment can seldom be fully exploited by a single individual or research group. Public access to the datasets provides an opportunity to generate novel information by combining data from separate experiments. Availability of data is also critical for planning experiments or to cross-validate existing experimental data. Policies and recommendations have and are being developed to deal with the practice and ethics of data sharing (http://datasharing.net). Such regulations will inevitably be faced by those who would consider publishing results from large scale mRNA profiling experiments in high impact journals. Submission of raw, properly described, expression data to one of the major publicly accessible databases; Gene Expression Omnibus (GEO, http://www.ncbi.nlm.nih.gov/geo/) *(27)*, or ArrayExpress (http://www.ebi.ac.uk/arrayexpress/) *(28)* is therefore required.

Promoting the sharing of high quality, well annotated data within the life sciences community is one of the activities of The Microarray Gene Expression Data (MGED) Society *(29)*. The society's major focus is on development and distribution of the standards for microarray and other large scale experiment data annotation. The best known project pursued by this group is MIAME, which stands for "Minimum Information About a Microarray Experiment" *(30)*. It describes what is needed to enable the unambiguous interpretation of the results of an experiment and, if necessary, how to accurately reproduce the entire experiment.

Accumulating concerns regarding reproducibility and quality of microarray data has been addressed by another initiative, the MicroArray Quality Control (MAQC) project. Under this project, sets of experiments were performed in different institutions to assess the level of "inter-platform consistency" (cited from *31*). Projects like GeneNetwork (www.genenetwork.org) *(32)* and MetNet (http://metnet.vrac.iastate.edu) *(33)* are excellent examples of the very welcome trend to integrate microarray along with a variety of other biological data into a common knowledgebase.

5. Final Words

With appropriately designed experiments that are focussed on addressing clear biological questions, gene expression profiling, largely through correlation analysis, excels at providing leads for further investigation. However, it should be emphasized that even if the number of potentially false "leads" is somehow minimized, the results of such correlation analyzes do not imply causality regarding the identified genes and the inferred biological process. As a result, most agree that this holistic technology is simply a first step in the detailed, and most often reductionist, analysis of a biological process or response. All agree that the technology is immensely powerful—in the right hands.

References

1. Stoughton RB (2005) Applications of DNA microarrays in biology. Annu Rev Biochem 74:53–82
2. Schena M (2003) Microarray analysis. Wiley-Liss, New Jersey, USA.
3. Eisen MB, Spellman PT, Brown PO, Botstein D (1998) Cluster analysis and display of genome-wide expression patterns. Proc Natl Acad Sci U S A 95(25):14, 863–14868
4. Allison DB, Cui X, Page GP, Sabripour M (2006) Microarray data analysis: from disarray to consolidation and consensus. Nat Rev Gen 7:55–65
5. Eriksson ME, Millar AJ (2003) The Circadian Clock. A plants best friend in a spinning world. Plant Physiology 132:732–738
6. Harmer SL, Hogenesch JB, Straume M, Chang HS, Han B, Zhu T, Wang X, Kreps JA, Kay SA (2000) Orchestrated transcription of key pathways in Arabidopsis by the circadian clock. Science 290:2110–2113
7. Galbraith DW, Birnbaum K, (2006) Global Studies of Cell Type-Specific Gene Expression in Plants. Annu Rev Plant Biol 57:451–475
8. Birnbaum K, Shasha DE, Wang JY, Jung JW, Lambert JM, Galbraith DW, Benfey PN (2003) A gene expression map of the Arabidopsis root. Science 302(5652):1956–1960
9. Schena M, Shalon D, Davis RW, Brown PO (1995) Quantitative monitoring of gene expression patterns with a complementary DNA microarray. Science 270(5235):467–70
10. Detailed information related to different aspects of the Affymetrix Genechip Technology, including, relevant references, platform design, instrumentation, reagents and analytical tools, can be found at: http://www.affymetrix.com/. And www.affymetrix.com/support/technical/manual/expression_manual.affx
11. Fodor SP, Read JL, Pirrung MC, Stryer L, Lu AT, Solas D (1991) Light-directed, spatially addressable parallel chemical synthesis. Science 251(4995):767–773
12. Irizarry RA et al (2003) Exploration, normalization, and summaries of high density oligonucleotide array probe level data. Biostatistics 4(2):249–264
13. Causton HC, Quackenbush J, Brazma A (eds.) (2003) Analysis of gene expression data matrices. In: Microarray gene expression data analysis. Blackwell, Oxford, UK. pp. 71–75

14. Leonhardt N, Kwak JM, Robert N, Waner D, Leonhardt G, Schroeder JI (2004) Microarray expression analyses of arabidopsis guard cells and isolation of a recessive abscisic acid hypersensitive protein phosphatase 2C mutant. Plant Cell 16:596–615

15. Vanneste S, Rybel BD, Beemster GTS, Ljung K, De Smet I, Van Isterdael G, Naudts M, Iida R, Gruissem W, Tasaka M, Inzé D, Fukaki H, Beeckman T (2005) Cell cycle progression in the pericycle is not sufficient for solitary root/IAA14-mediated lateral root initiation in *Arabidopsis thaliana*. Plant Cell 17:3035–3050

16. Mazzitelli L, Hancock RD, Haupt S, Walker PG, Pont SDA, McNicol J, Cardle L, Morris J, Viola R, Brennan R, Hedley PE, Taylor MA (2006) Coordinated gene expression during phases of dormancy release in raspberry (Rubus idaeus L.) buds. J Exp Bot 58(5):1035–1045

17. Caldo RA, Nettleton D, Wise RP (2004) Interaction-dependent gene expression in Mla-specified response to barley powdery mildew. Plant Cell 16(9):2514–2528

18. Damerval C, Maurice A, Josse JM, de-Vienne D (1994) Quantitative trait loci underlying gene product variation: a novel perspective for analyzing regulation of genome expression, Genetics 137:289–301

19. Jansen RC, Nap JP (2001) Genetical genomics: the added value from segregation. Trends Genet 17(7):388–391

20. Williams RW (2006) Expression genetics and the phenotype revolution. Mamm Genome 17(6):496–502

21. Rockman MV, Kruglyak L (2006) Genetics of global gene expression. Nat Rev Genet 7(11):862–872

22. Doerge RW (2002) Mapping and analysis of quantitative trait loci in experimental populations. Nat Rev Genet 3(1):43–52

23. West MAL, Kim K, Kliebenstein DJ, van Leeuwen H, Michelmore RW, Doerge RW, St.Clair DA (2007) Global eQTL mapping reveals the complex genetic architecture of transcript level variation in arabidopsis genetics. Genetics 106.06497

24. Druka A, Muehlbauer G, Druka I, Caldo R, Baumann U, Rostoks N, Schrelber A, Wise R, Close TC, Kleinhofs A, Graner A, Schulman A, Langridge P, Sato K, Hayes P, McNicol J, Marshall DF, Waugh R (2006) An atlas of gene expression from seed to seed through barley development. Funct Integr Genomics 6(3):202–21

25. Luo ZW, Potokina E, Druka A, Wise R, Waugh R, Kearsey MJ (2007) SFP genotyping from Affymetrix arrays is robust but largely detects cis-acting expression regulators. Genetics 176(2):789–800

26. Schadt EE, Lamb J, Yang X, Zhu J, Edwards S, GuhaThakurta D, Sieberts SK, Monks S, Reitman M, Zhang C, Lum PY, Leonardson A, Thieringer R, Metzger JM, Yang L, Castle J, Zhu H, Kash SF, Drake TA, Sachs A, Lusis AJ (2005) An integrative genomics approach to infer causal associations between gene expression and disease. Nat Genet 37(7):710–717

27. Barrett T, Suzek TO, Troup DB, Wilhite SE, Ngau W, Ledoux P, Rudnev D, Lash AE, Fujibuchi W, Edgar R (2006) NCBI GEO: mining tens of millions of expression profiles – database and tools update. Nucleic Acids Res 33:D562–6

28. ArrayExpress (http://www.ebi.ac.uk/arrayexpress/)

29. Ball CA, Brazma A (2006) MGED standards: work in progress. OMICS 10(2):138–144

30. Brazma A, Hingamp P, Quackenbush J, Sherlock G, Spellman P, Stoeckert C, Aach J, Ansorge W, Ball CA, Causton HC, Gaasterland T, Glenisson P, Holstege FCP, Kim IF, Markowitz V, Matese JC, Parkinson H, Robinson A, Sarkans U, Schulze-Kremer S, Stewart J, Taylor R, Vilo J, Vingron M (2001) Minimum information about a microarray experiment (MIAME) – toward standards for microarray data. Nat Genet 29(4):365–37

31. Shi L et al (2006) The MicroArray Quality Control (MAQC) project shows inter- and intraplatform reproducibility of gene expression measurements. Nat Biotechnol 24(9):1151–1161

32. Chesler EJ, Lu L, Wang J, Williams RW, Manly KF (2004) WebQTL: rapid exploratory analysis of gene expression and genetic networks for brain and behavior. Nat Neurosci 7(5):485–486

33. Yang Y, Engin L, Wurtele ES, Cruz-Neira C, Dickerson JA (2005) Integration of metabolic networks and gene expression in virtual reality. Bioinformatics 21(18):3645–3650

15

Comparative Genomic Hybridization in Clinical and Medical Research

Peng-Hui Wang, Yann-Jang Chen, and Chi-Hung Lin

1. Introduction

Cytogenetic research has had a major impact on the field of medicine, especially in oncology and reproductive medicine, providing an insight into the frequency of chromosomal abnormalities that occur during gametogenesis, embryonic development, and tumor development (1). This is well emphasized by the continuing focus on genetic abnormalities that are associated with, as well as probably responsible for, tumor origin, tumor progression, spontaneous abortions, and congenital anomalies. However, information on recurrent chromosomal aberrations in solid tumors and in some hematological cancer is still limited. The growth of solid tumor in culture for cytogenetic analysis is poor and is compounded by low mitotic indices (2). Often the specimens are contaminated with bacterial and other microbial agents and might contain large regions of necrotic tissue. In addition, the major clone that does grow might not reflect its true representation in the tumor in vivo, where multiple subclones exist with complex chromosomal alterations, making identification of primary genetic changes difficult. Furthermore, solid-tumor metaphase chromosomes often have poor morphology (1). A newly described molecular-cytogenetic technique that does not rely on growth of the tumor in culture might well accelerate the rate at which perturbed chromosomal regions can be cytogenetically identified and molecular-genetically characterized in solid tumors (2). In the past decade, fluorescence *in situ* hybridization (FISH) has significantly improved the cytogenetic analysis of tumors. FISH uses specific chromosomal probes, usually composed of cloned fragments of DNA (3). These probes will anneal only to their matching complementary DNA sequences on target chromosomes and can accurately detect and target one specific gene or chromosome region at a time.

However, the application of FISH in cytogenetic analysis leaves the majority of the genome unexamined (4). Now, these limitations can be circumvented through the use of molecular cytogenetic approaches referred to as new FISH-based technologies, including reverse FISH, multiplex FISH (M-FISH), spectral karyotyping (SKY), comparative genomic hybridization (CGH)

From: *Molecular Biomethods Handbook, 2nd Edition.*
Edited by: J. M. Walker and R. Rapley © Humana Press, Totowa, NJ

analysis, and matrix or microarray-CGH (M-CGH) *(4)*. These technologies have bridged the gap between molecular genetics and conventional cytogenetics. The combination of traditional cytogenetic techniques with molecular-genetic methodologies has added a new and powerful dimension to human genetics. Although the information derived using reverse FISH is highly informative, the procedure is technically demanding and requires specialized micromanipulation equipment to microdissect the region of interest from abnormal chromosomes *(3)*. Among these technologies, CGH has provided an unparalleled insight into the nature of chromosome imbalance in disease development and progression. CGH-based technology is able to discover and map genomic regions for chromosomal gains or losses in a single experiment without any prior information on the chromosomal aberration in question *(5)*. This ability addresses many of the deficiencies of FISH and conventional cytogenetic analyses. CGH produces a map of DNA sequence copy number changes as a function of chromosomal location throughout the entire genome *(6)*. In a typical CGH experiment, genomic DNA from tumor and normal tissue is separately labeled with different fluorochromes (green color for tumor and red for normal control); these differently labeled DNA probes are hybridized simultaneously to metaphase chromosome spreads prepared from normal individuals *(7)*. In addition to different fluorochromes for labeling (in the direct method), haptens (in the indirect method) are also frequently used as labeling dyes because of their flexibility and cost-efficiency. CGH is also performed with differentially labeled normal DNA as a reference standard for data analysis. Detailed analysis is performed using a sensitive monochrome cooled charge-coupled device (CCD) camera and automated image analysis software. Regions of loss or gain of DNA sequences are seen as changes in the ratio of the two fluorescence intensity ratio profiles along the target chromosomes. Thus, gene amplification or chromosomal duplication in the tumor DNA produces an elevated green-to-red ratio, and deletions of chromosomal loss cause a reduced ratio *(8–11)*. This chapter will focus on the technique of CGH and its modifications and will review the genetic perturbations revealed by CGH for a number of tumor types and its potential application in clinical practice.

2. Method

Using schematic representation, it is easy to understand that the basis of the CGH procedure involves competitive *in situ* hybridization of differentially labeled tumor DNA and normal reference DNA to normal human metaphase spreads (see **Fig. 15.1**). The CGH approach does no require mitotic tumor cells, so fresh, frozen, and paraffin-embedded tissues can be examined. In addition, only a small amount (less than 500 ng) of genomic DNA is needed for a whole-genomic analysis. However, to use CGH to determine the true incidence of chromosome abnormality in human embryos (for reproductive medicine) and to develop CGH protocols compatible with preimplantation genetic diagnosis (PGD), several modifications to existing methods are necessary, because a single cell contains only 5–10 pg of DNA. Consequently, the DNA content of the cell must be amplified before use for CGH. We can achieve the approx 40,000-fold amplification necessary using a polymerase

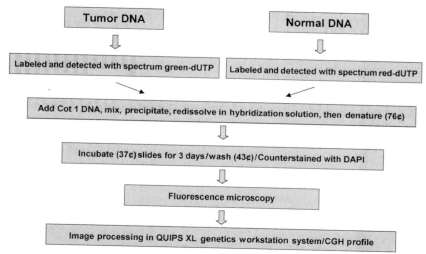

Fig. 15.1. Flowchart for CGH analysis. First, equal amounts (500 ng) of tumor DNA is labeled with green fluorochrome-conjugated nucleotide, such as Spectrum green–dUTP or fluorescence isothiocyanate–dUTP (FITC–dUTP) by nick translation, whereas reference DNA from peripheral lymphocytes of normal male or female donors is labeled with red fluorochrome-conjugated nucleotide, such as Spectrum red–dUTP or Texas red–dUTP. The sizes of the probes are optimized to a range from 500 bp to 2 kb. The labeled DNA (200 ng) is mixed with 10 μg of unlabeled human Cot-1 DNA for blocking ubiquitous repetitive sequences commonly detected on the centromeric and heterochromatic regions; then, it is ethanol precipitated and redissolved in 10 μl hybridization solution. The resulting probe mixture is denatured at 76°C for 7 min and reannealed at 37°C for 1 h. Metaphase chromosomes are also denatured at 76°C in 70% formamide solution for 3–4 min. The denatured probe mixture is dropped onto the metaphase chromosome slide, covered with a cover slip, sealed with rubber cement, and then allowed to hybridize by incubating the slide in a moist chamber at 37°C for 3 d. After hybridization, the slides are washed twice with 50% formamide with 2× SSC at 43°C for 10 min, followed by three changes with PN buffer at room temperature, 10 min each for removing the unbound probe. The slides are counterstained with diamidino-2- phenylindole (DAPI) and mounted in Vectashield mounting medium. Fluorescence signals from the hybridized chromosomes are captured and analyzed using CGH analysis software, such as the QUIPS XL Genetics Workstation system. Typically, 6–10 sets of metaphase chromosomes from one sample slide are observed under a fluorescence microscope equipped with a cooled CCD camera. The filter system consists of a triple-bandpass beam splitter, a triple-bandpass emission filter, and three single-bandpass excitation filters mounted on a computer-controlled filter wheel. This design allows collection of sequential, properly registered images from three fluorescence channels. The ratio profile of green (tumor) to red (control) fluorescence intensity is plotted as a function of locations along individual chromosomes using software. Data from 6–10 captured metaphases are pooled to obtain an averaged ratio profile for each sample (or patient). Genomic aberrations, such as gains (amplification) or losses (deletion), at certain chromosome regions are defined by setting the thresholds at 1.2 and 0.80, respectively

chain reaction (PCR)-based strategy to enzymatically copy the single-cell genome multiple times. The amplification is so efficient that sufficient DNA can be generated from a single cell for numerous subsequent PCR analyses, as well as for CGH *(3,12)*. Detailed methodological reviews can be found at http://www.nhgri.nih.gov/DIR/LCG/CGH/technology.html and http://www.utoronto.ca/cancyto/ or in several excellent articles *(2–4,6,13–19)*.

2.1. Normal Metaphase Preparation

Normal metaphase slides are prepared from phytohematoglutinin-stimulated peripheral blood lymphocyte cultures from a healthy individual. Cells are arrested in mitosis by colchicines, harvested, treated with hypotonic KC1, and fixed in methanol/acetic acid. The cells are dropped onto slides in such a way that chromosomes from mitotic cells are nicely spread *(18)*.

2.2. The Procedure of CGH

Study DNA can be obtained by any type of DNA isolation that yields high-molecular-weight DNA that is suitable for use in CGH. Normal DNA for use as a reference can be taken from blood lymphocytes from any healthy man. DNAs are extracted in phenol–chloroform using standard protocols. The extracted DNA concentrations are estimated by spectrophotometric measurement. Before beginning any labeling, the quality of the DNA must be assessed. In fact, after labeling, it is strongly suggested that the quality of the DNA be assessed again. Take a 1-µg sample of the DNA and run it on a 1% ethidium bromide stained gel. The criteria for the DNA include the following: (1) the sample must be of high molecular weight, (2) the DNA should also be quantified using an accurate spectrophotometer or a DyNA Quant 2000 fluorometer, and (3) the DNA should be dissolved in water, not TE buffer.

A successful CGH relies on the labeling of equal amounts of the high-quality DNA that is to be tested against the normal reference DNA. Test and reference DNAs are differentially labeled, and it is apparent that the size of the DNA before and after labeling is an important consideration in the overall success of the assay *(13)*. It is suggested that the labeling scheme be switched and the experiment repeated to ensure that the results are consistent.

Labeled DNAs should range in size from 500 bp to 2 kb to achieve optimal hybridization. In some cases, very high-molecular-weight DNA requires mechanical shearing before labeling, and in others, the extracted DNA can be labeled as is *(13)*. Labeling can be used with biotinylated and digoxigenin-conjugated deoxynucleotides, which require secondary detection steps before visualization posthybridization, or be used with directly fluorochrome-conjugated deoxynucleotides, which can be visualized, and require fewer posthybridization signals. **Table 15.1** lists the commonly used fluorochromes and their spectral characteristics. Nick translation is the method of choice for labeling the DNAs, because of its ability to regulate the nicking activity of DNAase I relative to the synthesizing activity of DNA polymerase I to achieve optimally sized fragments *(2)*. For applications on paraffin-embedded material, two publications described protocols for preparation, labeling, detection, and optimizing universal in vitro amplification of genomic DNA *(20,21)*. DOP-PCR proved to be the most effective method for amplifying and labeling genomic DNA from microdissected tissue areas *(19)*.

Table 15.1 Fluorescent dyes commonly used for CGH.

Fluorochrome	Color	Absorbance (nm)	Emission (nm)
DAPI	Blue	350	456
FITC	Green	490	520
Spectrum green	Green	497	524
Rhodamine	Red	550	575
Spectrum red	Red	587	612
Texas red	Red	595	615

As described in **Fig. 15.1**, the procedure of CGH is briefly summarized as follows: (1) differentially label the DNAs; (2) precipitate, denature, and hybridize the DNAs; (3) posthybridization washes and detection steps; (4) fluorescence microscopy and image analysis. The result is demonstrated as **Fig. 15.2 A,B**.

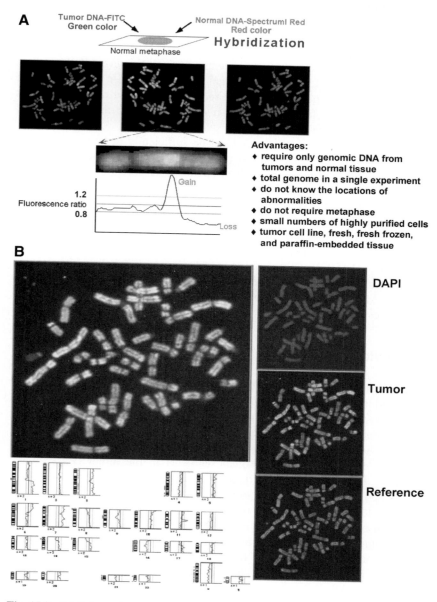

Fig. 15.2. (**A**) Schematic representation showing a summary of CGH at a glance. CGH offers many advantages in detecting unknown genomic imbalances from materials of interest. (**B**) Quantification of fluorescence intensity is depicted. The values of the fluorescence intensity ratio are drawn as a function of their positions along the individual chromosomes (curved lines). Ratio values less than the threshold value of 0.8 (red line to the right of the central black line) are considered gene deletions, whereas ratio values >1.2 (green line to the right of the central black line) are indicative of gene amplifications. The potential regions of loss and gain abnormalities are also marked (red and green bars); losses are shown at the left and gains at the right of the chromosome ideograms

2.3. Troubleshooting

The first ethanol–salt precipitation serves to remove the dNTPs that are not incorporated in the labeling reaction. To prevent loss of the labeled DNA, an excess of salmon sperm DNA (50 µg of salmon sperm DNA for each 1 µg of labeled DNA) is precipitated with the labeled DNA such that any loss of DNA from the precipitation procedure comes mainly from the salmon sperm DNA rather than the labeled DNA.

The best recovery of DNA results from leaving the DNA/salt/ethanol mixture at –20°C overnight before centrifugation. However, if this is not possible, 1 h at –70°C will give a decent recovery. In order to determine the amount of salmon sperm that is required, as well as the amount of water needed to yield the final concentration of 10 ng/µl, the actual amount of labeled probe must be determined.

On the one hand, chromosomes must be sufficiently denatured to permit hybridization of labeled DNAs, but, on the other hand, they must retain their morphology for unequivocal identification during karyotyping. A protocol for optimized chromosome preparations and hybridization conditions has been reported elsewhere *(13)* which provides a guideline for troubleshooting in CGH experiments (criteria for acceptable CGH images, control experiments, quality assurance, and interpretation of ratios). Such troubleshooting is now facilitated by commercially available and standardized CGH reagents required for CGH analysis (e.g., reference metaphase spreads, labeling kits, labeled nucleotides, and labeled reference DNAs) and control tumor DNAs (labeled and unlabeled MPE 600 DNA from a breast cancer cell line) with defined chromosomal imbalances that must be visible with CGH analysis.

3. Applications

Comparative genomic hybridization is a FISH-based technique that can detect gains and losses of whole chromosomes and subchromosomal regions. Often, CGH is based on a two-color, competitive FISH of differentially labeled tumor and reference DNA to normal metaphase chromosomes and can scan the whole genome without prior knowledge of specific chromosomal abnormalities *(4)*. CGH accounts for all chromosomal segments in the tumor cell genome, including those present in marker chromosomes whose origin cannot be determined by conventional karyotyping. Application of the CGH procedure has permitted the identification of recurrent imbalances in a wide variety of human diseases, and so far, more than 1500 articles have been published on CGH, with approx 90% reporting the use of CGH in delineating cytogenetic changes in cancer specimens (http://www3.ncbi.nlm.nih.gov/entrez/query.fcgi). About 6% of CGH articles have dealt with technical aspects and only a limited number have described the application of CGH in a clinical cytogenetics setting *(1)*.

3.1. Tumor Genetics

Cancer is a complex disease occurring as a result of a progressive accumulation of genetic aberrations and epigenetic changes that enable an escape from normal cellular and environmental controls *(4)*. Neoplastic cells might have numerous acquired genetic abnormalities, including aneuploidy, chromosomal rearrangements, amplifications, deletions, gene rearrangements, and loss-of-function or gain-of-function mutations *(4)*. These genetic abnormalities lead to the abnormal behavior common to all enoplastic cells, including the dysregulation of growth, lack of contact inhibition, genomic instability, and a propensity for metastases. The genes affected by aberrations in cancers are often divided into two main categories: genes that have gain-of-function (amplification) known as oncogenes, and genes that have loss-of-function (inactivation) known as tumor suppressor genes. The tumor suppressor genes often need a complete loss of function in both alleles because the chromosomes are often paired. More than 100 genes have been reported to be related to tumor development and/or tumor progression. Gene amplification is an essential mechanism of oncogene activation, in addition to structural alterations, loss of control mechanisms, insertional mutagenesis, and chromosome translocations *(22)*.

The power of CGH has been clearly proven, since the first published article by Kallioniemi et al. in 1992, as a tool to characterize chromosomal imbalances in neoplasias *(5)*. The number of studies concerning solid tumors and hematological cancers is impressive. Many excellent review articles or websites (e.g., http://www.helsinki.fi/~lgl_www/CMG.html, which contains the chromosomal locations of recurrent DNA copy number changes in 73 tumor types from 283 reports) have been found that summarize the chromosomal imbalances detected by CGH in solid tumors and in hematological diseases *(19,22–25)*. The majority of studies focus on specific types of tumor, with tumor development, progression, clinical correlation, prediction of response to therapy, and disease-free survival in a given population, with the presence of infection *(25)*. For example, Wang suggested that genes located at 6q27 might play a crucial role in the early events of ovarian tumor development and that there is a continuum in the progression model of ovarian neoplasia and the high frequency of gene amplification at 20q12-q13.2, indicating that the overpresentation of these genes might play a crucial role in the pathogenesis of ovarian cancer *(26)*. In fact, several of the copy-number changes in ovarian cancers might be explained by known abnormalities in the genes involved in ovarian tumorigenesis (loss of 17pter-q21 and *p53*, gain on 17q and amplification of *HER2/Neu/erbB2*, amplification on 8q24 and *myc*, and gain at 3q26.3 and amplification of the p110 catalytic subunit of PI3K), which provide unique targets. The *p53* tumor suppressor has been explored as a target for gene therapy in ovarian cancer, and *HER2/neu/erB2* is being targeted by antibody-mediated therapy (herceptin) and E1A-mediated gene therapy. In the study of ovarian cancer samples from Kudoh et al., the researchers demonstrated that the presence of an increased copy number at 1q21 and 13q13 correlate with a lack of response to a chemotherapy regimen consisting of cisplatin, doxorubicin, and cyclophosphamide *(27)*. Therefore, identification and characterization of the genes driving the copy-number abnormalities detected by CGH might provide new therapeutic targets in ovarian cancer, which might directly affect tumor cell growth or alter sensitivity to chemotherapy *(28)*.

In addition to the application of CGH for studying solid tumors, CGH also contributes to the knowledge of chromosomal alterations in hematological diseases such as leukemia and lymphomas. With the application of CGH in lymphoma, gene amplifications are also often seen *(19,25,29)*. Struski et al. further suggested the indications of CGH in hemopathies, including (1) a normal karyotype (a proliferation of normal cells to the detriment of tumor cells during the cell culture), (2) failure of the karyotype (low proliferative potential as multiple myeloma), and (3) uninterpretable metaphases because of poor quality (e.g., acute lymphoid leukemia) and complex karyotypes (e.g., lymphoma) *(25)*.

Because CGH recognizes only proportional changes in copy number, the ratio profiles do not indicate the absolute copy-number change. For example, Knuutila et al. found in diploid and near-diploid cells that a ratio of 1.5 indicates at least a 100% increase in the copy number of an entire chromosome arm or of a region of a chromosome band, but the threshold is not reached when the increase is only 50% (e.g., chromosomal trisomy) *(22)*. In addition, when a DNA copy number increase is restricted to a small chromosome area representing, for example, the amplification of a single gene, the copy number increase should be 10-fold or higher *(220)*.

3.2. Clinical Cytogenetics

Comparative genomic hybridization has also been useful in clinical cytogenetics and has facilitated the identification and characterization of intrachromosomal duplications, deletions, unbalanced translocations, and marker chromosomes in prenatal, postnatal, and preimplantation samples *(3,30–33)*. CGH is also useful in revising incorrectly assigned karyotypes. The ability of CGH to define more precisely the chromosomal material comprising marker chromosomes and unbalanced rearrangements has helped to further define the critical chromosomal regions that are associated with adverse phenotypic outcomes, thus providing prognostic information for genetic counseling *(31)*. This information is also beneficial to prenatally ascertaining cases of marker chromosomes, as it might provide couples with a means to make rational and informed decisions concerning the pregnancy. CGH is also powerful in advancing molecular cytogenetics in the area of evaluating mental retardation *(33)*. CGH has two major uses in the analysis of mental retardation, including the further characterization of unbalanced karyotypes as detected by routine banding analysis, such as additions, duplications, deletions, trans-locations, markers, or complex aberrations, and the screening for "hidden" chromosome aberrations in patients with apparently normal karyotypes.

Figure 15.3A–D illustrates a case of congenital anomaly that was diagnosed prenatally using amniocentesis performed at the gestational age of between 14 and 20 wk. We first identified the patient as probably having an abnormal chromosome, involving chromosome 1 and another chromosome (perhaps chromosome 5 or chromosome 13), using the conventional karyotyping method. Then, we used CGH to find the possibly abnormal area—deletion of 1q terminal and amplification of 13q. Based on the findings of CGH, we suspected that the translocation chromosome might be involved with chromosome 1 and chromosome 13. Finally, we used FISH to confirm the diagnosis, using whole-chromosome and specific telomere probes.

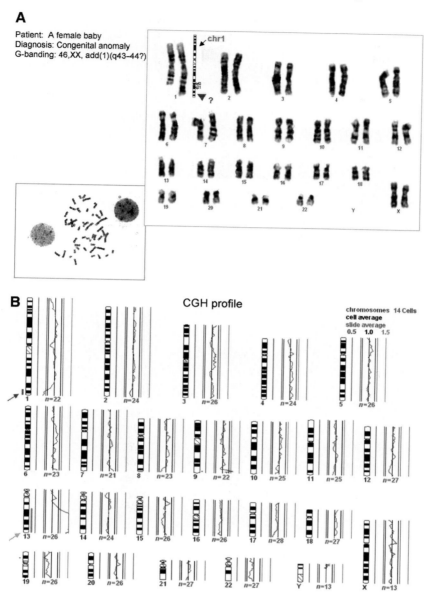

A

Patient: A female baby
Diagnosis: Congenital anomaly
G-banding: 46,XX, add(1)(q43–44?)

B   CGH profile

Fig. 15.3. The application of molecular cytogenetic tools in detecting the chromosome aberrations in a case with congenital anomaly. (**A**) Traditional G-banding analysis finds an abnormal chromosome with additional materials in the terminal end of one chromosome 1q. However, the origin of this material is unable to be determined by G-banding. (**B**) CGH is then performed and shows genomic changes with 1q terminal loss and 13q gain. (**C**) FISH with chromosome painting probes 5 and 13 (chromosome 5 painting probe is used as an internal control) is performed and shows the additional material in chromosome 1q terminal is from chromosome 13q. (**D**) FISH with 13q and 1q telomere probes is also done and detects the deletion of terminal region in one of chromosome 1. All of these FISH studies confirm the finding by CGH analysis and give us a clearer picture about this chromosome aberration.

C

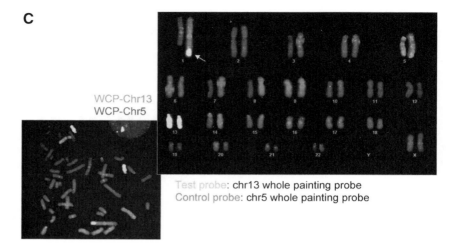

WCP-Chr13
WCP-Chr5

Test probe: chr13 whole painting probe
Control probe: chr5 whole painting probe

D

Test probe1: chr1 telomeric probe (green signal)
Test probe2: chr13 telomeric probe (red signal)

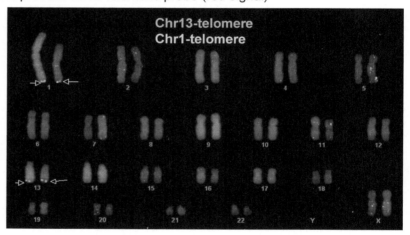

Fig. 15.3. (continued)

4. Conclusion

Methods for chromosomal analysis have become increasingly powerful, benefiting enormously from the fusion of traditional cytogenetic techniques and molecular genetics. This has not only led to advances in clinical diagnosis but has also provided markers for the assessment of prognosis and disease progression. CGH might be among the most significant methodological advances and has overcome many of the technical limitations that beset earlier cytogenetic methods, allowing detailed chromosomal data to be obtained from a variety of tissues that were previously considered problematic (2). CGH has been employed for the ascertainment of chromosomal duplications, amplifications, and deletions that contribute to neoplastic transformation, revealing the chromosomal location of tumor suppressor genes and oncogenes that are central to disease development or progression and can also identify new prognostic markers. However, it should be noted that CGH has limitations. It cannot detect balanced chromosomal abnormalities such as translocations, inversions, or point mutations. In addition, pericentromeric, telomeric and heterochromatic regions cannot be evaluated, and 1p32-pter, 16p, 19, and 22 could lead to a false-positive interpretation *(22)*. Chromosomal imbalances must be present in about 50% of cells to be detected, which means that CGH requires that tumor specimens be relatively free of surrounding normal tissue. Finally, the sensitivity and resolution of conventional chromosome-based CGH is likely limited to changes that are 5–10 Mb *(19,20)*, although thresholds of detection for amplification might be lower (2 Mb) compared to those of detection for deletion (10–20 Mb) *(13)*. As an example, an amplicon located at 19p, which contains *AKT2*, is frequently present in ovarian cancer cells but is too small to be detected by classical CGH *(18)*. Similarly, the frequency of copy-number abnormalities at 3q is greater when it is analyzed by FISH with region-specific probes than when it is assessed by chromosome-based CGH *(34)*. Because the limitations of CGH for the genetic characterization of cancer are mainly in the use of metaphase chromosomes as hybridization targets, its resolution is at the chromosomal banding level *(22)*. Thus, a new technology—array technology adapted to CGH, designated M-CGH *(35–38)*—will allow the resolution to increase from a cytogenetic level to a molecular level. For M-CGH, chromosome preparations are substituted by sets of well-defined genomic DNA fragments microarrayed on solid support to serve as hybridization targets *(39)*. Thus, genomic imbalances are detected with much higher resolution, allowing copy-number changes to be associated with individual loci and genomic markers. This approach is much more demanding than the widespread application of DNA microarrays for the detection of gene expression patterns, because it requires the reliable detection of subtle differences in the fluorescence ratios of test and control genomes (e.g., the diagnosis of alterations can rely on a ratio of difference smaller than 0.1); also, the complexity of the labeled total genomic DNA probe sequence pool is several orders of magnitude higher than that of a cDNA pool *(39)*. These requirements can be met using genomic DNA fragments cloned in bacterial, P1-derived, or yeast artificial chromosome (BAC, PAC, and YAC) vectors *(35,36)*. Recently, M-CGH has improved significantly, because a ligation-mediated PCR BAC labeling method has improved the signal-to-noise ratios, and clone density has also been increased *(40)*. Current human CGH arrays have a 1-Mb resolution (about 3,000 features), whereas cDNA arrays are already routinely made at 10,000–15,000 features per slide *(38)*.

Importantly, copy-number abnormalities detected by classical CGH might reflect a sum of multiple distinct small areas of copy-number abnormality. M-CGH, because of its increased ability to resolve areas of copy-number abnormalities, might exhibit an improved predictive value and also facilitate the identification of the gene or genes driving specific genomic amplifications or deletions. M-CGH is also likely to be more robust and less tedious than classical chromosome-based CGH.

In the future, the continuing improvement of CGH, such as the use of a standard reference interval instead of a fixed interval *(41)*, or related techniques, such as M-CGH, will allow large-scale screening of abnormal changes of chromosomes in diseases and continue to provide a better understanding of cancer.

Of most importance, the establishment of a pattern of genetic abnormalities for each tumor type should offer a precise histological diagnosis and assist in the prediction of which chemotherapeutic drugs will be most effective in the treatment of a given type of cancer and a single-array-based CGH experiment in a basic science laboratory could provide copy number and expression information from all human genes and a more focused DNA chip in the clinical diagnostic laboratory could assess all the specific chromosomal loci, genes, and signaling pathways involved in a given disease.

Acknowledgments: We greatly appreciate the technical support of supervisor Dr. Jeremy A. Squire at the Department of Laboratory Medicine and Pathobiology, University of Toronto, Toronto, Ontario, Canada (website: http://www.uto-ronto.ca/cancyto/), Miss Wen-Yuann Shyong at the Taipei Veterans General Hospital, and Dr. Wen-Ling Lee at the Department of Medicine, Cheng-Hsin Rehabilitation Center, Taipei, Taiwan. The work, which took place in the authors' laboratories, has been supported by the National Science Council (NSC 92-2314-B-075-115) and Taipei Veterans General Hospital.

References

1. Patel AS, Hawkins AL, and Griffin CA (2000) Cytogenetics and cancer. Curr Opin Oncol 12:62–67
2. Houldsworth J, Chaganti RSK (1994) Comparative genomic hybridization: an overview. Am J Pathol 145:1253–1260
3. Wells D, Levy B (2003) Cytogenetics in reproductive medicine: the contribution of comparative genomic hybridization (CGH). BioEssays 25:289–300
4. Boultwood J, Fidler C (eds) (2002) Molecular analysis of cancer, Humana, Totowa, NJ
5. Kallioniemi A, Kallioniemi OP, Sudar D, et al (1992) Comparative genomic hybridization for molecular cytogenetic analysis of solid tumors. Science 258: 818–821
6. Baksara BR, Pei J, Testa JR (2002) Comparative genomic hybridization analysis. In: Boultwood J, Fidler C (eds) molecular analysis of cancer. Humana, Totowa, NJ, pp. 45–65
7. Wang PH, Shyong WY, Lin CH, et al (2002) Analysis of genetic aberrations in uterine adenomyosis using comparative genomic hybridization. Anal Quant Cytol Histol. 24:1–6
8. du Manoir S, Schrock E, Bentz M, et al (1995) Quantitative analysis of comparative genomic hybridization. Cytometry 19:27–41
9. Piper J, Rutovitz D, Sudar D, et al (1995) Computer image analysis of comparative genomic hybridization. Cytometry 19:10–26
10. Lundsteen C, Maahr J, Christensen B, et al (1995) Image analysis in comparative genomic hybridization. Cytometry 19:42–50
11. du Manoir S, Kallioniemi OP, Lichter P, et al. (1995) Hardware and software requirements for quantitative analysis of comparative genomic hybridization. Cytometry 19:4–9
12. Wells D, Sherlock JK, Handyside AH, and Delhanty JD (1999) Detailed chromosomal and molecular genetic analysis of single cells by whole genome amplification and comparative genomic hybridization. Nucleic Acids Res. 27: 1214–1218
13. Kallioniemi OP, Kallioniemi A, Piper J, et al (1994) Optimizing comparative genomic hybridization for analysis of DNA sequences copy number changes in solid tumors. Genes Chromosomes Cancer 10:231–243

14. Isola J, Devries S, Chu L, Ghazvini S, and Waldman F (1994) Analysis of changes in DNA sequence copy number by comparative genomic hybridization in archival paraffin-embedded tumor samples. Am J Pathol 145:1301–1308

15. Choo KHA (1994) Methods in molecular biology: in situ hybridization protocols. Humana, Totowa, NJ

16. Kallioniemi A, Kallioniemi OP, Piper J, et al (1994) Detection and mapping of amplified DNA sequences in breast cancer by comparative genomic hybridization. Proc Natl Acad Sci USA 91:2156–160

17. Kirchhoff M, Gerdes T, Rose H, Maahr J, Ottesen AM, Lundsteen C (1998) Detection of chromosomal gains and losses in comparative genomic hybridization analysis based on standard reference intervals. Cytometry 31:163–173

18. Tachdjian G, Aboura A, Lapierre JM, Vigie F (2000) Cytogenetic analysis from DNA by comparative genomic hybridization. Ann Genet 43:147–154

19. Zitzelsberger H, Lehmann L, Wemer M, and Bauchinger M (1997) Comparative genomic hybridisation for the analysis of chromosomal imbalances in solid tumours and haematological malignancies. Histochem Cell Biol 108:403–417

20. James L, Varley J (1996) Preparation, labeling and detection of DNA from archival tissue sections suitable for comparative genomic hybridization. Chromosome Res 4:163–164

21. Kuukasjarvi T, Tanner M, Pennanen S, Karhu R, Visakorpi T, Isola J (1997) Optimizing DOP-PCR for universal amplification of small DNA samples in comparative genomic hybridization. Genes Chromosomes Cancer 18:94–101

22. Knuutila S, Bjorkqvist A, Autio K, et al (1998) DNA copy number amplifications in human neoplasms. Am J Pathol 152:1107–1123

23. Knuutila S, Aalto Y, Autio K, et al (1999) DNA copy number losses in human neoplasms. Am J Pathol 155:683–694

24. Knuutila S, Autio K, Aalto Y (2000) Online access to CGH data of DNA sequence copy number changes. Am J Pathol 157:689–690

25. Struski S, Doco-Fenzy M, Comillet-Lefebvre P (2002) Compilation of published comparative genomic hybridization studies. Cancer Genet Cytogenet 135:63–90

26. Wang N (2002) Cytogenetics and molecular genetics of ovarian cancer. Am J Med Genet 115:157–163

27. Kudoh K, Takano M, Koshikawa T, et al (1999) Gains of 1q21-q22 and 13q12-q14 are potential indicators for resistance to cisplatin-based chemotherapy in ovarian cancer patients. Clin Cancer Res 5:2526–2531

28. Mills GB, Schmandt R, Gershenson D, Bast RC (1999) Should therapy of ovarian cancer patients be individualized based on underlying genetic defects? Clin Cancer Res 5:2286–2288

29. Werner CA, Dohner H, Joos S, et al (1997) High-level DNA amplifications are common genetic aberrations in B-cell neoplasms. Am J Pathol 151:335–342

30. Bryndorf T, Kirchhoff M, Rose H, et al (1995) Comparative genomic hybridization in clinical cytogenetics. Am J Hum Genet 57:1211–1220

31. Levy B, Dunn TM, Kaffe S, Kardon N, Hirschhom K (1998) Clinical applications of comparative genomic hybridization. Genet Med 1:4–12

32. Levy B, Dunn TM, Kern JH, Hirschhorn K, Kardon NB (2002) Delineation of the dup5q phenotype by molecular cytogenetic analysis in a patient with dup5q/del 5p (cri du chat). Am J Med Genet 108:192–197

33. Xu J, Chen Z (2002) Advances in molecular cytogenetics for the evaluation of mental retardation. Am J Med Genet 117:15–24

34. Shayesteh L, Lu Y, Kuo WL, et al (1999) PIK3CA is implicated as an oncogene in ovarian cancer. Nat Genet 21:99–102

35. Pinkel D, Segraves R, Sudar D, et al (1998) High resolution analysis of DNA copy number variation using comparative genomic hybridization to microarrays. Nature Genet 20:207–211

36. Solinas-Toldo S, Lampel S, Stilgenbauer S, et al (1997) Matrix-based comparative genomic hybridization: biochips to screen for genomic imbalances. Genes Chromosomes Cancer 20:399–407

37. Pollack JR, Perou CM, Alizadeh AA, et al (1999) Genome-wide analysis of DNA copy-number changes using cDNA microarrays. Nature Genet 23:41–46

38. Armour JAL, Barton DE, Cockbum DJ, Taypor GR (2002) The detection of large deletions or duplications in genomic DNA. Hum Mut 20:325–337

39. Wessendorf S, Fritz B, Wrobel G, et al (2002) Automated screening for genomic imbalances using matrix-based comparative genomic hybridization. Lab Invest 82: 47–60

40. Snijders AM, Nowak N, Segraves R, et al (2001) Assembly of microarrays for genome-wide measurement of DNA copy number. Nature Genet 29:263–264

41. Kirchhoff M, Gerdes T, Rose H, Maahr J, Ottesen AM, Lundsteen C, (1998) Detection of chromosomal gains and losses in comparative genomic hybridization analysis based on standard reference intervals. Cytometry 31:163–173

16

Subtractive Hybridization

Craig Winstanley

1. Introduction

Subtractive hybridization involves the subtraction of a test DNA sample (the TESTER) from a reference DNA sample (the DRIVER), and the subsequent identification of those sequences present in the DRIVER DNA but absent from the TESTER DNA. The nature of the DNA samples varies depending on the specific application, but the two samples would normally share high levels of identity, thus lending extra significance to the differences between them. Subtractions fall into two major categories: (a) subtraction among closely related genomic DNA samples leading to the identification of genetic variations; (b) subtraction among cDNA samples generated from RNA isolated from cells exposed to different conditions, leading to the identification of differentially expressed genes.

2. Principles of Subtractive Hybridization

The basic steps in subtraction involve: (1) the isolation of the two closely related DNA samples (genomic or cDNA generated following RNA extraction); (2) digestion or shearing of DNA into fragments of a more manageable size; (3) the incorporation of either a label or a specific "adaptor" sequence to enable subsequent differentiation between TESTER and DRIVER DNA; (4) hybridization of the two denatured DNA samples with an excess of the DRIVER (reference) DNA; (5) separation and identification of those TESTER sequences that remained single stranded because of the absence of complimentary sequence in the driver DNA.

A method for genomic subtraction, used for the isolation of DNA absent in deletion mutants of yeast, was first reported in 1990 (*1*). Genomic subtraction incorporated the main features of subtractive hybridization. Genomic DNA was isolated from two closely-related sources and hybridized in such a way that those sequences common to both DNA samples would be removed, leaving only TESTER-specific sequences. Finally, those sequences unique to one of the sources were isolated and identified. This initial study involved the removal from wild-type

From: *Molecular Biomethods Handbook, 2nd Edition.*
Edited by: J. M. Walker and R. Rapley © Humana Press, Totowa, NJ

DNA (TESTER) of sequences present in the genomes of both yeast wild-type and a deletion mutant (DRIVER). DNA corresponding to the deleted region was enriched in the TESTER by allowing a mixture of denatured wild-type and biotinylated mutant DNA to reassociate. Avidin-coated beads were used to remove biotinylated sequences. The subtraction process was repeated several times. In each cycle unbound wild-type DNA from the previous round was hybridized with fresh biotinylated deletion mutant (DRIVER) DNA. After each cycle any TESTER DNA that was also present in the DRIVER DNA was removed using avidin-coated beads. Eventually short oligonucleotide sequences (adaptors) were ligated to the unbound DNA from the final cycle, containing the TESTER-specific sequences. Following the ligation, the recovered DNA was amplified by using an oligonucleotide primer designed to bind adaptor sequence in the polymerase chain reaction (PCR). Amplified DNA was then used to probe TESTER and DRIVER DNA samples to identify those sequences genuinely subtracted (only present in TESTER DNA).

Although this methodology has been amended subsequently, the principles of subtractive hybridization remain the same. A typical scheme for subtractive hybridization is presented in **Fig. 16.1**. Before hybridization of TESTER and DRIVER DNA, the samples are generally cleaved either by ultrasonication or by digestion with restriction enzymes. It is important to ensure that TESTER DNA sequences are short to minimize the number of hybrid sequences containing both TESTER-specific DNA and DNA shared by the TESTER and DRIVER. Despite containing potentially useful information, such hybrid sequences may be removed because of those regions that hybridize with the DRIVER. Thus, genuine TESTER-specific sequences could be lost. In the scheme presented in **Fig. 16.1** the TESTER DNA is digested with a frequently cutting restriction enzyme, such as *Sau*3AI, whilst the DRIVER DNA is fragmented by mechanical shearing. In the example shown, *Sau*3AI can be used to cleave the adaptors and facilitate cloning into a vector cleaved with *Bam*HI, an enzyme which produces complimentary ends.

To facilitate the removal of those TESTER sequences also present in the DRIVER DNA, the DRIVER DNA should be present in excess. To enrich for TESTER-specific sequences, it may be necessary to repeat the subtraction. It is important that a method should be available for the separation of nonhybridizing TESTER DNA from other sequences in the mixture. This can be achieved by a number of approaches. A biotin-based approach for selective enrichment of specific DNA sequences was reported as early as 1986 *(2)*. The original method for genome subtraction can be improved by the modification of both TESTER and DRIVER DNA before hybridization. In one approach, adaptors were ligated to the TESTER DNA whilst the DRIVER DNA was labeled with biotin, both before hybridization *(3)*. Following hybridization, hybrids containing DRIVER DNA could be removed by the capture of biotin using beads coated with streptavidin. As in the initial study, adaptor sequences were targeted for PCR amplification of those remaining sequences unique to the TESTER DNA.

Often, the output from a subtractive hybridization experiment is a mixed PCR product. PCR amplicons can be cloned directly using one of the many commercial vectors available, or digested using the relevant restriction enzyme (for example, *Sau*3AI) before cloning. This enables the production of a subtracted library of sequences present in the TESTER DNA but absent

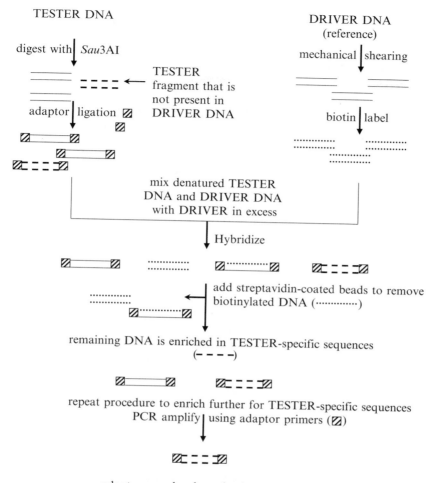

Fig. 16.1. Generalized scheme of subtractive hybridization

from the DRIVER DNA. It cannot be assumed that all sequences at this stage are genuinely subtracted. Such sequences can be identified by using DNA from clones in the subtracted library as probes against TESTER and DRIVER DNA samples.

Other strategies have also been employed to identify TESTER-specific sequences. For example, poly(A)-tailing of the TESTER DNA with terminal transferase and asymmetrical amplification after subtraction was used in a study to identify *L. monocytogenes*- specific sequences *(4)*. Another strategy involved PCR amplification of TESTER and DRIVER sequences before hybridization *(5)*. Different adaptors were ligated to *Sau*3AI-digested TESTER and DRIVER sequences to facilitate the PCR amplification steps. A further addition to the strategy was the inclusion of dUTP instead of dTTP in the DRIVER DNA PCR mixture. This enabled the removal of any contaminating DRIVER DNA following hybridization by digestion with uracil DNA glycosylase *(5)*.

3. Representational Difference Analysis

Representational difference analysis (RDA) is a variation on the subtractive hybridization technique designed to improve efficiency *(6,7)*. In particular, subtractive hybridization among genomic DNAs from higher organisms was inefficient because of the complexity of such genomes. In RDA PCR amplification is carried out on both TESTER and DRIVER DNAs before hybridization. This is achieved by ligating adaptors to the ends of restriction-digested fragments and using PCR primers designed to target the adaptor sequences. Because the majority of DNA fragments will be too large to amplify, this has the effect of reducing the sequence complexity and increasing the efficiency of subsequent subtractive hybridizations. Before proceeding further, the adaptors are removed from the amplified TESTER and DRIVER DNAs by restriction digestion.

RDA also incorporates the idea of "difference enrichment." Before each round of RDA, "long" oligonucleotide adaptors are ligated to the TESTER DNA fragments. A short oligonucleotide is used to improve the efficiency of this ligation. However, the "short" oligonucleotides are not covalently attached and dissociate at elevated temperatures. A round of RDA starts by mixing the TESTER DNA with an excess of DRIVER DNA, followed by denaturation and reassociation of the mixture. PCR amplification is then carried out using primers designed to the "long" oligonucleotides. Homoduplexes of TESTER-specific sequences will contain the primer-binding sites on both ends and are thus selectively amplified. Following digestion of the amplified products and the ligation of new (different) adaptors, reassociation and selective hybridization are repeated. Further rounds can be carried out if necessary. RDA has been combined with the use of cDNA library arrays to enable the simultaneous identification of differentially expressed genes *(8)*. This was achieved by using the "difference products" obtained using RDA directly as hybridization probes on cDNA arrays.

4. Suppression Subtractive Hybridization

The most common strategy for subtractive hybridization currently is suppression subtractive hybridization (SSH), which was first reported in 1996 *(9)*. The availability of commercial kits for SSH (BD Biosciences-Clontech) make it the most accessible version of the technique available to researchers *(10,11)*. The kits can be used with as little as 0.5–2 µg of polyA$^+$-RNA or 2 µg bacterial genomic DNA for both TESTER and DRIVER samples as starting material. Using SSH, rare transcripts can be enriched over 1,000-fold. A general outline of the SSH method is presented in **Fig. 16.2**. In SSH the TESTER DNA is digested using a restriction enzyme (such as *Rsa*I) and separated into two portions. A different oligonucleotide adaptor sequence is then ligated to the 5′ ends of each portion. Next, the two portions are hybridized separately to DRIVER DNA (in excess). Any TESTER sequences that hybridize with the DRIVER DNA should be "mopped up" leaving only TESTER-specific single-stranded sequences. Subsequently the two portions are mixed and hybridized together, allowing homologous single-stranded TESTER DNAs to hybridize. Thus, only those sequences unique to the TESTER will have different adaptors present on each strand. These sequences are detected by PCR amplification using primers designed to bind to adaptor sequences. The key to the success of this method is that sequences containing identical adaptor

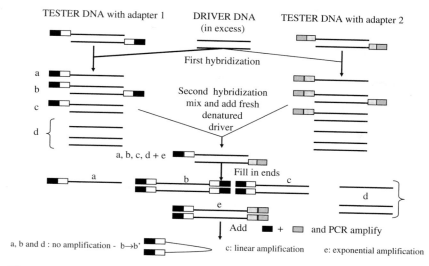

Fig. 16.2. Supression subtractive hybridization

sequence at both ends are less susceptible to PCR amplification. This is because a secondary structure forms to prevent primer annealing. This "suppression" effect ensures that those sequences carrying different adaptors at each end will amplify preferentially. The PCR products are cloned into a suitable vector to produce a subtracted DNA library. In reality the suppression is not entirely effective, but the method should lead to >50% of clones containing TESTER-specific sequences.

The efficacy of SSH for analyzing genetic differences among related strains of *Helicobacter pylori* has been tested using two genome sequenced strains *(12)*. Most of the 7% of genomic differences between the two strains were detected using four parallel subtractions with different restriction enzymes. Overall 95% of the unique open reading frames in each strain were identified using SSH. The study also demonstrated that as TESTER-specific sequences become limiting the proportion of repeat fragments increases.

It should be noted with all of the subtractive hybridization methods that the optimal hybridization temperature varies depending on the % (G+C) content of the DNAs being used. For example, bacterial genomes with a high % (G + C) content (65–70%), such as *Burkholderia* spp. *(13)* or *Pseudomonas aeruginosa (14)* require a higher hybridization temperature (approximately 73°C) than the 63°C recommended in the SSH kit manual (BD Biosciences-Clontech). Conversely, we have found improved results using low % (G+C) content (30–35%) bacterial genomes, such as *Campylobacter jejuni*, by lowering the hybridization temperature to 58°C (unpublished data).

SSH, like all subtractive hybridization techniques, can generate large numbers of anonymous sequences. Software is available for the handling, storage and analysis of such sequences *(15)*. The normal approach to analyzing the output data from genomic subtractions would be firstly to screen for genuinely subtracted sequences. When the chosen DRIVER strain has already been sequenced this is a relatively simple procedure. As an alternative DNA hybridization using TESTER and DRIVER DNA is required. Secondly, BLASTN and BLASTX searches of the database can be used to identify any matches for the genuinely subtracted sequences. Finally, it may be necessary to screen a panel of strains to determine the wider distribution of sequences. This can involve PCR amplification, hybridization techniques, or a combination of both.

5. Applications of Subtractive Hybridization

5.1. Genomic DNA Subtractions

There are many examples of the application of subtractive hybridization to the study of genetic variation, especially in microbiological research. A comprehensive list is beyond the scope of this chapter. However, some examples are given in **Table 16.1**. These include the discovery of new viruses (*16–18*). Subtractive hybridization has also been particularly useful for the identification

Table 16.1. Some example applications of subtractive hybridization to study genome variations.

DNA source	Application	References
Viruses		
KSHV (HHV-8)	Discovery of Kaposi's sarcoma-associated herpesvirus	*(30)*
EBV	Demonstrated Epstein-Barr virus related gastric cancer	*(31)*
Calicivuruses	Identification of novel calicivirus in walrus	*(32)*
GB hepatitis agent	Identification of GB viruses A and B	*(33)*
TTV	Identification of Torque teno virus	*(34)*
Bacteria		
Aeromonas hydrophila	Identification of genomic islands implicated in virulence	*(35)*
Burkholderia pseudomallei	Identification of genomic island implicated in virulence; Development of a typing scheme	*(36); (13)*
Chlamydia psittaci	Strain-specific diagnostic probe	*(37)*
Escherichia coli	Identification of genes specific to uropathogenic *E. coli*	*(38)*
Klebsiella pneumoniae	Identification of genomic island implicated in virulence	*(39)*
Listeria monocytogenes	Probes for diagnostic purposes	*(4)*
Neisseria spp.	Identification of genomic islands implicated in virulence	*(40)*
Pseudomonas aeruginosa	Strain-specific diagnostic probes	*(14,41)*
Salmonella spp.	Identification of genomic islands implicated in virulence	*(42)*

of markers specific to individual bacterial strains or clones (**Table 16.1**). In addition, subtractive hybridization has played an important role in the identification of transposable elements, integrated bacteriophages, and genomic islands implicated in bacterial virulence. Although it might seem that the advent of high-throughput sequencing and the consequent large expansion of the whole bacterial genomes database may have superseded this particular application of subtractive hybridization, the fact is that those strains chosen for sequencing are often not representative of the diversity present amongst natural populations. Many studies have demonstrated that subtractive hybridization still has a role to play in extending our knowledge of this diversity *(19–21)*. The method has also been applied to the study of metagenomics, using the microbiota of the rumen *(22)*. Subtractive hybridization techniques have also been used to search for genomic variations in higher organisms. For example, RDA has been proposed as a tool in the search for new tumor suppressor genes *(23)*.

Typically SSH and other methods for subtractive hybridization identify mainly short DNA fragments (<1 kb), some of which frequently yield "no significant hits" when BLASTN and BLASTX database searches are performed. Once a sequence has been identified and confirmed to be TESTER-specific, it is often desirable to extend it and analyze flanking genomic DNA. This may allow identification of complete ORFs or of neighboring ORFs that match database sequences. There are several methods for extending DNA fragments into unknown flanking regions, a procedure known as genome walking. These include inverse PCR amplification *(24)* and 'unpredictably primed PCR' *(25)*. Inverse PCR amplification involves digestion of the genomic DNA with a restriction enzyme followed by ligation to circularize the restriction fragments. PCR amplification primers are designed to read out in opposite directions from the known sequence. The method relies on finding restriction fragments that are small enough to yield a PCR amplicon. Siebert et al. *(26)* first reported the use of the suppression PCR effect in genome walking. This method of genome walking involves the ligation of adaptor sequences to restriction fragments and subsequent PCR amplification with 1 primer targeting a region within the known sequence and the second primer targeting the ligated adapter. Again the method may be unsuccessful if the distance to the next restriction enzyme cutting site is too great. Often this distance is not known. The chances can be increased by using several different restriction enzymes in parallel experiments. This approach now forms the basis of the BD Biosciences Clontech Genomewalker kit, where four different restriction enzymes are used.

5.2. Differentially Expressed Genes

Subtractive hybridization enables a comparison of gene expression among samples. The only difference in this approach is that complementary DNA (cDNA) must first be obtained following isolation of mRNA, or total RNA for bacteria. There are many examples where subtractive hybridization techniques have been used to identify differentially expressed genes. **Table 16.2** gives some examples relating to humans, plants, fish, and bacteria. The technique has proved particularly valuable in the search for disease-related genes *(27)* including those with a potential role in cancer *(28)*.

Table 16.2. Some example applications of subtractive hybridization to study differential gene expression.

	Application	References
Human		
	Differential expression in neuroblastoma cells	*(43)*
	Differential expression in idiopathic pulmonary arterial hypertension	*(44)*
	Characterization of genes associated with different phenotypes of bladder cancer cells	*(45)*
	Differential expression in prostrate cancer cells	*(46)*
	Differentially expressed genes associated with lung cancer	*(47)*
	Differential expression in a colon carcinoma cell line	*(48)*
	Identification of genes differentially expressed in hepatocellular carcinoma	*(49)*
Plants		
Wheat	Expression of genes during plant development	*(50)*
Tobacco	Expression of genes associated with resistance to infection	*(51)*
Fish		
Arctic salmon	Expression of genes associated with resistance to infection	*(52)*
Sea bass	Expression of genes associated with adaptation to salinity	*(53)*
Mussels	Identification of genes responsive to pollutants	*(54)*
Flounder	Identification of genes responsive to pollutants	*(55)*
Bacteria		
Mycobacterium tuberculosis	Identification of virulence genes	*(56)*
Mycobacterium avium	Identification of genes expressed following phagocytosis	*(57)*
Salmonella typhimurium	Identification of genes expressed following phagocytosis	*(58)*
Pseudomonas aeruginosa	Identification of drug-resistance genes	*(59)*

6. Summary

Subtractive hybridization still represents a relatively simple, cost-effective method for identifying variations among genomic DNA samples and differentially expressed genes. Although other techniques, such as high-throughput sequencing, microarrays, and proteomics offer attractive alternatives, they are often not viable options for many laboratories.

There is now a wealth of nucleotide sequence data from the genomes of bacterial pathogens (http://www.tigr.org/tdb/mdb/mdbcomplete.html) and comparative analysis of bacterial genomes is providing valuable information about how pathogens adapt and evolve. Detailed comparisons among related bacteria can now be achieved on a scale hitherto beyond reach *(29)*. However, although in some cases the choice of strain has included highly virulent or epidemic strains, many of the bacterial genomes sequenced are from strains that were chosen on the basis of common laboratory use. There are examples of comparative sequencing studies in which the genomes of close relatives have been targeted. However, it is unreasonable to expect genome sequencing to provide all the answers unless every strain of interest is targeted. Since two close relatives would share the majority of their genomes in common, whole genome sequencing can be a wasteful and expensive approach. For that reason, subtractive hybridization still has an important role to play.

Similarly, although microarray and proteomics technologies are becoming increasingly available, there is still an important role for subtractive hybridization in the identification of differentially expressed genes. Whereas microarray and proteomics are expensive and require specialist expertise and equipment, subtractive hybridization can be carried out in most laboratories where experience in the use of basic molecular techniques is available.

References

1. Straus D, Ausubel FM (1990) Genomic subtraction for cloning DNA corresponding to deletion mutations. Proc Natl Acad Sci U. S. A 87:1889–1893
2. Welcher AA, Torres AR, Ward DC (1986) Selective enrichment of specific DNA, cDNA and RNA sequences using biotinylated probes, avidin and copper-chelate agarose. Nucleic Acids Res 14:10,027–10,044
3. Schmidt KD, Schmidt-Rose T, Romling U, Tummler B (1998) Differential genome analysis of bacteria by genomic subtractive hybridization and pulsed field gel electrophoresis. Electrophoresis 19:509–514
4. Wu FM Muriana PM (1995) Genomic subtraction in combination with PCR for enrichment of Listeria monocytogenes-specific sequences. Int J Food Microbiol 27:161–174
5. Bjourson AJ, Stone CE, Cooper JE (1992) Combined subtraction hybridization and polymerase chain reaction amplification procedure for isolation of strain-specific Rhizobium DNA sequences. Appl Environ Microbiol 58:2296–2301
6. Lisitsyn N, Lisitsyn N, Wigler M (1993) Cloning the differences between two complex genomes. Science 259:946–951
7. Lisitsyn NA (1995) Representational difference analysis: finding the differences between genomes. Trends Genet 11:303–307
8. Geng M, Wallrapp C, Muller-Pillasch F, Frohme M, Hoheisel JD, Gress TM (1998) Isolation of differentially expressed genes by combining representational difference analysis (RDA) and cDNA library arrays. Biotechniques 25:434–438
9. Diatchenko L et al (1996) Suppression subtractive hybridization: a method for generating differentially regulated or tissue-specific cDNA probes and libraries. Proc Natl Acad Sci U S A 93:6025–6030
10. Winstanley C (2002) Spot the difference: applications of subtractive hybridisation to the study of bacterial pathogens. J Med Microbiol 51:459–467
11. Rebrikov DV, Desai SM, Siebert PD, Lukyanov SA (2004) Suppression subtractive hybridization. Methods Mol Biol 258:107–134
12. Agron PG, Macht M, Radnedge L, Skowronski EW, Miller W, Andersen GL (2002) Use of subtractive hybridization for comprehensive surveys of prokaryotic genome differences. FEMS Microbiol Lett 211:175–182
13. Duangsonk K, Gal D, Mayo M, Hart CA, Currie BJ, Winstanley C (2006) Use of a variable amplicon typing scheme reveals considerable variation in the accessory genomes of isolates of Burkholderia pseudomallei. J Clin Microbiol 44:1323–1334
14. Smart CH et al (2006) Development of a diagnostic test for the Midlands 1 cystic fibrosis epidemic strain of Pseudomonas aeruginosa. J Med Microbiol 55:1085–1091
15. Weckx S, De Rijk R, Van Broeckhoven C, Del Favero J (2004) SSHSuite: an integrated software package for analysis of large-scale suppression subtractive hybridization data. Biotechniques 36:1043–1045

16. Allander T, Emerson SU, Engle RE, Purcell RH, Bukh J (2001) A virus discovery method incorporating DNase treatment and its application to the identification of two bovine parvovirus species. Proc Natl Acad Sci U S A 98:11,609–11,614

17. Endoh D et al (2005) Species-independent detection of RNA virus by representational difference analysis using non-ribosomal hexanucleotides for reverse transcription. Nucleic Acids Res 33:e65

18. Ambrose HE, Clewley JP (2006) Virus discovery by sequence-independent genome amplification. Rev Med Virol 16:365–383

19. Golubov A, Heesemann J, Rakin A (2003) Uncovering genomic differences in human pathogenic Yersinia enterocolitica. FEMS Immunol Med Microbiol 38:107–111

20. Purdy A, Rohwer F, Edwards R, Azam F, Bartlett DH (2005) A glimpse into the expanded genome content of Vibrio cholerae through identification of genes present in environmental strains. J Bacteriol 187:2992–3001

21. Shen S, Mascarenhas M, Morgan R, Rahn K, Karmali MA (2005) Identification of four fimbria-encoding genomic islands that are highly specific for verocytotoxin-producing Escherichia coli serotype O157 strains. J Clin Microbiol 43:3840–3850

22. Galbraith EA, Antonopoulos DA, White BA (2004) Suppressive subtractive hybridization as a tool for identifying genetic diversity in an environmental metagenome: the rumen as a model. Environ Microbiol 6:928–937

23. Hollestelle A, Schutte M (2005) Representational difference analysis as a tool in the search for new tumor suppressor genes. Methods Mol Med 103:143–159

24. Ochman H, Gerber AS, Hartl DL (1988) Genetic applications of an inverse polymerase chain reaction. Genetics 120:621–623

25. Dominguez O, Lopez-Larrea C (1994) Gene walking by unpredictably primed PCR. Nucleic Acids Res 22:3247–3248

26. Siebert PD, Chenchik A, Kellogg DE, Lukyanov KA, Lukyanov SA (1995) An improved PCR method for walking in uncloned genomic DNA. Nucleic Acids Res 23:1087–1088

27. Wang X, Feuerstein GZ (2000) Suppression subtractive hybridisation: application in the discovery of novel pharmacological targets. Pharmacogenomics 1:101–108

28. Muller-Hagen G, Beinert T, Sommer A (2004) Aspects of lung cancer gene expression profiling. Curr Opin Drug Discov Devel 7:290–303

29. Frase CM, Eisen J, Fleischmann RD, Ketchum KA, Peterson S (2000) Comparative genomics and understanding of microbial biology. Emerg Infect Dis 6:505–512

30. Chang Y et al (1994) Identification of herpesvirus-like DNA sequences in AIDS-associated Kaposi's sarcoma. Science 266:1865–1869

31. Mita H, Itoh F, Toyota M, Hinoda Y, Imai S, Imai K (2000) Isolation of the Epstein-Barr virus in scirrhous gastric cancer by efficiency-monitored representational difference analysis. Tumour Biol 21:249–257

32. Ganova-Raeva L, Smith AW, Fields H, Khudyakov Y (2004) New Calicivirus isolated from walrus. Virus Res 102:207–213

33. Simons JN et al (1995) Identification of two flavivirus-like genomes in the GB hepatitis agent. Proc Natl Acad Sci U S A 92:3401–3405

34. Nishizawa T, Okamoto H, Konishi K, Yoshizawa H, Miyakawa Y, Mayumi M (1997) A novel DNA virus (TTV) associated with elevated transaminase levels in posttransfusion hepatitis of unknown etiology. Biochem Biophys Res Commun 241:92–97

35. Zhang YL, Ong CT, Leung KY (2000) Molecular analysis of genetic differences between virulent and avirulent strains of Aeromonas hydrophila isolated from diseased fish. Microbiology 146(Pt 4):999–1009

36. Reckseidler SL, DeShazer D, Sokol PA, Woods DE (2001) Detection of bacterial virulence genes by subtractive hybridization: identification of capsular polysaccharide of Burkholderia pseudomallei as a major virulence determinant. Infect Immun 69:34–44

37. Creelan JL, Bjourson AJ, Meehan BM, McCullough SJ (1999) Characterisation of strain-specific sequences from an abortifacient strain of ovine Chlamydia psittaci using subtraction hybridisation. FEMS Microbiol Lett 171:17–25

38. Janke B, Dobrindt U, Hacker J, Blum-Oehler G (2001) A subtractive hybridisation analysis of genomic differences between the uropathogenic E. coli strain 536 and the E. coli K-12 strain MG1655. FEMS Microbiol Lett 199:61–66

39. Lai YC, Yang SL, Peng HL, Chang HY (2000) Identification of genes present specifically in a virulent strain of Klebsiella pneumoniae. Infect Immun 68:7149–7151

40. Perrin A, Nassif X, Tinsley C (1999) Identification of regions of the chromosome of Neisseria meningitidis and Neisseria gonorrhoeae which are specific to the pathogenic Neisseria species. Infect Immun 67:6119–6129

41. Parsons YN, Panagea S, Smart CH, Walshaw MJ, Hart CA, Winstanley C (2002) Use of subtractive hybridization to identify a diagnostic probe for a cystic fibrosis epidemic strain of Pseudomonas aeruginosa. J Clin Microbiol 40:4607–4611

42. Emmerth M, Goebel W, Miller SI, Hueck CJ (1999) Genomic subtraction identifies Salmonella typhimurium prophages, F-related plasmid sequences, and a novel fimbrial operon, stf, which are absent in Salmonella typhi. J Bacteriol 181:5652–5661

43. Liu Z et al (2006) GM1 up-regulates Ubiquilin 1 expression in human neuroblastoma cells and rat cortical neurons. Neurosci Lett 407:59–63

44. Edgar AJ, Chacon MR, Bishop AE, Yacoub MH, Polak JM (2006) Upregulated genes in sporadic, idiopathic pulmonary arterial hypertension. Respir Res 7:1

45. Yang YC, Li X, Chen W (2006) Characterization of genes associated with different phenotypes of human bladder cancer cells. Acta Biochim Biophys Sin (Shanghai) 38:602–610

46. Rauhala HE, Porkka KP, Tolonen TT, Martikainen PM, Tammela TL, Visakorpi T (2005) Dual-specificity phosphatase 1 and serum/glucocorticoid-regulated kinase are downregulated in prostate cancer. Int J Cancer 117:738–745

47. Xiao W et al (2005) Differentially expressed genes associated with human lung cancer. Oncol Rep 14:229–234

48. Orian-Rousseau V et al (2005) Genes upregulated in a metastasizing human colon carcinoma cell line. Int J Cancer 113:699–705

49. Dong XY et al (2004) Identification of genes differentially expressed in human hepatocellular carcinoma by a modified suppression subtractive hybridization method. Int J Cancer 112:239–248

50. Jin Y, Tashpulatov AS, Katholnigg H, Heberle-Bors E, Touraev A (2006) Isolation and characterisation of two wheat beta-expansin genes expressed during male gametophyte development. Protoplasma 228:13–19

51. Szatmari A et al (2006) Characterisation of basal resistance (BR) by expression patterns of newly isolated representative genes in tobacco. Plant Cell Rep 25:728–740

52. Matejusova I et al (2006) Gene expression profiles of some immune relevant genes from skin of susceptible and responding Atlantic salmon (Salmo salar L.) infected with Gyrodactylus salaris (Monogenea) revealed by suppressive subtractive hybridisation. Int J Parasitol 36:1175–1183

53. Boutet I, Long Ky CL, Bonhomme F (2006) A transcriptomic approach of salinity response in the euryhaline teleost, Dicentrarchus labrax. Gene 379:40–50

54. Brown M, Davies IM, Moffat CF, Craft JA (2006) Application of SSH and a macroarray to investigate altered gene expression in Mytilus edulis in response to exposure to benzo(a)pyrene. Mar Environ Res 62 Suppl:S128–S135

55. Sheader DL, Williams TL, Lyons BP, Chipman JK (2006) Oxidative stress response of European flounder (Platichthys flesus) to cadmium determined by a custom cDNA microarray. Mar Environ Res 62:33–44

56. Dasgupta N et al (2000) Characterization of a two-component system, devR-devS, of Mycobacterium tuberculosis. Tuber Lung Dis 80:141–159

57. Plum G, Clark-Curtiss JE (1994) Induction of Mycobacterium avium gene expression following phagocytosis by human macrophages. Infect Immun 62:476–483

58. Morrow BJ, Graham JE, Curtiss R, III (1999) Genomic subtractive hybridization and selective capture of transcribed sequences identify a novel Salmonella typhimurium fimbrial operon and putative transcriptional regulator that are absent from the Salmonella typhi genome. Infect Immun 67:5106–5116

59. Westbrock-Wadman S et al (1999) Characterization of a Pseudomonas aeruginosa efflux pump contributing to aminoglycoside impermeability. Antimicrob Agents Chemother 43:2975–2983

17

Fluorescence In Situ Hybridization

Jane Bayani and Jeremy A. Squire

1. The Contribution of Chromosomal Analysis to the Study of Disease

Methodological advances have played a central role in our conceptual understanding of the genetic basis of human diseases such as cancer. They have also had a direct bearing on the integration of genetic techniques into routine clinical practice, as it is essential that assays can be performed quickly and often, on small biopsies obtained from patients. Chromosomes must be obtained from actively dividing cells as they are recognized in preparations of metaphase cells by their size and shape, and by the pattern of light and dark bands observed after staining by specific procedures. Methods for improving the yield and quality of dividing cells has allowed for a more precise definition of chromosomal aberrations in tumors, as well as the identification of previously undetected constitutional rearrangements associated with certain types of congenital syndromes.

The analysis of chromosomes is known as cytogenetics, and the process enables gross alterations of the entire genome to be assessed at once, and provides data on populations of cells. It has played a major role in the definition of specific classes of genetic diseases, and is used routinely in the clinical assessment of leukemias and lymphomas, since good quality preparations can be obtained routinely after immediate processing of a biopsy specimen or following a few days of in vitro tissue culture. Chromosome preparations are far more difficult to obtain from solid tumors, and more complex culture methods may be necessary to grow the tumor cells so that adequate numbers of metaphase cells are available for cytogenetic analysis. Furthermore, insufficient material may be available from solid tumors, since minimally invasive techniques are often employed to obtain samples for diagnosis.

Fluorescence in situ hybridization (FISH) was introduced as early as 1977 *(1)*, but was not implemented as a mainstream genetic or research tool until 1988 by Lichter et al. *(2)*. Akin to southern blotting methods, a DNA fragment containing the locus/gene of interest is labeled using a molecule detectable through antibody reactions or directly with a fluorescently conjugated

From: *Molecular Biomethods Handbook, 2nd Edition.*
Edited by: J. M. Walker and R. Rapley © Humana Press, Totowa, NJ

nucleotide substrate. This fluorescently labeled DNA constitutes the "FISH probe" to be used in the hybridization reaction. When double-stranded DNA is heated, the complementary strands separate (denature) to form single-stranded DNA. Given suitable conditions, the separated complementary regions of DNA can join together to re-form a double-stranded molecule. This renaturation process is called *hybridization*. The process is highly faithful, and when extensive hybridization has occurred, the resulting DNA duplex is very stable. DNA strands that are not highly complementary will not hybridize to one another or will interfere with complementary strand hybridization. In the case of the FISH assay, hybridization takes place to metaphase chromosomes or chromatin in interphase nuclei fixed on a glass slide (**Fig. 17.1**). Following a typical overnight hybridization based on the complimentary base pair relationship of DNA, the hybridized slide is carried through a series of

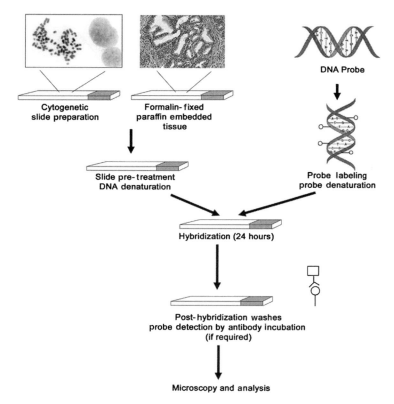

Fig. 17.1. Schematic representation of the basic FISH protocol. The target DNA may be a cytogenetic specimen or paraffin embedded tissue. Shown are examples of a metaphase spread from a tumor showing more than the normal 46 chromosomes and interphase nuclei; as well as a representation of a tissue section derived from a prostate carcinoma. The probe is labeled either directly with a fluorochrome or indirectly with a hapten (depicted as open circles bound to the DNA). The target DNA and labeled probes are processed, denatured and brought together during the hybridization process. The following day, the unbound probe is washed from the slide and, if required, the indirectly-labeled probe is detected with antibodies conjugated to a fluorochrome as illustrated through the symbolized antigen–antibody reaction. The slides are finally counterstained and mounted in an antifade medium and ready for microscopy

posthybridization washes to remove any unbound probe. Antibodies conjugated to fluorchromes or dyes against the hapten (used to label the DNA) are allowed to incubate on the slides. The excess antibodies are removed through detergent washes and the DNA is counterstained and mounted in an antifade medium. The slides could then be visualized by fluorescence microscopy. Hybridization signals are seen as small points of light located on chromosomes or on interphase nuclei.

In the 1990s, the early phases of the developing Human Genome Project involved significant mapping of newly discovered genes to human chromosomes. Major improvements in cloning strategies, fluorescent imaging and the use of different fluorochromes and dyes allowed for the development of FISH probes with a high level of sensitivity and specificity for both the normal mapping of genes as well as the abnormal mapping patterns of genes/chromosomal loci within tumor genomes. Mapping of these novel sequences to a specific chromosome band provided clues about which of the many genes at a particular genomic location might be affected by chromosome alterations or other cytogenetic abnormalities seen in human diseases or in cancer cells. Since there are on average between 30 and 60 genes per chromosome band, precise gene mapping by FISH was very important *(2,3)*. In the last 10 years FISH has been increasingly applied not only to metaphase preparations derived from normal human cells such as blood, but also to cellular specimens used to analyze various types of tumors *(4,5)* More advanced variations of the basic FISH technique (discussed further in the Applications sections) include Comparative Genomic Hybridization (CGH) *(6)*, Spectral Karyotyping (SKY) *(7)*, MFISH *(8)* and MBanding *(9)*.

This chapter will cover the principles of FISH including the fixation procedure for cytogenetic preparations, probe labeling, hybridization, post-hybridization washes and analysis. The applications of FISH with particular emphasis on the use of recent advances of this technique in the analysis of cancer will then be presented.

2. Methods

Fluorescence in situ Hybridization (FISH) is a multi-stepped process and is schematically depicted in **Fig. 17.1**. This process brings together a cytogenetic specimen or sample derived from tumor tissue, with the labeled probe in a hybridization reaction. It is then processed through post-hybridization washes and, if required, antibody incubations for detecting haptens linked to the DNA probe. Haptens are molecules that can react with antibodies, with the most commonly used haptens including biotin and digoxigenin. The antibodies used in the FISH procedure have a fluorescent tag present so they can be readily detected by fluorescence microcopy. The methods below describe the techniques for processing cultures derived from primary specimens as well as various types of tumor tissues for FISH. The reader is encouraged to refer to detailed protocols outline by Bayani and Squire *(10)* for a more comprehensive discussion of FISH-based techniques as well as other sources *(11)*.

FISH assays may use different target DNA substrates, but all require the hybridization of a labeled DNA containing the chromosomal locus or target gene of interest. There are different classes of FISH probes used to

Table 17.1. Typical FISH-based assays.

FISH Assay	Applications
Locus-specific FISH	Copy number status. Rearrangement or translocation status. Applicable to metaphase and interphase cells. Applicable to cytogenetic suspension and FFPE tissues.
Centromere-specific FISH	Copy number status. Applicable to metaphase and interphase cells. Applicable to cytogenetic suspension and FFPE tissues.
Multi-Color FISH (MFISH), Spectral Karyotyping (SKY) or Multi-Color Band (MFISH) Analysis	Copy number status. Rearrangement or translocation status. Intrachromosomal rearrangement. Applicable to metaphase cells only.
Metaphase Comparative Genomic Hybridization (CGH)	Net copy number status. Rearrangement or translocation status.
Telomere FISH	Determining telomere length associated with cell. aging and telomere erosion. Applicable to metaphase and interphase cells. Applicable to cytogenetic suspension and FFPE tissues.

answer both specific and more general questions (**Table 17.1**). Depending on the type of FISH analysis being conducted, a commercially labeled DNA probe may exist for the chromosomal locus or specific gene of interest and labeled either directly with a fluorochrome (and called a "directly-labeled probe"), or with a hapten (and called an "indirectly-labeled probe"). The use of commercially-labeled probes possessed the advantage of having been verified for optimal quality and consistency over in-house probes. However, as in the case of many research laboratories, a FISH probe must be created in-house.

To make a FISH probe the DNA segment or gene of interest will usually have been inserted into a bacterial virus or plasmid to facilitate its manipulation and propagation to sufficient quantities for labeling. At present Bacterial Artificial Chromosomes (BACs) are the most popular cloned forms of genomic DNA used for FISH probes. BACs can accommodate inserts that are larger (200 kb) than some of the previous vector systems, and can produce a stronger FISH signal.

Typical labeling strategies include nick translation or labeling through polymerase chain reaction (PCR) methods. Nick translation involves the simultaneous actions of two enzymes: DNase I and DNA polymerase I. DNAse I randomly nicks the DNA fragment in each strand of the double-stranded DNA molecule. DNA polymerase I (derived from *Escherichia coli*), with its three activities: exonuclease function, removing bases in the 5' to 3' direction; polymerase function that adds nucleotides from the 3' nick site; and the 3' to 5' proof reading function; incorporates the "label," whether indirectly using a hapten(biotin-d**X**TP or digoxigenin-d**X**TP: where "**X**" denotes one of the four nucleotides—adenine, guanine, cytosine, thymine) or directly (i.e., fluorescein-d**X**TP or rhodamine-d**X**TP). Nick translation can be applied to all cloned DNA sources. PCR-labeling employs multiple rounds of template denaturation, primer annealing and template replication, facilitated by *Taq* polymerase. Primers serve as the DNA "anchors" that start the newly synthesize strands against the DNA template in the reaction. Primers are variable and may include sequence specific primers to amplify targeted fragments; vector sequence primers to amplify and label cloned DNA; and/or universal primers. Compared to nick translation, which requires mg of starting DNA, PCR-labeling requires only ng of template. The resulting size of the labeled DNA probe ranges from 200–500 bp that can be assessed by running a small sample of the labeled probe on a 2% ethidium bromide DNA staining agarose gel. The labeled DNA is then ethanol precipitated in the presence of excess unlabeled sonnicated salmon sperm DNA (50:1) as well as unlabeled human COT-1 DNA (10:1). The excess of salmon sperm DNA prevents the loss of the labeled probe during the precipitation process whereas the human COT-1 DNA serves to suppress the presences of naturally occurring repeated sequences within the human genome. The labeled probe can either be resuspended in water or in a hybridization buffer, consisting of 50–60% formamide, 2× SSC and 10% dextran sulfate; and stored at −20°C unit ready for use. Both indirectly and directly labeled probes can be stored for several months. A well-labeled probe will produce a bright and specific signal with minimal to no background fluorescence.

2.1. Fluorescence In Situ Hybridization to Cytogenetic Specimens

2.1.1. Preparing a Cytogenetic Specimen

The first karyotypes were made from peripheral lymphocytes by Hungerford et al. in 1959 *(12)*, using a primitive squash technique. Later Moorhead et al. *(13)* published the method for air drying peripheral blood chromosomes, using methanol:acetic acid. The basic protocol for preparing cells for metaphase analysis has not change much in the last 50 years. Classical FISH analysis involves the short term culture of the test specimen—typically peripheral blood, skin fibroblasts, amniocytes, tumor biopsies or established cell lines; which are processed to produce a cytogenetic suspension that yields both metaphase spreads and interphase nuclei.

This process involves the treatment of dividing cells in either a short-termed culture, as is the case of primary specimens taken from the patient; or from established cultures, such as immortalized cell lines; with a mitotic spindle inhibitor, such as colcemid *(14)*. Through mitotic disruption, the dividing cells are arrested at metaphase where the chromosomes are most tightly coiled and able to be easily identifiable by size, shape, and banding pattern. The concentration and exposure time to colcemid can vary depending on the type of cell being used and on the mitotic activity of the culture; but typically involves 1–2 h of treatment. Following treatment, the cells are pelleted by centrifugation and resuspended in a hypotonic solution of potassium chloride (0.075 M). The hypotonic treatment causes the cells to become swollen and the resulting concentration gradient stretches the cell membrane. Should the hypotonic treatment occur too quickly, the cell membranes may burst yielding "chromosome soup." Too little swelling will prevent the membranes from adequately releasing the chromosomes from the confines of the cell membrane and permitting them to spread. Gradual and repeated fixation with a 3:1 methanol:acetic acid fixative helps to maintain this state until the cell is forced to flatten out when applied to the slide. When completely fixed, the cells can be stored pelleted and under fixative at −20°C almost indefinitely.

Slide making is very much an "art." Successful slide making consists of the application of the fixed cell suspension to a glass slide, resulting in a genomic target that yields well-spread chromosomes with minimal cytoplasmic debris (15). This technique requires the addition of the fixed cells to the slide such that the chromosomes housed within the swollen nuclear membrane burst out when the cell comes in contact with the slide. The consensus of many experienced cytogeneticists is that the relative humidity in the room where slides are made is the most critical parameter for slide making. Determining the best conditions for slide making requires frequent tests conditions and trips to a phase contrast microscope. In many state-of-the-art cytogenetics laboratories, a humidity and temperature controlled unit, about the size of a fume hood, has been used to establish the correct humidity and temperature for slide making. The storing of cytogenetic slides is also subjective. Some laboratories simply store at room temperature, whereas other store slides at −20°C (in, or free of ethanol) and still others store in desiccants. Each laboratory will need to determine the best storage conditions. However, if there is remaining cytogenetic suspension, fresh slides can always be made as needed.

2.1.2. Pretreatment of the Cytogenetic Slide

The first step of FISH is the pre-treatment and denaturation of the target DNA. As already discussed, the target DNA may come from a cytogenetic slide specimen or a histologically prepared tissue section (ie. formalin-fixed, paraffin embedded tissue section). The quality of metaphase preparations varies according to the cell type, culturing conditions, harvesting conditions (i.e., colcemid, hypotonic and fixation parameters), as well as the slide making conditions and the age of the slide. Thus the quality of the target DNA influences the success of FISH, just as much as the quality of the probe.

Cytogenetic slides are generally used a few days after being made, ensuring that the cells have completely dried and have begun to "age." Artificial aging techniques such as treatment in 2× SSC at 37°C for several hours; or heat treatment of the slide, ranging from 37°C to 90°C for several hours or several minutes, respectively; have been employed. Whether artificially or naturally aged, the slides are usually treated with a protease such as pepsin or proteinase K, to remove any cytoplasmic debris that might inhibit the access of the probe to the DNA. This pre-treatment also helps to minimize the background that might result from the incubation with antibodies (if the probe is not directly-labeled). Because pepsin is a gentler protease than proteinase K, most FISH protocols will employ its use. Following the protease treatment, the slide is washed briefly in 1× PBS before being passed through a dehydrating ethanol series (70%, 90%, and 100%) and allowed to air-dry. Once dry, the slides are processed through a denaturation step in a 70% formamide/2×SSC solution for 2 min at 72°C. The use of formamide allows the melting (denaturing) of DNA to occur at lower temperatures. The slides are then immediately placed in 70% ethanol, through to 100% ethanol, to maintain the single stranded, denatured state of the DNA on the slide. The slide is then allowed to air-dry and is ready for hybridization with the denatured, labeled DNA probe.

2.1.3. Labeled Probe Preparation and Denaturation

The labeled DNA probe is resuspended in a hybridization buffer consisting of 50–60% formamide/2× SSC and 10% dextran sulphate. If a commercial probe is being used, the investigator should follow the manufacturer's instructions. Anywhere from 200–500 ng of labeled probe can be used per slide. Like the target DNA, the DNA probe must also be denatured. This is accomplished by heat denaturing the probe at 75°C for 5 min. Because the DNA may contain repetitive sequences that could result in cross-hybridization and background, the probe should be allowed to undergo a pre-annealing step for about an hour at 37°C. During this process, the unlabeled human COT-1 DNA anneals with repetitive sequences at a faster rate than unique sequences.

2.1.4. Hybridization of the Denatured Cytogenetic Slide to the Denatured Labeled Probe

After the cytogenetic slide has been pre-treated and denatured, and the probe has been denatured and preannealed, the two components are brought together. The probe is applied to the slide, cover slipped and sealed with rubber cement. The slide is then place in a container containing a slightly dampened paper towel or gauze to create some humidity, and allowed to hybridize overnight at 37°C.

2.1.5. Posthybridization Washed and Probe Detection

Following the overnight hybridization, unbound probe must be removed from the slide. If the probe was labeled with a hapten, the application of primary, secondary or tertiary antibodies are required to visualize the probe. In the case of directly labeled probes, a series of washes to remove unbound probe is required. Both will be discussed here.

There are numerous methods of washing unbound probes and the method described below uses a "rapid method" of wash and eliminates the use of hazardous formamide in large quantities. Traditional FISH experiments make use of formamide washes carried out at 42–45°C at a 50% content in 2× SSC, optimized to only remove probe that has not hybridized to its target sequences, or to very weakly hybridized probe (11). The subsequent stringency and detergent washes also serve to remove any remaining unbound probe and antibodies. The choice of detergent is subjective, largely based on the preference and experience of the investigator. The most commonly used detergents include Tween-20, NP-40, IPEGAL, SDS and Triton X-100 (16) and are used in varying concentrations, temperatures and times. If the probe is indirectly labeled (i.e., using biotin or digoxigenin), an antibody system will be required, and many commercial sources for antibodies raised in the appropriate host and conjugated to fluorchromes already exist and optimized for FISH.

The "rapid wash" protocol is applicable to both cytogenetic preparations and to FFPE-tissues. Following the overnight hybridization at 37°C, the coverslips are removed from the slides and placed in a 2 min incubation at 72°C in a detergent solution (i.e., 0.3% NP-40/0.1× SSC), followed by a less stringent wash at room temperature for 5–10 min (i.e., 0.1% NP-40/2× SSC). If the probe was directly labeled, the slide would simply be counterstained with DAPI (which stains the DNA blue) typically in an antifade medium (to prevent the quenching of the fluorescent signal). If the probe was indirectly labeled, the appropriate antibody treatments would be required, with the final antibody conjugated to a dye or fluorochrome (16). Each antibody treatment lasts for approximately 30 min at 37°C and should be accompanied by a blocking step before each antibody application. The blocking solution typically consists of some concentration of bovine serum albumen (BSA) to reduce the non-specific binding of the antibodies, and reducing background and noise. Thus the use of an indirectly labeled probe results in a post-hybridization wash that is considerably longer, when compared to directly-labeled probes. Following the final antibody treatment, the slide is counterstained with DAPI and mounted in antifade. The slides may be stored at 4°C for short-term storage, or at −20°C for long-term storage and may still hold fluorescent signals for up to a year after hybridization.

2.2. Fluorescence in situ Hybridization to Formalin-Fixed Paraffin Embedded Tissues (FFPE)

For many investigations, viable material for short-termed culture is not available, thus metaphase analysis is not possible. In such cases interphase nuclei are almost certainly present in a clinical sample, but special techniques are required to prepare and analyze these specimens for FISH procedures. When a clinical laboratory receives a piece of human tissue for pathological analyses, the sample is preserved in a fixative called formalin and then embedded in liquid wax that will solidify as a rectangular block suitable for sectioning and microscopy. Such paraffin blocks are widely used since most pathology laboratories routinely archive all formalin-fixed paraffin embedded (FFPE) tissue for future retrospective studies. Thus, interphase cytogenetics (i.e., the interrogation of interphase nuclei), has been amenable to FISH and can provide the same information as metaphase analysis, depending on the nature of the specific question being asked. Typically FFPE tissues are cut into 5 micron sections and mounted onto charged microscope slides and heat treated.

2.2.1. Pretreament of FFPE Tissue Sections

Before the labeled probe can be applied to the tissue, the paraffin must be removed to allow access of the probe to the target DNA. The slide is passed through a series of xylene incubations to dissolve away the wax, followed by dehydration in an ethanol series (70%, 90%, and 100%), then air dried. The tissue is then treated with a protease, either pepsin or proteinase K (or in some cases, both), with the time, concentration and temperature of treatment established depending on the type of tissue, age of the specimen and thickness of the section. The slide is once again passed through a dehydrating ethanol series and allowed to air dry. At this point the slide awaits the addition of the probe, where both are codenatured.

2.2.2. Codenaturation of the Target DNA and Labeled DNA Probe

For FFPE-FISH, the probe is applied to the pre-treated FFPE tissue, cover-slipped and sealed with rubber cement, and placed on a temperature controlled hot-plate/slide warmer/oven and co-denatured at 80°C for 10 min. The pre-annealing step is generally not carried out since the hybridization efficiency is generally lower in paraffin embedded tissues, thus cross-hybridization signals are generally less problematic than in cytogenetic preparations. Following the codenaturation step, the slides are allowed to hybridize at 37°C overnight.

2.2.3. Posthybridization Washes and Probe Detection

Following hybridization, the FFPE-tissues are processed in a similar fashion as the hybridized cytogenetic preparations described above.

2.3. Microscopy and Analysis

After the counterstain and antifade solution have been applied to the slides, they are ready to be visualized. Many of today's fluorescent microscopes are equipped with basic imaging software to capture images for further analysis. The success of a FISH experiment not only lies in the most efficient labeling of DNA probes, slide pre-treatment and hybridization, but also the quality and choice of filters used to visualize the fluorescent signals. Using the wrong filters to visualize the fluorochromes used in the experiment will cause difficulties in signal scoring and interpretation. Depending on the nature of the experiment and the scientific question being asked, the reader is strongly encouraged to find a recent publication of a similar study to determine the best way to obtain and interpret the results of the experiment. Generally, all areas of the slide should show uniformity in signal strength. There should be high signal to background intensities, meaning that the FISH signal intensity should be consistently greater than background intensity in the regions of the slide chosen for analysis. If the background signals are equivalent to signals in the nuclei then your counts will be skewed and the results biased

3. Application of FISH-Based Assays

Although there are now many sophisticated applications of FISH (**Table 17.1**), the most fundamental question FISH can answer is: *What is the status of my chromosomal locus/gene within the targeted genome?* The answer can be classified into four general categories:

Is the chromosomal locus/gene of interest:

1) Present in **normal** copies (i.e., two copies per cell).
2) Present in more than normal copies (i.e., more than two copies) – and considered "gained" or "amplified."
3) Missing copies (i.e., less than two copies)—and considered "deleted."
4) Correctly mapped to its chromosomal location—if not the locus/gene is considered "translocated."

This fundamental question can be applied to all aspects of routine cytogenetics as well as research applications of cytogenetics.

3.1. FISH for Gene Mapping

The first applications of FISH were to determine the chromosomal mapping locations of genes that were cloned through other molecular assays (**Fig. 17.2A**). In this way, the cloned DNAs were labeled and hybridized to normal human metaphase slides and their chromosomal locations identified *(17)*. This permitted the physical mapping of genes and provided investigators important insights into the relationships between the chromosomal location and proximity to other genes within the genome. FISH mapping was not only restricted to the human genome, but was also applied to the mouse genome *(18,19)*.

3.2. Clinical Genetics and Clinical Cancer Cytogenetics

The use of FISH in clinical genetics ranges from its uses in in vitro fertilization *(20,21)* to routine prenatal screening of amniocytes *(22)*. These include

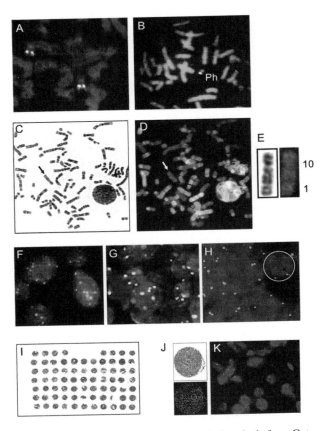

Fig. 17.2. Examples of Metaphase and Interphase FISH analysis from Cytogenetic preparations and FFPE-tissues. **A**. Mapping of BAC clones to human chromosome 19q13.3. This example shows the mapping location of two labeled BAC clones (red and green) that co-localized to the expected 19q13.3 region of the human genome. **B**. Example of the Ph chromosome in a CML specimen. Shown are the results of metaphase FISH analysis using probes for the BCR gene located on chromosome 22q (red) and for the ABL gene on 9q (green). The co-localization of the green and red signals confirms the presence of the Ph chromosome. **C–E**. Example of SKY analysis on a human ovarian primary tumor. In **C**, the DAPI counterstaining has been inverted to mimic the conventional banding patterns of chromosomes enabling identification. **D**. shows the hybridization of the 24-color probe cocktail to the metaphase spread and reveals that in addition to the excess of chromosomes over the normal 46, numerous chromosomal rearrangements are present and recognized by the change of color along the length of a continuous chromosome. In a normal karyotype, each chromosome posses a specific fluorescence signature, which is uniform along the length of the chromosome. **E**. shows the presence of an abnormal chromosome composed of a rearranged chromosome 10 and a portion of chromosome 1. **F**. Interphase FISH analysis using a multi-color centromere specific probe cocktail identifies the presence of more than two copies of the specified chromosomes per nucleus, indicating an abnormal genome. **G**. Interphase FISH analysis detecting amplification of the EGFR gene (red) in a lung tumor section. Normal cells contain only two copies of a gene. In this case, the mass of red signal indicates several hundred copies of this gene per cell. **H**. Interphase FISH analysis detecting the deletion of 1 copy of the PTEN gene (red) in a prostate cancer tissue section. Once cell is highlighted and shows two normal copies of the centromere of chromosome 10 (green), but only 1 copy of the PTEN gene (red). **I–K**. Tissue Microarray Analysis (TMA). **I**. Shown is a hematoxylin and eosin (H&E) stained section of a TMA. **J**. An enlargement of 1 of the tissue cores that has been "FISHed" with probes for PTEN (red) and centromere 10 (green). The blue core represents the same core counterstained with DAPI following FISH analysis. **K**. A further enlargement of a region of the core shows the deletion of the PTEN gene in many of the cells

the use of centromere-specific probes for chromosome 21 to confirm Downs syndrome (23), when standard Giemsa banding (G-banding) analysis fails; the use of locus specific probes to identify chromosomal alterations associated with Prader Willi/Angelman's syndrome (24); Cri Du Chat (25); DiGeorge Syndrome (26). More recently FISH was used to characterize patients affected with 22q11 deletion syndrome that is associated with congenital and later onset conditions including schizophrenia (27).

Clinical cancer cytogenetics has greatly benefited from the use of FISH analysis, since many short-term cultures derived from diseased cells produce poor quality metaphase spreads making standard G-banding difficult. Such is the case for many of the hematopoetic malignancies. Molecular studies have identified recurrent chromosomal abnormalities associated with specific types of leukemias (http://cgap.nci.nih.gov/Chromosomes/Mitelman), and this has permitted the development of gene-specific probes for the identification of these recurrent chromosomal abnormalities. The most well-known common recurrent chromosomal aberration is the Philadelphia chromosome (Ph) in chronic myelogenous leukemia (CML) (28). The Ph chromosome results from the translocation between chromosomes 9 and 22, causing the fusion of the ABL (9q34) and BCR (22q11) genes (**Fig. 17.2B**). The use of is specific chromosomal alteration makes it possible to interrogate both metaphase and interphase cells for diagnosis as well as for the on-going monitoring for residual disease and recurrence (29). Another common application of FISH in routine clinical cancer cytogenetics is the detection of gene amplification of Her2/Neu in breast carcinomas (30,31). Although gene amplification is typically a sign of late stage, and poor clinical outcome (32), it has been recently shown that women with Her2/Neu amplification showed a better response to trastuzumab (33).

3.3. Advanced Molecular Cancer Cytogenetics

Most cancers have an abnormal chromosomal content characterized by changes in chromosomal structure and number. In general, chromosomal aberrations are more numerous in malignant tumors than in benign ones, and the karyotypic complexity and cellular heterogeneity observed is often associated with poor prognosis. One of the challenges facing cancer researchers today is to understand how cancer cells acquire genomes with such a high degree of complexity (34), and to determine in what way these changes may be functionally significant. To investigate the chromosomal basis of disease, sophisticated FISH-based assays have been developed and include metaphase comparative genomic hybridization (CGH); multicolor FISH assays such as spectral karyotyping and MBanding analysis to augment the analysis generated by traditional FISH assays (also reviewed by Speicher and Carter (35)).

Comparative genomic hybridization (CGH) was first introduced in 1992 (6) and is described as a FISH-based that determines net gain or loss of genomic material in a given test DNA, without the need for fresh material required for short-term culture and chromosome analysis. Normal reference DNA and the tumor/test DNA is differentially labeled and hybridized to normal metaphase spreads. The normal DNA and tumor/test DNA is detected with the use of different fluorochromes (i.e., green and red) and visualized by fluorescence microscopy. Metaphase spreads are karyotyped by inverted DAPI banding, and the average green:red ratio (tumor/test:normal) is calculated. Regions of genomic gain in the tumor are expressed as an increase in green:red ratio, whereas regions that are lost in the tumor are expressed as a decrease in green:red ratio. Regions that are normal maintain a 1:1 ratio. High-level amplifications can be readily seen as a spike at a specific chromosomal locus and are generally ratios that exceed 1.5. The major advantage of CGH as compared to other cytogenetic methods (i.e., chromosome banding, FISH) is the fact that instead of metaphase chromosomes or interphase nuclei, only a few micrograms of genomic DNA is required from the cells or tissue to be studied. CGH has been an important tool in determining the net chromosomal changes across a number of neoplasms, (reader should refer to the Progenetix CGH database (http://www.progenetix.de/~pgscripts/progenetix/Aboutprogenetix.html) as well as the NCBI hosted database (http://www.ncbi.nlm.nih.gov/sky/)). CGH has also allowed investigators to identify regions of the genome that may contain putative oncogenes and tumor suppressor genes in many tumors including ovarian cancers (36), osteosarcomas (37) and brain tumors (38). In the past 5 years, array-based CGH methods have been used more prominently to provide higher resolution analysis of the genome, however metaphase CGH is still widely used in many laboratories.

In addition to copy number changes within the tumor genome, structural rearrangements play a large role in tumorigenesis (39). Large and small structural chromosomal aberrations are often difficult to determine with certainty using conventional cytogenetic banding methods alone (40). The problems that can typically arise in both clinical and cancer cytogenetics are the presence of structural chromosome aberrations with unidentifiable chromosomal regions, or very complex chromosomes (sometimes called "marker chromosomes") in which no recognizable banding pattern exists. Although locus-specific probes and whole chromosome paints may be used in succession until the marker chromosome and its constituents can be identified, this strategy is both costly and time-consuming and may lead to the depletion of valuable patient samples. Advances in microscopy and image analysis have yielded 2–3 different methods of distinguishing the distinct fluorescence of a mixture of several chromosomal paints during sequential or a single image acquisition. Filter-based systems are generically termed Multicolor FISH (MFISH) (8) (although each supplier has their own modified acronym for this technique). The second more frequently used system, called Spectral Karyotyping (SKY) (7), uses image analysis based on Fourier transformation to spectrally analyze the differential fluorescence of each chromosome painting probe. Both the SKY and MFISH methods require the use of human whole chromosomal paints that are differentially labeled, so that each chromosome will have a unique combination of colors emitted following hybridization for identification purposes. Use of this entire genome, whole chromosomal painting method has revealed the true complexity of many tumor karyotypes (36,37,41–44) (**Fig. 17.2C–E**). Another multi-color approach is MBand (9), where specific bands along a chromosome are differentially labeled in a 4 or 5-color experiment. The probe is hybridized to the test metaphase, where the resulting hybridization pattern of the chromosome of interest is compared to the normal hybridization pattern previously established and stored within analysis software. This method has been useful for identifying intra-chromosomal rearrangements, including small deletions, inversions and intra-chromosomal duplication events (45–48). In addition, MBanding has been useful more accurately determining the specific region of chromosomal rearrangement.

These sophisticated FISH-based assays all complement simple FISH analysis that investigates the copy number of chromosomal loci or genes associated with disease and disease progression, typically in experiments that detect changes in the overall ploidy of the genome (**Fig. 17.2F**) gene amplification *(49,50)* (**Fig. 17.2G**), deletion *(51)* (**Fig. 17.2H**) and specific translocations or rearrangements *(52,53)*.

Understanding the causes of cancer, and identifying the characteristic cytogenetic alterations associated with the onset of neoplasia provides essential molecular diagnostic tools for the clinical laboratory. Other types of cytogenetic change may not be apparent at diagnosis, but may be acquired later on, when the cancer progresses to a more advanced phase of the disease. Such cytogenetic changes may be quite consistent in the latter phases of disease and they can be used as a reliable prognostic biomarker that tells clinicians to modify treatment to deal with the tumors' more aggressive behavior. Because cancer is a cellular disease of relentless genetic progression, it is often associated with specific molecular biological and histological change *(54)*. The ability to develop FISH-based cellular biomarkers that can detect the critical components of these established molecular "hallmarks of cancer" will provide a powerful basis for diagnosing, monitoring and predicting outcome and response to treatment. It is through this key concept that FISH-based analysis, particularly interphase-FISH, is becoming a critical and important tool in biomarker studies *(50)*. Due to the specificity of DNA as a probe, interphase FISH can be a sensitive, stabile and reproducible assay for the detection of genomic/gene deletion, amplification, specific translocations and global genomic instability. Furthermore, since FISH can be applied to both cytogenetic specimens and tissues embedded in paraffin section, the technique has been widely applied to tissue microarrays (TMAs) *(55)* (**Fig. 17.2I–K**) that afford the high-throughput screening of many tissues within one experiment and permits comparative analysis with histology.

4. Conclusions and Perspectives

Advances in chromosomal and cytogenetic analysis have occurred rapidly and have played a central role in the development of a conceptual understanding of human genetic diseases and cancer. Initial genetic analysis of tumors was limited to gross chromosomal abnormalities, but in recent years impressive progress in FISH analytical approaches have yielded a diversity of molecular cytogenetic methods to understand genomic alterations in the chromosomes of human cells. The range of analytical methods available in 2008 can address diverse genomic questions from identifying gross structural changes of chromosomes in the genome down to newer array methods that examine single-nucleotide differences. These high-resolution technologies are increasingly allowing us to understand the processes that are involved in normal genomic function and disease. Future analyses will be able to utilize minute amounts of DNA because of advances in whole genome amplification protocols, automated sample processing methodologies with continuing advances in imaging hardware and software platforms. The use FISH to analyze higher-order chromatin structure by 3D-imaging methods is an area of particular importance at present that will provide an understanding of the impact of changing genomic locations within the nucleus itself. Other developments of FISH technology will include more advanced and sophisticated ways of performing multicolor FISH analyses in a high-throughput format, to provide an increasing level of detail concerning the causes and consequences of chromosomal rearrangement in genetic syndromes and in cancer cells.

Acknowledgments: The authors wish to acknowledge all current and former members of the Squire and Zielenska Laboratories for their technical contributions (http://www.utoronto.ca/cancyto/). This work has been supported through funds from the National Cancer Institute of Canada (NCIC) and the Terry Fox Foundation, The Prostate Cancer Research Foundation of Canada (PCRFC), The Ontario Cancer Research Network (OCRN), The Canadian Foundation for Innovation (CFI), The James Fund for Neuroblastoma Research and The Princess Margaret Ovarian Cancer Foundation.

References

1. Rudkin GT, Stollar BD (1977) High resolution detection of DNA-RNA hybrids in situ by indirect immunofluorescence. Nature 265:472–473
2. Lichter P, Cremer T, Borden J, Manuelidis L, Ward DC (1988) Delineation of individual human chromosomes in metaphase and interphase cells by in situ suppression hybridization using recombinant DNA libraries. Hum Genet 80:224–234
3. Jang W, Yonescu R, Knutsen T, Brown T, Reppert T, Sirotkin K, Schuler GD, Ried T, Kirsch IR (2006) Linking the human cytogenetic map with nucleotide sequence: the CCAP clone set. Cancer Genet Cytogenet 168:89–97
4. Knutsen T, Gobu V, Knaus R, Padilla-Nash H, Augustus M, Strausberg RL, Kirsch IR, Sirotkin K, Ried T (2005) The interactive online SKY/M-FISH & CGH database and the Entrez cancer chromosomes search database: linkage of chromosomal aberrations with the genome sequence. Genes Chromosomes Cancer 44:52–64
5. Oliveira AM, French CA (2005) Applications of fluorescence in situ hybridization in cytopathology: a review. Acta Cytol 49:587–594
6. Kallioniemi A, Kallioniemi OP, Sudar D, Rutovitz D, Gray JW, Waldman F, Pinkel D (1992) Comparative genomic hybridization for molecular cytogenetic analysis of solid tumors. Science 258:818–821
7. Veldman T, Vignon C, Schrock E, Rowley JD, Ried T (1997) Hidden chromosome abnormalities in haematological malignancies detected by multicolour spectral karyotyping. Nat Genet 15:406–410
8. Speicher MR, Gwyn Ballard S, Ward DC (1996) Karyotyping human chromosomes by combinatorial multi-fluor FISH. Nat Genet 12:368–375
9. Chudoba I, Plesch A, Lorch T, Lemke J, Claussen U, Senger G (1999) High resolution multicolor-banding: a new technique for refined FISH analysis of human chromosomes. Cytogenet Cell Genet 84:156–160
10. Bayani J, Squire JA (2000) Chapter 22 cell biology of chromosomes and Nuclei. In: Current protocols in cell biology (Morgan, K.). John Wiley & Sons, Inc, Bethesda
11. Schwarzacher T, Heslop-Harrison P (2000) Practical in situ hybridization. Springer-Verlag, New York
12. Hungerford DA, Donnely A, Nowel A, Beck S (1959) The chromosome constitution of a human phenotypic intersex. Am J Hum Gen 11:215
13. Moorhead PS, Nowell PC, Mellman WJ, Battips DM, Hungerford DA (1960) Chromosome preparations of leukocytes cultured from human peripheral blood. Exp Cell Res 20:613–616

14. Barch MJ (1991) The ACT cytogenetics laboratory manual, 2nd edn Raven Press, New York

15. Henegariu O, Heerema NA, Lowe Wright L, Bray-Ward P, Ward DC, Vance GH (2001) Improvements in cytogenetic slide preparation: controlled chromosome spreading, chemical aging and gradual denaturing. Cytometry 43:101–109

16. Speel EJ (1999) Robert Feulgen Prize Lecture 1999. Detection and amplification systems for sensitive, multiple-target DNA and RNA in situ hybridization: looking inside cells with a spectrum of colors. Histochem Cell Biol 112:89–113

17. Squire J, Meurs EF, Chong KL, McMillan NA, Hovanessian AG, Williams BR (1993) Localization of the human interferon-induced, ds-RNA activated p68 kinase gene (PRKR) to chromosome 2p21–p22. Genomics 16:768–770

18. Matsuda Y, Harada YN, Natsuume-Sakai S, Lee K, Shiomi T, Chapman VM (1992) Location of the mouse complement factor H gene (cfh) by FISH analysis and replication R-banding. Cytogenet Cell Genet 61:282–285

19. Milatovich A, Hsieh CL, Bonaminio G, Tecott L, Julius D, Francke U (1992) Serotonin receptor 1c gene assigned to X chromosome in human (band q24) and mouse (bands D-F4). Hum Mol Genet 1:681–684

20. Liu J, Tsai YL, Zheng XZ, Baramki TA, Yazigi RA, Katz E (1998) Potential use of repeated fluorescence in situ hybridization in the same human blastomeres for preimplantation genetic diagnosis. Fertil Steril 70:729–733

21. Verlinsky Y, Cieslak J, Ivakhnenko V, Evsikov S, Wolf G, White M, Lifchez A, Kaplan B, Moise J, Valle J, Ginsberg N, Strom C, Kuliev A (1997) Prepregnancy genetic testing for age-related aneuploidies by polar body analysis. Genet Test 1:231–235

22. Daniel A, Wu Z, Darmanian A, Malafiej P, Tembe V, Peters G, Kennedy C, Ades L (2004) Issues arising from the prenatal diagnosis of some rare trisomy mosaics – the importance of cryptic fetal mosaicism. Prenat Diagn 24:524–536

23. Romana SP, Tachdjian G, Druart L, Cohen D, Berger R, Cherif D (1993) A simple method for prenatal diagnosis of trisomy 21 on uncultured amniocytes. Eur J Hum Genet 1:245–251

24. Leana-Cox J, Jenkins L, Palmer CG, Plattner R, Sheppard L, Flejter WL, Zackowski J, Tsien F, Schwartz S (1994) Molecular cytogenetic analysis of inv dup(15) chromosomes, using probes specific for the Prader-Willi/Angelman syndrome region: clinical implications. Am J Hum Genet 54:748–756

25. Pettenati MJ, Hayworth R, Cox K, Rao PN (1994) Prenatal detection of cri du chat syndrome on uncultured amniocytes using fluorescence in situ hybridization (FISH). Clin Genet 45:17–20

26. Driscoll DA (2001) Prenatal diagnosis of the 22q11.2 deletion syndrome. Genet Med 3:14–18

27. Weksberg R, Stachon AC, Squire JA, Moldovan L, Bayani J, Meyn S, Chow E, Bassett AS (2006) Molecular characterization of deletion break-points in adults with 22q11 deletion syndrome. Hum Genet 6:837–845

28. Rowley JD (1973) Letter: A new consistent chromosomal abnormality in chronic myelogenous leukaemia identified by quinacrine fluorescence and Giemsa staining. Nature 243:290–293

29. Landstrom AP, Tefferi A (2006) Fluorescent in situ hybridization in the diagnosis, prognosis, and treatment monitoring of chronic myeloid leukemia. Leuk Lymphoma 47:397–402

30. Hanna W (2001) Testing for HER2 status. Oncology 61 Suppl 2:22–30

31. Hicks DG, Tubbs RR (2005) Assessment of the HER2 status in breast cancer by fluorescence in situ hybridization: a technical review with interpretive guidelines. Hum Pathol 36:250–261

32. Slamon DJ, Clark GM, Wong SG, Levin WJ, Ullrich A, McGuire WL (1987) Human breast cancer: correlation of relapse and survival with amplification of the HER-2/neu oncogene. Science 235:177–182

33. Ross JS, Fletcher JA, Bloom KJ, Linette GP, Stec J, Symmans WF, Pusztai L, Hortobagyi GN (2004) Targeted therapy in breast cancer: the HER-2/neu gene and protein. Mol Cell Proteomics 3:379–398

34. Balmain A, Gray J, Ponder B (2003) The genetics and genomics of cancer. Nat Genet 33 Suppl:238–244

35. Speicher MR, Carter NP (2005) The new cytogenetics: blurring the boundaries with molecular biology. Nat Rev Genet 6:782–792

36. Bayani J, Brenton JD, Macgregor PF, Beheshti B, Albert M, Nallainathan D, Karaskova J, Rosen B, Murphy J, Laframboise S, Zanke B, Squire JA (2002) Parallel analysis of sporadic primary ovarian carcinomas by spectral karyotyping, comparative genomic hybridization, and expression microarrays. Cancer Res 62:3466–3476

37. Zielenska M, Bayani J, Pandita A, Toledo S, Marrano P, Andrade J, Petrilli A, Thorner P, Sorensen P, Squire JA (2001) Comparative genomic hybridization analysis identifies gains of 1p35 approximately p36 and chromosome 19 in osteosarcoma. Cancer Genet Cytogenet 130:14–21

38. Bayani J, Pandita A, Squire JA (2005) Molecular cytogenetic analysis in the study of brain tumors: findings and applications. Neurosurg Focus 19:E1

39. Bayani J, Selvarajah S, Maire G, Vukovic B, Al-Romaih K, Zielenska M, Squire JA (2006) Genomic mechanisms and measurement of structural and numerical instability in cancer cells. Semin Cancer Biol 1:5–18

40. Bayani JM, Squire JA (2002) Applications of SKY in cancer cytogenetics. Cancer Invest 20:373–386

41. Bayani J, Zielenska M, Pandita A, Al-Romaih K, Karaskova J, Harrison K, Bridge JA, Sorensen P, Thorner P, Squire JA (2003) Spectral karyotyping identifies recurrent complex rearrangements of chromosomes 8, 17, and 20 in osteosarcomas. Genes Chromosomes Cancer 36:7–16

42. Beheshti B, Karaskova J, Park PC, Squire JA, Beatty BG (2000) Identification of a high frequency of chromosomal rearrangements in the centromeric regions of prostate cancer cell lines by sequential giemsa banding and spectral karyotyping. Mol Diagn 5:23–32

43. Singh SK, Hawkins C, Clarke ID, Squire JA, Bayani J, Hide T, Henkelman RM, Cusimano MD, Dirks, PB (2004) Identification of human brain tumor initiating cells. Nature 432:396–401

44. Squire JA, Arab S, Marrano P, Bayani J, Karaskova J, Taylor M, Becker L, Rutka J, Zielenska M (2001) Molecular cytogenetic analysis of glial tumors using spectral karyotyping and comparative genomic hybridization. Mol Diagn 6:93–108

45. Lim G, Karaskova J, Beheshti B, Vukovic B, Bayani J, Selvarajah S, Watson SK, Lam WL, Zielenska M, Squire JA (2005) An integrated mBAND and submegabase resolution tiling set (SMRT) CGH array analysis of focal amplification, microdeletions, and ladder structures consistent with breakage-fusion-bridge cycle events in osteosarcoma. Genes Chromosomes Cancer 42:392–403

46. Lim G, Karaskova J, Vukovic B, Bayani J, Beheshti B, Bernardini M, Squire JA, Zielenska M (2004) Combined spectral karyotyping, multicolor banding, and microarray comparative genomic hybridization analysis provides a detailed characterization of complex structural chromosomal rearrangements associated with gene amplification in the osteosarcoma cell line MG-63. Cancer Genet Cytogenet 153:158–164

47. Selvarajah S, Yoshimoto M, Park PC, Maire G, Paderova J, Bayani J, Lim G, Al-Romaih K, Squire JA, Zielenska M (2006) The breakage-fusion-bridge (BFB) cycle as a mechanism for generating genetic heterogeneity in osteosarcoma. Chromosoma 6:459–467

48. Vukovic B, Beheshti B, Park PC, Lim G, Bayani J, Zielenska M, Squire JA Correlating breakage-fusion-bridge events with the over-all chromosomal

instability and in vitro karyotypic evolution in prostate cancer. Cytogenet Genome Res 1–2:1–11

49. Squire JA, Thorner P, Marrano P, Parkinson D, Ng YK, Gerrie B, Chilton-Macneill S, Zielenska M (1996) Identification of MYCN copy number heterogeneity by direct FISH analysis of neuroblastoma preparations. Mol Diagn 1:281–289

50. Tsao MS, Sakurada A, Cutz JC, Zhu CQ, Kamel-Reid S, Squire J, Lorimer I, Zhang T, Liu N, Daneshmand M, Marrano P, da Cunha Santos G, Lagarde A, Richardson F, Seymour L, Whitehead M, Ding K, Pater J, Shepherd FA (2005) Erlotinib in lung cancer – molecular and clinical predictors of outcome. N Engl J Med 353:133–144

51. Yoshimoto M, Cutz JC, Nuin PA, Joshua AM, Bayani J, Evans AJ, Zielenska M, Squire JA (2006) Interphase FISH analysis of PTEN in histologic sections shows genomic deletions in 68% of primary prostate cancer and 23% of high-grade prostatic intra-epithelial neoplasias. Cancer Genet Cytogenet 169:128–137

52. Kolomietz E, Al-Maghrabi J, Brennan S, Karaskova J, Minkin S, Lipton J, Squire JA (2001) Primary chromosomal rearrangements of leukemia are frequently accompanied by extensive submicroscopic deletions and may lead to altered prognosis. Blood 97:3581–3588

53. Yoshimoto M, Joshua AM, Chilton-Macneill S, Bayani J, Selvarajah S, Evans AJ, Zielenska M, Squire JA (2006) Three-color FISH analysis of TMPRSS2/ERG fusions in prostate cancer indicates that genomic microdeletion of chromosome 21 is associated with rearrangement. Neoplasia 8:465–469

54. Kelloff GJ, Lippman SM, Dannenberg AJ, Sigman CC, Pearce HL, Reid BJ, Szabo E, Jordan VC, Spitz MR, Mills GB, Papadimitrakopoulou VA, Lotan R, Aggarwal BB, Bresalier RS, Kim J, Arun B, Lu KH, Thomas ME, Rhodes HE, Brewer MA, Follen M, Shin DM, Parnes HL, Siegfried JM, Evans AA, Blot WJ, Chow WH, Blount PL, Maley CC, Wang KK, Lam S, Lee JJ, Dubinett SM, Engstrom PF, Meyskens FL, Jr, O'Shaughnessy J, Hawk ET, Levin B, Nelson WG, Hong WK (2006) Progress in chemoprevention drug development: the promise of molecular biomarkers for prevention of intraepithelial neoplasia and cancer – a plan to move forward. Clin Cancer Res 12:3661–3697

55. Braunschweig T, Chung JY, Hewitt SM (2005) Tissue microarrays: bridging the gap between research and the clinic. Expert Rev Proteomics 2:325–336

18

Quantitative Trait Locus Mapping to Identify Genes for Complex Traits in Mice

Jonathan D. Smith

1. Introduction

Let us say you performed a survey of five inbred mouse strains by following their body weight over time after feeding them a high fat diet. You identify three strains that became obese, whereas two strains did not. How can you identify the genes that are responsible for the different outcomes of these strains? One can apply the method of quantitative trait locus (QTL) mapping to identify the chromosomal region (locus) of a gene, or genes, that have an effect on a trait. This mapping is the first step in the identification of the responsible gene by a method that is referred to as positional cloning. In this chapter, the focus will be on the use of QTL mapping to identify genes for complex traits in mice; although, QTL mapping can be applied to any experimental system in which there is meiotic recombination and different inbred strains are available. A complex trait is a phenotype, such as body weight, that is influenced by several genes and the environment. An inbred strain contains individuals that are genetically homozygous at each locus, and thus all individuals within a strain are genetically identical. Two inbred strains may differ from each other at millions of places throughout their genomes. The goal of QTL mapping is to find the region where those differences have an effect on the phenotype. This chapter will discuss QTL mapping theory and methods, as well as several applications and emerging technology.

2. Methods and Applications

2.1. QTL Theory and Planning

The theory behind the most basic form of QTL mapping is based upon intercrossing two inbred strains. The mouse genome consists of 19 pairs of autosomes (non sex-determining chromosome) and the X and Y chromosomes. In the example shown in **Fig. 18.1**, we are intercrossing stain A (shown with a black chromosome pair) with strain B (shown with a white chromosome pair). The initial F_1 (filial generation 1) mice are true hybrids, with each individual

From: *Molecular Biomethods Handbook, 2nd Edition.*
Edited by: J. M. Walker and R. Rapley © Humana Press, Totowa, NJ

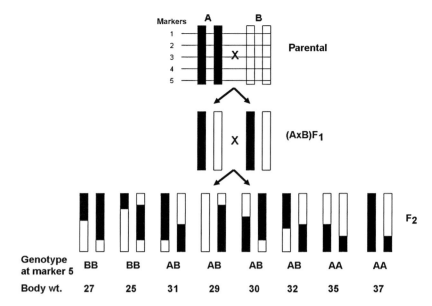

Fig. 18.1. Diagram of genetic heterogeneity in an F_2 cohort derived from a strain intercross. Strain A is shown with a black chromosome pair, and strain B with a white chromosome pair. The position of five strain polymorphic markers are shown. The F_1 generation contains individuals that are genetically identical to each other for their autosomes. Owing to meiotic recombination, each individual of the F_2 generation is genetically distinct. Below the representative eight F_2 subjects' chromosome pair is the genotype for marker 5, and the simulated body weight data after feeding a high fat diet

inheriting one black and one white chromosome. Thus all F_1 individuals are genetically identical to each other for their autosomes, and this generation is not informative as to the location of genes affecting a trait. The F_1 mice are then brother-sister mated to generate the F_2 progeny. During meiosis to generate haploid eggs and sperm, recombination takes place on the autosomes (and X chromosomes in females), most commonly with 1 recombination per chromosome, although 0 and 2 recombination events are also observed. This recombination during gemetogenesis in the F_1 parents yields chromosomes in their F_2 offspring that can have linear stretches of A and B parental origins. Thus, each F_2 mouse is unique genetically, inheriting a different patchwork arrangement of parental alleles along its genome. To derive the QTL map, each F_2 mouse is individually phenotyped (body weight measured in our example) and subjected to a genome scan that determines which one of the possible three genotypes (AA, AB, or BB) was inherited at each of hundreds to thousands of strain polymorphic markers at intervals along each autosome and the X chromosome. In the example shown in **Fig. 18.1**, the genome scan data for 1 chromosome is graphically represented for eight male F_2 mice, along with their body weights. There appears to be a correlation, such that the mice that have the BB genotype for marker 5 have the lowest body weights, whereas the mice that are AB for that marker have intermediate body weights, and the mice that are AA for that marker have the highest body weights. The statistical analysis of the genotype-phenotype correlations is performed by the use of QTL software, which will lead to the identification of loci in which the inheritance of parental alleles correlates with the phenotypes, as well as an indication of the strength of this correlation. The final output of a QTL study is a graph of the 19 autosomes and X chromosome in which a score for the correlation is plotted along the genome (**Fig. 18.2B**). Peaks represent loci in which a gene resides that affect the trait.

So, how do you go about planning and performing a QTL study, and how do you identify the responsible gene within a QTL that you have identified? Generally, one starts by performing a strain survey to find two parental inbred strains that have a markedly different trait. One can now look up many different traits of inbred mice online at the Mouse Phenome Database (http://phenome. jax.org/pub-cgi/phenome/mpdcgi?rtn=docs/home). However, the trait you may want to study may not be present in wild type mice, so you may want to cross a mutant (or genetically engineered) strain onto several inbred strains. By use of the marker assisted backcrossing method (*1*) or by simply backcrossing for ten generations, one can isolate strains that are >99.9% identical to the recipient strain, but retain the mutation selected for at each generation. One caveat of this strategy is that genes closely linked to the mutation will remain from the donor strain, and these may affect the phenotype. The next step involves characterizing the phenotype in a cohort of mice from each parental strain and from the hybrid F_1 generation. If the hybrid mice have a phenotype identical to one of the parental strains, then the allele or alleles from that parental strain are dominant, and the strain intercross should be performed by crossing the F_1 hybrids back to the recessive parental strain to generate a backcross N_2 cohort, rather than an F_2 cohort. If the F_1 hybrids have an intermediate phenotype (as in **Fig. 18.2A**), then it means that the major genes act in a codominant (additive) manner, or that there are many genes involved with various modes of inheritance, and an F_2 cohort should be bred for the QTL mapping. How large of a N_2 or F_2 cohort is required for QTL mapping? Clearly, the larger the cohort, the more power there is to detect QTL loci, and the loci detected will have increased statistical significance. Cohorts between 200 and 600 are common in mouse studies and have adequate power to identify QTL for complex traits. The phenotype distribution in the F_2 cohort can also be informative. If there is a bimodal distribution with a 3:1 ratio of mice in the two peaks, this would imply that there is 1 major gene affecting the trait, and that one strain's allele is dominant and the other strain's allele is recessive. If there is a clear trimodal distribution with a 1:2:1 ratio, this would imply that there is a major gene with a codominant effect on the trait. However, it is common to see a broad variation in the phenotype of the F_2 cohort, covering both parental phenotypes, with no clear modal distribution (as in **Fig. 18.2A**). This implies that there are several genes affecting the phenotype.

2.2. Performing a QTL Study

It is useful to try to capture as much phenotypic information about each F_2 mouse as possible, as phenotypes can be tested for correlations with each other, and each phenotype can be used as the quantitative trait in QTL mapping. For example, instead of only getting loci for body weight, you can also get loci for plasma cholesterol, triglycerides, free fatty acids, abdominal fat pad weight, liver weight, etc. It is crucial to record the sex of each subject, as sex can be either an additive or interactive covariate, and many QTLs are

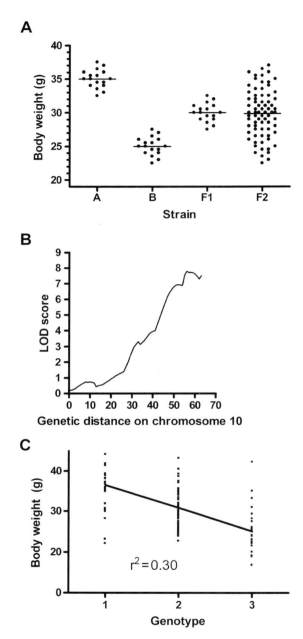

Fig. 18.2. QTL mapping. **A**. Simulated body weight data for male mice of strain A, strain B, and the F_1 and F_2 generations derived from the strain intercross. **B**. Simulated QTL peak for body weight on the distal end of chromosome 10. **C**. Linear regression of the simulated data was used to determine that body weight in the F_2 male cohort fit a codominant model for the marker nearest the LOD peak on chromosome 10. Genotypes 1, 2, and 3 refer to mice with AA, AB, and BB alleles of this marker. The r^2 value indicates that 30% of the body weight variance in the male F2 cohort is associated with the genotype at this 1 marker

found in only males or females. Upon sacrifice of each mouse, tissue must be obtained to prepare genomic DNA. Tail tip or spleens are commonly taken, and spare tissue is frozen away so that independent DNA preparations can be made should a sample run out or be of low quality. The next step is to perform a genome scan for each F_2 mouse. This is routinely done by PCR amplification across strain polymorphic microsatellite repeats (simple dinucleotide repeats), and running the products out on acrylamide or agarose gels, or by capillary electrophoresis. These markers can be found by searching the Mouse Genome Informatics database online at http://www.informatics.jax.org/. Generally 100–200 markers are used yielding an average interval of 20–10 cM among markers (cM, centimorgan, is a unit of genetic distance with 1 cM = 1% recombination frequency). This yields sufficient resolution to generate QTL maps. However, this can be laborious, and a newer method is available via the use of mouse SNP (single nucleotide polymorphism) chips. We have used this method and obtained ~2000 informative markers between two inbred strains, yielding a marker on average every 1 cM *(2)*. Genotypes should be examined to make sure that they are in Hardy Weinberg equilibrium (if not, it is likely that the genotype assay was not valid), and to make sure that the markers show on average 1 recombination per chromosome (double recombinants around a single marker are suspicious and may be erroneous).

The next step is to perform the QTL analysis. For this you will have to download software. Three of the most commonly used freely available packages are Mapmaker (http://www.broad.mit.edu/ftp/distribution/software/mapmaker3/) *(3)*, Map Manager QTX (http://www.mapmanager.org/mmQTX.html) *(4)*, and r/qtl (http://www.biostat.jhsph.edu/~kbroman/qtl/) *(5)*. Each package will utilize the genotypic and phenotypic data and the multipoint linkage mapping method to produce an interval map using either LOD or LRS units to show the location of the QTLs on the mouse genome (for a full review of QTL statistics, see *6*). The LOD score is the logarithm of the odds favoring linkage, thus a LOD score of 3 has a 1,000-fold odds of that the locus is linked to the phenotype. The LRS score is a likelihood ratio statistic, and it is ~4.6 × the LOD score. Some QTL software programs can also look for gene–gene interactions or epistasis. Even looking at only two genes at once breaks an F_2 cohort into nine genotype groups, thus even larger sample sizes may be required for detecting significant levels of epistasis with a low false discovery rate. Before QTL statistical analysis, one should determine if the phenotypic data is normally distributed, and if it is not, log transformation should be considered. The QTL analysis should be performed with both sexes combined using sex as an additive or interactive covariate and in both sexes separately. After running the data through the software and obtaining the interval map with LOD peaks, one must determine if a LOD peak is significant. Lander and Kruglyak have defined criteria for genome-wide significance for QTLs after estimated correction for multiple testing, referring to those with $p < 0.001$ as highly significant, $p < 0.05$ as significant, and $p < 0.63$ as suggestive *(7)*. However, permutation analysis, in which the phenotypic data is randomly scrambled, can give an empirical level of significance based upon the real data set, which is probably better than using estimated whole genome corrections for multiple testing *(8)*.

Let us return to our sample data in **Fig. 18.2**. Strain A and B males have average body weights of 35 and 25 g, respectively. You found that the F_1 strain had an average body weight of 30 g, and thus you breed an intercross F_2 cohort.

The average weight of the F_2 mice is also 30 g, but the phenotype overlaps both parental strains and the coefficient of variance is much greater than observed in the F_1 cohort. The degree of variance in the trait that is due to genetic variation, rather than to environmental or stochastic effects, can be estimated by comparing the phenotypic variance in the F_2 (genetically heterogeneous) cohort with the F_1 (genetically homogenous) cohorts using the following equation: (variance$_{F2}$ – variance$_{F1}$)/ variance F_2 *(9)*. For the example shown in **Fig. 18.2A**, 62% of the variance in the F_2 cohort is genetically determined. Next, perform a genome scan, and input the genetic and phenotypic data into a QTL software program. **Figure 18.2B** shows the results on chromosome 10, where there is a peak LOD score of ~8 at 60 cM near the distal end. You perform a permutation analysis and you found that this peak has a genome wide *p* value of <0.001, highly significant. Congratulations, you mapped a novel QTL for body weight in response to a high fat diet.

Does your QTL overlap with other known QTLs for body weight? To estimate the confidence interval of the locus one can use the 1-LOD or 1.5-LOD drop-off interval. One simply determines the cM region encompassed by the peak LOD minus 1 (or 1.5) LOD units. Next, one can determine the inheritance model, dominant/recessive versus codominant, and the % of the phenotypic data associated with the QTL. This is best accomplished via linear regression. For the codominant model, all of the mice with AA genotype at the marker closest to the QTL peak are coded as 1, all of the AB mice are coded as 2, and all of the BB mice are coded as 3. These values are used in an *xy* plot along with the phenotypic data and liner regression can be used to calculate r^2, the correlation coefficient. For the dominant models, repeat this analysis twice more, once with the AA and AB mice coded as 1 and BB coded as 2 (A dominant) and once with AA coded as 1 and AB and BB coded as 2 (B dominant). The largest of the three r^2 values defines the model that best fits the data, and this r^2 value equals the % of the phenotypic variance associated with the QTL. For our example in **Fig. 18.2C**, the codominant model fit the data best, with 30% of the variance associated with the QTL on the distal end of chromosome 10. Finally, one needs to name the QTL, and this can be done by following the rules of and submission to the Mouse Nomenclature Committee (http://www.informatics.jax.org/mgihome/nomen/).

There are other ways to find QTL loci in addition to breeding F_2 or N_2 cohorts. These include the use of panels of recombinant inbred strains *(10)*, chromosome substitution strains (also called consomic strains) *(11)*, and congenic strains *(12)*. One can phenotype a panel of these strains and perform a QTL analysis without the need for genotyping, as the genotypes have already been ascertained for the different strains. The use of a high density genome scan via a SNP chip may can lead to a smaller confidence interval for a QTL than obtained by a traditional genome scan using microsatellite markers *(2)*, and in this case this interval is limited by recombination rather than by marker density. Thus, it may be useful to breed F_3 or F_4 cohorts for QTL mapping by high density genome scan, which will increase recombination frequency and should result in even smaller QTL intervals.

2.3. Confirmation and Fine Mapping

Once a QTL interval is identified, one must confirm it and attempt to identify the responsible gene. Although an independent strain intercross can be used to

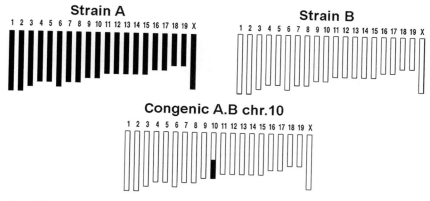

Fig. 18.3. Diagram of a congenic strain that contains the body weight QTL interval on chromosome 10 donated from strain A on the strain B recipient genetic background

confirm a QTL, this does not help in identifying the responsible gene. Thus, most investigators breed interval specific congenic strains in which one region of the genome is maintained by the donor genotype whereas the rest of the genome is of the recipient genotype. **Figure 18.3** shows an interval specific congenic strain in which the distal end of chromosome 10 is derived from strain A, whereas the rest of the genome is derived from strain B. To generate this congenic strain an F1 mouse was backcrossed multiple generations to parental strain B, at each generation selecting progeny for further backcrossing that retain heterozygosity over the QTL interval. After ten generations of backcrossing (N10) the congenic strain should on average contain 99.9% recipient genotype, outside of the selected QTL interval. Alternatively, speed congenics can be obtained after 5–6 generations of backcrossing, and selecting with markers not only within the QTL interval, but also across the whole genome to find the best progeny for subsequent backcrosses *(1)*. Initially the congenic strain is heterozygous for the two strains across the selected interval, but these mice can be brother sister mated to generate a cohort for progeny testing that contain 0, 1, or 2 copies of the donor strain allele. Formal proof of the QTL is obtained if at least one of these types of progeny has a statistically significant different phenotype from the other types of progeny.

Typically, the initial QTL interval will cover ~30 cM, or about 60 Mb. To narrow down the region for candidate gene testing, one must perform fine mapping. This involves identifying a set of markers across the QTL interval and then further backcrossing of the congenic strain to select progeny in which recombination occurred within the interval. Further breeding will generate a set of partially overlapping subcongenic strains. Progeny testing is then performed and can lead to QTL interval of 1 cM or less containing 1–2 Mb of DNA. This interval may contain only one gene or perhaps 10–20 genes, which are all candidates for the causative gene.

2.4. Candidate Gene Testing

How can one prove if a specific candidate gene is the causative gene? This issue has been addressed previously *(13,14)*, and both circumstantial evidence as well as more direct evidence can lead to varying levels of confidence.

The first step in identifying the causative gene is to sequence coding and regulatory regions of the candidate genes to identify strain specific polymorphisms in the gene that might affect the protein function or expression level. If the gene product is known to effect a pathway involved in the phenotype, or expressed in the correct cell types, this is also useful information. In vitro functional studies can be performed after transfections of mammalian cells, or after bacterial expression and purification, to see if the strain specific protein isoforms have altered enzymatic activity, regulation, or binding of other proteins or ligands. The above evidence is circumstantial, but it can be convincing if strong enough. The gold standard for direct in vivo evidence is allele replacement, where gene knock-in would replace the strain A allele with the strain B allele. However, this is not readily feasible. Gene knock-in technology uses embryonic stem (ES), which have only been successfully derived from 129 and C57BL/6 strains. Thus, if the QTL was identified using other mouse strains it may not be possible to use this method unless one is prepared to backcross the replacement onto a different strain. More commonly, one can test the candidate gene by over and/or under expression. Over expression can be performed by making a transgenic mouse. This can be achieved through the use of a cDNA minigene, or a BAC derived genomic construction. The effect of overexpression of the transgene on the phenotype can be ascertained. To test for the effect of a protein coding polymorphism, one can make constructions containing the alternate alleles, and test the expression levels in several independent transgenic lines to select strains with equivalent expression. These strains can then be subjected to phenotypic testing to prove whether the protein polymorphism affects the trait. Under expression is tested by creating a knock out, also through the use of ES cells; thus, it may be necessary to breed the knock out onto the strains used for QTL mapping. There are now available several large public libraries of ES cell clones containing knock outs for thousands of mouse genes, obtained through gene trapping insertional mutagenesis *(15)*. Thus, if a candidate gene has been knocked out in this way, it is possible to obtain the knockout mice fairly simply, without the need for creating a gene targeting vector and selecting recombinant ES cell clones. An alternative way to knock down expression of a candidate gene in vivo is through the use of RNA interference (RNAi). Although, the methods for use of RNAi in vivo are still being developed, this method avoids the problem of the effect of closely linked genes being transmitted during back crossing of a gene knockout; and, this method was recently used to verify a candidate gene that modifies for type I diabetes *(16)*.

2.5. Shortcut to Candidate Gene Identification: eQTLs

Although, mapping and fine mapping mouse QTLs is time consuming, laborious, and expensive, it is also fairly straight forward, with a high probability of success. It is the identification of the responsible gene that is more difficult and often much more time consuming, and luck (specific recombinants) may play a significant role. However, there is a shortcut that has proven to be quite useful to identify candidate genes, even before fine mapping, and this involves the use of expression microarrays. Even when expression arrays were just being developed, their use enabled the identification of the CD36 gene as responsible for a QTL associated with insulin resistance and fatty acid metabolism in isolated adipocytes from the spontaneous hypertensive rat *(17)*. Microarrays covering most of the known mouse expressed transcripts are available, and these can very useful in the gene identification process. First, one must collect tissue from the F_2 or N_2 cohort for RNA preparation, and which tissue to take is an important consideration. For body weight, one might take adipose tissue, liver, or the brain. However, it may be preferable to actually isolate a pure cell type, such as adipocytes, before making the RNA. All complex tissues or organs, or for that matter pathological tissue samples, are a collection of various cell types. It is quite possible that the costly gene expression data might be no more informative than a simple histological assay. For example, if large fat pads in obese mice lead to inflammation and more leukocytes than in the small fat pads of the thin mice, this would result in an increased level of expression of leuko-cyte expressed genes in the obese mice. This might be informative, but if this result is a consequence rather than a cause of obesity, it might lead down a false avenue of investigation. Laser capture microdissection can be used to circum-vent this problem, and examine a more homogeneous cell population *(18)*.

Once the tissue has been selected, RNA prepared, and gene expression data obtained, there are two main ways in which this data can be evaluated. One is by simple correlation analysis, where the expression of each transcript is correlated to the phenotype (body weight in our example) and the transcripts with the best correlations are examined to see if any happen to map to a body weight QTL. This analysis is easily done in a spread sheet and it is quite pow-erful in quickly identifying candidate genes before fine mapping. The second method is to use the expression level of each of the thousands of expressed transcripts as a quantitative trait, and use the existing genome scan data to identify expression QTLs (eQTLS) for the expression level of each transcript. For example, Schadt et al. examined liver RNA in a cohort of 111 F2 mice generated from intercrossing the C57BL/6 and DBA/2 strains *(19)*. They identified eQTLs for ~4300 transcripts with a LOD score >4.3. Of these about 1/3 were cis eQTLs, where the transcript mapped to the location of the eQTL, and 2/3 were trans eQTLs, where the transcript mapped outside of the eQTL region. And, as had been previously observed in yeast crosses *(20)*, the eQTLs were not randomly distributed. There were several hotspots or regions that had trans eQTLs for hundreds of transcripts, where presumably a key transcription factor or signal-transduction pathway gene resides that is polymorphic among the parental strains *(19)*. To identify candidate genes, one can then look for transcripts with either cis or trans eQTLs that map to the phenotypic QTL. In this way, it may be possible to identify gene expression pathways involved in the phenotype. For example, if gene Z, whose expression is highly correlated with body weight maps to the body weight QTL, and has a cis eQTL at that position, it may be possible to find additional genes with trans eQTLs at the same locus whose expression is correlated (or inversely correlated) with the expression of gene Z. Expression of these additional genes may be directly affected by the expression of gene Z, and play a downstream role in adipose physiology. Some eQTLs are conserved across different tissues and for these the choice of tissue is less important, for example 15% of the eQTLs detected independently in rat kidney and fat were common to both tissues *(21)*. The use of these genetic-genomic methods is now widely accepted to be a key shortcut in identifying candidate genes and metabolic pathways involved in complex traits.

2.6 Confounding Issues

The QTL method has yielded hundreds of loci for complex traits, but only a handful of genes have been successfully isolated thus far. The use of the gene expression microarray data will probably accelerate this pace; however, there are constraints that may make rapid progress difficult to achieve. For example, in one recent study a 1 cM genomic interval in the plant Arabidopsis that was not known to contain any QTLs for growth rate was examined in detail. Two growth rate QTLs were found within a 210-kb region, and both showed epistasis, such that their effects depended upon the genetic background (22). The amount of complexity in such a small genomic interval suggests that there may be overwhelming complexity of the genetic architecture of complex traits, making it very difficult to identify the genes responsible for much of the genetic-associated variation in these traits, particularly if many of these effects are epistatic in nature and thus harder to identify. Using the set of 22 chromosome substitution strains, where each strain contains one A/J strain chromosome on the C57BL/6 background, Nadeau and colleagues found that 17 of these strains have an altered level of diet induced obesity compared to the C57Bl/6 strain, with the cumulative effects much greater than that observed between the two parental strains (11). Even within one of these chromosome substitution strains, where QTL can be readily mapped, and subcongenic strains easily made, multiple loci effecting diet induced obesity are being found (Joe Nadeau, personal communication). This seems to confirm what was observed in the Arabidopsis study, there may be too many QTLs for some complex traits, with nonadditive and unknown levels of gene-gene and gene-environment interactions.

2.7. Cross Species QTLs

What is the significance of a rodent QTL for human complex traits such as susceptibility to common diseases? QTLs for a complex trait in mice and rats often overlap with the syntenous region of human chromosomes that by linkage analysis are thought to harbor genes for the same complex trait (23,24). These so-called cross species QTLs suggest that the rodent and human genes (called orthologs) are active in their respective species to modify disease severity or susceptibility. For example, Jacob and colleagues have described 15 clusters of blood pressure related QTLs from several rat strain intercrosses (25). Many of these QTLs seem to be conserved across species, as seven mouse blood pressure QTLs and five of six known human blood pressure QTLs map to syntenic chromosomal regions with the rat QTL clusters. The information obtained from the identification of a rodent gene for a complex trait may be useful in two ways. First, human genetic variation in the orthologous gene can be probed by association studies to see if common human genetic variation is associated with a complex trait such as common disease susceptibility. As an example, human genetic variation in the TNSF4 gene (the human ortholog of the gene responsible for an atherosclerosis QTL in mice) was found to be associated with coronary artery disease (26). Second, new pathways involved in disease pathogenesis may be uncovered through rodent QTL studies, and human genetic variation in several genes involved in the pathway can be probed by association studies. As an example, the identification of genetic variation in the 5-lipoxygenase gene that affects atherosclerosis in mice strengthened the interest in and helped select the ALOX5AP (FLAP) gene as a candidate within a heart attack associated locus on human chromosome 13 *(27,28)*. Thus, it appears that mouse and rat QTLs studies are informative in discovering human complex trait genes.

References

1. Markel P, Shu P, Ebeling C et al (1997) Theoretical and empirical issues for marker-assisted breeding of congenic mouse strains. Nat Genet 17:280–284
2. Smith JD, Bhasin JM, Baglione J et al (2006) Atherosclerosis susceptibility loci identified from a strain intercross of apolipoprotein E-deficient mice via a high-density genome scan. Arterioscler Thromb Vasc Biol 26:597–603
3. Lander ES, Green P, Abrahamson J et al (1987) MAPMAKER: an interactive computer package for constructing primary genetic linkage maps of experimental and natural populations. Genomics 1:174–181
4. Manly KF, Cudmore RH, Jr, Meer JM (2001) Map Manager QTX, cross-platform software for genetic mapping. Mamm Genome 12:930–932
5. Broman KW, Wu H, Sen S, Churchill GA (2003) R/qtl: QTL mapping in experimental crosses. Bioinformatics 19:889–890
6. Broman KW (2001) Review of statistical methods for QTL mapping in experimental crosses. Lab Anim (NY) 30:44–52
7. Lander E, Kruglyak L (1995) Genetic dissection of complex traits: guidelines for interpreting and reporting linkage results. Nat Genet 11:241–247
8. Churchill GA, Doerge RW (1994) Empirical threshold values for quantitative trait mapping. Genetics 138:963–971
9. Green EL (1966) in *Biology of the Laboratory Mouse*. McGraw-Hill, New York, N.Y.
10. Churchill GA, Airey DC, Allayee H et al (2004) The Collaborative Cross, a community resource for the genetic analysis of complex traits. Nat Genet 36: 1133–1137
11. Singer JB, Hill AE, Burrage LC et al (2004) Genetic dissection of complex traits with chromosome substitution strains of mice. Science 304:445–448
12. Davis RC, Schadt EE, Smith D J et al (2005) A genome-wide set of congenic mouse strains derived from DBA/2J on a C57BL/6J background. Genomics 86:259–270
13. Glazier AM, Nadeau JH, Aitman TJ (2002) Finding genes that underlie complex traits. Science 298:2345–2349
14. Abiola O, Angel JM, Avner P et al (2003) The nature and identification of quantitative trait loci: a community's view. Nat Rev Genet 4:911–916
15. Nord AS, Chang PJ, Conklin BR et al (2006) The International Gene Trap Consortium Website: a portal to all publicly available gene trap cell lines in mouse. Nucleic Acids Res 34:D642–D648
16. Kissler S, Stern P, Takahashi K et al (2006) In vivo RNA interference demonstrates a role for Nrampl in modifying susceptibility to type 1 diabetes. Nat. Genet 38:479–483
17. Aitman TJ, Glazier AM, Wallace CA et al (1999) Identification of Cd36 (Fat) as an insulin-resistance gene causing defective fatty acid and glucose metabolism in hypertensive rats. Nat Genet 21:76–83
18. Trogan E, Choudhury RP, Dansky HM et al (2002) Laser capture microdissection analysis of gene expression in macrophages from atherosclerotic lesions of apolipoprotein E-deficient mice. Proc Natl Acad Sci U. S. A 99:2234–2239
19. Schadt EE, Monks SA, Drake TA et al (2003) Genetics of gene expression surveyed in maize, mouse and man. Nature 422:297–302
20. Brem RB, Yvert G, Clinton R, Kruglyak L (2002) Genetic dissection of transcriptional regulation in budding yeast. Science 296:752–755

21. Hubner N, Wallace CA, Zimdahl H et al (2005) Integrated transcriptional profiling and linkage analysis for identification of genes underlying disease. Nat Genet 37:243–353

22. Kroymann J, Mitchell-Olds T (2005) Epistasis and balanced polymorphism influencing complex trait variation. Nature 435:95–98

23. Vitt U, Gietzen D, Stevens K et al (2004) Identification of candidate disease genes by EST alignments, synteny, and expression and verification of Ensembl genes on rat chromosome 1q43–54. Genome Res 14:640–50

24. Wang X, Ishimori N, Korstanje R et al (2005) Identifying novel genes for atherosclerosis through mouse-human comparative genetics. Am J Hum Genet 77:1–15

25. Stoll M, Kwitek-Black AE, Cowley AW, Jr et al (2000) New target regions for human hypertension via comparative genomics. Genome Res. 10:473–82

26. Wang X, Ria M, Kelmenson PM et al (2005) Positional identification of TNFSF4, encoding OX40 ligand, as a gene that influences atherosclerosis susceptibility. Nat Genet 37:365–372

27. Mehrabian M, Allayee H, Wong J et al (2002) Identification of 5-lipoxygenase as a major gene contributing to atherosclerosis susceptibility in mice. Circ Res 91:120–126

28. Helgadottir A, Manolescu A, Thorleifsson G et al (2004) The gene encoding 5-lipoxygenase activating protein confers risk of myocardial infarction and stroke. Nat Genet 36:233–239

cDNA Microarrays

Phillip G. Febbo

1. Background and Theory of cDNA Microarrays

1.1. Overview

Clinicians and scientists are limited in their ability to understand human disease and cellular biology by the technologies available to measure the state of the organism or cell. For millennia, scientists have studied human biology and disease based on anatomical observations; for centuries, decisions have been based on microscopic observations, and over the past several decades, decisions have been based on the status of specific genes associated with disease. In the mid-1990s, cDNA microarray technology emerged that simultaneously measured the expression of thousands of genes *(1–5)* These expression microarrays have rapidly evolved to cover most of the 34,000 genes in the human genome *(6)* and now offer clinicians and scientists an unprecedented level of detail through which they can observe human disease and cellular biology.

The central position of gene expression in cellular homeostasis makes it a provocative window through which to view cellular biology *(7)* From the genetic and epigenetic events that cause disease come profound changes in the cell biology that are reflected in the global pattern of gene expression *(8).* These changes can then be analyzed to identify specific target genes of particular interest *(9)* or to implicate cellular processes with mechanistic import *(10)*.

Scientists and clinicians have seized on the new modality of cDNA microarrays to assay and observe cellular biology. Investigators began applying microarrays to single-cell organisms and have advanced up the phylogenetic tree. They began with very simple experimental designs in simple model systems and have progressed to large, multifaceted experiments in complex models. As the technology has developed, so too have the methods by which to analyze and interpret data of increasing complexity generated by microarrays.

1.2. RNA Expression

RNA stands between DNA and protein in the central dogma of life proposed by Francis Crick *(11)* Although the majority of messenger RNA species have no

From: *Molecular Biomethods Handbook, 2nd Edition.*
Edited by: J. M. Walker and R. Rapley © Humana Press, Totowa, NJ

direct role in cellular metabolism, the relative abundance of each gene's transcript can reflect the identity and state of each cell. Thus, accurately measuring the pattern of expression across all genes (herein referred to as the "transcriptome" *(12)* is a potential mechanism by which to assay cellular biology.

Messenger RNA (mRNA) comprises approx 1% of total cellular RNA but is the template for protein translation and the major focus of expression analysis. The posttranscriptional addition of a poly-A tail (3′ polyadenylation) to the majority of mature mRNA species is used opportunistically to process samples for microarrays, thereby enabling a broad representation of the transcriptome. The product resulting from mRNA processing for microarrays (henceforth referred to as target) depends on the microarray platform with the two most common forms being single-stranded complementary DNA (cDNA) following reverse transcription of mRNA and antisense RNA (aRNA) resulting from in vitro transcription of a double-stranded cDNA template.

Two key features of target synthesis are critical to the successful microarray analysis. First, the resulting target must be in a form that can hybridize to its complementary sequence. In general, the target is single stranded and not too heavily laden with large macromolecules so as to interfere with complementary basepair binding. In addition, the final target is often fragmented to shorter lengths to minimize secondary structure that can significantly affect complementary binding. Second, the target must be detectable when bound to its complementary sequence. Although this is achieved by incorporating radioactive isotopes or fluorescent-dye-labeled nucleotides into the final synthesis of target, a balance must be struck between successful detection and steric hindrance of complementary binding. However, through the judicious use of radioactive labeling or methods of fluorescent signal amplification, successful labeling of the target results in sensitivities in the attomolar range.

1.3. cDNA Microarrays

Once a labeled target is synthesized from mRNA, microarrays are used to detect the relative abundance of each transcript. The platforms upon which DNA arrays have been made range from the earliest having cDNA clones on Nylon filters to silicon wafers that use photolithography to create oligonucleotides of known sequence. In general, microarray detection of a labeled target differs from previous broad surveys of gene expression (e.g., SAGE *(13)* and differential display *(14)* in that the curated platform of the microarray allows immediate identification of genes differentially expressed whereas previous techniques required intensive cloning and sequencing efforts.

The two major platforms currently in use for large-scale expression analysis are spotted microarrays and synthesized microarrays. Spotted microarrays are created by adhering individual species from curated cDNA libraries onto a glass slide. Each spotted microarray element is a known cDNA assigned to a specific location on a two-dimensional surface. Synthesized oligonucleotide microarrays use chemistry to create a grid of unique oligonucleotides (called features) complementary to known genes *(5)*

Each platform has advantages and disadvantages, but all use the basic chemistry of sequence-specific hybridization. After a labeled target is hybridized to the microarray, the amount of radioactivity or fluorescence at each location on the microarray (signal) is determined. Because the intensity of signal at any location is dependent on many variables, microarray determination of expression is relative not absolute. Although this is obvious with the dual-hybridization approach applied to most spotted arrays, it is equally true for synthesized arrays. Thus, detection of a gene on a microarray is almost meaningless unless evaluated in the context of a well-designed experiment or previously subjected to rigorous analysis to understand the correlation between detected expression and absolute expression.

1.4. Microarray Data Analysis

With the high-density organization of spotted elements or features on microarrays, the expression data representing the transcriptome is sizable and complex. Successful analysis of data generated from microarrays involves (1) an assessment of microarray staining quality, (2) normalization of expression across microarrays in an experiment to minimize technically introduced variation, (3) exclusion of genes not detected as being expressed or without expression variation, and (4) expression analysis. Here, expression analysis is defined as the application of computational algorithms in order to find structure within complex expression patterns.

Although the computational approaches applied to expression analysis have ranged from the very simple (e.g., fold difference in mean expression of genes between classes of samples) to the very complex (e.g., support vector machines), there are two basic approaches to expression analysis: supervised and unsupervised analysis. During supervised analysis, sample identifiers are used to assess the correlation between gene expression and sample characteristics. In unsupervised analysis, no sample identification is provided during analysis.

The computational tools for microarray analysis have advanced along with the technology to measure gene expression. The computational demands engendered by technologies assaying a cell's transcriptome required the assembly of collaborative investigative teams to successfully design, implement, and analyze data generated from expression arrays. These multidisciplinary teams create an exciting environment within which important discoveries are being made and represent a paradigm for the future application of other genomic technologies.

2. Practical Steps Involved in cDNA Microarrays

As outlined above, cDNA microarray analysis involves study design, RNA isolation, target synthesis, microarray hybridization and scanning, data processing, and data analysis. This section discusses the practical steps of cDNA microarray analysis and highlights areas of particular importance to foster a strong conceptual foundation. The specifics of each step involved in cDNA microarray analysis will evolve along with the continued advancement of technology platforms. However, many of the challenges involved in effective study design, such as RNA isolation, target synthesis, microarray development, microarray hybridization and scanning, and analysis will remain consistent and these are discussed below.

2.1. Study Design

Although there are no hard and fast rules for the successful design of microarray studies, some general guidelines should be kept in mind when planning an experiment. First, microarrays include probes for tens of thousands of genes and, thus, create experiments where there are significantly more variables (i.e., genes) than experimental samples. This challenges standard methods of evaluation and interpretation and requires specific approaches during the experimental design *(15)*. Additionally, study design also has to anticipate the significant biologic and technical variation inherent to most experimental systems and RNA processing. While this topic has been reviewed in detail elsewhere *(16)*, the important elements for study design are discussed below.

In general, the number of samples required for expression analysis will be dependent on the specific question being addressed and the experimental "system" being used *(17)*. As the anticipated difference in gene expression across an experiment increases, the number of samples required decreases. Similarly, for well-controlled experimental systems where biological variability can be minimized, fewer samples are required than for experiments using primary clinical samples. Other significant factors influencing study design are the specific array platform to be used and the anticipated methods of analysis *(17)*.

Although methods have been proposed for sample size calculation in classification models *(18,19)*, there is generally insufficient *a priori* knowledge upon which to base accurate sample size estimates. Practically, it is often most helpful to review the literature to determine how many samples were required to perform a successful microarray experiment in a similar system.

For in vitro cell-based experiments, triplicate samples for each experimental condition are generally sufficient. Collection of samples over a time-course can significantly help identify genes with small but reproducible expression changes in response to a stimulus but late time-point untreated (or vehicle-treated) controls are necessary. The best experiments have internal control genes that are followed in parallel on the same cells for which expression will be measured through a technique independent of microarrays.

For clinical samples, it is often impractical to perform duplicate or triplicate analysis on each sample. In addition, the effects of tissue heterogeneity, differences in specimen handling, and biological variability are likely to affect final expression patterns more than technically introduced variation during target preparation, and resources are better spent obtaining additional unique samples than duplicating samples. All of the factors mentioned can obfuscate expression data in clinical samples and, in general, mandate larger sample sizes for experiments using primary samples than those using cell-culture systems.

A critical part of the design of spotted arrays is choosing the appropriate control sample that serves as a common reference for all of the test samples. There are alternative design schemes for dual-hybridization techniques, but the use of a single standard reference is most common. In general, an RNA sample pooled from many cell lines or samples is used to provide optimal coverage of genes present on the array. Alternatively, it has been suggested that pooling a small number samples with diverse expression could result in higher-quality expression data *(20)*.

2.2. RNA Isolation

cDNA microarray analysis begins with RNA isolation. Currently, fresh cells or rapidly frozen tissue are required for genomewide expression analysis. Great care must be taken to minimize RNA degradation, as RNase activity is ubiquitous and introduces uninformative changes in the measured transcriptome.

Many methods of RNA isolation are compatible with microarray analysis. The best methods preserve mRNA transcript length, minimize DNA contamination, and result in relatively concentrated RNA in solution without excessive salt or protein contaminants. Prior to target synthesis, if an investigator is relatively new to RNA isolation techniques, it is best to view the RNA (approx 0.5 µg) after separation on a 1% denaturing agarose gel. Specifically, high-quality RNA samples should have clear and sharp 18S and 28S ribosomal RNA bands and a diffuse smear representing the less abundant mRNA species of variable lengths. Diffuse ribosomal bands or heavy smears close to the gel-loading wells can indicate RNA degradation or sample contamination, respectively, and the RNA from these samples is likely to yield poor quality expression data and should not be used. Although there are alternative means to assess RNA quality, there is no gold standard and the simple method mentioned here is generally sufficient.

Standardizing the amount of input RNA across experiments is important regardless of the microarray platform subsequently used. Additionally, more RNA is not always better. Excessive starting RNA can saturate the target preparation reactions and negatively affect yield. The amount of total RNA required depends on the specific protocol but ranges from as low as approx 50 ng *(21)* to as much as 15 µg *(22)*.

There is great interest in applying microarrays to paraffin-embedded tissue samples because of the relative scarcity of frozen tissue compared to paraffin-embedded tissue. Formalin fixation of tissue prior to paraffin embedding, routinely used to process surgical specimens, crosslinks and fragments RNA. As a result, RNA isolated from paraffin-embedded specimens tends to be of very short length and would not pass the quality assessment discussed above. Standard techniques for labeling RNA prior to microarray analysis are ineffective and resultant expression data quality is poor. Novel approaches, including targeted multiplexed reverse transcription-polymerase chain reaction (RT-PCR), redesign of microarrays to bias probes to the 3′ end of gene transcripts, and new enzymological approaches, will be tested rigorously over the next few years. If these prove successful in generating high-quality expression data, they are likely to rapidly replace existing techniques for tissue-based projects.

In the end, prior to starting target synthesis, the required amount of RNA should be in a standardized volume of solution. Excessive vacuum concentration should be avoided and an RNA pellet should never be allowed to fully air-dry. Although it might seem trivial, beginning with high-quality, contaminant-free RNA is a critical step in microarray analysis and its importance cannot be overstated.

2.3. Target Synthesis

There are a myriad of specific protocols for target preparation. The specific protocol used will depend on the amount of starting RNA and the microarray platform used. When relatively unlimited RNA is available, a target for spotted arrays is created by directly incorporating aminoallyl into the first cDNA strand synthesis from approx 2 µg of mRNA or approx 100 µg of total RNA *(23)*. The fluorescent dyes (Cy3 or Cy5) are subsequently covalently bound to the aminoallyl linkers to label the product. Oligo-dT or random hexamer primers are used to prime cDNA synthesis and second- or third-generation reverse transcriptases are used to allow cDNA synthesis at higher temperatures that minimize secondary RNA structure and maximize cDNA length. The resulting product is processed and column purified to remove RNA and unbound dye and concentrate the labeled cDNA product. A detailed description of this protocol can be found at http://cmgm.stanford.edu/pbrown/protocols/index.html.

Synthesized arrays take advantage of in vitro transcription to amplify the RNA transcript number and to create a labeled product of the correct complementation to the designed features on the arrays. Briefly, single-stranded cDNA is synthesized from RNA using a oligo-dT primer that also includes a T7 polymerase site. Double-stranded cDNA (dscDNA) is created using a combination of RNase H to digest the RNA from the RNA/DNA duplex, DNA polymerase to create the second strand, and DNA ligase to complete the phosphate backbone of the second strand. The dscDNA can subsequently be used with T7 mediated in vitro transcription (IVT) to create antisense RNA (aRNA). During IVT, biotin-labeled nucleotides (bio-UTP and bio-CTP) are incorporated into the aRNA for eventual detection on the microarrays. Specifics for this protocol can be found at http://www.affymetrix.com/support/technical/other/cdna_protocol_manual.pdf.

When RNA is of very limited quantity, methods of RNA amplification can be applied to obtain a sufficient target for expression analysis. Again, there are a number of methods commercially available and more are in development. The most common method of RNA amplification involves sequential rounds of dscDNA synthesis and IVT *(24).* For this protocol, the first round of cDNA synthesis and IVT proceeds similar to that outlined above but biotinlabeled nucleotides are not incorporated into the aRNA. Instead, the aRNA is used as a template for an additional round of cDNA synthesis. Because of the antisense orientation of the aRNA, random hexamers are used to prime first-strand cDNA synthesis, and the oligo-dT primer with the T7 polymerase start site is used to create the dscDNA. This sequential method significantly increases the target yield and makes it feasible to obtain expression data from only 50 ng of total RNA. There is some cost to amplification; the lengths of the amplified target decrease with each round and the signal intensity diminishes. This cost has to be balanced with the practicality of obtaining increased amounts of RNA for an experiment.

2.4. Microarray Design

2.4.1. Spotted Arrays

There are significant but surmountable technical challenges to the reproducible creation of cDNA arrays because of sequence specific differences between the individual cDNAs, differences in the lengths of cDNA species, and the chemistry of fixing cDNA to surfaces. These technical challenges necessitate a dual-hybridization approach (test sample and control sample) in order to obtain reproducible expression data from cDNA arrays (see the following section).

Most recently, investigators have switched to spotting short oligonucleotides of similar length onto glass slides. Spotted oligonucleotide arrays have greater specificity and sensitivity *(25)* than the cDNA arrays but still require a dual-hybridization approach.

2.4.2. Synthesized Arrays

The quaternary genetic code allows for the development of small oligonucleotide probes that are highly specific to genes of interest. Using complemenary sequence hybridization is at the backbone of this technology. As such, the chemistry around minimizing secondary structure while maintaining strand integrity and minimizing mutational events is critical to cDNA array technology. Additionally, incorporating sufficient controls so as to account for non-specific hybridization ("cross-hybridization") is also critical for success.

Synthesized oligonucleotide microarrays (i.e., Affymetrix) do not require a dual-hybridization approach but are only available commercially. In this process, chemical masking is combined with nucleic acid synthesis to create a grid of unique 25-mer oligonucleotides (5). The chemical precision of the process (adapted from the synthetic process of microprocessors) abrogates the need for the hybridization of a control and a test sample on each microarray. However, as the detection of each gene is dependent on the success of the synthesized probes and primary structure of the gene, expression should still be viewed as relative rather than absolute. Although test and control samples are not required for the same array, understanding the expression of any single gene will require that results from several samples to be compared.

2.5. Microarray Hybridization and Scanning

The labeled target is hybridized to either spotted or synthesized microarrays and scanned to generate the expression data. Hybridization occurs at temperatures around 60°C in a buffer that minimizes nonspecific binding of target to probe and maximizes signal intensity for true hybridization. Hybridization buffer contains a combination of competing unlabeled DNA, salts, and serum that minimizes secondary structure of nucleic acids and saturates sites likely to bind nonspecifically with nucleic acids. After several hours of hybridization, the arrays are washed with buffers of variable stringency to remove excess, unbound target.

A laser is used to excite and measure the emission of the fluorescent moieties incorporated into the target to determine the amount of target bound to each microarray element. For spotted arrays, two-color excitation and emission is measured, whereas with synthetic microarrays, only a single emission is measured. The end result for both array platforms is a data file with fluorescence intensity at each coordinate on the grid of the microarray. These fluorescence intensities are subsequently used to calculate expression for each gene represented on the array.

2.6. Data Processing

The first step in data analysis is calculating gene expression from the emission intensity for each element on the microarray. For spotted arrays, the intensity of the test sample dye is divided by the intensity of the reference sample. A log2(ratio) value reflects the fold difference in expression for the gene in the test sample compared to the reference sample. Because these values can be dependent on fluorescence intensity, log2(ratio) are often normalized using a locally weighted linear regression (lowess) (26).

For synthetic arrays, dual hybridization is not performed and gene expression is determined by the difference in staining intensity between matched and mismatched probes. The matched probes are perfectly complementary to the gene of interest, whereas the mismatched probe differs by one nucleic acid in the 13th position. Staining intensity at the matched probe is used to represent specific hybridization and staining at the mismatched probe is considered non-specific. Currently, the MAS5 software provided with Affymetrix microarrays determines gene expression by performing a ranking statistic for the difference in hybridization between each of the 11 pairs of matched and mismatched probe sets for each gene. Based on the values and consistency between the 11 sets of probes, the software will assign a confidence call (Present, Absent, Moderate) and a value. Alternative methods have been proposed to obtain expression values from synthetic arrays (27) and this remains an active area of research.

Once expression values are assigned for each gene on the array, all of the arrays from the experiment are brought together for analysis. Array-to-array differences in overall fluorescence intensity are somewhat unavoidable during the staining, washing, and scanning of arrays. Because of this, microarrays are often scaled together (also referred to as normalized) to minimize the effect of this variation on subsequent analysis (reviewed in **ref.** 28). Most approaches to array normalization assume that overall microarray intensity should be equal across an experiment and use linear adjustments to make equal median or mean expression for each array in an experiment. A few examples of alternative strategies to normalize microarray data include intensity-based (26) nonlinear (29), and rank-invariant (30) normalization techniques. Although this process might appear trivial, there can be profound effects on subsequent analysis (31) Simple linear scaling can decrease true differential expression between samples if cells within an experiment differ significantly with respect to their global transcriptional activity. Scaling can also artificially accentuate variations in gene expression if an array of poor quality and poor overall staining is included because of the high scaling factors required (32). Thus, integral to the scaling together of microarrays in an experiment is quality assessment (33). Again, there are multiple methods with which to assess the quality of each individual microarray (30,34,35). The critical element of quality assessment is identifying microarrays (or regions of microarrays) that are of poor quality and need to be excluded from subsequent analysis. The specific approach and execution of quality assessment is dependent on platform and experimental design.

2.7. Expression Analysis

Expression analysis applies computational methods to find informative structure within the data generated from microarrays. One of Albert Einstein's quotes anticipated the basic approach of expression analysis: "Out of clutter, find Simplicity, from discord, find Harmony. In the middle of difficulty lies opportunity." However research in the field should keep another important quote from Einstein in mind: "Make everything as simple as possible but no simpler." Although some experiments can be successfully analyzed with very simple analysis, the complexity of the data generated by microarrays often mandate sophisticated analytic approaches. Because of this, microarray technology has forged strong collaborations between biologists and computational analysts and has helped foster a new field of computational biology.

As mentioned, there are two basic approaches to expression analysis, supervised and unsupervised analysis. Each has its strengths and weaknesses and these will be discussed along with specific examples.

2.7.1. Unsupervised Analysis

Unsupervised analysis imports no knowledge about the samples being analyzed other than the expression data. This type of analysis is least biased and most likely to define structure in a dataset that is novel and not based on *a priori* knowledge or assumptions about the question being addressed. Examples of unsupervised analysis include hierarchical clustering *(36)* and self-organized maps *(37)*. Although the least biased, unsupervised methods of analysis are the most susceptible to technical variation. Global differences between in vitro transcription batches or differences in the cellular components comprising clinical samples can dominate the structure detected by unsupervised means. Thus, more subtle phenotypes are often lost during unsupervised analysis because of competing expression structure.

Initially, most unsupervised analytic techniques lacked a measure against which to determine how different the actual results are compared to that expected by chance alone. One approach to determining the significance of discovered clusters is to annotate each gene on the microarray with characteristics (e.g., gene ontology (GO) information) and then determine the likelihood of having a number of genes sharing the same GO terms within any specific subcluster *(38)*.

2.7.2. Supervised Analysis

Supervised analysis imports information associated with each sample that is used to analyze microarray data. This analysis is less sensitive to technical artifact provided the samples were processed together or in a randomized manner. However, these methods are also sensitive to overfitting because of the large number of variables (genes). Basically, the sample information is used to identify genes with correlating expression patterns. Many measures of correlation have been applied, including fold change, t-tests, Z-tests, Pearson's correlation coefficient, and a variant of a signal-to-noise (S2N) metric *(22)*, just to name a few. While most of these measures of correlation to test for statistical significance, alternative means of assessing significance are generally required because of multiple hypothesis testing and the lack of independence of gene expression between some genes on the microarray.

Permutation testing is one means by which investigators have started to assess the significance of associations between gene expression and sample characteristics. In this method, after the degree of correlation between gene expression and the sample characteristic of interest is established, sample identification is randomized. Such randomization breaks any true structure between gene expression and the characteristic of choice. The same methods are then applied to the data after randomized identifications and the degree of correlation between gene expression and the same characteristic is again calculated. This process is repeated n times. The results are then combined and the experimental data are compared to the aggregate results from n random permutations. If the experimental correlation is stronger than that found with the randomized data at a frequency of 0.05 (or another predetermined level of significance), then statistical significance is inferred.

This is one example of a commonly used methodology; alternatives exist and there will be continued evolution in the statistical methods used to assess the significance between gene expression and sample characteristics to make discovery. Whereas the specifics are less important, it is critical to understand that sophisticated methods are often required in order to properly account for the multiple-hypothesis testing problem. However, the best test of a finding during supervised (or unsupervised) analysis is to determine if the same structure discovered in an initial dataset is present in an independent dataset, this is called validation (see **Section 2.8**).

Both unsupervised and supervised methods continue to be developed. There are very interesting methods being applied to microarray data in order to identify gene copy number changes *(39)*, biological pathway activity *(10,39)*, drug sensitivity *(40)*, and many other applications. Many recent computational approaches use the expression of sets of genes rather than single genes in order to limit the effects of biological and technical variability and such approaches seem to hold great promise *(41)*. As computational approaches to microarray data continue to evolve, it will be very interesting to see if this field continues to diversify into a practically limitless number of options or into a relatively set number of accepted standards.

2.8. Validation

Once a complex genomic pattern is associated with disease behavior, validating the model becomes of prime importance *(42)*. If the goal of an experiment is to identify specific marker genes associated with an experimental or clinical feature, validation confirms differential gene expression independent of the microarray analysis. Although there is no "gold standard," quantitative RT-PCR has been widely adopted as the most appropriate method to validate differential expression of a single gene. Alternatively, some investigators look at protein expression to validate genes identified by microarrays. Although not directly confirming the microarray results, finding changes in protein expression for a marker gene lends additional support to importance of the identified gene.

If expression analysis develops a model from gene expression predicting phenotype or clinical outcome, validation demands that a model, developed in a training set, be applied without changes to an independent set of tumors (none of which were used during the training of the model) and accurately reproduce the preliminary findings *(43)*. Although this represents the ideal, investigators often resort to alternative means of validation because of limited access to clinical specimens and a desire to maximize the information obtained from those that are available *(44)*.

Cross-validation, leave-one-out, and bootstrapping are different mechanisms to perform resubstitution estimates of a model's error rate and represent internal validation *(45–47)*. Routinely used, these methods maximize disease sampling by allowing investigators to use all available samples to train and test a model *(47–51)*. While decreasing the risk of overfitting, resubstitution approaches tend to underestimate the true error rate of a model *(44)* and further validation on independent samples is required prior to clinical application.

Applying internally validated models on independent samples obtained from different experiments, laboratories, or locations is a more stringent validation test. The application of genomic models across laboratories or clinics help determine if developed models remain accurate despite differences in tissue collection, tissue processing, and data acquisition. In addition, with many datasets becoming publicly available, investigators can often use these datasets to determine if genes associated with a specific phenotype are similarly correlated in an independent dataset.

2.9. Complementary Analysis

Expression analysis is one window through which to view the biology of cells. There is intense investigation ongoing to combine the complex data from microarrays from that generated using other platforms. Data from methods to broadly assay the DNA alterations in an individual (genomic) or in disease (somatic), including single-nucleotide polymorphism *(52)* and comparative genomic hybridization microarrays *(8)*, can complement RNA expression data and result in novel discoveries. With the evolution and maturation of proteomics, certainly combining serum- or tissue-based patterns of protein expression with RNA expression holds promise. Finally, other rich sources of complex data such as the literature can be used to complement our analysis of microarray data *(39)*. These analyses face significant challenges with respect to gene annotation and statistical interpretation, but such combined approaches are likely to typify the next wave of array-based discoveries.

In conclusion, from start to finish, expression analysis works to identify marker genes or gene patterns correlating with cellular biology or disease characteristics. Like other methods, microarray analysis requires scientific experimental design and rigorous execution. The complexity of data generated often mandates sophisticated computational analysis previously outside the realm of the biological sciences. To handle the complexity of analysis and facilitate reproducibility, standards of laboratory practice need to be established and some have already been proposed, if not widely accepted *(53)*. However, as with past technological advances, the community of scientific investigators has risen to meet these challenges. As the challenges of microarray analysis discussed above have been met, this powerful investigational tool has been focused on addressing basic and clinical questions examples of which are discussed below.

3. Applications of cDNA Microarrays (Clinical/Medical)

Microarrays have contributed significantly to the genomics revolution over the past decade and will continue to play an important role in our understanding of cellular biology. In some settings, cDNA microarrays will be remain a tool for basic discovery; in others, microarrays will be directly applied to patient care. At this point, it is easy to forecast a lasting role for microarrays but impossible to accurately anticipate specific applications. Although a complete review of the important literature demonstrating the use of cDNA microarrays in biomedical and clinical research is not possible given space limitations, here we highlight recent examples of microarrays applications within biomedical and clinical research and discuss future directions.

3.1. Biological Discovery

The ability to simultaneously measure tens of thousands of genes in cellular systems offers an unbiased approach to improving our understanding of the basic biology underlying important cellular functions or phenotypes. Expression analysis has improved our understanding of the molecular mechanisms that are necessary and/or sufficient for specific, well-defined phenotypes. Early studies applied microarray analysis to describe the global transcriptional activity during replication in yeast *(54)* synchronized proliferation of fibroblasts *(55)*, and controlled hematopoietic differentiation *(56)* and identified sets of genes whose coordinate expression were associated with basic cellular processes such as mitosis and differentiation. These and many additional studies have demonstrated that systems with robust biology, profound domain knowledge, and strong in vitro models can be interrogated and analyzed using cDNA microarrays in order to make new discoveries.

Although rigorous scientific methods are required to generate informative expression patterns, microarray data are often viewed as hypothesis generating and significant work goes into validating observations and definitively testing novel hypotheses with more standard laboratory methodologies *(42)*. Functional validation of genes identified via microarray experiments has become commonplace in laboratories and there are thousands of manuscripts reporting the use of microarrays to identify candidate genes in a biological system.

Because of the rigor required to validate even simple associations, many unexpected yet intriguing findings lack true validation. Often, the optimistic experimental goals of mapping all of the important pathways associated with a complex cellular trait are reduced to the identification and further exploration of one or a few genes not previously known to be involved with the studied phenotype. Initial aspirations of using microarrays to comprehensively map the molecular pathways underlying complex cellular phenotypes was not immediately realized and continues to be a challenge *(57)*.

As cDNA microarray technology and associated computational analysis continue to improve, investigators have focused on more complex systems including multicellular organisms. Developmental transcriptional maps of *Caenorhabditis elegans (58,59)*, *Drosophila melanogaster (60–62)*, and *Danio rerio* (zebrafish) *(63)* have been derived using microarrays in order to understand the temporal relationships of gene expression in organisms. Data from organism-based studies have subsequently been combined to identify interspecies transcriptional similarities. For example, Stuart et al. used data from 3182 microarrays to identify genes with coordinate RNA expression conserved across species and successfully inferred gene function based on shared expression *(64)*. In a similar approach, McCarroll et al. identified sets of genes with expression commonly associated with aging in both worms and flies *(65)*.

Gene expression patterns have also been interrogated to implicate drug mechanism. In a seminal paper, Hughes et al. used microarrays to interrogate the expression patterns from 300 yeast experiments involving either gene mutation or chemical treatment *(66)*. In this work, the function of previously uncharacterized genes could be inferred from the expression similarity between yeasts with these genes mutated and other yeast cultures harboring mutations in functionally characterized genes and or exposed to chemicals affecting specific pathways *(66)*. The use of global gene expression as a phenotype with which to infer function for genes or chemicals is an approach that holds great promise *(67)*. In a recent example underscoring the potential of this approach, Stegmaier et al. used microarrays to identify a signature for therapy-induced differentiation in human leukemia cells and then used the signature to identify novel differentiation-causing agents from a screen of 1,739 compounds *(68)*.

3.2. Medical/Clinical Applications

Microarrays are now a frequent element of laboratory-based biomedical investigation. However, along with biomedical discovery, there is great hope that microarrays will improve medical care. Microarrays have been applied to clinical medicine in order to better understand the underlying biology and physiology, to identify marker genes for specific disease behavior, and to improve disease prognosis and treatment response prediction. Here, we will review some of the early applications of microarrays to clinical disease. It is worth noting that the application of microarrays to cancer currently dominates the literature because of the ability to obtain tumor tissue for analysis. However, other fields of medicine are currently applying microarray analysis to address fundamental biological, pathological, and clinical questions and a more diverse literature will be forthcoming.

3.2.1. Diagnosis

cDNA arrays have been applied to primary human samples of complex phenotypes in order to identify candidate marker genes for disease, to discover molecular classes of diseases, and to molecularly describe clinical behavior. Early on, it became clear that tissue- and cancer-specific patterns of expression existed. In an early seminal article, Golub et al. found strong expression differences between the two major forms of leukemia, acute myeloblastic leukemia (AML) and acute lymphoblastic leukemia (ALL), using microarrays *(22)*. In that article, the investigators could accurately predict the identity of an unknown sample (either AML and ALL) based on gene expression alone. This work has been extended in ALL and distinct expression patterns associated with the common chromosomal abnormalities underlying leukemia have been identified *(69)*. Thus, global expression patterns were found to underlie both histological and genetic distinctions in leukemia.

Large differences in global gene expression also exist between different types of solid tumor and lymphoma. For solid tumors, gene expression can re-establish histological differences between solid tumors from different organs with an accuracy of approx 80% *(70,71)*. The genes found to best discriminate between tumor types were often tissue-specific rather than tumor-specific and poorly differentiated tumors continue to be difficult to classify *(71)*.

Gene expression can easily classify follicular lymphomas from diffuse large B-cell Tymphomas (DLBCL) *(72)* and can further separate diffuse B-cell lymphomas into two classes likely based on their origin within lymph nodes: germinal center B-like and activated B-like DLBCL *(73)*.

Investigators also applied microarrays to detect gene expression differences between normal tissues and cancers derived from those tissues in order to identify novel markers for cancer detection or diagnosis. Profound differences in gene expression have been found between normal and tumor tissue for breast, prostate, ovarian, lung, brain, gastric, esophageal, and most other forms of cancer *(47,74–78)*. In a specific example, two groups simultaneously used microarrays to identified a gene over expressed in prostate tumors compared to normal tumors called α-methylacyl coenzyme A racemase (*AMACR*) and validated their results using immunohistochemistry *(79,80)*. Some clinical pathologists now use *AMACR* to help diagnose cancer in prostate biopsies, representing a successful evolution from microarray discovery to clinical application.

Although other examples exist for microarray-derived diagnostic tissue-based tests, there have been no novel serological tests yet introduced into the clinic based on a gene expression experiment. For any gene, there are many biochemical and cellular processes between mRNA expression in a cell and protein circulating in the blood. This has likely contributed to the difficulty in translating microarray data to novel serological tests but work is ongoing and it is likely that some candidates will be successfully translated to the clinic as blood-based diagnostic tests.

Investigators have also used microarrays to detect gene expression changes associated with the genetics of cancer. As mentioned above, gene expression changes have been found that correlate with the major chromosomal abnormalities in ALL *(69)*. Similarly, breast cancer tumors harboring mutations in the *BRCA1* and *BRCA2* cancer predisposition genes also have distinct gene expression signatures measured by microarrays *(81)*.

In addition to recapitulating known histological or genetic traits of disease, microarrays have identified previously unrecognized molecular subclasses for some solid tumors. Gene expression not only separates the different major types of lung cancer (e.g., small cell vs adenocarcinoma) but can also subclassify the most common form of lung cancer, adenocarcinoma of the lung *(82,83)*. Specifically, gene expression analysis identified a subgroup within adenocarcinomas that expressed neuroendocrine marker genes and had worse survival compared to the other groups *(83)*. In a similar example, gene expression identified a new subgroup of tumors (MLL) from within cases of leukemia with very similar morphology but remarkably different clinical behavior *(84)*.

There are also very good examples of investigators using microarrays to assess gene expression differences between normal and diseased tissues that do not focus on cancer. Investigators have used microarrays to identify gene expression changes associated with heart failure *(85)*. diabetes *(10)*, inflammatory diseases mellitus *(86)*, diabetic nephropathy *(87)*, multiple sclerosis *(88,89)*, and many others. Most of these studies apply microarrays in order to better understand the biology underlying disease and to identify potential diagnostic markers of disease. Often, a major challenge is determining the most appropriate "normal" tissue with which to compare the diseased tissue. For example, whereas the robust immune response causes damage to normal tissues in some inflammatory diseases, the gene expression changes caused by the inflammation is likely to overwhelm expression changes because of the root cause of the disease. Similarly, the cellular architecture of diseased tissues is often different than the corresponding normal tissue (i.e., atherosclerotic plaques vs normal arterial intima) and expression changes might be more related to the tissue composition than disease pathogenesis. In analyzing this literature, it is very important to keep these points in mind.

Mootha et al. combined excellent design with novel computation in order to investigate the metabolic implications of diabetes mellitus *(10)*. These investigators processed skeletal muscle biopsies from normal and diabetic patients for microarray analysis. On the first analysis, there were little differences between the sets of muscle biopsies with respect to histology and supervised analysis of gene expression. Specifically, there were no individual genes with statistically significant expression differences between normal or diabetic muscle. However, when a novel computational method was applied called gene set enrichment analysis (GSEA), there was a significant decrease in the expression of genes involved in oxidative phosphorylation which are also high at sites of glucose disposal.

Be it cancer or other human disease, microarray analysis can redefine diseases from clinical and pathological collections of findings to molecular entities. Thus, differentiating disease diagnosis based on organ site might start to hold less weight than common underlying biology. The potential for this approach might be realized in anticipating disease outcome and choosing therapy. Diagnosing cancers based on specific pathway activation rather than tissue of origin might allow more effective prognosis and treatment than the diagnostic classifications used currently. While provocative, such musing is preliminary and what has been demonstrated with respect to disease prognosis and treatment choice using microarrays will be discussed below.

3.2.2. Prognosis

Diagnosis and prognosis often are related in medicine. However, whereas diagnosis focuses on the current disease state, prognosis focuses on the future behavior of disease in the context of the individual. Investigators have applied microarray analysis to assess if gene expression patterns correlate with disease outcome and have met with some success.

Oncologists remain optimistic that by understanding the biology and genetics of an individual's tumor, they will be able to accurately predict outcome. Microarrays have identified gene expression patterns that are associated with disease progression and/or patient survival in breast cancer (*90–93*), prostate cancer (*47,94*), lymphoma (*95,96*), lung cancer (*83*), and some brain tumors (*50*) among others. Outcome can be defined as recurrence following definitive surgery, development of metastasis, or death from disease. Regardless, the preliminary success of the studies mentioned above suggests that gene expression changes within localized tumors can anticipate recurrence, metastasis, and possibly death from disease.

Interestingly, although most studies focused on specific types of cancer, expression differences between local and metastatic tumors (of multiple cancer types) were also used to predict outcome (*97*). In this report, Ramaswamy et al. applied a gene expression signature comprised of genes differentially expressed between local and metastatic tumors to successfully predict outcome in breast, prostate, and a type of brain tumor but not in lymphoma, again supporting the idea that some local tumors are preprogrammed for recurrence or progression following local therapy and that microarray analysis can measure this programming and anticipate outcome.

Breast cancer is the disease furthest along with respect to the clinical application of microarrays. As touched upon above, two independent groups have found that microarray analysis can predict the development of metastasis and survival in women initially diagnosed with localized disease (*90,92*) and one group has validated their results in a larger cohort of women with disease (*93*). Today, clinical trials are ongoing that test how these predictive models derived from microarrays compare to standard risk stratification using clinical and pathological features of breast cancer. Even without clinical trials demonstrating the usefulness of these genomic tests, at least two companies are now offering microarray-based testing for women diagnosed with localized breast cancer (http://www.genomichealth.com). These tests are expensive and need to be compared to standard prognostic methods before they should be used broadly, but they have the potential to significantly improve our ability to identify patients with high- or low-risk disease so as to optimize management.

Noncancer diseases have been studied with respect to the ability of microarrays to anticipate the disease course, although this area of investigation remains less well developed. There is some evidence that expression analysis can model the progression of heart failure (98,99), Parkinson's disease (100), kidney disease (101), and lung injury (102), among others, but these studies largely involve laboratory models of disease and little has been directly tested on human disease. That being said, strong expression patterns associated with a variety of diseases are being identified and subsequently tested on specimens collected from patients in clinical trials.

3.2.3. Treatment Choice

For a patient diagnosed with a disease, it is helpful for physicians to be able to anticipate the severity and natural history of the disease. However, for patients found to have aggressive disease by conventional or molecular means, it becomes critical for investigators to optimize therapy. Microarrays, by assaying the underlying biology of disease processes, have the potential to anticipate response to specific therapies.

The best examples to date are also in oncology. As cancer chemotherapy is toxic and has profound side effects, only those patients likely to respond would ideally be treated. Breast cancer expression patterns were found to correlate with sensitivity to two different types of chemotherapy: a taxane (103) and anthracyclines (104). The subclass of leukemia detected by microarrays (MLL) was subsequently found to be sensitive to agents inhibiting one of the genes (FLT3) detected as over expressed by microarrays (105).

In the future, it is possible that treatment choice will be determined by the molecular biology of the disease as measured by microarrays and other genomic techniques rather than clinical or histopathological features. It is premature to feel confident that microarray-based tests will be used to determine individualized treatment but the work performed so far supports this possibility.

4. Future Directions

As cDNA microarray technology and analysis continue to improve, it is important to understand the critical steps that currently limit our ability to map complex cellular phenotypes using expression analysis and apply microarrays clinically as biomedical assays. Initially, the number of genes analyzed was thought to be critical, with more genes denoting better microarrays. However, current cDNA technologies are very close to comprehensively covering the approx 25,000–30,000 genes in the human genome and current technologies likely represent a sufficient sampling of the human transcriptome. Also, the ability to measure thousands of genes simultaneously initially outpaced our analytic tools. However, after recruiting scientists from fields outside of biology, the development of tools for expression analysis is now in step with microarray technology.

It is more likely that our inability to use microarrays for disease diagnosis, prognosis, and treatment has more to do with sampling size, gene annotation, and the onerous work of functional validation than with any single technical limitation. Microarray experiments remain expensive and, as such, experimental designs have to be limited. Access to less expensive technologies and the ability to combine data from different microarray platforms will add significantly to our ability to identify important mechanisms active in complex phenotypes.

However, even with great annotation and larger experiments, RNA expression alone might not sufficiently assay a disease state to allow accurate disease prediction. For a comprehensive picture of disease, it is likely that multiple genomic technologies will have to be brought together. It is clear that the developing proteomic technologies together with the DNA-based arrays measuring allelic loss or gain will provide complementary information to expression analysis. Data from disease tissues (i.e., tumors) as well has the host will be combined in the future in order to obtain a full description of disease state.

Microarrays are now a fundamental part of basic biomedical laboratory practice. Early evidence suggests they have a role in clinical medicine, and work over the next decade will test the full potential of this novel technique to influence how we treat patients.

References

1. Schena M et al (1995) Quantitative monitoring of gene expression patterns with a complementary DNA microarray. Science 270(5235):467–470
2. Lipshutz RJ, et al (1995) Using oligonucleotide probe arrays to access genetic diversity. Biotechniques 19(3):442–447
3. Chu S, et al (1998) The transcriptional program of sporulation in budding yeast. Science 282(5389):699–705
4. Wodicka L, et al (1997) Genome-wide expression monitoring in Saccharomyces cerevisiae. Nature Biotechnol 15(13):1359–1367
5. Lockhart DJ, et al (1996) Expression monitoring by hybridization to high-density oligonucleotide arrays. Nature Biotechnol 14(13):1675–1680
6. Baltimore D (2001) Our genome unveiled. Nature 409:814–816
7. Hanahan D, Weinberg RA (2000) The hallmarks of cancer. Cell 100(1):57–70
8. Pollack JR, et al (2002) Microarray analysis reveals a major direct role of DNA copy number alteration in the transcriptional program of human breast tumors. Proc Natl Acad Sci USA 99(20):12,963–12,968
9. Varambally S, et al (2002) The polycomb group protein EZH2 is involved in progression of prostate cancer. Nature 419(6907):624–629
10. Mootha VK, et al (2003) PGC-lalpha-responsive genes involved in oxidative phosphorylation are coordinately downregulated in human diabetes. Nature Genet 34(3):267–273
11. Crick F (1970) Central dogma of molecular biology. Nature 227(258):561–563
12. Velculescu VE, et al (1997) Characterization of the yeast transcriptome. Cell 88(2):243–251
13. Velculescu VE, et al (1995) Serial analysis of gene expression. Science 270(5235): 484–487
14. Liang P, Pardee AB (1992) Differential display of eukaryotic messenger RNA by means of the polymerase chain reaction. Science 257(5072):967–971
15. Kerr MK and Churchill GA (2001) Statistical design and the analysis of gene expression microarray data. Genet Res 77(2):123–128
16. Churchill GA (2002) Fundamentals of experimental design for cDNA microarrays. Nature Genet 32 (Suppl):490–495
17. Simon R, Radmacher MD, Dobbin K (2002) Design of studies using DNA microarrays. Genet Epidemiol 23(1):21–36

18. Mukherjee S, et al (2003) Estimating dataset size requirements for classifying DNA microarray data. J Comput Biol 10(2):119–142

19. Van Der Laan MJ, Bryan J (2001) Gene expression analysis with the parametric bootstrap. Biostatistics 2(4):445–61

20. Yang IV, et al (2002) Within the fold: assessing differential expression measures and reproducibility in microarray assays. Genome Biology 3:62.1–62.12

21. Ma XJ, et al (2003) Gene expression profiles of human breast cancer progression. Proc Natl Acad Sci USA 100(10):5974–5979

22. Golub TR, et al (1999) Molecular classification of cancer: class discovery and class prediction by gene expression monitoring. Science 286(5439):531–537

23. Perou CM, et al (2000) Molecular portraits of human breast tumours. Nature 406(6797):747–752

24. Baugh LR, et al (2001) Quantitative analysis of mRNA amplification by in vitro transcription. Nucleic Acids Res 29(5):E29

25. Barrett JC, Kawasaki ES (2003) Microarrays: the use of oligonucleotides and cDNA for the analysis of gene expression. Drug Discov Today 8(3):134–141

26. Yang YH, et al (2002) Normalization for cDNA microarray data: a robust composite method addressing single and multiple slide systemic variation. Nucelic Acids Res 30(4):e15

27. Li C, Wong WH (2001) Model-based analysis of oligonucleotide arrays: expression index computation and outlier detection. Proc Natl Acad Sci USA 98(1):31–36

28. Quackenbush J (2002) Microarray data normalization and transformation. Nature Genet 32 (Suppl):496–501

29. Workman C et al (2002) A new non-linear normalization method for reducing variability in DNA microarray experiments. Genome Biol 3(9):research0048

30. Tseng GC, et al (2001) Issues in cDNA microarray analysis: quality filtering, channel normalization, models of variations and assessment of gene effects. Nucleic Acids Res 29(12):2549–2557

31. Hoffmann R, Seidl T, Dugas M (2002) Profound effect of normalization on detection of differentially expressed genes in oligonucleotide microarray data analysis. Genome Biol 3(7):p. research0033

32. Hautaniemi S, et al (2003) A novel strategy for microarray quality control using Bayesian networks. Bioinformatics 19(16):2031–2038

33. Smyth GK, Yang YH, Speed T (2003) Statistical issues in cDNA microarray data analysis. Methods Mol Biol 224:111–136

34. Jenssen TK, et al (2002) Analysis of repeatability in spotted cDNA microarrays. Nucleic Acids Res 30(14):3235–3244

35. Gollub J, et al (2003) The Stanford Microarray Database: data access and quality assessment tools. Nucleic Acids Res 31(1):94–96

36. Eisen MB, et al (1998) Cluster analysis and display of genome-wide expression patterns. Proc Natl Acad Sci USA 95(25):14,863–14,868

37. Tamayo P, et al (1999) Interpreting patterns of gene expression with self-organizing maps: methods and application to hematopoietic differentiation. Proc Natl Acad Sci USA 96(6):2907–2912

38. Zhong S, Li C, Wong WH (2003) ChipInfo: Software for extracting gene annotation and gene ontology information for microarray analysis. Nucleic Acids Res. 31(13):3483–3486

39. Jenssen TK, et al (2001) A literature network of human genes for high-throughput analysis of gene expression. Nature Genet. 28(1):21–28

40. Butte AJ, et al (2000) Discovering functional relationships between RNA expression and chemotherapeutic susceptibility using relevance networks. Proc Natl Acad Sci USA 97(22):12,182–12,186

41. Nevins JR, et al (2003) Towards integrated clinico-genomic models for personalized medicine: combining gene expression signatures and clinical factors in breast cancer outcomes prediction. Hum Mol Genet 12:(Epub 8/19/03)

42. Chuaqui RF, et al (2002) Post-analysis follow-up and validation of microarray experiments. Nature Genet 32 (Suppl):509–514

43. Slonim DK (2002) From patterns to pathways: gene expression data analysis comes of age. Nature Genet 32 (Suppl):502–508

44. Dougherty E (2001) Small sample issues for microarray-based classification. Comp Function Genom 2:28–34

45. Kerr MK, Churchill GA (2001) Bootstrapping cluster analysis: assessing the reliability of conclusions from microarray experiments. Proc Natl Acad Sci USA 98(16):8961–8965

46. Azuaje F (2003) Genomic data sampling and its effect on classification performance assessment. BMC Bioinformatics **4(1)**, 5

47. Singh D, et al (2002) Gene expression correlates of clinical prostate cancer behavior. Cancer Cell 1(2):203–209

48. Dyrskjot L, et al (2003) Identifying distinct classes of bladder carcinoma using microarrays. Nature Genet 33(1):90–96

49. Nutt CL, et al (2003) Gene expression-based classification of malignant gliomas correlates better with survival than histological classification. Cancer Res 63(7): 1602–1607

50. Pomeroy SL, et al (2002) Prediction of central nervous system embryonal tumour outcome based on gene expression. Nature 415(6870):436–442

51. Shipp MA, et al (2002) Diffuse large B-cell lymphoma outcome prediction by gene-expression profiling and supervised machine learning. Nature Med 8(1):68–74

52. Stickney HL, et al (2002) Rapid mapping of zebrafish mutations with SNPs and oligonucleotide microarrays. Genome Res 12(12):1929–1934

53. Brazma A, et al (2001) Minimum information about a microarray experiment (MIAME)-toward standards for microarray data. Nature Genet 29(4):365–371

54. Spellman PT, et al (1998) Comprehensive identification of cell cycle-regulated genes of the yeast *Saccharomyces cerevisiae* by microarray hybridization. Mol Biol Cell 9(12):3273–3297

55. Iyer VR, et al (1999) The transcriptional program in the response of human fibroblasts to serum. Science 283(5398):83–87

56. Le Naour F, et al (2001) Profiling changes in gene expression during differentiation and maturation of monocyte-derived dendritic cells using both oligonucleotide microarrays and proteomics. J Biol Chem 276(21):17920–17931

57. Quackenbush J (2003) Genomics. Microarrays—guilt by association. Science 302(5643):240–241

58. Kim SK, et al (2001) A gene expression map for *Caenorhabditis elegans*. Science 293(5537), 2087–2092

59. Walhout AJ, et al (2002) Integrating interactome, phenome, and transcriptome mapping data for the C. elegans germline. Curr Biol 12(22):1952–1958

60. White KP, et al (1999) Microarray analysis of *Drosophila* development during metamorphosis. Science 286(5447):2179–2184

61. Jin W, et al (2001) The contributions of sex, genotype and age to transcriptional variance in *Drosophila melanogaster*. Nature Genet 29(4):389–395

62. Arbeitman MN, et al (2002) Gene expression during the life cycle of *Drosophila melanogaster*. Science 297(5590):2270–2275

63. Ton C, et al (2002) Construction of a zebrafish cDNA microarray: gene expression profiling of the zebrafish during development. Biochem Biophys Res Commun, 296(5):1134–42

64. Stuart JM, et al (2003) A gene-coexpression network for global discovery of conserved genetic modules. Science 302(5643):249–255

65. McCarroll SA, et al (2004) Comparing genomic expression patterns across species identifies shared transcriptional profile in aging. Nature Genet 36(2):197–204

66. Hughes TR, et al (2000) Functional discovery via a compendium of expression profiles. Cell 102(1):109–126

67. Schadt EE, Monks SA, Friend SH (2003) A new paradigm for drug discovery: integrating clinical, genetic, genomic and molecular phenotype data to identify drug targets. Biochem Soc Trans 31(2):437–443

68. Stegmaier K, et al (2004) Gene expression-based high-throughput screening (GE-HTS) and application to leukemia differentiation. Nature Genet 36(3):257–263

69. Yeoh EJ, et al (2002) Classification, subtype discovery, and prediction of outcome in pediatric acute lymphoblastic leukemia by gene expression profiling. Cancer Cell 1(2):133–143

70. Su AI, et al (2001) Molecular classification of human carcinomas by use of gene expression signatures. Cancer Res 61(20):7388–7393

71. Ramaswamy S, et al (2001) Multiclass cancer diagnosis using tumor gene expression signatures. Proc Natl Acad Sci USA 98(26):15,149–15,154

72. Chan WC, Huang JZ (2001) Gene expression analysis in aggressive NHL. Ann Hemato. 80 (Suppl. 3):B38–B41

73. Alizadeh AA, et al (2000) Distinct types of diffuse large B-cell lymphoma identified by gene expression profiling. Nature 403(6769):503–511

74. Ono K, et al (2000) Identification by cDNA microarray of genes involved in ovarian carcinogenesis. Cancer Res 60(18):5007–5011

75. Sallinen SL, et al (2000) Identification of differentially expressed genes in human gliomas by DNA microarray and tissue chip techniques. Cancer Res. 60(23): 6617–6622

76. Lu J, et al (2001) Gene expression profile changes in initiation and progression of squamous cell carcinoma of esophagus. Int J Cancer 91(3):288–294

77. Mori M, et al (2002) Analysis of the gene-expression profile regarding the progression of human gastric carcinoma. Surgery 131(1 Suppl):S39–S47

78. Jiang Y, et al (2002) Discovery of differentially expressed genes in human breast cancer using subtracted cDNA libraries and cDNA microarrays. Oncogene 21(14):2270–2282

79. Rubin MA, et al (2002) Alpha-Methylacyl coenzyme A racemase as a tissue biomarker for prostate cancer. JAMA 287(13):1662–1670

80. Luo J, et al (2002) Alpha-methylacyl-CoA racemase: a new molecular marker for prostate cancer. Cancer Res 62(8):2220–2226

81. Hedenfalk I, et al (2001) Gene-expression profiles in hereditary breast cancer. N Engl J Med 344(8):539–548

82. Garber ME, et al (2001) Diversity of gene expression in adenocarcinoma of the lung Proc Natl Acad Sci USA 98(24):13,784–13,789

83. Bhattacharjee A, et al (2001) Classification of human lung carcinomas by mRNA expression profiling reveals distinct adenocarcinoma subclasses. Proc Natl Acad Sci USA 98(24):13,790–13,795

84. Armstrong SA, et al (2002) MLL translocations specify a distinct gene expression profile that distinguishes a unique leukemia. Nature Genet 30(1):41–47

85. Yussman MG, et al (2002) Mitochondrial death protein Nix is induced in cardiac hypertrophy and triggers apoptotic cardiomyopathy. Nature Med 8(7):725–730

86. Heller RA, et al (1997) Discovery and analysis of inflammatory disease-related genes using cDNA microarrays. Proc Natl Acad Sci USA 94(6):2150–2155

87. Baelde HJ, et al (2004) Gene expression profiling in glomeruli from human kidneys with diabetic nephropathy. Am J Kidney Dis 43(4):636–650

88. Whitney LW, et al (1999) Analysis of gene expression in mutiple sclerosis lesions using cDNA microarrays. Ann Neurol 46(3):425–428

89. Chabas D, et al (2001) The influence of the proinflammatory cytokine, osteopontin, on autoimmune demyelinating disease. Science 294(5547):1731–1735

90. van't Veer LJ, et al (2002) Gene expression profiling predicts clinical outcome of breast cancer. Nature 415(6871):530–536

91. West M, et al (2001) Predicting the clinical status of human breast cancer by using gene expression profiles. Proc Natl Acad Sci USA 98(20):11,462–11,467

92. Huang E, et al (2003) Gene expression predictors of breast cancer outcomes. Lancet 361(9369):1590–1596

93. van de Vijver MJ, et al (2002) A gene-expression signature as a predictor of survival in breast cancer. N Engl J Med 347(25):1999–2009

94. Henshall SM, et al (2003) Survival analysis of genome-wide gene expression profiles of prostate cancers identifies new prognostic targets of disease relapse. Cancer Res 63(14):4196–4203

95. Li S, et al (2001) Comparative genome-scale analysis of gene expression profiles in T cell lymphoma cells during malignant progression using a complementary DNA microarray. Am J Pathol 158(4):1231–1237

96. Wright G, et al (2003) A gene expression-based method to diagnose clinically distinct subgroups of diffuse large B cell lymphoma. Proc Natl Acad Sci USA 100(17):9991–9996

97. Ramaswamy S, et al (2003) A molecular signature of metastasis in primary solid tumors. Nature Genet 33(1):49–54

98. Blaxall BC, et al (2003) Differential myocardial gene expression in the development and rescue of murine heart failure. Physiol Genom 15(2):105–114

99. Ueno S, et al (2003) DNA microarray analysis of in vivo progression mechanism of heart failure. Biochem Biophys Res Commun 307(4):771–777

100. Youdim MB, et al (2002) Early and late molecular events in neurodegeneration and neuroprotection in Parkinson's disease MPTP model as assessed by cDNA microarray; the role of iron. Neurotox Res 4(7–8):679–689

101. Eikmans M, et al (2002) RNA expression profiling as prognostic tool in renal patients: toward nephrogenomics. Kidney Int 62(4):1125–1135

102. Leikauf GD, et al (2002) Acute lung injury: functional genomics and genetic susceptibility. Chest 121(3 Suppl.):70S–75S

103. Chang JC, et al (2003) Gene expression profiling for the prediction of therapeutic response to docetaxel in patients with breast cancer. Lancet 362(9381):362–369

104. Faneyte IF, et al (2003) Breast cancer response to neoadjuvant chemotherapy: predictive markers and relation with outcome. Br J Cancer 88(3):406–412

105. Armstrong SA, et al (2003) Inhibition of FLT3 in MLL. Validation of a therapeutic target identified by gene expression based classification. Cancer Cell 3(2): 173–183

20

Mapping Techniques

Simon G. Gregory

1. Introduction

In 1920, German botanist Hans Winkler first used the term *genome*, reputedly by the fusion of GENe and chromosOME, in order to describe the complex notion of the entire set of chromosomes and all of the genes contained within an organism. A great deal of progress has since been made in the elucidation of the complex molecular interactions that underlie cellular functioning and the syntenic relationship between organisms at a nucleotide level.

The basis for these advances was the characterization of the structure of DNA by Watson and Crick in 1953 (*1*) and the realization that DNA could be decoded to provide a guide to genetic inheritance. This underpinned the concept of genetics and provided scientists with the opportunity to explore and quantify the nature and extent of the biological information passed on from one generation to the next. The characterization of biological inheritance permitted the elucidation of what it was that was being encoded and how it could determine biochemical function. Finally, extending from elucidation of the mechanisms behind inheritance of monogenic diseases, scientists are beginning to grasp how sequence is also involved in complex interactions, occasionally under the influence of environmental factors, to contribute to many (but still not all) diseases.

The speed at which the vast amount of human sequence data were generated can be attributed to the evolution of strategies and techniques developed to map and sequence organisms such as bacteria (*2*) yeast (*3*) and the nematode worm (*4*) The availability of such an evolutionary diverse collection of species, with the addition of the mouse (*5*) and other complex multicellular organisms, has also enabled comparisons to be made at a nucleotide level.

The first genomes that were characterized were relatively small by current standards, bacteriophage ΦX174, 5 kb (*6,7*) and bacteriophage λ, 48 kb (*8*) – but they provided the underlying techniques and strategies that are being used for the more complex organisms currently being studied. Chain termination sequencing, developed by Sanger (*8*) is a synthetic method in which nested sets of labeled fragments are generated in vitro by a DNA polymerase reaction.

From: *Molecular Biomethods Handbook, 2nd Edition.*
Edited by: J. M. Walker and R. Rapley © Humana Press, Totowa, NJ

Because the method is highly sensitive and robust, it has been amenable to biochemical optimization, producing long, accurate sequence reads, and also to automation, which was necessary for large-scale application of the technique. In these respects, it differed from the method of Maxam and Gilbert (9) which necessitated production of all of the labeled material prior to chemical degradation to form the sequence ladders of nested fragments. As a result, the Sanger method has remained the technique by which the majority of genomic sequence from a variety of complex organisms is presently being generated (see **Fig. 20.1**). However, neither method is capable of generating single reads of greater than 2–300 nucleotides, limited in part by the sequence production itself and partly by the ability to separate the sequence by gel electrophoresis at single-base resolution (even today, sequencing read lengths approaching 1 kb are rare).

The assembly of larger tracts of DNA therefore required the development of methods to reassemble a consensus sequence from multiple individual reads. Two approaches were adopted for this; first, the construction of physical maps of restriction fragments using sequence-specific restriction enzymes to order and orientate large segments of DNA from which individual units were selected for sequencing; second, the use of the information gained from each individual sequence read to order and orient each segment relative to overlapping neighbors, which required the development of advanced computer programs to make the task possible on all but the smallest scale.

A further modification of the latter was made by Anderson (10) who developed the random shotgun strategy to elucidate the mitochondrial genome, involved using a random fragmentation process by partial DNAse I digestion (11). This removed the dependence on sequence-specific restriction enzymes while still relying on sequence-based assembly of contiguous tracts of overlapping reads. The random shotgun approach, in which genomic DNA is randomly sequenced in similarly sized segments and then assembled simultaneously to provide a representation of the genomic template, provided the basis of the strategies used to assemble sequences of large inserts cloned in

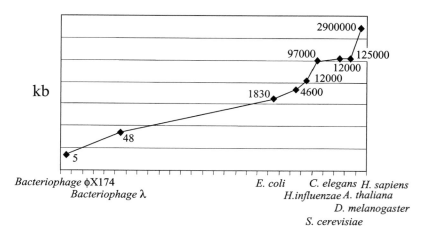

Fig. 20.1. A plot of the near-logarithmic increase in the complexity of genomic mapping and sequencing; from the first full genomic sequence of bacteriophage φK174 in 1977 to the completed human genome in April 2003

plasmids, lambda phage, and cosmid vectors *(12)*, and also the later bacterial artificial chromosome (BAC) and P1-derived artificial chromosome (PAC) clones *(13)*. The same random shotgun strategy was adopted to sequence the 1.8-Mb genome of the bacterium *Haemophilus influenzae (14)*. Although the whole-genome shotgun sequencing approach has proven itself to be a successful strategy for the rapid assembly of smaller genomes, there are doubts as to whether this strategy is suitable for assembling the sequence of complex organisms.

The generation of a physical map, in which the genome is divided into bacterial clone units of 40–200 kb and assembled into contiguous stretches (contigs) of overlapping clones, is a process analogous to the sequence contig assembly process. In contrast to sequence assembly, however, the information used to compare individual clones and identify overlaps of a physical map (e.g., the *Caenorhabditis elegans (4)* and *Saccharomyces cerevisiae (3)* genome projects) use a one-dimensional fingerprint prepared by separating restriction fragments from a limit digest of each cloned DNA by electrophoresis. Overlaps between clones were detected on the basis of partially (or completely) shared fingerprint patterns. An alternative approach to identify overlapping relationships between clones was to test clones for the presence of characterized markers. Overlaps between clones could be identified on the basis that they shared a single copy sequence. The presence of the sequence was identified using a specific hybridization probe or polymerase chain reaction (PCR) assay. Given a physical map of overlapping clones, individual clones can then be selected from the map to provide maximum genomic coverage with minimal redundancy. These clones permit specific regions to be targeted for further investigation and, in particular, for the determination of the complete DNA sequence separately from other clones within the physical map. Because the source of the genomic sequence is limited to an individual clone, problems encountered with sequence assemblies are greatly reduced compared to the corresponding whole-genome assemblies.

At the time of their inception, the physical maps of the *C. elegans (4)* and *S. cerevisiae (3)* genomes were constructed to enhance the molecular genetics of the respective organisms by facilitating the cloning of known genes and to serve as an archive for genomic information. However, the data associated with the construction of the clonal physical maps–even with good alignment to the genetic map—carried only a tiny proportion of information present *(16)* within the genome. Consequently, a minimum tile path of the 30-kb cosmid and 15-kb lambda clones, used to build the physical maps of the *C. elegans* and *S. cerevisiae*, respectively, were subcloned into M13 phage vectors (1.3–2 kb insert size) and sequenced on a per-clone basis. The physical maps of the two genomes *(2)(15)*, and subsequently of *Drosophila melanogaster (17)*, and human *(12)*, used restriction enzyme fragments in various ways to overlap clonal units for the construction of genomewide physical maps.

2. Mapping the Human Genome

The human genome is contained within 22 autosomes (numbered from 1–22, largely according to size) and two sex chromosomes, X and Y (female XX and male XY). Chromosomes are punctuated with centromere structures that are either located close to chromosome ends (acrocentric), toward a chromosome end (submetacentric), or centrally between ends (metacentric). The initial size estimate of the genome, 3,200 Mb, was based largely on cytometric measurements *(18)* and has since been revised to 2,900 Mb in light of the higher-resolution human draft sequence analysis *(19)* and is supported by observed sizes of completed chromosome sequences that suggested that the earlier figures were overestimates *(20–22)*. The construction of a map of the human genome was an important step toward understanding and characterizing the sequence contained within it, as it provided a means by which all of the features could be ordered and partitioned, and the task of detailed characterization and sequencing could be divided up into manageable segments.

2.1. Cytogenetic Mapping

The treatment of metaphase chromosome spreads with trypsin digestion and Giemsa staining creates differential chromosome banding patterns. The generation of light (R-bands) and dark (G-bands) bands by Giemsa staining is reliant on nucleotide content, and the staining pattern therefore reflects the base composition and correlates other properties of the different regions (see **Fig. 20.2**). However, the maximum genome-wide resolution was limited to an 850-genomewide banding pattern *(23)* The recognition of characteristic banding patterns of chromosomal regions provided the basis for much of the early characterization of chromosome aberrations (duplications, deletions, and translocations) that were associated with clinical phenotypes *(24–26)*.

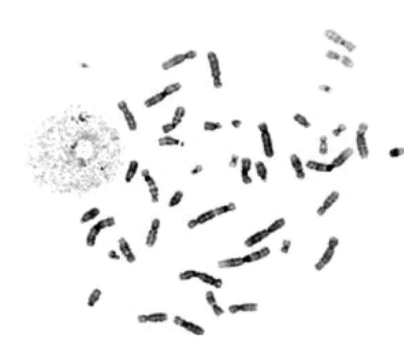

Fig. 20.2. Giemsa staining of human metaphase chromosomes (G-banding)

The ability to hybridize labeled probes containing specific sequences, and to detect their location on metaphase chromosome by autoradiographic or fluorescent detection techniques (fluorescence *in situ* hybridization (FISH)) *(27)* revolutionized cytogenetic mapping. Typically, FISH has used cloned DNA as the template for the generation of a fluorescently labeled PCR probe for hybridization to genomic DNA. The signal emitted by the fluorescent nucleotide contained within the probe is detected by using epifluorescence microscopy. Initially, the location of the probe relative to the metaphase banding pattern provided an approximate map position for the sequence represented by the probe. Pairs of markers, labeled with different fluorochromes, could be simultaneously placed relative to the cytogenetic banding and also ordered with respect to each other. The use of pairs of differentially labeled markers in combination with a third reference marker enabled FISH to be applied to chromosomal DNA in a less condensed state (in interphase nuclei). Although no banding pattern can be obtained in interphase DNA, the decondensed state of the chromatin relative to metaphase chromosomes means that increased levels of resolution could be obtained, as probes were better separated. An interprobe distance of 1–5 Mb can be resolved using metaphase FISH, 0.1–1.0 Mb by interphase FISH *(28)*, and 5 kb by FISH using mechanical pretreatment to extend DNA into fibers *(29)*.

2.2. Genetic Mapping

Genetic maps use the likelihood of recombination between adjacent markers during meiosis to calculate intermarker genetic distances, and from this to infer a physical distance. The closer two landmarks are together on a chromosome, the less likelihood there is of a recombination event occurring between, with the opposite being true for markers that are further apart. The calculation of distance and, therefore, the metric on which the genetic map is based is the length of the chromosomal segment that, on average, undergoes one exchange with a sister chromatid during meiosis, the Morgan (M). Therefore, a 1% recombination frequency is equivalent to 1 centimorgan (cM), and because the human genome covers 3,000 cM and contains approx 3,000 Mb, 1 cM is approximately equivalent to 1 Mb. However, recombination is known to be nonrandom, which can lead to a level of inaccuracy *(30)* in inferring physical distances from measurements of genetic recombination.

The inherent limitation of primary genetic maps was the lack of availability of polymorphic markers between which genetic distances could be calculated. This was ameliorated in part by the suggested use of restriction fragment length polymorphisms (RFLPs), identified by Kan and Dozy *(31)* for the construction of a genomewide genetic linkage map *(32)*. The first such map *(33)* was limited in its usefulness, however, because of RFLPs have a maximum heterozygosity of 50% and the low level of resolution of the 403 characterized polymorphic markers, including 393 RFLPs, covering the genome. The identification of hypervariable regions, which showed multiallelic variation *(34)* provided a new source of markers for genetic mapping. The variable regions contained short (11–60 bp) variable number tandem repeats (VNTRs) which showed allelic variation. However, these minisatellite markers *(35)* and VNTRs *(36)* were shown to cluster at chromosome arms and were not inherently stable *(37)*. The identification of microsatellite markers (containing dinucleotide, trinucleotide or tetranucleotide repeats) greatly facilitated the generation of genetic maps. They were proven to be widely distributed throughout the genome, showed allelic variation *(38,39)*, and were amenable to PCR amplification *(40)* by sequence-tagged-site screening *(41)*. In a relatively short period of time, a number of genetic maps were published with increasing marker density and resolutions, culminating in the most recent deCODE genetic map that contains 5,136 markers genotyped across 1257 meioses *(42)* (see **Table 20.1**).

2.3. Radiation Hybrid Mapping

The utilization of somatic cell hybrids to maintain human genomic fragments, such as whole chromosomes or chromosomal regions, permits the generation of another form of mapping resource to be generated the radiation hybrid map. The modification of a technique that fragmented human chromosomes by irradiation and that were then rescued by fusion to rodent cells *(47)* prompted Cox et al. *(48)* to propose that radiation hybrid (RH) mapping could be applied to the construction of long-range maps of mammalian chromosomes.

The premise of the technique is similar to that of the genetic map; that is, the more closely related two markers are within the genome, the less likelihood there is of a radiation-induced break between them in a reference panel of cell lines and, hence, the less likely is their segregation to different chromosomal locations based on the association of the markers to different sets of fragments. As the presence of two markers within a radiation fragment gives no indication to their physical distance, a panel of radiation hybrids was required. By estimating the frequency of breakage and, thus, the distance between two markers, it is possible to determine their order. The unit of map distance is the centiray (cR) and represents a 1% probability of breakage between two markers for given a radiation dose. Unlike the level of information garnered from a genetic marker, which may or may not be informative within a varying number of meioses, the RH marker is either positive or negative for a DNA fragment, effectively digitizing PCR results. Any amplifiable single-copy sequence can therefore be placed in a RH map. The RH mapping technique has been used for the construction of high-resolution gene maps *(49,50)* and has also been used to supplement the construction of chromosome physical maps *(51)*.

Table 20.1. A comparison of marker content within genetic maps.

No. of markers	Ref.
100	*(43)*
813	*(44)*
2066	*(45)*
5840	*(46)*
5264	*(30)*
5136	*(42)*

2.4. Physical Mapping

The generation of a physical map relies upon the construction of an ordered and orientated set of clone-based contigs. The term *contig* was coined by Staden *(52)* to refer to a contiguous set of overlapping segments that together represent a consensus region. These segments can be sequence, or clones, whose overlapping relationship is defined by information in common to each pair of overlapping segments. Performing a pairwise comparison of the dataset associated with each segment identifies the overlaps. Similarities that are statistically significant indicate the presence, and sometimes the extent, of overlap. Bacterial clone contigs are the most convenient route for the sequence generation of larger genomes. They present a means of coordinating physical mapping and, because of the way in which they are constructed, provide an optimal set of clones (the tile path) for sequencing.

2.4.1. YAC Maps

The main benefit of using yeast artificial chromosomes (YACs) for the construction of a physical map is that the insert size (up to 2 Mb) results in the coverage of large regions of the genome with relatively few clones. Green and Olson *(53)* used YACs to construct a physical map across the cystic fibrosis region on human chromosome 7 by overlapping YACs by sequence-tagged sites (STS) content data. Chromosome-specific *(54,55)* and genome wide YAC maps have also been published *(56,57)*. Although STS content mapping is the most frequently used method to generate YAC contigs, techniques such as repeat-mediated fingerprinting, either by *Alu*-PCR *(58)* or by repeat content hybridization *(43)*, have also been used. The advantages of using YACs are, however, offset by the relative difficulty of constructing YAC libraries and analyzing the cloned DNA compared to the use of bacterial cloning systems. Many YAC clones have also been found to be chimeric (i.e., to contain fragments derived from noncontiguous parts of genomic DNA being cloned) *(59–61)* Rather than being used as a primary sequence resource, YACs came more generally to be used to support the construction of detailed landmark maps and to underpin sequence-ready bacterial clone maps *(62,63)*. Recently, YACs have been used to facilitate gap closure in the bacterial clone maps by linking contigs *(64)* The links are identified by STS content mapping. In these cases, the YACs have been sequenced directly.

2.4.2. Bacterial Clone Maps

In contrast to YACs, bacterial clone libraries are easier to make and the cloned DNA is more easily manipulated. Chimerism is low *(65,66)* and the supercoiled recombinant DNA can be purified readily from the host DNA. An important factor influencing the construction of bacterial clone contigs is the available genomic resources. Whereas the *C. elegans* and *S. cerevisiae* maps utilized total genomic 30-kb cosmid and 15-kb lambda libraries, in sevenfold and five-fold coverage, respectively, current bacterial clone contig construction uses large-insert P1-derived artificial chromosome (PAC) *(66)* and bacterial artificial chromosome (BAC) *(65)* libraries. Each BAC or PAC clone typically contains an insert of 100–300 kb and maps have been constructed from a greater than 15-fold genomic clone coverage.

Two types of strategy were used for the construction of sequence-ready bacterial maps of the human genome: the hierarchical strategy and the whole-genome fingerprinting approach. The hierarchical strategy was based on the use of well- characterized publicly available markers at a target density along the length of a chromosome, 15 markers/Mb. The use of RH and/or genetic mapped markers, in the form of gene fragments (expressed sequence tags (ESTs)), polymorphic microsatellite markers used for genetic mapping, and markers designed from flow-sorted small insert libraries, allowed for a region or chromosome-specific strategy for map construction and sequence generation (see **Fig. 20.3A–D**). The whole-genome fingerprinting approach of map construction relied on the *in silico* assembly of fingerprints generated from the restriction digest of large-insert bacterial clones from total-genomic PAC or BAC libraries. This process generated substantial amounts of genomic coverage, but contigs lacked order and orientation without the supplementation of a subset of the publicly available markers used in the hierarchical strategy (see **Fig. 20.3E–F**). Ultimately, it was a combination of both techniques that were used for the construction of sequence-ready maps of the human genome. The assimilation of both sets of data generated an estimated >98% coverage of the coding (euchromatic) portion of the human genome and acted as the resource for the generation of high-quality finished sequence data (see **Fig. 20.3G**).

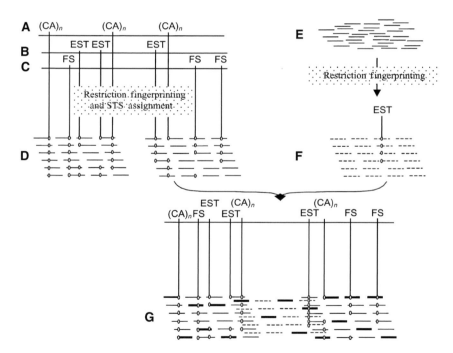

Fig. 20.3. A representation of the two strategies used to construct sequence-ready bacterial clone maps of the human genome. The hierarchal method utilizes polymorphic genetic markers $(CA)_n$ **(A)**, expresses sequence tags (ESTs) **(B)**, and markers generated by sequencing small insert libraries (FS) **(C)** that have been RH mapped and screened across genomic libraries. Restriction fingerprinting and STS assignment is performed in parallel prior to data assimilation in FPC **(D)**. The whole-genome fingerprinting approach uses restriction digest fingerprinting of a 15-fold redundant genomic library **(E)**, including some marker data, to establish bacterial clone coverage **(F)**. Data from both of these techniques is combined to generate contiguous map coverage **(G)**, to provide a resource for the selection of a minimum tile path clones (bold lines)

The relative uniformity of the physical map, coupled with the use of markers from the RH and genetic maps in its construction, permits a high-resolution comparison to be made among the three types of map. Algorithms used to construct the RH map assume random distribution of breaks along the length of the chromosome. However, experimental data (*50*) have shown that the high retention rate, coupled with variation of DNA fragment sizes (in comparison to the rest of the chromosome), results in an overestimation of the centiray distances between markers adjacent to chromosome centromeres. From the perspective of the genetic map, it has been proven that there are large variations in the rate of recombination along the length of a chromosome (*19*). For example, recombination rates at telomeres are greater than within chromosome arms, which are, in turn, greater than regions adjacent to the centromere. The improved resolution of markers on the physical map therefore enables correct ordering of markers with respect to their locations on the RH map and permits the separation of markers previously binned within the same genetic interval on the genetic map (see **Fig. 20.4**).

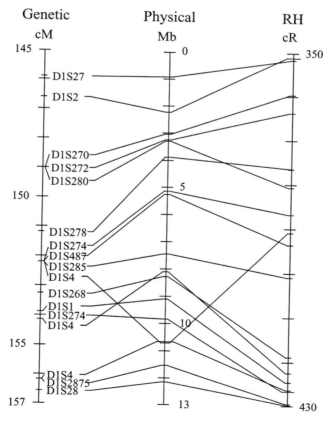

Fig. 20.4. A comparison of marker distribution among genetic, physical, and RH maps in a 12-Mb region of chromosome 1. Only markers that were present on all three maps have been represented

The next phase in the evolution of physical map construction was driven by the availability of ordered genomic sequence. Conservation of sequence and long-range order between organisms that are sufficiently closely related means that the genome of one species can act as the template upon which a physical map of another can be built and, in doing so, elucidate the homologous relationship between them (*67*). The success of the comparative physical mapping approach was demonstrated by the construction of a clone map of the mouse genome using the assembled human genome sequence as a template (*68*). In this study, the human genomic sequence was used to align stringently assembled BAC fingerprint contigs by matching mouse BAC end sequences (BESs) to their corresponding locations in the human genome. Ordered and orientated contigs (previously assembled by fingerprinting) were subsequently joined following further fingerprint analysis and the addition of available genetic and RH markers (see **Fig. 20.5**). The availability of BESs from a highly redundant fingerprint assembly of BAC clones and using the strategy outlined above, greatly simplified the process of contig assembly, as the majority of the 7,500 contigs generated in the first fingerprinting phase were juxtaposed correctly relative to each other on the basis of homology between the two genomes. As a result, 7,500 × 7,500 possible joins (more than 56 million) was reduced to analysis of <10,000 putative joins. This permitted the construction of a physical map covering 98% of the 2,500 Mb mouse genome, contained within 296 contigs, in approx 12 mo. The same approach could be adopted for any genome for which there is sufficient sequence homology to allow alignment of BESs (or equivalent sequence tags), plus sufficient homology between the template genome and the genome under study. The approach has important

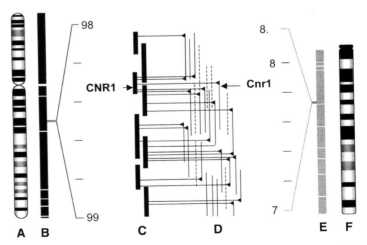

Fig. 20.5. Construction of the physical map of the mouse genome using the human genomic sequence. The generation of finished sequence from large-insert bacterial clones (**C**), originating from the physical map (**B**) of human chromosome 6 (**A**) provided the template for the alignment of end sequences of mouse BACs (**D**) that had previously been assembled into fingerprint contigs. Contig assembly using the described strategy resulted in rapid assembly of sequence-ready contig coverage (**E**) of the mouse genome, including mouse chromosome 4 (**F**)

applications for genomes where the full genome sequence is anticipated and also (perhaps even more importantly) it is a cost-effective way to provide access to regions of a genome for which there are no plans to generate genomic sequence on any scale.

Although the construction of a physical map, and therefore a clone-by-clone approach, proved successful for the generation of human sequence, are physical maps required given the possible contribution of a whole-genome shotgun (WGS) approach to sequencing complex organisms? The main advantages of WGS are that the production of data is very rapid, can be highly automated, avoids cloning biases of BAC systems, and is very cost-effective. The assembly inherent from the sequence alignment also provides important mapping information that is unbiased by additional experimental mapping systems or procedures. Although it remains true that WGS in isolation has disadvantages that prevent completion of either the map or finished sequence of a large genome, the possibility of combining the advantages of both approaches has been explored. A hybrid strategy emerged from the *Drosophila* project, and has since been adopted for the mouse genome. Sevenfold WGS coverage was generated from subcloned plasmids of varying sizes, which, when assembled with BESs, generated 96% coverage of the euchromatic portion of the mouse genome. This estimate was derived by assessing the amount of WGS coverage provided, which matched 187 Mb of finished mouse sequence. For a second, independent estimate, a genomic alignment of a curated collection of cDNAs to the WGS assembly was also used. This alignment included 96.4% of cDNA bases. Paired-end reads from large-insert plasmids and BACs provided the scaffold upon which the assembled whole-genome shotgun sequence was ordered and orientated, and it simultaneously integrated BAC clones into the sequence. A tiling path of BAC clones from the physical map is currently being used for directed finishing of the draft genomic sequence. The physical map helped to assemble the sequence scaffold, and the WGS data increased the rate of clone-based finishing *(5)*.

If WGS sequence data can accurately place BACs via their BESs within the sequence assembly, is a restriction fingerprint database actually required? The answer is probably yes. Whereas BES localization within a WGS assembly facilitates a more optimal minimum tiling path selection, overlaps within fingerprinting contigs can link sequence assemblies (as reported by the assembly of the mouse WGS sequence *(5)*. Assembling plasmid and BAC end sequences in the WGS assembly generated 377 anchored 'supercontigs'. This number was reduced to 88 when two or more sequence supercontigs were localized within a single restriction fingerprint contig. The overlaps generated by fingerprint analysis may also be able to resolve errors in the genomic assembly, where, for example, low copy repeats may have resulted in a compression of the sequence assembly. The proven success of assembling genomewide physical maps, the cost of constructing a >15-fold genomic BAC library, and the ease with which genomewide fingerprint databases can be assembled has led to the construction of several genomic fingerprint databases (see **Table 20.2**). Whereas genomewide fingerprint maps will facilitate the large-scale characterization of many varied species, the construction of small region-specific sequence-ready maps will continue to be important for detailed interspecies sequence comparisons *(67)*.

Table 20.2. Species-specific genomic fingerprint databases.

Organism	Ref.
A. thaliana	*(69)*
Rice	*(70)*
H. sapiens	*(15)*
M. musculus	*(68)*
R. rattus	http://www.bcgsc.ca/lab/mapping
C. neoformans	http://www.bcgsc.ca/lab/mapping
Bovine	http://www.bcgsc.ca/lab/mapping
G. aculeatus	http://www.bcgsc.ca/lab/mapping
Porcine	http://www.nps.ars.usda.gov/
D. rario	http://www.sanger.ac.uk/Projects/D_rerio/
Soybean	http://hbz.tamu.edu/soybean.html

3. Computational Genomics

3.1. In Silico Gene Prediction

The in silico prediction of genes within the genomic sequence utilizes characteristic sequence motifs associated with genes. Unlike prokaryotic organisms, in which genes are located as a single tract of DNA, complex organisms, from yeast onward, contain genes that are usually segmented by introns of noncoding sequence *(71,72)*. The spliceosome recognizes sequence motifs within the intron that leads to their excision, usually a GT dinucleotide at the 5′ end of an intron (splice donor), an AG dinucleotide at the 3′ end (splice acceptor), and an internal branch point *(73)*. Localizing the site of translation initiation within genomic sequence, unlike the transcription start sites, which are predicted on the basis of the combined occurrence of CpG islands and TATA boxes flanked by regions of C-G motifs, has been facilitated by the identification of a consensus motif within the genomic sequence. The translation start site, usually an ATG, is typically found in a consensus (GCC$^A/_G$CCATGG), which includes the two bases that exert the strongest effect: a G at the first base after the translation start, ATG, and a purine (preferably an A) that is located three nucleotides upstream *(74)*. The identification of stop codons (TGA, TAA, or TAG) and polyadenylation signals *(75)*, most commonly as AATAAA *(76)* has helped define the 3′ ends of genes within genomic sequence.

Whereas initial computer programs were developed to identify single exons (e.g., GRAIL *(77)* and HEXON *(78)*), more recently developed programs attempt to identify complete gene structures. These programs, GENSCAN *(79)* and FGENESH *(80)* predict individual exons based on codon usage and sequence signals and assemble these putative exons into candidate gene structures. The greatest problem associated with using *in silico* gene prediction programs to identify coding structures within genomic sequence is the number of over predictions that are generated. Although setting low prediction thresholds might identify all genes, the gene structures will be generated with low specificity *(81)*. The estimated total number of genes contained within the human genome has varied considerably according to the technique that was used to evaluate it and the data that were available at the time. Estimates have been based variously on average genome and gene size, the number of observed CpG islands (and the proportion associated with genes), redundant and nonredundant EST sequences and, finally, chromosome specific totals, comparative analysis and genomewide sequence analysis (see **Table 20.3**).

3.2. Sequence Analysis

Although computer programs have been written to predict a number of features associated with coding sequences, the alignment of experimental data is critical to the validation of predicted structures. Programs such as CLUSTALW *(87)*, which is used to align multiple nucleotide or protein sequences, DOTTER *(88)*, which uses pairwise local sequence alignment strategy, and PipMaker *(89)*, which graphically represents the percentage identify between two sequences, are useful for inferring structural and functional conservation by sequence homology. Sequence homology searching can also be performed using SSAHA *(90)*, Exonerate (Slater, unpublished), and BLAT *(91)*, which permits homology sequences to be identified within gigabases of DNA. BLAST (basic local alignment search tool), which measures the local similarity between two sequences *(92,93)*, is the primary method for identifying protein and DNA sequence similarities prior to incorporation of the features into project-specific AceDB databases (http://www.acedb.org/) or genome browsers. One of the major advantages of using BLAST for sequence alignment is the flexibility with which nucleotide and amino acid sequences can be aligned (see **Table 20.4**).

Whereas BLAST alignment of human mRNA, EST, and protein sequences to predict coding structures provides a primary level of support, predicted features can also be supported by alignments with sequence from other organ-

Table 20.3. Genes in the human genome.

Dataset	Gene no.	Date	Ref. or source
Hypothetical	100,000	1992	*(72)*
CpG islands	80,000	1993	*(82)*
EST clusters	60,000–70,000	1994	*(83)*
Unigene clusters	92,000	1996	*(49)*
Gene sequences	140,000	1999	IncyteGenomics[a]
Chromosome 22 sequence	43,000–61,000	1999	*(20)*
Chromosomes 22 and 21 sequence	44,000	2000	*(21)*
Tetraodon sequence	28,000–34,000	2000	*(84)*
ESTs in dbEST	120,000	2000	*(85)*
EST and mRNA	35,000	2000	*(86)*
Draft sequence	31,000	2001	*(19)*

[a]Press release available at http://incyte.com/company/news/1999/genes.shtml.

Table 20.4. Sequence queries available using BLAST alignment.

Program	Query	Database	Comparison
blastn	DNA	DNA	DNA level
blastp	Protein	Protein	Protein level
blastx	DNA	Protein	Protein level
tblastn	Protein	DNA	Protein level
tblastx	DNA	DNA	Protein level

Source: Adapted from Brenner, S. E., Chothia, C., and Hubbard, T. J. (1998) Assessing sequence comparison methods with reliable structurally identified distant evolutionary relationships. *Proc. Natl. Acad. Sci. USA 95*, 6073–6078.

isms for comparison (comparative sequence analysis). The identification of sequences that are conserved between species is important because sequences that contain elements that are potentially functional are more likely to retain their sequence than nonfunctional segments, under the constraints of natural selection during evolution. The evolutionary distance between species is an important consideration. Sequence comparisons between closely related species may facilitate the identification of gene structures and regulatory elements but if the evolutionary distance between the species is relatively small, these sequences may be obscured by nonfunctional sequence conservation. Therefore, a variety of species, including more distantly related species, might be required to identify potential functional sequences using the comparative approach.

The identification of conserved sequences by comparative analysis has focused on the identification of noncoding regions *(94–96)* and protein coding regions *(97–99)* between human and mouse genomes. The alignment of sequence from multiple organisms has also been used to identify upstream regions that may affect gene expression *(100)*. Although comparative sequence analysis may not identify all control regions associated with a gene, conserved regions may be identified that would be a candidate for further experimental investigation *(101)*. The availability of large tracts of human genomic sequence has necessitated the development of databases (genome browsers) that provide a framework upon which the enormous amount of data associated with the human genome can be stored and displayed. The three main databases, Ensembl, developed at the Wellcome Trust Sanger Institute and the European Bioinformatics Institute (http://www.ensembl.org/Homo_sapiens/), the University of California Santa Cruz (UCSC) genome browser (http://genome.cse.ucsc.edu/), and the NCBI browser (http://www.ncbi.nlm.nih.gov/mapview/map_search.cgi?taxid=9606) each contain information pertaining to physical maps, chromosome-specific sequence assemblies, aligned mRNAs and ESTs, cross-species homologies, single-nucleotide polymorphisms (SNPs), and repeat elements. The development of generic genome browsers, as such as those hosted by Ensembl, makes possible the rapid identification of homologous sequences between comparative organisms and, in doing so, assist in identifying conserved features that might be of some functional significance.

4. Conclusions

The generation of genetic, RH and physical maps of the human genome have provided a means by which the genome's various components can be partitioned and characterized, in addition to acting as the basis for identifying segregating regions of inheritance that are associated with disease-causing genes. The construction of a sequence-ready physical map of the human genome has been central to the production of a high-quality finished genomic sequence, an essential facet of the complete identification all coding and regulatory features contained within.

In the future, substantial efforts will be made to fully characterize all of the genes in the human genome. These studies will result in a fuller understanding of the specificity and range of biochemical structures and functions that are encoded in the human genome sequence. In general, there is likely to remain a distinction between the study of functions encoded at the DNA level, which affect gene expression via transcriptional control, and the study of functions reflected at the protein level following translation, taking into account posttranslational modifications (processes which are largely genetically determined). Without a genic catalog, functional studies are necessarily limited to the investigation of a specific target a gene, a protein, or a disease. These approaches are an essential part of fully interpreting the genome, as they provide a means by which hypotheses can be experimentally tested and which produce valid and supplementary results. However, the production of a complete gene catalog (if completion can indeed be measured or achieved) will provide the raw material for modeling whole systems. The extensive use of computational biology to suggest how such complex systems are made up of their interacting components will, in itself, enable predictions to be made of the system model. These predictions can be tested, both to determine the validity of the modeled system and to test the success of the methods used to derive the system.

A more complete knowledge of biochemical processes will yield a better understanding of complex disease and how it should be treated. At present, our knowledge is primarily based on monogenic diseases. As the problem is reduced to a single gene, hypotheses for function can be tested by biochemical assays, protein structural studies, experimental knockouts, or the study of naturally occurring mutants. The approach to complex disease centers on a similar approach (i.e., trying to identify the one or few dominant genetic factors that contribute the most significant effect to the overall phenotype). However, there is a realization that these genetic factors might not fully explain the observed phenotype and that a proportion of the remaining factors might not be identified. In tl l lhese instances, a comprehensive knowledge of the systems involved will be more informative than the approach of complex disease genetics, both in how the phenotype arises and how it might be possible to intervene more effectively. This is potentially a true long-term value of the genome sequence and its interpretation in a biochemical, biological, and genetic context, for the advancement of medicine in the future.

References

1. Watson JD, Crick F (1953) A structure for deoxyribose nucleic acid. Nature 171:171
2. Kohara Y, Akiyama K, Isono K (1987) The physical map of the whole E. coli chromosome: application of a new strategy for rapid analysis and sorting of a large genomic library. Cell 50:495–508
3. Olson MV, Dutchik JE, Graham MY et al (1986) Random-clone strategy for genomic restriction mapping in yeast. Proc Natl Acad Sci USA 83:7826–7830
4. Coulson A, Sulston J, Brenner S, Karn J (1986) Toward a physical map of the genome of the nematode Caenorhabditis elegans. Proc Natl Acad Sci USA 83:7821–7825
5. Mouse Genome Sequencing Consortium (2002) Initial sequencing and comparative analysis of the mouse genome. Nature 420:520–562
6. Sanger F, Air GM, Barrell BG et al (1977) Nucliotide sequence of bacteriophage phi X174 DNA. Nature 265:687–695
7. Sanger F, Coulson, AR, Friedmann T et al (1978) The nucleotide sequence of bacteriophage phiX174. J Mol Biol 125:225–246
8. Sanger F, Coulson AR, Hong GF, Hill D F, and Petersen GB (1982) Nucleotide sequence of bacteriophage lambda DNA. J Mol Biol 162:729–773
9. Maxam AM, Gilbert W (1977) A new method for sequencing DNA. Proc Natl Acad Sci USA 74:560–564
10. Anderson S (1981) Shotgun DNA sequencing using cloned DNase I-generated fragments. Nucleic Acids Res 9:3015–3027
11. Anderson S, Bankier AT, Barrell BG et al (1981) Sequence and organization of the human mitochondrial genome. Nature 290:457–465.
12. McPherson JD, Marra M, Hillier L et al (2001) A physical map of the human genome. Nature 409:934–941
13. Burke DT, Carle GF, Olson MV. (1987) Cloning of large segments of exogenous DNA into yeast by means of artificial chromosome vectors. Science 236:806–812
14. Fleischmann RD, Adams MD, White O et al (1995) Whole-genome random sequencing and assembly of Haemophilus influenzae Rd Science 269:496–512
15. Arabidopsis Genome Initiative (2000) Analysis of the genome sequence of the flowering plant Arabidopsis thaliana. Nature 408:796–815
16. Kim UJ, Shizuya H, de Jong, PJ, Birren B, and Simon MI (1992) Stable propagation of cosmid sized human DNA inserts in an F factor based vector. Nucleic Acids Res 20:1083–1085
17. Hoskins RA, Nelson CR, Berman BP et al (2000) A BAC-based physical map of the major autosomes of Drosophila melanogaster. Science 287:2271–2274
18. Morton NE. (1991) Parameters of the human genome Proc Natl Acad Sci USA 88:7474–6
19. International Human Genome Sequencing Consortium (2001) Initial sequencing and analysis of the human genome. Nature 409:860–921
20. Dunham I, Shimizu N, Roe BA et al (1999) The DNA sequence of human chromosome 22. Nature 402:489–495
21. Hattori M, Fujiyama A, Taylor TD et al (2000) The DNA sequence of human chromosome 21. Nature 405:311–319
22. Deloukas P, Matthews LH, Ashurst J et al (2001) The DNA sequence and comparative analysis of human chromosome 20. Nature 414:865–871
23. Bickmore WA, Sumner AT (1989) Mammalian chromosome banding—an expression of genome organization. Trends Genet 5:144–148
24. Pinkel D, Landegent J, Collins C et al (1988) Fluorescence in situ hybridization with human chromosome-specific libraries:detection of trisomy 21 and translocations of chromosome 4. Proc Natl Acad Sci USA 85:9138–9142

25. Tkachuk DC, Westbrook CA, Andreeff M et al (1990) Detection of bcr-abl fusion in chronic myelogeneous leukemia by in situ hybridization. Science 250:559–562

26. Dauwerse JG, Kievits T, Beverstock GC et al (1990) Rapid detection of chromosome 16 inversion in acute nonlymphocytic leukemia, subtype M4: regional localization of the breakpoint in 16p. Cytogenet Cell Genet 53:126–128

27. Pinkel D, Straume T, Gray JW (1986) Cytogenetic analysis using quantitative, high-sensitivity, fluorescence hybridization. Proc Natl Acad Sci USA 83:2934–2988

28. Wilke CM, Guo SW, Hall BK et al (1994) Multicolor FISH mapping of YAC clones in 3p14 and identification of a YAC spanning both FRA3B and the t(3;8) associated with hereditary renal cell carcinoma. Genomics 22:319–326

29. Heiskanen M, Karhu R, Hellsten E, Peltonen L, Kallioniemi OP, Palotie A (1994) High resolution mapping using fluorescence in situ hybridization to extended DNA fibers prepared from agarose-embedded cells. Biotechniques 17:928–929, 932–933

30. Dib C, Faure S, Fizames C et al (1996) A comprehensive genetic map of the human genome based on 5,264 microsatellites. Nature 380:152–154

31. Kan YW, Dozy AM (1978) Polymorphism of DNA sequence adjacent to human beta-globin structural gene: relationship to sickle mutation. Proc Natl Acad Sci USA 75:5631–5635

32. Botstein D, White RL, Skolnick M, Davis RW (1980) Construction of a genetic linkage map in man using restriction fragment length polymorphisms. Am J Hum Genet 32:314–331

33. Donis-Keller H, Green P, Helms C et al (1987) A genetic linkage map of the human genome. Cell 51:319–337

34. Wyman AR, White R (1980) A highly polymorphic locus in human DNA. Proc Natl Acad Sci USA 77:6754–6758

35. Jeffreys AJ, Wilson V, Thein SL (1985) Hypervariable 'minisatellite' regions in human DNA. Nature 314:67–73

36. Nakamura Y, Leppert M, O'Connell P et al (1987) Variable number of tandem repeat (VNTR) markers for human gene mapping. Science 235:1616–1622

37. Royle NJ, Clarkson RE, Wong Z, and Jeffreys, AJ (1988) Clustering of hypervariable minisatellites in the proterminal regions of human autosomes. Genomics 3:352–360

38. Litt M, Luty JA (1989) A hypervariable microsatellite revealed by in vitro amplification of a dinucleotide repeat within the cardiac muscle actin gene. Am J Hum Genet 44:397–401

39. Weber JL, May PE (1989) Abundant class of human DNA polymorphisms which can be typed using the polymerase chain reaction. Am J Hum Genet 44:388–396

40. Saiki RK, Gelfand DH, Stoffel S et al (1988) Primer-directed enzymatic amplification of DNA with a thermostable DNA polymerase. Science 239:487–491

41. Olson M, Hood L, Cantor C, Botstein D (1989) A common language for physical mapping of the human genome. Science 245:1434–1435

42. Kong A, Gudbjartsson DF, Sainz J et al (2002) A high-resolution recombination map of the human genome. Nature Genet 31:241–247

43. Cohen D, Chumakov I, Weissenbach J (1993) A first-generation physical map of the human genome. Nature 366:698–701

44. Weissenbach J, Gyapay G, Dib C et al (1992) A second-generation linkage map of the human genome. Nature 359:794–801

45. Gyapay G, Morissette J, Vignal A et al (1994) The 1993–1994 Genethon human genetic linkage map. Nature Genet 7:246–339

46. Murray JC, Buetow KH, Weber JL et al (1994) A comprehensive human linkage map with centimorgan density. Cooperative Human Linkage Center (CHLC). Science 265:2049–2054

47. Goss SJ, Harris H (1975) New method for mapping genes in human chromosomes. Nature 255:680–684

48. Cox DR, Burmeister M, Price, ER, Kim S, Myers RM (1990) Radiation hybrid mapping: a somatic cell genetic method for constructing high-resolution maps of mammalian chromosomes. Science 250:245–250

49. Schuler GD, Boguski MS, Stewart EA et al (1996) A gene map of the human genome. Science 274:540–546

50. Deloukas P, Schuler GD, Gyapay G et al (1998) A physical map of 30,000 human genes. Science 282:744–746

51. Mungall AJ, Edwards CA, Ranby SA et al (1996) Physical mapping of chromosome 6: a strategy for the rapid generation of sequence-ready contigs. DNA Sea 7:47–49

52. Staden R (1980) A new computer method for the storage and manipulation of DNA gel reading data. Nucleic Acids Res 8:3673–3694

53. Green ED, Olson MV (1990) Chromosomal region of the cystic fibrosis gene in yeast artificial chromosomes: a model for human genome mapping. Science 250:94–98

54. Chumakov IM, Le Gall I, Billault A et al (1992) Isolation of chromosome 21-specific yeast artificial chromosomes from a total human genome library. Nature Genet 1:222–225

55. Foote S, Vollrath D, Hilton A, Page DC (1992) The human Y chromosome: overlapping DNA clones spanning the euchromatic region. Science 258:60–66

56. Chumakov IM, Rigault P, Le Gall I et al (1995) A YAC contig map of the human genome. Nature 377:175–297

57. Hudson TJ, Stein LD, Gerety SS et al (1995) An STS-based map of the human genome. Science 270:1945–1954

58. Coffey AJ, Roberts RG, Green ED et al (1992) Construction of a 2.6-Mb contig in yeast artificial chromosomes spanning the human dystrophin gene using an STS-based approach. Genomics 12:474–484

59. Green ED, Riethman HC, Dutchik JE, Olson MV (1991) Detection and characterization of chimeric yeast artificial-chromosome clones. Genomics 11:658–669

60. Bates GP, Valdes J, Hummerich H et al (1992) Characterization of a yeast artificial chromosome contig spanning the Huntington's disease gene candidate region. Nature Genet 1:180–187

61. Slim R, Le Paslier D, Compain S et al (1993) Construction of a yeast artificial chromosome contig spanning the pseudoautosomal region and isolation of 25 new sequence-tagged sites. Genomics 16:691–697

62. Collins JE, Cole CG, Smink LJ et al (1995) A high-density YAC contig map of human chromosome 22. Nature 377:367–379

63. Bouffard GG, Idol JR, Braden VV et al (1997) A physical map of human chromosome 7: an integrated YAC contig map with average STS spacing of 79 kb. Genome Res 7:673–692

64. Coulson A, Huynh C, Kozono Y, Shownkeen R (1995) The physical map of the Caenorhabditis elegans genome. Methods Cell Biol 48:533–550

65. Shizuya H, Birren B, Kim UJ et al (1992) Cloning and stable maintenance of 300-kilobase-pair fragments of human DNA in Escherichia coli using an F-factor-based vector. Proc. Natl. Acad. Sci. USA 89:8794–8797

66. Ioannou PA, Amemiya CT, Garnes J et al (1994) A new bacteriophage P1-derived vector for the propagation of large human DNA fragments. Nature Genet 6:84–89

67. Thomas JW, Prasad AB, Summers TJ et al (2002) Parallel construction of orthologous sequence-ready clone contig maps in multiple species. Genome Res 12:1277–1285

68. Gregory SG, Sekhon M, Schein J et al (2002) A physical map of the mouse genome. Nature 418:743–750

69. Marra M, Kucaba T, Sekhon M et al (1999) A map for sequence analysis of the Arabidopsis thaliana genome. Nature Genet 22:265–270

70. Tao Q, Chang Y-L, Wang J et al (2001) Bacterial artificial chromosome-based physical map of the rice genome constructed by restriction fingerprint analysis. Genetics 158:1711–1724

71. Tilghman SM, Tiemeier DC, Seidman JG et al (1978) Intervening sequence of DNA identified in the structural portion of a mouse beta-globin gene Proc Natl Acad Sci USA 75:725–729

72. Gilbert W (1978) Why genes in pieces? Nature 271:501

73. Moore MJ, Sharp PA (1993) Evidence for two active sites in the spliceosome provided by stereochemistry of pre-mRNA splicing. Nature 365:364–368

74. Kozak M (1987) An analysis of 5'-noncoding sequences from 699 vertebrate messenger RNAs. Nucleic Acids Res 15:8125–8148

75. Kessler MM, Beckendorf RC, Westhafer MA, Nordstrom JL, (1986) Requirement of A-A-U-A-A-A and adjacent downstream sequences for SV40 early polyadenylation. Nucleic Acids Res 14:4939–4952

76. Beaudoing E, Freier S, Wyatt JR, Claverie JM, Gautheret D (2000) Patterns of variant polyadenylation signal usage in human genes. Genome Res 10:1001–1010

77. Uberbacher EC, Xu Y, Mural RJ (1996) Discovering and understanding genes in human DNA sequence using GRAIL. Methods Enzymol 266:259–281

78. Solovyev VV, Salamov AA, Lawrence CB (1994) Predicting internal exons by oligonucleotide composition and discriminant analysis of spliceable open reading frames. Nucleic Acids Res 22:5156–5163

79. Burge C, Karlin S (1997) Prediction of complete gene structures in human genomic DNA J Mol Biol 268:78–94

80. Solovyev VV, Salamov AA, and Lawrence CB (1995) Identification of human gene structure using linear discriminant functions and dynamic programming. Proc Int Conf Intel Syst Mol Biol 3:367–375

81. Guigo R, Agarwal P, Abril JF, Burset M, Fickett JW (2000) An assessment of gene prediction accuracy in large DNA sequences. Genome Res 10:1631–1642

82. Antequera F, Bird A(1993) Number of CpG islands and genes in human and mouse. Proc Natl Acad Sci USA 90:11,995–11,999

83. Fields C, Adams MD, White O, Venter JC (1994) How many genes in the human genome? Nature Genet 7:345–346

84. Roest-Crollius H, Jaillon O, Bernot A et al (2000) Estimate of human gene number provided by genome-wide analysis using Tetraodon nigroviridis DNA sequence. Nature Genet 25:235–238

85. Liang F, Holt I, Pertea G, Karamycheva S, Salzberg SL, Quackenbush J (2000) Gene index analysis of the human genome estimates approximately 120,000 genes. Nature Genet 25:239–240

86. Ewing B, Green P (2000) Analysis of expressed sequence tags indicates 35,000 human genes. Nature Genet 25:232–234

87. Thompson JD, Higgins DG, Gibson TJ (1994) CLUSTAL W: improving the sensitivity of progressive multiple sequence alignment through sequence weighting, position-specific gap penalties and weight matrix choice. Nucleic Acids Res 22:4673–4680

88. Sonnhammer EL, Durbin R (1995) A dot-matrix program with dynamic threshold control suited for genomic DNA and protein sequence analysis. Gene 167:GC1–GC10

89. Schwartz S, Zhang Z, Frazer KA et al (2000) PipMaker—A web server for aligning two genomic DNA sequences. Genome Res 10:577–586

90. Ning Z, Cox AJ, Mullikin JC (2001) SSAHA: a fast search method for large DNA databases. Genome Res 11:1725–1729

91. Kent WJ (2002) BLAT—the BLAST-like alignment tool. Genome Res 12, 656–664

92. Altschul SF, Gish W, Miller W, Myers EW, Lipman DJ (1990) Basic local alignment search tool. J Mol Biol 215:403–410

93. Altschul SF, Madden TL, Schaffer AA et al (1997) Gapped BLAST and PSI-BLAST: a new generation of protein database search programs. Nucleic Acids Res 25:3389–3402

94. Hardison R, Slightom JL, Gumucio DL, Goodman M, Stojanovic N, Miller W (1997) Locus control regions of mammalian beta-globin gene clusters: combining phylogenetic analyses and experimental results to gain functional insights. Gene 205:73–94

95. Koop BF, Hood L (1994) Striking sequence similarity over almost 100 kilobases of human and mouse T-cell receptor DNA. Nature Genet 7:48–53

96. Hardison R, Slightom JL, Gumucio DL, Goodman M, Stojanovic N, Miller W (1997) Locus control regions of mammalian beta-globin gene clusters: combining phylogenetic analyses and experimental results to gain functional insights. Gene 205:73–94

97. Makalowski W, Zhang J, Boguski MS (1996) Comparative analysis of 1196 orthologous mouse and human full-length mRNA and protein sequences. Genome Res 6:846–857

98. Ansari-Lari MA, Oeltjen JC, Schwartz S et al (1998) Comparative sequence analysis of a gene-rich cluster at human chromosome 12p13 and its syntenic region in mouse chromosome 6. Genome Res 8:29–40

99. Jang W, Hua A, Spilson SV, Miller W, Roe BA, Meisler MH (1999) Comparative sequence of human and mouse BAC clones from the mnd2 region of chromosome 2p13. Genome Res 9:53–61

100. Gottgens B, Barton LM, Gilbert JG et al (2000) Analysis of vertebrate SCL loci identifies conserved enhancers. Nature Biotechnol 18:181–186

101. Pennacchio LA, Olivier M, Hubacek JA et al (2001) An apolipoprotein influencing triglycerides in humans and mice revealed by comparative sequencing. Science 294:169–173

21

Single Nucleotide Polymorphisms

Nameeta Shah

1. Introduction

The particular order of the 4 different bases: adenine (A), thymine (T), cytosine (C), and guanine (G) that are present in DNA, arranged along the sugar-phosphate backbone of DNA is called its sequence; the DNA sequence specifies the exact genetic instructions required to create a particular organism with its own unique traits. The complete set of instructions for making an organism is called its genome. The size of the genome varies from several thousand bases in yeast to 3 billion in human. Genomes of individuals from same species are highly similar with minor variations, e.g., human genomes are known to differ in 1 basepair per 1,000 basepairs *(1)*. A variation that occurs when a single nucleotide in a genome is altered is called single nucleotide polymorphism (SNP). An alteration of the sequence ACCCGGTACT to AACCGGTACT consists of 1 SNP at position 2 where base C is altered to base A. Each individual has many SNPs creating a unique DNA pattern for that person. This fact is being used in DNA testing which has revolutionized forensic science for crime solving. SNPs are of particular interest for expanding our understanding of human disease and henceforth development of drugs. Huge efforts are ongoing for identification of SNPs that are cause of a disease or make an individual genetically predisposed to a disease. With current high throughput technologies it has become possible to sequence genomes or parts of genome of large number of healthy and diseased population. Comparison of SNPs from different population groups will enable the scientific community to identify SNPs that are disease causative mutations from millions of SNPs, of which majority are normal variations. In addition, SNPs are used extensively in efforts to study the evolution of microbial populations in the newly emerging area of environmental genomics. Rest of the section reviews few definitions that are essential in understanding underlying theory of application of SNPs.

Crossing-over—Source of majority of SNPs is crossing-over. Crossing-over is part of a complicated process which can occur during meiosis. During meiosis, the precursor cells of the sperm or ova must multiply and at the same time reduce the number of chromosomes to one full set. During the early stages

From: *Molecular Biomethods Handbook, 2nd Edition.*
Edited by: J. M. Walker and R. Rapley © Humana Press, Totowa, NJ

of cell division in meiosis, when homologous chromosomes pair up, exchange of DNA segments between them may occur. This exchange or recombination produces genetic variations in germ cells.

Genotype—The genotype is the specific genetic makeup (the specific genome) of an individual, in the form of DNA sequence. It could refer to only one locus or to an entire genome.

Haplotypes—Genetic variants in close proximity tend to be inherited together. For example, any individual with base A on chromosome 7 at location 300 instead of G will always have base T on chromosome 7 at location 4,000 and base G on chromosome 7 at location 4,500. Given the base at chromosome 7 at location 300, it is possible to infer bases at other two locations. These regions of linked variants are known as haplotypes. Haplotype may refer to the whole genome or a part of it. Different parts of genomes have different number of haplotypes in a given population but this number in reality is orders of magnitude smaller than the total number of theoretically possible haplotypes.

Linkage Disequilibrium (LD)—Linkage disequilibrium describes a situation in which some combinations of alleles or genetic markers occur more or less frequently in a population than would be expected from a random formation of haplotypes from alleles based on their frequencies. Nonrandom associations between genes at different loci are measured by the degree of linkage disequilibrium (LD).

2. SNP Detection Techniques

There are numerous methods and variety of platforms available for SNP detection ranging from detecting few SNPs to genome-wide detection.

2.1. Restriction Fragment Length Polymorphism (RFLP)

RFLP technique is generally used to test presence of certain known disease associated risk alleles or in forensic science for identification. DNA of every individual consists of small DNA sequences known as restriction sites. Restriction enzymes are endonucleases that can identify particular restriction sites and they cut the DNA at these sites generating restriction fragments. The restriction fragments are then separated according to length by agarose gel electrophoresis which provides a pattern of bands. The resulting gel may be enhanced by Southern blotting. As DNAs from different individuals rarely have the same array of restriction sites and intersite distances, a unique pattern of bands is generated. Presence of disease risk alleles is tested by comparing the band pattern with patterns of known alleles.

2.2. The SNPlex™ Genotyping System (Applied Biosystems)

The SNPlex system (http://docs.appliedbiosystems.com/pebiodocs/04360856.pdf) combines multiplex PCR amplification and genotyping into a single reaction enabling simultaneous genotyping of up to 48 SNPs against a single biological sample. In order to specify which DNA to amplify, "primers" are used. The primers are DNA sequences that recognize a nonrepeated sequence at 5' and 3' ends of the DNA region that is to be amplified, and which are used by the DNA polymerase that does the actual copying. For PCR amplification, one probe, i.e., single-stranded oligonucleotide complementary to a segment of 20–60 nucleotides between the two primers is added to the reaction. For genotyping two probes that have discriminating nucleotide at 3' end that can hybridize to a given polymorphic sequence in an allele-specific manner are added to a single PCR reaction. A fluorescent reporter or fluorophore (e.g., 6-carboxyfluorescein, acronym: *FAM*, or tetrachlorofluorescin, acronym: TET) and quencher (e.g., tetramethylrhodamine, acronym: TAMRA, of dihydro-cyclopyrroloindole tripeptide "minor groove binder," acronym: MGB) are covalently attached to the 5' and 3' ends of each of the probes, respectively. The close proximity between fluorophore and quencher attached to the probe inhibits fluorescence from the fluorophore. During PCR, as DNA synthesis commences, the 5' to 3' exonuclease activity of the DNA polymerase degrades that proportion of the probe that has annealed to the DNA template. Degradation of the probe releases the fluorophore from it and breaks the close proximity to the quencher, thus relieving the quenching effect and allowing fluorescence of the fluorophore. After the DNA has been copied, the new DNA molecules are separated by size, by gel electrophoresis. The genotype of that SNP is determined by comparing the fluorescent signal for each of the two allele-specific reporter dyes.

2.3. iPLEX Assay (Sequenom)

iPLEX genotyping assay from Sequenom is based on single-base extension (SBE) technique (http://www.sequenom.com/Assets/pdfs/appnotes/8876-006.pdf). The SBE method begins by amplifying an area of DNA containing a known or suspected SNP. Then a primer is synthesized directly upstream from the SNP. After the primer has been synthesized, then the SBE method is performed. The primer anneals to the amplified template and is extended by one terminating base that may or may not be labeled depending on the platform used. iPLEX uses molecular weight differences of single base extension products. In this case, the single base extension reaction, outlined above, is run with unlabeled ddNTPs, resulting in two extension products of different molecular weights based on the allele incorporated. The reaction is analysed by MALDI-TOF mass spectrometry analysis and peak heights are indicative of the genotype. Multiplexing of up to 29 polymorphic sites is possible on this system.

2.4. GoldenGate Genotyping Assay (Illumina)

The GoldenGate Assay allows for a high degree of multiplexing, up to 1536 SNPs during the extension and amplification steps (http://www.illumina.com/downloads/GOLDENGATEASSAY.pdf). The DNA sample used in this assay is activated for binding to paramagnetic particles. Assay oligonucleotides, hybridization buffer, and paramagnetic particles are then combined with the activated DNA in the hybridization. Three oligonucleotides are designed for each SNP locus. Two oligos are specific to each allele of the SNP site, called the Allele-Specific Oligos (ASOs). A third oligo that hybridizes several bases downstream from the SNP site is the Locus-Specific Oligo (LSO). All three oligonucleotide sequences contain regions of genomic complementarity and universal PCR primer sites; the LSO also contains a unique address sequence that targets a particular bead type. During the primer hybridization process, the assay oligonucleotides hybridize to the genomic DNA sample bound to paramagnetic particles. Because hybridization occurs prior to any amplification steps, no amplification bias can be introduced into the assay. Following hybridization, several wash steps are performed, reducing noise by removing excess and mis-hybridized oligonucleotides. Extension of the appropriate ASO and ligation of the extended product to the LSO joins information about the genotype present at the SNP site to the address sequence on the LSO. These joined, full-length products provide a template for PCR using universal PCR primers P1, P2, and P3. Universal PCR primers P1 and P2 are Cy3- and Cy5-labeled. After downstream-processing the single-stranded, dye-labeled DNAs are hybridized to their complement bead type through their unique address sequences. The genotypes are determined by the relative fluorescence of the two labels observed for each bead.

2.5. SNPStream Assay (Orchid Cellmark/Beckman Coulter)

The SNPStream genotyping assay is based on the technique of SBE described above. In this assay dideoxy nucleotides are added with each ddNTP for each SNP allele labeled with a different fluorescent color. For example, for a C/T SNP, the ddCTP is labeled with Bodipy-Fluorescein and the ddTTP is labeled with the fluorophore TAMRA. The mix containing the hybridized primers and labeled dideoxy nucleotides are extended one base into the target SNP. These single-base extended products are hybridized to a plate that contains, in each well, an array of oligonucleotides complementary to each of the extension primer tags used. Upon hybridization of the extension product to its complementary tag, the 2-color fluorescence of each spot within each well is determined. Each SNP is identified by its position within the array and genotypes are determined by the relative 2-color fluorescence observed at each position.

2.6. Genome-Wide Human SNP Array 5.0 (Affymetrix)

With the Affymetrix Genome-Wide Human SNP Array 5.0 it is possible to genotype 500,568 SNPs (http://www.affymetrix.com/products/arrays/specific/genome_wide/genome_wide_quickprodinfo.affx). For genome-wide genotyping multiplex PCR becomes technically difficult as the number of SNPs increases. An alternative approach is to reproducibly amplify a subset of the human genome through a genome complexity reduction step. The reduced genome is of sufficient complexity to contain thousands of SNP loci, yet not so complex as to prevent the analysis of these SNPs. Affymetrix uses adaptor-PCR method to create a reduced-complexity genome for SNP analysis. Briefly, genomic DNA is digested with restriction endonuclease *Xba*I. Adaptors are ligated to all size fragments, but after adaptor PCR, only fragments in 400–800 bp size range are preferentially amplified. This amplified product represents about 2% of the whole human genome. These are biotin labeled by TdT (terminal deoxyribonucleotide transferase) mediated end-labeling, followed by array hybridization and scanning. Twenty-five mer-probes are synthesized corresponding to both of the two possible alleles at each SNP within amplified *Xba*I fragments. Owing to the nature of the genome-complexity reduction approach, it can be scaled to higher levels of SNP genotyping by simply altering the restriction enzyme or PCR conditions to create a higher complexity subset and a greater number of amplified SNPs.

2.7. Infinium Genotyping Assay (Illumina)

Currently, the Infinium assay is capable of analysing over 550,000 SNPs distributed in an exon-centric manner across the genome (http://icom.illumina.com/General/Products/SNP/pdf/INFINWKFLOW.pdf). The Infinium Whole-Genome Genotyping Assay is designed to interrogate a large number of SNPs at unlimited levels of loci multiplexing. The DNA sample used for this assay is isothermally amplified, a non-PCR approach. The amplified product is then fragmented by a controlled enzymatic process. After alcohol precipitation and resuspension, the BeadChip is prepared for hybridization in the capillary flow-through chamber; samples are applied to BeadChips and incubated overnight. The amplified and fragmented DNA samples anneal to locus-specific 50-mers (covalently linked to 1 of over 200,000 bead-types) during the hybridization step. One of two bead-types corresponds to each allele per SNP locus. After hybridization, allelic specificity is conferred by enzymatic extension. Products are subsequently fluorescently stained. The intensities of the beads' fluorescence are detected by the Illumina BeadArray Reader, and the relative signal observed for each pair of beads is used to determine the genotype of each SNP.

2.8. Resequencing

Completion of a single version of the human genome *(2,3)* has now provided the substrates for direct comparison of individuals in both health and disease. Ideally, to better understand the genetic contributions to severe diseases, one would obtain the entire human genome sequence for all disease-carrying individuals for comparison to unaffected control groups. While these complete data sets are not readily obtainable today, a strategy that is currently approachable is the re-sequencing of a large set of appropriate candidate genes in individuals with a given disease to screen for potential causative/susceptibility alleles. This technique is specifically used to detect unknown SNPs. Pros and cons of different SNP detection techniques are described in *(4)*.

3. Applications

Major application areas in which SNPs are used are disease understanding and identity and paternity tests in forensic science.

3.1. Linkage Studies

Linkage studies are done to identify regions of the genome linked with a particular disease by genotyping individuals of families with diseased members. During meiosis there is crossing-over between maternal and paternal homologous chromosomes. If the material that is exchanged has different alleles then the resultant product is a recombination of those alleles. Alleles in close proximity are likely to be inherited together, i.e., co-segregate. Linkage studies exploit the fact that as the disease-related gene segregates through a family, alleles in its close proximity co-segregate in affected individuals. All family members are genotyped for polymorphic markers distributed across the genome. Family members tend to share large fragments of inherited DNA, as a result of which as less as 500 markers may be enough for gross mapping of the chromosomal region associated with the disease. Segregation of the disease in a family is compared to the segregation of each marker. Depending on the model of the disease, a logarithm of the odds (LOD) score is computed for each marker to assess if it co-segregates with the disease. A good review of statistical methods to estimate linkage is presented in *(5)*. Finer mapping of the region can then be obtained by placing additional markers in the linked region *(6)* or candidate genes within the linked region can be selected for further analyses.

Linkage studies have been more successful in identifying genes in Mendelian diseases (chronic granulomatous disease, the X-linked muscular dystrophies, cystic fibrosis, Fanconi anemia etc. *(7)*), which are rare, high risk diseases than in finding disease loci in complex multifactorial genetic disorders. One of the largest genetic linkage studies till date was done to identify autism risk loci *(8)*. The Autism Genome Project Consortium collected samples from ~1400 families comprising of different ethnicities that had at least two individuals with autism spectrum disorder (ASD). They performed 18 linkage analyses using all samples and 18 using families of European ancestry. Two major risk loci identified in subsets of the dataset were 11p12-p13 region and gene NRXN1 which functions in cell recognition and cell adhesion and may play a role in formation or maintenance of synaptic junctions and may mediate intracellular signaling. DNA samples were genotyped using Affymetrix 10k SNP arrays.

3.2. Association Studies

Association studies test for linkage which measures the relative frequency with which a particular SNP occurs together with (i.e., is associated with) the disease of interest in a population. Association studies in which unrelated individuals are genotyped are fundamentally different in design from linkage studies.

3.2.1. Direct Association Studies

In direct association studies, putative SNPs are genotyped in a population with a particular disease and each SNP is tested for association to disease risk. Typically, the genotyped SNPs are in the coding region (cSNPs) and cause an amino acid to change, there by possibly changing the protein structure. SNPs could also be in the regulatory region of the gene which may affect gene expression. To conduct this type of studies it is essential to have a comprehensive list of functional variants of candidate genes. This information can be obtained from existing SNP databases or performing re-sequencing of the candidate genes. A genetic polymorphism in Catechol O-methyltransferase (COMT) gene, which plays an important role in the metabolism of catecholamines, catecholestrogens and catechol drugs, has been implicated as a possible risk factor for neuropsychiatric disease. Shield et al. *(9)* resequenced the human COMT gene using DNA samples from 60 African-American and 60 Caucasian-American subjects to comprehensively identify SNPs associated with the disease. Candidate genes can be identified using linkage analysis, microarray gene expression analysis, comparative genomics, knowledge of development and physiology, etc. Majority of the SNPs linked with Mendelian diseases are found in the coding regions that make the resultant protein a functional variant or nonfunctional, which is a direct cause for the disease. Based on this knowledge and the possibility of SNPs for complex multi-gene disorders showing a similar trend *(7)*, this study design has intriguing potential. Number of possible cSNPs is several orders of magnitude smaller than the total number of SNPs. Recent public efforts to comprehensively identify cSNPs have made it possible to conduct genome-wide direct association studies. A recent genome-wide association study was performed using 19,779 cSNPs in 735 individuals with Crohn disease and 368 controls *(10)* using SNPlex arrays. Disease association was found to a SNP in the autophagy-related 16-like 1 gene (ATG16L1).

Identification of SNPs in promoter region of genes that controls the gene's expression is also a promising pursuit, which is still in its infancy. A recent study *(11)* considered association of two promoter variants of the gene lipo-protein lipase (LPL), a pivotal enzyme in lipoprotein metabolism, to obesity and type 2 diabetes. The SNPs were genotyped in population in southern India using RFLP. They identified 1 variant to be associated with obesity and another to be protective against both obesity and type two diabetes.

3.2.2. Indirect Association Studies

Indirect association studies differ from direct ones in the fact that identified SNPs may not be the direct cause for the disease. Polymorphic markers for such studies are placed densely in the region of interest. The hypothesis is that if the risk SNP exists then it will either be directly genotyped or in strong LD with one of the genotyped markers. One of the caveats of this method is that you may miss an association if none of the genotyped SNPs are in LD with the risk SNP. This is becoming less of a concern with the expanding HapMap, which is a catalog of common genetic variants that occur in human beings. The HapMap provides information on tag SNPs, the SNPs when genotyped will uniquely identify a haplotype so that one can infer alleles at other locations. The advantage of this method is no prior knowledge of functionally important SNPs is required and it is easy to obtain large number of case samples from unrelated individuals with the particular disease. The disadvantage is higher number of polymorphic markers is required as unrelated individuals are unlikely to share a large number of contiguous alleles. With advancement in SNP array technology and completeness of publicly available databases, advantages will far outweigh disadvantages of indirect association studies.

Genes responsible for regulating life span and aging are suspected for their tumorigenic contribution based on the resemblance of high risk of developing cancer to accelerated aging. A recent study speculating the association of *WRN* gene, responsible for regulating life span and aging, with breast tumorigenesis examined SNPs in 935 primary breast cancer patients and 1,545 healthy controls *(12)*. All the samples were obtained from Taiwanese population, which was selected because of its homogenous genetic background providing advantages for studying the effects of subtle genetic variations, SNPs. They used data from HapMap to identify markers to be genotyped in the candidate gene. The data showed three blocks to be genetically homogenous in Taiwanese population, and linkage disequilibrium between SNPs was much stronger than that in other populations. Five markers from three blocks, evenly distributed throughout the entire gene, were genotyped. Genotyping was carried out using Taqman assays from Applied Biosystems. One SNP in *WRN* was identified as significantly associated with breast cancer risk.

Genome-wide association studies have now become feasible with availability of high density SNP arrays. A systematic search for the variants associated with Type 2 diabetes mellitus, a common complex disease was recently done by testing 392,935 single-nucleotide polymorphisms in a French case–control cohort *(13)*. They used Illumina Infinium Human1 BeadArrays, which assay 109,365 SNPs chosen using a gene-centred design; and Human Hap300 BeadArrays, which assay 317,503 SNPs chosen to tag haplotype blocks identified by the Phase I HapMap. There were 59 SNPs, showing significant association with the disease in genome-wide study, which were tested on a larger cohort using the Sequenom iPlex assay. They identified four SNPs containing variants that confer type 2 diabetes risk. These loci include a nonsynonymous polymorphism in the zinc transporter *SLC30A8,* which is expressed exclusively in insulin-producing β-cells, and two linkage disequilibrium blocks that contain genes potentially involved in β-cell development or function (*IDE–KIF11–HHEX* and *EXT2–ALX4*).

Even when genome-wide studies are possible, there are statistical difficulties arising due to multiple hypotheses testing. A good review of this issue and possible solutions are presented in *(14)*.

3.2.3. *Pool-Based Genome-Wide Association Studies*

Genotyping of individual samples for genome-wide association (GWA) studies may be cost-prohibitive. A low cost alternative is to use pooled DNA samples of disease and control groups for genotyping. Success of this method depends on whether the associated alleles are major or modest risk. A recent study suggests that pooling-based GWA studies can be used as a first step for determining whether major genetic associations exist in diseases with high heritability *(15)*. In their study, the authors report the development and validation of experimental methods, study designs, and analysis software for pooling-based genome-wide association (GWA) studies that use high-throughput single-nucleotide-polymorphism (SNP) genotyping microarrays. They apply these methods to data with known associated risk alleles and successfully identify associations for rare single gene disease (sudden infant death with dysgenesis of the testes syndrome), common complex disease (Alzheimer disease) and rare complex disease (progressive supranuclear palsy) across multiple genotyping platforms. Comparisons of different types of studies and their suitability for performing genome-wide associations studies is presented in *(16)*.

3.3. Functional Analysis

Once disease-risk associated alleles in functional regions of genes or in conserved noncoding regions that might cause significant changes in gene expression are identified, the next logical step is to understand how these variants change the transcript leading to changes in protein expression and structure. This understanding can provide insight into how functions of biochemical pathways are affected by disease-causative genetic variants. Two recent studies performed functional analysis of mutations found in SOS1 gene (encodes a RAS-specific guanine nucleotide exchange factor) associated with Noonan syndrome, which is a developmental disorder characterized by short stature, facial dysmorphia, congenital heart defects and skeletal anomalies *(17,18)*. Noonan syndrome is caused by dysregulated RAS-MAPK signaling. Based on the knowledge of biochemistry of RAS-MAPK signaling SOS1 gene was a suspect in both studies. Putative disease-causative SNPs in this gene were identified using re-sequencing and its functional implications were studied. In both studies gain-of-function mutations in this gene were implicated in the disease. The functional analysis revealed a new mechanism by which upregulation of the RAS pathway profoundly changes human development.

3.4. SNPs in Forensic Science

SNP patterns across the whole of human genome are unique to an individual. It is not practical to sequence the whole genome for the purpose of identification or kinship test done in forensic science but what is approachable is genotyping a few (from 10 to a few hundred) highly polymorphic SNPs that makes misidentification highly unlikely or impossible in reality. In addition, SNPs are better suited for the analysis of highly degraded DNA, since the distance between the primer binding sites can be designed to be very short. Finding such polymorphic SNPs for assessment purposes is not a problem because of the public SNP databases. With advancement in technologies for obtaining DNA and genotyping, the throughput potential of SNPs offers significant time and cost advantages. Study by Lee et al. reports selection of 24 highly informative SNP markers for human identification and paternity analysis in Korean population and gives insight into the methods for selecting such markers (*19*).

3.5. Environmental Genomics

Our oceans, soil and air contain thousands of microbes about which we know nothing. Microbial communities are vital in the functioning of all ecosystems; however, most microorganisms are uncultivated, and their roles in natural systems are unclear. Earlier it was not possible to sequence an environmental sample but with advent of shotgun sequencing it is possible to do so (*20,21*). Analysis of such data can provide insight into complex ecosystems and discovery of new species. Such knowledge can then be extended to devise better treatments for environmentally hazardous substances. In this newly emerging area called environmental genomics, SNPs are analyzed to study the evolution of co-occurring microbial populations. Study by Tyson et al. sequenced a sample taken from an acid mine drainage (outflow of acidic water) site and identified presence of various species and genes. Analysis of the gene complement for each organism revealed the pathways for carbon and nitrogen fixation and energy generation, and provided insights into survival strategies in an extreme environment. SNPs analysis of the *Ferroplasma* type II genome revealed it to be a composite from three ancestral strains that have undergone homologous recombination to form a large population of mosaic genomes.

4. Additional Resources

4.1. Online Learning about SNPs Research

1. http://snp.wustl.edu/
2. http://www.ncbi.nlm.nih.gov/About/primer/snps.html

4.2. Databases

1. NCBI dbSNP http://www.ncbi.nlm.nih.gov/projects/SNP/
2. The SNP consortium Ltd. http://snp.cshl.org/about/
3. JG SNP http://www.tmgh.metro.tokyo.jp/jg-snp/english/E_top.html
4. The International HapMap Project http://www.hapmap.org/
5. OMIM™ - Online Mendelian Inheritance in Man™ http://www.ncbi.nlm.nih.gov/entrez/query.fcgi?db=OMIM
6. Human Genome Mutation Database (HGMD) http://www.hgmd.cf.ac.uk/ac/index.php
7. Cancer Genome Anatomy Project Genome Annotation Initiative (CGAP-GAI) http://lpgws.nci.nih.gov/cgap-gai/

4.3. Statistical Methods for Genome-Wide Association Studies

1. A tutorial on statistical methods for population association studies *(22)*.
2. Detection of Gene x Gene Interactions in Genome-Wide Association Studies of Human Population Data *(23)*.
3. Detecting multiple associations in genome-wide studies *(14)*.

4.4. Online Resources on Forensic Science

1. http://www.isfg.org/
2. http://www.snpforid.org/
3. http://snp.wustl.edu/snp-research/forensics/

4.5. Online Resources on Environmental Genomics

1. http://www.venterinstitute.org/research/
2. http://www.jgi.doe.gov/whoweare/microbialecology.html

References

1. Sachidanandam R et al (2001) A map of human genome sequence variation containing 1.42 million single nucleotide polymorphisms. Nature 409:928–933
2. Venter JC et al (2001) The sequence of the human genome. Science 291:1304–1351
3. Lander ES et al (2001) Initial sequencing and analysis of the human genome. Nature 409:860–921
4. Engle LJ, Simpson CL, Landers JE (2006) Using high-throughput SNP technologies to study cancer. Oncogene 25:1594–1601
5. Elston RC, Anne Spence M (2006) Advances in statistical human genetics over the last 25 years. *Stat Med* 25:3049–3080
6. Larson GP et al (2005) Genetic linkage of prostate cancer risk to the chromosome 3 region bearing FHIT. Cancer Res 65:805–814
7. Botstein D, Risch N (2003) Discovering genotypes underlying human phenotypes: past successes for mendelian disease, future approaches for complex disease. Nat Genet 33:228–237
8. The Autism Genome Project Consortium (2007) Mapping autism risk loci using genetic linkage and chromosomal rearrangements. Nat Genet Advanced online publication
9. Shield AJ, Thomae BA, Eckloff BW, Wieben ED, Weinshilboum RM (2004) Human catechol *O*-methyltransferase genetic variation: gene resequencing and functional characterization of variant allozymes. Mol Psychiatry 9:151–160

10. Hampe J et al (2007) A genome-wide association scan of nonsynonymous SNPs identifies a susceptibility variant for Crohn disease in ATG16L1. Nat Genet 39:207–211

11. Radha V, Vimaleswaran KS, Ayyappa KA, Mohan V (2007) Association of lipoprotein lipase gene polymorphisms with obesity and type 2 diabetes in an Asian Indian population. Int J Obes (Lond) 13:13

12. Ding SL, Yu JC, Chen ST, Hsu GC, Shen CY (2007) Genetic variation in the premature aging gene WRN: a case-control study on breast cancer susceptibility. Cancer Epidemiol Biomarkers Prev 16:263–269

13. Sladek R et al (2007) A genome-wide association study identifies novel risk loci for type 2 diabetes. Nature 445:881–885

14. Dudbridge F, Gusnanto A, Koeleman BP (2006) Detecting multiple associations in genome-wide studies. Hum Genomics 2:310–317

15. Pearson JV et al (2007) Identification of the genetic basis for complex disorders by use of pooling-based genomewide single-nucleotide-polymorphism association studies. Am J Hum Genet 80:126–139

16. Carlson CS, Eberle MA, Kruglyak L, Nickerson DA (2004) Mapping complex disease loci in whole-genome association studies. Nature 429:446–452

17. Tartaglia M et al (2007) Gain-of-function SOS1 mutations cause a distinctive form of Noonan syndrome. Nat Genet 39:75–79

18. Roberts AE et al (2007) Germline gain-of-function mutations in SOS1 cause Noonan syndrome. Nat Genet 39:70–74

19. Lee HY et al (2005) Selection of twenty-four highly informative SNP markers for human identification and paternity analysis in Koreans. Forensic Sci Int 148:107–112

20. Venter JC et al (2004) Environmental genome shotgun sequencing of the Sargasso Sea. Science 304:66–74

21. Tyson GW et al (2004) Community structure and metabolism through reconstruction of microbial genomes from the environment. Nature 428:37–43

22. Balding DJ (2006) A tutorial on statistical methods for population association studies. Nat Rev Genet 7:781–791

23. Musani SK et al (2007) Detection of gene x gene interactions in genome-wide association studies of human population data. Hum Hered 63:67–84

Gene/Protein Sequence Analysis
A Compilation of Bioinformatic Tools

Bernd H. A. Rehm and Frank Reinecke

1. Introduction

The advent of automated high throughput DNA sequencing methods has strongly enabled genome sequencing strategies, culminating in determination of the entire human genome *(1,2)*. An enormous amount of DNA sequence data are available and databases still grow exponentially (see **Fig. 22.1**). Analysis of this overwhelming amount of data, including hundreds of genomes from both prokaryotes and eukaryotes, has given rise to the field of bioinformatics. Development of bioinformatic tools has evolved rapidly in order to identify genes that encode functional proteins or RNA. This is an important task, considering that even in the best studied bacterium *Escherichia coli* more than 30% of the identified open reading frames (ORFs) represent hypothetical genes with no known function. Future challenges of genome-sequence analysis will include the understanding of diseases, gene regulation, and metabolic pathway reconstruction. In addition, a set of methods for protein analysis summarized under the term *proteomics* holds tremendous potential for biomedicine and biotechnology *(141)*. The large number of bioinformatic tools that have been made available to scientists during the last few years has presented the problem of which to use and how best to obtain scientifically valid answers *(3)*. In this chapter, we will provide a guide for the most efficient way to analyze a given sequence or to collect information regarding a gene, protein, structure, or interaction of interest by applying current publicly available software and databases that mainly use the World Wide Web. All links to services or download sites are given in the text or listed in **Table 22.1**; the succession of tools is briefly summarized in **Fig. 22.2**.

2. Software Tools for Bioinformatics

In the first part of this chapter, software tools will be described that mainly use algorithms and are based either on very short-sequence comparisons, physical or chemical properties of molecules, or statistics. A second group of software

From: *Molecular Biomethods Handbook, 2nd Edition.*
Edited by: J. M. Walker and R. Rapley © Humana Press, Totowa, NJ

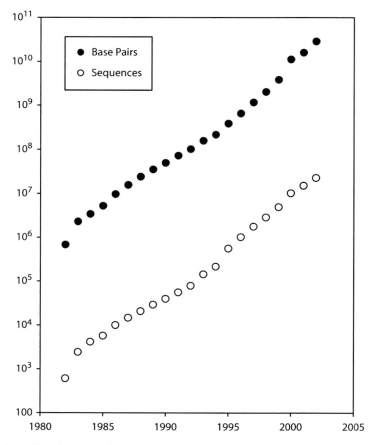

Fig. 22.1. Development of stored DNA-sequence information in GenBank from 1982 to 2002 (●, base pairs; ○, sequences) (From http://www.ncbi.nlm.nih.gov/Genbank/genbankstats.html)

relies mainly on databases and will be discussed below. As so-called integrated methods are evolving and becoming more and more popular, it is difficult to divide programs into these two groups.

There are many programs routinely used to generate contiguous DNA sequences from raw data obtained from high- throughput sequencers, to assign quality scores to each base, remove contaminating sequences (such as vector DNA), and provide the means to link sequences containing applications. First, base- callers like Phred *(4,5)* extract raw sequences from raw data. There are also contig assemblers like Phrap (University of Washington, http://bozeman.mbt.washington.edu/phrap.docs/phrap.html) or CAP3 *(6)* that assemble fragments to contigs and packages like consed *(7)* or GAP4 *(8)*, which are used to finish sequencing projects. These programs are not explained in detail here.

Any DNA region that can be assigned a function is of special interest. The sequence elements that can be found within them include promoters and various transcription factor-binding sites, ribosome-binding sites, start and stop codons, splice sites, and so forth. These are referred to as signals. Methods to detect them are termed *signal sensors*. In contrast, extended

Table 22.1. Compilation of links to bioinformatic services and software.

Program	Link
Gene Finding	
AMIGene	http://www.genoscope.cns.fr/agc/tools/amigene/index.html
Critica	http://www.ttaxus.com
EasyGene	http://www.cbs.dtu.dk/services/EasyGene
EUGENE'HOM	http://genopole.toulouse.inra.fr/bioinfo/eugene/EuGeneHom/cgibin/ EuGeneHom.pl
GeneFizz	http://pbga.pasteur.fr/GeneFizz
GeneMark.hmm2	http://opal.biology.gatech.edu/GeneMark/gmhmm2_prok.cgi
GeneMarkS	http://opal.biology.gatech.edu/geneMark/genemarks.cgi
GeneScan	http://genes.mit.edu/GENSCAN.html
Genie	http://www.soe.ucsc.edu/~dkulp/cgi-bin/genie
Glimmer	http://www.cs.jhu.edu/labs/compbio/glimmer.html
GlimmerM	http://www.tigr.org/tdb/glimmerm/glmr_form.html
Grail	http://compbio.ornl.gov/Grail-1.3
HMMgene	http://www.cbs.dtu.dk/services/HMMgene
ORF-Finder	http://www.ncbi.nlm.nih.gov/gorf/gorf.html
Procrustes	http://www-hto.usc.edu/software/procrustes
Veil	http://www.cs.jhu.edu/labs/compbio/veil.html
ZCURVE	http://tubic.tju.edu.cn/ZCURVE
Signal Finding	
MatInspector	http://transfac.gbf.de/cgi- bin/matSearch/matsearch.pl
PromotorScan	http://bimas.dcrt.nih.gov/molbio/proscan
SignalScan	http://bimas.dcrt.nih.gov/molbio/signal
TRANSFAC	http://transfac.gbf.de/TRANSFAC
Sequence Alignment	
CLUSTALW	ftp://ftp-igbmc.u-strasbg.fr/pub/ClustalW
	http://www.ebi.ac.uk/clustalw
CLUSTALX	ftp://ftp-igbmc.u-strasbg.fr/pub/ClustalX
DbClustal	http://igbmc.u- strasbg.fr/DbClustal/dbclustal.html
HMMER	http://hmmer.wustl.edu
T-COFFEE	http://www.ch.embnet.org/software/TCoffee.html
Phylogeny	
PAUP	http://onyx.si.edu/PAUP
GCG package	http://www.gcg.com
PHYLIP	http://evolution.genetics.washington.edu/phylip.html
Phylodendron	http://iubio.bio.indiana.edu/treeapp
Tree View	http://taxonomy.zoology.gla.ac.uk/rod/treeview.html
Protein Properties and Structure	
DAS	http://www.sbc.su.se/~miklos/DAS
ExPASy	http://www.expasy.org
META PP	http://cubic.bioc.columbia.edu/predictprotein/submit_meta.html
PredictProtein	http://cubic.bioc.columbia.edu/predictprotein
TMHMM	http://www.cbs.dtu.dk/services/TMHMM-2.0
TMpred	http://www.ch.embnet.org/software/TMPRED_form.html
Database Searching	
NCBI BLAST	http://www.ncbi.nlm.nih.gov/BLAST
WUBLAST	http://blast.wustl.edu
Protein Families and Motifs	
BLOCKS	http://www.blocks.fhcrc.org
InterPro	http://www.ebi.ac.uk/interpro/scan.html

(continued)

Table 22.1. (continued)

Program	Link
Pfam	http://www.sanger.ac.uk/Software/Pfam
PRINTS	http://www.biochem.ucl.ac.uk/bsm/dbbrowser/PRINTS
PROSITE	http://www.expasy.org/prosite
SMART	http://smart.embl-heidelberg.de
Protein Structure	
CATH	http://www.biochem.ucl.ac.uk/bsm/cath
PDB	http://www.pdb.org
SCOP	http://scop.mrc-lmb.cam.ac.uk/scop
Structure Modeling	
CPHmodels	http://www.cbs.dtu.dk/services/CPHmodels
ESyPred3D	http://www.fundp.ac.be/urbm/bioinfo/esypred
Geno3D	http://www.geno3d-pbil.ibcp.fr
SWISS-MODEL	http://swissmodel.expasy.org
Protein Interaction	
BIND	http://binddb.org
CAPRI	http://capri.ebi.ac.uk
DIP	http://dip.doe-mbi.ucla.edu/dip/Main.cgi
Genome Analysis	
COG	http://www.ncbi.nlm.nih.gov/COG
NCBI Genomes	http://www.ncbi-nlm.nih.gov/genomes
SNPs and Expression Profiling	
cSNP	http://csnp.unige.ch
dbSNP	http://www.ncbi.nlm.nih.gov/Entrez
GEO	http://www.ncbi.nlm.nih.gov/geo

and variable-length regions, such as exons and introns, are termed *contents*. These are recognized by methods that can be called content sensors (*9*). It is a major challenge to find the functional sites responsible for gene structure, regulation and transcription. Computational methodology for finding genes and other functional sites in genomic DNA has evolved significantly over the past years (*10–20*).

2.1. Gene-Finding Methods

The most basic signal sensor is a simple consensus sequence or an expression that describes a consensus sequence together with allowable variations. Sophisticated types of signal sensor, such as neural nets, are extensively used (*21,22*). The most important content sensors are programs that predict coding regions (*23*). In prokaryotes, genes are identified simply by looking for long ORFs. However, these relatively simple methods cannot be transferred to higher eukaryotes. In order to discriminate coding against noncoding regions in eukaryotes, exon content sensors use statistical models of the nucleotide frequencies (*24*) and dependencies present in codon structures. The most commonly used statistical models are known as Markov models. Neural nets are used to combine several coding hints together with signal sensors for the flanking splice sites in exon detectors (*22*). Other content sensors include those for CpG sites (regions that often occur at the beginning of genes, where the dinucleotide CG appears more frequently than in the rest of the genome and

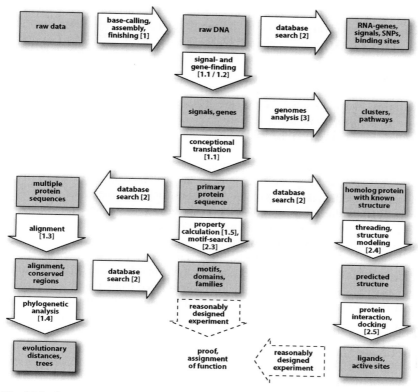

Fig. 22.2. Succession of programs during assignment of function to DNA or proteins. Arrows indicate action of bioinformatic tools, detailed descriptions can be found in the chapter given in brackets

sensors for repetitive DNA such as human ALU sequences *(25)*. The latter sensors are often used as masks or filters that completely remove the repetitive DNA, leaving the remaining DNA to be analyzed.

The statistical signals that signal and content sensors try to localize are usually weak, and there are usually dependencies between signals and contents, such as the possible correlation between splice-site strength and exon size *(26)*. During the past decade, several systems that combine signal and content sensors have been developed in an attempt to identify complete gene structures. The first program using linguistic rules and a formal grammar for the arrangement of certain signals required for gene prediction was GenLang *(27)*. As with most integrated gene-finders to date, GenLang uses dynamic programming to combine potential exon regions and other scored regions and sites into gene prediction with a maximal total score *(13,16,28)*. These models are called hidden Markov models (HMMs). Gene-finding HMMs can be viewed as stochastic versions of the gene structure grammars. Early gene-finding HMMs included EcoParse for *E. coli* *(29)*–also recently used in the annotation of the *Mycobacterium tuberculosis* genome *(30)*–and Xpound *(31)*, Veil *(32)*, and HMMgene *(16)* for the human genome *(13)*. More recent programs include GeneMark HMM *(33)*, GLIMMER *(34)*, and Critica *(35)*.

Different programs specializing in special detectable differences between coding and noncoding regions have been developed recently. EasyGene *(20)* and AMIGene *(36)* apply statistical methods on predicted ORFs of prokaryotes, ZCURVE *(19)* concentrates on nucleic acid distribution for bacterial or archaeal genomes. GeneMarkS is an improved version of GeneMark, which has been applied to identify genes in the genomes of *Bacillus subtilis* and *E. coli* with the highest accuracy described to date *(37)*. Even physical properties of DNA are used to predict genes: GeneFizz *(38)* compares the physics-based structural segmentation between helix and coil domains. Measuring the spectral rotation based on a process termed discrete Fourier transform (DFT) has proven to be capable of predicting genes in *Saccharomyces cerevisiae* *(39)*. A slightly more general class of probabilistic models, called generalized HMMs or (hidden) semi- Markov models, has roots in GeneParser *(40)* and is more fully developed in Genie *(41)* and, subsequently, GenScan *(42)*. The above gene-finders predict gene structure based only on general features of genes, rather than using explicit comparisons to known genes and their corresponding proteins, or auxiliary information such as expressed sequence tag (EST) matches. Some gene-finding systems combine multiple statistical measures with protein database homology searches performed using the predicted gene or deduced protein *(11,15,43)*. This homology approach was developed by Gelfand et al *(44)* and is used by EUGENE'HOM *(45)* or Procrustes *(15)*, which uses a "spliced alignment" algorithm, similar to a Smith–Waterman algorithm *(46)*, to derive a putative gene structure by aligning the DNA to a partial protein homolog of the gene to be predicted. Instead of inventing and approving yet another gene-finding program, there are several approaches to combining different existing algorithms using advantages of each program to eliminate disadvantages inherent to each single method *(47)*.

2.2. Signal-Finding Bioinformatics Methods

There is a tremendous variety of software exploiting various ways to identify structural genes in a DNA sequence, and as already outlined, there are more elements present than just structural genes. Some gene-finding approaches presented above already consider bases outside the start and stop codons, but there are specialized resources, namely MatInspector *(48)* and SignalScan *(49)*, to find transcription factor-binding sites using a relatively small database called TRANSFAC *(50)*. Another program designed to find putative eukaryotic polymerase II promoter sequences in primary sequence data is PromotorScan *(51)*.

2.3. Sequence-Alignment Methods

An alignment refers to the procedure of comparing two or more sequences by looking for a series of individual characters or character patterns that are found in the same order in the sequences. To align sequences, identical or similar characters are grouped in the same column, whereas nonidentical characters can either be placed in the same column, resulting in a mismatch, or opposite a gap in one of the other sequences. In an optimal alignment, mismatches and gaps are distributed in such a way that matches are maximized. Two types of sequence alignment have been recognized. In a global alignment, an attempt is made to align the entire sequences with as many characters as possible.

In a local alignment, stretches of sequence with the highest density of matches are given the highest priority, thus generating one or more islands of matches in the aligned sequences and producing totally mismatching regions. Alignments are the working principle of programs (e.g., BLAST) that search similar sequences by successively aligning a query with an entire sequence database; they are also useful for determining the evolutionary distance between homologous sequences of different origin.

2.3.1. Multiple-Sequence Alignment

Comparison of multiple sequences can reveal gene functions that are not evident from simple sequence homologies. As a result of genome-sequencing projects, new sequences are often found to be similar to several uncharacterized sequences, defining whole families of novel genes with no obvious function. However, such a family enables the application of efficient alternative similarity search methods. Software packages are now available that derive profiles from multiple-sequence alignments. Profiles incorporate position-specific scoring information that is derived from the abundance of a given residue in an aligned column. Because sequence families preferentially conserve certain critical residues and motifs, this information should allow more sensitive database searches. Most new profile software are based on statistical HMMs. Much more comprehensive reviews of the literature on profile HMM methods are available elsewhere (12,28,52–55). ClustalW is a well-supported and frequently used free program capable of dealing with large numbers of sequences at high processing speeds as compared to other alignment algorithms, and it is available for Macintosh, Windows, and various UNIX systems (56). There is also a graphical user interface–ClustalX (57). However, for sequences with less than 30% identity, the program T-COFFEE might be used, which is more accurate than the progressively aligning ClustalW, but slower. Once the family is defined, obtaining an acceptable multiple-sequence alignment is usually straightforward. Multiple alignments can either be generated from FASTA format files (using a ClustalW supporting website) or from DbClustal, which produces a BLAST output in which the family members can be selected and the multiple alignment subsequently produced. It is important to inspect the alignment in the graphical display of ClustalX to make sure that it appears consistent. The alignment can also be saved in multiple-sequence format (MSF), which can be read by other software for further analysis (e.g., careful editing, trimming, coloring, shading, and printing). GeneDoc available for Windows (www.psc.edu/biomed/genedoc) offers many of these editing features (58).

2.4. Phylogenetic Analysis

Phylogenetic trees can be constructed based on multiple alignments. In rooted trees, the ancestral state of the organisms, or genes, being studied is shown at the bottom of the tree, and the tree branches, or bifurcates, until it reaches the terminal branches, tips, or leaves at the top of the tree. An unrooted tree is a less intuitive, more abstract concept. Unrooted trees represent the branching order, but do not indicate the root, or location, of the last common ancestor. Ideally, rooted trees are preferable, but almost every phylogenetic reconstruction algorithm provides an unrooted tree. Molecular sequence analysis is a field in its infancy and an inexact science in which there are few analytical tools that are truly based on general mathematical and statistical principles. Consequently, many phylogenetic trees reconstructed from molecular sequences are incorrect. This is mainly caused by the following:

1. Incorrect sequence alignments.
2. The failure to properly account for site-to-site variation (all sites within sequences can evolve at different rates).
3. Unequal rate effects (the inability of most tree-building algorithms to produce good phylogenetic trees when genes from different taxa in the tree have evolved at different rates).

Of the three pitfalls, alignment artifacts are potentially the most serious. A new algorithm, paralinear (logdet) distances *(59,60)*, provides a simple, but rigorous, mathematical solution for the third pitfall. For a discussion of many other useful algorithms currently available, including maximum parsimony likelihood and other distance methods, see **refs. *61*** and ***62***. Sequence alignments should be carefully checked before calculating evolutionary trees. There are several programs to help calculate trees from genome data. The best known software for reconstructing trees is the program PAUP (phylogenetic analysis using parsimony), which is part of the GCG sequence analysis package that supports logdet analysis. PAUP is user friendly and comprehensive. PHYLIP/Phylodendron are further well-known packages that contain a large variety of routines, including several that incorporate the latest theoretical developments. A stand-alone software package available for many computer platforms for viewing, editing, rearranging, and printing trees is TreeView *(63, 64)*.

2.5. Protein Properties and Structure Prediction

Protein sequences allow extensive calculations that help to assign function, to predict topology (subcellular localization, spanning of membranes) and structure, and to find sites that are likely to be cleaved or modified; interaction or catalytic mechanisms can be simulated. Bioinformatic resources on the WWW range from the determination of the molecular weight to complex threading and three-dimensional (3D) prediction algorithms. A huge list of tools can be found on the ExPASy proteomic tools homepage *(65)*. Because of the great variety of programs available, several of these single tools have been integrated into one interface. Examples are PredictProtein *(66)* or META PP *(67)*. These integrate resources such as SignalP *(68)*, which predicts the presence and location of signal peptide cleavage sites in amino acid sequences from different organisms–NetOglyc [predictions of mucin type *O*-glycosylation sites in mammalian proteins *(69–71)*, NetPhos [predicting potential phosphorylation sites at serine, threonine or tyrosine residues in protein sequences, *(72)*, NetPico [predictions of cleavage sites of picornaviral proteases *(73)*, and ChloroP [predicting chloroplast transit peptides and their cleavage sites *(74)*. Secondary structure prediction is performed by JPRED *(75)*; transmembrane helices are identified using TMHMM *(76)*, TopPred *(77,78)*, and DAS *(79)*. Structural databases are searched to detect similarities between remote homolog proteins too weak to be inferred from simple sequence alignment techniques by FRSVR *(80,81)* and SAM-T02 *(82)* but the detection of remote homologs represents a problem to be solved because most of the results returned are supposedly wrong. Results should be checked very carefully. Homology modeling is also covered by META PP, applying both SWISS-MODEL *(83–85)* and CPHmodels *(86)* described in the following section.

3. Databases

A database is any collection of data or information that is specially organized for rapid search and retrieval by a computer. To cope with not only the vast amount of sequence information but also other experimental data, biological databases have been set up and are updated continuously. For biological data such as information about a protein's sequence, structure, modification, or interaction, software tools have been developed that enable searching, comparing, and retrieving these stored data.

3.1. Matching Algorithms

Basic queries like finding a key word in an article employ simple pattern-matching algorithms that do not need a statistical evaluation of the result. Bioinformatic tools started like this and most tools apply algorithms that match a query against all targets in a database, taking into account the degree and type of mismatches or gaps *(87)*. Deciding whether the observed degree of structural likeness is significant and, therefore, a hint toward functional identity is a task for statistical methods based on special biological matrices *(88,89)*. These matrices are crucial to considering the biological nature of the data. According to structural relevance, varieties in certain amino acid residues, for example, are decisive, whereas other differences can be negligible.

Sequence database matching has proven to be a remarkably useful method for assigning a function to an unknown sequence. If sequence similarity to one or more database sequences, whose function is already known, is obtained, the unknown sequence can be inferred to have the same function, biochemical activity, or structure. The strength of these inferences depends on the strength of the similarity. As a rough rule, if more than 25–30% of a protein sequence is identical in an alignment, then the sequences are homologous *(90)*. RNA genes are usually much more conserved, which is the reason why they represent suitable markers for phylogenetic analyses. Functional DNA sequences like promoters or other regulatory regions are significantly shorter than genes encoding enzyme proteins or RNA, making them hard to identify by means of sequence comparison or alignment. Identification and assignment of genes, as well as the functional and structural classification of proteins, is performed based on similarity of sequence and/or properties such as motifs or structurally conserved regions. Because DNA sequences are variable in the third base position of the codon, protein-sequence analysis is the more valuable approach. In general, sequence analysis requires the comparison of sequences from unknown genes or proteins with those of known function deposited in databases. However, the sequences of homologous proteins can diverge greatly over time, whereas the structure or function of the same proteins has diverged only slightly. Conversely, proteins with similar folds can exhibit completely different functions. However, much can be deduced about an unknown protein when significant sequence similarity is detected with a well-studied protein.

Alignment provides a powerful tool to compare related sequences, and the alignment of two residues could reflect a common evolutionary origin or represent common structural and/or catalytic roles, not always reflecting an evolutionary process.

3.1.1. Substitution Matrices and Alignment Scores

To identify the most valuable alignments, the standard procedure is to assign scores to them. For each pair of letters that can be aligned, a substitution score is chosen. The complete set of these scores is called a substitution matrix [PAM (91) and BLOSUM (92)]. Additionally, scores are chosen for gaps, which consist of one or more adjacent nulls in one sequence aligned with letters in the other. Because a single mutational event can insert or delete more than one residue, a long gap should be penalized only slightly more than a short gap. Accordingly, affined gap costs, which charge a relatively large penalty for the existence of a gap and a smaller penalty for each residue it contains, have become the most widely used gap-scoring system. The quality of sequence comparison depends very much on the choice of appropriate substitution and gap scores. In brief, for ungapped alignments, the alignment score of a given pair of residues i and j depends on the fraction q_{ij} of true alignment positions in which these paired residues tend to appear (88). Accordingly, the design of a good substitution matrix is based on estimating the target frequencies q_{ij} accurately. However, the target frequencies depend on the degree of evolutionary divergence between the related sequences of interest. Therefore, a series of matrices tailored to varying degrees of evolutionary divergence are required (88,91,92). This was the intention in constructing the PAM and BLOSUM series of amino-acid-substitution matrices. These matrices are generally used unmodified for gapped local and global alignment. There is no widely accepted theory for selecting gap costs that requires adjustment for individual similarity searches (93).

3.1.2. Alignment Scores and E Values

To test the biological relevance of a global or local alignment of two sequences, one needs to know how the value of an alignment score can be expected to occur by chance. Current versions of the FASTA and BLAST search programs report the raw scores of the alignments they return, as well as assessments of their statistical significance based on the extreme value distribution. Most simply, these assessments take the form of E values. The E value for a given alignment depends on its score, as well as the lengths of both the query sequence and the database sequence searched. It represents the number of distinct alignments with equivalent or superior scores that might have been expected to occur only by chance. The smaller the E value, the more likely that the alignment is significant and not occurring by chance (88,89,94).

3.1.3. Filtering Database Sequences

Many DNA and protein sequences contain regions of highly restricted nucleic acid and amino acid compositions and regions of short elements repeated many times. The standard alignment models and scoring systems were not designed to capture the evolutionary processes that led to these low-complexity regions. As a result, two sequences containing compositionally biased regions can receive a very high similarity score that reflects this bias alone. For many purposes, these regions are not relevant and can obscure other important similarities. Therefore, programs that filter low-complexity regions from query or database sequences will often turn a useless database search into a valuable one. For this reason, the NCBI BLAST server will remove such sections in proteins using a program termed SEG *(95)*. Although these programs automatically remove the majority of problematic matches, some problems invariably occur. Furthermore, masking might preclude interesting hits. Therefore, it is useful to adjust the masking parameters or turn filtering off completely.

3.1.4. Database Searching

Fundamentally, performing a database search is a very simple operation: A query sequence is aligned with each of the sequences in a database and a score describing the degree of likeness is calculated using a suitable matrix. Nevertheless, sequence comparison procedures should be applied carefully. The design of a BLAST database search requires consideration of the kind of information one hopes to obtain about the query sequence of interest *(96)*. A major constraint of database searching is that it only reveals similarity and might not indicate function. Therefore, it is better to use data that describe the natural situation as accurately as possible (e.g., comparing 3D structures of proteins with each other). This is because 3D structures rather than the primary sequence is conserved during evolution processes. However, in most cases, the information will consist of a primary sequence alone. One should, nonetheless, compare deduced protein sequences rather than DNA if the query DNA is likely to encode for a protein. This also enables the detection of remote homologs *(97)*. In DNA comparisons, there is noise from the rapidly mutated third-base position in each codon and from comparisons of noncoding frames. In addition, amino acids have chemical characteristics that allow degrees of similarity to be assessed, rather than simple recognition of identity or nonidentity. DNA versus DNA comparison (BLASTN program) is typically used to find identical regions of sequence in a database. One should apply this search to find RNA-encoding or regulatory regions and/or to discover whether a protein-encoding gene has been previously sequenced or contains splice junctions. Briefly, protein-level searches are valuable for detecting evolutionarily related genes, whereas DNA searches are best for locating nearly identical regions of sequence. The following should be considered when designing a database search:

1. Search a large current database (SWISS-Prot, EMBL, and Genebank).
2. Compare relevant data.
3. Filter query for low-complexity regions.
4. Interpret scores with *E* values.
5. Recognize that most homologs are not found by pairwise sequence comparison.
6. Consider slower and more powerful methods, but use iterative programs with great caution (iterative programs might indicate homology, which is not related to function).

3.2. Sequence Databases

Protein-homology searches are usually performed employing the nr (nonredundant) sequence database at the NCBI (National Center for Biotechnology Information) website. The nr database combines data from several sources, removes redundant identical sequences, and yields a collection with nearly all known proteins. A frequent update of the NCBI nr database guarantees that the most recent and complete database is used. Obviously, a search will not identify a sequence that has not been included in the database and, as databases are growing so rapidly, use of a current database is essential. Several specialized databases are also available, each of which is a subset of the nr database. One might also wish to search DNA databases at the protein level. Programs can do so automatically by first translating the DNA in all six reading frames and then making comparisons with each of these translations. The nr database, which contains the most publicly available DNA sequences, is useful to search when hunting for new genes; identified genes in this database would already be in the protein nr database. Because of the different combinations of queries and database types, there are several variants of BLAST *(87,89,90)*. The BLAST programs can be run via the Internet or they can alternatively be downloaded from an ftp site to run locally. Another option is to use the FASTA package *(97)*. The FASTA program is slower but can be more effective than BLAST. The package also contains SSEARCH, an implementation of the rigorous Smith–Waterman algorithm, which is slow but the most sensitive. Iterative programs such as PSI-BLAST require extreme care in their operation because they can provide misleading results; however, they have the potential to find more homologs than purely pairwise methods. The effectiveness of any alignment program depends on the scoring systems it employs *(88,92,93)*.

3.3. Protein Family and Motif Databases

There are several collections of amino-acid-sequence motifs that indicate particular structural or functional elements. Web-based searches of these collections with a newly identified sequence allow reasonably confident functional predictions to be made. A variety of genome- and cDNA-sequencing projects is producing raw sequence data at a breathtaking speed, creating the need for a large-scale functional classification effort. On a smaller scale, the average molecular biologist can also be faced with a new sequence without any a priori functional knowledge. Any hint as to whether the newly identified gene encodes a transcription factor, a cytoskeletal protein, or a metabolic enzyme would certainly help to interpret the experimental results and would suggest a direction for subsequent investigations.

3.3.1. Protein versus Domain Classification

The first step is usually a database search with BLAST or a similar program. Optimally, the BLAST output would show a clear similarity to a single, well-characterized protein spanning the complete length of the query protein. However, in the worst case, the output list would fail to show any significant hit. In reality, the most frequent result is a list of partial matches to assorted proteins, most of them uncharacterized, with the remainder having dubious or even contradictory functional assignments. Much of this confusion is caused by the modular architecture of the proteins involved. An analysis of known 3D protein structures reveals that, rather than being monolithic, many of them contain multiple folding units. Each unit (domain) has its own hydrophobic core and has most of its residue–residue contacts internally. In order to fulfill these conditions, independent domains must have a minimum size of approx 50 residues unless stabilized by metal ions or disulfide bridges. Analysis of protein sequences contradicts this structural observation. Sequence pairs frequently exhibit localized regions of similarity, whereas the rest of the proteins are totally dissimilar. Folding independence for all of these so-called homology domains has not been demonstrated experimentally. For protein classification, it is important to note that the homology domains also frequently harbor independent functions. Some domains have enzymatic activity, others bind to small messenger molecules, and others specifically bind to DNA, RNA, or proteins. A multidomain protein can, therefore, have more than one function and belong to more than one protein family or class. For this reason, most of the current approaches to protein functional classification focus on domains rather than complete proteins.

3.3.2. The Protein Superfamily Assignment

Efforts have been undertaken to group protein sequences into families and superfamilies. The various approaches differ in their degree of automation, their comprehensiveness, their focus on complete proteins or protein domains, and the methodology applied. Some of these efforts are aimed exclusively at the classification of existing sequence data. Others go one step further and aim to extract the essential features from sequence families and to store them in the form of domain or motif descriptors, which can then be used for searches with user-supplied protein sequences. These searches exert high sensitivity, which has proven to be most useful for the functional assignment of unknown proteins. A parallel development, which will be discussed later, is the classification of protein 3D structures. A comprehensive discussion of this topic can be found in **refs. *98*** and ***99***. Some of the most popular collections, which consider the modular nature of proteins, are briefly discussed. The PROSITE pattern library was one of the pioneering efforts in collecting descriptors for important protein motifs with biological relevance *(100,101)*. A PROSITE pattern does not describe a complete domain or even protein, but just tries to identify the functionally most important residue combinations, such as the catalytic site of an enzyme. All motifs are accompanied by extensive documentation, including references. However, the short patterns do not contain enough information to yield statistically significant matches in the large and growing protein databases. Consequently, a certain number of false-positive hits is to be expected when carrying out a database search, and any hit reported after scanning the PROSITE database with a sequence has to be treated with appropriate caution. To solve these restrictions, the PROSITE pattern library has been supplemented since 1995 by the PROSITE profile library *(101)*. Generalized profiles are at an intermediate position between a sequence-to-sequence comparison and the matching of a regular expression to a sequence *(102)*. The ProDom database was the first comprehensive collection of complete protein domains *(103,104)*. It is derived from SWISS-PROT, and the domains are denoted only by cluster numbers and do not contain any biological annotation. Moreover, the automatically determined domain boundaries are unreliable and the associated search methods are not very sensitive. Pfam, which is derived from ProDom, contains HMMs, which are conceptually related to the PROSITE profiles *(53,105)*. The Pfam models typically span complete protein domains and can be searched with the HMMER package or on a web-based server. The current release of Pfam (10.0) contains 6,190 families *(106)*. Similar to the PROSITE profiles, the Pfam models are refined iteratively, starting from clear homologs and incorporating increasingly distant family members in the process. Because of their information-rich descriptors, both collections are able to detect even very distant instances of a protein motif that are rarely found by any other method. Because Pfam models and PROSITE profiles can be interconverted *(102)* combination searches are available at InterPro *(107,108)*. The current release of InterPro (7.0) contains 8547 entries describing 6416 families, 1902 domains, 163 repeats, 26 active sites, 20 binding sites, and 20 posttranslational modifications. The use of this integrated service is therefore recommended, although there are still some specialized databases that are not covered. MEROPS *(109)* is a catalog and classification system of enzymes with proteolytic activity (peptidases or proteases).

NIFAS is a Java applet, which retrieves domain information from the Pfam database and uses ClustalW to calculate a tree for a given domain and to enable visual analysis of domain evolution in proteins. Consideration of the evolution of certain domains might be important for functional annotation of modular proteins and for understanding the function of individual domains *(110)*. SMART (simple modular architecture research tool) allows the identification and annotation of genetically mobile domains and the analysis of domain architectures. The SMART database is an independent collection of HMMs (domain families)–660 in version 3.5–focusing on protein domains related to signaling, extracellular, and chromatin-associated proteins *(111–113)*. These domains are extensively annotated with respect to phyletic distributions, functional class, tertiary structure, and functionally important residues. Domains found in the nr protein database as well as search parameters and taxonomic information are stored in a relational database system. User interfaces to this database allow searches for proteins containing specific combinations of domains in defined taxa. BLOCKS *(114)* and PRINTS *(63,115)* are two motif databases that represent protein or domain families by several short, ungapped multiple alignment fragments. The current release of BLOCKS (13.0) contains 8,656 blocks representing 2,101 groups, which are derived from PROSITE patterns. The blocks for the BLOCKS database are made automatically by looking for the most highly conserved regions in groups of proteins documented in the PROSITE database. The Internet-based versions of the PROSITE and SWISS-PROT databases that are used are located at the ExPASy molecular biology web-server of the Geneva University Hospital and the University of Geneva. The blocks created by Block Maker are created in the same manner as the blocks in the BLOCKS database but with sequences provided by the user. Results are reported in a multiple-sequence alignment format and in the standard Block format for searching. PRINTS is a compendium of protein fingerprints. A fingerprint is a group of conserved motifs used to character-ize a protein family; its diagnostic power is refined by iterative scanning of a composite of SWISS-PROT+SP-TrEMBL. Usually the motifs do not over-lap, but are separated along a sequence, although they might be contiguous in 3D space. Fingerprints can encode protein folds and functionalities more flexibly and powerfully than can single motifs, their full diagnostic potency deriving from the mutual context afforded by motif neighbors. BLOCKS and PRINTS can be searched with the same programs at the website InterPro (see above). Domains important in signal transduction are likely to be found with the PROSITE profiles or SMART; Pfam emphasizes extracellular domains, and the PROSITE patterns are good at identifying enzyme classes by their active-site motif. Recently, a unified protein family resource, MetaFam, was generated to support the general classification efforts (*116*). MetaFam is a protein family classification built up from 10 publicly accessible protein family databases (Blocks + DOMO, Pfam, PIR-ALN, PRINTS, PROSITE, ProDom, PROTOMAP, SBASE, and SYSTERS). Meta-Fam's family "supersets" are created automatically by comparing families between the databases. However, the number of available single and combined domain descriptors should not be overestimated as a quality criterion, as the databases and the associated search methods differ in generality and sensitivity. The most promising approach to predicting the exact function of a protein is to find its characterized ortholog from a different species or a well-conserved paralog that fulfills a related but different function (*117*). In addition, the databases contain large amounts of incorrect annotated sequences.

3.4. Protein Structure Databases

The complexity and sophistication of biological molecular interactions are astonishing. In this context, it is essential to develop bioinformatic tools that reliably allow the prediction of protein structure, as the structure determines interaction with all kinds of small molecules (substrates, activators, repressors, drugs) and other proteins (either specific as in natural multiprotein complexes or unspecific), consequently revealing the protein's function. In the near future, representative structures for most water-soluble protein domains will be available, which will allow modeling and classification of related sequences to provide structures for all gene products. However, elucidating the function of all gene products in vivo will be a long-term challenge for biologists. The emphasis will shift to understanding of principles and control of biological function and the interactions between molecules. A 3D model of a protein can help one to understand the "docking" of ligands and proteins, which is essential to enable their rational design or modification to efficiently discover drug targets or design new drugs targeting both proteins in pathogens and disease-related human proteins.

3.4.1. Structure Classification

The Protein Data Bank, a computer-based archival file for macromolecular structures, was founded under the term "Brookhaven National Laboratory Protein Data Bank" (BNL PDB) in 1977 (*118*). Today, the PDB repository for the processing and distribution of 3D biological macromolecular structure data contains over 22,053 entries in a standardized file format that can be browsed and searched online (*119*). There are several projects taking data from PDB for further analysis. The SCOP (*120*) database aims to provide a detailed and comprehensive description of the structural and evolutionary relationships among all proteins whose structure is known, including all entries in PDB. It is available as a set of tightly linked hypertext documents, which make the large database comprehensible and accessible. SCOP uses three different major levels of hierarchy: family (clear evolutionarily relationship), superfamily (probable common evolutionary origin), and fold (major structural similarity). A similar approach is realized in the CATH database (*121,122*), which is also a hierarchical domain classification of protein structures in the PDB but only crystal structures solved to resolution better than 3.0 Å are considered, together with nuclear magnetic resonance (NMR) structures. CATH employs four major levels in this hierarchy: class, architecture, topology (fold family), and homologous superfamily.

3.4.2. Structure Modeling

Three-dimensional structure prediction (modeling) of proteins produces reliable results only using the "homology modeling" approach, which generally consists of four steps:

1. Data banks searching to identify the structural homolog.
2. Target-template alignment.
3. Model building and optimization.
4. Model evaluation.

SWISS-MODEL is a server for automated comparative homology modeling of 3D protein structures. It pioneered the field of automated modeling starting in 1993 (123) and is the most widely used free web-based automated modeling facility today. In 2002, the server computed 120,000 user requests for 3D protein models. SWISS-MODEL provides several levels of user interaction through its Internet interface (124). In the "first approach mode," only an amino acid sequence of a protein is submitted to build a 3D model. Template selection, alignment, and model building are performed completely automated by the server. In the "alignment mode," the modeling process is based on a user-defined target–template alignment. Complex modeling tasks can be handled with the "project mode" using Deep View (125), the Swiss-PdbViewer (available for PC, Macintosh, Linux and SGI, downloadable from http://www.expasy.org/spdbv), an integrated sequence-to-structure workbench. All models are sent back via e-mail with a detailed modeling report. WhatCheck analyses and ANOLEA evaluations are provided optionally. Similar homology modelers are CPHmodels (86), Geno3D (126), and ESyPred3D (127).

3.5. Protein Interaction Databases

Protein-protein interactions play important roles in nearly every event that takes place in a cell. The Biomolecular Interaction Network Database (BIND) is a database designed to store full descriptions of interactions, molecular complexes, and pathways (128). An Interaction record is based on the interaction between two objects. An object can be a protein, DNA, RNA, ligand, or molecular complex. The description of an interaction encompasses cellular location, experimental conditions used to observe the interaction, conserved sequence, molecular location of interaction, chemical action, kinetics, thermodynamics, and chemical state and can be accessed through a BLAST search against the database to gather information on the interactions of the query sequence stored in BIND (128). The DIP database (129) catalogs experimentally determined interactions between proteins. It combines information from a variety of sources to create a single, consistent set of protein–protein interactions.

3.5.1. Protein–Protein Interaction Prediction and Docking

The protein–protein or protein–ligand docking problem started to fascinate biophysical chemists and computational biologists almost 30 yr ago (130,131). Given the 3D structures of two interacting proteins, a docking algorithm aims to determine the 3D structures of the complex by rotating and translating the proteins, generating a large number of candidate complexes in the computer, and to select favorable ones. Docking procedures are tested first on protein–protein complexes taken from the Protein Data Bank, mostly protease-inhibitor and antigen-antibody complexes. The CAPRI experiment *(132)*, inspired by the CASP (Critical Assessment of Structure Prediction) algorithm was given atomic coordinates for protein components of several target complexes. The predicted interactions were assessed by comparison to x-ray structures and show significant success on some of the targets. However, the prediction failed with others, and progress is still needed before large-scale predictions of protein–protein interactions can be made reliably. The docking of small molecules and proteins is reviewed in **ref.** *133*

4. Bioinformatics Genomics and Medical Applications

4.1. Genome Analysis and Databases

Most software tools and databases presented above can be used with any kind of DNA or protein sequence. The availability of complete genome sequences of hundreds of more or less related organisms (mainly prokaryotes) allows additional approaches leading the assignment of function to thus far unknown genes and proteins that are not possible with just a subset of a genome. There are also a number of medically related databases such as OMIM (Online mendelian inheritance in man), which contains information regarding inherited and other diseases. Furthermore, attempts to correlate data regarding particular diseases are also being developed, such as the Cancer Genome Anatomy Project, which is a database of known mutations in genes arising in particular tissues.

4.2. Comparative Genomics

Methods requiring complete genome sequences include 1) mapping and alignments of entire genomes of closely related organisms to identify clusters and functional units. 2) metabolic pathway reconstruction to identify missing links and assign function (which is of special biotechnological interest), and 3) comparison of entire genomes of closely related organisms with a different phenotype. The latter technique is suitable for detecting genes that might contribute to virulence toward humans or plants. It is, therefore, of special interest for medical science, the pharmaceutic industry, and agriculture. By means of subtracting the entire genome of a harmless bacterium (e.g., a *Bacillus* strain) from the genome of a closely related virulent bacterium (e.g., *Bacillus anthracis*), genes that are not related to virulence are eliminated. This procedure yields candidates that are probably responsible for the pathogenic phenotype of *B. anthracis* *(134,135)* or might be suitable for use as vaccines *(136)*. As a consequence, these genes represent promising targets for specific drugs against the virulence system of *B. anthracis* without affecting apathogenic strains. The described comparison can be performed using predicted genes only; more accurate results are obtained comparing expression profiles or applying proteomics.

Comparisons of entire genomes reveal clusters that are conserved. Clusters of orthologous groups of proteins (COGs) were delineated by comparing protein sequences encoded in 43 complete genomes, representing 30 major phylogenetic lineages. Each COG consists of individual proteins or groups of paralogs from at least three lineages and, thus, corresponds to an ancient conserved domain. The COG database *(137,138)* provides a phyletic pattern search web page that is available to facilitate the creation of a specific filter that, as being applied to the COGs, can filter out a COG set that will comply with the condition specified in the query.

4.3. Pharmacogenomics

Pharmacogenomics is the study of how an individual's genetic inheritance affects the body's response to drugs. The term comes from the words pharmacology and genomics and is, thus, the intersection of pharmaceuticals and genetics. Pharmacogenomics holds the promise that drugs might one day be tailor-made for individuals and adapted to each person's own genetic makeup. Environment, diet, age, lifestyle, and state of health can influence a person's response to medicines, but understanding an individual's genetic makeup is thought to be the key to creating personalized drugs with greater efficiency and safety. Pharmacogenomics combines traditional pharmaceutical sciences such as biochemistry with annotated knowledge of genes, proteins, and single-nucleotide polymorphisms.

The anticipated benefits of pharmacogenomics are as follows:

1. More powerful medicines (by a therapy more targeted to specific diseases).
2. Better, safer drugs (doctors will be able to analyze a patient's genetic profile and prescribe the best available drug therapy from the beginning).
3. More accurate methods of determining appropriate drug dosages (dosages on weight and age will be replaced with dosages based on a person's genetics).
4. Advanced screening for disease (knowledge of a particular disease susceptibility will allow careful monitoring, and treatments can be introduced at the most appropriate stage to maximize their therapy).
5. Better vaccines (vaccines made of genetic material, either DNA or RNA, promise all the benefits of existing vaccines without all the risks).
6. Improvements in the drug discovery and approval process (pharmaceutical companies will be able to discover potential therapies more easily using genome targets),
7. Decrease in the overall cost of health care.

The explosion in both single-nucleotide polymorphism (SNP) and microarray data generated from the human genome project has necessitated the development of a means of cataloging and annotating (briefly describing) these data so that scientists can more easily access and use it for their research. Database repositories for both SNP (dbSNP) and microarray (GEO) data are available at the NCBI. These databases include either descriptive information about the data within the site itself (GEO) or links to NCBI and external information resources (dbSNP). Access to these data and information resources allows scientists to more easily interpret data that will be used not only to help determine drug response but to study disease susceptibility and conduct basic research in population genetics.

4.3.1. SNP Databases

A key aspect of human genome research and pharmacogenomics is associating sequence variations with heritable phenotypes. The most common variations are SNPs, which occur approximately once every 100–300 bases. Because SNPs are expected to facilitate large-scale association genetics studies, there has recently been great interest in SNP discovery and detection. The cSNP database specializing on human chromosome 21 is a joint project between the Division of Medical Genetics of the University of Geneva Medical School and the Swiss Institute of Bioinformatics, which offers BLAST and text searches to explore their data. In collaboration with the National Human Genome Research Institute, the National Center for Biotechnology Information has established the dbSNP database (*139*) to serve as a central repository for both single-base nucleotide subsitutions and short deletion and insertion polymorphisms. Once discovered, these polymorphisms could be used by additional laboratories, using the sequence information around the polymorphism and the specific experimental conditions. The data in dbSNP are integrated with other NCBI genomic data and are accessible by the same tools as other NCBI databases.

4.3.2. Expression Profiling

The Gene Expression Omnibus (GEO) is a gene expression and hybridization array data repository, as well as a curated, online resource for gene expression data browsing, query, and retrieval. GEO was the first fully public high-throughput gene expression data repository and became operational in July 2000 (*140*). There are several ways to deposit and retrieve GEO data. The search facilities "Gene profiles," "Dataset," and "Sequence BLAST" are powerful and link to the well-known Entrez-Interface, including accession links to relevant genes and proteins.

References

1. Venter JC, et al (2001) The sequence of the human genome. Science 291:1304–1351
2. Lander ES, et al (2001) Initial sequencing and analysis of the human genome. Nature 409:860–921
3. Rehm BH(2001) Bioinformatic tools for DNA/protein sequence analysis, functional assignment of genes and protein classification. Appl Microbiol Biotechnol 57:579–592
4. Ewing B, Hillier L, Wendl MC, Green P (1998) Base-calling of automated sequencer traces using phred. I. Accuracy assessment. Genome Res 8:175–185
5. Ewing B, Green P (1998) Base-calling of automated sequencer traces using phred. II. Error probabilities. Genome Res 8:186–194
6. Huang X, Madan A (1999) CAP3: A DNA sequence assembly program. Genome Res 9:868–877
7. Gordon D, Abajian C, Green P (1998) Consed: a graphical tool for sequence finishing. Genome Res 8:195–202
8. Staden R (1996) The Staden Sequence Analysis Package. Mol Biotech 5:233–241
9. Staden R (1984) Computer methods to locate signals in nucleic acid sequences. Nucleic Acids Res 12:505–519
10. Claverie JM (1997) Computational methods for the identification of genes in vertebrate genomic sequences. Hum Mol Genet 6:1735–1744
11. Guigo R (1997) Computational gene identification: an open problem. Comput Chem 21:215–222
12. Krogh A (1998) In: Salzberg SL, Searls D, Kasif S (eds) Computational methods in molecular biology. Elsevier, Amsterdam
13. Krogh A (1998) In: Bishop MJ (ed) Guide to human genome computing, 2nd edn. Academic, New York, pp. 261–274
14. Delcher AL, Harmon D, Kasif S, White O, Salzberg SL (1999) Improved microbial gene identification with GLIMMER. Nucleic Acids Res 27:4636–4641

15. Guigo R, Agarwal P, Abril JF, Burset M, Fickett JW (2000) An assessment of gene prediction accuracy in large DNA sequences. Genome Res 10:1631–1642

16. Krogh A (2000) Using database matches with for HMMGene for automated gene detection in Drosophila. Genome Res 10:523–528

17. Shibuya T, Rigoutsos I (2002) Dictionary-driven prokaryotic gene finding. Nucleic Acids Res 30:2710–2725

18. Pedersen JS, Hein J (2003) Gene finding with a hidden Markov model of genome structure and evolution. Bioinformatics 19:219–227

19. Guo FB, Ou HY, Zhang CT (2003) ZCURVE: a new system for recognizing protein-coding genes in bacterial and archaeal genomes. Nucleic Acids Res 31: 1780–1789

20. Larsen TS, Krogh A (2003) EasyGene – a prokaryotic gene finder that ranks ORFs by statistical significance. BMC Bioinformat 4:21

21. Gelfand MS (1995) Prediction of function in DNA sequence analysis. J Comput Biol 2:87–115

22. Sherriff A, Ott J (2001) Applications of neural networks for gene finding. Adv Genet 42:287–297

23. Fickett JW (1996) Finding genes by computer: the state of the art. Trends Genet 12:316–320

24. Zhang CT, Wang J, Zhang R (2002) Using a Euclid distance discriminant method to find protein coding genes in the yeast genome. Comput Chem 26:195–206

25. Bajic VB, Seah SH (2003) Dragon gene start finder: an advanced system for finding approximate locations of the start of gene transcriptional units. Genome Res 13:1923–1929

26. Zhang MQ (1998) Statistical features of human exons and their flanking regions. Hum Mol Genet 7:919–932

27. Searls DB (1992) The linguistics of DNA. Am Sci 80:579–591

28. Durbin R, Eddy S, Krogh A, Mitchison G (1998) Biological sequence analysis: probabilistic models of proteins and nucleic acids. Cambridge University Press, Cambridge

29. Krogh A, Mian IS, Haussler D (1994) A hidden Markov model that finds genes in E. coli DNA. Nucleic Acids Res 22:4768–4778

30. Cole ST, Brosch R, Parkhill J, et al (1998) Deciphering the biology of Mycobacterium tuberculosis from the complete genome sequence. Nature 393: 537–544

31. Thomas A, Skolnick M (1994) A probabilistic model for detecting coding regions in DNA sequences. IMA J Math Appl Med Biol 11:149–160

32. Henderson J, Salzberg S, Fasman K (1997) Finding genes in DNA with a hidden Markov model. J Comput Biol 4:127–141

33. Lukashin AV, Borodovsky M (1998) GeneMark hmm: new solutions for gene finding. Nucleic Acids Res 26:1107–1115

34. Salzberg SL, Pertea M, Delcher AL, Gardner MJ, Tettelin H (1999) Interpolated Markov models for eukaryotic gene finding. Genomics 59:24–31

35. Badger JH, Olsen GJ (1999) CRITICA: coding region identification tool invoking comparative analysis. Mol Biol Eyol 16:512–524

36. Bocs S, Cruveiller S, Vallenet D, Nuel G, Medigue C (2003) AMIGene: annotation of microbial genes. Nucleic Acids Res 31:3723–6

37. Besemer J, Lomsadze A, Borodovsky M (2001) GeneMarkS: a self-training method for prediction of gene starts in microbial genomes. Implications for finding sequence motifs in regulatory regions. Nucleic Acids Res 29:2607–2618

38. Yeramian E, Jones L (2003) GeneFizz: a web tool to compare genetic (coding/non-coding) and physical (helix/coil) segmentations of DNA sequences. Gene discovery and evolutionary perspectives. Nucleic Acids Res 31:3843–3849

39. Kotlar D, Lavner Y (2003) Gene prediction by spectral rotation measure: a new method for identifying protein-coding regions. Genome Res 13:1930–1937

40. Snyder E, Stormo G (1995) Identification of protein coding regions in genomic DNA. J Mol Biol 248:1–18

41. Reese MG, Eeckman FH, Kulp D, Haussler D (1997) Improved splice site detection in Genie. J Comput Biol 4:311–323

42. Burge C, Karlin S (1997) Prediction of complete gene structures in human genomic DNA. J Mol Biol 268:78–94

43. Xu Y, Uberbacher EC (1997) Automated gene identification in large-scale genomic sequences. J Comput Biol 4:325–338

44. Gelfand MS, Mironov AA, Pevzner PA (1996) Gene recognition via spliced sequence alignment. Proc Natl Acad Sci USA 93:9061–9066

45. Foissac S, Bardou P, Moisan A, Cros MJ, Schiex T (2003) EUGENE'HOM: a generic similarity-based gene finder using multiple homologous sequences. Nucleic Acids Res 31:3742–3745

46. Smith TE, Waterman MS (1981) Identification of common molecular subsequences. J Mol Biol 147:195–197

47. Yada T, Takagi T, Totoki Y, Sakaki Y, Takaeda Y (2003) DIGIT: a novel gene finding program by combining gene-finders. Pac Symp Biocomput 8:375–387

48. Quandt K, Frech K, Karas H, Wingender E, Werner T (1995) MatInd and MatInspector – new fast and versatile tools for detection of consensus matches in nucleotide sequence data. Nucleic Acids Res 23:4878–4884

49. Prestridge DS (1991) SIGNAL SCAN: a computer program that scans DNA sequences for eukaryotic transcriptional elements. CABIOS 7:203–206

50. Wingender E, Chen X, Hehl R, et al (2000) TRANSFAC: an integrated system for gene expression regulation. Nucleic Acids Res 28:316–319

51. Prestridge DS (1995) Predicting Pol II Promoter Sequences Using Transcription Factor Binding Sites. J Mol Biol 249:923–932

52. Eddy SR (1996) Hidden Markov models. Curr Opin Struct Biol 6:361–365

53. Eddy SR (1998) Profile hidden Markov models. Bioinformatics 14:755–763

54. Baldi R, Brunak S (1998) Bioinformatics: the machine learning approach. MIT Press, Boston, MA

55. Korenberg MJ, David R, Hunter IW, Solomon JE (2000) Automatic classification of protein sequences into structure/function groups via parallel cascade identification: a feasibility study. Ann Biomed Eng 28:803–811

56. Thompson JD, Higgins, DG, Gibson TJ (1994) CLUSTAL W: improving the sensitivity of progressive multiple sequence alignment through sequence weighting, position-specific gap penalties and weight matrix choice. Nucleic Acids Res 22:4673–4680

57. Thompson JD, Gibson TJ, Plewniak F, Jeanmougin F, Higgins DG (1997) The CLUSTAL X windows interface: flexible strategies for multiple sequence alignment aided by quality analysis tools. Nucleic Acids Res 25:4876–4882

58. Nicholas KB, Nicholas HB, Jr, Deerfield DW, II (1997) GeneDoc: analysis and visualization of genetic variation. EMBNEW NEWS 4:14

59. Lake JA (1994) Reconstructing evolutionary trees from DNA and protein sequences: paralinear distances. Proc Natl Acad Sci USA 91: 1451–1459

60. Lockhart PJ, Steel MA, Hendy MD, Penny D (1994) Recovering evolutionary trees under a more realistic model of sequence. Mol Biol Evol 11:605–612

61. Brocchieri L (2001) Phylogenetic inferences from molecular sequences: review and critique. Theor Popul Biol 59:27–40

62. Stewart CB (1993) The powers and pitfalls of parsimony. Nature 361:603–607

63. Attwood TK, Beck ME, Flower DR, Scordis P, Selley JN (1998) The PRINTS protein fingerprint database in its fifth year. Nucleic Acids Res 26:304–308

64. Page RD (1996) Tree View: an application to display phylogenetic trees on personal computers. Comput Appl Biosci 12:357–358

65. Gasteiger E, Gattiker A, Hoogland C, Ivanyi I, Appel RD, Bairoch A (2003) ExPASy: the proteomics server for in-depth protein knowledge and analysis. Nucleic Acids Res 31:3784–3788

66. Rost B (1996) PHD: predicting one-dimensional protein structure by profile based neural networks. Methods Enzymol 266:525–539

67. Eyrich VA, Rost B (2003) META-PP: single interface to crucial prediction servers. Nucleic Acids Res 31:3308–3310

68. Nielsen H, Engelbrecht J, Brunak S, von Heijne G (1997) Identification of prokaryotic and eukaryotic signal peptides and prediction of their cleavage sites. Protein Eng 10:1–6

69. Hansen JE, Lund O, Tolstrup N, Gooley AA, Williams KL, Brunak S (1998) NetOglyc: Prediction of mucin type O-glycosylation sites based on sequence context and surface accessibility. Glycoconjugate J 15:115–130

70. Hansen JE, Lund O, Rapacki K, Brunak S (1997) O-glycbase version 2.0 – a revised database of O-glycosylated proteins. Nucleic Acids Res 25:278–282

71. Hansen JE, Lund O, Rapacki K, et al (1995) Prediction of O-glycosylation of mammalian proteins: specificity patterns of UDP-GalNAc:-polypeptide N-acetyl-galactosaminyltransferase. Biochem J 308:801–813

72. Blom N, Gammeltoft S, Brunak S (1999) Sequence- and structure-based prediction of eukaryotic protein phosphorylation sites. J Mol Biol 294:1351–1362

73. Blom N, Hansen J, Blaas D, Brunak S (1996) Cleavage site analysis in picornaviral polyproteins: discovering cellular targets by neural networks. Protein Sci 5:2203–2216

74. Emanuelsson O, Nielsen H, von Heijne G (1999) ChloroP, a neural network-based method for predicting chloroplast transit peptides and their cleavage sites. Protein Sci 8:978–984

75. Cuff JA, Barton GJ (1999) Evaluation and improvement of multiple sequence methods for protein secondary structure prediction. Proteins 34:508–519

76. Sonnhammer ELL, von Heijne G, Krogh A (1998) A hidden Markov model for predicting transmembrane helices in protein sequences, In proceedings of the sixth intern conference on intelligent systems for molecular biology, (ISMB98), pp175–182

77. von Heijne G (1992) Membrane protein structure prediction, hydrophobicity analysis and the positive-inside rule. J Mol Biol 225:487–494

78. Karplus K, Barrett C, Hughey R (1998) Hidden markov models for detecting remote protein homologies. Bioinformatics 14:846–856

79. Cserzo M, Wallin E, Simon I, von Heijne G, Elofsson A (1997) Prediction of transmembrane alpha-helices in procariotic membrane proteins: the dense alignment surface method. Protein Eng 10:673–676

80. Fischer D, Eisenberg DA (1996) Fold recognition using sequence-derived properties. Protein Sci 5:947–955

81. Elofsson A, Fischer D, Rice DW, LeGrand S, Eisenberg DA (1996) Study of combined structure-sequence profiles. Folding Design 1:451–461

82. Karplus K, Karchin R, Draper J, et al (2003) Combining local-structure, fold-recognition, and new-fold methods for protein structure prediction. Proteins 53(Suppl 6):491–496

83. Peitsch MC (1995) Protein modelling by E-mail. BioTechnology 13:658–660

84. Peitsch MC (1996) ProMod and Swiss-Model: internet-based tools for automated comparative protein modelling. Biochem Soc Trans 24:274–279

85. Guex N, Peitsch MC (1997) SWISS-MODEL and the Swiss-PdbViewer: an environment for comparative protein modelling. Electrophoresis 18:2714–2723

86. Lund O, Frimand K, Gorodkin J, et al (1997) Protein distance constraints predicted by neural networks and probability density functions. Protein Eng 10:1241–1248

87. Altschul SF, Gish W, Miller W, Myers EW, Lipman DJ (1990) Basic local alignment search tool. J Mol Biol 215:403–410

88. Altschul SF (1991) Amino acid substitution matrices from an information theoretic perspective. J Mol Biol 219:555–565

89. Altschul SF, Gish W (1996) Local alignment statistics. Methods Enzymol. 266:460–480

90. Rost B, Schneider R, Sander C (1997) Protein fold recognition by prediction-based threading. J Mol Biol 270:471–480

91. Dayhoff MO, Barker WC, Hunt LT (1983) Establishing homologies in protein sequences. Methods Enzymol 91:524–545

92. Henikoff S, Henikoff JG (1992) Amino acid substitution matrices from protein blocks. Proc Natl Acad Sci USA 89:10,915–10,919

93. Pearson WR (1995) Comparison of methods for searching protein sequence databases. Protein Sci 4:1145–1160

94. Karlin S, Altschul SE (1990) Methods for assessing the statistical significance of molecular sequence features by using general scoring schemes. Proc Natl Acad Sci USA 87:2264–2268

95. Wootton JC (1994) Non-globular domains in protein sequences: automated segmentation using complexity measures. Comput Chem 18:269–285

96. Altschul SF, Madden TL, Schäffer AA, et al (1997) Gapped BLAST and PSI-BLAST: a new generation of protein database search programs. Nucleic Acids Res 25:3389–3402

97. Pearson WR, Lipman DJ (1988) Improved tools for biological sequence comparison. Proc Natl Acad Sci USA 85:2444–2448

98. Martin AC, Orengo CA, Hutchinson EG, et al (1998) Protein folds and functions. Structure 6:875–884

99. McGuffin LJ, Bryson K, Jones DT (2001) What are the baselines for protein fold recognition? Bioinformatics 17:63–72

100. Bairoch A (1991) PROSITE: a dictionary of sites and patterns in proteins. Nucleic Acids Res 19:2241–2245

101. Bairoch A, Bucher P, Hofmann K (1997) The PROSITE database, its status in 1997. Nucleic Acids Res 25:217–221

102. Bucher P, Karplus K, Moeri, N, Hofmann K (1996) A flexible motif search technique based on generalized profiles. Comput Chem 20:3–23

103. Sonnhammer EL, Kahn D (1994) Modular arrangement of proteins as inferred from analysis of homology. Protein Sci 3:482–492

104. Corpet F, Gouzy J, Kahn D (1998) The ProDom database of protein domain families. Nucleic Acids Res 26:323–326

105. Sonnhammer EL, Eddy SR, Durbin R (1997) Pfam: a comprehensive database of protein domain families based on seed alignments. Proteins 28:405–420

106. Bateman A, Birney E, Cerruti L, et al (2002) The Pfam protein families database. Nucleic Acids Res 30:276–280

107. Apweiler R, Attwood TK, Bairoch A, et al (2001) The InterPro database, an integrated documentation resource for protein families, domains and functional sites. Nucleic Acids Res 29:37–40

108. Mulder NJ, Apweiler R, Attwood TK, et al (2003) The InterPro Database, 2003 brings increased coverage and new features. Nucleic Acids Res 31:315–8

109. Rawlings ND, O'Brien E, Barrett AJ (2002) MEROPS: the protease database. Nucleic Acids Res 30:343–346

110. Storm CE, Sonnhammer EL (2001) NIFAS: visual analysis of domain evolution in proteins. Bioinformatics 17:343–348

111. Schultz J, Milpetz F, Bork P, Ponting, CP (1998) SMART, a simple modular architecture research tool: identification of signaling domains. Proc Natl Acad Sci USA 95:5857–5864

112. Schultz J, Copley RR, Doerks T, Ponting CP, Bork P (2000) SMART: a web-based tool for the study of genetically mobile domains. Nucleic Acids Res 28:231–234

113. Letunic I, Goodstadt L, Dickens NJ, et al (2002) Recent improvements to the SMART domain-based sequence annotation resource. Nucleic Acids Res 30:242–244

114. Pietrokovski S, Henikoff JG, Henikoff S (1996) The Blocks database—a system for protein classification. Nucleic Acids Res 24:197–200

115. Attwood TK, Flower DR, Lewis AP, et al (1999) PRINTS prepares for the new millennium. Nucleic Acids Res 27:220–225

116. Silverstein KA, Shoop E, Johnson JE, Retzel EF (2001) MetaFam: a unified classification of protein families. I. Overview and statistics. Bioinformatics 17:249–261

117. Yuan YP, Eulenstein O, Vingron M, Bork P (1998) Towards detection of orthologues in sequence databases. Bioinformatics 14:285–289

118. Bernstein FC, Koetzle TF, Williams GJ, et al (1977) The Protein Data Bank. A computer-based archival file for macromolecular structures. Eur J Biochem 80:319–324

119. Berman HM, Westbrook J, Feng Z, et al (2000) The Protein Data Bank. Nucleic Acids Res 28:235–242

120. Murzin AG, Brenner SE, Hubbard T, Chothia C (1995) SCOP: a structural classification of proteins database for the investigation of sequences and structures. J Mol Biol 247:536–540

121. Orengo CA, Michie AD, Jones S, Jones DT, Swindells MB, Thornton JM (1997) CATH—a Hierarchic classification of protein domain structures. Structure 5:1093–1108

122. Pearl FMG, Lee D, Bray JE, Sillitoe I, Todd AE, Harrison AP, Thornton JM, Orengo CA (2000) Assigning genomic sequences to CATH. Nucleic Acids Res 28:277–282

123. Peitsch MC, Jongeneel V (1993) A 3- dimensional model for the CD40 ligand predicts that it is a compact trimer similar to the tumor necrosis factors. Int Immunol 5:233–238

124. Schwede T, Kopp J, Guex N, Peitsch MC (2003) SWISS-MODEL: an automated protein homology-modeling server. Nucleic Acids Res 31:3381–3385

125. Guex N, Peitsch MC (1997) SWISS-MODEL and the Swiss-Pdb Viewer: an environment for comparative protein modeling. Electrophoresis 18:2714–2723

126. Combet C, Jambon M, Deleage G, Geourjon C (2002) Geno3D: automatic comparative molecular modelling of protein. Bioinformatics 18:213–214

127. Lambert C, Leonard N, De Bolle X, Depiereux E (2002) ESyPred3D: prediction of proteins 3D structures. Bioinformatics 18:1250–1256

128. Bader GD, Betel D, Hogue CW (2003) BIND: the Biomolecular Interaction Network Database. Nucleic Acids Res 31:248–250

129. Xenarios I, Rice DW, Salwinski L, Baron MK, Marcotte EM, Eisenberg D (2000) DIP: The Database of Interacting Proteins. Nucleic Acids Res 28:289–291

130. Levinthal C, Wodak SJ, Kahn P, Dadivanian AK (1975) Hemoglobin interaction in sickle cell fibers. I. Theoretical approaches to the molecular contacts. Proc Natl Acad Sci USA 72:1330–1334

131. Wodak SJ, Janin J (1978) Computer analysis of protein-protein interaction. J Mol Biol 124:323–342

132. Janin J, Henrick K, Moult J, et al (2003) CAPRI: a Critical Assessment of PRedicted Interactions. Proteins 52:2–9

133. Taylor RD, Jewsbury PJ, Essex JW (2002) A review of protein-small molecule docking methods. J Comput Aided Mol Des 16:151–166

134. Read TD, Peterson SN, Tourasse N, et al (2003) The genome sequence of Bacillus anthracis Ames and comparison to closely related bacteria. Nature 423:81–86

135. Ivanova N, Sorokin A, Anderson I, et al (2003) Genome sequence of Bacillus cereus and comparative analysis with Bacillus anthracis. Nature 423:87–91

136. Smith DR (1996) Microbial pathogen genomes - new strategies for identifying therapeutics and vaccine targets. Trends Biotechnol 14:290–293

137. Tatusov RL, Koonin EV, Lipman DJ (1997) A genomic perspective on protein families. Science 278:631–637

138. Tatusov, RL, Natale DA, Garkavtsev IV, et al (2001) The COG database: new developments in phylogenetic classification of proteins from complete genomes. Nucleic Acids Res 29:22–28

139. Wheeler DL, Church DM, Federhen S, et al (2003) Database resources of the National Center for Biotechnology. Nucleic Acids Res 31:28–33

140. Edgar R, Domrachev M, Lash AE (2002) Gene Expression Omnibus: NCBI gene expression and hybridization array data repository. Nucleic Acids Res 30:207–210

141. Rehm BHA, Reinecke F (2004) Evaluation of proteomic techniques: applications and potential. Curr Proteomics 1:103–111

Part B

Protein and Cell Methods

23

Protein Electrophoresis

David Sheehan and Siobhan O'Sullivan

1. Introduction

Amino acid side-chains of proteins (as well as some groups added by posttranslational modification, e.g., phosphates) confer charge characteristics. Only at the pH value represented by their isoelectric point (pI) do proteins lack charge. In fact, this charge is responsible for protein solubility in aqueous solution. When placed in an electric field of field strength E, proteins will freely move towards the electrode of opposite charge. However, they move at quite different and individual rates depending on their physical characteristics and the experimental system used (**Fig. 23.1**). The velocity of movement, v, of a charged molecule under these conditions depends on variables described by Eq. 1;

$$v = \frac{E \cdot q}{f} \tag{1}$$

The frictional coefficient, f, describes frictional resistance to mobility and depends on factors such as protein mass (M_r), degree of compactness, matrix porosity and buffer viscosity. The net charge, q, is determined by the number of positive and negative charges in the protein arising from charged side-chains and post-translational modifications such as deamidation, acylation, or phosphorylation. Equation 1 implies that molecules will move faster as their net charge increases, the electric field strengthens or as f decreases (a function of molecular mass/shape). Molecules of similar net charge separate due to differences in frictional coefficient whereas molecules of similar mass/shape may differ widely from each other in net charge. Consequently, electrophoresis is a high resolution technique.

The electric field is established by applying a voltage, V, to a pair of electrodes separated by a distance, d (**Fig. 23.1**), resulting in an electrical field of strength E;

$$E = \frac{V}{d} \tag{2}$$

Current is carried between the electrodes by the buffer that also maintains constant pH. The most commonly-used buffer systems in protein electrophoresis

From: *Molecular Biomethods Handbook, 2nd Edition.*
Edited by: J. M. Walker and R. Rapley © Humana Press, Totowa, NJ

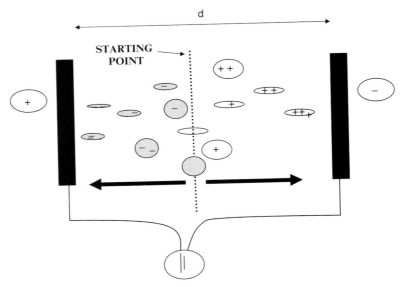

Fig. 23.1. Physical basis of electrophoresis. Molecules move in an electric field (strength E) as determined by their net charge, M_r, and shape. Smaller and more heavily charged species move with a greater velocity whereas proteins of identical charge separate because of their differing shape

are Tris-Cl or Tris-glycine. Buffers are held in reservoirs connected to each electrode and provide a constant supply of ions to the electrophoresis system throughout the separation.

Ohm's law relates V to current, I, by electrical resistance, R;

$$V = R \times I \tag{3}$$

We might predict that increasing V would result in much faster migration of molecules due to greater current. However, large voltages result in significant power generation mainly dissipated in the form of heat. The power (in Watts) generated during electrophoresis is given by Eq. 4.

$$W = I^2 \times R \tag{4}$$

Heat generation is undesirable because it leads to loss of resolution (convection of buffer causes mixing of separated proteins), a decrease of buffer viscosity (decreases R) and, in extreme cases, structural breakdown of thermally-labile proteins. A decrease in R means that, under conditions of constant voltage, I will increase during electrophoresis in turn leading to further heat generation (Eq. 3). In practice, constant voltage conditions are used in most electrophoresis experiments but, for certain applications, a constant power supply may be used that maintains W during the experiment allowing V to change (Eq. 4). In general, conditions are selected that are adequate to separate samples in a reasonable time-frame but that avoid extensive heating.

Because E may vary widely among different experimental formats, the electrophoretic mobility, μ, of a sample is defined as;

$$\mu = \frac{v}{E} \tag{5}$$

Combining this with Eq. 1 shows that;

$$\mu = \frac{E \times q}{E \times f} = \frac{q}{f} \tag{6}$$

That is, proteins migrate based on the ratio of net charge to frictional coefficient. Because f is strongly mass-dependent for classes of biopolymers of similar shape (e.g., globular proteins), differences in μ approximate closely to differences in charge/mass ratio.

This is an incomplete description of protein electrophoresis because it excludes possible interaction of proteins with the support medium (e.g., gels), charge suppression on the protein surface or effects of the buffer composition. Thus, protein electrophoresis is largely an empirical technique. High resolution mobility data can be obtained by comparison with standard molecules of similar charge-density and shape. However, it is not usually possible to make direct measurements (as compared to comparative measurements) of M_r or shape from electrophoretic mobilities alone due to lack of detailed information on variables involved in the process. Although most proteins behave predictably in electrophoresis, there are examples of proteins of different charge/mass comigrating or of similar charge/mass separating due to differences in their electrophoretic mobility.

2. Methods

Electrophoresis was originally performed in solution, but most modern protein electrophoresis is performed in gel networks (1). Hydrated gels allow a wide variety of mechanically-stable experimental formats such as vertical electrophoresis in slab gels or electrophoresis in tubes or capillaries. Their mechanical stability also facilitates postelectrophoretic manipulation making further experimentation possible. Gels used in protein electrophoresis are chemically unreactive and interact minimally with proteins during electrophoresis allowing separation based on physical rather than chemical differences among sample components. Highly-controlled procedures allow formation of gels of a narrow range of porosity that will allow only molecules of a defined maximum mass to pass through whereas excluding proteins with larger M_r. Increasing/decreasing the size of these pores alters the mass that can be selected by the gel. The most common gel used in protein electrophoresis is formed by polymerisation of acrylamide (**Fig. 23.2**). Inclusion of a small amount of acrylamide crosslinked by a methylene bridge (N,N'-methylene bisacrylamide) forms a crosslinked gel with a highly-controlled porosity that is mechanically strong and chemically inert. For separation of proteins, the ratio of acrylamide: N,N'-methylene bisacrylamide is usually 40:1. Such gels are suitable for high resolution separation of proteins across a large mass range (**Table 23.1**). A wider range of M_r in an individual gel is achieved with gradient gels, in which a gradient of polyacrylamide (e.g. 5–20%) is formed.

In practice, protein samples are loaded into "wells" formed in polyacrylamide that are approximately 1 cm deep. If electrophoresis was performed at a continuous pH, protein bands at the end of the experiment would be at least 1 cm thick i.e., resolution would be extremely low. High resolution

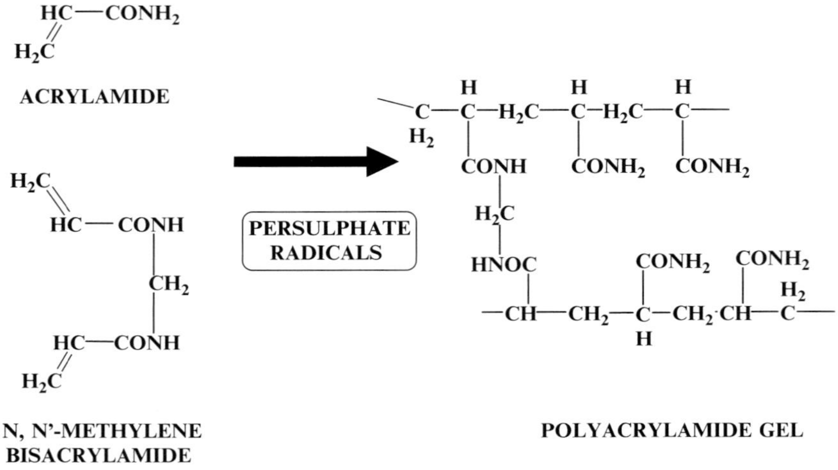

Fig. 23.2. Acryalide polymerises in the presence of persulphate radicals to form polyacrylamide. *N,N'*-methylene bisacrylamide introduces crosslinks between the polyacrylamide strands

Table 23.1. Range of separation of proteins in polyacrylamide gels of differing polyacrylamide concentration.

Acrylamide conc. (%)	Separation range (kDa)
5	>1,000
8	300–1,000
12	50–300
15	10–80
20	5–30

in polyacrylamide gel electrophoresis (PAGE) arises from the fact that the experiment is performed in a "discontinuous" system consisting of two gels (stacking and resolving) held at pH 6.9 and 8–9, respectively (**Fig. 23.3**). The stacking gel concentrates samples into thin bands or "stacks" that then accumulate at the interface between the two gels before separation. This gel has a low polyacrylamide concentration (3–5%), low ionic strength and a pH near neutrality. The resolving gel, by contrast, has a higher polyacrylamide concentration (8–20%), higher ionic strength and an alkaline pH. This gel achieves separation of sample molecules stacked at the interface. The lower ionic strength of the stacking gel causes higher electrical resistance and hence higher E in this gel compared to the resolving gel. At a given V, samples have higher mobility in the stacking compared to the resolving gel (Eq. 1).

Sample is applied to the stacking gel in sample buffer containing Tris-glycine at pH 8–9. At this pH, glycine exists in the form of a mixture of anion and zwitterion because the pK for deprotonation of $-NH_3^+$ is approx 9.6;

$$NH_3^+ - CH_2\text{-}COO^- \leftrightarrow NH_2\text{--}CH_2\text{--} COO^- + H^+ \qquad (7)$$

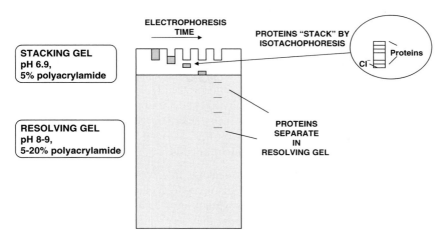

Fig. 23.3. Discontinuous polyacrylamide gel electrophoresis. Sample is loaded in a small "well" in the polyacrylamide stacking gel. It is concentrated into a thin layer by isotachophoresis through the stacker and concentrates at the intergel interface. The proteins then separate from each other in the resolving gel as sharply defined bands

Zwitterion form   Anion form

As the sample enters the stacking gel at pH 6.9, the balance of this equilibrium shifts strongly towards the uncharged zwitterion form that has no electrophoretic mobility. To maintain a constant I, a flow of anions is necessary. At pH 6.9, most proteins are anionic and these, together with chloride, replace glycinate as mobile ions. In practice, proteins become "sandwiched" between chloride (high mobility) and a small amount of glycinate ions (low mobility) as they move quickly through the stacking gel, unimpeded by the large pores. This phenomenon of "sandwiching" among ions of different electrophoretic mobility is called "isotachophoresis." Chlorine is a strongly electronegative atom that moves towards the anode with much greater velocity than any other species present. This band of anions leaves behind it a zone of low conductivity. As this passes through the rest of the sample, molecules in the sample become sorted on the basis of their charge from most to least negatively charged. Simultaneously, they are concentrated based on this charge discrimination. This stacks the sample into a number of thin layers. When this front of ions reaches the interface with the resolving gel (pH 8–9) however, the glycinate ion concentration increases dramatically (Eq. 7) and now carries the bulk of the current. At the same time, protein ions encounter a higher concentration of polyacrylamide with a narrow pore size and a more alkaline pH. The thin stacks of protein therefore separate in this gel depending on their mass/charge and shape characteristics.

Once separated in an electrophoresis experiment, the gel can be stained in a variety of ways *(2)*. Coomassie blue is a standard stain that detects most proteins. Silver staining is more sensitive and detects low-abundance bands. Examples of more specific staining are represented by activity stains (see the following) and stains specific for particular categories of proteins such as glycoproteins. A further set of applications is made possible by transferring proteins from the gels to membranes producing a protein "blot" that can be probed with antibodies, stained or otherwise processed.

2.1. Native Electrophoresis

Polyacrylamide is a suitable environment for the electrophoretic separation of proteins under native conditions in which proteins are regarded as being in their natural, biologically-active form. They separate based on intrinsic charges of groups located on the protein surface (1). Each protein has a characteristic mobility in a nondenaturing system determined by a combination of these charges combined with physical characteristics such as M_r and shape.

2.2. SDS Polyacrylamide Gel Electrophoresis

Proteins are held together by noncovalent, interactions such as hydrogen bonds and salt bridges. These can be disrupted to denature proteins and then to separate them electrophoretically by denaturing electrophoresis. Such experiments are useful with proteins because they have an especially varied range of tertiary structures. Electrophoretic mobility in denaturing conditions is altered in comparison to that in nondenaturing conditions. This results from altered charge and/or shape because the polypeptide now migrates as an unstructured monomer through the gel. Any biological activity or quaternary structure associated with the sample components is lost in denaturing electrophoresis.

A possible denaturation strategy is offered by the chaotropic agent, urea (3), which has the useful property that, whilst itself possessing zero net charge, it is nonetheless a polar molecule with unequal internal charge distribution. High concentrations of urea interrupt protein hydrogen bonds, leading to complete disruption of secondary, tertiary and quaternary structure. Urea renders polypeptides highly water-soluble but, because it is uncharged, it does not migrate in electric fields. Proteins therefore migrate in urea as determined by their net intrinsic charge, despite the fact that they are denatured under these conditions.

The detergent sodium dodecyl sulphate (SDS) contains a 12-carbon hydrophobic chain and a polar sulphated head and is also a powerful denaturant of protein structure. The hydrophobic chain intercalates into hydrophobic parts of the protein by detergent action, disrupting tertiary structure. The sulphated head remains in contact with water, maintaining the solubility of the detergent-protein complex. This disrupts the folded structure of single polypeptides as well as subunit–subunit (i.e., quaternary structure) and protein-membrane interactions. SDS coats proteins more or less uniformly with a "layer" of negative charge. They therefore always migrate towards the anode when placed in an electrical field, regardless of their original intrinsic charge. The negative charge gives a charge-density largely independent of the primary structure or M_r of the polypeptide. For this reason, there is a close relationship between mobility of SDS-protein complexes in polyacrylamide gels and the protein M_r. This is called SDS PAGE, the most widely-used form of protein electrophoresis (4).

SDS PAGE has a number of important limitations. It is assumed that proteins migrate as perfect spheres with a uniform charge-distribution. Proteins deviating from a globular shape (e.g., fibrous proteins) or proteins binding above- or below-average amounts of SDS may behave nonideally and inaccurate M_r estimates might result. It is therefore important to compare unknown proteins to appropriate standards in SDS PAGE (i.e., globular unknowns with globular standards and fibrous unknowns with fibrous standards). M_r values estimated by this technique are often referred to as "apparent M_r" because they depend on comparison with other proteins rather than on direct measurement. Post-translational modifications can also alter protein mobility in SDS PAGE gels (e.g., SDS does not bind to sugar so glycoproteins migrate slower in SDS PAGE).

2.3. Isoelectric Focusing

The net charge on a protein varies with pH. This is a reflection of differences in amino acid sequence and/or post-translational modification. Under standard experimental conditions and in the absence of extensive chemical modification, pI may be regarded as a constant property of a protein. We can determine pI experimentally by isoelectric focusing (IEF). This involves formation of a stable pH gradient *(5)*. It is technically difficult to achieve this with buffer components because they would simply diffuse together in free solution. Ampholytes are synthetic, low M_r heteropolymers of oligoamino and oligocarboxylic acids. Various combinations of amino and carboxylic acid groups allow synthesis of a wide range of polymers each possessing a slightly different pI. When a mixture of ampholytes is placed in an electric field, each migrates to its individual pI value where it acts as a local buffer, thus forming a pH gradient.

An alternative to the use of free ampholytes is provided by immobilized pH gradients *(6)*. This involves the use of acrylamide derivatives (immobilines) that contain weak acid or base groups. The acid groups have pK values of 3.6–4.6 whereas basic groups have pKs of 6.2, 7.0, 8.5, or 9.3. At least one each of the acid and alkaline immobilines are mixed together in the presence of acrylamide monomers to form a polyacrylamide gel. By varying the identity and number of immobilines from the two categories available, a variety of pH gradients may be generated. A particular advantage of these gradients over those formed with free ampholytes is that they can cover a very narrow pH-range allowing finer resolution among similar pI values. Such gradients can now be localised on plastic strips that are commercially available and that result in highly reproducible pH gradients.

2.4. Capillary Electrophoresis

It was pointed out above that high values of V lead to considerable heat generation in electrophoresis and this places an effective upper limit of 300–500 V on most protein electrophoresis separations. However, performance of electrophoresis in very thin capillaries, with small internal volumes and relatively large surface areas, enables use of V up to values of 5–50 kV because heat is efficiently dissipated. This is the basis of capillary electrophoresis (CE), a major analytical application of protein electrophoresis *(7)*. The glass capillary used in CE has an inner-diameter of 10–100 μm, an external diameter of 300 μm and a typical length of 10–100 cm. This gives an included volume for separation that is approximately a thousand times smaller than that of a conventional protein electrophoresis gel. The capillary may be filled with a buffer (free solution CE) with a polyacrylamide gel or a noncrosslinked linear polymer (gel electrophoresis CE or capillary gel electrophoresis). All of the electrophoresis applications so far described in this chapter such as IEF, non-denaturing electrophoresis, and SDS PAGE are possible in CE. Small sample volumes (nL) and loadings (Attomoles) are typical of CE.

Because a major component of glass used in capillaries is negatively-charged silica, a layer of counter-ions such as Na^+ and H^+ assemble along its interior surface that, in turn, attracts a hydration layer of water. During electrophoresis, the positively-charged Na^+/H^+ ions are electrophoretically attracted towards the cathode carrying the hydration layer with them. This phenomenon, called electroosmotic flow, has a particular significance in CE due to the extremely small internal volume of the capillary (7). The hydration layer represents a major fraction of the water contained within the capillary. Electroosmotic flow is therefore quantitatively particularly important in CE. It is strongly pH-dependent being up to ten times faster at low than at high pH. Simultaneously, samples also experience electrophoretic flow (i.e., positively charged ions are attracted to the cathode, negatively charged ions to the anode). The precise mobility of an individual ion will therefore be the result of a combination of these two flows. Positively charged ions will tend to flow toward the cathode as a result of both electroosmotic and electrophoretic flow whereas uncharged components will move towards the cathode in response to electroosmotic flow only. Negatively charged ions will move either towards the cathode or the anode depending on the relative strength of the two flows.

This gives rise to some apparent paradoxes because uncharged molecules move in a CE system (in most electrophoresis systems they experience no movement) and negatively-charged ions can move towards the cathode in such systems (which seems to contradict electrostatic attraction). By varying pH and hence the strength of electroosmotic flow, separation of individual components can be optimised in CE. If it is desired to carry out separations on the basis of differences in electrophoretic flow alone, it is possible to coat the inner surface of the capillary to remove ionic interactions. Such interactions may be undesirable in separation of proteins.

3. Applications

3.1. Native Electrophoresis

3.1.1. Protein Mass Determination by Nondenaturing Electrophoresis

Nondenaturing electrophoresis allows determination of protein native M_r. Because mobility is strongly affected by mass and shape, it is possible to compare the mobility of a protein of unknown mass with a series of standards of similar shape but known M_r. This mobility is measured in nondenaturing gels of differing polyacrylamide concentration. The mobility of each protein is measured and expressed as R_f. A plot of log R_f for each standard protein versus % polyacrylamide is then made (it is necessary to use a minimum of five different polyacrylamide concentrations for accurate results) (**Fig. 23.4**). The negative slope of these plots is the retardation coefficient, K_r, for that protein as;

$$K_r = - (\text{slope}) \tag{8}$$

In the case of globular proteins, there is a linear relationship between K_r and the Stokes radius. A plot of K_r versus M_r generates a standard curve from which native M_r may be estimated. These data complement mass estimates from other techniques (e.g., gel filtration) and are especially useful when only small amounts of protein are available. Combining such measurements with M_r estimates from SDS PAGE (see below) allows protein quaternary structure to be determined.

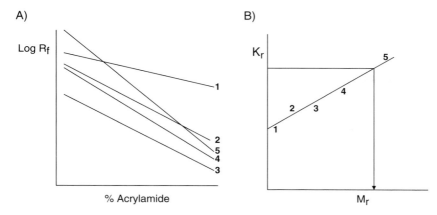

Fig. 23.4. Determination of native M_r by nondenaturing electrophoresis. (**A**) The mobility (R_f) of proteins of known M_r are estimated in nondenaturing gels of differing percentages. The retardation coefficient (K_r) is calculated as the negative slope of this line for each protein. (**B**) K_r is plotted against M_r to generate a standard curve. Based on the K_r of the unknown protein (arrow) a value for M_r can be calculated

3.1.2. Activity Staining

Proteins generally retain biological activity in nondenaturing electrophoresis. Thus, catalytic activity of enzymes can be used as a specific stain, a process called "activity staining." An artificial substrate is converted to an insoluble, coloured product by the enzyme-catalysed reaction. The location of the protein in the gel can be visualised by observation of the insoluble (and therefore precipitated) product. Because a single enzyme may go through many thousands of catalytic cycles in a few minutes, very tiny amounts of enzyme can be visualised.

Particular activity stains are available for groups of enzymes sharing a common catalytic process such as dehydrogenases (they reduce tetrazolium to produce formazan that is insoluble) *(8)*. By selecting substrates specific for a particular dehydrogenase (e.g., succinate for succinate dehydrogenase, malate for malate dehydrogenase) highly individual staining for dehydrogenases can be achieved with essentially the same staining procedure. This can be useful in identifying which band among several visible on a nondenaturing gel is the band representing the enzyme of interest and is especially useful in demonstrating the presence of multiple enzymes catalysing a particular chemical reaction in biological extracts. Activity-stained nondenaturing gels are called zymograms and these may be used to characterise cell-types, tissues, individuals and populations on the basis of isoenzyme expression.

3.1.3. Counting Protein Thiols

Protein thiols react quantitatively with iodoacetic acid. This confers an extra negative charge on each cysteine. Conversely, reaction with iodoacetamide results in no net charge change (**Fig. 23.5**). By treating a protein with an increasing ratio of iodoacetic acid:iodoacetamide, progressively more negative charges can be introduced to the protein ranging from 0 to n, the number of protein thiols. Mixing all the samples together across this ratio generates a "ladder" of bands with the number of bands equating to $n + 1$.

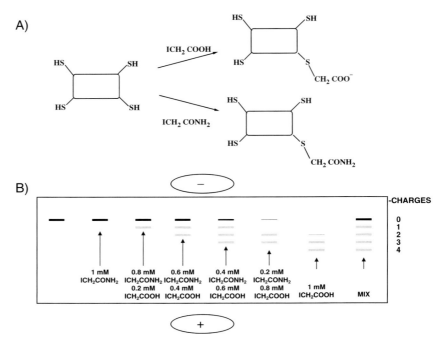

Fig. 23.5. Counting protein thiols in native gels. (**A**) Iodoacetic acid reacts with protein thiols to introduce a negative charge. This species will migrate further towards the anode than the original protein. Iodoacetamide reacts with thiols but does not add an extra negative charge. (**B**) Treating protein with 1 mM iodoacetic acid introduces four negative charges whereas treatment with 1 mM iodoacetamide introduces no negative charges. Altering the ratio of iodoacetic acid to iodoacetamide generates a series of charge variants dependant on n. Electrophoresis of samples from across this gradient reveals a "ladder" of these variants. Counting the bands gives $n + 1$

3.2. SDS PAGE

3.2.1. M_r Determination by SDS PAGE

SDS PAGE allows determination of subunit M_r by comparison with standard proteins because a plot of mobility versus log M_r forms a standard curve (**4**). Insights to aspects of protein structure can be obtained by varying this simple experiment (**Fig. 23.6**). Two subunits linked by disulphide bridges will migrate as a single species under nonreducing conditions while migrating as individual subunits in reducing conditions. Inclusion of a reducing agent (e.g., 2-mercaptoethanol) in sample and running buffer facilitates this comparison. The reducing gel might reveal two subunit M_r values, whereas the nonreducing gel would give a larger M_r corresponding to that of the intact protein, the sum of the values for the individual subunits. Pretreatment of proteins with crosslinking agents such as dimethyl suberimidate allows crosslinking between adjacent subunits containing the common amino acid lysine (**Fig. 23.6**). Such crosslinking experiments can reveal structural associations among subunits in oligomeric proteins by comparing M_rs of crosslinked to noncrosslinked subunits.

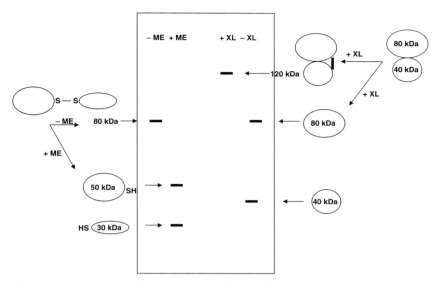

Fig. 23.6. Insights to protein structure from SDS PAGE. A protein consisting of 50 and 30 kDa subunits linked by a disulphide bridge will migrate as 80 kDa under nonreducing conditions (–ME; 2-mercaptoethanol absent) and as two bands of 50 and 30 kDa, respectively, under reducing conditions (+ME; 2-mercaptoethanol present). Similarly, two subunits (80 and 40 kDa) that are structurally associated can be chemically crosslinked (+XL) so a single polypeptide of 120 kDa is visible in SDS PAGE. In the absence of crosslinker (–XL) two bands of 80 and 40 kDa, respectively are visible

3.2.2. Determination of Disulphide Bridge Patterns by Diagonal Gels

Some proteins contain disulphide bridges that are formed in the endoplasmic reticulum in a reaction catalysed by protein disulphide isomerase. This is a key aspect of protein folding. The pattern of protein disulphides in a protein extract can be altered by processes such as oxidative stress. A means of studying this is offered by first carrying out SDS PAGE in nonreducing conditions (**Fig. 23.7**). The entire gel track is excised, exposed to reducing buffer and electrophoresed orthogonally under reducing conditions (*9*). Proteins lacking disulphides migrate identically under reducing and nonreducing conditions forming a diagonal. Proteins with intermolecular disulphide bridges migrate in the second dimension as individual polypeptides and therefore migrate below the diagonal. Proteins with intramolecular disulphide bridges have a less compact molecular structure and migrate more slowly in reducing conditions appearing as bands above the diagonal. In this way, it is possible in a single experiment to distinguish nondisulphide bridged proteins with those containing intrachain or interchain disulphides.

3.2.3. Two-Dimensional SDS PAGE

SDS PAGE and IEF can be combined in a technique called 2-dimensional electrophoresis (2D SDS PAGE) (*6,10*). This avails of the fact that proteins may have identical M_r or identical pI but rarely share the same value for both parameters. In modern practice, pH gradients immobilised on plastic strips are used for the IEF dimension. After focusing, the strips are equilibrated in SDS PAGE sample buffer and electrophoresed orthogonally through an SDS

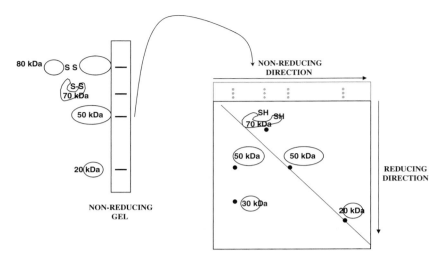

Fig. 23.7. Diagonal gel electrophoresis. Proteins migrate in nonreducing SDS PAGE with disulphide bridges intact. If the entire gel track is then excised, exposed to reducing buffer and laid across a second SDS PAGE gel in reducing conditions, proteins lacking disulphide bridges migrate identically as in non reducing conditions and thus form a diagonal (dashed line). Proteins containing interchain disulphides run as separate polypeptides (e.g., 50 kDa and 30 kDa) in reducing conditions. These appear below the diagonal. Proteins with intrachain disulphides have a less compact structure in reducing conditions and thus migrate above the diagonal

PAGE gel. When stained, the gel usually contains hundreds of distinct spots, each corresponding to a single protein. 2D SDS PAGE is a key technique in proteomics because it allows comparison of the protein complement of matched biological sample. Thus, a protein present in one sample but absent in the other can be recognised. New staining and image analysis technologies allow quantitative data to be obtained from such comparisons. Spots of interest can be further characterised and identified by direct N-terminal sequencing or by mass spectrometry techniques. See p 367 for a typical 2-D gel.

Acknowledgements: Work in our laboratory is supported by the Irish Research Council for Science Engineering and Technology, Programme for Research in Third Level Institutions and the Health Research Board of Ireland.

References

1. Righetti PG (2005) Electrophoresis: The march of pennies, the march of dimes. J Chromatog A 1079:24–40
2. Westermeier R, Marouga R (2005) Protein detection methods in proteomics research. Biosci Reports 25:19–32
3. Girardet JM, Miclo L, Florent S, Molle D Gaillard JL (2006) Determination of the phosphorylation level and deamidation susceptibility of equine beta-casein. Proteomics 6:3707–3717
4. Laemmli UK (1970) Cleavage of structural proteins during the assembly of the head of bacteriophage T4. Nature 227:680–685
5. Radola BJ (1973) Isoelectric focusing in layers of granulated gels 1. Thin layer isoelectric focusing of proteins. Biochim Biophys Acta 295:412–428

6. Görg A, Boguth G, Obermaier C, Weiss W (1998) Two dimensional electrophoresis of proteins in an immobilized pH 4-12 gradient. Electrophoresis 19:1516–1519.

7. Ghosal S (2004) Fluid mechanics of electroosmotic flow and its effect on band broadening in capillary electrophoresis. Electrophoresis 25:214–228

8. Seymour JL, Lazarus RA (1989) Native gel activity stain and preparative electrophoretic method for the detection and purification of pyridine nucleotide-linked dehydrogenases. Analytical Biochem 178:243–247

9. Molinari M, Helenius A (2002) Analyzing cotranslational protein folding and disulfide formation by diagonal sodium dodecyl sulfate polyacrylamide gel electrophoresis. Methods in Enzymol. 348:35–42

10. O'Farrell P (1975) High-resolution two-dimensional electrophoresis of proteins. J Biol Chem 250:4007–4021

24

Protein Blotting

Patricia Gravel

1. Introduction

Protein blotting, also known as Western blotting refers to the transfer of electrophoresed proteins from the polyacrylamide gel electrophoresis (SDS-PAGE
or 2-dimensional PAGE [2D-PAGE]) to an adsorbent membrane that binds the
eluted macromolecules ("the blot"). This method was first described in 1979
by Towbin et al. *(1)*.

Electrophoretic transfer uses the driving force of an electric field to elute
proteins from gels. This method is fast, efficient and maintains the high resolution of the protein pattern. Different probes can be used to react with the
transferred proteins on the blot:

- antibody for the identification of the corresponding antigen,
- lectin for the detection of glycoproteins,
- ligand for the detection of blotted receptor components, etc.

Western transfer with subsequent immunodetection has found wide application in the fields of life sciences and biochemistry. The blotted proteins
can efficiently be detected and characterized, especially those that are of low
abundance.

The blot is also widely used with various techniques of protein identification, from which the measurement of protein mass (mass spectrometry)
or determination of the protein sequence (*N*-terminal Edman degradation,
C-terminal sequence or amino acid analysis).

The power of protein blotting lies in its ability to provide simultaneous resolution of multiple immunogenic proteins within a sample. The blot analysis generally
requires small amount of reagents, the transferred proteins on membrane can be
stored for many weeks before their use and the same blot can be used for multiple
successive analyses.

This chapter summarizes the different methods (1) to transfer proteins from
gel to membrane (Section 2.1) and (2) to detect proteins on blots (Section 2.2).
Several applications of the protein blotting technique are presented in Section
3 of this chapter.

From: *Molecular Biomethods Handbook, 2nd Edition.*
Edited by: J. M. Walker and R. Rapley © Humana Press, Totowa, NJ

2. Methods

2.1. Efficiency of Protein Blotting

Two principal factors affect the efficiency of protein blotting: (1) the elution efficiency of proteins out of the gel matrix and (2) the efficiency of binding by the membrane.

2.1.1. Elution Efficiency of Proteins and Techniques Used

The efficient transfer of proteins from the gel to a solid membrane support depends greatly on the acrylamide concentration of the gel, the ionic strength and the pH of the buffer, the additional constituents of the transfer buffer such as sodium-dodecyl-sulfate (SDS) and methanol *(2)*, and the molecular mass of the proteins transferred. In a general way, the lower the percentage of acrylamide and cross-linker, the easier the transfer will be. The use of thinner gels allows a faster and more complete transfer. Methanol increases the binding capacity of matrix presumably by exposing hydrophobic protein domains, so that they can interact with the matrix. When there is SDS in transfer buffer (up to 0.1% w/v), the proteins are negatively charged and elute efficiently from the gel. High molecular-weight (MW) proteins blot poorly from SDS-PAGE or 2D-PAGE, which leads to low levels of detection on immunoblots. However, the transfer of high MW proteins can been facilitated with heat, special buffers and partial proteolytic digestion before transfer *(3,4)*.

Protein transfer from gel electrophoresis to membrane has been achieved in three different ways: simple diffusion, vacuum-assisted solvent flow and electrophoretic elution *(5)*. This later method is the most common and efficient and will be summarized here below. There are currently two main configurations of electroblotting apparatus *(6)*:

1. tanks of buffer with vertically placed wire or plate electrodes (wet transfer) and
2. semi-dry transfer with flat-plate electrodes (see **Fig. 24.1**). The name semi-dry transfer refers to the limited amount of buffer that is confined to the stacks of filter paper.

Semi-dry blotting requires considerably less buffer than the tank method, the transfer from single gels is simpler to set up, it allows the use of multiple transfer buffers and it is reserved for rapid transfers because the use of external cooling system is not possible. Nevertheless, both techniques have a

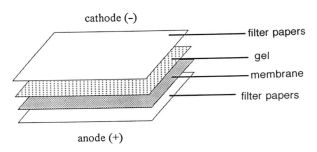

Fig. 24.1. Assembly of a horizontal electroblotting apparatus for a semi-dry transfer with flat-plate electrodes

high efficacy and the choice between the two types of transfer is a matter or preference.

2.1.2. Binding to the Membrane

The binding capacity is mainly determined by the character of the membrane but also by the transfer buffer composition *(7,8)*.

Nitrocellulose, PVDF (polyvinylidene difluoride), activated paper, or activated nylon have been used successfully to bind transferred proteins. Nitrocellulose was the first matrix used in electroblotting and is still the support used for most experiments. It has a high binding capacity, it is not expensive and the nonspecific protein binding sites are easily and rapidly blocked. However, the proteins are not covalently bound and small proteins tend to move through nitrocellulose membranes and only a small fraction of the total amount actually binds.

PVDF membranes are advantageous because of high protein binding capacity, physical strength and chemical stability. Most commonly used protein stains and immunochemical detection systems are compatible with PVDF membranes. In addition, replicate lanes from a single gel can be obtained and used for different purposes, along with Western analysis (*N*-terminal sequencing, proteolysis-peptide separation-internal sequencing, etc.). PVDF membranes can be stained with Coomassie brilliant blue (CBB), allowing excision of proteins for *N*-terminal sequencing.

The efficacy of the Western blot using semi-dry method that uses a simple buffer system is illustrated in **Fig. 24.2** *(6)*. Human plasma proteins (120 µg) were separated by 2-D PAGE, transferred on PVDF membrane and stained with Coomassie blue (**Fig. 24.2B**). The blot pattern is compared to the Coomassie blue staining of the same protein sample before transfer from 2-D PAGE (**Fig. 24.2A**). The resolution, shape and abundance of protein spots on membrane are comparable to the 2-D polyacrylamide gel pattern.

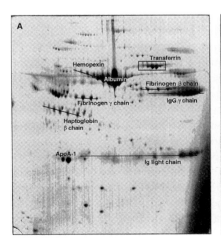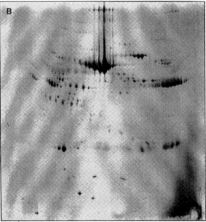

Fig. 24.2. Plasma proteins separated by 2-dimensional polyacrylamide gel electrophoresis and (**A**) stained with Coomasie Brilliant Blue R250 or (**B**) transferred to PVDF membrane using the semi-dry system (2 h, 15 V) with Towbin buffer diluted 1:2 in water and stained with Coomasie Blue

Several protocols have been developed from the basic electroblotting procedure to improve the amount of protein transferred and retained on the membrane. A review has been published recently *(9)*.

Whatever the membrane used, exceeding its binding capacity tends to reduce the signal eventually obtained on blots. For 2-D PAGE, the best recovery and resolution of proteins are obtained when loading 120 ug of human plasma or platelet proteins *(10)*.

2.2. Protein Detection

After blotting, the proteins are present in an accessible state, bound to the solid matrix of the membrane. They may be assayed for enzymatic function *(11)*, chemical reactivity *(12)* or amino acid sequence *(13)*. However, protein blotting is most often followed by reaction of the bound proteins with antibodies, before detection with antibody-specific labeled probes (immunoblotting). Another interesting probe is lectin, a class of carbohydrate-binding proteins, to discriminate and analyze the glycan structure of glycoproteins transferred to membranes (lectin blotting) *(10)*.

The following section described the protein stains, the immunodetection of antigens and the glycoprotein analysis using lectin blotting.

2.2.1. General Proteins Stains

It is often necessary to visualize the transferred proteins to allow exact alignment of bands (if the blot is obtain following SDS-PAGE) or spots (if 2-D PAGE is used) and to control the quality of the transfer. Staining refers to the reversible or irreversible binding by the proteins of a colored organic or inorganic chemical.

The proteins may be stained before or after the electrotransfer. Initially, the stains used for visualization of proteins in gels were also used for nitrocellulose membrane, typically Coomassie blue or amido black *(14)*, although these stains cannot be used with nylon membranes because the charged nature of the membrane results in very high levels of background staining *(15)*.

One problem with the staining before Western blotting is the longer staining time required with proteins contained in the gel matrix.

Staining on blots (after the Western blotting) often represents the preliminary step for specific detection/characterization procedures. *N*-terminal sequencing requires permanent staining stains; Coomassie blue has been routinely used with nitrocellulose membrane and amido black with PVDF membrane. Conversely, immunological and affinity reagents require reversible stains (colorimetric dyes such as direct blue 71, copper iodide, metal chelates or fluorescent dye).

The common limitation of protein staining, before or after the electrotransfer, is the reduction in immunoreactivity of the membrane-bound proteins. This may be caused by the blocking of antibody-binding by the protein-bound stain proteins or to the denaturing effects of solvent during the staining process *(16)*.

Proteins have also been detected after immunoblotting onto membrane supports directly by use of fluorescent labels (fluorescamine, coumarin), various silver staining methods *(17)* and colloidal particles such as gold, silver, copper, iron, or India ink *(18)*.

2.2.2. Specific Immunodetection of Antigens

After transfer, unused macromolecular binding sites of the membrane must be blocked to prevent nonspecific adsorption of probe molecules. The selection of a blocking solution from the wide range available, together with the temperature and duration of the blocking incubation, may affect the level of background staining *(19)*. The majority of blocking solutions are protein-based. Buffered solutions of skimmed milk or casein are widely used and effective.

Two methods are commonly used for detecting proteins, after the addition of primary antibody to protein blots that have been blocked: radioactive and enzyme-linked reagents.

With Western blotting, the proteins transferred are in a highly denatured state, which may prevent the reaction of the majority of antibodies, except those that react with conformation-insensitive epitopes to bind *(20)*. This illustrates the importance of using polyclonal antibodies that contain multiple epitopes of a protein, some of which are likely to be denaturation-resistant. It is commonly found that monoclonal antibodies fail to react in Western blotting.

Different modifications of the electrophoresis technique have also been developed to retain more of the native protein structure and therefore increase the immunoreactivity, for example avoid the use of sulphydryl reagent, reduction or omission of SDS *(21,22)*.

2.2.3. Specific Stains of Glycoproteins Using Lectin Blotting

Glycoproteins result from the covalent association of carbohydrate moieties (glycans) with proteins. The enzymatic glycosylation of proteins is a common and complex form of post-translational modification. It has been established that glycans perform important biological roles including: stabilization of the protein structure, protection from degradation, control of protein solubility, of protein transport in cells and of protein half-life in blood. They also mediate the interactions with other macromolecules and the recognition and association with viruses, enzymes and lectins *(23,24)*.

Carbohydrate moieties are known to play a part in several pathological processes. Alterations in protein glycosylation have been observed, for example, with the membrane glycoproteins of cancer cells, with the plasma glycoproteins of alcoholic patients and patients with liver disease, with the glycoproteins in human brains from patients with Alzheimer disease, inflammation and infection. These changes provide the basis for more sensitive and more discriminative clinical tests *(25–29)*.

Lectins are carbohydrate-binding proteins that can bind specifically and non-covalently to a certain sugar sequence in oligosaccharides and glycoconjugates. Their restricted binding capacity is the basis not only for recognition of glycoproteins but also an indirect way for accessing the composition of their glycan moieties. In most cases, they bind more strongly to oligosaccharides (di, tri, and tetra saccharides) than to monosaccharides *(30,31)*. Many lectins recognize terminal nonreducing saccharides, whereas others also recognize internal sugar sequences. For example, concanavalin A binds to internal and nonreducing terminal α-mannosyl groups, whereas lectins from *Sambucus nigra* and from *Maackia amunrensis* show affinity for specific types of sialic acid linkages. Together, these later lectins can detect most glycoproteins of animal origin because all antennae of the glycans from these sources ending with sialic acid residues. See Gravel et al. (2002) *(31)* for a review of the specificity of lectins for glycans and for the description of a protocol for the detection of glycoproteins on nitrocellulose membrane using biotinylated lectins and avidin conjugated with horseradish peroxidase or with alkaline phosphatase. **Figure 24.3A** below shows

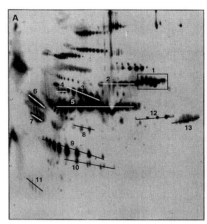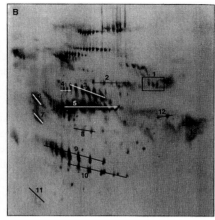

Fig. 24.3. Glycoprotein blot pattern of 2-D PAGE separation of plasma proteins (120 μg) probed with WGA (specific for *N*-acetylglucosamine and neuraminic acid) and (**A**) revealed with chemiluminesence (15 s film exposure) and (**B**) with NBT/BCIP (20 min for the development of the color reaction). Because most of the glycoproteins in plasma contain one or more N-linked glycans with at least two *N*-acetylglucosamine residues, the use of WGA allows a general staining of N-linked glycoproteins. (1) transferrin, (2) IgM μ-chain, (3) hemopexin, (4) α1-β-glycoprotein, (5) IgA α-chain, (6) α1-antichymotrypsin, (7) α2-HS-glycoprotein, (8) fibrinogen γ-chain, (9) haptoglobin β-chain, (10) haptoglobin cleaved β-chain, (11) apolipoprotein D, (12) fibrinogen β-chain, (13) IgG γ-chain

the plasma glycoprotein signals (using the above method, i.e., high-resolution 2-D PAGE followed by lectin blotting method on nitrocellulose membrane) detected with wheat germ agglutinin (WGA, specific for *N*-acetylglucosamine and neuraminic acid) and generated on a film after chemiluminescence detection. **Figure 24.3B** shows an identical blot stained with nitro blue tetrazolium/bromochloro-indolyl phosphate (NBT/BCIP). The same pattern of glycoprotein subunits are revealed by both methods but the chemiluminescent detection system shows higher sensitivity (about 10-fold) than NBT/BCIP staining. Albumin, which does not contain any carbohydrate moiety, represents a negative protein control in all blots (blank area below the IgM μ–chain [protein identified by number 2 in **Fig. 24.3**]).

Lectins do not have an absolute specificity and therefore can bind with different affinities to a number of similar carbohydrate groups. Despite this limitation, lectin probes do provide some information as to the nature and composition of oligosaccharide substituents on glycoproteins. Their use together with blotting technique provides a convenient method of screening complex protein samples for abnormalities in the glycosylation of the component proteins. See Section 3 for the application of this technique to identify carbohydrate-deficient transferrin from plasma sample of alcoholic patients.

3. Applications

Presently, there is an intense interest in applying proteomics (a new science that focuses on the study of proteins: their roles, their structures, their localization, their interactions, and other factors) to marker identification of different disease.

Proteomic approaches to this end include comparative analysis of protein expression in normal and abnormal tissues to identify aberrantly expressed proteins that may represent novel markers. Various tools from the high-resolution 2D-PAGE to liquid chromatography and mass spectrometric analysis, Western blotting and immunodetection have been applied to biomarker development.

3.1. Autoantibodies to Tumor Antigens

The analysis of serum for autoantibodies against tumor proteins, using among other methods, the Western-blotting technique, has been accomplished in several ways. A large number of tumor antigens that elicit autoantibodies have been identified by screening gene expression library with patient sera (32). Proteomics has provided an alternative approach to expression library screening and is increasingly used for tumor antigen identification. The interest of a proteomic approach to tumor antigen identification is that it allows proteins and peptides in their modified states, as they occur in cells, to be analyzed for antigenicity. Given that proteins are subject to post-translational modifications that may be immunogenic, notably glycosylation, antibodies to epitope that result from such post-translational modifications can be preserved and detected with proteomics techniques. The standard proteonomic tools are 2D-PAGE, Western blotting and mass spectrometry. With 2D gels, proteins in tumor cell lysates are first separated and then transferred onto membranes that are incubated with subject sera. Proteins that specifically react with antibodies in cancer patients sera are then identified by mass spectrometry. This strategy, which uses the Western-blotting method, was applied to the identification of new breast cancer markers (33).

3.2. Carbohydrate-Deficient Transferrin as a Biomarker of Chronic Alcohol Intake

Excessive alcohol consumption is a common problem in society and medical practice. There is a need for a diagnostic tool for the detection of excessive alcohol consumption in unselected medical populations. Carbohydrate deficient transferrin, also called CDT, in the plasma during chronic alcohol exposure is a well-known protein alteration and is the result of multiple alterations of glycosylation (34). It represents the lack of negatively charged terminal sialic acid residues. The use of this alteration as a new, sensitive and specific marker of chronic alcohol consumption is still controversial. Further studies in a large number of patients, are needed.

Using 2-dimensional gel electrophoresis combined with lectin blotting techniques, it was possible to screen plasma proteins from alcoholics and cirrhotic patients for abnormalities in protein patterns and glycosylation. The identification and confirmation of different protein alterations associated with both diseases were possible (hypergammaglobulinemia, decrease in albumin, decrease of haptoglobin spots). In addition, glycosylation abnormalities in transferrin, haptoglobin and α-1 antitrypsin of alcoholic patients were demonstrated as additional spots (in the 2-D gel pattern) at the basic (cathodic) end of the pH gradient. The additional spots represent carbohydrate deficient glycoproteins caused by the loss of some negatively charged sialic acid residues (34), which leads to a lower global chemical charge (35). The high-resolution 2-D PAGE combined with lectin blotting proved useful to visualize, in a single experiment, different changes (of charge and molecular weight) associated to the glycosylation modifications of proteins.

3.3. HIV Diagnostic Tests

Current methods available for diagnosis of HIV infection have improved the care of many patients at risk for HIV infection or currently infected with the virus. All HIV diagnostic tests are based upon (i) the detection of one or more of the molecules that make up an HIV virus particle or (ii) the detection of the antibodies that human hosts make against HIV particles. The goal of most HIV diagnostic test is to detect HIV infection as early as possible, to ensure the safety of patients and early counseling and treatment. The different test can detect host antibodies specific to the virus or can directly detect the HIV.

Enzyme immunoassay (EIA) is the standard method used to screen a patient for antibodies to HIV. The antibodies detected are primarily of the immunoglobulin G (IgG) subtype. To minimize the risk of reporting false-positives, a confirmatory test should be conducted before the release of a positive result of a screening test. The assay commonly used is the Western blot, in which the patient's antibodies (in blood sample) are incubated with the HIV viral antigen and allowed to complex. The different protein complexes are then loaded into a gel matrix and separated by SDS-PAGE. Following transferred of proteins into a membrane, radiolabeled antibodies to the protein bands can be detected using autoradiography *(36,37)*.

3.4. Diagnosis of Prion Diseases

Transmissible spongiform encephalopathies (TSEs) encompass a group of fatal neurodegenerative diseases in animals and man, which can be transmitted experimentally to laboratory rodents and primates. About 75% of human prion diseases are sporadic forms of Creutzfeldt-Jakob disease. Clinical symptoms of TSEs include dementia and loss of movement co-ordination. In the 1980s, it was established that a common hallmark of TSEs was the accumulation of an abnormal isoform of the host-encoded prion protein (PrP) in the brains of affected animals and humans. Prion diseases are difficult to diagnose using conventional methods such as Polymerase Chain Reaction (PCR), serology or cell culture assays. This is because the infectious agent (prion) lacks a nucleic acid component and consists solely of an abnormally folded conformer of the normal host protein PrP that the infected organism does not recognize as foreign. Laboratory diagnosis of TSEs is further complicated by the uneven distribution of TSE agents in body tissues, mainly in the nervous system tissues, and low amount in easily accessible body fluids (blood or urine). That is why prion disease is usually confirmed by postmortem histopathological examination of brain tissue. The only reliable molecular marker for prion disease is the PrP^{sc}, an abnormal isoform of the host-encoded prion protein that accumulates in the brains of affected animals and humans.

Presently the most widely used diagnostic tests of TSEs in Europe (8 million bovine spongiform encephalopathies tests are performed per year), approved by national authorities, are a Western-blotting method and an ELISA *(38,39)*. The Western-blot assay is based on the postmortem immunochemical detection of PrP^{sc} in brain tissue. In this assay, a size shift (i.e., reduction of molecular weight caused by digestion of the *N*-terminus of PrP^{sc}) is directly visible and constitutes a specificity criterion for a positive assay. The other criterions are the presence of a typical 3-band pattern (caused by different glycosylation forms of PrP) and the presence of a PrP-immunoreactive signal. Commercially available Western-blot kits exist for this assay.

3.5. Diagnosis of Various Infections

In the last decade, the rate of introduction of immunoblotting into the repertoire of assay for the serodiagnosis of parasitic infections has been increasing. Several Western-blot kits are commercially available for the diagnosis of infections, such as *Cysticercosis* infection, Lyme disease, *Schistosomiasis* infection, etc.

Cysticercosis is a chronic disease worldwide resulting from infection with the parasite *Taenia solium*, the pork tapeworm. The infection is endemic in various countries (parts of Southeast Asia, Africa, Mexico, Latin America, Eastern Europe, etc.). The disease is transmitted by the ingestion of food that has been contaminated with *T. solium* eggs. The organisms enter the bloodstream and encyst and develop in the central nervous system and other tissue. This infection can be very difficult to diagnose owing to the wide range of symptoms that often resemble to epilepsy or migraine headaches. In addition, the observed cross-reactivity of *Cysticercosis* patient's sera with antigens of other parasites has limited the accuracy of serological methods such as ELISA (Enzyme-Linked Immunosorbent Assay). The Western blot is an appropriate tool to confirm the presence of antibodies to *T. solium* (sensitivity of 95% and specificity of 100%). Once diagnosed, this infection may be effectively treated with drugs.

The commercialized kit is composed of strips of nitrocellulose membrane containing purified *T. solium* glycoprotein antigens (separated previously according to their molecular weight by SDS-PAGE). The strip is incubated with the patient's serum or plasma sample, containing antibodies, if the patient is infected. *T. solium* antibody/protein complexes are then detected by adding goat anti-human immunoglobulin-alkaline phosphatase conjugate. By adding the substrate of the enzyme, the complexes are revealed and appeared as colored bands.

The same principle is applied to the other industrially produced strips for Western blots used in the diagnosis of many other infections.

References

1. Towbin H, Staehelin T, Gordon J (1979) Electrophoretic transfer of proteins from polyacrylamide gels to nitrocellulose sheets: procedure and some applications. Proc Natl Acad Sci USA 76:4350–4354
2. Sanchez JC, Ravier F, Pasquali C, Frutiger S, Bjellqvist B, Hochstrasser DF, Hughes GJ (1992) Improving the detection of proteins after transfer to polyvinylidene difluoride membranes. Electrophoresis 13:715–717
3. Bolt MW, Mahoney PA (1997) High-efficiency blotting of proteins of diverse sizes following sodium dodecyl sulfate-polyacrylamide gel electrophoresis. Anal Biochem 247:185–192
4. Kurien BT, ScoWeld RH, (2002) Heat-mediated, ultra-rapid electrophoretic transfer of high and low molecular weight proteins to nitrocellulose membranes. J Immunol Methods. 266:12–133
5. Kurien BR, ScoWeld RH (1997) Multiple immunoblots after non-electrophoretic bidirectional transfer of a single SDS-PAGE gel with multiple antigens. J Immunol Methods 205:91–94

6. Gravel P (2002) Protein blotting by the semi-dry method. In: Walker JM (ed) Protein protocol handbook, chapter 40. Humana, Totowa, NJ, pp 321–334

7. Gershoni JM, Palade GE (1983) Protein blotting: principles and applications. Anal Biochem 131:1–15

8. Jungblut P, Eckerskorn C, Lottspeich F et al (1990) Blotting efficiency investigated by using two-dimensional electrophoresis, hydrophobic membranes and proteins from different sources. Electrophoresis 11:581–588

9. Kurien BT, Scofield RH (2006) Western blotting. Methods 38:283–293

10. Gravel P, Golaz O, Walzer C, Hochstrasser DF, Turler H, Balant LP (1994) Analysis of glycoproteins separated by two-dimensional gel electrophoresis using lectin blotting revealed by chemiluminescence. Anal Biochem 221:66–71

11. Kanellis AK, Solomos T, Mattoo AK (1989) Visualization of acid phosphatase activity on nitrocellulose filters following electroblotting of polyacrylamide gels. Anal Biochem 179:194–197

12. Gershoni JM, Bayer EA, Wilcheck M (1985) Blot analyses of glycoconjugates: enzyme-hydrazide: a novel reagent for the detection of aldehydes. Anal Biochem 146:59–63

13. Kennedy TE, Wager-Smith K, Barzilai A et al (1988) Sequencing proteins from polyacrylamide gels. Nature (London). 336:499, 500

14. Lin W, Kasamatsu H (1983) On the electrotransfer of polypeptides from gels to nitrocellulose membranes. Anal Biochem 128:302–311

15. Pluskal MG, Przekop MB, Kavonian MR et al (1986) Immobilon™ PVDV transfer membrane. A new membrane substrate for Western blotting of proteins. Biotechniques 4:272–283

16. Tracey RP, Monkovic D, Adrianorivo A et al (1987) The effect of prestaining before immunoreaction during electroblotting of proteins. Electrophoresis 8:350–355

17. Merril CR (1987) In: Chrambach A, Dunn M, Radola B (eds) Advances in electrophoresis, vol. 1. VCH Publishers, Weinheim, Germany, pp 111–139

18. Patton WF, Lam L, Su Q et al (1994) Metal chelates as reversible stains for detection of electroblotted proteins:application to protein microsequencing and immunoblotting. Anal Biochem 220:324–329

19. Hauri HP, Bucher K (1986) Immunoblotting with monoclonal antibodies: importance of the blocking solution. Anal Biochem 159:386–389

20. Chapsal JM, Pereira L (1988) Characterization of epitopes on native and denatured forms of herpes simplex virus glycoproteins B. Virology 164:427–434

21. Birk HW, Koepsell H (1987) Reaction of monoclonal antibodies with plasma membrane proteins after binding on nitrocellulose: renaturation of antigenic sites and reduction of non-specific antibody binding. Anal Biochem 164:12–22

22. Cohen GH, Isola VJ, Kuhns J et al (1986) Localization of discontinuous epitopes of herpes simplex virus glycoprotein D: use of a nondenaturing (« native »gel) system of polyacrylamide gel electrophoresis couples with Western blotting. J Virol 60: 157–166

23. Rademacher TW, Parekh RB, Dwek RA (1988) Glycobiology. Annu Rev Biochem 57:785–838

24. Berger EG, Buddecke E, Kamerling JP, Kobata A, Paulson JC, Vliegenthart JFG (1982) Structure, biosynthesis and functions of glycoprotein glycans. Experientia 38:1129–1158

25. Turner GA (1992) N-Glycosylation of serum proteins in disease and its investigation using lectins. Clin Chim Acta 208:149–171

26. Stibler H, Borg S (1981) Evidence of a reduced sialic acid content in serum transferrin in male alcoholics. Alcohol Clin Exp Res 5:545–549

27. Thompson S, Turner GA (1987) Elevated levels of abnormally-fucosylated haptoglobins in cancer sera. Br J Cancer 56:605–610

28. Takahashi M, Tsujioka Y, Yamada T et al (1999) Glycosylation of microtubule-associated protein tau in Alzheimer's disease brain. Acta Neuropathol 97:635–641
29. Guevara J, Espinosa B, Zenteno E. et al. (1998) Altered glycosylation pattern of proteins in Alzheimer disease. J Neuropathol Exp Neurol 57:905–914
30. Goldstein IJ Poretz RD (1986) Isolation, physicochemical characterization, and carbohydrate-binding specificity of lectins. In: Liener IE, Sharon N, Goldstein IJ (eds) The lectins: properties, functions and applications in biology and medicine. Academic Press, Orlando. pp 235–247
31. Gravel P (2002) Identification of glycoproteins on nitrocellulose membranes using lectin blotting. In: Walker JM (ed) Protein protocol handbook, chapter 106. Humana, Totowa, NJ, pp 779–793
32. Stockert E, Jager E, Chen YT et al (1998) A survey of the humoral immune response of cancer patients to a panel of human tumor antigens. J Exp Med 187:1349–1354
33. Le Naour DE, Misek MC, Krause L et al (2001) Proteomics-based identification of RS/DJ-1 as a novel circulating tumor antigen in breast cancer. Clin Cancer Res 7:3328–3335
34. Stibler H (1991) Carbohydrate-deficient transferrin in serum: a new marker of potentially harmful alcohol consumption reviewed. Clin Chem 37:2029–2037
35. Gravel P, Walser C, Aubry C et al (1996) New Alterations of Serum Glycoproteins in Alcoholic and Cirrhotic Patients Revealed by High Resolution Two-Dimensional Gel Electrophoresis. Biochem Biophys Res Comm 220:78–85
36. Golsby RA, Kindt TJ, Osborne BA (2000) AIDS and other immunodeficiencies. In: Kuby immunology, 4th edn. W.H. Freeman and Company, NewYork, pp. 467–496
37. Paul SM, Grimes-Dennis J, Burr CK et al (2003) Rapid diagnostic testing for HIV : clinical implications. NJ Med 100 (Suppl 9):11–14
38. Schaller O, Fatzer R, Stack M et al (1999) Validation of a Western immunoblotting procedure for bovine PrP(Sc) detection and its use as a rapid surveillance method for the diagnosis of bovine spongiform encephalopathy (BSE). Acta Neuropatho 98:4373
39. Kübler E, Oesch B, Raeber AJ (2003) Diagnosis of prion diseases. Br Med Bull 66:267–279

25

Capillary Electrophoresis of Proteins

Mark Strege

1. Introduction

1.1. Capillary Electrophoresis of Proteins

Capillary electrophoresis (CE) is a separation technique that combines aspects of both gel electrophoresis and high performance liquid chromatography (HPLC). As is the case for gel electrophoresis, the separation in CE is based upon differential migration in an electrical field. Like HPLC, the detection of the migrating sample analytes may be monitored on-line or postcolumn/capillary for both quantitation and characterization, thereby eliminating the need for labor-intensive staining and destaining. The CE separation may take place within free solution or in the presence of a viscous gel medium. Since its initial description by Hjerten in 1967 (1), CE techniques analogous to most conventional electrophoretic methods have been demonstrated, including zone electrophoresis, displacement electrophoresis (isotachophoresis), isoelectric focusing, and molecular sieving separations. Data presentation and analysis are also similar to HPLC in that the detector output can be displayed as an "electropherogram" representing peaks on a baseline, and can therefore be integrated by area or height to provide quantitation. In contrast to conventional gel electrophoresis where multiple samples are run in parallel fashion on one gel, in CE (as in HPLC) a single sample is injected into the end of a capillary and a sample set is run in serial fashion. Electroosmotic flow (EOF), a phenomenon caused by a high-density charged surface such as that present in a uncoated fused silica capillary, is an additional force with which analytes can be transported down the capillary in the presence of an electrical field via plug-flow, resulting in very high efficiencies (i.e., narrow peaks).

For the analysis of small molecules, the success of CE has been limited by poor reproducibility owing to capillary wall-analyte interactions, variable EOF, and limited detection sensitivity. In the world of biopolymers, however, the story has been quite different as CE has achieved significant success for the enhancement of separation methods traditionally performed through the use of gels. The most notable example is the adaptation of CE for use in the multichannel DNA sequencers that were employed for the sequencing

From: *Molecular Biomethods Handbook, 2nd Edition.*
Edited by: J.M. Walker and R. Rapley © Humana Press, Totowa, NJ

of the human genome in less than 2 yr. Lesser publicized but equally success-ful has been the application of CE as a replacement for gel electrophoresis analyses of protein therapeutics in the biopharmaceutical industry. Several major biopharmaceutical companies have developed and validated CE protein methods according to ICH and FDA guidelines for control and release of marketed products. This chapter will focus primarily upon three CE protein analysis techniques that have become routinely employed: (1) the use of CE for free solution analysis of glycoproteins (2) the use of CE as a replacement for sodium dodecyl sulfate-polyacrylamide gel electrophoresis (SDS-PAGE), and (3) the use of CE as a replacement for gel isoelectric focusing.

1.2. Capillary Electrophoresis Instrumentation

CE separates analytes within the lumen of a small bore (typically ≤ 50 mcm) capillary filled with a buffer solution. A schematic of a CE system is presented in **Fig. 25.1**. The capillary is immersed in electrolyte-filled reservoirs into which are also inserted electrodes connected to a high voltage power supply. Sample is introduced into the inlet end of the capillary opposite the detector window via a brief application of positive pressure or electrical potential, and separation occurs as the analytes migrate the length of the capillary toward the outlet end. As separated components pass by the detector window an electrical signal is sent to a data system. Conventional commercial CE instruments (first marketed in the 1990s) use individual fused silica capillaries that are enclosed within a thermostatically controlled chamber, interfaced with an autosampler holding sample and buffer vials of typically 10 mcL–10 mL volume, and mounted within a detection system (typically a UV absorbance detector). Recently chip-based instruments for the analysis of biopolymers have been introduced by several companies. These systems employ microfabricated

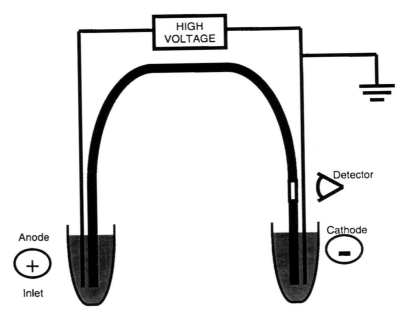

Fig. 25.1. Schematic of a capillary electrophoresis system

devices with channels etched into substrates such as glass and plastics for facilitation of electrically driven separations. Kits for specific applications, including protein separations, are provided with each of these commercial instruments.

1.3. Free Zone Electrophoresis

The basis of separation by electrophoresis is differential migration of analyte molecules in the presence of an applied electric field. The electrophoretic migration velocity (v) will depend upon the magnitude of the electric field (E) and the electrophoretic mobility (μ) of the analyte:

$$v = \mu E \tag{1}$$

In a buffer solution at a given pH, the mobility of the analyte is expressed by:

$$\mu = z/6\pi\eta r \tag{2}$$

Where z is the net charge of the analyte, η is the viscosity of the medium, and r is the Stoke's radius of the protein. Therefore, mobility will increase directly with increasing charge and inversely with molecular weight (because the Stoke's radius is based upon molecular mass). Considering field strength and migration time, mobility can be represented by:

$$\mu = (L/t_m)(L_{tot}/V) \tag{3}$$

where L is the distance from the inlet to the detection point (the "effective capillary length"), t_m is the time required for the analyte to reach the detection point (migration time), V is the applied voltage, and L_{tot} is the total length of the capillary. In a bare silica capillary, the velocity of an analyte as it passes through the capillary will also be heavily dependent upon the magnitude of the EOF. EOF is a phenomenon observed when an electrical potential is applied to a solution within a capillary with fixed charges present on the capillary walls, as is the case facilitated by the ionization of silanol groups on the surface of fused silica (silanols are weakly acidic and ionize at pH values >pH 3). An electrical double layer is formed when hydrated cations in solution associate with the ionized surface silanols. Upon application of an electrical field, the mobile outer cation layer moves toward the cathode, creating a net flow of bulk liquid in the capillary, as depicted in **Fig. 25.2**. The magnitude of the EOF is highly dependent upon the charge density of the capillary wall and the pH of the buffer medium. Because it is a chemically driven rather than physically driven flow (as is provided by a mechanical pump in HPLC), the EOF has proven to be difficult to control run-to-run and in many protein applications it has proven advantageous to take measures to minimize or completely eliminate it through the use of coated capillaries and/or viscous buffer mediums.

1.4. Capillary Electrophoresis SDS-PAGE (CE-SDS-PAGE)

Capillary gel electrophoresis is a modification of traditional gel electrophoresis to the capillary format, where CE is performed in the presence of a hydrophilic polymer solution that provides a polymer gel medium. Capillary gel electrophoresis separates molecules according to their size, and separation media include noncrosslinked polymers such as linear polyacrylamide, polyethylene

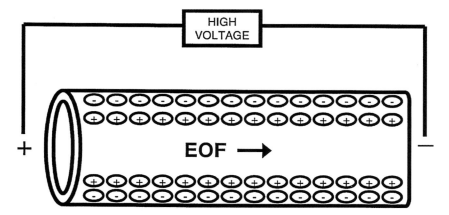

Fig. 25.2. Electroosmotic flow in an uncoated fused silica capillary

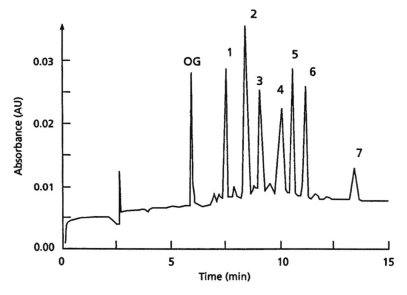

Fig. 25.3. CE-SDS-PAGE separation of a protein test mixture. Peaks are represented as follows: OG, Orange-G tracking dye, 1 = β-lactoglobulin (MW 14,200), 2 = carbonic anhydrase (MW 29,000), 3 = ovalbumin (MW 45,000), 4 = bovine serum albumin (MW 66,000), 5 = phosphorylase B (MW 97,400), 6 = β-galactosidase (MW 116,000), 7 = myosin (MW 205,000). Reproduced with permission from **ref.** *29*

glycol, and cellulose derivatives. The entangled polymer network inside the capillary serves as a molecular sieve in which smaller molecules migrate faster than large molecules. The polymer network also provides the benefits of reduction of both the solute diffusion rate and the adsorption of solute to the capillary wall, thereby increasing efficiency and facilitating the use of relatively short capillaries. A CE-SDS-PAGE separation of a protein test mixture is displayed in **Fig. 25.3**.

SDS-PAGE has for years served as a critical tool for monitoring product purity, detecting specific minor impurities, and evaluating lot-to-lot consistency of protein products. However, its limitations include the fact that the technique is labor intensive and time consuming (typically taking one full day to run the gel, stain it, and destain it). SDS-PAGE has also been considered at best a semi-quantitative technique because the staining process is not linear and protein-dependent. The addition of SDS-PAGE to the CE format has addressed these limitations. In addition to the attributes of capillary gel electrophoresis described above, in CE-SDS-PAGE, on-line UV absorbance or fluorescence detection provides quantitative information and the entire analysis process can be fully automated.

1.5. Capillary Isoelectric Focusing (CE-IEF)

Conventional gel-based isoelectric focusing suffers from the same limitations already described for SDS-PAGE, and because of these issues scientists within the biopharmaceutical industry have embraced CE-IEF. The major applications of CE-IEF in the biopharmaceutical industry are the determination of protein isoelectric point (pI) and the monitoring of protein charge heterogeneity. Separation in CE-IEF is based on differences in the pI of sample components rather than differences in electrophoretic mobility. A mixture of zwitterionic polymers known as ampholytes is used to generate a pH gradient inside the capillary during focusing. Focusing takes place as positively charged ampholytes migrate toward the cathode and negatively charged ampholytes migrate toward the anode, resulting in an increase in pH at the cathode end of the capillary and a decrease in pH at the anode end. When an ampholyte reaches its pI and is no

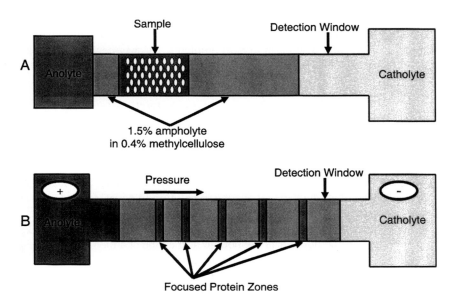

Fig. 25.4. Diagram of a CIEF separation using simultaneous pressure/voltage mobilization. (**A**) catholyte is backflushed past the detection point and a sample plug is introduced into the coated capillary. (**B**) focusing of the sample is complete and the sample components are driven toward the detector by a low pressure rinse (high voltage is applied during this step)

longer charged, its migration ceases and a stable pH gradient is formed. During focusing, analyte molecules migrate in similar fashion and eventually encounter a pH where they possess zero net charge and cease to migrate. For successful focusing, the pH of the electrolyte at the cathode must be higher than the pIs of all the basic ampholytes and the pH of the electrolyte at the anode must be lower than the pIs of all the acidic ampholytes. CE-IEF is also most effective in the absence of electroosmotic flow, conditions that are typically facilitated through the use of coated capillaries. In CE-IEF, the width of a solute zone is represented by the variance of a Gaussian distribution:

$$\sigma^2 = (D/E)(d(\text{pH})/d\mu_{app})(dx/d(\text{pH})) \qquad (4)$$

Smaller variance, which results in a sharper zone, is favored by high field strength (E), a low diffusion coefficient (D), and high values of $d\mu_{app}/d(\text{pH})$ (the rate of change of mobility with pH) and $d(\text{pH})/dx$ (the slope of the pH gradient). For a complete separation of two solutes, a difference between the two pIs must be greater than 4σ. A diagram demonstrating a CIEF separation using simultaneous pressure/voltage mobilization in a coated capillary is displayed in **Fig. 25.4**.

2. Methods

2.1. Free Zone Electrophoresis of Oligosaccharides

Free zone electrophoresis has been extensively applied for the characterization of therapeutically relevant complex glycoproteins and monoclonal antibodies through the separation profiling of the oligosaccharides present in these macromolecules. Carbohydrates present a challenge for CE analysis because they have poor UV absorbance, and neutral sugars demonstrate electrophoretic mobility under only extremely basic conditions. Derivatization with a charged fluorophore provides a solution to both problems. An overview of the conditions for the enzymatic release, chemical derivatization, and analysis of oligosaccharides is described below.

1. An appropriate volume of protein solution is transferred to a conical polypropylene tube and evaporated to dryness in a vacuum centrifuge without applying heat.
2. The release of the oligosaccharides from the native protein is accomplished through reconstitution of the protein in the presence of glycanase enzyme solution (buffered to provide optimal enzymatic activity), followed by incubation of the reconstituted solution in a water bath for a set period of time.
3. Following incubation, the protein solution is centrifuged briefly to make sure that all of the liquid is at the bottom of the tube and then is transferred to a microconcentration tube containing a molecular weight cut-off membrane. The tube is centrifuged to separate free oligosaccharides that will pass through the membrane from the protein that will be retained.
4. The oligosaccharide solution is transferred to a polypropylene tube and evaporated to dryness without applying heat.
5. The dried sample is reconstituted in fluorescent labeling reagent solution. After all labeling reagents have been added, the solution is incubated in a water bath for a set period of time.

6. The reaction tube is removed from the water bath and centrifuged briefly to make sure that all of the liquid is at the bottom of the tube. The derivatization reaction is quenched, and the sample is diluted in CE separation buffer.

7. The analysis is performed in CE separation buffer inside a bare silica capillary or a coated capillary. Prior to each injection, a bare silica capillary must first be conditioned via sequential rinsing of water, dilute HCl, dilute base, water, and finally separation buffer. Migration and separation of the analytes takes place upon application of high voltage, and typically requires 5–10 min.

8. Oligosaccharides are identified through spiking with reference standards. When standards are not available, the analytes may be identified through the observation of peak behavior and intensities upon treatment with exoglycosidases of known specificity.

2.2. Capillary Electrophoresis SDS-PAGE (CE-SDS-PAGE)

The analysis of monoclonal antibodies is a common application of CE-SDS-PAGE within the biopharmaceutical industry. Cell culture development, recovery process design, formulation development, stability studies, and product characterization are examples of development applications, whereas in-process monitoring and lot release analyses may support manufacturing. Below is an overview of a typical procedure employed for the preparation and analysis of proteins by CE-SDS-PAGE. The sample preparation is equivalent to that used for conventional gel SDS-PAGE.

1. The protein sample is mixed with a buffer containing SDS and (if appropriate) a reducing agent such as mercaptoethanol. The mixture is heated for a few minutes at elevated temperature, and then allowed to cool to room temperature.

2. Prior to injection, the capillary is washed with dilute base and acid solutions, the buffered polymer solution is then loaded into the capillary, and the capillary ends are dipped into wash solutions to wash off the residual viscous polymer solution.

3. The sample is introduced into capillary inlet via a brief application of an electric potential, and then the separation is performed. The separation typically requires 10–15 min.

2.3. Capillary Isoelectric Focusing (CE-IEF)

Because gel-based IEF suffers from the same limitations as those described for SDS-PAGE, many IEF applications within the biopharmaceutical industry have been converted into the capillary format. Below are described the steps necessary for performing CE-IEF.

1. The protein sample is mixed with the ampholyte solution and the capillary is filled with this mixture.

2. One end of the capillary is immersed in an analyte solution (such as dilute phosphoric acid), whereas the other end is immersed in catholyte (typically dilute sodium hydroxide).

3. A stable pH gradient is formed upon application of high voltage via the migration of the ampholytes, with proteins migrating to and focusing as narrow bands within the region of the capillary where they possess zero net charge. This step typically requires several minutes.

4. CE instruments that possess a whole-column imaging detector (such as a CCD camera) can record all protein zones within the capillary prior to the discontinuation of the voltage. Other instruments that use on-capillary detection at a fixed point along the capillary require mobilization of the protein bands across the detection point. Mobilization can be accomplished by pressurizing the capillary inlet or applying a vacuum to the outlet, or by changing the composition of either the analyte or catholyte to affect a pH gradient shift with time.

3. Applications

3.1. Free Zone Electrophoresis of Oligosaccharides

Glycoproteins are macromolecules that are generally composed of a common polypeptide chain but vary in their carbohydrate moieties, resulting in a population of closely related glycosylation variants often known as glycoforms. The carbohydrate groups are covalently attached to the polypeptide backbone through the amide nitrogen of an asparagine residue (*N*-glycosylation) or through an *O*-linkage with a serine, threonine, and sometimes a hydroxyproline residue (*O*-glycosylation). Glycosylation is often a critical determinant in many properties of glycoproteins, and this is particularly important in the case of therapeutic glycoproteins because the biological activity, clearance rate, immunogenicity, solubility, and stability may be significantly affected by the type of oligosaccharide attached to the protein.

Serving as a quantitative and automated enhancement to traditional slab gel techniques, CE has demonstrated great use for glycopeptide and oligosaccharide mapping and also for the establishment of the glycoprotein heterogeneity of the intact protein. Excellent reviews of the progress made in this specific area have been published *(2–4)*.

An effective approach for the analysis of oligosaccharides by CE has been the combination of CE with laser-induced fluorescence (LIF) detection. To enable fluorescence, oligosaccharides released from the protein core are labeled with fluorescent molecules via reductive amination using a fluorescent amino compound and sodium cyanoborohydride. Among the agents useful for labeling, 8-aminopyrene-1, 3, 6-trisulfonic acid (APTS) has demonstrated excellent use. CE methods reported by Ma and Nashabeh *(5)* and Patrick et al. *(6)* used derivatization with APTS for carbohydrate analysis. In the former study, both oligosaccharides and monosaccharides were analyzed in coated capillaries using reversed polarity for the purposes of monitoring the glycan distribution in rhuMab production and for gaining insight into the post-translational modifications occurring in the cell culture. In the latter investigation, bare silica capillaries were found to provide resolution of various galactose positional isomers, including those from different linkage configurations present within monoclonal antibodies. Structures of typical aspargine-linked (*N*-linked) biantennary oligosaccharides present on antibodies are indicated in **Fig. 25.5**, and an electropherogram produced from the ATPS-derivatized oligosaccharides released from an antibody is displayed in **Fig. 25.6**. A recent investigation by Ma et al. employed ATPS derivatization to analyze *N*-linked oligosaccharides on a recombinant IgG1 Mab and also to quantitate terminal monosaccharides *(7)*. Another fluorophoric agent, 5-amino-2-naphthalenesulfonic acid, was also

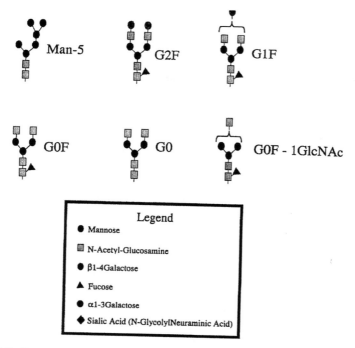

Fig. 25.5. Structures of typical asparagines-linked (N-linked) biantennary oligosaccharides present on the antibodies. Reproduced with permission from **ref. 6**

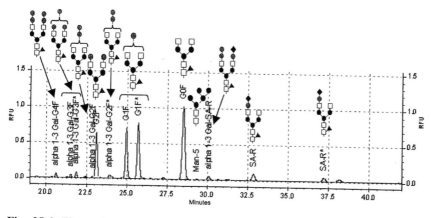

Fig. 25.6. Electropherogram produced from the APTS-derivatized oligosaccharides released from an Mab. The symbols are as described in the legend to **Fig. 25.5**, and common nomenclature is also included. Reproduced with permission from **ref. 6**

used to chemically modify N-linked oligosaccharides from a glycoprotein. Kamoda et al. employed both APTS and 3-aminobenzoic acid to derivatize carbohydrate chains released from therapeutic antibodies via glycoamidase, and found the accuracy of the two methods to be comparable (8). Sialo-N-glycans in glycoproteins have also been analyzed by CE in free solution in the presence of surfactants via a technique known as micellar electrokinetic capillary chromatography (MECC) (9). In this study, the glycans were labeled with 1-phenyl-3-methyl-5-pyrazolone (PMP) derivatives and were sensitively detected simply by UV absorbance detection. Laboratory protocols describing the characterization of oligosaccharides derived from complex carbohydrates and glycoproteins and analyzed by CE with LIF detection have been outlined by Chen (10). The use of CE-MS for the determination of carbohydrates has also been reported (11) The advantage of CE-MS for this application is the fact that derivatization is not required and molecular weight information may be acquired on-line for rapid analyte characterization.

Free zone CE has also been applied effectively for the characterization of intact glycoproteins. Early work in the area of the application of CE for the profiling of monoclonal antibody heterogeneity was performed by Hoffstetter-Kuhn et al. (12). In these studies, the presence of borate in the separation buffer induced complex formation with carbohydrate chains on the protein and resulted in resolution of glycoforms not possible in phosphate buffer. The technique was successfully applied for the evaluation of both batch-to-batch consistency in production and formulation stability. In two reports, a highly heterogeneous macromolecule, α1-acid glycoprotein, was resolved into its glycoforms by free zone CE using coated capillaries and acidic buffers (13,14) As an adjunct to these separations, N-glycosidase F-released carbohydrate chains were also analyzed following derivatization with APTS or 3-aminobenzoic acid. In one study, CE fractions containing each glycoform in its nearly pure state were collected and subsequently analyzed by matrix assisted laser desorption time-of-flight mass spectrometry (14). The results provided basic information on the contribution of carbohydrate chains to the separation mechanisms of glycoforms by CE.

A clinical application of CE for the quantitative separation of glycoprotein isoforms that has received significant attention has been the determination of carbohydrate-deficient transferrin (CDT). CDT is currently considered to be the best available marker for the diagnosis of chronic alcoholism. An article by Wuyts and Delanghe reviewed a variety of analytical methods that have been developed for determination of CDT, and suggested the advantages of free zone CE in comparison to the other techniques (15). CE in the presence of strong electroosmotic flow facilitated full resolution of the transferrin isoforms in a short analysis time, and genetic transferrin variants were easily detected, thereby avoiding false-positive results.

Glycosylation is one of the most important post-translational events for proteins because it affects their functions in health and disease, playing significant roles in various information traffics for intracellular biological events. The interaction between carbohydrate chains and the proteins that recognize them has been a target to understand the biological roles of glycosylation. A review of the applications of CE for various kinds of studies related to carbohydrate-protein binding has been recently published (16) In one set of investigations, capillary affinity electrophoresis (CAE) methods to study carbohydrate-protein interactions were based upon high resolution separations of fluorescent-labeled carbohydrates by free zone CE with LIF detection in the presence of carbohydrate-binding proteins over a range of concentrations (17). The techniques facilitated simultaneous determination of carbohydrate chains, binding specificity of the constituent carbohydrate chains to specific proteins, and kinetic data reflecting the association constant of each carbohydrate. Nakajima et al. also reported the use of CAE to screen for carbohydrate-binding proteins in plant extracts (18).

3.2. Capillary Electrophoresis SDS-PAGE (CE-SDS-PAGE)

Monoclonal antibodies are one specific class of glycoprotein that is of current interest as both immunodiagnostics and therapeutic agents. The specificity of antibodies for target analytes has made them highly attractive for use in immunoassays because they provide a means for high sensitivity and selectivity for analyte detection at low concentrations and in the presence of complex matrices. Within the biopharmaceutical industry, antibodies can be used directly as drugs or indirectly as delivery systems. Therefore, a significant need has existed for analytical techniques for the characterization and quantitation of these biomolecules, and CE is one of several techniques that have demonstrated effective applications within this field.

Synagis® is a monoclonal antibody that has been developed for prevention of Respiratory Syncytial Virus infection in infants, and the development, optimization, and validation of a capillary gel electrophoresis (CGE) method for support of commercial production of this compound has been reported by Schenerman and Bowen (*19*). The CGE electropherograms of process matrices were directly compared to SDS-PAGE densitometry scans, as were those of the reference standard and bulk drug substance (see **Fig. 25.7**), and the parameters of specificity, linearity, range, accuracy, repeatability, intermediate

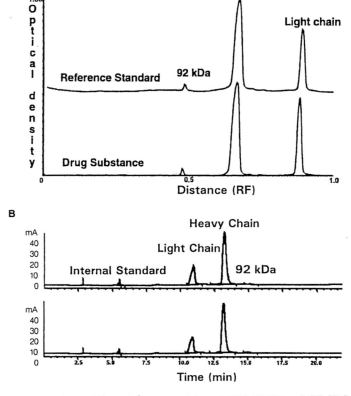

Fig. 25.7. Comparison of Synagis® separated by gel SDS-PAGE and CE-SDS-PAGE. (**A**) Gel SDS-PAGE densitometry scan obtained using a charge-coupled device camera. (**B**) CE-SDS-PAGE. Reproduced with permission from **ref.** *19*

precision, reproducibility, robustness, sensitivity, and system suitability were validated. These parameters were identical to those required by the ICH for the validation of HPLC methods, but it is important to note that appropriate acceptance criteria specific to the CGE method were investigated and set prior to the formal validation through the use of pilot studies. In a separate report, it was determined that preparation steps such as sample concentration, reduction, and centrifugation-diafiltration had a significant impact upon the reliability and robustness of the CGE method *(20)*. These sample preparation conditions were optimized for use in a protein purity method. In summary, the authors found that the CGE method could be validated to the same level of assurance as a typical HPLC method, and the CGE method validation was approved by the FDA for routine testing of Synagis®.

A similar approach was employed by Lee et al. who used CGE to quantitate murine immunoglobulin Gs (IgGs) *(21)*. A primary focus of this study was the enhancement of quantitative reproducibility through the use of a subclass of IgG as an internal standard. The fact that the reference standard was nearly identical to the analytes of interest ensured that both compounds exhibited the same assay precision so that their peak-area ratio (analyte: internal reference) remained constant. Through this approach, intra- and interday RSD values were lowered from >10% to <2% for peak-area ratio reproducibility.

Ma and Nashabeh used CGE to perform a variety of studies for characterization of a recombinant human monoclonal antibody (rhuMab) *(5)*. In accordance with **ref.** *19* mentioned earlier, these investigators found that the preparation of the sample (specifically the incubation of the protein with SDS at high temperature) had a very marked effect upon the CGE separation profile. The robustness of the SDS-binding step was found to be optimal at a temperature of 60°C. Quantitative CGE purity analyses of samples from a chromatographic purification enabled optimization of that step within the production process. The authors also determined that under nonreducing conditions, the CE electropherogram depicted a characteristic fingerprint of the various rhuMab size-variants generated by different combinations of light and heavy chains. Successful separations of antibody fragments in glycosylated, nonglycosylated, and polyethylene glycol-derivatized states were also achieved. Examples of the practical applications of CE-SDS-PAGE for process monitoring and product monitoring of rhuMab and recombinant protein biotherapeutics have been presented *(22–24)*. CE-SDS-PAGE was demonstrated to be a convenient and rapid method to profile the purification process, compare purification processes, and provide a fingerprint of the bulk drug that was helpful for determining purity and lot-to-lot consistency. The practical advantages and limitations of the method for process and product monitoring were discussed in these reports, and comparisons with analyses by other techniques, such as HPLC and conventional SDS-PAGE, were provided.

Miniaturization of gel electrophoresis, widely used in biomolecule analysis, has attracted much attention as it holds the promise of significantly reducing the analysis time and the amounts of sample needed, and has the potential to be automated and portable. As mentioned in the Introduction, chip-based instruments and separation kits for the analysis of biopolymers are commercially available, but research in this field continues to be active. Recent applications include the work of Nagata et al. who used SDS and linear polyacrylamide buffer solutions and polyethylene glycol-coated polymethyl methacrylate polymer microchips to achieve protein (21–116 kDa) separations over 3 mm channel lengths within 8 s *(25)*. The simultaneous electrophoretic separation of both native and SDS-complexed proteins on a single microchip within 20 min was demonstrated by Tsai et al. *(26)*. The microchannel array with self-contained electrodes prevented inter-channel cross-contamination and provided opportunities for analysis of many different protein samples during a single electrophoretic run. In another study, a photopatterning technique was used to cast in situ crosslinked polyacrylamide gel in a microchannel to perform SDS-PAGE *(27)* A fluorescent protein marker mixture covering a MW range of 20–200 kDa was separated in less than 30 s using less than 2 mm of channel length.

Another approach that has been developed for high-throughput protein analyses is the use of multiplexing (parallel separations run simultaneously through the use of multiple capillaries), as had been previously developed and implemented for DNA sequencing. Luo et al. reported the use of a commercially available instrument for the parallel analysis of 96 protein samples using UV absorbance detection and a 30 min separation time *(28)*. The sizing accuracy and repeatability of the multiplexed system was found to compare to conventional SDS-PAGE while providing a significant increase in throughput and automation.

Although linear polyacrylamide has been established as the most popular gel matrix for CE-SDS-based separations, investigations of the sieving matrices employed for protein separations have continued. An excellent review of the history of capillary gel electrophoresis authored by Guttman provides an overview of the gel matrices that have been used for CE separations *(29)*. Most recently, Lu et al. compared a variety of polymer sieving agents for protein separations and found replaceable cross-linked polyacrylamide to facilitate optimal resolution over a wide protein size range (4–300 kDa) *(30)*.

Novel 2-dimensional (2D) CE separation systems for proteins have been reported by Liu et al. *(31)*. In these systems, a porous glass membrane or a piece of dialysis hollow-fiber membrane was employed as the interface for on-line combination of CIEF and CE-SDS-seiving in a manner similar to gel-based 2D PAGE. Proteins were focused and separated in first dimension CIEF based on differences in isoelectric points. In the latter report, focused protein zones were transferred to the dialysis hollow-fiber interface, where proteins complexed with SDS. The negatively charged proteins were electromigrated and further resolved by their differences in size using the second dimension in which dextran solution was employed for facilitation of sieving. The feasibility and orthogonality of the 2D system were demonstrated via the separation of hemoglobin and protein mixtures from rat lung cancer cell excretions. CE-SDS-PAGE and CIEF have also been combined in a microchip format to provide 2D separations in less than 30 s *(27)*.

3.3. Capillary Isoelectric Focusing (CIEF)

CIEF has become an important tool for the quality assurance of biotherapeutics and also for proteome analysis. The critical performance parameters of this technique are the precisions of the isoelectric point values and the analyte peak areas. An investigation of CIEF reproducibility performed by Graf and Waetzig demonstrated that 0.5% RSD could be obtained for pI determination over the course of 106 repeated analyses, but peak area results demonstrated poor reproducibility (3–15% RSD) *(32)*. Reproducibility was determined to be primarily limited by the effects of protein adsorption to the capillary walls. The use of coated capillaries reduced the adsorption by 50% relative to bare silica capillaries, but could not prevent it completely. Another challenge for CIEF analysis is the focusing of extremely acidic or basic proteins, because the pH gradient facilitated by the most commonly used ampholyte mixtures covers the range of pH 3–10. Proteins such as lysozyme, cytochrome C, and pepsin with pIs > 10 or < 3 require special techniques, such as that proposed by Yang et al. *(33)*. In this study, a novel instrumental configuration was employed that made use of a sampling capillary as a bypass fixed to the separation capillary to achieve successful CIEF of these analytes.

Because the isoelectric point is an effective indicator of charge heterogeneity existing within a protein population, CIEF has proven to be an effective tool for the evaluation of glycoproteins. The comprehensive protein charge distribution is based upon a combination of the heterogeneity in the protein backbone and in the carbohydrates added during post-translational modification.

To investigate the origins of the charge heterogeneity of a proprietary glycoprotein, Ma and Nashabeh employed carboxypeptidase-B and neuraminidase to remove the C-terminal lysine residue and the sialic acids, respectively *(5)*. The CIEF profiles before and after digestion are displayed in **Fig. 25.8**. It is clear from these profiles that the majority of the charge heterogeneity in this protein was caused by the sialic acid distribution, although it was also evident that significant variability was also present in the intact protein in response to variability in the C-terminal lysine processing.

CIEF was applied for the analysis of recombinant human tumor necrosis factor receptor (p75) Fc fusion protein (rhu TNFR:Fc), an antibody marketed as Enbrel® *(34)*. The protein contained three N-linked glycosylation sites and multiple *O*-linked glycosylation sites, all of which are occupied with typical mammalian oligosaccharide structures. **Figure 25.9** displays a comparison between the analysis of rhu TNFR:Fc by slab gel IEF and CIEF, and both profiles reveal the complexity of the glycosylation isoform profile. CIEF was applied for the assessment of the desialylation of the protein by neuraminidase and also for the qualitative monitoring of variations in the isoform distribution in response to changes introduced into the rhu TNFR:Fc manufacturing process.

An ideal detection method for CIEF is whole-column-imaging because it facilitates real-time monitoring and direct visualization of the separation process. In whole-column-imaging detection (WCID), a short (3–6 cm) capillary is used as a separation capillary. The detection technique has been commercialized *(35)*, and experience and practice has proven that WCID permits the direct observation of the IEF focusing dynamics and greatly accelerates analysis speed. A whole-column-imaging CIEF separation of α-human chorionic gonadotrophin with two peptide pI markers is displayed in **Fig. 25.10**. Recently a coupling method of solid-phase microextraction (SPME) and CIEF with laser-induced fluorescence WCID was developed for the analysis of proteins, and was applied to the analysis of extracellular phycoerythrins from cultured cyanobacteria at the nanomolar level *(36)*.

A major area of interest involving CIEF is the integration of the technique with mass spectrometry. The combination of the two powerful separation/analysis methods has been especially attractive for the analysis of complex protein mixtures. The advantages of this approach include a high peak capacity in the

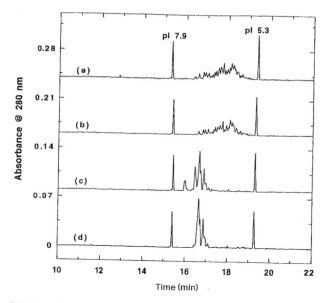

Fig. 25.8. CIEF profiles of glycoprotein obtained before or after different enzymatic digestions: (**a**) intact; (**b**) carboxypeptidase B; (**c**) neuraminidase; (**d**) carboxypeptidase B and neuraminidase. Reproduced with permission from **ref. 5**

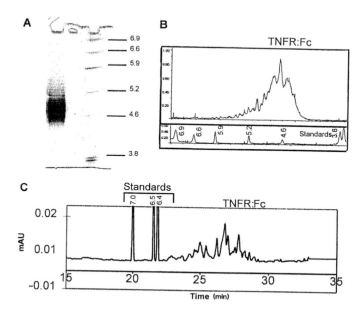

Fig. 25.9. Comparison of the rhuTNFR:Fc IEF slab gel with isoform profile generated by CIEF. Panel A shows a Coomassie stained IEF gel of rhuTNFR:Fc with standards (Novex pre-cast gel pI range 3.5–7.0). Panel B shows a densitometer scan of the IEF gel. Panel C shows a CIEF electropherogram of rhuTNFR:Fc injected at 0.35 mg/mL with 2% wide range ampholytes (Ampholine pH 3.5–9.5), 0.2% methylcellulose, and 2.5% TEMED. Reproduced with permission from **ref. 34**

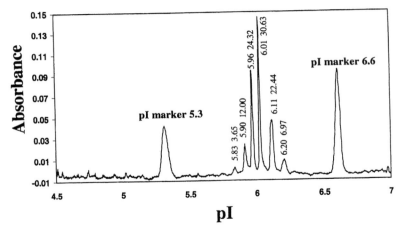

Fig. 25.10. Whole-column imaging CIEF results of an α-hCG sample with two Biomarkers. Carrier ampholyte, pH 4.0–7.0. Reproduced with permission from **ref. 35**

CIEF separation (resolution better than 0.02 isoelectric point units) and high sensitivity caused by the large amounts of sample injected into the capillary combined with the focusing effect. In contrast to multidimensional HPLC separations, the use of CIEF as a first dimension provides isoelectric point information useful for protein identification in database searches. There have been two major limitations to CIEF-MS interfacing, (1) the need to remove ampholytes prior to introduction of the pH gradient into the MS to prevent ion suppression and fouling of the ionization source, and (2) ion suppression of low-abundance proteins that comigrate with high-abundance proteins. Various approaches have been implemented to address these limitations. Two reviews on this subject have recently been published (37,38).

CIEF coupled with electrospray ionization (ESI) mass spectrometry provides a liquid-based alternative to traditional 2D-PAGE (a technique limited by sensitivity and throughput). To overcome the limitations of CIEF-MS interfacing, a reversed phase liquid chromatographic (RPLC) step was inserted between CIEF and MS (39). In this work, CIEF was performed with a micro-dialysis membrane-based cathodic cell that also facilitated fraction collection, followed by a wash to remove ampholytes and analysis by RPLC-MS. Using this approach, protein detection at the low-femtomole level was demonstrated with little or no interference from ampholyte. The instrumental configuration described in this report enabled the analysis of seven fractions taken from a complex mixture in the range of pI 3–10 to be completed by RP-HPLC in 2 h. Other researchers have employed CIEF-ESI-MS for the quantitative analysis of peptides and proteins through the use of 1% Pharmalyte 3–10 as ampholyte and a sheath liquid containing water, methanol, and acetic acid (40). The method was validated for linearity, accuracy, repeatability, and the limit of detection was 0.22 μM (about 10-fold lower than that obtained via UV absorbance detection). A third approach for avoiding ionization interferences from ampholytes was demonstrated through CIEF-MS in the absence of ampholytes (41). Under these conditions, however, the analyte ions were not focused at their pIs and electrophoretic mobility was observed, resulting in low separation efficiencies.

The capabilities of CIEF-based multidimensional separations for performing proteome analyses from minute samples create new opportunities in the pursuit of biomarker discovery. Recent advances in the online integration of CIEF with nano-RPLC for achieving high-resolution peptide and protein separations prior to mass spectrometry analysis have been reviewed, along with potential applications to tissue proteomics *(42)*. Extensions of this work were reported for the direct integration of CIEF with ESI-MS *(43,44)*. The optimization of protein identification (via proteomics database searching) from digests analyzed by CIEF-MS has also been described *(45)*. Off-line coupling of CIEF with matrix-assisted laser desorption/ionization time-of-flight (MALDI-TOF) mass spectrometry has been used for the analysis of human blood serum *(46)*. In this work, serum proteins were initially separated by CIEF, and fractions of the isoelectric focusing separation were eluted sequentially to a MALDI-TOF MS sample target. Both pI and mass information were obtained from the complex biological sample, similar to traditional 2D techniques, and the platform was faster, more automatable, and simpler than 2D gel techniques for proteomics studies.

References

1. Hjerten S (1967) Free Zone Electrophoresis. Chromatogr Rev 9:122
2. Kakehi K, Kinoshita M, Nakano M (2002) Analysis of glycoproteins and the oligosaccharides thereof by high performance capillary electrophoresis – significance in regulatory studies on biopharmaceutical products. Biomed Chromatogr 16:103–115
3. Tran TT, Cabanes-Macheteau M, Taverna M (2002) Analysis of glycoproteins and their glycopeptide and glycan fragments by electrophoresis and capillary electrophoresis. In: El Rassi Z (ed) Carbohydrate analysis by modern chromatography and electrophoresis. journal of chromatography library vol. 66 Elsevier, Amsterdam, pp 777–785
4. Thibault P, Honda S (eds) (2004) Capillary electrophoresis of carbohydrates. Humana, Totowa, NJ
5. Ma S, Nashabeh W (2001) Analysis of protein therapeutics by capillary electrophoresis. Chromatographia Suppl. 53:S75–S89
6. Patrick JS, Rener BP, Clanton GS, Lagu AS (2004) Analysis of neutral N-linked oligosaccharides from antibodies using free-solution capillary electrophoresis in bare fused-silica capillaries. In: Strege MA, Lagu AS, (eds) Methods in molecular biology, vol. 276: capillary electrophoresis of proteins and peptides. Humana, Totawa, NJ, pp 137–152
7. Ma S, Lau W, Keck R, Briggs J, Jones A, Moorhouse K, Nashabeh W (2005) Capillary electrophoresis of carbohydrates derivatized with fluorophoric compounds. In: Smales C, James D (eds) Methods in molecular biology, vol. 308: therapeutic proteins. Humana, Totowa, NJ, pp 397–409
8. Kamoda S, Nomura C, Kinoshita M, Nishiura S, Ishikawa R, Kakehi K, Kawasaki N, Hayakawa T (2004) Profiling analysis of oligosaccharides in antibody pharmaceuticals by capillary electrophoresis. J Chromatogr A 1050:211–216
9. Suzuki S, Tanaka R, Takada K, Inoue N, Yashima Y, Honda, A, Honda S (2001) Analysis of sialo-N-glycans in glycoproteins as 1-phenyl-3-methyl-5-pyrazolone derivatives by capillary electrophoresis. J. Chromatogr. A 910:319–329
10. Chen F (2003) Characterization of Oligosaccharides from Starch, Dextran, Cellulose, and Glycoproteins by Capillary Electrophoresis. In: Thibault P, Honda S (eds) Methods in molecular biology, vol. 213: capillary electrophoresis of carbohydrates. Humana, Totawa, NJ, pp 105–120

11. Bateman K, White R, Yaguchi M, Thibault P (1998) Characterization of protein glycoforms by capillary-zone electrophoresis-nanoelectrospray mass spectrometry. J Chromatogr A 794:327–344

12. Hoffstetter-Kuhn S, Alt G, Kuhn R. (1996) Profiling of oligosaccharide-mediated microheterogeneity of a monoclonal antibody by capillary electrophoresis. Electrophoresis 17(2):418–422

13. Kakehi K, Kinoshita M, Kawakami D, Tanaka J, Sei K, Endo K, Oda Y, Iwaki M, Masuko T (2001) Capillary electrophoresis of sialic acid-containing glycoprotein. Effect of the heterogeneity of carbohydrate chains on glycoform separation using an α-acid glycoprotein as a model. Anal Chem 73:2640–2647

14. Sei K, Nakano M, Kinoshita M, Masuko T, Kakehi K (2002) Collection of glycoprotein molecular species by capillary electrophoresis and the analysis of their molecular masses and carbohydrate chains. J Chromatogr. A 958: 273–281

15. Wuyts B, Delanghe J (2003) The analysis of carbohydrate-deficient transferring, marker of chronic alcoholism, using capillary electrophoresis. Clin Chem Lab. Med. 41(6):739–746

16. Honda S, Taga A (2003) Studies of carbohydrate-protein interaction by capillary electrophoresis. Methods Enzym 362:434–454

17. Nakajima K, Oda Y, Kinoshita M, Kakehi K (2003) Capillary affinity electrophoresis for the screening of post-translational modification of proteins with carbohydrates. J Prot Res 2(1):81–88

18. Nakajima K, Kinoshita M, Oda Y, Masuko T., Kaku H, Shibuya N, Kakehi K (2004) Screening method of carbohydrate-binding proteins in biological sources by capillary affinity electrophoresis and its application in tulip bulbs. Glycobiology 14(9):793–804

19. Schenerman M, Bowen S (2001) Optimization, validation, and use of capillary gel electrophoresis for quality control testing of Synagis®, a monoclonal antibody. Chromatographia Suppl 53:S66–S74

20. Schenerman M, Bowen S (2001) Optimizing sample preparation for capillary gel electrophoresis. LC-GC 19(2):190–198

21. Lee H, Chang S, Fritsche E (2002) Rational approach to quantitative sodium dodecyl sulfate capillary gel electrophoresis of monoclonal antibodies. J Chromatogr A 947:143–149

22. Brooks S, Sydor W, Guariglia L, Obara J, Mengisen R (2003) Process and product monitoring of recombinant DNA-derived biopharmaceuticals with high-performance capillary electrophoresis. J. Cap. Electrophoresis 8(5–6):87–99

23. Klyushnichenko V (2004) Capillary electrophoresis in the analysis and monitoring of biotechnological processes. In: Strege MA, Lagu AS (eds) Methods in molecular biology, vol. 276: capillary electrophoresis of proteins and peptides. Humana, Totawa, NJ, pp 77–120

24. Good D, Cummins-Bitz S, Fields R, Nunnally B (2004) Capillary electrophoresis of proteins in a quality control environment. In: Strege MA, Lagu AS (eds) Methods in molecular biology, vol. 276: capillary electrophoresis of proteins and peptides. Humana, Totawa, NJ, pp 121–136

25. Nagata H, Tabuchi M, Hirano K, Baba Y (2005) High-speed separation of proteins by microchip electrophoresis using a polyethylene glycol-coated plastic chip with a sodium dodecyl sulfate-linear polyacrylamide solution. Electrophoresis 26: 2687–2691

26. Tsai S, Loughran M, Suzuki H, Karube I (2004) Native and sodium dodecyl sulfate-capillary gel electrophoresis of proteins on a single microchip. Electrophoresis 25:494–501

27. Han J, Singh A (2004) Rapid protein separations in ultra-short microchannels: microchip sodium dodecyl sulfate-polyacrylamide gel electrophoresis and isoelectric focusing. J Chromatogr A 1049:205–209

28. Luo S, Feng J, Pang H (2004) High-throughput protein analysis by multiplexed sodium dodecyl sulfate capillary gel electrophoresis with UV absorption detection. J Chromatogr A 1051:131–134

29. Guttman A (2004) The evolution of capillary gel electrophoresis: from proteins to DNA sequencing. LCGC North America 22(9):896–904

30. Lu J, Liu S, Pu Q (2005) Replaceable cross-linked polyacrylamide for high performance separation of proteins. J Prot Res 4:1012–1016

31. Liu H, Yang C, Yang Q, Zhang W, Zhang Y (2005) On-line combination of capillary isoelectric focusing and capillary non-gel sieving electrophoresis using a hollow-fiber membrane interface: a novel two-dimensional separation system for proteins. J Chromatogr B 817:119–126

32. Graf M, Waetzig H (2004) Capillary isoelectric focusing-reproducibility and protein adsorption. Electrophoresis 25(17):2959–2964

33. Yang C, Zhang W, Zhang J, Duen J, Zhang Y (2005) Protocol of capillary isoelectric focusing to separate extremely acidic and basic proteins. J Sep Science 28(1):78–86

34. Jochheim C, Novick S, Balland A, Mahan-Boyce J, Wang WC, Goetze A, Gombotz W (2001) Separation of enbrel (rhuTNFR:Fc) isoforms by capillary isoelectric focusing. Chromatographia Suppl 53:S59–S65

35. Wu J, Wu X, Huang T, Pawliszyn J (2004) Analysis of proteins by CE, CIEF, and microfluidic devices with whole-column-imaging detection. In: Strege MA, Lagu AS (eds) Methods in molecular biology, vol. 276: capillary electrophoresis of proteins and peptides. Humana, Totawa, NJ, pp 229–252

36. Liu Z, Pawliszyn J (2005) Coupling of solid-phase microextraction and capillary isoelectric focusing with laser-induced fluorescence whole column imaging detection for protein analysis. Anal Chem 77(1):165–171

37. Wehr T (2005) Coupling capillary isoelectric focusing with mass spectrometry. LCGC North America (Suppl.): 80–85

38. Martinovic S, Pasa-Tolic L, Smith R (2004) Capillary isoelectric focusing-mass spectrometry of proteins and protein complexes. In: Strege MA, Lagu AS (eds) Methods in molecular biology, vol. 276: capillary electrophoresis of proteins and peptides. Humana, Totawa, NJ, pp 291–304

39. Zhou F, Johnston M (2005) Protein profiling by capillary isoelectric focusing, reversed-phase liquid chromatography, and mass spectrometry. Electrophoresis 26(7–8):1383–1388

40. Kuroda Y, Yukinaga H, Kitano M, Noguchi T, Nemati M, Shibukawa A, Nakagawa T, Matsuzaki K (2005) On-line capillary isoelectric focusing-mass spectrometry for quantitative analysis of peptides and proteins. J Pharm Biomed Anal 37(3):423–428

41. Storms H, van der Heijden R, Tjaden U, van der Greef J (2004) Capillary isoelectric focusing-mass spectrometry for shotgun approach in proteomics. Electrophoresis, 25(20):3461–3467

42. Wang Y, Balgley B, Lee C (2005) Tissue proteomics using capillary isoelectric focusing-based multidimensional separations. Expert Rev. of Proteomics 2(5):659–667

43. Wang Y, Rudnick P, Evans E, Li J, Zhuang Z, DeVoe D, Lee C, Balgley B (2005) Proteome analysis of microdissected tumor tissue using a capillary isoelectric focusing-based multidimensional separation platform coupled with ESI-tandem MS. Anal. Chem. 77(20):6549–6556

44. Wang Y, Balgley B, Rudnick P, Evans E, DeVoe D, Lee C (2005) Integrated capillary isoelectric focusing / nano-reversed phase liquid chromatography coupled with ESI-MS for characterization of intact yeast proteins. J Prot Res 4(1):36–42

45. Storms H, van der Jeijden R, Tjaden U, van der Greef J (2005) Optimization of protein identification from digests as analyzed by capillary isoelectric focusing-mass spectrometry. J Chromatogr B 824(1–2):189–200

46. Crowley T, Hayes M (2005) Analysis of human blood serum using the off-line coupling of capillary isoelectric focusing to matrix-assisted laser desorption/ionization time of flight mass spectrometry. Proteomics 5(14):3798–3804

26

Autoradiography and Fluorography

Bronwen M. Harvey

1. Introduction

Autoradiography is a technique widely used in biology and medicine. It uses a photographic emulsion to visualize molecules that are radioactively labeled. The technique provides a convenient method of detection, giving an accurate representation of the distribution of the label within a sample. The image is often referred to as the autoradiograph or autoradiogram.

The image is generated through the radioactive decay of the labeled ligand that is bound to a protein and/or nucleic acid found within a tissue or cell or held on an insert solid support (see **Table 26.1**). For example, it can be used to:

- Identify a specific protein from a mixture separated by polyacrylamide electrophoresis *(1)* and held on a support: Western blotting *(2)*.
- Identify nucleic acid fragments separated by gel electrophoresis held on a support: Southern blotting *(3)*, Northern blotting *(4)*.
- Identify the distribution of nucleic acids in a tissue section: in situ hybridization *(5,6)*.
- Identify the cellular location of a radioactive drug product introduced into a metabolic pathway in vivo *(7)*.

The first autoradiograph was obtained accidentally in 1867 when Niepce de St Victor observed the blackening of a silver chloride and silver iodide emulsion by uranium nitrate. The first biological experiments were undertaken in 1924 and involved the analysis of the distribution of polonium in biological specimens, although the development of autoradiograph as a biological technique did not start until the mid twentieth century following the development of photographic emulsions using silver halides. The quality and accuracy of the image depends on many factors including the autoradiographic technique, the radioisotope employed, the photographic medium used to record the image and the photographic process itself.

Autoradiography can be further divided into microautoradiography and macroautoradiography. The former involves the use of liquid emulsions into which a sample is dipped, following exposure and development of

From: *Molecular Biomethods Handbook, 2nd Edition.*
Edited by: J. M. Walker and R. Rapley © Humana Press, Totowa, NJ

Table 26.1. Autoradiography methods used with Life Science applications.

Application	Result required	Label	Method
Southern/Northern blots	High speed and sensitivity	^{32}P	Preflash and screens at −70°C
	Accurate quantification		
Plaque/Colony lifts	Maximum speed and sensitivity	^{32}P	Screens at −70°C
	Optimum resolution	$^{33}P/^{35}S$	Direct autoradiography
Slot blots	High speed and sensitivity	^{32}P	Preflash and screens at −70°C
	Accurate quantification		
	Maximum speed and sensitivity	^{32}P	Screens at −70°C
Dideoxy sequencing	High speed	^{32}P	Direct autoradiography
	Optimum resolution and maximum speed for difficult sequences	^{35}S	Direct autoradiography
	Good resolution and speed for routine work	^{35}S	Direct autoradiography
Cycle sequencing	Optimum resolution and maximum speed for difficult sequences	^{33}P	Direct autoradiography
	Good resolution and speed for routine work	^{33}P	Direct autoradiography
Protein synthesis	Maximum speed	$^{35}S/^{14}C/^{3}H$	Preflash and screens at −70°C
	Optimum resolution	^{125}I	Indirect autoradiography

the photographic emulsion silver atoms/grains are visualized under a light microscope. Kodak's NTB-2 and NTB-3, and Hypercoat™ LM-1 (GE Healthcare) are examples of liquid emulsions currently in use. Emulsions such as Hypercoat™ EM-1 with small grain sizes are suitable for electron microscope imaging. Macroautoradiography involves the use of x-ray or radiographic films to create permanent images that replicate the distribution of a radioisotope within sample. Many vendors provide suitable autoradiography film including Fuji, GE Healthcare (Hyperfilm™), and Kodak Inc (X-Omat™ and BioMax™).

The macroautoradiographic procedure and sharpness of the resulting image depends heavily on the isotopes characteristics. The mode of decay, the energy associated with the decay and the half-life are all important properties to consider along with the amount of radioactivity associated with the specimen all affect the autoradiograph.

2. Radioisotopes

The nuclei of radioactive isotopes are unstable, they disintegrate or decay to produce a new daughter atom. Isotopes for any particular element vary slightly in their atomic mass, although the number of electrons is constant and all have the same chemical properties. The later characteristic is an important consideration in the formation and integration of radioactively labeled ligands. Isotopes typically used in Life Science applications are identified in **Table 26.2**.

Table 26.2. Commonly used isotopes in life science applications.

Isotopes	Emission	Energy (MeV[max.])	Half-life
^{3}H	Weak β	0.019	12.4 yr
^{14}C	Weak β	0.159	5730 yr
^{35}S	Weak β	0.167	87.4 d
^{33}P	Weak β	0.249	25.4 d
^{32}P	Weak β	1.709	14.3 d
^{125}I	X-ray	0.027	60 d
	γ-ray	0.035	
	Auger electrons	0.030	

2.1. Characteristics of the Different Types of Radiation

During radioactive decay alpha particles, beta particles or gamma rays are the principal emissions.

2.1.1. α Particles

Alpha (α) particles are positively charged, and consist of two protons and two neutrons. These particles are emitted by radioactive nucleic such as uranium and radium. They are capable of producing many ionizations throughout their short path length. The energy of an α particles varies, high energy particles being emitted from larger nuclei, however even those with associated high energy have low speeds. As a result of their charge and large mass α particles are easily absorbed making them unsuitable for autoradiography applications.

2.1.2. β Particles

Beta (β) particles are high energy electrons (β-) or positron (β+) and have different energies, even those produced from the same isotope. This energy distribution is important in determining the resolution of the image produced in macroautoradiography. Emitted β particles have long path length and fewer ionizations that decrease in energy with distance compared to α particles. The path itself is random and the particle can be easily deflected from its course. The particles are also absorbed by the matter they penetrate. Absorbance is dependant on the density and thickness of the absorbing material as well as the energy of the particle. This is an important consideration in selecting the isotope to use (see **Table 26.1**). Beta particles produced by ^{35}S and ^{14}C will have most of their radiation absorbed by the photographic emulsion closest to the sample, as a result demonstrate good image resolution. Low-energy emitting isotopes, such as ^{3}H provided they reach the emulsion give better resolution. This is in contrast to high-energy emissions given by isotopes like ^{32}P, which can pass through the sample and emulsion. The resolution of an image depends not only on the path length of the radioactive emission but also the photographic emulsion grain size.

2.1.3. γ-Rays

X-ray and gamma (γ) ray are two names for the same electromagnetic radiation. A γ-ray is a discrete quantity of energy without mass or charge propagated as a wave. It is distinguished from an x-ray as it is not produced as a result of electron bombardment of a metal target in a vacuum. This type of radiation is more penetrating than either α or β particles but γ-rays contain less energy. In elements with low atomic numbers (< 50), Auger electrons that have an energy similar to ^{3}H are produced as a result of the emission being absorbed by the same atomic electron shell.

3. The Photographic Process

3.1. Latent Image Formation

Photographic emulsions are a clear matrix of gelatine, in which are embedded crystals of a silver halide usually a bromide (8). In the case of film, the emulsion is cast as a thin layer on a clear solid support or base, and in most cases the emulsion is protected by an antiscratch layer. The base layer may be coated with the emulsion on one or both sides.

The crystals of silver halide, also known as the grain of the emulsion conventionally forms an eight-surface solid cube of silver and halide. Sensitive or faster films contain larger grains. Larger grains however are prone to a 'grainy' effect that leads to an image with poor resolution. Therefore films of this type are not suitable for those applications where good resolution is required. In recent years, companies such as Kodak have used crystals of silver halides that are flatter and more tubular in shape (9). So called T-grain emulsions demonstrate greater speed, for a similar total amount of silver, as the flatter shape intercepts more light without an increase in the graininess of the film.

A photographic emulsion does not generate a perfect crystal lattice. The silver ions that do not occupy a crystal position are important in the formation of the image. Relatively, the number of these interstitial silver ions is small compared to the total number. In addition there are distortions or dislocations in the uniform crystal caused by contaminants in the gelatine or molecules produced by various side reactions during emulsion formation. These imperfection sites or faults are important in image formation. In the more usual photographic process, the response of an emulsion is to light, when a photon of light of energy greater than a certain minimum value strikes the emulsion it is absorbed in a silver halide crystal. This action releases an electron from a halide ion. Should the freed electron strike a fault it becomes trapped. The now negatively charged trap attracts the positively-charged silver ion resulting in the deposition of an atom of silver. This sequence of events can occur many times in a single trap causing an aggregation of silver atoms. This aggregate forms the latent image. The latent image is converted to a visible image by the process of 'development'. The presence of silver atoms makes the whole grain susceptible to the reducing action of the developer.

A single atom of silver however is relatively unstable breaking down easily to an electron and a positive silver ion. Therefore the interval between the formation of the first silver atom and the arrival of the second photon is important. Without timely arrival of the second photon of light energy, the energy associated with the first is wasted. Successive hits are extremely unlikely in situations where light levels are low. As a result photographic emulsions are disproportionately insensitive at low intensities of light. With an increase in the intensity of light comes an increase in the efficiency of the process described. To produce a developable image, each silver halide grain will require energy from approximately five photons.

There is a fundamental difference between the response of a photographic emulsion to light and its response to ionizing radiation. In the latter the silver halide crystal is exposed to the electrons resulting from an absorption event. The electron can transmit hundreds of times more energy through the crystals or gains than a photon of light. The number of grains exposed per interaction can vary from one grain per 10 KeV of ionizing radiation to 50 or more grains for a 1-MeV emission. However, with the higher energies there is a low probability of an interaction that transfers the total energy to the grains. Also higher-energy electrons pass out of an emulsion before all their energy is dissipated. It is estimated for high energy emissions, that 5–10 grains are made developable per interaction. In this type of autoradiography (direct) at low levels of exposure each increment of exposure results in the same number of grains becoming developable. Therefore there is a direct relationship between the density or blackness of the image and exposure. Only when the exposure becomes so great that appreciable energy is wasted on grains already exposed does the linear relationship break down. This characteristic allows quantification studies to be carried out using direct autoradiography. Practically this is generally limited to two or three orders of magnitude.

Weak β emissions such as those from ^3H and ^{14}C may be absorbed by the sample before reaching the emulsion and hence do not contribute to latent image formation. This quenching can also be overcome with the use of scintillator that is allowed to penetrate the sample before it is exposed to the photographic emulsion. Refer to the Section 5 on indirect autoradiography.

3.2. The Development Process

The development process is key to the formation of permanent image. However the process of development also affects image quality, imaging stability as well as film drying.

During development of a photographic emulsion the silver halide is reduced to metallic silver. Typically used developing agents include hydroquinone and phenidone, often a mixture of developers are used, these can provide for a superior image. The development reaction is speeded up by the presence of the metallic silver in the latent image. The latent image acts as an electron conducting bridge by which electrons from the developing agent reach the silver ion. Electrons are easily given up to an exposed crystal but not an unexposed crystal. The electrons combine with the silver ion in the crystal neutralising the positive charge producing an atom of silver.

A typical developing solution consists of several components each of which has a purpose. For good image quality it is important to mix developing components well and in the correct order using a good quality diluent where concentrates are used. An alkali with strong buffering capacity is required owing to the liberation of hydrogen ions that accompanies the development process. Lower capacity buffering agents result in poor developer shelf life with frequent replenishment being required. The presence of a preservative prevents oxidation of the developing agents, thereby prolonging its life. Commonly sulphite salts are used for the purpose. The preservative also reacts with the reaction products of the development process maintaining the development rate and preventing staining of the photographic layer when film is used. Hence the ratio of preservative to developer is critical to performance. An antifog agent assists in producing good quality images, typically bromide is used. These agents decrease the concentration of silver ion in solution, protecting unexposed crystals from the action of the developer thereby sustaining the latent image produced during exposure. Antifog agents therefore affect the development rate and the amount of film blackening (density). Hardeners frequently used in automatic processes limit film swell and help to protect the film from processing artefacts. Glutaraldehyde is the commonest hardener in use. Developers may also contain solvents to kept the developing agent in solution and a sequestering agent that counters the adverse effect of impurities are often introduced in the water used to prepare the developer from its concentrate. Water quality is therefore important in generating good quality images.

Following development the image must be stabilized or fixed. The fixing stage dissolves any nonmetallic silver halide and renders the emulsion transparent; the emulsion at this stage is soft and easily damaged. Film antiscratch layers serve to protect the film at this stage as well as during exposure manipulations. Fixing agents stop the development process. Thiosulphates are the most common fixing agents. As with the developer, fixing solutions contain a preservative, a sulphide usually, to prevent oxidation and prolong the solution's shelf life. The hardener, commonly an aluminium salt, protects the film from damage and helps accelerate the drying process. Buffering agents maintain a constant pH and, as with the developer, affects the fixative replenishment rate. Sequestering agents prevent the formation of aluminium hydroxide that lead to improper drying of the film.

Between each of the steps and before drying, washing is required to remove residual chemicals. A good washing technique with good quality water helps to eliminate artefacts, prevents contamination of the fixative with developer, removes excessive fix, and enhances the stability of the image as well as promoting drying. Like the development and fixation steps, washing is sensitive to time and temperature.

It is important to follow the manufacturers' instructions for the preparation, use and storage of developers and fixatives. Most type of x-ray film can be processed by hand or automatically using a film processor. However, different films will often require different lengths of processing. Film lacking antiscratch layers are not suitable for automatic processing and care must be taken during hand processing to prevent film artefacts.

4. Direct Autoradiography

Coating photographic emulsions on to a support producing an "x-ray film" is the most commonly available autoradiography product. In principle there are two type of x-ray film, the direct type and the screen type, although most x-ray films are suitable for both techniques, refer to **Table 26.1**. Direct films are suitable for use with the isotopes ^{33}P, ^{35}S, ^{14}C, and ^{3}H provided their emissions are not absorbed by the sample. Direct autoradiography is the method of choice where resolution is more important than sensitivity. The lack of an antiscratch layer may improve sensitivity particularly when used with weaker β emitters such as ^{3}H. The sample should be held as close as possible to the film to maximize spatial resolution. Exposure occurs at room temperature although −20/−70°C exposure are advantageous for wet samples as freezing avoids diffusion of the radioactive label. The resulting images are quantifiable. Most films are double-coated but the disadvantage of this type of film structure is reduced resolution compared to single-coated film. In the case of medium energy β-emitters, for example ^{35}S and ^{14}C as most of the energy is absorbed close to the sample, the second layer does not contribute significantly to the image.

Liquid photographic emulsions are also available to the researcher these products are particularly useful when working with tissue sections and/or layers of cultured cells. In this case the sample is dipped into the liquid emulsion under dark room conditions where it is allowed to solidify before an appropriate period of exposure. The procedure decreases the distance between the sample and the silver grains in the emulsion thus increasing sensitivity and resolution. The whole specimen is subjected to development and fixation process, this results in deposits of silver appearing embedded within the specimen. The morphology of the tissue and the signal from the radioactive probe can therefore be viewed simultaneously in a light or electron microscope *(10)*.

Screen-type films are ideal for use indirect autoradiography as they are designed to respond to light, usually light in the blue and ultraviolet range of the spectrum. However some are optimized to match the green emissions. It is therefore important to ensure films are matched to the wavelength of light produced in order to optimize performance.

5. Indirect Autoradiography

In this technique *(11)* emitted ionizing energy is converted to light by means of a scintillator. The scintillator, which can be an inorganic or organic molecule, emits many hundreds of photons of light when excited by a single β particle or γ ray.

5.1. Fluorography

The process of indirect autoradiography is achieved using fluorography, when the sample is impregnated with the scintillator. Fluorography helps overcome the problem of quenching within the sample, because the photon of light is capable of travelling further than the original β particles. This technique is ideal for use with the lower energy β emitters such as ^{33}P, ^{35}S, and ^{14}C. Exposures must occur at $-70°C$ *(12)* to maximize the effect of the scintillator. Because of dispersion effects image resolution is adversely affected with this technique therefore is not suitable for those application where resolution is important. Scintillators include 2,5-diphenyloxazole (PPO) *(1,13)*, sodium salicylate *(14)* and the commercially available branded reagents including Amplify™ (GE Healthcare), Fluoro-Hance™ (Research Products International), and EA-wax(GenTaur), refer to **Table 26.3** for some protocol details.

5.2. Intensifying Screens

Placing a screen, usually referred to as intensifying screens, incorporating a scintillator behind the film to which the sample is directly applied allows the highly energetic emissions that pass straight through the film, without transferring their energy to the crystal lattice, to be converted to light (see **Fig. 26.1**). For conventional intensifying screen to bear benefits, radiation from the

Table 26.3. Polyacrylamide gel fluorography protocols.

Method	PPO in DMSO	PPO in glacial acetic acid	Sodium salicylate	Amplify™
Fixing advisable	Yes	No	Yes	Yes
Recommended fixer/ time	Acetic acid: 2 vol Methanol: 9 vol Water: 9 vol 1 h	-	Acetic acid: 2 vol Methanol: 9 vol Water: 9 vol 30 min	7%(v/v) acetic acid 30 min
Presoak required	2 × 30 min in DMSO	1 × 5 min in glacial acetic acid	1 × 30 min in water	None
Scintillant cocktail	4× gel volume of 22.2% (w/v) PPO in DMSO	4× gel volume of 20% (w/v) PPO in glacial acetic acid	10× gel volume of 1 M sodium salicylate pH 5.0–7.0	4x gel volume of Amplify, as supplied™
Time to impregnate	3 h	1.5 h	0.5 h	0.3–0.5 h
Rinses	1 h in 20x gel volume of water	1 × 30 min in water	None	None
Drying	Under vacuum, 1 h	Under vacuum at 70°C 3–5 h	Under vacuum at 80°C 1 h	Under vacuum at 70–80°C 1 h

PPO, 2,5-diphenyloxazole; DMSO, dimethyl sulphoxide.
The information is appropriate for gels up to 1-mm thick. Thicker gels may require longer incubation times.

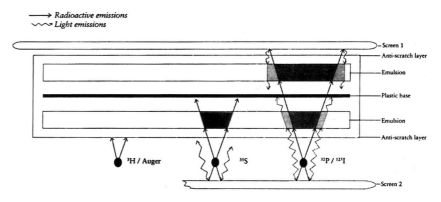

Fig. 26.1. Use of intensifying screens: a compromise between sensitivity gain and resolution loss

radioisotope must have an energy greater than 0.4 MeV. This allows the β energy to reach the intensifying screen. These screens are therefore limited to use with, ^{32}P and ^{125}I *(15)*, i.e., those with associated high energy β particles. The radioisotopes such a ^{14}C, ^{35}S, ^{33}P and ^{3}H lack sufficient energy to penetrate the base and/or the second emulsion layers. Unfortunately it is these lower energy radioisotopes that would benefit most from the action of intensifying screen. Intensifying screens contain an inorganic phosphor; calcium tungstate ($CaWO_4$) is the commonest form that produces blue light. Terbium-activated rare-earth oxysulphides such as lanthanum oxysulphide produce green light. The performance of the screen will vary with the coverage and thickness of the phosphor in the screen as well as the phosphor grain size and its purity.

The photons produced from the bombardment of the intensifying screen by β particle or γ rays produces the photographic image, which is superimposed on the radiographic image. Use of a film/screen system increases the sensitivity of the film, and helps overcome the problem of under-representation at low light intensities *(16)*. Often the use of two screens offers little benefits over the use of one as sample usually obscures one of the screens. The conversion of radiation to light decreases image resolution and the different responses of the emulsion to radiation and light means that unlike direct autoradiography quantification is only possible after preflashing (see Section 6). Reducing the temperature during exposure helps stabilize the latent image, by reducing thermal reversion of the silver atom there by stabilizing the excited silver halide crystals, increasing the time available to capture the second photon of energy. The optimal temperature for stable latent image formation is between –60 and –80°C. Hence exposure using this technique occurs at –70°C, the effect of intensifying screens at room temperature is minimal. The difference between latent image formation between light and ionizing radiation means that the reducing the temperature during direct autoradiography has no effect on sensitivity when this technique is used.

The recent introduction of gadolinuium oxysulphide:terbium (GOS) screens, which emit in the green range of the spectrum, have improved the performance of green light intensifying screen. This benefit has been provided by Kodak who in 1995 introduced the GOS phosphor in their TranScreen™ system *(17)*. This patented system helps eliminates absorbance by the film support and offers reduced exposure times when used in combination with T-grain BioMax™ film to which it is matched. TranScreen LS intensifying screens provide improved resolution with all types of β-particles. The TranScreen™ HE intensifying screen has a thicker layer of phosphor converts more of the high energy emissions offering an improvement in sensitivity compared to a conventional system.

6. Preflashing

The relationship between the amount of radioactivity and blackening of the film is not linear. Preflashing can help overcome under-representation at low levels of light or ionizing radiation; there is no effect for large amounts. As a technique it can be used in those circumstances where the use of low temperature exposures as required with intensifying screen are not possible. These include chemiluminescence *(18,19)* detection where the use of the low temperatures would significantly affect the light producing enzymatic reaction, see **Fig. 26.2**. Preflashing increases the sensitivity for the low signals giving the film a greater linear response, allowing accurate quantification over a wider range if required.

The film is pre-exposed to an instantaneous flash of light prior to the sample's exposure to the film. This flash of light allows for at least two conversions of silver ions to atoms with the silver halide crystal. As a result, the reversible stage of latent image formation is overcome. Obviously, the conditions for preflashing require careful optimisation (see **Fig. 26.3**). Preflashing the film, so that its absorbance at 450 mm after development is

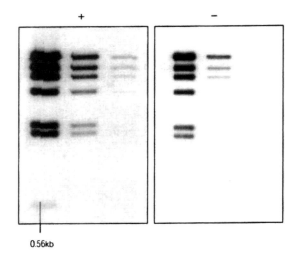

Fig. 26.2. Lambda Hind III digest (10-fold dilution) ECL™ (GE Healthcare Ltd) detected and exposed to Hyperfilm™ ECL (GE Healthcare Ltd). Note the presence of the 0.56 Kb fragment after preflashing, demonstrating increased sensitivity following this procedure

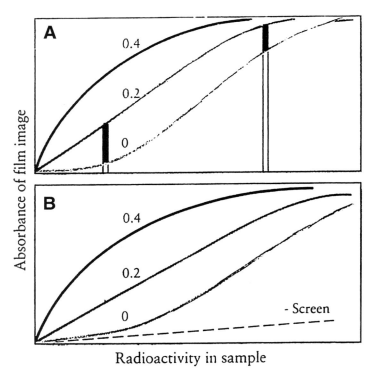

Fig. 26.3. Preflashing requirement for pre-exposure to obtain a linear response of film to light from **(A)** a ^{3}H fluorography or **(B)** ^{32}P with an intensifying screen. Preflashing absorbance of 0, 0.2 or 0.4 U above the absorbance of the unflashed film are shown. The vertical bars in (A) illustrate how the effect of preflashing is easily under estimated when it is assessed only with large amounts of radioactivity

increased by 0.1–0.2 absorbance units compared to the control, effectively introduces a stable pair of silver atoms per crystal. Preflashing above this range will disproportionately increase the film's responses to low levels of light. The effect of preflashing is greater for longer exposure times. The flash of light must be short, 1 ms is sufficient, and the light source should be of appropriate intensity and wavelength. These conditions are provided by most photographic flash units.

7. Storage and Handling of Autoradiographic Products

The storage and handling of autoradiographic products is important for achieving high quality reproducible results. Film products and emulsions must be stored away from penetration radiation at temperatures between 10 and 20°C in humidity between 30 and 50%. Storing the film upright and avoiding stacking avoids film artefacts. It is important to remove the film gently from its box or the exposure device/cassette, rapid movement can cause a static discharge leading to blemishes on the film. Some vendors provide film inter-leaved with paper or alternatively individual sheets of film sealed in light-tight envelopes that give maximum protection. These film envelopes are particularly useful for the infrequent user.

In the darkroom ensure the area is protected from white light penetration. Ensure the proper safelight conditions are available. Improper bulb wattage, filter type and distance between the safelight and the photographic emulsion will fog film or result in high levels of background in applications using liquid emulsions.

8. Filmless Autoradiography

Limitations in image quality and detection of low levels of radioactive labeling have prompted development of a number of image capture systems with improved resolution and/or sensitivity. Digital autoradiography is now well established in many areas of Life Science research.

PhosphorImager devices such as Storm™ and Typhoon™ (GE Healthcare) are instruments designed for the Life Science research. These instruments utilize storage phosphor autoradiography (20), originally described by Kodak. A re-useable screen, made from europium:barium fluorobromide (Eu:BaFBr) for example, is used instead of film. The screen, cleared by exposure to visible light, is able to capture quantitative data from the radio-labeled sample. The technique differs from intensifying screens in that rather than producing light in response to ionizing radiation these screens store a portion of the energy in the form of a trapped electrical charge within the phosphor material. The distribution of these trapped charges mirrors the distribution of radioactive label within the sample. The exposure to ionizing radiation results in the oxidation of Eu(2+) to Eu(3+) and a reduction of BaFBr to BaFBr⁻. When the exposed screen is irradiated with light of an appropriate wavelength (633 nm) from a helium-neon laser the trapped charges recombine releasing a photon of blue light (590 nm) that is collected simultaneously to provide a quantitative representation of the sample.

9. Appendix: Working Safely with Radioactive Materials *(21)*

This advice does not replace any instruction or training in your establishments, local rules or advise from your Radiation Protection Adviser.

In general, compounds labeled with low energy emitters may be handled safely in the small quantities found in most research and teaching laboratories with only modest precautions. When handling high energy β emitters, such as ^{32}P or γ-labeled compounds further precautions are necessary. Although radiation protection can be a complex subject, it is possible to simplify it to ten basic things you should do–golden rules.

1. Understand the nature of the hazard and get practical training. Never work with unprotected cuts or breaks in the skin. Never use any mouth-operated equipment. Always store compounds under the conditions recommended. Label all containers, clearly indicating nuclide, compound, specific activity, total activity, date and name of the user. Containers should be properly sealed and shielded.

2. Plan ahead to minimize the time spent handling radioactivity. To check your procedure, do a dummy run of your procedures without radioactivity. The shorter the time the smaller the dose.

3. Distance yourself appropriately from the sources of radiation doubling the distance from the source quarters the radiation dose (inverse square law).

4. Use appropriate shielding for the radiation. One centimetre of Perspex will γ stop all β emissions, but beware of Bremsstrahlung radiation from high energy emitters. Use suitable thickness of lead for γ emitters or x-rays.

5. Contain radioactive materials in define work areas. Always keep active and inactive work separate, preferably by maintaining rooms to be used solely for radioactive work. Always work over a spill tray and work in a ventilated enclosure.

6. Wear appropriate protective clothing and dosimeter. Local rules will define what dosimeters should be worn.

7. Monitor the work area frequently for contamination control. In the event of a spill follow a prepared contingency plan: Verbally warn all people in the vicinity. Restrict unnecessary movement into and through the area. Report the spill to the radiation protection supervisor/advisor. Treat the contaminated personnel first. Follow a clean up protocol.

8. Follow the local rules and safe ways of working. Do not eat, drink, smoke or apply cosmetics in an area where radioactivity is handled. Use paper handkerchiefs and dispose of the appropriately. Never pipet radioactive solutions by mouth. Always work carefully and tidily.

9. Minimize the accumulation of waste and dispose of it by an appropriate route. Use the minimum quantity of radioactivity needed for the investigation. The disposal of radioactive material is subject to statutory control. Be aware of the requirements and use only an authorized route for disposal.

10. After completion of the work, monitor yourself, wash and monitor again. Report to the local supervisor if contamination is found.

Acknowledgments: Figures reproduced from a "Guide to Autoradiography" and Efficient detection of Biomolecules by Autoradiography, Fluorography and Chemiluminescence. Review booklet 23. GE Healthcare UK Ltd, Amersham Place, Little Chalfont, Buckinghamshire, HP7 9NA, England.

References

1. Bonner WM, Laskey RA (1974) Film detection method for tritium-labeled proteins and nucleic acids in polyacrylamide gels. Eur J Biochem 46:83–88
2. Towbin H, Staehelin T, Gordin J (1979) Electrophoretic transfer of proteins from polyacrylamide gels to nitrocellulose sheets: procedure and some applications. Proc Natl Acad Sci USA 76:4530–4354
3. Southern EM (1975) Detection of specific sequences among DNA fragments separated by gel electrophoresis. J Mol Bio 98:503–517
4. Alwine JC, Kemp DJ, Stark GR (1977) Method for detection of specific RNAs in agarose gels by transfer to diazobenzyloxymethyl-paper and hybridisation with DNA probes. Proc Natl Acad Sci USA 74:5350–5354
5. Pardue ML, Gall JG (1969) Formation and detection of RNA-DNA hybrid molecules in cytological preparations. Proc Natl Acad Sci USA 63:378–383
6. Jin L, Lloyd RV (1997) In-situ methods and applications J. Clin Lab. Anal. 11(1): 2–9.
7. Clark CR, Hall MD (1986) Hormone receptor autoradiography: recent developments. Trends in Biochem Sci 11:95–199
8. Rogers A (1979) Techniques of Autoradiography, 3rd edn. Elsevier Amsterdam.
9. Steinfield R, McLaughlin W, Vizard D, Bundy D (1994) Advances in autoradiography; a new film brings quality improvements. The biotechnology report. London UK. Campden Publishing Ltd, UK, pp.147–149
10. Pickel VM, Beaudet A (1984) In: Polak JM, Varndell M (eds) Immunolabelling for Electron microscopy. Elsevier, Oxford, UK
11. Laskey RA Efficient detection of Biomolecules by Autoradiography, Fluorography and Chemiluminescence. Review booklet 23. GE Healthcare UK Ltd, Amersham Place, Little Chalfont, Buckinghamshire, HP7 9NA, England
12. Luthi U, Waser PG (1966) Thin layer fluorography of tritium labelled compounds. Adv Tracer Methodol 3:149–155
13. Skinner MK, Griswold MD (1983) Fluorographic detection of radioactivity in polyacrylamide gels with 2,5-diphenyloxazole in acetic acid and its comparison with existing procedures Biochem J 209:281–284
14. Chamberlain JP (1979) Fluorographic detection of radioactivity in polyacrylaminde gels with water-soluble fluor, sodium-salicylate. Anal Biochem 98:132–135
15. Laskey RA, Mills AD (1977) Enhanced autoradiographic detection of ^{32}P and ^{125}I using intensifying screens and hypersensitized film. FEBS Letters 82:314–316
16. Swanstrom R, Shank P (1978) X-ray intensifying screen greatly enhance detection by autoradiography of the radioactive isotopes ^{32}P and ^{125}I. Anal Biochem 86: 184–192
17. Kodak A universal intensifying screen system for enhanced detection of low and high energy isotopes. KSI_IC0005-07/05, 2003
18. Whitehead TP, Thorpe GHG, Carter CJN, Groucutt C, Kricka LJ (1983) Enhanced luminescence procedure for sensitive determination of peroxidase-labelled conjugated in immunoassay. Nature 305:158,159
19. Schaap AP, Akhavan-Tafti H, Romano LJ (1989) Chemiluminescent substrate for alkaline phosphatase, application to ultrasensitive enzyme-linked immunoassays and DNA probes. Clin Chem 35:1863–1864
20. Kanekal S, Sahai A, Jones RE, Brown DJ (1995) Storage-phosphor autoradiography: A rapid and highly sensitive method for spatial imaging and quantification of radioisotopes. J Pharma and Tox Methods 33(3):171–178

21. Extracts from Safe and Secure. A guide to working safely with radioactive compounds. GE Healthcare UK Ltd, Amersham Place, Little Chalfont, Buckinghamshire, HP7 9NA, England

27

Mass Spectrometry of Proteins and Peptides

Kenneth G. Standing

1. Introduction

In the last few years, mass spectrometry (MS) has emerged as a major tool for the identification and characterization of peptides and proteins. It is now possible to measure proteins of masses >100 kDa to an accuracy of a few Da, and to measure the masses of peptides with an accuracy of a few mDa. As a result, the information yielded by an MS measurement is highly specific. In addition, MS has extremely high sensitivity, often in the femtomole (10^{-15} mole) range, so it is a method that is suitable for the analysis of trace amounts of sample.

Mass spectrometry relies on the properties of charged particles moving under the influence of electric and magnetic fields, so the species studied must be ions (charge ze) rather than molecules. Most MS experiments are performed on positive ions, which can be formed either by the removal of one or more electrons from each molecule, or by the addition of one or more cations, usually protons. Consequently, the first step in any mass measurement is to transfer the molecule into the gas phase and to ionize it; what is actually measured then is the ratio of molecular mass to charge (m/z).

Most biological samples are mixtures of a number of compounds, so their m/z spectra can be very complex. Moreover, even pure compounds yield a number of peaks in their m/z spectra, corresponding to various values of charge z, and to the distribution of isotopes in the compound. The main isotope effect in organic compounds is caused by the ~1.1% ^{13}C in natural carbon. For example, **Fig. 27.1** shows the m/z spectra of two singly charged peptide ions. In **Fig. 27.1A** the most abundant peak in the spectrum is the "monoisotopic" peak at 1053.587 Da (see definitions in **Table 27.1**), corresponding to the ions containing only the most abundant isotopes. For larger molecules, such as the peptide shown in **Fig. 27.1B**, the distribution is shifted upwards, and the monoisotopic peak is no longer the largest one. As the molecular mass increases still further, the probability that *all* atoms in the molecule consist of the most abundant isotopes decreases, so the monoisotopic peak continues to decrease until finally (at >15 kDa) it is usually too small to observe.

From: *Molecular Biomethods Handbook, 2nd Edition.*
Edited by: J. M. Walker and R. Rapley © Humana Press, Totowa, NJ

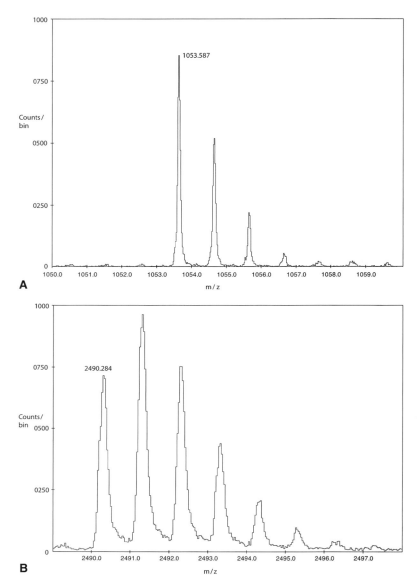

Fig. 27.1. A. MALDI-TOF spectrum of the singly-charged ions from the peptide HIPEFVRR (citrate synthase, amino acid residues 283–290). The chemical composition of the compound is $C_{48}H_{76}N_{16}O_{11}$, so the nominal mass of the singly protonated ion $(M+H)^+$ is 1053 Da (see definitions in **Table 27.1**). The values of $(M+H)^+$ corresponding to the monoisotopic mass are: 1053.587 Da (measured), and 1053.596 Da (calculated from the known chemical composition). The calculated *average* value of $(M+H)^+$ is 1054.241 Da, about 0.06% greater than its monoisotopic mass. Doubly charged ions $(M+2H)^{++}$ would be expected to appear at m/z ~528 (far below the present scale), but are not observed above background (intensity <0.3% of the singly-charged peaks). Note that in this case the probability that *all* carbons in the molecule are 12C is only ~$(0.989)^{48}$ ~0.588. **B**. MALDI-TOF spectrum of the singly-charged ions from the peptide [ALVLIAFAQYLQQCPFEDHVK] from human protein P02768 (Serum Albumin Precursor). The monatomic ion has measured $m/z = 2490.284$ (calculated $m/z = 2490.286$), and average $m/z = 2491.888$

Table 27.1. Some Definitions.

The atomic unit of mass, called u or Dalton (Da), is $1/12^{th}$ the mass of the ^{12}C atom.

The nominal mass of a molecule is calculated from the integral mass of the most abundant isotopes of its constituents, i.e., H = 1, C = 12, N = 14, O = 16 etc.

The monoisotopic mass of a molecule is calculated from the exact mass of the most abundant isotopes of its constituents, i.e., ^{1}H = 1.007825, ^{12}C = 12.000000, ^{14}N = 14.003074, ^{16}O = 15.994915, ^{32}S = 31.972070 etc.

The average mass of a molecule is calculated from the average mass of its constituents, weighted for abundance, i.e., H = 1.00794, C = 12.011 etc.

2. Methods of Ionization

Most peptides and proteins are polar, involatile, and thermally unstable, so the classical methods of ion production (evaporation, followed by electron bombardment) provide little information about molecular structure, since they usually break up the molecule into small pieces *(1)*. This situation changed dramatically about twenty years ago with the development of new ionization techniques, notably matrix-assisted laser desorption/ionization (MALDI), and electrospray ionization (ESI) – techniques that are especially well adapted to the analysis of large biomolecules.

In MALDI, the analyte is deposited on a solid surface, usually in vacuum, along with a considerable excess of "matrix," and bombarded with a series of pulses from a laser (**Fig. 27.2**). The matrix serves to absorb energy from the laser pulse, and the resulting strong heating serves to eject an expanding plume of matrix + analyte from the target surface. Reactions in the plume between the analyte molecules and the matrix ionize the analyte molecules. This process yields mostly singly charged ions, so the determination of mass from *m/z* is not usually a problem.

In electrospray ionization (ESI), shown schematically in **Fig. 27.3**, the analyte is dissolved in a suitable liquid to form a dilute acidic solution. In this solution proteins are usually unfolded, with most of their basic sites protonated. Multicharged droplets of the solution are extracted at atmospheric pressure from the electrospray needle by the application of a high voltage (a few kV) to the needle. In a typical configuration, the resulting electric field accelerates them towards a heated capillary, then through a series of small apertures into regions at progressively reduced pressure until they finally enter the high vacuum region of the mass spectrometer. During this process, ions may be produced either by ejection from a droplet, or as the residue of a droplet after evaporation of the solvent. The resulting shower of ions generally consists of a mixture of highly charged ions of various charges (**Fig. 27.4A**).

Nevertheless, the determination of charge state and molecular mass is still straightforward. Consider any two *adjacent* peaks in the electrospray spectrum, with measured *m/z* values μ_1 and μ_2. If we assume that these peaks correspond to charges z and $(z - 1)$, the measurement yields the equations $\mu_1 = m/z$ and $\mu_2 = m/(z - 1)$; i.e., two equations in two unknowns (*m* and *z*). Thus both *m* and *z* are determined; [$m = \mu_1\mu_2/(\mu_2 - \mu_1)$ and $z = \mu_2/(\mu_2 - \mu_1)$].

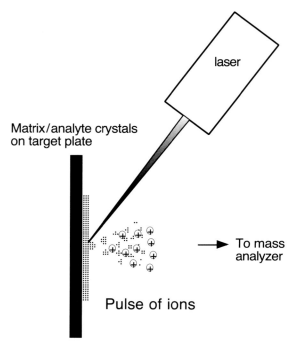

Fig. 27.2. Schematic diagram of a MALDI source. The most frequently used laser is a nitrogen UV laser running at 20 to 100 Hz, giving ~3 ns pulses at a wavelength of 337 nm. Common matrices are α-cyano-4-hydroxycinnamic acid (favored for peptides), and 2,5-dihydroxybenzoic acid (favored for proteins)

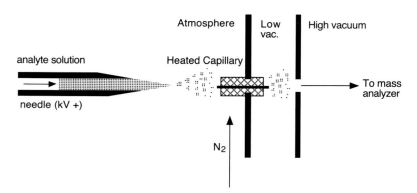

Fig. 27.3. Schematic diagram of an ESI source. Typical parameters: aqueous solution of 50% acetonitrile or methanol, 1% acetic acid; spray rate ~0.25 μL/min for electrospray, ~20 nL/min for nanospray

In practice, a "deconvolution" algorithm based on the same principle, but taking all the electrospray peaks into account, is used to calculate the overall best mass value from the resultant mass spectrum (**Fig. 27.4B**).

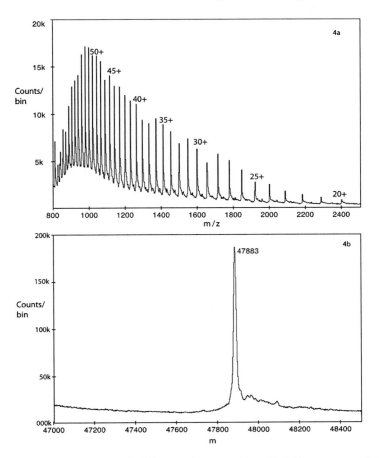

Fig. 27.4. A. ESI spectrum of wild type citrate synthase; $9\,\mu M$ in aqueous solution, 50% methanol, 1% acetic acid. Note that *each* of the multicharged peaks in the spectrum is a superposition of an isotope distribution like the one in **Fig. 27.1**, but here unresolved. **B**. Deconvoluted spectrum (i.e., the mass spectrum) corresponding to the ESI spectrum of **Fig. 27.3**; measured mass 47,883 Da, average mass calculated from the known composition 47,885 Da

3. Mass Spectrometers

There have also been significant advances in instrumentation in recent years. Mass spectrometers serve to separate charge-bearing molecules according to their values of m/z, and thus to measure their masses if the charge state is known. Classical methods used magnetic sector mass spectrometers, which gave high mass accuracy but poor sensitivity, and were not well adapted to the new ionization methods.[1] They have now been almost entirely replaced by other instruments such as time-of-flight (TOF), quadrupole, and ion resonance mass spectrometers.

---

[1] Earlier developments are described in **ref. *1***.

3.1. Time-of-Flight Mass Spectrometer

An instrument that is well adapted to MALDI measurements is the time-of-flight (TOF) mass spectrometer (2). In its simplest form (**Fig. 27.5**), ions are produced by MALDI from an analyte deposited on a conducting target surface at potential V, and are accelerated to energy zeV by the electric field between the target and a parallel grid at ground potential. The ion flight time in the field-free region between the grid and detector determines the ion speed v, and therefore its ratio of mass to charge; i.e., the ion kinetic energy $mv^2/2 = zeV$, so $m/z = 2eV/v^2 = 2eVt^2/L^2$, where t is the flight time over the field-free path length L. In practice, the defining time is measured from the time that the pulsed laser fires to the time that the ion is detected, and the value of m/z is determined from the equation $m/z = (at + b)^2$, where the constants a and b are calculated from the m/z values measured for two ions of known mass. This takes approximate account of the flight time from target to grid, and other small effects. It is important to note that a TOF instrument measures ions of all m/z values without scanning.

A more sophisticated TOF instrument is shown in **Fig. 27.6** (3). It incorporates an electrostatic ion mirror that can produce a retarding electric field. If this field is turned off, the instrument acts as a simple linear TOF spectrometer, in which the ions are registered in detector 1. This mode of operation is often preferred for measurements of large proteins.

When the electric field in the mirror is turned on, it reverses the ion direction and corrects for initial spreads in ion energy, i.e., an ion of lower than normal energy will spend more time in the field-free region than one of normal energy, but less time in the mirror. If the electric field in the mirror is adjusted to the correct value these two times almost compensate each other, so the instrument corrects for variations in the energy of ions from the source, and thus improves the resolution (3). This mode of operation is usually favored for measurements on peptides.

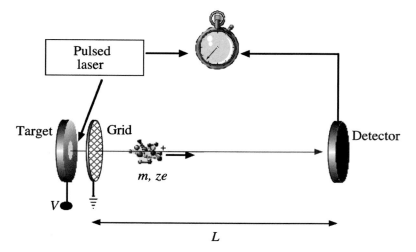

Fig. 27.5. Schematic diagram of a simple TOF mass spectrometer. The detector is normally a microchannel plate. The "clock" is usually an electronic time-to-digital converter, capable of measuring the flight time to an accuracy of a few ns

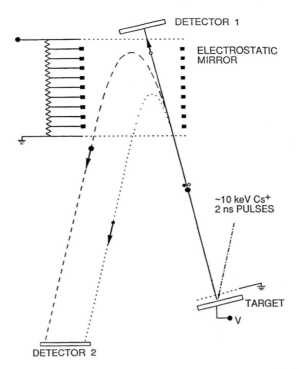

DETECTOR 1

ELECTROSTATIC
MIRROR

~10 keV Cs⁺
2 ns PULSES

TARGET

V

DETECTOR 2

Fig. 27.6. Schematic diagram of an early reflecting TOF instrument *(3)*. In this instrument's original form, analyte ions were produced as secondary ions by bombardment by ~10 keV Cs⁺ ions, as shown, but the instrument was converted later to use MALDI ions. Here, the angle between the secondary ion path and the spectrometer axis has been exaggerated for the sake of clarity; the actual angle was ~1.4°. The dashed line shows the path of a typical parent ion. If a parent ion decays along the flight path (metastable or "post-source" decay), it normally produces two products – a neutral and a charged daughter; the neutral will follow the solid line (a straight path) and can be registered in detector 1; the dotted line shows the path of the corresponding charged daughter, which is registered in detector 2

3.2. Quadrupole Mass Spectrometers

3.2.1. Linear Quadrupole Mass Filter

In contrast to the TOF spectrometer, which is most easily adapted to a pulsed ion source, the linear quadrupole is most compatible with a continuous ion source, such as electrospray *(4)*. **Fig. 27.7** shows a schematic diagram of a linear quadrupole mass filter; it consists of four rods, ideally hyperbolic, but usually cylindrical in practice. When DC voltages U_0 and alternating voltages $V_0 \cos \omega t$ (typical frequencies 700 kHz to a few MHz) are applied to the rods as indicated, focusing forces act in the transverse directions, yielding a motion described by the Mathieu equation, which depends on parameters a_u and q_u *(4)*. The motion may be stable (an oscillation about the central axis), or unstable, in which case the ions will escape radially. A typical region of stability (ABC) is illustrated in **Fig. 27.8**. If no DC voltage is applied ($U_0 = 0$, so $a_u = 0$), the motion is unstable for high values of q (beyond point C on the diagram), i.e., for low values of m/z. Thus ions are lost if their m/z values are too low, but

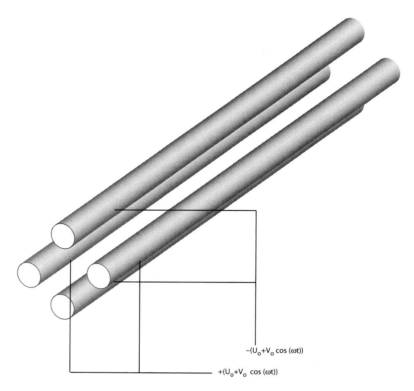

−(U₀+V₀ cos (ωt))

+(U₀+V₀ cos (ωt))

Fig. 27.7. Schematic diagram of a linear quadrupole mass filter

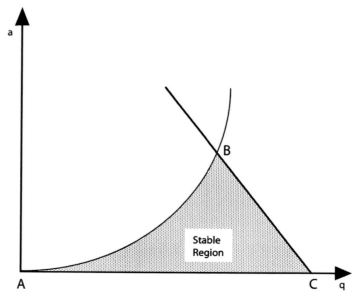

Fig. 27.8. Behavior of ions in the quadrupole mass filter. The behavior depends on the values of the Mathieu parameters a_u and q_u, $a_u = (8/r_0^2\omega^2)$ (ze/m) U_0, and $q_u = (4/r_0^2\omega^2)$ (ze/m) V_0, where r_0 is a geometrical parameter. The motion is stable only for values of a_u and q_u that lie within the region ABC

the instrument acts as an ion guide for ions with m/z values beyond the cutoff, since their motion is stable.

If an additional DC potential U_0 is applied to the rods, the range of ze/m that can undergo stable motion is restricted, particularly near the upper tip B of the stability diagram, so the device serves as a mass filter; i.e., only ions with a limited *range* of m/z values will be stable. **Fig. 27.9** shows the stability regions for several values of m/z as a function of U_0 and V_0, as well as a "scan line." If the values of U_0 and V_0 are varied along the scan line, successively larger values of m/z will be selected, so the instrument serves as a scanning mass spectrometer.

3.2.2. Quadrupole Ion Traps

Another important instrument that makes use of quadrupole electric fields is the 3-dimensional quadrupole ion trap, a versatile tool for measuring mass spectra *(4)*. It consists of three hyperbolic electrodes, (a ring and two endcaps), whose cross-section is shown in **Fig. 27.10**. The instrument is symmetrical about the z axis. An electrostatic ion gate is pulsed so as to inject ions into the trap through a hole in one of the end caps. Again there is a region of stability for oscillations within the trap, described by a slightly more complicated version of the Mathieu equation. All ions are stored in the trap while m/z analysis is performed. Collisions with helium gas (pressure ~1 mtorr) within the trapping volume damp the ion motion, and thus improve the mass resolution by reducing the ion kinetic energy and contracting the trajectories to the centre of the trap. Once the ions are trapped, and possibly manipulated,

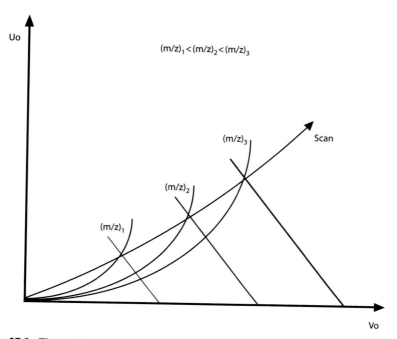

Fig. 27.9. The stability regions for several values of m/z are shown as a function of U_0 and V_0 (for constant $\omega\omega$ as well as a "scan line." If the values of U_0 and V_0 are varied along the scan line, successively larger values of m/z will be selected

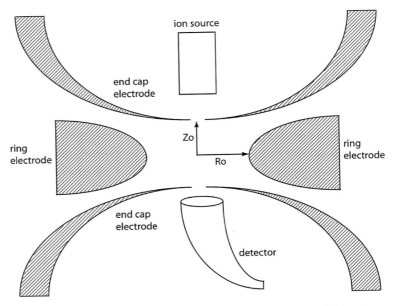

Fig. 27.10. Schematic cross-section of the 3D quadrupole ion trap. The endcaps and the ring are symmetrical about the z axis

they can be ejected sequentially through a hole in the other endcap into an electron multiplier detector. An important strength of this device is its ability to perform multiple stages of mass spectrometry in a single instrument, greatly increasing the information obtainable from a given analyte (see the following). The instrument is also robust and very sensitive, as ions can be accumulated in the trap for a considerable length of time, but most versions suffer from limited mass accuracy.

Linear ion traps have recently been put on the market (*4*). Their configuration is similar to the geometry of the linear quadrupole, but with additional electrodes to permit trapping. They have the advantage of larger ion storage capacity than the 3D traps.

3.3. Resonance Instruments

3.3.1. Fourier Transform Ion Cyclotron Resonance (FTICR) Mass Spectrometers (5)

An ion charge ze moving in a plane perpendicular to a constant magnetic field B feels a Lorentz force ($zev \times B$). It traces a circle whose radius r can be obtained by equating the Lorentz force to the centripetal force mv^2/r., i.e., $zevB = mv^2/r$. The periodic time T for this motion is given by $T = 2\pi r/v = 2\pi m/zeB$, so the frequency of oscillation is $f = 1/T = (B/2\pi) ze/m$. Thus measurement of the oscillation frequency f determines the value of m/z when the field strength B is known. Note that all ions of given m/z have the same oscillation frequency independent of their energy.

Ion cyclotron motion may be rendered spatially coherent (and thus observable) by the application of a spatially uniform rf electric field (excitation) at the same frequency as the ion cyclotron frequency (i.e., "resonant" with it).

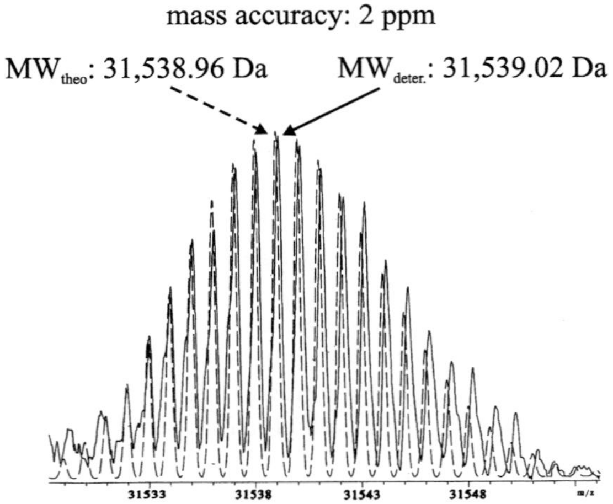

mass accuracy: 2 ppm

$MW_{theo.}$: 31,538.96 Da $MW_{deter.}$: 31,539.02 Da

Fig. 27.11. Deconvoluted FTICR-MS spectrum from cytidine deaminase (CDA), obtained with a Bruker 9.4 T Apex QqFTICR. The spectrum obtained (solid line) is superimposed on the predicted spectrum (dashed line), calculated from the isotopic distribution of CDA derived from the known elemental composition. The most abundant mass measured (31,539.02 Da) agrees with the calculated mass (31,538.96 Da) within 2 ppm. From C. Borchers, private communication, as described in **ref. 6**

The ICR (time-domain) signal results from induction (detection) of an oscillating "image" charge on two opposed parallel electrodes. A frequency-domain spectrum (convertible to a mass-domain spectrum) is obtained by Fourier transformation of the digitized time-domain ICR signal.

FTICR instruments have unexcelled mass resolution and mass accuracy; see **Fig. 27.11** for example. However, their performance improves with increasing magnetic field B, and is optimized only for high magnetic field. Consequently they use large superconducting magnets, making the cost of these instruments considerably higher than most other types of mass spectrometer.

3.3.2. The Orbitrap

This relatively new device traps ions in a cylindrically symmetric electrostatic field between two curved electrodes *(7,8)*. Ions circle the central electrode and also undergo oscillations in the axial direction. The frequency of the oscillations determines the value of *m/z* for the trapped ions. It appears that this device may offer real competition to the FTICR instruments for the highest resolution and mass accuracy.

3.4. Protein and Peptide Sequencing

Perhaps the most important use of mass spectrometry for analysis of peptides and proteins has been the determination of their primary structure, i.e., their amino acid sequence *(9)*. If the corresponding nucleotide sequence has been deposited in one of the standard databases, it defines the protein sequence, so the initial problem is simply the identification of the particular protein examined. There may be modifications that are not defined by the nucleotide sequence in the database, e.g., mutations in a different sample, or post-translational modifications, but at least the basic structure of the protein is defined. However, if the nucleotide sequence is not in the database, "de novo" sequencing is required *(10)*, which is much more difficult, as no template is available.

The standard method of analyzing a protein (bottom-up sequencing) first breaks up the molecule by the action of an enzyme, usually trypsin, which cleaves the amino acid chain at the C-terminal end of either arginine or lysine. The tryptic fragments produced by this digestion are then examined in a mass spectrometer. The resulting list of *m/z* values (mass fingerprinting, or mass mapping) may be sufficient to identify the protein, as long as the sequence is contained in the standard databases *(9)*.

If mass mapping fails to identify the protein, it is necessary to break up the enzymatic fragments, usually by collisions with gas molecules, and measure the masses of the daughter ions produced *(9,11)*, usually designated an MS/MS measurement. This process is carried out in a tandem mass spectrometer. Some instruments, for example the 3D ion trap, allow such measurements to be performed sequentially in a single instrument. Others require the use of a pair of separate spectrometers, as described below.

3.5. Tandem Mass Spectrometers

These spectrometers evolved in order to obtain more detailed information than the overall mass values provided by a simple *m/z* measurement. Tandem (in space) measurements are typically carried out in two *m/z* analyzers in series. The first analyzer selects a given parent (precursor) ion, which is broken up, usually by collisions in a gas cell. The daughter (product) ions are measured in a second mass spectrometer.

3.5.1. The Triple Quadrupole

This instrument consists of three quadrupoles in series in a configuration Q1q2Q3—two quadrupole mass filters, Q1 and Q3, with an RF quadrupole ion guide q2 between them *(12)*. When a mixture of molecules is fed into the quadrupole mass filter Q1, it selects a parent ion, which is fed into a gas cell that is surrounded by the RF quadrupole q2. Collisions with the gas molecules break up the parent ion, and the daughter ions are focused towards the axis by the quadrupole field of q2. Q3 selects daughter ions, one species at a time, and feeds them to a detector. The instrument is simple and robust, and it has become a workhorse for small molecule measurements. However, its efficiency is reduced by the need to scan both Q1 (parent ion scan) and Q3 (daughter ion scan).

3.5.2. The Quadrupole–Time-of-Flight Mass Spectrometer

The need for double scanning in a triple quadrupole instrument has stimulated the search for alternatives. A popular solution calls for the final quadrupole to be replaced by a time of flight instrument. As in the triple quadrupole, Q1 selects the parent ion, which is broken up by collisions with the gas in the ion guide q2. However, Q3 is now replaced by the TOF spectrometer, which is capable of measuring the entire daughter ion spectrum without scanning, thus enhancing the efficiency. For this reason, the QqTOF instrument has also become a favorite device for MS/MS measurements, both for ESI and MALDI peptide ions *(13,14)*.

For optimum efficiency, it is necessary to cool the ions by gas collisions in an additional quadrupole ion guide q0 before injection into Q1, thus producing a configuration q0Q1q2TOF. Such instruments also benefit greatly from

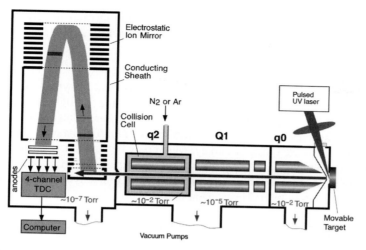

Fig. 27.12. Schematic diagram of a hybrid quadrupole–TOF mass spectrometer with an ion mirror and orthogonal injection. In this instrument ions are cooled by gas collisions in q0, mass-selected in Q1, and broken up by collisions with the gas in q2. The quadrupole q2 injects slow ions perpendicular to the TOF axis into the storage region of the modulator. The resulting ion "sausage" is then accelerated in the axial direction by pulses applied to electrodes below and above the storage region, and subsequently by a DC voltage in the accelerator. The pulses provide the required "start" signals for measuring the flight time. The m/z values for the resulting daughter (product) ions are measured in the reflecting TOF section

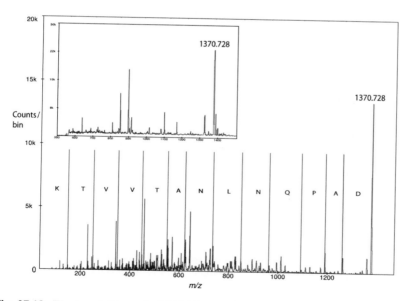

Fig. 27.13. The insert shows the MALDI m/z spectrum of the coat protein from the plant virus TriMV. The main part of the figure shows a daughter ion spectrum (MS/MS spectrum) resulting from collisional-induced dissociation of the parent ion with $m/z =$ 1370.28, shown in the insert. This corresponds to the peptide DAPQNLNATVVTK, amino acid residues 044 to 056 of TriMV

"orthogonal injection," i.e., injection into the TOF instrument perpendicular to its axis *(15)*. Such an instrument is shown in **Fig. 27.12**, and a typical daughter ion spectrum is shown in **Fig. 27.13**.

3.5.3. Other Tandem Configurations

More recent alternatives are the TOF/TOF instrument, in which both parent and daughter mass selection are carried out by time of flight *(16)*, and the quadrupole FTICR spectrometer, in which *m/z* measurements of the daughter ions are carried out in an FTICR instrument *(17)*. The latter is capable of providing very high mass accuracy, which may be sufficient to enable "top-down" sequencing, i.e., breaking up the protein itself, without enzymatic digestion. Similar properties may be obtainable from a hybrid linear quadrupole trap–orbitrap hybrid instrument *(8)*.

3.6. Coupling to Other Separation Methods

Although mass spectrometry has the ability to resolve a very large number of biomolecular species, it still may still be insufficient to unravel the components in a complex mixture. Coupling to other separation methods may therefore be necessary, particularly for mass spectrometers with limited resolving power. The most common coupling is with high performance liquid chromatography (HPLC) *(18)*.

References

1. McClosky JA (ed) (1990) Methods in enzymology, vol. 193: mass spectrometry. Academic Press, New York, N.Y. pp. 1–960
2. Cotter RJ (1997) Time-of-flight mass spectrometry: instrumentation and applications in biological research. American Chemical Society
3. Tang X, Beavis R, Ens W, Lafortune F, Schueler B, Standing KG (1988) A Secondary Ion Time-of-Flight Mass Spectrometer with an Ion Mirror. Int J Mass Spectrom Ion Processes 85:43–67
4. March RE, Todd JFJ (2005) Quadrupole ion trap mass spectrometry, 2nd edn., John Wiley and Sons, Hoboken, NJ
5. Marshall AG, Hendrickson CL, Jackson GS (1998) Fourier transform ion cyclotron resonance mass spectrometry: a primer. Mass Spectrom Rev 17:1–35
6. Borchers CH, Marquez VE, Schroeder GK, Short SA, Snider MJ, Speir JP, Wolfenden R (2004) Fourier transform ion cyclotron resonance MS reveals the presence of a water molecule in an enzyme transition-state analogue complex. Proc Natl Acad Sci U S A. 101:15,341–15,3415
7. Makarov A (2000) Electrostatic axially harmonic orbital trapping: a high-performance technique of mass analysis. Anal Chem 72:1156–1162
8. Scigelova M, Makarov A (2006) Orbitrap mass analyzer – overview and applications in proteomics. Proteomics 6 Suppl:2 16–21
9. Kinter M, Sherman, NE (2000) Protein sequencing and identification using tandem mass spectrometry. Wiley-Interscience, New York, NY
10. Standing KG (2003) Peptide and protein de novo sequencing by mass spectrometry. Curr Opin Struct Biol 13:595–601
11. Wysocki VH, Resing KA, Zhang Q, Cheng G (2005) Mass spectrometry of peptides and proteins. Methods 35:211–222
12. Yost RA, Boyd RK (1990) Tandem mass spectrometry: quadrupole and hybrid instruments. In: (McClosky JA (ed) Methods in enzymology, vol. 193: mass spectrometry. Academic Press, New York, NY, pp 154–200

13. Chernushevich IV, Loboda AV, Thomson BA (2001) An introduction to quadrupole-time-of-flight mass spectrometry. J Mass Spectrom 36:849–865

14. Ens W, Standing KG (2005) Hybrid quadrupole time-of-flight mass spectrometers for analysis of biomolecules. In: Burlingame AL (ed) Methods in enzymology, vol. 402: biological mass spectrometry. pp 49–78

15. Chernushevich IV, Ens W, Standing KG. (1999). Orthogonal Injection TOFMS for Analyzing Biomolecules. Anal Chem 71:452A–461A

16. Vestal ML, Campbell JM (2005) Tandem time-of-flight mass spectrometry. In: Burlingame AL (ed) Methods in enzymology, vol. 402: biological mass spectrometry. pp. 79–108

17. Jebanathirajah JA, Pittman JL, Thomson BA, Budnik BA, Kaur P, Rape M, Kirschner M, Costello CE, O'Connor PB (2005). Characterization of a new qQq-FTICR mass spectrometer for post-translational modification analysis and top-down tandem mass spectrometry of whole proteins. J Am Soc Mass Spectrom 16:1985–1999

18. Ferguson PL, Smith RD (2003) Proteome analysis by mass spectrometry. Annu Rev Biophys Biomol Struct 32:399–424

28

Post-Translational Modifications
of Proteins

Christoph Kannicht and Birte Fuchs

1. Introduction

Post-translational modifications (PTMs) of proteins are referred to as chemical modifications or cleavage of the protein after its translation. The protein's polypeptide chain may be altered by proteolytic cleavage, formation of disulfide bonds or covalent attachment of phosphate, sulfate, alkyl groups, lipids, carbohydrates, polypeptides, and others (1,2). Though some covalent modifications, e.g., *N*-glycosylation, occur cotranslationally at the nascent polypeptide chain, the term "post-translational modifications" is commonly used to cover both, co- and post-translational modifications, for reasons of simplicity. The majority of all proteins undergo PTMs: For example around 30% of all proteins found in a mammalian cell exist in a phosphorylated state, and nearly all circulating plasma proteins are glycosylated.

PTMs can influence charge, hydrophobicity, conformation, immunological properties, stability, turnover, localization, and activity of a protein (3,4). The biological function of many proteins are influenced by their PTMs: Specific oligosaccharide structures are involved in L-selectin-mediated lymphocyte homing and recruitment (5), signalling cascades are turned on and off by the reversible addition and removal of phosphate (6) and ubiquitination plays an important role in the intracellular protein degradation (7), to name just a few arbitrary examples. Please note, that not every PTM does necessarily alter the functional properties of a protein. Nevertheless, full understanding of a specific protein structure–function relationship requires detailed information not only on its amino acid sequence – which is determined by the corresponding DNA/mRNA sequence – but also on the presence and structure of its PTMs.

Proteomic research and the rising number of therapeutic proteins have significantly increased the focus on PTMs of proteins during the past 10 yr. The successful research in the field of "genomics" has led to knowledge of the complete human DNA sequence and the genome of several organisms. The fact that around 25,000 human genes encode about 1 million different proteins – mainly generated by alternative splicing and PTMs – emphasizes the importance of PTMs and the analysis thereof (8). Proteomic research describes the expression levels of proteins related to a defined cell or tissue

From: *Molecular Biomethods Handbook, 2nd Edition.*
Edited by: J. M. Walker and R. Rapley © Humana Press, Totowa, NJ

status *(9)*. As measurement of the mRNA, the "transcriptome," does not allow prediction of the level of protein expression of a cell at a specific state, direct measurement of the expressed proteins is mandatory. It will be incomplete without knowledge of the PTMs of those proteins.

Therapeutic proteins, either isolated from human plasma or recombinantly expressed in different expression systems, have to be thoroughly investigated, monitored during production and documented for registration with respect to their PTMs to ensure product quality.

How is the detection and analysis of PTMs of proteins generally accomplished? First of all, they change the molecular weight of the protein. Consequently, mass spectrometry has become a core technique for identification and characterization of PTMs *(10,11)*. Even the automatic detection of PTMs of known mass in proteolytic digests of proteins by coupled liquid chromatography MS–MS systems has become possible.

Secondly, a number of modifications as acylation, alkylation, carboxymethylation, phosphorylation, sulfation, carboxylation, or siaylation can lead to charge-dependent changes to a protein. Thus, these modifications result in p*I*-shifts in the first dimension of 2-dimensional-gel electrophoresis (2D-GE) *(12)*. Consequently, 2D-GE has become another very important tool for separation of protein mixtures and protein isoforms. It is frequently applied for detection of PTMs, either for protein purification for further characterization, or associated with selective staining for detection of different PTMs *(13)*. However, one has to be aware, that protein-modifications as methionine oxidation or protein alkylation may also occur during sample preparation or during analysis *(14)*.

General strategies for detection and analysis of PTMs typically include (i) selective purification of proteins comprising specific PTMs *(15)*, (ii) prefractionation of proteins prior to analysis by 2D chromatography *(16)*, (iii) mass spectrometric analysis after protease cleavage *(17)* and (iv) chemical or enzymatic release and subsequent analysis of the respective modification. Finally, web-based protein databases give information on protein modifications and allow the prediction of PTMs on yet uncharacterized proteins, based on the fact that PTMs occur at specific amino acids, amino acid sequences or specific 3D-structures of the protein, respectively *(18,19)*.

In general, PTMs of proteins can be classified according to their chemistry or the targeted amino acid. They can be subdivided into reversible or irreversible reactions, enzymatic or nonenzymatic reactions, according to their subcellular location or functional aspects of the modification. The organization of the method chapter considers both, the frequency and the chemical nature of the particular PTM, but still remains a bit arbitrary. Not all known, but the most important PTMs and the methods for their characterization are covered in order to keep the chapter concise.

2. Methods

2.1. Proteolytic Cleavage

The mass difference resulting from proteolytic cleavage, e.g., of the *N*-terminal signal peptide, during activation of zymogens, inactivation of enzymes or simply from proteolytic degradation can be detected by 1- or 2D-GE, or determined by mass spectrometry (MS). The exact cleavage site can be analyzed by automated chemical *N-* or *C-*terminal sequencing, depending on its location. Direct mass determination by MS and comparison with either the measured or the theoretical mass of uncleaved protein offers information on the exact mass of the segregated peptide. Provided that the amino acid sequence of the protein is known, the exact cleavage site can be deducted. If MS of the entire protein is difficult because of size or charge, proteolytic cleavage by typically trypsin and subsequent determination of the apparent masses of the resulting peptides by MS can be applied to define the cleavage site *(20)*.

2.2. Disulfide Bridges

Disulfide bonds in proteins are built by oxidation of the sulfhydryl (-SH) groups provided by the amino acid cysteine. They play important roles in stabilizing 3-dimensional structure and modulating bioactivity of the cystinyl proteins. The determination of disulfide bond linkage therefore is an integral part of structural characterization of proteins *(21)*.

There are different strategies for identification of free cysteine residues and assignment of disulfide bonds in proteins, which involve the cleavage of the protein backbone, isolation and subsequent sequencing of the cystinyl peptides *(22,23)*. A method for assignment of disulfide bonds in proteins is described by Wu et al. using chemical cleavage and MS *(24)*. This method involves two steps, (1) the identification of free cysteine residues and (2) the disulfide bond mapping by partial reduction and cyanylation-induced chemical cleavage. For proteins containing both, sulfhydryls and disulfide bonds, the first step serves to determine the number and location of sulfhydryl groups.

1. The identification of free cysteine residues by mass-mapping of cyanylation-induced cleavage products takes advantage of the selective chemical cleavage at cyanylated cysteinyl residues. In brief, the denatured original protein is cyanylated by 1-cyano-4-dimethylamino-pyridinium tetrafluoroborate (CDAP) and chemically cleaved by NH_4OH at free cyteine residues. The subsequent mass determination of the resulting cleavage products by MALDI-TOF MS and comparison with known theoretical cleavage peptides deducted from the known amino acid sequence of the protein allows to determine the number and location of free cysteine residues *(25)*. Note that each derivatizable sulfhydryl group will cause a 26-Da mass shift.

2. For assignment of disulfide bonds in proteins, the protein sample is denatured by guanidine-HCl and partially reduced by addition of 1/10 molar Tris(2-carboxyethyl)-phosphine hydrochloride (TCEP) with respect to the proteins cysteine content. The experimental conditions of the reduction step–such as incubation time, temperature, and stoichiometry of reducing agents–are chosen to preferably obtain singly-reduced isoforms of the protein. Subsequently, the nascent sulfhydryl groups are cyanylated and chemically cleaved as described above. The cleavage of the different singly reduced protein species results in a set of accordingly different peptides, depending on the location of the reduced disulfide bonds. The cleavage products are consecutively separated by reversed-phase (RP) chromatography, and the molecular weights of the fractionated peptides are determined by MALDI-TOF MS. Comparison with the theoretical molecular weight of peptides from the known sequence of the protein, again corrected by the mass shift caused by reduction and cyanylation, allows the identification of the disulfide bonds locus.

2.3. Phosphorylation

The reversible attachment of a phosphate group to serine-, threonine-, or tyrosine residues of proteins through kinase enzymes is one of the most frequent PTMs determining the protein function. Phosphorylation plays an important role in many biological pathways and cellular processes, including signal transduction, cell cycle regulation or the degree of enzyme activity *(26)*. The determination of phosphorylation sites therefore is essential for a deeper understanding of cellular regulation and – since aberrant phosphorylation events are known to occur in many diseases – the definition of potential new drug targets *(27)*.

Despite recent technology advances in MS, the determination of phosphorylation sites remains challenging: The classical chemical sequencing approach (Edman degradation) is restrained because of the insolubility of the phosphoamino acid products and the necessity to obtain highly purified phosphopeptides, and MS is complicated due to low signal intensities disappearing into the background because of the low stoichiometry of phosphorylation and the low ionization efficiency of phosphopeptides *(28)*. Several approaches are known to enhance the detection level, e.g., (1) chemical replacement of the phosphate group by other functionalities that enhance ionization efficiency and MS/MS fragmentation behaviour, e.g., via β-elimination and subsequent Michael addition, (2) affinity enrichment of phosphorylated species, e.g. by immobilized metal-affinity chromatography (IMAC) on Fe^{3+} or Ga^{3+} as well as ZrO_2 or TiO_2 matrices, however, the enrichment is rarely specific and acidic peptides are likely to be enhanced as well *(29,30)*. (3) Alternatively, peptides phosphorylated on tyrosine can be purified using anti-P-Tyr-antibodies. No antibodies with good specificity for P-Ser and P-Thr are available so far. Phosphorylated proteins can be sensitively detected in 2D-gels by phosphoprotein-specific fluorescent staining down to less than 10 ng for a monophosphorylated protein *(31)*. Briefly, gels are washed with water after fixation and subsequently incubated with Pro-Q Diamond phosphoprotein stain for around 1–2 h. Images are recorded with digital imagers equipped with adequate excitation and emission filters.

MS-based methods are the methods of choice for the identification of phosphorylation sites; however, biochemical pre-fractionation and enrichment protocols will be needed to produce suitable samples in the case of low-stoichiometry phosphorylation. A state-of-the-art approach to determine phosphorylation sites in a peptide mixture is described by Weise and Lenz using LC–MS/MS (direct coupling of a liquid-chromatography system to a mass spectrometer) involving In-Gel reduction, alkylation and tryptic protein digestion followed by the detection of phosphorylated peptides, and analysis of the phosphopeptides sequence. In short, SDS-PAGE separated Coomassie-stained gel bands are excised, destained and dehydrated. Cysteine bridges are reduced with dithiothreitol (DTT) followed by alkylation of free cysteines using iodacetamide, and the protein mixture is subjected to tryptic digestion. The peptides are extracted and dissolved in loading solvent for nanoflow liquid chromatography (nano-LC), usually composed of formic acid in acetonitrile:water mixtures, and subjected to LC–MS/MS analysis. Phosphorylated peptides are detected using a precursor ion scan for m/z 79 (PO_3^-) in negative detection mode: Phosphopeptides selectively detected by precursor ion scanning are subsequently fragmented by collision-induced dissociation (CID) with ion scanning in negative-ion mode in a production experiment to establish their sequence and the site of phosphorylation. The data is analysed by database search.

2.4. Sulfation

Covalently sulfated proteins are formed by protein sulfotransferase action. Tyrosine *O*-sulfation is the most abundant PTM on tyrosine residues and occurs almost exclusively on secreted and trans-membrane proteins. It is thought to serve as a key modulator of protein-protein interaction, being involved in various biological processes including hemostasis regulation, leukocyte trafficking, modulation of proteolytic processing and secretory pathways *(32)*.

For determining tyrosine *O*-sulfation various biochemical methods are available, encompassing radioactive labelling with ^{35}S-isotope, Edman sequencing with trifluoracetic acid (TFA) hydrolysis, amino acid analysis of ^{3}H-labelled tyrosines via complete alkaline hydrolysis [e.g., with $Ba(OH)_2$], peptide mapping using HPLC and MALDI-MS for analysis of cleaved peptides or separation methods like HPLC, SDS-PAGE or thin layer chromatography (TLC) under alkaline conditions. The extreme instability of the sulfotyrosine-containing peptide/ sulfoesters severely affects all aspects of "classical" MS analyses, but combining enrichment procedures with recent developed fields of MS electron capture dissociation (EDC), electron transfer dissociation (ETD) or electron detachment dissociation (EDD), sulfation sites can be located. Bundgaard et al. provide methods for the establishment of sulfation specific antisera and suited chromatographic systems for the analysis of tyrosine sulfation *(33)*. Using the change in physical and chemical protein properties by introducing sulfation, chromatographic techniques are suitable to separate sulfated and nonsulfated forms, e.g., ion-exchange chromatography (IEC) or reversed-phase high performance liquid chromatographie (RP-HPLC) under neutral pH conditions. Additionally, various proteinases are available, e.g., trypsin or the endoproteinases LysC, GluC, AspN, for analysis of the peptide before and after digestion followed by separation via chromatography to reveal the presence of sulfated tyrosine. Peptides can be eluted with a linear gradient of trifluoroacetic acid (TFA) or ammonium acetate (NH_4Ac) via RP-HPLC, whereas the separation in the NH_4Ac-system is more pronounced. Compared to the nonsulfated forms, sulfated peptides elute earlier because of the loss of hydrophobicity through the introduction of the sulfate group.

2.5. Glycosylation

Glycosylation denotes the covalent attachment of saccharides to proteins occurring co- and post-translational during synthesis within the endoplasmic reticulum (ER). This includes proteins that reside in the ER as well as membrane and secreted proteins, and occurs at the carboxamino nitrogen of asparagine residues (*N*-linked glycosylation) or at the hydroxyl side chains of serine and threonine residues (*O*-linked glycosylation). Oligosaccharide structures alter the physical protein properties due to their steric dimensions and highly hydrophilic character. Glycoproteins can exist in different isomeric and diverse branching forms, resulting in three-dimensional complexity associated with diverse biological functions. Glycosylation can serve various functions, like proper protein folding, stability, cell–cell adhesion, subcellular addressing, immune response, cancer cell masking, injury, and inflammation, or function as selective ligand *(34,35)*. This does not necessarily mean, that a specific biological function can be assigned to the glycan moiety of every glycoprotein *(36,37)*. In contrast to *O*-linked glycosylation, biosynthesis of *N*-linked oligosaccharides results in a common core structure *(38)*. For this reason, and because *N*-linked oligosaccharides can be removed from the glycoprotein by a specific peptide *N*-glycosidase, this chapter on characterization of protein glycosylation is subdivided into analysis of *N*- and *O*-glycosylation. In addition, detection of protein glycosylation and description of carbohydrate composition analysis, which apply for both, *N*- and *O*-glycosylation, are arranged in front of these chapters.

2.5.1. Detection of Protein Glycosylation

The general question, if a protein is glycosylated or not, can be examined by specific fluorescent staining, specific binding of lectins, or monitoring of characteristic masses resulting from fragmentation. For instance, glycosylated proteins can be detected in 2D-gels by selectively fluorescent staining *(39)*. The fluorescent dye Pro-Q Emerald enables direct detection of glycoproteins in gels *(40)*. In brief, the gel is washed in acetic acid and subsequently incubated in an oxidizing solution. After an additional washing of the gel with acetic acid, it is incubated in Pro-Q Emerald dye solution for 2 h or overnight in the dark. Then the gel is washed again with acetic acid prior to image analysis. The fluorescence-stained glycoproteins are detected by a laser scanner or a digital imaging system using the appropriate excitation and emission filters. The interesting thing with these kind of fluorescent staining method is, that they allow sequential staining of the phosphorylated, glycosylated and all proteins in one 2D-gel and hence provide an important tool for proteomic research *(41)*. Another approach for detection of glycoproteins after separation in 2D-GE is application of lectin to blotted proteins *(42)*. Thereby the proteins are transferred to a nitrocellulose membrane by electro-blotting after GE. The membrane is incubated with digoxygenin-labeled lectins to let them bind to the respective glycoproteins. Subsequently, peroxidase-labeled anti-digoxigenin antibodies are bound to the lectins and the glycoproteins are visualized by a chemiluminescence substrate. Images are recorded through digital imaging. The use of MS and selective ion monitoring for detection of protein glycosylation is described below in the section on characterization of protein *N*-glycosylation.

2.5.2. Carbohydrate Composition Analysis

The carbohydrate composition analysis is similar to amino acid analysis of proteins. It simply provides information on the type and relative amount of the monosaccharides, of which the protein-bound or already purified oligosaccharides are composed. In principle, the carbohydrate composition analysis implements acidic hydrolysis of the oligosaccharides, purification and labeling of the resulting monosaccharides and subsequent chromatographic separation, detection and quantification. The acidic hydrolysis is typically done using TFA or HCl. The hydrolytic conditions, i.e., acidic strength, temperature and hydrolysis time, are specifically chosen for quantification of either sialic acids or neutral monosaccharides. Separation and detection of monosaccharides can be performed by anion-exchange chromatography using pulsed amperometric detection (HPAE-PAD) without prior labeling *(43)*. Alternatively, monosaccharides or sialic acid resulting from hydrolysis can be labeled by fluorescent dyes *(44)*. Subsequent separation and detection can be performed by RP chromatography and highly sensitive fluorescence detection *(45)*. For both chromatographic methods, identification of the monosaccharides is done by assignment of their (relative) retention times to the respective monosaccharide standards. Quantification is obtained by comparison of resulting peak areas to those of concomitantly derivatized and analyzed monosaccharide standards.

2.5.3. N-Linked Glycosylation

Biosynthesis of *N*-glycosylated proteins involves several enzymatic steps in assembly, arrangement and maturation, resulting in heterogeneous glyco-protein populations with multiple glycoforms of the same protein. *N*-linked glycosylation can be divided into two major saccharide types (1) high-mannose oligosaccharides and (2) complex oligosaccharides. Oligosaccharides are attached to Asp by oligosaccharyltransferase, which recognizes the consensus sequence Asn-X-Ser/Thr. Characterization of *N*-linked glycosylation of glyco-proteins can be done by application of a set of different approaches, depending on the desired information and the available sample amount *(46)*. In-depth analysis of the *N*-linked glycosylation of a glycoprotein should provide information on the exact structure, i.e., their monosaccharide composition and sequence, types of glycosidic linkages within the oligosaccharide chain and their occurrence at specific binding sites within the glycoprotein. In general, *N*-glycans are released from glycoproteins by enzymatic hydrolysis using a specific enzyme, the peptide-N4-(acetyl-β-glucosaminyl)-asparagine amidase (PNGase F). PNGase F cleaves asparagine linked oligosaccharides from glycoproteins except oligosac-charides containing alpha(1,3)-linked core fucose commonly found on plant glycoproteins. The resulting oligosaccharides successively are either fluores-cence labeled and separated by different chromatographic approaches *(47)*, or characterized directly by MS. Separated oligosaccharides are frequently further analyzed by enzymatic sequence analysis or MS for their exact structure *(48)*. Advances in MS allow the direct analysis of site-specific glycosylation from tryptic peptides by RP chromatography directly coupled to electrospray ioniza-tion mass spectrometry (LC/ESI-MS) *(49)*. In brief, the glycoprotein is reduced, alkylated and subsequently digested with trypsin. The resulting (glyco-)peptides are separated by microbore RP chromatography directly coupled to ESI-MS. Glycopeptide-containing fractions are identified by selective ion monitoring (SIM), i.e., by searching for characteristic masses resulting from fragmentation of oligosaccharides. The type of oligosaccharide is deducted from identification of characteristic mass differences within the fragmentation pattern of the mass spectra. Please note, that interpretation of MS data takes advantage of the common core-structure and both, limited possible types of glycosidic linkages and type of monosaccharides within *N*-linked glycans *(50)*.

Other common methods for characterization of *N*-linked glycans are HPAE-PAD *(51)*, fluorophore assisted carbohydrate electrophoresis (FACE) *(52)*, lectin chromatography *(53)*, sequential exoglycosidase digestion *(54,55)* and nuclear magnetic resonance (NMR) *(56)*.

Chromatographic methods are used either for purification of single oli-gosaccharides, or for identification of oligosaccharides by comparison of relative retention times with known standard oligosaccharides. Sequential exoglycosidase digestion can be applied to purified oligosaccharides or oli-gosaccharide mixtures. The principal concept of this method is the application of highly specific exoglycosidases with known cleavage specificity for the type of monosaccharide, anomeric configuration, type of linkage and branching. The number of cleaved monosaccharides after a certain exoglycosidase detection step can be monitored either by MS, size-exclusion chromatography, or GE *(57)*. For example, occurrence of a specific structural oligosaccharide motive within the oligosaccharide moiety of a glycoprotein can be achieved by enzymatic cleavage of the *N*-linked glycans, purification of the *N*-glycans, stepwise application of specific exoglycosidases, and determination of the oligosaccharide masses by MALDI-TOF MS *(58)*.

2.5.4. O-Linked Glycosylation

O-linked glycosylation starts with the addition of monosaccharides generally at the hydroxyl side of Thr and Ser residues, typically resulting in disaccharide and branched trisaccharide glycoproteins *(59)*. In contrast to *N*-linked oligosaccharides – which are attached to a specific consensus sequence – no such particular sequence motif is found for *O*-glycosylation *(60)*. The probability of mucin-type *O*-glycosylation can be predicted using a web-based tool (http://www.cbs.dtu.dk/services/NetOGlyc) relying on a number of corresponding, known binding sites *(61)*.

Moreover, *O*-linked glycans do not share a common core structure like *N*-linked glycans, and unfortunately there is no single endoglycosidase available for enzymatic hydrolysis of all *O*-linked glycans. *O*-linked glycosylation can be characterized from tryptic digests by MS as described for *N*-linked glycosylation above *(62)*. For detailed analysis, *O*-linked glycans can be released from glycoproteins chemically using beta-elimination by incubation with a mixture of NaOH and $NaBH_4$. The oligosaccharides are released as alditols and can be subjected to further analysis after neutralization, removal of boric acid and further purification by chromatographic desalting steps *(63)*. Principally, analysis of *O*-linked oligosaccharides after their cleavage from the protein involves the same steps as described for *N*-glycans above: Labelling, fractionation by anion-exchange-, amino-bonded phase-, or RP chromatography, capillary electrophoresis, enzymatic sequence analysis, MS and NMR *(64)*.

2.6. O-GlcNAc

The addition of *O*-linked *N*-acetylglucosamine (*O*-GlcNAc) to target proteins has an exceptional position within the glycosylation of proteins and thus is discussed separately from *N*- and *O*-glycosylation. *O*-GlcNAc is a transient modification, which is involved in several cellular functions as transcription, translation, nuclear transport and cell signalling *(65)*. Many proteins of the nucleus, cytoskeleton, cytoplasm, and the cytosolic tail of membrane proteins are dynamically modified at their serine and threonine hydroxyl groups by the covalent attachment of *O*-linked *β*-*N*-acetylglucosamine monosaccharides. Like many PTMs, *O*-GlcNAc is often prevalent on low-abundance regulatory proteins affecting diverse cellular processes, ranging from nutrient sensing to the regulation of proteasomal degradation and gene silencing, and is known to be associated with diseases such as cancer, neurodegenerative diseases and diabetes *(66)*.

Several methods are available for the identification of *O*-GlcNAc-modified proteins: tritium-labeling, enrichment with lectins or antibodies, chemical tagging by metabolic labeling or BEMAD (*β*-elimination followed by Michael addition with DTT), chemoenzymatic derivatization with enrichment using affinity methods and MS along with capillary electrophoresis and HPLC separation of the released glycan fragments *(67,68)*, sequential digestion by specific glycosidases *(69,70)* followed by analysis of the remaining oligosaccharide chain by MS or application of electron capture dissociation MS technique combined with Wheat Germ Agglutination affinity chromatography *(71)*.

Nevertheless, many of these techniques are time consuming and require practical expertise and expensive technical and analytical equipment. An immunological detection method using *O*-GlcNAc specific antibodies is extensively described by Ahrend et al. *(72)* comparing the application of the mouse monoclonal antibody RL2 against *O*-GlcNAc modified pore complexes and mouse monoclonal antibody CTD 110.6 against the synthetic peptide YSPTS(*O*-GlcNAc)PSK *(73)* in ELISA, 1D and 2D Western blots as well as immunohistochemical analysis using Cy-2 conjugated second anti-mouse antibodies. However, this method cannot provide detailed information on, e.g., sites of *O*-GlcNAc modifications.

2.7. Glycosylphosphatidylinositols

Multiple cell surface proteins of lower and higher eukaryotes contain complex glycolipid structures, the glycosylphosphatidylinositol (GPI), at their C-terminus *(74)*. Besides their functionality as an anchor to the outer layer of the plasma membrane, GPIs have been described to be involved in signalling for protein sorting in epithelial cells, signal transduction, immune responses, and pathology of infectious diseases. The biosynthesis of GPIs, their transfer to proteins and their subsequent processing are exhaustively reviewed elsewhere *(75)*.

The experimental characterization of GPI-anchored membrane proteins includes fractionation of membrane proteins, followed by cleavage with phosphatidylinositol-specific phospholipase C to solubilize GPI-anchored proteins, concentration of the released proteins and analyses by denaturing gel electrophoresis and subsequent MS for peptide identification *(76)*. Futhermore, Azzouz et al. *(77)* describe various protocols to identify and analyse GPI-biosynthesis intermediates and GPI-anchor precursors exemplified for the malaria parasite *Plasmodium falciparum* depending on metabolic labelling techniques using radioactive GPI-precursor molecules, organic solvent extraction, and chemical cleavage or GPI-specific phospholipases. Briefly, GPIs are identified using nitrous acid deamination (HNO_2), enzymatic cleavage with phosphatidylinositol-specific phospholipase C (PI-PLC) and glycosylphosphatidylinositol-specific phospholipase D (GPI-PLD). The structural characterization results from analysis of hydrophilic fragments and neutral core-glycans, whereas former can be analyzed using size exclusion chromatography and via dephosphorylation, deamination or reduction generated core-glycans by high pH anion exchange chromatography. Hydrophobic fragments of GPIs metabolically labeled with fatty acids are investigated by thin-layer chromatography (TLC). The predicted structures of GPI-glycans can be verified by exoglycosidase treatment.

2.8. Fatty Acid Modifications

Numerous eukaryotic or virus proteins undergo covalent modifications with the attachment of fatty acids that help to target the modified proteins to particular membranes. Four major types of lipid anchors appended enzymatically to proteins by distinct modification strategies are known: (1) at the *N*-terminus (*N*-myristoylation), (2) the *C*-terminus (glycosyl phosphatidylinositol [GPI] anchor), and (3) at cysteine thiolates proximal to membrane surfaces (*S*-acetylation/ Palmitoylation and *S*-phenylation) *(78–80)*, upon which the *N*-myristoylation in contrast to the other three types occurs cotranslational.

Various methods for the detection of fatty acid modification are available; e.g., acid hydrolysis and detection with gas chromatography/mass spectrometry (GC/MS), RP-HPLC or LC/MS *(81,82)*. Analysis of *S*-acetylation is usually done by site-directed mutagenesis of cysteine residues and subsequent expression of wild type and mutant proteins in vertebrate cells.

Veit et al. describe the evaluation of *S*-acylated proteins by metabolic labeling of palmitoylated proteins with ^{3}H-palmitate *(83)*, involving transient expression of recombinant proteins with the Vaccinia virus/T7-RNA polymerase system and the analysis of bound fatty acids via acid hydrolysis of ^{3}H-palmitate-labeled proteins from gel slices with extraction of released fatty acids with hexane and thin-layer chromatography (TLC) to separate fatty acid species. Furthermore, the determination of a possible turnover of protein-bound fatty acids is introduced by two different methods, whereas deacylation is visible as a decrease in the ^{3}H-palmitate labeling with increasing chase time, estimating the half-life of fatty acid cleavage. Yet another approach is available: the PCR overlap extension method, which is based on the fact that sequences added to the 5'-end of a PCR primer become incorporated into the end of the resulting molecule. By adding the appropriate sequences, a PCR amplified segment can be made to overlap sequences with another segment. In the second PCR this overlap serves as a primer for extension resulting in a recombinant molecule. Once a nonpalmitoylated mutant has been created, it can be used for functional studies to determine the role of the fatty acids in the life cycle of the protein. For the analysis of cell free palmitoylation enzyme reactions are used: The acceptor protein is incubated with the acyldonor ^{3}H-Pal-CoA in the presence or absence of an enzyme source. The samples are then subjected to SDS-PAGE and fluorography to check for incorporation of ^{3}H-palmitate.

2.9. Acetylation and Methylation

Post-translational methylation of proteins most commonly involves one-carbon transfer at nitrogen (*N*-methylation) or oxygen atoms (*O*-methylation) or of nucleophilic side chains *(84)* adding hydrophobicity and/or effecting protein charge. Mono-, di-, and trimethylated side chains exist and possess different protein properties. *N*-methylations are permanent and can occur on lysine-, histidine-, argenine-, glutamine-, and asparagine residues, whereas *O*-methylation can be hydrolysed and is found at glutamate- and aspartate side chains creating methyl esters. Methylations are also found at cysteine residues (*S*-methylation) or at arginine and glutamine side chains (*C*-methylation) of methyl coenzyme M reductase from methanogenic bacteria *(85)*.

Historically, protein methylation was determined using protein hydrolysis adding radiolabeled carbon, and amino acid analysis of liberated *N*-methyl amino acid, which remains stable under acid hydrolysis, whereas *O*-carboxymethyl amino acids are sensitive to hydrolysis and therefore not detected. Nowadays, the most useful tool for the analysis of methylated proteins is MS, where the introduction of each CH$_3$-moiety results in an increase of 14 mass units at the side chain undergoing methylation.

Protein acetylation occurs with donor substrate acyl coenzyme A (acyl CoA) at nucleophilic protein side chains for two distinct biological purposes: (1) the irreversible cotranslationally N-terminal acetylation in about 80–90 % of higher eukaryotic proteins with mostly yet unknown biological significance and (2) the through N-deacetylase enzymes reversed regiospecific N-acetylation of particular lysine side chains basically of histones and transcription factors, affecting selective gene transcription and chromatin structure. The N-acetylation of histones can be detected by MS, with an increase of 42 mass units for each acetyl group introduced, or by use of radioactive labeled acetyl CoA as cosubstrate to monitor protein covalent radioactivity, as well as via N-acetyllysine-specific antibodies in chromatin immunoprecipitation (ChIP) assays for qualitative detection of acetylated histone levels.

A detailed description for the analysis of methylation and acetylation exemplified for ribosomal proteins of *Escherichia coli* using matrix-assisted laser desorption/ionization time-of-flight (MALDI-TOF) and *Caulobacter crescentus* by electrospray ionization quadrupole time-of-flight (ESI-QTOF) MS is given by Arnold et al. *(86)*. The methodological procedure involves bacteria growth with subsequent cell lysis using grinding or a French Press followed by gradient centrifugation with a sucrose cushion to enrich the ribosomal proteins. Adjacent MALDI-TOF MS is carried out using a sinapinic acid matrix solution mixed with through the addition of TFA acidified ribosomal proteins. Masses obtained by MALDI-TOF are compared with masses calculated from the amino sequence of known proteins to determine PTMs. Alternatively, LC ESI-TOF MS in chromatography media of aqueous acetonitrile mobile phases and total ion chromatogram (TIC) mode for MS followed by mass deconvolution can be used. The protein identities and proposed PTMs are deduced by comparison of deconvoluted masses and protein masses calculated from the proteome sequence. Confirmation of protein identities and proposed modifications is gained through enzymatic analysis.

2.10. Ubiquitination

The covalent addition of the 8 kDa, 76-amino acid polypeptide ubiquitin to the ε-amino group of lysine side chains of cellular proteins is a common PTM. Polyubiquitination for instance leads to protein turnover via the ubiquitin-proteasome system, but independently (mono)ubiquitination provides an appropriate tool to regulate cellular processes, like cell division, signal transduction, differentiation as well as quality control *(87)*. Aberrant ubiquitination is associated with some diseases including neurodegenerative disorders, pathologies of the inflammation system and certain malignancies.

MS exhibits the method of choice for determining protein ubiquitination, sometimes with prior enrichment of His-tagged ubiquitinylated proteins using Ni-affinity chromatography. After tryptic digestion of purified proteins, peptides can be separated by multidimensional chromatography followed by MS analysis, e.g., ESI-MS/MS *(88)*. MS can be applied for the analysis of ubiquitination when (1) the intact protein is ubiquitinated, (2) the target protein and the attached ubiquitin exhibit coelectrophoretic migration, and (3) there is a mass shift of an ubiquitinated peptide relative to the non-ubiquitinated peptide. Parker et al. *(89)* describe the application of MS techniques for these three cases involving immune-affinity purification of the ubiquitinated protein prior to MALDI-MS analysis, in-gel digestion of separated proteins followed by protein identification via MALDI-MS or LC–MS/MS. Proteolytic cleavage using trypsin or gluC generates characteristic 'tails' on the ubiquitinated lysine, resulting in peptide mass shifts of around 114 Da during MS allowing distinction from unmodified peptides. Determination of the ubiquitination site is carried out using MS/MS sequencing.

2.11. SUMOylation

In higher eukaryotes, ubiquitin is joined by about ten protein homologues – ubiquitin-like proteins (Ubls) – among them *s*mall *u*biquitin-like *mo*difiers (SUMOs) are one of the best characterized. SUMOylation takes place between the *C*-terminal glycine residue of SUMO and the ε-amino group of the target protein, modifying diverse cellular functions including control of transcription factors, regulation of protein stability, nucleo-cytoplasmatic trafficking, cell-cycle regulation, as well as maintenance of genome integrity and transcription, resulting in a potentially involvement in cancer development, progression, and metastasis *(90)*.

Since steady state SUMOylation levels are very low, determination mostly involves a three-step process of affinity purification, proteolytic digestion, and analysis by tandem MS *(91)*, using the possibility of *N*-terminal tagging of SUMOylated proteins for purification purposes subsequently to expression. A methodological approach is given by Pichler et al. *(92,93)*, involving enrichment of SUMO1 conjugates indicative for HeLa cell lines by stable expression of polyhistidine-tagged SUMO1 using immobilized metal ion affinity based chromatography (IMAC) on Ni^{2+} beads under denaturing conditions, followed by detection of SUMOylated proteins by immunoblot analysis. After in vitro SUMOylation enhancement using a small fragment of SUMO E3 ligase RanBP2, peptide identification is done by MS analysis. An automated pattern recognition tool (SUMmOn) to determine modified peptides and SUMOylation sites is described by Pedrioli et al. *(94)*.

2.12. Protein ISGylation

Protein ISGylation is another ubiquitin-like conjugation system, whereas interferon stimulated gene 15 (ISG15), a 15 kDa protein composed of two tandem repeats of ubiquitin-like domains, is attached to proteins of vertebrates via a pathway similar to ubiquitination *(95)*. The gene encoding ISG15 is induced by interferons, viral infection or exposure of cells to lipopolysaccharide (LPS). ISG15 can act as free polypeptide in immunoregulatory properties or through modification of target proteins (ISGylation) with signal transduction, protein conjugation and extracellular cytokine activity *(96,97)*.

The determination of ISGylated proteins usually involves affinity purification and detection via Western blot analysis or identification via MS. A detailed experimental procedure is given by Takeuchi et al. *(98)* involving plasmid transfection with, i.e., Flag-tagged ISG15 expression plasmid into HeLa cells, immunoprecipitation-based affinity purification of ISGylated proteins using agarose beads with immobilized anti-Flag-tag M2 antibodies, and detection via SDS-PAGE and Western Blot analysis. To identify ISGylated proteins, MALDI-TOF/TOF MS or HPLC-ES Q-TOF MS/MS subsequently to tryptic protein digestion after enrichment of ISGylated proteins via ISG15 immunoaffinity purification can be used.

2.13. γ-Glutamate and β-Hydroxyaspartate

Post-translational hydroxylation of amino acid side chains in proteins is very uncommon, but occurs in one of the most abundant eukaryotic protein, collagen (proline or lysine hydroxylation), as well as on epidermal growth factor-like domains of secreted proteins in blood coagulation factors (vitamin K-dependent factors VIII, IX, and X), thrombomodulin, protein C and S, and LDL-receptors. In these cases, hydroxylation takes place on asparagines/ aspartates at the β-CH_2 group, resulting in the production of β-OH-Asn/Asp side chains leading to large conformational changes determining their function, e.g., in blood coagulation *(99,100)*. Additionally, vitamin K-dependent coagulation proteins are irreversibly carboxylated at the γ-CH_2 loci of glutamate side chains producing γ-carboxyglutamyl side chains (Gla) generating high-affinity ligands for cations, especially for calcium ions *(101)*.

A reliable method for the analysis of β-hydroxyaspartate and γ-glutamate in proteins is given by Castellino et al., using protein hydrolysis with KOH (Gla-determination) or 6*N* HCl (for hydroxyaspartate determination) followed by amino acid derivatization with ortho-phthalaldehyde (OPA)/ ethanethiol (ET) prior to ion exchange HPLC with isocratic elution at 47°C for hydroxyaspartate and RP-HPLC on C8 column for Glu, determining modified proteins in comparison to standard preparations.

2.14. Amidation/Deamidation

Some proteins – like eukaryotic peptide hormones, neurotransmitters, or growth factors – are found with C-terminal NH_2-groups generated by hydroxylation of the C-terminal glycine residue of the precursor protein *(102,103)*, resulting in biological active peptides. The α-amidation completes the peptide biosynthesis and is essential for full biological activity of the protein, e.g., signal transduction or receptor binding *(104)*.

For the determination of α-amidated peptides the radioimmunoassay (RIA) and MS provide useful tools. Detailed protocols for the analysis of α-amidation involving antibody production and radiolabeling of RIA peptides with Na^{125}iodine, are given by Mueller et al., also discussing techniques for identification and verification of α-amidated peptides like HPLC, Western blot analysis, MS using MALDI-TOF and in vivo models to study the biological function *(105)*.

2.15. Use of Web-Based Databanks and Tools

The increasing availability of Internet resources for querying, predicting and comparing PTMs to date provide a useful tool in proteomics. Various bio-informatic applications are collected in a special issue of Proteomics *(106)*, including *inter alia* publications on the Unimod database *(107)* for the use of protein modifications in MS applications as well as an excellent review using the Swiss-Prot/Mod-Prot database *(108)* for the prediction of common PTMs. Further information for the use of databases to obtain an overview on cellular processes underlying sequence variety and structural diversity is excessively reviewed by Boeckmann et al. *(109)* using the UniProtKB/Swiss-Prot protein knowlegebase or by Ivanisenko et al. *(110)* executing the PROSITE database for querying or searching of PTMs in protein sequences available via the EyPASy proteomics server www.expasy.ch, the PDBSiteScan for 3D structuring and the ProMoST program to calculate isoelectric point, molecular mass and PTM isoforms providing also substantial web resources including references related to protein PTM sites. **Table 28.1** provides a listing of available databases and proteomic tools, but it is not exhaustive.

Table 28.1. Proteomics databases and post-translational modification prediction tools.

Name	Tool	Web reference
ExPASy	Database	www.expasy.ch
Swiss-Prot	Database	www.expasy.org/sprot/, www.ebi.ac.uk/ swissprot/
UniProt	Database	www.expasy.uniprot.org/
NCBI	Database	www.ncbi.nlm.nih.gov/
SRS	Database	www.expasy.org/srs/ and srs.ebi.ac.uk
ExPASy tools	Sulfation, Glycosylation, Peptide mass…	www.expasy.ch/tools/
Center for biological sequence analysis	Database	www.cbs.dtu.dk/
RESID	Annotations a nd structures of PTMs	www.ebi.ac.uk/RESID and www.ncifcrf.gov/ RESID
PROSITE	Protein families and domains	us.expasy.org/prosite/
PDBSite	3D structures	wwwmgs.bionet.nsc.ru/mgs/gnw/pdbsite/
ChloroP	Prediction of chloroplast transit peptides	www.cbs.dtu.dk/services/ChloroP/
LipoP	Prediction of lipoproteins and signal peptides in Gram negative bacteria	www.cbs.dtu.dk/services/LipoP/
MITOPROT	Prediction of mitochondrial targeting sequences	ihg.gsf.de/ihg/mitoprot.html
PATS	Prediction of apicoplast targeted sequences	gecco.org.chemie.uni-frankfurt.de/pats/ pats-index.php
PlasMit	Prediction of mitochondrial transit peptides in Plasmodium falciparum	gecco.org.chemie.uni-frankfurt.de/plasmit/ index.html
Predotar	Prediction of mitochondrial and plastid targeting sequences	www.inra.fr/predotar/
PTS1	Prediction of peroxisomal targeting signal 1 containing proteins	mendel.imp.univie.ac.at/mendeljsp/sat/pts1/ PTS1predictor.jsp
SignalP	Prediction of signal peptide cleavage sites	www.cbs.dtu.dk/services/SignalP/
NetAcet	Prediction of N-acetyltransferase A (NatA) substrates (in yeast and mammalian proteins)	www.cbs.dtu.dk/services/NetAcet/
NetOGlyc	Prediction of O-GalNAc (mucin type) glycosylation sites in mammalian proteins	www.cbs.dtu.dk/services/NetOGlyc/
NetNGlyc	Prediction of N-glycosylation sites in human proteins	www.cbs.dtu.dk/services/NetNGlyc/

Table 28.1. (continued).

Name	Tool	Web reference
OGPET	Prediction of *O*-GalNAc (mucin-type) glycosylation sites in eukaryotic (non-protozoan) proteins	ogpet.utep.edu/
DictyOGlyc	Prediction of GlcNAc *O*-glyco-sylation sites in Dictyostelium	www.cbs.dtu.dk/services/DictyOGlyc/
YinOYang	*O*-beta-GlcNAc attachment sites in eukaryotic protein sequences	www.cbs.dtu.dk/services/YinOYang/
big-PI Predictor	GPI modification site prediction	mendel.imp.univie.ac.at/sat/gpi/gpi_server.html
DGPI	Prediction of GPI-anchor and cleavage sites	129.194.185.165/dgpi/
GPI-SOM	Identification of GPI-anchor signals by a Kohonen Self Organizing Map	gpi.unibe.ch/
Myristoylator	Prediction of N-terminal myris-toylation by neural networks	expasy.org/tools/myristoylator/
NetPhos	Prediction of Ser, Thr and Tyr phosphorylation sites in eukaryotic proteins	www.cbs.dtu.dk/services/NetPhos/
NetPicoRNA	Prediction of protease cleavage sites in picornaviral proteins	www.cbs.dtu.dk/services/NetPicoRNA/
NMT	Prediction of *N*-terminal *N*-myristoylation	mendel.imp.univie.ac.at/myristate/SUPLpredictor.htm
PrePS	Prenylation Prediction Suite	mendel.imp.ac.at/sat/PrePS/index.html
Sulfinator	Prediction of tyrosine sulfation sites	expasy.org/tools/sulfinator/
SUMOplot	Prediction of SUMO protein attachment sites	www.abgent.com/doc/sumoplot
TermiNator	Prediction of *N*-terminal modifi-cation	www.isv.cnrs-gif.fr/terminator2/index.html
Phospho.ELM	Phosphorylation	phospho.elm.eu.org
Phosphorylation site DB	Phosphorylation	vigen.biochem.vt.edu/xpd/xpd.htm
DSDBASE	Disulphide bonds	www.ncbs.res.in/~faculty/mini/dsdbase/dsdbase.html
O-GLYCBASE	Glycosylation	www.cbs.dtu.dk/databases/OGLYCBASE/
IMP Bioinfor-matics group	Lipidation	mendel.imp.ac.at/mendeljsp/index.jsp

3. Applications

Taking into consideration that the overwhelming majority of proteins undergo posttranslational modifications, it becomes clear that the analysis of such modifications is an essential tool for biochemistry.

In general, they can be divided into functional and nonfunctional modifications. PTMs without direct biological function nevertheless contribute to the protein's physicochemical properties. The definition of the structure of a protein mostly requires analysis of its PTMs beside characterization of its primary, secondary and tertiary structure. Virtually, all methods listed above are applied for characterization of posttranslational modified proteins. The importance of characterization of PTMs with biological function is immediately comprehensible, as they are involved e.g., in cell–cell interaction, fertilization, protein half-life, protein targeting, protein degradation, signal transduction, and many others.

A NCBI PubMed search using the terms "protein," "posttranslational modification," and "function" results in more than 20.000 hits, of which around 3,500 are reviews on this subject. Moreover, analysis of PTMs is essential for proteomic research, the development of new drugs and for the production, registration, and monitoring of therapeutic pharmaceutical proteins.

The increasing interest in two of the most important and abundant PTMs and their characterization within proteomic research is reflected by use of the terms "phosphoproteomics" and "glycomics." Phosphoproteomics describes the analysis of the sites and amount of protein phosphorylation under different biological conditions (111). Typical examples are the investigation of signal transduction (112) or the characterization of functional protein networks (113) and their dynamic alteration during physiological and pathophysiological processes in platelets (114). Glycomics, i.e., investigation of structure and function of oligosaccharides, may deal with drug development (115) or development of analytical tools for detection of diseases (116), just to mention some examples. Glycoengineering, i.e., the directed modification of the glycosylation of, or the artificial attachment of polymers to therapeutic proteins, demand analytical tools for their characterization as well (117,118).

The definition of PTMs is an essential part of the characterization of therapeutic proteins for approval, and during the approval process for biosimilars (119). The exact structure of a protein pharmaceutical cannot be defined without knowledge of all PTMs. In their guidance Q6A for the pharmaceutical industries, the International Conference on harmonisation of technical requirements for registration of pharmaceuticals for human use (ICH) states, that "For desired product and product-related substances, details should be provided on primary, secondary and higher-order structure; posttranslational forms (e.g., glycoforms); biological activity, purity, and immunochemical properties, when relevant." Consequently, almost each and every PTM of a protein is of concern for the regulatory agencies. The test specifications and acceptance criteria are further specified by guideline Q6B. For example, concerning the glycosylation of proteins "… the carbohydrate content (neutral sugars, amino sugars, and sialic acids) is determined. In addition, the structure of the carbohydrate chains, the oligosaccharide pattern (antennary profile) and the glycosylation site(s) of the polypeptide chain is analyzed, to the extent possible." Eventually, the required analytical data on PTMs depend on known functional importance of a certain modification and the availability of appropriate analytical methods for its characterization. Thus, the requirements may change with the development of new, sensitive methods for analysis of PTMs.

In the case of recombinant proteins, the PTMs depend on both, the type of host cell line (120,121) and specific cell culture conditions like temperature or ammonium ion- and glucosamine concentration (122,123). James et al. demonstrate the influence of host cell type on the N-glycosylation of recombinant human interferon-gamma expressed in Chinese hamster ovary cells, baculovirus-infected Sf9 insect cells and the mammary gland of transgenic mice by application of enzymatic hydrolysis of *N*-linked glycans by PNGaseF, fluorescent labeling of the released *N*-glycans, and subsequent characterization of the oligosaccharides by anion-exchange chromatography, MALDI-MS and ESI-MS. A detailed strategy for monitoring the glycosylation of therapeutic glycoproteins for consistency during production by HPLC of fluorescence labeling of oligosaccharides is given by Dhume et al. *(124)*.

There are far more applications for the characterization of PTMs, whose detailed description would certainly go far beyond the scope of this chapter. Nevertheless, due to the influence on diverse cellular processes, examination of PTMs is crucial for understanding protein structure-function relationship. Further advances in the development of even more sensitive methods for the analysis of PTMs will certainly lead to new insights into their biological impact in the future.

References

1. Graves DJ, Martin BL, Wang JH (1994) Co- and posttranslational modification of proteins: chemical principles and biological effects. Oxford University Press, Oxford

2. Walsh CT (2006) Posttranslational modification of proteins: expanding nature's inventory. Roberts and Company Publishers, Greenwood Village, CO

3. Miklos GLG, Maleszka R (2001) Protein functions and biological contexts. Proteomics 1:169–178

4. Gooley AA, Packer NH (1997) The importance of protein co- and posttranslational modifications in proteome projects. In: Proteome research: new frontiers in functional genomics. Springer-Verlag Berlin Heidelberg New York, pp. 65–91

5. Mitoma J, Bao X, Petryanik B, Schaerli P, Gauguet J-M, Yu SY, Kawashima H, Saito H, Ohtsubo K, Marth JD, Khoo K-H, von Andrian UH, Lowe, J. B. and Fukuda, M. (2007) Critical functions of N-glycans in L-selectin-mediated lymphocyte homing and recruitment. Nature Immunol 8:409–418

6. Cohen P (2000) The regulation of protein function by multisite phosphorylation: a 25 year update. Trends Biochem Sci 25:596–601

7. Ciechanover A (2006) Intracellular protein degradation: from a vague idea thru the lysosome and the ubiquitin-proteasome system and onto human diseases and drug targeting. Exp Biol Med 7:1197–1211

8. Boeckmann B, Blatter M-C, Famiglietti L, Hinz U, Lane L, Rochert B, Bairoch A (2005) Protein variety and functional diversity: Swiss-Prot annotation in its biological context. C. R. Biologies 328:882–899

9. Williams KL, Hochstrasser DF (1997) Introduction to the proteome. In: Proteome research: new frontiers in functional genomics. Springer-Verlag Berlin Heidelberg New York, pp. 1–12

10. Godovac-Zimmermann J, Brown LR (2001) Perspectives for mass spectrometry and functional proteomics. Mass Spectrometry Rev 20:1–57

11. Mann M, Jensen ON (2003) Proteomic analysis of post-translational modifications. Nat Biotechnol 21:255–261

12. Zhu K, Zhao J, Miller FR, Barder TJ, Lubman DM (2005) Protein pI shifts due to posttranslational modifications in the separation and characterization of proteins. Anal Chem 77:2745–2755

13. Wu J, Lenchik NJ, Pabst MJ, Solomon SS, Shull J, Gerling IC (2005) Functional characterization of two-dimensional gel-separated proteins using sequential staining. Electrophoresis 26:225–237

14. Hamdan M, Galvani M, Righetti PG (2001) Monitoring 2-D gel induced modifications of proteins by MALDI-TOF mass spectrometry. Mass Spectrometry Rev 20:121–141
15. Schroeder MJ, Webb DJ, Shabanowitz J, Horwitz AF, Hunt DF (2005) Methods for the detection of paxillin post-translational modifications and interacting proteins by mass spectrometry. J. Proteome Res 4:1832–1841
16. Nilsson CL, Davidsson P (2000) New separation tools for comprehensive studies of protein expression by mass spectrometry. Mass Spectrometry Rev 19:390–397
17. James P (2001) Proteome research: mass spectrometry. Springer-Verlag Berlin, Heidelberg
18. Farriol-Mathis N, Garavelli JS, Boeckmann B, Duvaud S, Gasteiger E, Gateau A, Veuthey AL, Bairoch A (2004) Annotation of post-translational modifications in the Swiss-Prot knowledge base. Proteomics 4:1527–1550
19. Blom N, Sicheritz-Pontén T, Gupta R, Gammeltoft S, Brunak S (2004) Prediction of post-translational glycosylation and phosphorylation of proteins from the amino acid sequence. Proteomics 4:1633–1649
20. Rune M (2006) Mass spectrometry data analysis in proteomics. Humana Press, Totowa
21. Creighton TE (1984) Disulfide bond formation in proteins. In: Wold, F, Moldave, K (eds) Methods in Enzymology, vol. 107. Academic, San Diego, CA, pp. 305–329
22. Smith DL, Zhou Z (1990) Strategies for locating disulfide bonds in proteins. In: Methods in Enzymology, vol. 193. McCloskey JA (ed) Academic, New York, pp. 374–389
23. Hirayama K, Akashi S (1994) Assignment of disulfide bonds in proteins. In: Matsuo, T, Caprioli RM, Gross ML, Seyama Y (eds) Biological mass spectrometry: present and future, Wiley, New York, pp. 299–312
24. Wu J, (2008) In: Kannicht C (ed) Methods in molecular biology, vol. 446: Posttranslational modifications of proteins Humana, Totowa, NJ, pp. 1–20
25. Wu J, Gage DA, Watson, JT (1996) A strategy to locate cysteine residues in proteins by specific chemical cleavage followed by matrix-assisted laser desorption/ionization time-of-flight mass spectrometry. Anal Biochem 235:161–174
26. Reinders J, Lewandrowski U, Möbius J, Wagner Y, Sickmann A (2004) Challenges in mass spectrometry-based proteomics. Proteomics 4:3686–3703
27. Weise C, Lenz C, (2008) Identification of Protein Phosphorylation Sites by Advanced LC-ESI_MS/MS Methods, In: Kannicht C (ed) Methods in molecular biology, vol. 446, Posttranslational modifications of proteins Humana, Totowa, NJ, pp. 33–46
28. Steen H, Jebanathirajah JH, Rush J, Morrice N, and Kirschner, MW (2006) Myths, facts, and the consequences for qualitative and quantitative measurements. Molecular & Cellular Proteomics 5:172–181
29. see ref 27
30. see ref 14
31. Steinberg TH, Agnew BJ, Gee K.R, Leung W.-Y, Goodman T, Schulenberg B, Hendrickson J, Beechem JM, Haugland, RP, Patton WF (2003) Global quantitative phosphoprotein analysis using multiplexed proteomics technology. Proteomics 3:1128–1144
32. Monigatti F, Hekking B, Steen H (2006) Protein sulfation analysis – A primer. Biochim Biophys Acta 1764:1904–1913
33. Bundgaard JR, Sen JW, Johnsen AH, Rehfeld JF (2008) Analysis of tyrosine-O-sulfation. In: Kannicht C (ed) Methods in molecular biology , vol. 446, Posttranslational Modifications of Proteins. Humana, Totowa, NJ, pp. 47–66
34. Walsh CT (2006) Protein Glycosylation In: Posttranslational Modifications of Proteins: expanding nature's inventory, Roberts and Company Publishers, Greenwood Village, CO, pp. 281–316

35. Mechref YH, Novotny MV (2002) Structural investigations of glycoconjugates at high sensitivity. Chem Rev 102: 321–369
36. Varki A (1993) Biological roles of oligosaccharides: all of the theories are correct. Glycobiology 3:97–130
37. Varki A (2006) Nothing in glycobiology makes sense, except in the light of evolution. Cell 126:841–845
38. Kornfeld R, Kornfeld S (1985) Assembly of asparagine-linked oligosaccharides. Annu Rev Biochem 54:631–664
39. Miller I, Crawford J, Gianazza E (2006) Protein stains for proteomic applications: which, when, why? Proteomics 6:5385–5408
40. Hart C, Schulenberg B, Steinberg TH, Leung WY, Patton WF (2003) Detection of glycoproteins in polyacrylamide gels and on electroblots using Pro-Q Emerald 488 dye, a fluorescent periodate Schiff-base stain. Electrophoresis 24:588–598
41. Wu J, Lenchik NJ, Pabst MJ, Solomon SS, Shull J, Gerling IC (2005) Functional characterization of two-dimensional gel-separated proteins using sequential staining. Electrophoresis 26:225–237
42. Löster K, Kannicht C (2008) 2-Dimensional-Electrophoresis – detection of glycosylation and influence on spot pattern, In: Kannicht C (ed) Methods in molecular biology, vol. 446, Posttranslational modifications of proteins. Humana, Totowa, NJ, pp. 199–214.
43. Davies MJ, Hounsell EF (1998) HPLC and HPAEC of oligosaccharides and glycopeptides. In: Hounsell EF (ed) Methods in molecular biology, glycoanalysis protocols Humana Press, Totowa, NJ, pp. 79–100
44. Anumula KR (2006) Advances in fluorescence derivatization methods for high-performance liquid chromatographic analysis of glycoprotein carbohydrates. Anal Biochem. 350:1–23
45. Saddic NG, Dhume ST, Anumula KR (2008) Carbohydrate composition analysis of glycoproteins by HPLC using highly flourescent anthranilic acid (AA) tag. In: Kannicht C (ed) Methods in molecular biology, vol. 446: Posttranslational modifications of proteins. Humana, Totowa, NJ, pp. 1215–1230
46. Geyer H, Geyer R (2006) Strategies for analysis of glycoprotein glycosylation. Biochim Biophys Acta 1764:1853–1869
47. Hounsell EF (1998) Glycoanalysis Protocols, 2nd edn. Humana Press, Totowa, NJ.
48. Harvey DH (2001) Identification of protein-bound carbohydrates by mass spectrometry. Proteomics 1:311–328
49. Medzihradszky KF (2008) Characterization of site-specific N-glycosylation, In: Kannicht C (ed) Methods in molecular biology, vol. 446: Posttranslational modifications of proteins. Humana, Totowa, NJ, pp. 1293–1316
50. Trombetta ES (2003) The contribution of N-glycans and their processing in the endoplasmic reticulum to glycoprotein biosynthesis. Glycobiology 13:77R–91R
51. Townsend RR, Hardy MR (1991) Analysis of glycoprotein oligosaccharides using high-pH anion exchange chromatography. Glycobiology 2:139–147
52. Kumar HP, Hague C, Haley T, Starr CM, Besman MJ, Lundblad RL, Baker D (1996) Elucidation of N-linked oligosaccharide structures of recombinant human factor VIII using fluorophore-assisted carbohydrate electrophoresis. Biotechnol Appl Biochem 24:207–216
53. Kobata A (1994) Affinity chromatography with use of immobilized lectin columns. Biochem Soc Trans 22:360–364
54. Kobata A (1979) Use of endo- and exoglycosidases for structural studies of glycoconjugates. Anal Biochem 100:1–14
55. Tyagarajan K, Forte JG, Townsend RR (1996) Exoglycosidase purity and linkage specificity: assessment using oligosaccharide substrates and high-pH anion-exchange chromatography with pulsed amperometric detection. Glycobiology 6:83–93

56. Fu D, Chen L, O'Neill RA (1994) A detailed structural characterization of ribonuclease B oligosaccharides by 1H NMR spectroscopy and mass spectrometry. Carbohydr Res 261:173–186

57. Kannicht C, Grunow D, Lucka L (2008) Enzymatic sequence analysis of N-Glycans by exoglycosidase cleavage and mass spectrometry – Detection of Lewis X structures. In: Kannicht C (ed) Methods in molecular biology, vol. 446, Posttranslational modifications of proteins. Humana, Totowa, NJ, pp. 255–266

58. Lucka L, Fernando M, Grunow D, Kannicht C, Horst AK, Nollau P, Wagener, C (2005) Identification of Lewisx structures of the cell adhesion molecule CEACAM1 from human granulocytes. Glycobiol 15:87–100

59. Van den Steen P, Rudd PM, Dwek, RA, Opdenakker G (1998) Concepts and principles of O-linked glycosylation. Crit Rev Biochem Mol Biol 33:151–208

60. Hounsell EF, Davies MJ, and Renouf DV (1996) O-linked protein glycosylation structure and function. Glycoconj J 13:19–26.

61. Julenius K, Mølgaard A, Gupta R, Brunak S (2005) Prediction, conservation analysis and structural characterization of mammalian mucin-type O-glycosylation sites. Glycobiology 15:153–164

62. see ref. 49

63. Calvete JJ, Sanz J (2008) Analysis of O-Glycosylation. In: Kannicht C (ed) Methods in Molecular Biology, vol. 446: Posttranslational modifications of proteins. Humana, Totowa, NJ, pp. 1281–1292

64. Mechref Y, Novotny MV (2002) Structural investigations of glycoconjugates at high sensitivity. Chem Rev 102:321–369

65. Hanover JA (2001) Glycan-dependent signaling: O-linked N-acetylglucosamine. FASEB J. 15:1865–1876

66. Khidekel N, Ficarro SB, Peters EC, Hsieh-Wilson LC (2004) Exploring the O-GlcNAc proteome: Direct identification of O-GlcNAc-modified proteins from the brain. Proc Natl Acad Sci 101:13132–13137

67. see ref. 64

68. see ref. 66

69. Rudd PM, Mattu TS, Zitzmann N, Metha A, Colominas C, Hart E, Opdenakker G, Dwek RA (1999) Glycoproteins: Rapid sequencing technology for N-linked and GPI anchor glycans. Biotechnol Genet Eng Rev 16:1–21

70. Rudd PM, Colominas C, Royle L, Murphy N, Hart E, Merry AH, Hebesteit HF, Dwek RA. (2001) A high-performance liquid chromatography based strategy for rapid sensitive sequencing of N-linked oligosaccharide modifications to proteins in sodium dodecyl sulphate polyacrylamide electrophoresis gel bands. Proteomics 1:285–294

71. Vosseller K, Trinidad JC, Chalkley RJ, Specht CG, Thalhammer A, Lynn AJ, Snedecor JH, Guan S, Medzihradszky KF, Maltby DA, Schoepfer R, Burlingame AL (2006). O-linked N-acetylglucosamine proteomics of postsynaptic density preparations using lectin weak affinity chromatography (LWAC) and mass spectrometry. Mol. Cell. Proteomics 5:923–934

72. Ahrend M, Käberich A, Fergen M-T, Schmitz B (2008) Immunochemical methods for the rapid screening of the O-glycosidically linked N-acetylglucosamine modification of proteins. In: Kannicht C (ed) Methods in molecular biology, vol. 446, Posttranslational modifications of proteins. Humana, Totowa, NJ, pp. 267–280

73. Comer FI, Vosseller K, Wells L, Accavitti MA, Hart GW (2001). Characterization of a mouse monoclonal antibody specific for O-linked N-acetylglucosamine. Anal Biochem 293:169–177

74. Walsh CT (2006) Protein Lipidation. In: Posttranslational modifications of proteins: expanding nature's inventory. Roberts and Company Publishers, Greenwood Village, CO, pp. 171–202

75. Orlean P, Menon AK (2007) GPI anchoring of protein in yeast and mammalian cells or: how we learned to stop worrying and love glycophospholipids. J Lipid Res. 48:993–1011

76. Elortza F, Nuhse TS, Foster LJ, Stensballe A, Peck SC, Jensen ON (2003) Proteomic analysis of glycosylphosphatidylinositol-anchored membrane proteins. Mol Cell Proteomics 2:1261–1270

77. Azzouz N, Gerold P, Schwarz RT. (2008) Metabolic labeling and structural analysis of glycosylphosphatidylinositols from parasitic protozoa. In: Kannicht C (ed) Methods in molecular biology, vol.446, Posttranslational modifications of proteins Humana, Totowa, NJ, pp. 183–198

78. see ref. 74

79. Bijlmakers MJ, Marsh M (2003) The on-off story of protein palmitoylation. Trends Cell Biol 13, 32–42

80. Glomset JA, Gelb MH, Farnsworth CC (1990) Prenyl proteins in eukaryotic cells: A new type of membrane anchor. Trends Biochem. Sci 15:139–142

81. see ref 1

82. Lottspeich F, Zorbas H (1998) Lipidanalytik in Bioanalytik Spektrum Akademischer Verlag GmBH Heidelberg Berlin, pp. 537–568

83. Veit M, Ponimaskin E, Schmidt MFG (2008) Analysis of S-Acylation of Proteins. In: Kannicht C (ed) Methods in molecular biology, vol. 446, Posttranslational Modifications of Proteins Humana, Totowa, NJ, pp. 163–183

84. Walsh CT, (2006) Protein methylation and protein N-acetylation, in Posttranslational modifications of proteins: expanding nature's inventory, Roberts and Company Publishers, Greenwood Village, CO, pp. 121–170

85. Ermler U, Grabarse W, Shima, S, Goubeaud M, Thauer RK (1997) Crystal structure of methyl-coenzyme M reductase: The key enzyme of biological methane formation. Science 278:1457–1462

86. Arnold RJ, Running W, Reilly JP (2008) Analysis of methylation, acetylation and other modifications in bacterial ribosomal proteins. In: Kannicht C (ed) Methods in molecular biology, vol. 446, Posttranslational modifications of proteins. Humana, Totowa, NJ, pp. 151–162

87. Mukhapadhyay D, Riezman H (2007) Proeasome-independent functions of ubiquitin in endocytosis and signaling. Science 315:201–205

88. Denison C, Kirkpatrick DS, Gygi SP (2005) Proteomic insights into ubiquitin and ubiquitin-like proteins. Current Opinion Chem Biol 9:69–75

89. Parker CE, Warren MRE, Mocanu V, Greer SF, Borchers CH (2008) Mass spectrometric determination of protein ubiquitination, In: Kannicht C (ed) Methods in molecular biology, vol. 446, Posttranslational modifications of proteins. Humana, Totowa, NJ, pp. 109–130.

90. Kim KI, Baek SH (2006) SUMOylation code in cancer development and metastasis. Mol Cells 22:247–253

91. see ref. 88

92. Pichler A (2008) Analysis of SUMOylation, In: Kannicht C (ed) Methods in molecular biology, vol. 446, Posttranslational modifications of proteins. Humana, Totowa, NJ, pp. 131–138

93. Pichler A, Knipscheer P, Saitoh H, Sixma TK, Melchior F (2004) The RanBP2 SUMO E3 ligase is neither HECT- nor RING-type. Nat Struct Mol Biol 11: 984–991

94. Pedrioli PG, Raught B, Zhang XD, Rogers R, Aitchison J, Matunis M, Aebersold R (2006) Automated identification of SUMOylation sites using mass spectrometry and SUMmOn pattern recognition software. Nat Methods 3:533–539

95. Loeb KR, Haas AL (1992) The interferon-inducible 15-kDa ubiquitin homolog conjugates to intracellular proteins. J Biol Chem 267:7806–7813

96. Staub O (2004) Ubiquitylation and isgylation: overlapping enzymatic cascades do the job. Sci STKE 245:pe43

97. Giannakopoulos NV, Luo J-K, Papov V, Zou W, Lenschow DJ, Jacobs BS, Borden EC, Li J, Virgin HW, Zhang D-E (2005) Proteomic identification of proteins conjugated to ISG15 in mouse and human cells. Biochem Biophys Res Commun 336:496–506

98. Takeuchi T, Yokosawa H (2008) Detection and analysis of protein ISGylation In: Kannicht C (ed) Methods in molecular biology, vol. 446, Posttranslational modifications of proteins. Humana, Totowa, NJ, pp. 139–150

99. Walsh CT (2006) Postranslational hydroxylation of proteins, in Posttranslational Modifications of Proteins: expanding nature's inventory, Roberts and Company Publishers, Greenwood Village, CO, pp. 331–348

100. Castellino FJ, Ploplis VA, Zhang L (2008) Gamma-Glutamate and β-Hydrosyaspartate. In: Kannicht C (ed) Methods in molecular biology vol. 446, Posttranslational modifications of proteins Humana, Totowa, NJ, pp. 85–94

101. Furie B, Bouchard BA, Furie BC (1999) Vitamin K-dependent biosynthesis of γ-carboxyglutamic acid. Blood 93: 1798–1808

102. Walsh CT (2006) Protein carboxylation and amidation. In: Posttranslational modifications of proteins: expanding nature's inventory, Roberts and Company Publishers, Greenwood Village, CO, pp. 435–460

103. Bradbury AF, Smyth DG (1991) Peptide amidation. Trends Biochem Sci 3: 112–115

104. Eipper BA, Milgram SL, Husten EJ, Yun H, Mains RE (1993) Peptidylglycine (alpha)-amidating monooxygenase: A multifunctional protein with catalytic, processing, and routing domains. Protein Sci 4:489–497

105. Mueller GP, Driscoll WJ (2008) α-amidated peptides: approaches for analysis. In: Kannicht C (ed) Methods in molecular biology, vol. 446, Posttranslational modifications of proteins Humana, Totowa, NJ, pp. 167–184

106. Appel RD, Bairoch A (2004) Post-translational modifications: a challenge for proteomics and bioinformatics. Proteomics 6:1525–1526

107. Creasy DM, Cottrell JS (2004) Unimod: Protein modifications for mass spectrometry. Proteomics 6:1534–1536

108. Farriol-Mathis N, Garavelli JS, Boeckmann B, Duvaud S, Gasteiger E, Gateau A, Veuthey AL, Bairoch A (2004) Annotation of post-translational modifications in the Swiss-Prot knowledge base. Proteomics. 6, 1537–1550

109. Boeckmann B, Blatter M-C, Famiglietti L, Hinz U, Lane L, Roechert B, Bairoch, A (2005) C.R. Biologies 328: 882–899

110. Ivanisenko VA, Afonnikov DA, Kolchanov NA (2008) Web-based computational tools for the prediction and analysis of posttranslational modifications of proteins. In: Kannicht C (ed) Methods in molecular biology, vol. 446, Posttranslational modifications of proteins Humana, Totowa, NJ, pp. 363–384.

111. Johnson SA, Hunter T (2004) Phosphoproteomics finds its timing. Nature Biotechnology 22: 1093–1094

112. Morandell S, Stasyk T, Grosstessner-Hain K, Roitinger E, Mechtler K, Bonn GK, Huber LA (2006) Phosphoproteomics strategies for the functional analysis of signal transduction. Proteomics 6:4047–4056

113. Blagoev B, Ong S-E, Kratchmarova I, Mann M (2004) Temporal analysis of phosphotyrosine-dependent signaling networks by quantitative proteomics. Nature Biotechnology 22:1139–1145

114. Zahedi RP, Begonia AJ, Gambaryan S, Sickmann A (2006) Phosphoproteomics of human platelets: A quest for novel activation pathways. Biochim Biophys Acta 1764:1963–1976

115. Gesslbauer B, Kungl AJ (2006) Glycomic approaches toward drug development: therapeutically exploring the glycosaminoglycanome. Curr Opin Mol Ther. 8: 521–528

116. Miyamoto S (2006) Clinical applications of glycomic approaches for the detection of cancer and other diseases. Curr Opin Mol Ther. 8:507–513

117. Sinclair AM, Elliott S (2005) Glycoengineering: the effect of glycosylation on the properties of therapeutic proteins. J Pharm Sci 94:1626–1635

118. Gregoriadis G, Jain S, Papaioannou I, Laing P (2005) Improving the therapeutic efficacy of peptides and proteins: a role for polysialic acids. Int J Pharm 300:125–130

119. Walsh G, Jefferis R (2006) Post-translational modifications in the context of therapeutic proteins. Nat Biotechnol 24:1241–1252

120. James DC, Freedman RB, Hoare M, Ogonah OW, Rooney BC, Larionov OA, Dobrovolsky VN, Lagutin OV, Jenkins N (1995) N-glycosylation of recombinant human interferon-gamma produced in different animal expression systems. Nature Biotechnology 13:592–596

121. James DC, Goldman MH, Hoare M, Jenkins N, Oliver RW, Green BN, Freedman RB (1996) Posttranslational processing of recombinant human interferon-gamma in animal expression systems. Protein Sci 5:331–340

122. Gawlitzek M, Valley U, Wagner R (1998) Ammonium ion and glucosamine dependent increases of oligosaccharide complexity in recombinant glycoproteins secreted from cultivated BHK-21 cells. Biotechnol Bioeng 57:518–528

123. Bollati-Fogolin M, Forno G, Nimtz M, Conradt HS, Etcheverrigaray M, Kratie R (2005) Temperature reduction in cultures of hGM-CSF-expressing CHO cells: effect on productivity and product quality. Biotechnol Prog 21:17–21

124. Dhume ST, Saddic GN, Anumula KR (2008) Monitoring glycosylation of therapeutic glycoproteins for consistency by HPLC using highly fluorescent anthranilic acid (AA) tag. In: Kannicht C (ed) Methods in molecular biology, vol. 446, Posttranslational modifications of proteins Humana, Totowa, NJ, pp. 317–332

29

Protein Microarray Technology

Charlotte H. Clarke and Eric T. Fung

1. Introduction

Protein microarrays are increasingly utilized to better understand the expression patterns and function of proteins in various disease states. Additionally, their use in diagnostics holds great promise for applications in clinical medicine. The term "protein array" is used loosely to describe a technology founded on a number of classic protein assays that have been modified to function in a miniaturized environment with a common goal of enabling sensitive and reproducible, high throughput, multiplexed sample analysis. Similar to a gene array, a protein array is produced by immobilizing many (up to hundreds) of individual biomolecules in a defined pattern onto a solid surface for parallel analysis of samples in a high-throughput fashion. Generally, arrays consist of multiplexing on a planar surface, in contrast to multiplexing on beads, which is the basis for technologies such as xMAP® (Luminex). However, in contrast to DNA or RNA microarrays, the inherently diverse nature of proteins in biological systems makes it more difficult to achieve the same level of reproducibility for protein arrays as for gene arrays. A number of preanalytical and analytical variables must be identified and addressed to obtain meaningful and reproducible protein array data. In addition, because proteomes are characterized by protein expression across a large dynamic range, a common problem for most protein array technologies is sample complexity, which is being addressed via sample preparation methodologies performed before array binding. Frequently, the use of arrays in proteomic studies may include any of the following strategies: 1) antibody recognition of sample proteins, 2) chromatographic profiling of sample proteins, 3) expression of cDNA libraries, 3) in-situ tissue immuno- recognition, 4) protein function analysis (e.g., kinase), 5) protein–protein, nucleic acid or other molecule interaction or 6) protein domain–protein interaction. In this chapter, we will introduce the more common protein microarray technologies as well as challenges and considerations necessary for successful proteomic array studies.

The design of current protein arrays ranges from the utilization of a substrate with immobilized, spatially addressed biomolecules (a flat surface such as a coated microscope glass slide, microwells or arrays of beads) to

From: *Molecular Biomethods Handbook, 2nd Edition.*
Edited by: J. M. Walker and R. Rapley © Humana Press, Totowa, NJ

chemically modified surfaces (e.g., ProteinChip arrays). The immobilized biomolecules can include oligonucleotides or photoaptamers (single-stranded nucleic acids with high affinity to proteins), antibodies, proteins, peptides, carbohydrates, and other small molecules; whereas, a chromatographic substrate provides binding environments for proteins based on pH, hydrophobicity, or metal affinity. Since their inception in the late 1990s, protein array methods have continually undergone developmental changes and are substantially improved. Although technical challenges remain, the focused work of numerous laboratories has greatly advanced the understanding of many of the critical variables of array design and production. In general, protein array methodologies continue to be improved upon in four main categories: (1) formats of the protein array in terms of their applications, (2) sources of proteins used to generate the array, (3) surface and immobilization chemistry used to generate the protein array and (4) different methods used for the detection of protein activities on the array *(1)*. Automation of many steps of both microarray production and use is essential for reproducibility. The general scheme of a typical protein array experiment is shown in **Fig. 29.1.** A set of capture ligands is arrayed on a solid support. Following buffer washes

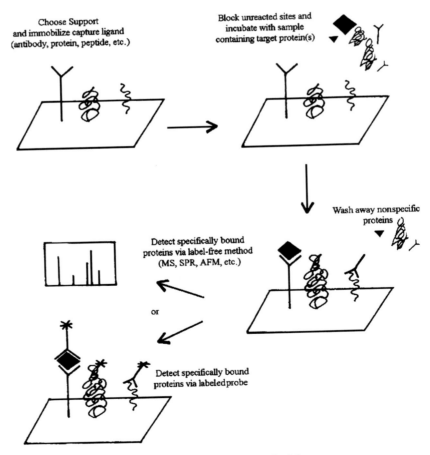

Fig. 29.1. General scheme of protein microarray methodology

and blocking of any unreacted surface sites, the array is then probed with a complex sample containing the counterparts of the capture molecules bound to the array. When an interaction occurs, a signal is revealed on the surface by a variety of detection techniques such as fluorescence, chemiluminescence or direct detection of the capture molecule *(15)*.

The collection of molecules arranged (or "arrayed") on the substrate can easily contain all the negative and positive controls associated with each specific probe that is also needed for thorough data analysis. Various sample types, including serum (or other bodily fluids), cell culture or tissue lysate, and conditioned culture media, can be incubated with a single slide containing the multiple antibodies or other probes. As with standard protein assaying methodologies, minimal nonspecific binding of biomolecules to the surface is one of the most important criteria for high quality micro array experiments. Detection of bound analytes is achieved by standard visualization methods (fluorescent or enzyme-linked reaction) that can employ direct labeling of the sample proteins, hapten molecule(s) or a secondary and/or tertiary antibody schema. The best choice of detection method is dependent on the particular array in question.

Antibody microarrays are common protein arrays in use today and are, in essence, a more high- throughput and efficient array-based version of a standard enzyme-linked immunosorbent assay (ELISA). Although retaining the specificity and quantitative characteristics of an ELISA, this technology also has the ability to make rapid, multiple, parallel, and more sensitive measurements of numerous analytes from a small volume of a single sample. Multiple antibodies can be attached onto a slide in a specified pattern via "printing" with a robot and normally contain as few as 20 or 30 up to several hundred different antibodies. Again, as with an ELISA, an antibody microarray will only be as good as each antibody/antigen pair. Therefore careful considerations must be taken into account concerning the quality (level of purification, concentration, specificity, etc.) of each antibody selected to measure the proteins of interest in each sample. Likewise, use of proper controls and generation of concentration curves are standard protocol.

The tissue microarray is a widely used, high-throughput platform for the analysis of proteins in fixed tissue specimens. Simply put, up to 500 sections (0.6–2.0 mm cores) of a fixed tissue (s) are attached to a substrate (slide) and incubated with a single probe (antibody, DNA, etc.) *(3)*. They are often used for target verification of results from cDNA micro arrays or expression profiling of tumors and tissues. Archival material can be used as well as freshly collected samples and both also yield histologic and cytologic detail not possible with other protein arrays. Although a tissue array does not replace the basic microscopic analysis of tissue histology or pathology, a well designed tissue array can replace the need to perform the same experiment over and over while also reducing the variability of experiments performed in multibatch mode. Mastering the method of tissue arraying is quite easy; however, getting the most out of a tissue microarray requires thoughtful planning and attention to detail before construction of the array. The goal of a tissue array is to present the pertinent tissue on the array. Therefore, different tissue types and disease states require different levels of accuracy in selecting the appropriate tissue from a donor block. Although some tissues can be cored from unmapped blocks, the optimal method to select the tissue for arraying from a donor block is to first map a hematoxylin and eosin (H & E) slide from the donor block *(3)*.

Although an antibody- based approach of sample "arraying" provides the means to measure the level of any list of known proteins, it is also possible to generate expression profiles of unknown protein species in a likewise high throughput, reproducible manner using chromatographic ProteinChip arrays. Depending on the array chemistry used, proteins can be retained on the array surface according to inherent protein characteristics (e.g., pI, hydrophobicity). Direct detection of the noncovalently bound analytes is made in a time of flight mass spectrometer (TOF-MS). This method allows for discovery of novel biomarkers of disease that might not be hypothesized to have a significant disregulation in the disease state and therefore, never measured by an antibody capture method.

2. Methods

2.1. Antibody Microarrays

2.1.1. Protocol Considerations

Substrates used for antibody microarrays are the "glue" that holds antibodies in a specified position during an assay. The type of substrate that can be used to cover a slide is varied and may include: poly-L-lysine- coating, aldehyde-coating, nitrocellulose, or a poly acrylamide-based HydroGel. It has been determined to be crucial to use an optimal slide coating for antibody immobilization, thus efforts have focused on determining the best coatings that offer high binding capacity, low auto-fluorescence, and a nondenaturing environment *(2)*.

Highly purified antibodies (e.g., the antibody is the major protein in the solution) work best in a microarray assay because a high concentration of contaminating proteins in the antibody solution usually results in a weakened or nonspecific signal. Therefore, antibodies only available as ascites fluid (fluid from the abdominal cavity of the animal used to produce the antibody) or antisera (animal serum containing antibodies) should be further purified before use. Additionally, although monoclonals known to work in ELISAs are preferred, polyclonals may also work well. High concentrations of agents that will interfere with antibody to substrate (surface) binding, such as excess glycerol or Tris-HCl (or amine containing buffers), must be avoided or removed if present. The concentration of antibody used during array printing has a recommended minimum range (300–500 µg/ml); however, higher concentrations may afford better results (e.g., increased signal intensity) if the amount of antibody expenditure is not a concern *(2)*.

If a direct-labeling method is used, the sample is processed (before incubation on the array) so that all proteins in the mixture are labeled with a hapten (e.g., biotin molecule) or fluorophore (a fluorescent molecule) that allows for subsequent detection. The simplicity of this method and the ability to incubate mixed samples on the same array (e.g., reference mixture labeled with a different color fluorophore) are advantageous. However, a disadvantage is increased background and decreased sensitivity as compared to amplification gained with the use of a secondary antibody *(2)*.

The choice of hapten for detection or dye for a secondary antibody will vary based on user. Fluorescent molecules appear to be the favorite for secondary labels as enzyme-linked amplification methods produce soluble products (e.g., horseradish peroxidase enzyme linked to the antibody will react with an added substrate to create a visible precipitate) that can diffuse away from the spot of origin and thus not be compatible with the microarray assay. Detection limits will depend on the antibodies used, the protein background in the sample, and the detection conditions. Generally, a direct-labeling method will allow detection of analytes in the low ng/mL range for targets in a serum background; whereas, a fluorescently tagged secondary antibody can give detection limits in the low pg/ml range *(2)*.

As part of the analysis of each array, a normalization factor should be calculated to bring the data from different microarrays onto a common scale. Normalization is used to eliminate some sources of variation in the data that can affect the measured protein expression levels. A normalization antibody should detect a purified protein spiked in to the samples or a protein normally found in the samples (such as IgG in serum). Likewise, quantitation of each protein is made based on a standard curve generated by binding of a known concentration of antigen bound to a particular antibody. Finally, reproducibility between replicate experiments is vital to the effectiveness of protein profiling experiments and should be monitored as a means to ensure good laboratory practice as well as assessing reagent quality (e.g., filter out unreliable antibodies). The reproducibility of each antibody can be assessed by calculating both the average coefficient of variation (CV) and the correlation between duplicate experiment sets *(2)*.

2.1.2. Antibody Microarray Method Overview

1. Antibody selection and preparation (e.g., make dilution for binding, removal of interfering substances if needed).
2. Preparation of slide with substrate (substrate will hold antibodies on slide).
3. Printing of microarray with antibodies (place antibodies in specific locations on slide).
4. Sample preparation and incubation on antibody-containing array.
5. Incubation with secondary detection agent (s) if necessary (e.g., detection antibody that recognizes target protein followed by fluorescent-tagged secondary antibody).
6. Data collection/analysis.

2.2. Tissue Microarrays

2.2.1. Protocol Considerations

Immediately after collection and before any processing, biological tissue must be "fixed" so that it remains in the state at which it existed at the time of collection. Depending on the fixative used, the proteins and molecules in both the cells and extracellular spaces of a tissue will become cross-linked or precipitated in clusters that render further biological activity impossible. Although there are variations of chemical fixative solutions, 10% formalin is the most common. Fixed tissue is then embedded in paraffin wax (all water is removed and replaced with paraffin) to give it support during subsequent handling. To create the array, a needle is used to remove "cores" of tissue from the wax-encased specimen termed the "donor block". Once the desired tissue has been dissected from the specimen, it is placed into a hole in a "recipient block" (made of low-melt paraffin) in a predetermined spatial arrangement (i.e., arrayed). The recipient block containing arrayed tissues is then sectioned with a microtome and each section mounted onto a slide before the paraffin is melted away to allow for labeling.

If the tissue to be arrayed is from an archive (samples collected at some time in the past and stored for later use), it is important to know the fixative that was used after collection, as different fixatives will require different experimental methods. Although it is possible to create an array of tissue processed in mixed fixatives, knowledge of these details is imperative for interpretation (3).

The more important aspects of tissue array design are 1) matching the individual core size to the total number of cores that will be used and 2) putting them into a user friendly design on the slide. The use of "subarrays" to organize tissue in some meaningful manner will significantly ease the work of the user analyzing the array by reducing the chance of getting "lost" on the slide. Suggested subarray sizes are therefore 3 × 3, 4 × 4, or 5 × 5 with 0.6 mm cores that can be viewed in its entirety with a 4× microscope objective. Considerations must be made about what tissue to place where on the array and are based on including the appropriate controls (benign disease, healthy normals, etc.) core size, over-sampling, and matched disease state and normal tissue pairing. The best advice is to anticipate as many questions that might be asked during analysis, e.g., is there nonspecific staining, is there endogenous biotin binding the label, etc., and include the necessary controls in the design to be able to answer them (3).

Oversampling a tissue is the attempt to deal with tissue heterogeneity by taking multiple samples (cores) from different areas of each tissue specimen. The number of cores necessary for complete representation may vary depending upon the specific tissue type and protein (s) measured. Core diameter used will give more or less information about the cellular architecture in one area. The biology of the tissue under study will ultimately determine the optimum balance to obtain between the two. It is important to note that there are some tissues and disease states that require extreme precision and accuracy during sampling, are challenging to adequately represent on an array or may not be amenable to representation on tissue arrays (3).

2.2.2. Tissue Microarray Method Overview

1. Array design (e.g., determine optimum physical layout of specimen cores within the array).
2. Mapping of donor tissue (e.g., H & E stained slide of the donor tissue can be used to determine optimum areas from which to take core samples).
3. Sampling of donor tissue (i.e., removing cores of the sample with a needle).
4. Arraying donor cores in recipient block.
5. Sectioning of the completed array (i.e., using a microtome to generate thin slices of the donor block that are then mounted onto a new slide).
6. Immunohistochemistry (or other labeling method as desired) to detect specific proteins/protein levels within each tissue sample on the array.
7. Data collection/analysis.

2.3. Chromatographic Surface Arrays (e.g., Seldi-TOF-MS)

2.3.1. Protocol Considerations

To decrease sample complexity and increase total number of proteins detected from a protein solution, it is common to perform some type of sample fractionation, e.g., anion-exchange fractionation, before binding on a ProteinChip© array. This principle can be applied to virtually any type of sample from serum to cell culture lysate to cerebrospinal fluid. It is then suggested that the same fraction be profiled on all surfaces at the same time so that the samples are not subjected to multiple freeze-thaw cycles.

The array surfaces and matrix (energy absorbing molecule needed for laser desorption–time-of-flight mass spectrometry detection) used to profile the samples is at the discretion of the user. However, it is suggested that each sample is arrayed on different protein binding surfaces (i.e. ionic exchange or hydrophobic retention) because each array surface will retain an overlapping subsets of proteins. Different matrices will also reveal different profiles.

The use of robotics (any type of automated liquid handler, e.g., Biomek or Tecan) for sample and array preparation will support high throughput sample processing while increasing reproducibility. It is possible to process 96 samples in each bioprocessor that holds 12 ProteinChip arrays and three or four bioprocessors can be processed during one run. All samples should be bound to arrays on duplicate spots and the arrays read (in a time-of-flight mass spectrometer) within a reasonably similar period of time following preparation.

2.3.2. ProteinChip Array Method Overview

1. Sample preparation (e.g., fractionation of the protein containing sample and/or dilution into binding buffers).
2. Binding of samples to array surfaces (i.e., allowing protein containing samples to bind to the chemically modified surface).
3. Selective buffer washes (e.g., pH or NaCl content used in the wash buffer will determine stringency of protein binding to a particular surface).
4. Addition of matrix (i.e., solution of energy absorbing molecules is applied to the ProteinChip surface containing bound proteins).
5. Data collection/analysis (i.e., spectra that indicate mass and relative quantity are generated after proteins are desorbed from the surface of the array in a time of flight mass spectrometer).

3. Applications

Microarrays of proteins and peptides are making it possible to screen numerous binding events in a parallel and high throughput fashion; therefore they are emerging as a powerful tool for proteomics research and clinical assays. The complex nature of the proteome, the wide dynamic range of protein concentration in biological samples and the critical role of optimized preparation of any type of array are essential concepts to address. Keeping these in mind, the possibilities for continued protein array use is exciting and promising. For a more in-depth study of protein microarray technologies, suggested reading would include a number of helpful review articles and books that cover the many types of microarrays including those not mentioned here (1,4–7).

Although method development is ongoing, meaningful protein microarray data is already a vital part of studies designed to better understand proteomes. Present research aimed at understanding the degree of changes in protein expression, post- translational protein modification and function and/or molecular interactions can be readily assessed at new levels via protein microarrays. A quick search of the literature will reveal numerous published studies presenting protein microarray data.

Protein phosphorylation is an especially important post-translational regulator of many processes inside cells. Complex signaling pathways can be regulated by multiple coordinated phosphorylation events; therefore, with a microarray, one has the ability to examine the phosphorylation states of multiple proteins and/or multiple samples in parallel. In a study of colorectal cancer, Lugli et al., *(8)* were interested in the diagnostic and prognostic value of phosphorylated ERK and phosphorylated AKT (two downstream molecules of the MAPK and PI3K/AKT pathways). Using tissue microarrays it was possible to measure these phosphorylated proteins in 1,420 colorectal cancer resection specimens simultaneously while correlating the findings with other relevant clinicopathologic features. Bowick et al., *(9)* report measuring protein phosphorylation and kinase activity to better understand the effect of virus infection on host-cell signaling in infected guinea pigs. The PepChip kinase assay system was used to assess the ability of cytoplasmic extracts of infected macrophages (from infected guinea pigs) to phosphorylate synthetic peptide kinase-substrates ex vivo. This particular microarray contains 2 × 1,176 peptides attached onto the surface of a 25 × 75mm slide. The peptides are substrates for possible phosphorylation events if the appropriate enzyme is available in the incubated sample (e.g., viral infected macrophages versus normal). In a variation of the antibody microarray, Akkiprik et al., *(10)* used a "reverse phase" microarray to study 40 different cell signaling proteins and their phosphoryation state in 14 different breast cancer cell lines. In this procedure, proteins from cell lysates were robotically spotted onto a coated glass slide. Specific antibodies were then used to detect the level of protein expression in these samples on each slide. Because of the density of the spots that can be included on one slide, multiple dilutions and replicates of each sample were incorporated into the design to increase the data robustness. This study allowed the investigators to identify important interactions between different signal transduction pathways, the apoptotic pathway, and the cell cycle pathway at the protein level in multiple breast tumor phenotypes.

Instead of measuring a single analyte for diagnostic or theranostic purposes, it has been suggested that multiple markers for a specific disease may be used together to improve diagnostic accuracy if the markers offer complementary discrimination information. Thus, the ability to efficiently screen putative markers in parallel, as enabled by protein microarrays, could allow an expansive characterization of alterations present in diseased patient samples.

The benefit of measuring multiple proteins via antibody array for the classification of cancer, benign or normal patient serum was reported by Orchekowski et al. *(11)* in the improvement in the classification accuracy of multiple markers relative to the use of single antibodies. Measuring 90 proteins in 140 samples, this study produced results that demonstrated a strategy for using antibody microarrays to profile proteins and identify candidate biomarkers. Data analysis resulted in the identification of previously unrecognized associations of serum proteins with pancreatic cancer and improved classification accuracy using combined measurements. However, it is stressed that a careful evaluation of factors that could introduce bias, such as low prevalence of disease often leading to use of combined sample sets, is important to avoid misleading results in biomarker research. In addition to quality control assessments of reagents, etc., statistical analysis of the effects of such variables as patient age and sample acquisition site may add confidence to the results. However, when available, the use of collections of complete larger sample sets with highly consistent collection and handling procedures would be expected to yield optimum results.

Rolland et al. *(12)* were interested in determining the prognostic power of two specific proteins, p53 and Bcl-2, combined, to indicate survival in breast cancer patients. Use of tissue microarray allowed for simultaneous measurement of the proteins in 819 cases of resected primary breast cancer. Though evidence suggests that these markers may have some independent prognostic power, the researchers found that combined analysis of p53 with Bcl-2 proved greater than the sum of the parts with biological significance; the presence of mutant p53 may be linked to loss of Bcl-2 and a subsequent synergistic increase in cellular proliferation. Zhang et al. *(13)* also demonstrated the multimarker approach in cancer diagnostics when reporting three significant markers of ovarian cancer from comparing the protein profiles from cancer, benign disease, and normal patient serum. The use of the Seldi ProteinChip array platform allowed the investigators to screen 500 serum samples in a high throughput, reproducible manner. As with Seldi, using a chemically defined substrate for protein retention rather than a known capture ligand (e.g., antibody), makes it possible to identify totally novel protein markers, including modified forms of known proteins, which may not be considered for study in a predetermined antibody array or may not have an antibody against it available.

Diagnostics for the determination of allergic reaction may also benefit from the use of microarray technology. Deinhofer et al. *(14)* developed a multiallergen assay, which contained recombinant allergen proteins printed onto a glass slide. The multiallergen test system presented in this study enables one to determine a patient's individual IgE reactivity profile against up to 400 individual allergens. One advantage of chip-based allergy diagnosis is that the IgE-reactivity profile to a large number of allergen components can be determined in a single test. However, it was noted that several problems, including high CV values (batch to batch variation), artificial signals owing to glass substrate defects, accumulation of dust particles on the surface, and partial or complete dehumidification leading to artificially increased signals, must be properly addressed before allergen chips can be used for routine testing.

Many of the microarrays used in the aforementioned and other proteomics studies are produced in-house by the researchers themselves or an institutional core facility; however, a wide variety are also available from commercial sources. A quick search on the internet will reveal the suppliers, cost, and type of protein microarray (s) available for purchase. These sites usually also contain a wealth of information regarding specific technological questions about the offered microarray products.

Protein microarrays are more commonly being used in biological laboratories for a host of research interests to advance our understanding of protein functions, protein–protein interactions and differential protein expression. Although, it is important to remember that protein microarray technology is not as straightforward as DNA technology, the protein microarray can be an excellent high-throughput tool used to examine a large collection of proteins simultaneously. It is an excellent method to discover previously unknown multifunctional proteins as well as to better understand well-known proteins. The future of microarray-based technologies for protein study is promising. With the continued momentum of the postgenomic era in biomedical research, proteomics and microarray-based technologies are playing increasingly greater roles and yeilding impressive results.

References

1. Chen G, Uttamchandani M, Lue R, Lesaicherre M, Yao S (2003). Array based technologies and their applications in proteomics. Current Topics Medicinal Chemistry 3:705–724
2. Haab B, Zhou H (2004) Multiplexed protein analysis using spotted antibody microarrays. In: Fung E (ed) Methods in molecular biology: protein arrays: methods and protocols. Humana Press. Vol. 264:33–45
3. Hewitt S (2004) Design, construction, and use of tissue microarrays. In: Fung E (ed) methods in molecular biology: protein arrays: methods and protocols. Humana Press. Vol. 264:61–72
4. Fung E (ed) (2004) Methods in molecular biology, volume 264: protein arrays, methods and protocols. Humana Press
5. Uttamchandani M, Wang J, Yao S (2006) Protein and small molecule microarrays: powerful tools for high throughput proteomics. Mol Biosyst 2 (1):58–68
6. Haab B (2006). Applications of antibody array platforms. Current Opinion Biotechnol 17 (4):415–421
7. Gulmann C, Sheehan K, Kay E, Liotta L, Petricoin C (2006). Array based proteomics: mapping of protein circuitries for diagnostics, prognostics, and therapy guidance in cancer. J Pathol 208:595–606
8. Lugli A, Zlobec I, Minoo P, Baker K, Tornillo L, Terracciano L, Jass J (2006). Role of the mitogen activated protein kinase and phosphoinositide 3- kinase/AKT pathways downstream molecules, phosphorylated extracellular signal – regulated kinase, and phosphorylated AKT in colorectal cancer–A tissue microarray based approach. Human Pathol 37:1022–1031
9. Bowick G, Fennewald S, Scott E, Zhang L, Elsom B, Aronson J, Spratt H Luxon B, Gorenstein D, Herzog N (2006). Identification of differentially activated cell-signaling networks associated with pichinde virus pathogenesis using systems kinomics. J Virol. Published Online Dec. 6
10. Akkiprik M, Nicorici D, Cogdell D, Jia Y, Hategan A, Tabus I, Yli-Harja O, Yu D, Sahin A, Zhang W (2006). Dissection of signalling pathways in fourteen breast cancer cell lines using reverse-phase protein lysate microarray. Technol Cancer Res Treatment. 5 (6):543–551
11. Orchekowski R, Hamelinck D, Li L, Gliwa E, VanBrocklin M, Marrero J, Vande Woude G, Feng Z, Brand R, Haab B (2005). Antibody microarray profiling reveals individual and combined serum proteins associated with pancreatic cancer. Cancer Res; 65 (23):11193–11202
12. Rolland P, Spendlove I, Madjid Z, Rakha E, Patel P, Ellis I, Durrant L (2006). The p53 positive Bcl-2 negative phenotype is an independent marker of prognosis in breast cancer. Int J Cancer Published Online Dec. 22
13. Zhang Z, Bast Jr, R, Yu Y, Li J, Sokoll L, Rai A, Rosenzweig J, Cameron B, Wang Y, Meng X, Berchuck A, van Haaften-Day C, Hacker N, de Bruijn H, van der Zee A, Jacobs I, Fung E, Chan D (2004). Three biomarkers identified from serum

proteomic analysis for the detection of early stage ovarian cancer. Cancer Res 64 (16):5882–5890

14. Deinhofer K, Sevcik H, Balic N, Harwanegg C, Hiller R, Rumpold H, Mueller M, Spitzauer S (2004). Microarrayed allergens for IgE profiling. Methods 32: 249–254

15. Cretich M, Damin F, Pirri G, Chiaria M (2006) Protein and peptide arrays: recent trends and new directions. Biomol Eng 23:77–88

30

Protein–Protein Interactions

Hae Ryoun Park, Lisa Montoya Cockrell, Yuhong Du, Andrea Kasinski,
Jonathan Havel, Jing Zhao, Francisca Reyes-Turcu, Keith D. Wilkinson, and Haian Fu

1. Introduction

Diverse cellular processes are mediated by dynamic networks of interacting
proteins in living organisms (1,2). These highly regulated protein–protein interactions determine cellular functions that are fundamental to life. As increasing numbers of protein complexes and interconnected protein networks are
revealed by a variety of experimental approaches, general principles underlying
protein–protein interactions and their roles in controlling cellular processes
have emerged. It appears that a general mode of protein–protein interaction is
mediated by a diverse group of specialized protein modules within individual
proteins (2). These protein modules often contain sequence motifs and structures conserved throughout evolution. The efficient regulation of many protein
interactions is achieved in part by posttranslational modification of a specific
protein motif, such as phosphorylation of a protein motif generating a new
binding site for other proteins. For example, Src homology 2 (SH2) domain
containing proteins specifically recognize protein motifs phosphorylated at
tyrosine. 14-3-3 proteins recognize various protein motifs only when they are
phosphorylated at a serine or threonine site (3). Through these tightly controlled mechanisms, protein–protein interactions form the backbone of various
signal transduction cascades that control vital cellular functions. One example
is the mitogen-activated protein kinase cascade composed of three tiers of
kinases, Raf-MEK-ERK (4). This kinase cascade is induced by a variety of
environmental signals and controls a number of cellular functions including
cell proliferation and differentiation. Because of their essential role in cellular
regulation, dysregulation of protein–protein interactions is associated with a
large number of human diseases, including cancer, neurodegenerative diseases,
and various metabolic diseases. Thus, identifying and studying protein complex
formation or dissociation is crucial for understanding general mechanisms that
govern normal cell growth and development as well as for targeting altered protein–protein interactions in diseases for drug discovery (5). Recent successes
in developing small molecule protein–protein interaction inhibitors strongly
support this line of research. This chapter focuses on methods for detecting and
monitoring protein–protein interactions.

From: *Molecular Biomethods Handbook, 2nd Edition.*
Edited by: J. M. Walker and R. Rapley © Humana Press, Totowa, NJ

Techniques for studying protein–protein interactions have been detailed in a number of specialized books *(6,7)*. These include various biochemical techniques for examining protein–protein interactions in vitro, biosensor based cell biology methodologies for monitoring protein–protein interactions in vivo, and some robust protein complex detection technologies for proteome exploration and high throughput screening incorporated into various drug discovery platforms. This chapter intends to highlight some basic methods frequently used in laboratories for studying protein interactions in vitro and in vivo. Some of these techniques are also used for proteomics studies and for high throughput screening purposes.

2. Methods

Protein–protein interactions are detected by a variety of techniques. Many of these techniques rely on the capturing of a target protein (bait) in a complex through an immobilized affinity reagent, such as an antibody. The first section will discuss these solid-phase based methods, including co-immunoprecipitation (co-IP) and affinity-tag based pull-down assays. Some transient protein–protein interactions are difficult to capture. The use of a chemical cross-linking approach coupled with co-IP or pull-down assays may be helpful to detect these transient protein–protein interactions *(8)*. The second section describes frequently used homogenous assays, which are often used for quantitative measurement of protein interactions and for high throughput screening purposes. The final section presents state-of-the-art techniques for monitoring protein–protein interactions in cells.

2.1. Solid Phase Affinity Chromatography-Based Methods

To detect a particular protein inside of cells or in test tubes, a reagent that can specifically recognize the protein of interest with high affinity is essential. High affinity reagents include antibodies that are specific for a native protein or a heterologous protein artificially tagged with a well defined epitope. Use of antibodies to capture the protein of interest and its associated protein partners is widely applied to detect protein interactions, which is termed coimmunoprecipitation (Co-IP; **Fig. 30.1A**). Other affinity reagents are also used for this purpose. Highly popular methods include the use of glutathione conjugated resin for isolation of glutathione *S*-transferase (GST)-tagged proteins and the use of nickel charged resin for isolation of hexahistidine (6 x His)-tagged protein complexes.

2.1.1. Coimmunoprecipitation

Co-IP utilizes specific antibodies to capture the protein of interest (bait) and proteins associated with the bait protein from a cell lysate pool *(9,10)*. Once isolated, the associated proteins are separated by SDS polyacrylamide gel electrophoresis (SDS-PAGE). Following this separation, the methods to detect the coprecipitating proteins are varied, but include mass spectroscopy, silver staining and Western blot *(11)*.

The most important component of co-IP is the antibody, which should have high affinity and specificity to the protein of interest. Antibodies are of two classes: monoclonal or polyclonal *(9)*. Monoclonal antibodies are produced

A. Coimmunoprecipitation

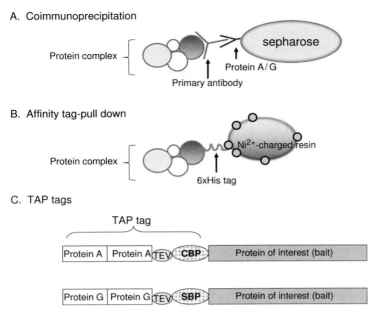

B. Affinity tag-pull down

C. TAP tags

Fig. 30.1. Schematic of solid phase based protein–protein interaction methods. (**A**) Co-immunoprecipitation. Primary antibodies are used to capture the antigen (bait) and its associated proteins in the complex. The sepharose beads are used to precipitate the captured antibody- antigen complex through conjugated secondary antibodies. (**B**) Affinity tag-based pull-down assays. A 6xHis-tagged protein is used as an example. The 6xHis tag fused to the bait protein has high affinity to nickle ions at the surface of activated sepharose beads. Nickle-charged resin captures 6xHis tagged bait protein and its associated proteins in the complex. (**C**) Tandem Affinity Purification (TAP) tags. Two representative TAP tags are shown.

by the fusion of isolated B lymphocytes with immortal cell cultures to form hybridomas. Each B lymphocyte produces antibodies to one specific epitope on an antigen, resulting in a hybridoma that produces antibodies to one particular epitope; hence its high specificity. Polyclonal antibodies are mixtures of antibodies that are produced when a susceptible animal is immunized with the antigen of interest. The resulting antibodies are specific to the antigen, but may recognize a variety of different epitopes on the antigen. Although the advantage of polyclonal antibodies is that they will tolerate subtle changes in the antigen due to the recognition of multiple antigen epitopes, monoclonal antibodies tend to be more specific. In co-IP, an antibody to a target protein is added to cell lysates. The bait protein complex captured by the antibody is precipitated by either protein A (from *Staphylococcus aureus*) or protein G (from *Streptococcus*) conjugated to sepharose resin. Both protein A and protein G have high affinity for a particular Fc domain in the immunoglobulin. An overview of the co-IP procedure and a commonly used method of detecting interacting proteins, Western blot, are described below.

1. Cells are seeded in appropriate amounts before the experiment. If necessary, proteins may be exogenously overexpressed by transfecting the cells with an epitope-tagged target gene.

2. Cells are lysed in a HEPES or Tris-HCl buffered lysis solution near neutral pH containing detergent and protease inhibitors (*see 12,13* for examples). Detergent selection is dependent on the strength of the protein–protein interaction under investigation. Typically used detergents include Nonidet-P40 and Triton-X 100. Lower concentrations are used when the target protein interaction is not very strong, while higher concentrations are utilized when the protein interaction affinity is high. Higher detergent concentrations are more stringent, reducing the amount of nonspecific binding.

3. Cell lysates are cleared by a centrifugation step (10 min, 16,110×g, microcentrifuge) at 4°C. This step removes cellular debris such as nuclear material, leaving the soluble protein lysate in the supernatant. Cells can also be disrupted by physical force in a Dounce homogenizer followed by centrifugation to obtain whole cell lysates. Whole cell proteins are extracted by a buffer with detergents such as Triton X-100.

4. The centrifuged lysates are further cleared with an appropriate amount of either Protein A or G sepharose. This step removes resin-protein A/G binding proteins, reducing non-specific interactions. After incubation, the sepharose resin is removed with a quick pulse microcentrifugation step, and the supernatant is transferred to a new tube.

5. To this newly cleared lysate, antibody specific for the protein of interest is added. The amount of antibody added depends on a number of factors, including the affinity of the antibody to the protein antigen, and the amount of antigen protein present in the lysate. This solution is rotated at 4°C, for 2 h to overnight. Following incubation with the antibody alone, protein A or G conjugated sepharose resin is added to isolate the antibody/protein complexes out of the lysate solution. Because of the rapidity and high affinity of protein A and G binding to the immunoglobulin protein, this incubation (4°C) usually needs not extend over 2 h.

6. After incubation, the protein A/G conjugated sepharose resin is collected with a quick pulse spin and is washed extensively with lysis buffer to remove non-specific interacting proteins. Following the last wash, the protein complex can be eluted from the protein A/G sepharose resin in various ways. For analytical detection of the associated proteins, a denaturing buffer containing SDS and a reducing agent such as DTT or β-mercaptoethanol is used to denature the proteins by boiling.

7. Protein samples are separated by SDS-PAGE. Following SDS-PAGE, the bait protein and the bait-associated proteins are revealed by various methods depending on the purpose and the abundance of the associated proteins. They can be directly visualized with staining methods, such as silver staining or Coomassie Blue staining. To detect a known protein in the complex, Western blot is used if the antibody is available. Proteins separated by SDS-PAGE are transferred onto a nitrocellulose or PVDF membrane. Interacting proteins are probed by Western blot, using specific antibodies. If sufficient amount of a unknown protein is available, the gel can be sliced and the protein eluted for mass spectroscopic analysis.

Co-IP allows investigators to study a protein without the need of exogenous overexpression, which may lead to undesired artifacts. Additionally, large protein tags such as GST can cause steric hindrance of protein–protein interactions in some cases. However, antibodies may not exist for certain proteins of interest. In this situation, the investigator can choose to use an antibody that specifically recognizes an epitope fused to the protein of interest. For example, antibodies are available for the commonly used protein tags c-Myc, FLAG, and hemagglutinin (HA). The protein of interest is then expressed in cells as a fusion with the epitope tag and immunoprecipitated with the corresponding antibody.

Several factors should be carefully considered when selecting antibodies for co-IP *(9)*. The specificity of the antibody for the antigen, or protein, is important to reduce nonspecific interactions. The affinity of the antibody for the target protein is also a crucial factor, as some antibody/antigen interactions are not strong enough for detection in co-IP experiments. Similarly, the abundance of the target protein can determine the success of co-IP. Proteins that have relatively low level of expression may not be detectable by typical co-IP methods. If this is the case, the investigator may exogenously overexpress the protein to increase its abundance in the cellular protein pool.

2.1.2. *Epitope Tag-Based Pull-Down Assays*

In many cases, high affinity antibodies are unavailable for specific proteins. With the completion of the genome sequences for a number of organisms including human, molecular biology approaches can be employed to add an epitope tag which is recognized by well characterized antibodies or specific affinity reagents. Widely used epitope tags include glutathione S-transferase (GST), 6xHis, FLAG, HA, and Myc epitopes. The epitope tagged proteins thus can be recognized by immobilized antibodies or specialized reagents, and the protein complex is isolated through solid phase affinity chromatography. GST-tag and 6xHis tag-based protein interaction methods are described below.

2.1.2.1. GST Pull-Down: One of the most practical and widely applied affinity chromatography methods to determine protein interactions is the GST pull-down. GST pull-down takes advantage of the high affinity of the glutathione-*S*-transferase for its substrate, glutathione. Typically, the bait protein is fused with GST through molecular cloning (see *(14)* for an example). The GST-tagged protein is isolated by applying glutathione-conjugated sepharose to the cell lysates to bind the GST. The sepharose is then washed and analyzed for proteins associated with the GST-tagged fusion protein. An overview of the GST pull-down procedure to detect protein interaction in mammalian cells is outlined next.

1. A GST-protein fusion is generated by cloning the cDNA of interest into a vector to generate an in-frame fusion with the GST gene. This expression plasmid is delivered into cells. Plasmids for expression either in *E. coli* or in mammalian cells have been used.
2. For mammalian cells, cell lysates are prepared after expression of the transfected plasmid in a lysis buffer as described in the Co-IP protocol.
3. Glutathione-conjugated sepharose resin is added to the cleared lysate.
4. This solution is rotated at 4°C. Usually, 2 h is adequate for the binding of GST-tagged proteins from the lysate to the glutathione-sepharose resin. However this incubation period may be adjusted as needed.
5. The resin is extensively washed with PBS or other wash buffer to minimize nonspecific interactions. The resulting resin is isolated by centrifugation.

The GST-tagged protein and its associated proteins are eluted and separated by SDS-PAGE and revealed either by direct staining or by specific antibodies in Western blot analysis.

2.1.2.2. 6xHis Pull-Down: The hexaHis-tag-based pull-down assay (6xHis pull-down) is a well-established affinity tag method used to determine physical interaction between two or more proteins **(Fig. 30.1B)**. The two basic elements for 6xHis pull-down assay are the availability of the bait protein tagged with six consecutive histidine residues and its associated protein (prey), either as a purified form or present in a mixture of cell lysates. The 6xHis-tagged bait protein is captured by an immobilized affinity ligand, either nickel ion or an anti-6xHis antibody, thereby allowing selective enrichment of the bait-prey protein complex. After extensive washing, the bait and the binding partners are eluted and detected as described next.

1. The gene encoding the bait protein is cloned into a prokaryotic or an neukaryotic expression vector harboring an six tandem histidine tag. Examples include pET15b for expression in *E. coli* and pDEST26 for expression in mammalian cells.
2. The 6xHis-tagged protein is expressed and purified from bacteria or mammalian cells. Often, it is unnecessary to purify 6xHis-tagged bait proteins for interaction assays; the protein lysate containing the 6xHis-tagged protein can be used as a bait source.
3. The 6xHis-tagged bait protein is incubated with a target protein. The target proteins may be purified proteins, proteins translated in vitro using cell-free expression systems, proteins in cell culture lysates, or proteins from tissue samples.
4. The nickel-chelating resin or anti-6xHis antibody-conjugated resin is added to the mix to capture the 6xHis-tagged bait along with its associated prey proteins.
5. The resin-bait-prey complex is washed under appropriate conditions in the presence of low concentrations of imidazole to remove nonspecifically bound proteins.
6. The bait protein and its interacting proteins are eluted with buffer containing a high concentration of imidazole. The isolated proteins are resolved by SDS-PAGE and detected by staining or Western blot with corresponding antibodies. If radioisotope labeled proteins are used, the associated proteins separated on SDS-PAGE will be visualized with radiography.

2.1.3. Tandem Affinity Purification

Affinity tags can be coupled together to improve the efficiency of protein complex recovery from a mixture of cell lysates. The key feature of the tandem affinity purification (TAP) technology is the use of two different affinity purification tags that are fused to the target protein of interest (bait) for a two step sequential affinity purification protocol *(15,16)*. Such a design allows the isolation of protein complexes under near physiological conditions for subsequent mass spectrometry analysis. One such TAP tag utilizes two immunoglobulin G (IgG)-binding domains of *Staphylococcus aureus* protein A, a cleavage site for tobacco etch virus (TEV) protease, and a calmodulin binding peptide (CBP) **(Fig. 30.1C)**. In this TAP, the bait protein is fused in-frame with the protein A_2-TEV-CBP tag. In the first step of the TAP purification, the protein A of the fusion protein is bound to IgG sepharose resin. The bound proteins are cleaved by the TEV protease, releasing the CBP-fusion protein. At the second step, the CBP-fusion is bound to calmodulin-coated beads in the presence of calcium and is eluted using EGTA. One of the advantages of the TAP method is the gentle washing conditions used with physiological buffers throughout the whole purification process, preventing the disruption of protein–protein interactions within the protein complexes of interest.

1. The N-terminal or C-terminal TAP tag is fused in-frame with the coding region of the bait protein in an appropriate expression vector *(16,17)*.
2. The TAP vector is introduced into recipient cells or organisms for transient or stable expression of the fusion protein *(18,19)*.
3. Total proteins are extracted from cells or organisms expressing the TAP-tagged target protein *(16)*.
4. Protein extracts are subjected to two successive purification steps based on the type of TAP systems used *(17)*. Three basic steps are involved. The first step is to capture the full length TAP-fusion protein. Besides the original design that uses IgG-sepharose for protein A tag, protein G tag has also been used in other TAP systems. In this case, IgG-sepharose is added to the cell lysate to precipitate protein A-or protein G-tagged fusion proteins. This step enriches the TAP-fusion population. Typically, the TAP system incorporates a protease cleavage site between the two tags. The most frequently used protease for this purpose is the TEV protease due to its high specificity and the absence of the protease in yeast and mammalian host cells. The second step is to release the second tag-fusion protein by adding TEV protease. The third step is to re-capture the fusion protein through the second tag. The second tag varies in different systems. For example, besides calmodulin-binding peptide, CBP, the streptavidin-binding peptide (SBP) has been incorporated in the GS-TAP system (**Fig. 30.1C**; *(20)*). In this step, either calmodulin sepharose or streptavidin sepharose is used to further purify the fusion protein complex depending on the type of tag used.
5. The retrieved proteins in the bait complexes are identified through mass spectrometry analysis *(21,22)*. For known proteins associated with the bait protein, Western blot with specific antibodies is used to monitor the presence of a particular protein in the complex.

2.1.4. Surface Plasmon Resonance

Surface plasmon resonance (SPR) is a technique that relies on an optical biosensor that can be used to quantify protein–protein interactions *(23–26)*. SPR occurs when light is reflected from a sensor chip at all angles except one where absorption occurs. The angle where light is absorbed is dependent on the refractive index of a thin layer at the surface of the sensor. Changes in the surface refractive index occur when a receptor binds to a ligand coupled to the sensor chip. SPR allows for monitoring, in real time, of a molecular interaction and thus provides a measurement for the association (k_a) and dissociation (k_d) rates of binding. This information is then used to calculate the affinity of the interaction (K_D) since the following relationship exists:

$$K_D = k_d / k_a$$

There are three main components in a SPR instrument. The first is the sensor chip which consists of a glass-covered thin layer of gold, whereby the ligand is immobilized onto the nonilluminated side of the film. The second is a sample delivery system used to deliver the receptor (analyte) to the ligand on the sensor chip. The third is a detector linked to a computer, which records the data in the form of a plot of SPR response (in RU units) versus time; this readout is called a sensogram. In a SPR experiment, buffer is first flowed over the chip surface to obtain a baseline. Next, the analyte is delivered to the surface and the instrument records the changes in the refractive index as the analyte binds to the ligand. These changes allow the direct measurement of the k_a of the interaction. Once steady-state is reached, buffer is passed over the surface again to record the dissociation rate of the interaction.

2.1.4.1. SPR Experiment Setup

1. There are many types of sensor chips which allow for different strategies to attach the ligand. A widely used chip is the CM5 from Biacore Inc., which contains a layer of carboxymethylated dextran matrix that extends about 100 nm into the flow cell and is surrounded by an aqueous environment. The carboxyl groups of the dextran layer allow the coupling of proteins via amine, thiol, and aldehyde groups. Other commercially available chips such as SA and NTA chips can be used to couple the ligand in a uniform orientation. In SA chips, streptavidin is linked to the carboxydextran layer to allow coupling of biotinylated proteins to the surface, while in NTA chips, nitrolotriacetic acid is used to couple 6*x*His-tagged ligands. Coupling of the ligand in a particular orientation can also be achieved by linking antibodies to the carboxymethylated dextran that recognize either an epitope on the protein or a protein tag such as FLAG, or GST (see description above).
2. If amine coupling is carried out, buffers containing primary amino groups, such as Tris, cannot be used *(23)*. In this case, HEPES and PBS buffers can be used. The first step used to couple a ligand via amine groups is to activate the surface with a mixture of NHS (*N*-hydroxysuccinimide) and EDC (*N*-ethyl-*N′*-dimethylaminopropyl-carbodiimide). Upon completion of activation, the ligand is passed across the surface for conjugation. Ethanolamine is then used to block the remaining sites.
3. An important consideration in deciding which of the two binding partners to couple to the chip is the molecular weight of the molecule. Since the SPR signal is proportional to the molecular weight of the bound molecule, it is desirable to attach the lowest molecular weight molecule to the sensor chip in order to obtain the strongest signal *(24)*.
4. High purity of both the ligand and the analyte is critical to obtain accurate measurements. Impurities in the sample preparations can cause errors in protein concentration as well as errors owing to nonspecific binding.
5. Surface regeneration: To dissociate the remaining bound analyte, the surface must be regenerated using conditions that might be deleterious to the ligand. It is therefore very important to test the activity of the ligand after treatment with these conditions. Regeneration conditions can include high salt, high or low pH, and detergent washes. Good regeneration is achieved when the signal is brought back to the baseline and the ligand is still active.

6. Controls included in an SPR experiment are control injections and measurement of a signal from an underivatized reference surface *(24,26)*. The control injections consist of running buffer, which contains everything except the analyte of interest. The reference surface is a chip that has undergone identical chemical treatment as the ligand surface except that it lacks the ligand. The use of control injections and a reference chip allow subtraction of noise generated by nonspecific binding, injection noise, and baseline drifts.

7. Data analysis: To obtain kinetic information, the analyte must be injected in a range of concentrations, between 1 n*M*–100 μ*M*. High analyte concentrations will provide information about the surface capacity since the surface will be saturated, while low analyte concentration will provide information about the association rate. Data from the control injection and reference surface must be subtracted from the raw data. All data sets are fit simultaneously to obtain k_a and k_d values, and surface capacity. This type of global analysis allows for good estimates of the kinetic parameters compared to nonlinear curve fitting of individual curves *(26)*. Software packages used to fit the data are BIAevaluation Version 3.0 (from Biacore) or CLAMP (www.core.utah.edu).

2.2. Homogeneous Protein–Protein Interaction Assays in Solution

2.2.1. Protein–Protein Proximity Assay

A number of methods have been described for detecting protein–protein interactions based on induced proximity. The signal generation in these methods relies on distance-dependent interaction of sensors, often fluorescent molecules coupled to the two interacting proteins. Förster (or Fluorescence) Resonance Energy Transfer (FRET) is a widely used such method *(27,28)*.

FRET is a photophysical effect where energy that is absorbed by one fluorescent molecule (donor) is transferred nonradiatively to a second fluorescent molecule (acceptor) *(27,29)*. Energy transfer from donor to acceptor fluorophores occurs when (i) the emission spectrum of the donor fluorophore significantly overlaps with the absorption spectrum of the acceptor fluorophore, (ii) the donor and acceptor transition dipole orientations are approximately parallel, and (iii) donor and acceptor molecules are in close proximity (typically 10–100 Å). The exceptional sensitivity and specificity of the FRET phenomenon is largely due to the sixth power dependence of energy transfer efficiency (*E*) on the distance (*R*) separating the donor and acceptor molecules as defined by the following equation *(27,29)*:

$$E = R_o^6/(R_o^6 + R^6)$$

where R_o (Forster distance) is defined as the separation distance between the donor and acceptor, for which the energy transfer efficiency is 50%. For a given donor–acceptor pair, R_o is a constant in space and time. In order to measure a reasonable FRET signal, the donor–acceptor separation should be comparable to this value of R_o. For example, at $R = R_o$, the transfer efficiency is 50% while this drastically reduces to 1.5% when $R = 2R_o$ (see *(27,29)* for detailed description).

The distance between a given donor and acceptor fluorophore pair can be decreased by attaching them to two interacting proteins (**Fig. 30.2A**). Thus,

A. FRET

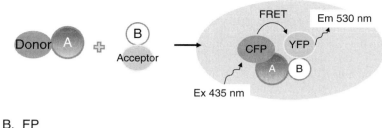

B. FP

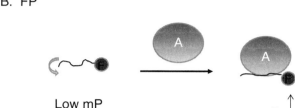

Fig. 30.2. Schematic of FRET and FP assays. (**A**) FRET. Interaction of protein A with protein B brings their coupled donor and acceptor fluorophores into proximity, leading to energy transfer. CFP and YFP are used as an example of a donor/acceptor pair. (**B**) FP. Rapidly rotating small molecule fluorophore gives low FP signal (low mP). The association of a relatively large molecule, such as a protein (A as shown), with the small molecule fluorophore slows down the motion of the fluorophore, leading to increased FP signal

these two interacting proteins, when coupled to the appropriate donor and acceptor fluorophores, can bring the two fluorophores into proximity and induce a FRET signal. Based on this principle, FRET methods have been designed for monitoring protein–protein interactions under a variety of conditions. When the spectral overlap, dipole orientation, and distance criteria are satisfied, the illuminated donor fluorophore-induced fluorescence emission from the acceptor is an indication of the interaction of two fluorophore-coupled proteins separated by <100 Å.

With the appropriate type of fluorophores, FRET can be used to monitor molecular interactions in vitro and in living cells. The widely used donor and acceptor fluorophore pairs for studying protein–protein interactions come from the auto-fluorescent proteins, green fluorescent protein (GFP) and its derivatives, which include CFP (cyan), YFP (yellow), BFP-GFP, and CFP-DsRed. Other pairs of fluorophores are often used for FRET measurements include Cy3-Cy5, europium-Cy5, and YFP-Cy3 (*27, 29*). Two methods for measuring FRET under in vitro or in vivo conditions are briefly described here.

2.2.1.1. In Vitro FRET Assay: Monitoring bimolecular interactions in vitro using FRET technology generally involves the following steps.

1. Label two interacting partners, such as protein or peptides, with a pair of FRET fluorophores to serve as the donor and acceptor. Europium and Cy5 or CFP and YFP are often used for this purpose. A number of methods are employed to couple fluorophores to proteins or peptides, which include (i) direct labeling with fluorophores through chemical reactions, (ii) indirect

labeling through fluorescently labeled conjugating agents, for example, europium chelate conjugated anti-6xHis antibody used for the labeling of 6xHis-tagged protein, and (iii) expressing fluorescent proteins fused to the test protein pair through genetic engineering with fluorophors such as CFP and YFP. These fusion proteins can be expressed in host cells and purified for in vitro use.

2. Mix labeled protein pair in a protein interaction buffer and incubate. Buffer used depends on the specific protein interaction under investigation. One general condition uses 50 mM HEPES (pH 7.4), 150 mM NaCl, and 0.1% bovine serum albumin.

3. Measure FRET signals using the appropriate settings corresponding to a particular fluorophor pair. There are a number of instruments for monitoring FRET signals in a microplate format (96-well or 384-well). These instruments offer high sensitivity and flexibility for FRET assays with different combinations of excitation and emission filter sets. For the europium-Cy5 pair, upon illumination at 330 nm, emission of the donor europium at 620 nm (F_{620nm}) and that of acceptor Cy5 at 665 nm (F_{665nm}) are recorded. For the CFP-YFP pair, upon excitation at 435 nm, emission spectrum of CFP at 480 nm and that of YFP at 530 nm are recorded.

4. Analyze FRET signals. FRET signal is expressed as the ratio between emission fluorescence of the acceptor and donor.

$$FRET = (F_{665nm(acceptor)}/F_{620nm(donor)}) \times 10^4 \text{ for the europium-Cy5 pair}$$

$$FRET = (F_{530nm(acceptor)}/F_{480nm(donor)}) \times 10^4 \text{ for the CFP-YFP pair}$$

2.2.1.2. FRET Assay in Cells

1. Construct expression vectors. The genes encoding test interacting protein pair are subcloned into appropriate expression vectors to generate fusion proteins, such as CFP-protein A (donor), YFP-protein B (acceptor).

2. Deliver FRET fusion genes into host cells. Mammalian cells, such as Cos7, on a slide or a culture plate, are transfected with expression vectors for CFP-protein A and YFP-protein B using efficient transfection reagent. Controls should be included, which include CFP-protein A only, YFP-protein B only, in addition to the test sample with both CFP-protein A and YFP-protein B. It will be valuable to include a test protein mutant that is defective in binding to the partner if available.

3. Incubate cells for 1–2 days to allow expression of fluorescent fusion proteins. Expression of fluorescent proteins can be monitored throughout the experiment.

4. Capture images of fluorescent cells with fluorescence microcopy. For live cell imaging, cells with expressed fluorescent proteins are placed under the viewing chamber and images are collected with corresponding excitation and emission filters for CFP and YFP. It is recommended that HEPES buffered medium without phenol red should be used for this purpose to decrease the background. Cells can also be fixed and mounted for image acquisition and analysis. Exposure time and light intensity of the camera settings should be adjusted to obtain images with maximum signal to background ratio.

5. Analyze data. Whole cell fluorescent images or regional images are analyzed for FRET signals. A number of methods have been developed to calculate the extent of FRET signals from changes in fluorescence intensity or lifetime (see *(27)* for details).

Besides FRET, other related technologies include Bioluminescence Resonance Energy Transfer (BRET) and the Amplified Luminescent Proximity Homogeneous Assay (AlphaScreen) *(30,31)*. BRET is based on the nonradiative transfer of energy between luminescent donor and fluorescent acceptor proteins. Renilla luciferase is often used as the luminescence donor, which catalyzes the degradation of coelenterazine, leading to luminescence signal. Upon energy transfer to the acceptor molecule due to protein–protein interaction induced proximity, the acceptor GFP or YFP, in turn, emits fluorescence. In this system, two test proteins fused to renilla luciferase and GFP, respectively, are examined under various conditions, such as in living cells. The AlphaScreen utilizes two types of beads coupled to two test proteins and so is only useful in vitro. Upon illumination, the donor beads release singlet oxygen, which excites the acceptor beads in their vicinity, leading to emission of fluorescence. The strict dependence of the energy transfer on the close proximity of the donor and acceptor beads allows the study of two interacting proteins conjugated to these beads (see *(32)* for an example).

2.2.2. Fluorescence Polarization

Fluorescence polarization (FP) is a highly sensitive method for the study of molecular interactions in solution *(33)*. This method can be used to measure association and dissociation between two molecules if one of the molecules is relatively small and fluorescent. When fluorescent small molecules (such as a small peptide) in solution are bound to bigger molecules (such as a protein), the rotational movement of the fluorophore becomes slower (**Fig. 30.2B**). When such a complex is irradiated with polarized light, much of the emitted light is also polarized because the complex moves slowly relative to the time it takes the excited fluorophore to emit a photon. Thus, the binding of a fluorescently labeled peptide to a protein can be monitored by the change in polarization.

1. Major components of an FP assay include a buffer with low fluorescence background and an appropriate fluorescently labeled ligand (tracer or probe). Frequently used buffers have neutral pH such as PBS or HEPES. The fluorescent tracers should be selected to attain sensitivity in a FP binding study. Molecular mass (i.e., molecular size and shape) of the analyte molecule is an important factor in FP measurement because molecular size is considered to be inversely proportional to the molecular motion in solution. When a fluorescent molecule with the molecular mass of tens of kDa binds a macromolecular substance, the FP value remains small. Therefore, fluorescently-tagged ligands having low molecular masses should be selected for the accurate analysis of the binding in the FP analysis. Tracers used in fluorescence polarization assays include a fluorescent dye conjugated to test peptides, drugs, or cytokines. They are synthesized by conjugating a fluorescent dye with a reactive derivative of the analyte. Typical fluorophores used in FP are fluorescein, rhodamine, and BODIPY dyes. The BODIPY dyes have longer excited-state lifetimes than fluorescein

and rhodamine, making their fluorescence polarization sensitive to binding interactions over a larger molecular weight range *(34)*.

2. Binding studies are carried out by mixing the fluorescently labeled tracer with its associated protein in a suitable buffer.

3. Fluorescence polarization measurements can be performed directly on a plate reader such as Analyst HT (Molecular Devices, Sunnyvale, CA). For rhodamine-labeled tracer, measurements are made with an excitation filter at 545 nm and emission filter at 610–75 nM. The dichroic filter (beam splitter) with a cutoff at 565 nm is used. Fluorescence polarization is defined as:

$$\text{Polarization} = P = (I_{\text{vertical}} - I_{\text{horizontal}})(I_{\text{vertical}} + I_{\text{horizontal}})$$

Where I_{vertical} is the intensity of the emission light parallel to the excitation light plane and $I_{\text{horizontal}}$ is the intensity of the emission light perpendicular to the excitation light plane *(33)*. All polarization values are expressed as the millipolarization units (mP).

Data analysis: The dynamic range of the FP assay, i.e., assay window, is defined as $mP_b - mP_f$, where mP_b is the recorded mP value for the specific binding in the presence of a particular protein concentration and mP_f is the recorded mP value for free tracer from the specific binding proteins *(35)*. Initially, the concentration of the fluorescently-labeled ligand is kept constant and the FP values are recorded by changing the concentrations of the binding protein. The FP value at each concentration is used to generate a binding isotherm for the calculation of association parameters such as *Kd* and maximal binding.

2.3. Protein Fragment Complementation Based Methods

2.3.1. Two-Hybrid Systems

The modular nature of a protein has been used to design methods that allow the detection of protein–protein interactions. For example, a transcription factor, such as Gal4, contains two functionally and structurally separable domains, a DNA-binding domain and a transcriptional activation domain. These two domains can be individually fused to two separate proteins. If these two fused proteins form a complex, this interaction brings the DNA-binding domain and the transcriptional activation domain into proximity and reconstitutes the function of Gal4 to activate the expression of a reporter gene *(36)*. In this way, the expression of a reporter gene, such as β-galactosidase, reflects the interaction of two proteins (**Fig. 30.3A**). One widely used method is the yeast two-hybrid system that measures protein interactions in yeast cells *(36)*. Other systems include two-hybrid systems using the bacterial host or mammalian cells *(6)*.

A number of yeast two-hybrid systems are available. The classical system developed utilizes the Gal4 transcription factor *(37)*. The *N*-terminal fragment (Gal4$_{1-147}$) of Gal4p carries the DNA-<u>b</u>inding <u>d</u>omain (BD) of the protein, while the C-terminal 112 residue fragment (Gal4$_{768-881}$) contains a transcription <u>a</u>ctivating <u>d</u>omain (AD). Fields and Song demonstrated that the reconstitution of these separate domains of the Gal4p protein through two interacting proteins leads to transcriptional activation of a Gal4-responsive promoter and the subsequent expression of a reporter gene *(36)*. Therefore, the separate BD and AD domains could potentially be fused to any two proteins. If the proteins interact, the transcription from reporter genes bearing GAL4-response

A. Two-hybrid system

B. PCA

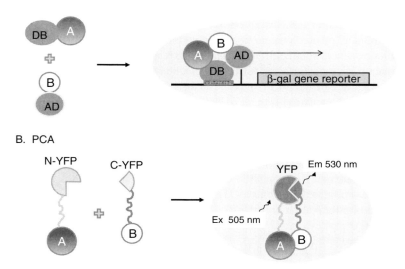

Fig. 30.3. Schematic of Two-hybrid system and Protein complementation assay (PCA). (**A**) A general yeast two- hybrid system. Two test proteins A and B are fused to a DNA binding domain (DB) and an activation domain (AD) of a selected transcription factor, respectively. The interaction of A and B brings AD and DB into proximity, leading to reconstitution of its transcriptional function and the expression of the reporter gene (β-galactosidase gene as shown) with the corresponding DNA bindging sequence (dotted box). (**B**) PCA. The fluorescent protein YFP is split into two parts, N-YFP and C-YFP. Two test interacting proteins are fused to N-YFP and C-YFP, respectively. The association of protein A and B brings N-YFP and C-YFP into proximity, allowing the refolding of a functional YFP. The fluorescence intensity of the refolded YFP reflects the interaction of A and B. Other reporter proteins are used, including luciferase, DHFR, TEV protein, and β-lactamase.

elements will reveal the interaction. The DNA binding domain in combination with the appropriate *cis* elements and an activation domain from other transcription factors, or selected artificial transcriptional activators, can also be employed in a similar manner. The Interaction trap is a modified version of the yeast Gal4-based two-hybrid system *(38)*. Interaction trap utilizes (i) the LexA DNA binding domain that can recognize the ColE1 LexA operator sequences in a *GAL1-lacZ* reporter gene and (ii) the selected B42 activation domain *(38)*. Two test proteins (a bait and a prey) are fused to LexA and B42, respectively (see *(38,39)* for examples). Interaction of the bait and the prey proteins then brings LexA close to B42, leading to the expression of LexA controlled *GAL1-lacZ* reporter gene.

1. The first step of this method is to clone a bait protein-coding gene into a two-hybrid system vector that generates a BD-bait fusion and to clone a prey coding gene into a vector that produce an AD-prey fusion. If the system is used to screen a library for new interacting partners, an appropriate cDNA library will be selected for the AD fusion partner.
2. Yeast host cells harboring the reporter gene are transformed with plasmids that express the BD-bait and AD-prey (or AD-cDNA library). For example,

Saccharomyces cerevisiae EGY48 (*MAT*a *trpl ura3 his3 LEU2::pLexAop-6LEU2*) is used as a host for the LexA-based system. For the protein/protein interaction analysis, EGY48 harboring a *lacZ* reporter is cotransformed with pEG202 derivatives and pJG4-5 derivatives by the lithium acetate method *(11)*.

3. Transformants are maintained in synthetic medium with glucose (2%) under selection for the *URA3*, *HIS3*, and *TRP1* containing expression plasmids (reporter, pEG202, and pJG4-5). Colonies are isolated for reporter gene expression analysis.

4. The expression of the reporter gene is evaluated. The expression of the lacZ gene is detected on indicator plates or quantified in a liquid medium assay. For a plate assay, colonies are patched onto synthetic medium plates containing galactose (2%), raffinose (1%), and X-gal to induce and detect the expression of the *lacZ* reporter gene. Positive expression induces blue color production. The time required for color development of positive interactions on X-gal selection plates ranges from 8 to 24 h. For the quantitative liquid assay, yeast transformants are grown overnight in the appropriate synthetic selecting medium to $A_{600} \sim 1.0$ before transferred to the galactose induction medium. After further induction, cells are permeabilized with chloroform and SDS *(11)*. Chlorophenyl-red-β-D-galactopyranoside is added as a chromogenic substrate. The amount of liberated chlorophenol red is detected with a spectrometer. Blue color formation on X-gal plates and the production of chlorophenol red indicate positive interaction of the test proteins.

5. For library screening to identify interacting proteins, positive transformants are selected. Library containing plasmids, such as pJG-cDNA library, are recovered from yeast cells and retested to eliminate false positives. Isolated plasmids are amplified in *E. coli*. The identities of the new interacting proteins are derived from DNA sequencing.

2.3.2. Protein Complementation Assay (PCA)

For detecting protein–protein interactions in living cells, the protein complementation assay (PCA) has been gaining increased attention. This method depends on the division of a monomeric "reporter" or "biosensor" protein into two separate, inactive components. These two components can be structurally reconstituted and refolded into a functional molecule upon association. This association of the two complementing fragments is driven by the interaction of two proteins. For example, the reporter protein is rationally fragmented into N- and C-terminal segments that independently do not exhibit any activity. The two fragments are genetically fused to two potential interaction partners. If the interaction occurs between the two proteins, the fragments are brought into proximity and able to complement each other through noncovalent interactions. The function of the fragmented but refolded protein is restored, leading to signal output (**Fig. 30.3B**).

An early description of this PCA-related technology is the ubiquitin-based split-protein sensor *(40)*. Here, Ubiquitin is split into two inactive fragments, which were fused to known interacting proteins. Upon interaction between these two proteins, the function of ubiquitin is restored by complementation of its fragments, leading to the cleavage of a reporter protein by ubiquitin-dependent proteases *(40)*. Many of the current reporter proteins are enzymes such as β-galactosidase, dihydrofolotate reductase, and β-lactamase *(41–43)*. Fluorescent complementation technologies have now been developed using both split yellow fluorescent protein (YFP) and green fluorescent protein (GFP), eliminating the need for incubation with substrates. *(44,45)* Although fluorescent protein complementation allows for direct spectroscopic read-outs, fluorescence-based approaches tend to suffer from slow development of fluorescence (folding) and background contributed by cellular auto-fluorescence. Bioluminescence assays, mainly split firefly and renilla luciferase, have been explored which give decreased background allowing for more sensitive quantification of signals *(46–48)*. A new PCA system has been described recently that uses *Gaussia* luciferase that gives rise to much improved luciferase signal *(49)*. Interestingly, the luciferase reporter has been coupled to the split TEV (tobacco etch virus) protease PCA system *(50)*. Reconstitution of the split TEV through fused interacting proteins is linked to either the cleavage and release of the active luciferase or the release of a transcription factor to activate the expression of the luciferase reporter gene. The availability of various reporters permits the use of the PCA method for a diverse array of applications. The specific readout varies depending on the type of the PCA system used. However, the use of the PCA method involves the following general steps.

1. Identify a reporter protein that gives high activity with low background upon re-association of the two fragmented segments. To illustrate the use of PCA, renilla luciferase is used as an example.
2. Design a strategy to split the reporter protein at a site that would allow maximum refolding and recovery of the protein activity. For renilla luciferase, one strategy uses renilla luciferase that is split after two consecutive glycine molecules at residue 229 to generate the N-terminal fragment (1–229). The C-terminal fragment begins with lysine 230 and continues through amino acid 311 *(51)*. Addition of glycine linkers to the region of the reporter that is fused to the gene of interest aids in the flexibility of the fragments allowing for more possibilities of interaction in vivo.
3. Amplify the DNA sequence for the N-and C-terminal fragments of renilla luciferase by PCR and subclone them into two separate expression vectors. Adding restriction sites on the primers will aid in cloning in subsequent steps. Using vectors that incorporates epitope tags (i.e., 6xHis, HA, or FLAG) will be useful for analyzing the expression of the fragments. Generating parent vectors where the segmented reporter is in frame with either the 5′ or 3′ portion of gene in question will aid in decreasing false negative results. Depending on where the interaction takes place on the proteins in question, the two portions of the reporter need to be in close enough proximity to find each other and restore proper enzyme function. This may only happen if the fusion is on either the N- or the C-terminal.
4. Make the fragmented renilla luciferase-target protein fusions. The interacting protein pair of interest are subsequently cloned into the two parent vectors in frame with the segmented reporter protein, generating two complementary PCA expression vectors. Consideration should be taken to introduce start and stop codons into the reporter as necessary. For example, if using the C-terminal reporter fragment fused to the N-terminal residue of the protein

of interest, a methionine must be incorporated at the beginning of the C-terminal reporter fragment to initiate translation.

5. Express PCA vectors in host cells. Mammalian cells are selected based on the experimental relevance for expression of PCA vectors. For example, Cos7 cells are transiently transfected with PCA vectors for their ease of transfection and their use for specific protein interactions in this in vivo environment. To verify expression, cells are lysed after growing for one to two days for analysis by Western blotting with an antibody specific to the test protein fusions or the introduced tags in the fusion proteins.

6. Monitor protein–protein interaction-induced luciferase activity. Lysates of PCA expression cells along with various control cells are used for luciferase activity assay in a luminescence plate reader or a standard luminometer *(41)*. Controls include protein pairs that do not interact or a mutant protein that fails to interact with the corresponding protein fusion. The expression of PCA plasmids in live cells can also be detected using a luminescence plate reader. Results are expressed as relative luciferase units (RLU) normalized to cell numbers or protein concentrations. Positive luciferase activity over the non-interacting protein pair control background is an indication of protein interaction.

3. Applications

3.1. Solid Phase Affinity Chromatography-Based Methods

3.1.1. Coimmunoprecipitation

Co-IP is a widely used method to determine if two proteins can bind to each other under native conditions. It is particularly important to use this method to confirm the physiological interaction of two proteins demonstrated by other means under artificial experimental conditions. One example of co-IP is the demonstration of the interaction between the TSC2 and 14-3-3 proteins *(52)*. Shumway et al. verified the interaction between these two proteins both with overexpressed and endogenous co-IP experiments. First, a c-Myc tagged version of the 14-3-3 protein was transiently expressed in cells. Lysates of these cells were subjected to co-IP, with an antibody to TSC2 to isolate TSC2 protein complexes, and reverse co-IP, with an antibody to the c-Myc tag to isolate Myc-14-3-3-associated protein complexes. Second, TSC2 antibody was used to co-IP endogenous TSC2, and associated endogenous 14-3-3, from cell lysates. All of the isolated protein interaction complexes were resolved by SDS-PAGE and determined by probing with specific antibodies in a Western blot.

One important consideration to meaningfully interpret co-IP results is the use of proper controls, extensively discussed by Phizicky and Fields *(53)*. One cause of false positive interactions is due to nonspecific binding of the antibody to the coprecipitated protein itself. To eliminate this possibility, the protein interaction should be demonstrated with the use of multiple antibodies derived from different sources, and recognizing different epitopes. If the interaction region on one or both proteins is known, mutations in this region which would disrupt protein–protein interactions are an efficient method to determine the specificity of the resulting interaction. For example, the K49E point mutation in the 14-3-3 protein results in a diminishment of 14-3-3's ability to bind to client proteins. This 14-3-3 K49E mutant is therefore a reliable tool to use when comparing binding results *(54)*. Likewise, if the amino acid sequence important for the protein interaction is known, a peptide corresponding to this sequence can be generated. The investigator can then include this control competitive peptide in the co-IP reaction, and can monitor if the peptide effectively competes with the protein interaction. This method was employed with the disruption of coimmunoprecipitated Raf/14-3-3 complex by difopein, a dimeric 14-3-3 peptide antagonist *(55)*.

Co-IP is an informative tool to identify and characterize protein interactions. It is both practical for studying known protein–protein interactions, and also useful for identifying new proteins associated with a bait protein recognized by the selected antibody. Co-IP enriches protein interaction complexes from cell lysate pools, allowing for extensive characterization of the resulting binding partners. Therefore, it is a valuable tool for proteomics analysis of the protein complex. An understanding of the basic principles of co-IP allows the investigator to discover novel protein interaction complexes which are regulated and occur under diverse sets of conditions.

However, we should realize that interacting proteins detected by co-IP from cell lysate may not represent direct association between these two proteins. Other in vitro assays are needed to confirm the nature of direct interaction with proper controls. Methods that can be routinely used to confirm direct protein–protein interactions include affinity pull-down assays using purified proteins described below, as well as protein overlay assays *(6)*.

3.1.2. Affinity Pull-Down Methods

Affinity pull-down assays with various tags allow for a quick and reliable isolation of tagged proteins from a mixture of cell lysates and analysis of proteins which co-purify with the tagged bait protein. Therefore, they can serve as both a confirmatory tool to verify previously suspected protein–protein interactions and a discovery tool to identify unknown protein–protein interactions. For confirmatory studies, they are used for determining whether two proteins directly bind to each other or through other proteins in the complex. These pull-down assays also provide a simple method to determine structure–function relationships to identify domains or residues that are responsible for the interaction. For discovery studies, any cellular or tissue lysates where the bait is functionally present are used as prey protein pools. Proteins associated with the tagged bait protein are isolated through affinity chromatography. The identities of the associated proteins are usually determined by mass spectrometry.

To determine direct protein–protein interactions, purified protein pairs are used. GST-tagged or 6xHis-tagged bait proteins can be used to show a direct interaction. Using this technique, the 6xHis-tagged ExoS ADP-ribosyltransferase protein was shown to bind 14-3-3 in a direct fashion *(56)*. The two purified proteins were mixed together, and were subjected to nickel-charged affinity chromatography to isolate 6xHis-protein complexes. To quantify the interaction, the amount of 14-3-3 eluted from the 6xHis-ExoS resin was determined. It was found that essentially molar equivalents of ExoS and 14-3-3 were reversibly bound to the affinity matrix while a ligand binding mutant of 14-3-3 or egg albumin was detected primarily in the unbound phase *(56)*. Further evidence in support of the direct interaction is provided by an alternative measure using surface plasmon resonance technology.

Another common application of the affinity pull-down is to verify an interaction and to define the structural determinants for the interaction. The source of the tagged proteins can be purified proteins from *E. coli*, mammalian cells, or other culture systems. Additionally, tagged proteins in a protein mix may be suitable under certain conditions because of the affinity chromatographic step used in the interaction assay. The target and prey proteins can be untagged native proteins from a variety of sources as long as a readout is available for the detection of the protein of interest. For example, radiography is used to detect the interaction of tagged proteins with a radiolabeled protein synthesized in an in vitro transcription/translation system *(57)*. Western blot is used for the detection of known interacting proteins with an available antibody (see below). An example of this is described by Bonnet et al. to identify the region of the PKR protein responsible for interaction with the IKK protein complex *(58)*. In this example, GST-tagged fragments of the PKR protein were expressed in *E. coli*. The GST-PKR protein fragments were captured from the bacterial lysates by glutathione-conjugated sepharose. The resulting GST-PKR protein fragments, bound to the glutathione sepharose, were incubated with mammalian cell lysates, allowing binding of GST-PKR to endogenous proteins. The resulting resin was washed and interacting proteins were analyzed by SDS-PAGE followed by Western blot with antibodies specific for IKK. Using this method, the PKR fragments that harbor IKK binding site were determined.

Affinity tagged pull-down assays have also been used for large scale protein–protein interaction assays. The GST-14-3-3 affinity column was used to carry out global proteomics analysis for identification of 14-3-3-associated proteins in different phases of the mammalian cell cycle *(59)*. This work has revealed 209 binding proteins in mitotic phase and 184 from the interphase 14-3-3 binding pool, emphasizing the significance of this affinity method. Similarly, the GST-tagged protein may be used to identify differentially regulated protein–protein interactions, coupled with the use of stable isotopic amino acids in cell culture (SILAC) technology *(60)*. In this example, combined cell lysates from EGF-stimulated versus unstimulated cells with SILAC were affinity-purified over the GST-tagged SH2 domain of a Grb2 fusion protein that specifically binds phosphorylated EGFR and Shc protein. This approach identified 28 EGFR/Shc-binding proteins selectively enriched upon EGF stimulation.

Owing to its high affinity for immobilized glutathione and the ease of manipulation, the GST-tag is widely used as a capture agent in various protein arrays for studying protein–protein interactions *(61)*. For instance, 5,800 proteins in the yeast proteome are individually tagged with GST and rapidly purified *(62)*. The GST-tagged proteins are individually printed onto slides at high density to form a yeast proteome microarray, which is used to screen for interacting proteins. For example, biotinylated calmodulin was used to screen the yeast proteome microarray, and the interacting proteins, were detected with Cy3-labeled streptavidin *(62)*. The affinity tags, such as GST, have an important role in spectral biosensor area for direct protein interaction detection, which may be applicable for high throughput screening purpose. The gold array chip with a glutathione surface is used to capture various GST-fusion bait proteins. Proteins that interact with the bait fused to GST are detected by the spectral SPR biosensor *(63)*. This method is likely to be useful for high through put screening purpose for isolation of protein–protein inter-action inhibitors.

Despite its powerful applications in a variety of platforms, some disadvantages of GST pull-down are noted. The GST protein itself is relatively large, approx 22 kDa and exists as a dimer. Because of its bulky size, it may sterically hinder the protein interactions of the fused protein. The GST protein is also prone to nonspecific interactions apart from the desired protein interactions that occur with the bait protein. Compared to other affinity tag-based pull-down techniques, 6xHis pull-down has its own advantages and disadvantages. The short histidine peptide is shown not to affect the naive conformation of bait proteins and thus maintains its partner binding activity. On the other hand, some endogenous proteins carry tandem histidine residues that might mimic the interaction with the 6xHis-tag, resulting in false positive results. Also, it is notable that affinity tag-based pull-down assays only represent the binding capacity of an exogenously expressed fusion protein in an artificial system. In vivo interaction remains to be further investigated by other techniques, which permit the formation of real protein complexes in a native environment, such as endogenous immunoprecipitation. Thus, co-IP and affinity tag based pull-down assays represent complementary category of methods for studying protein–protein interactions.

3.1.3. TAP

Protein–protein interactions require the isolation of protein complexes under non-denaturing conditions. Use of high affinity antibodies or affinity tags can allow a very high degree of purification, and preserve the protein complex and its biological activity. However, the number of highly specific antibodies or affinity tags is limited, and each when used alone is often inadequate for protein complex studies (64). To overcome this limitation, the TAP methods utilizing two consecutive affinity purification steps have been developed and have proven to be highly effective in the identification of protein complexes (15). The TAP system is useful in routine detection of protein–protein interactions. It is especially powerful for proteomics studies to reveal protein–protein interaction networks in a variety of organisms when coupled with mass spectrometry.

This TAP method was originally developed and successfully applied for interaction proteomics in yeast (15,65). Several variations on the TAP tag have been developed that may offer advantages for applications in mammalian cells (20,21,66–69). In one example, the CBP element was combined with two additional affinity tags, a 6xHis-tag, and three copies of the hemagglutinin epitope (MAFT) (66). The third affinity step would theoretically improve purity. In another, streptavidin binding peptide (SBP) tag replaces the CBP moiety or protein A and has several advantages (20). The SBP tag can avoid the use of calcium or EGTA. Another important advantage of the SBP tag is that a wide variety of streptavidin-conjugated materials and reagents are commercially available, which include plates, beads, enzymes, and fluorophores. Also, because SBP can be selectively eluted from streptavidin-conjugated resin by the addition of biotin, a high degree of purification can be achieved (64). In addition to the purity of protein complexes, Drakas et al isolated dramatically increased quantities of protein complexes by taking advantage of the strong biotin–streptavidin interaction (68).

The original design placed the TAP tag at the C-terminal end of the fusion protein (15). In the event that a C-terminal tag disrupts protein function, an

N-terminal TAP tag needs to be generated *(16)*. Protein overexpression may often lead to the formation of nonspecific and/or nonnatural protein interactions with host proteins. Ideally, the TAP-tagged protein should be expressed at low natural levels to replace the endogenous wild type gene. For example, the TAP tag was placed under the control of the native promoters in yeast for global gene expression and protein interaction analysis *(70)*. However, this is not always possible. Forler et al. developed an iTAP strategy, in which TAP approach is combined with suppression of the corresponding endogenous protein by RNAi *(67)*. It is recommended to use stable cell lines for the purification of interacting proteins rather than transiently overexpressed cells. Stable cell lines usually express moderate amount of proteins, and are less likely to produce artifacts due to overexpression and association with unnatural partners. In addition, a variety of modifications have been tried to improve the efficiency of TAP *(22,71)*. A recent description of a tag based on protein G and the streptavidin-binding peptide (GS-TAP) illustrates its efficient use in mammalian cells with increased protein-complex yield and improved specificity *(20)*.

Taken together, the choice of the appropriate number and/or type of TAP tags and the purification conditions depend on the nature of target proteins and the purpose of the designed experiments. It is expected that the TAP technology will find a broad application in dissecting interaction proteomics, the interactomes.

3.1.4. Surface Plasmon Resonance

SPR is another quantitative method that has a lot in common with pull-downs. That is, one component is immobilized while the other is in solution. It is amenable to rigorous analysis however since the steady-state level of binding is observed in real time and therefore does not suffer from elution of ligand when the beads are washed. Only analyte within a few angstroms of the surface gives rise to a signal and so only when the analyte is bound do we detect it. The method is widely applicable when binding constants are in the range of 10^{-5} to 10^{-10} *M*. The other advantage is that association and dissociation rates can be measured (Association rate constant (k_a): typically $10^3 - 5 \times 10^6$ $M^{-1}s^{-1}$ and Dissociation constant (k_d): typically $10^{-5} - 10^{-3}$ s^{-1}). Complications from restricted diffusion or rebinding of released analyte are easily detected by deviation from ideal sensorgrams.

An example is given in the recent studies on the specificity of binding of polyubiquitin to isolated UBA domains *(72)*. These domains bind ubiquitin in the micromolar range and exhibit selectivity as to the length and linkages of polyubiquitin chains. Binding constants for three different ubiquitin polymers interacting with sixteen different UBA domains revealed affinities varying from micromolar to millimolar and allowed the classification of the binding specificity of these domains into four classes. The binding specificity of the UBA domain is then predictive of the type of chain that it can interact with in the context of the physiological receptor and can offer important clues about the biological role(s) of the receptor.

3.2. Homogeneous Protein–Protein Interaction Assays in Solution

3.2.1. FRET

FRET is a unique and powerful technique to study protein–protein interactions, receptor-ligand interaction, protein conformational changes, and other molecular dynamics. It can be used to study bimolecular interaction in vitro, signal transduction pathways in vivo, and in high throughput screening for drug discovery.

FRET has been widely used to monitor protein–protein interaction in vitro. The most popular FRET pair for biological use is the CFP-YFP pair, which can be genetically fused with test proteins. For example, a FRET based assay was designed to monitor the interaction between BAD and 14-3-3ζ proteins in vitro and in vivo (73). The enhanced CFP was fused to BAD as a FRET donor and the enhanced YFP fused to 14-3-3ζ as an acceptor molecule. These two fusion proteins were purified and tested for their interaction as indicated by the FRET signal production. The interaction of 14-3-3 proteins with Bad is phosphorylation-dependent promoted by protein kinase A. In the absence of a kinase, mixing of the Bad-CFP and 14-3-3ζ-YFP only gave rise to a minimal change in fluorescence signal. However, when PKA-treated Bad-CFP was incubated with 14-3-3ζ-YFP, a significant decrease at 480 nm (CFP emission) and a significant increase at 535 nm (YFP emission) was observed, indicating a kinase induced interaction of Bad with 14-3-3ζ in vitro. The ratio of the YFP emission (535 nm) over CFP emission (480 nm) intensity was used to quantify the FRET signal.

A major advantage of using the CFP-YFP FRET pair is for examining protein–protein interactions in living cells. The association of Bad and 14-3-3ζ is used as an example for this application (73). Expression vectors for BAD-CFP and 14-3-3ζ-YFP were introduced into mammalian cells. The dynamic interaction between BAD-CFP and 14-3-3ζ-YFP was examined upon treatment of cells with both phosphorylation inhibitors or activators. The treatment of cells with staurosporine, a general inhibitor of protein kinases including PKA, significantly decreased the FRET signal intensity ($F_{535 nm}/F_{480 nm}$), suggesting the dissociation of BAD-CFP from 14-3-3ζ-YFP. On the other hand, increased phosphorylation induced by the treatment of cells with a phosphatase inhibitor, okadaic acid, drastically increased the FRET signal, indicating an increased association of BAD-CFP with 14-3-3ζ-YFP. By using the FRET method, it was demonstrated that association between BAD and 14-3-3ζ is regulated by the balance among multiple phosphorylation events on BAD. Thus, FRET allows the dynamic measurement of protein–protein interactions in a defined intracellular environment and the visualization of interactions in a specific subcellular location.

Many fluorescent compounds are widely used in FRET assays for quantification of protein–protein interactions. FRET is a useful technique, not only for the detection of molecular interactions in vitro and in vivo, but also for high-throughput screening (HTS). FRET assay offers tremendous advantage over other methods for HTS such as a nonradioactive format, ease of automation, excellent reproducibility, and low fluorescence interference from diverse compounds in HTS operations. For this purpose, the time-resolved FRET (TR-FRET) is particularly useful (74). In contrast to standard FRET assays, TR-FRET uses a long-lifetime lanthanide chelate as the donor molecule. Lanthanide chelates are unique in that their excited state lifetime (the average time that the molecule spends in the excited state after accepting a photon) can be on the order of a millisecond or longer. The lifetime of common fluorophores used in conventional FRET is typically in the nanosecond range. The use of long-lived lanthanides combined with time-resolved detection (a delay between excitation and emission detection) minimizes background fluorescence interference. It is important for screening of large compound libraries because autofluorecent compounds and scattered light may contribute to background fluorescence. The most commonly used lanthanides in TR-FRET assays for HTS are europium and terbium. The europium-Cy5, or allophycocyanin (APC) are frequently employed. For example, a homogeneous in vitro TR-FRET has been developed to study the ligand-dependent interaction of estrogen receptor (ERs) with various nuclear coactivators (75). The assay consists of FLAG-tagged ER ligand binding domain (ER-LBD), a biotinylated coactivator peptide, europium-labeled anti-FLAG antibody, and streptavidin-conjugated allophycocyanin (APC). Excitation of europium at 340 nm led to the emission of the FRET signal at 665 nm upon ER-LBD association with its APC-coupled coactivator peptide. In this study, the effect of various components on agonist-induced ER-LBD/coactivator interaction was examined. The TR-FRET assay was developed in a 384 well plate format for both mechanistic evaluation and HTS applications (75). For HTS, terbium offers some useful properties when used as the donor fluorophore in a TR-FRET assay. In particular, the terbium donor molecule can use common fluorophores such as rhodamine as the acceptor, which may simplify assay design and development.

3.2.2. FP

Fluorescence polarization is a versatile technique, and along with SPR is capable of measuring equilibrium binding constants. This simple technology has many applications, such as monitoring DNA–protein and DNA–DNA interactions, protein–protein interactions, protease assays, immunoassays, conformational changes of proteins, and cell biochemical studies (33). FP assays are homogeneous and so do not require a separation step or immobilization. Polarization values can be measured repeatedly and after the addition of reagents and operation is rapid and does not destroy the sample.

FP is often used for monitoring protein-peptide interactions in a homogeneous assay format. For example, a simple one-step "mix-and-measure" method has been developed that can be used to monitor the binding of the 14-3-3 protein with a variety of its client proteins (35). In this assay, purified GST-14-3-3 along with a rhodamine-labeled peptide derived from a well-studied 14-3-3 binding protein, Raf-1 was used. By increasing the amount of GST-14-3-3 proteins, polarization values progressively increased to reach saturation, suggesting that a greater fraction of fluorescent peptide was bound to the 14-3-3 protein. The maximum assay window (ΔmP = mP of bound peptide – mP of free peptide) reached ~150 mP with an estimated dissociation constant, K_d, of 0.41 ± 0.01 µM for the Raf peptide. This FP signal was likely due to the specific interaction of the Raf-1 peptide with 14-3-3 because Raf-1 peptide with GST alone did not induce FP signals. This assay has been used to compare the affinity of different isoforms of 14-3-3 for the Raf-1 peptide and to determine the structural requirement of 14-3-3 for Raf-1 binding. Similar assay formats can be designed for studying the interaction of a variety of proteins with their binding peptides.

Fluorescence polarization detection technology enables homogeneous assays suitable for HTS in 96/384 well format or even for ultraHTS in 1536 well format in the drug discovery field. The FP assay offers a simple one step "mix-and-measure" protocol, which is highly suitable for automated operation. For screening of a large number of compounds for molecular interaction modulators, competitive FP binding assays are used. Assay stability, sensitivity, and plate-to-plate variability are assessed before large scale HTS is performed. This type of assay has been used for many HTS operations *(76)*.

3.3. Protein Fragment Complementation Based Methods

3.3.1. Yeast Two-Hybrid Method

The yeast two-hybrid method is relatively simple to implement, requiring only the availability of the bait/prey gene cloned into suitable vectors, an AD-cDNA library (if for screening purpose), yeast host cells, and various media. This simplicity has led to the wide spread use of this technology. The power of this technology to reveal new interacting proteins without any prior knowledge makes it a particularly valuable tool to identify protein complexes and establish signaling networks in cells.

The primary and most popular application of the yeast two-hybrid system is to identify new proteins that interact with a known protein of interest. Numerous new interactions have been established using this method. In each case, the protein of interest, the bait, is used to screen an appropriate cDNA library expressed in *S. cerevisiae* for new interacting proteins *(6,11,37,38)*. The main weakness of this method is the generation of a large number of false positives. Therefore, it is important to include well defined negative and positive controls to decrease the number of false positives. For example, an unrelated bait protein, or an interaction-defective mutant of the bait is used to eliminate non-specific interacting proteins. Also, intracellular interaction in a protein complex may not necessarily indicates a direct association between two test proteins. Alternative methods using two purified proteins should be used to validate the interaction. Despite of these weaknesses, the yeast two-hybrid system remains the choice of many investigators for identifying new interacting proteins.

Using an interaction mating approach, the yeast two-hybrid method has been employed to study pairwised protein interactions in a group of proteins *(77)*. Because of its simplicity and the availability of the large genome data, the yeast two-hybrid system has been utilized for systematic mapping of protein–protein interactions to establish interactomes in model organisms. This application has led to the generation of interaction maps of model systems including the *S. cerevisiae* proteome and the partial human protein–protein interaction map *(78)*. These interactomes provide a framework upon which further methods will be used for validation and functional confirmation.

When two proteins are found to interact with each other, the yeast two-hybrid system can be used to define the interaction domains or residues. For example, deletion mutations are made to eliminate regions that are not involved in the interaction and narrow down the region of binding in the same system. Based on the known structural data, residues may be predicted and tested for their direct role in the interaction. For example, residues in the amphipathic groove of the 14-3-3 proteins, K49 and R56, are found to be important for Raf-1 interaction using the yeast two-hybrid system *(39)*. On the other hand, the reverse two-hybrid system can be used to screen for residues that are important for interaction *(6)*.

3.3.2. Protein Complementation Assays

PCA has an advantage over conventional techniques in that protein–protein interactions can be measured in living cells and monitored in real time *(45,47, 48,79,80)*. In addition, protein interactions may be detected in any subcellular compartment of the cell. The PCA technology can also be adapted to monitor protein–protein interactions in living animals in a noninvasive manner *(45)*. These benefits make PCA amendable to the study of protein–protein interactions as they relate to a wide range of novel applications in chemical genetics, proteomics research, and drug discovery.

While simple in concept and in practice, PCA has proven extremely useful in the study of a wide variety of highly complex protein–protein interactions. The appeal of PCA is derived from its ease of use, high sensitivity, and broad versatility. The interaction of virtually any pair of putative binding proteins can be monitored in the cellular environment with outputs ranging from fluorescence and luminescence to affinity for labeled small molecules and survival in selective growth media. PCA has proven effective in various applications, including the screening of large protein libraries for novel binding partners, elucidating the mechanisms of regulation unique to specific protein–protein interactions, and investigating the effects of pharmacological agents in cell and animal models. It is hoped that the following examples will provide an appreciation for the vast utility of PCA, while sparking the imaginations of current and future investigators.

The production of antibodies for use in a research laboratory can often be a long and arduous task, requiring the purification of antigen protein and the use of live animals for the production of immune serum. Therefore, much interest is currently focused on methods of high throughput antibody selection from large libraries; however, all currently available library screening methods center on extracellular selection and therefore require a second step to assess antibody function in the reductive cytosolic environment. Since PCA occurs entirely intracellularly and does not require the purification of target or binding proteins, it presents a convenient single-step approach to the selection and verification of high specificity antibodies *(81,82)*. A method using PCA for the one-round selection of a single-chain variable antibody fragment (scFv) specific for the c-Jun N-terminal kinase 2 (JNK2) was reported by Koch et al. *(82)*. Specifically, the murine dihydrofolate reductase (mDHFR) PCA system was used, wherein mDHFR was genetically cleaved and the complementary fragments were cloned into a JNK2 antigen-containing plasmid and a synthetic scFv library, respectively. *E. coli* cells were co-transformed with the plasmids and grown on selective media containing a specific inhibitor of bacterial DHFR. Therefore, only those bacteria containing fused mDHFR could reproduce, and intracellular antigen antibody interactions were selected for by colony formation. Since selection took place within the intracellular environment, both selection and verification of intracellular functionality were achieved simultaneously *(82)*.

Beyond widespread screening for the identification of novel protein binding partners, PCA can also be used to probe the more subtle regulatory complexities of specific protein binding pairs or complexes. Specifically, mDHFR PCA was used to confirm a novel activation mechanism of the erythropoietin receptor (EpoR) *(83)*. Erythropoietin (Epo) is a glycoprotein hormone that binds EpoR and induces the differentiation of erythroid progenitor cells into erythrocytes. Free EpoR was long thought to exist primarily as two monomers which associate upon ligand binding, resulting in autophosphorylation and the propagation of differentiation signals. However, some crystallographic data have indicated that free EpoR can exist in a dimeric, but conformationally restrained and inactive, configuration. This hypothesis was tested through PCA in which complementary fragments of mDHFR were genetically fused to each monomer of EpoR via peptide linkers of varying lengths. Interaction of the two monomers was monitored in the presence and absence of Epo by the introduction of fluorescein-labeled methotrexate (fMTX), which specifically binds full-length mDHFR. Therefore, retention of fMTX within the cell served as a reporter for EpoR inter-monomeric interaction. The short (5 nm) and long (30 nm) linkers were used to distinguish between ligand-induced interaction and interactions due to constitutive conformational proximity, respectively. The authors observed an interaction of EpoR monomers regardless of whether the linkers were short or long; however, for EpoR fusions with the short linkers the interaction was directly dependent upon the presence of Epo, whereas this interaction was constitutive and independent of Epo when the long linkers were used. These PCA results support the hypothesis that EpoR constitutively exists in a dimeric form, but that ligand binding induces an activating conformational rearrangement *(83)*.

Another example of PCA's utility in probing the details of protein–protein interactions involves the investigation of γ-aminobutyric acid transporter 1 (GAT1) oligomerization *(84)*. γ-aminobutyric acid (GABA) is the primary inhibitory neurotransmitter of the central nervous system. Its inhibitory activity is regulated in part by transport proteins such as GAT1, which mediate reuptake of GABA from the synapses. GAT1 is an oligomeric transmembrane protein that is a common anti-depressant and anti-convulsant pharmacological target. Amino acid residues critical to the efficient oligomerization of GAT1 were identified via a PCA in which complementary fragments of β-galactosidase were genetically fused to mutated and wild type GAT1 monomers. The resulting plasmids were cotransfected into cells, which were later fixed, lysed, and assayed for β-galactosidase enzymatic activity. Amino acids critical to the normal oligomerization of GAT1 were identified by observing which point mutations resulted in a decrease of β-galactosidase activity relative to non-mutated GAT1 monomers *(84)*. Similar approaches have been used in the investigation of homo-and heterodimerization of the immunologically relevant toll-like receptors (TLR) *(85)*.

In addition to providing a means of monitoring mechanistic details of protein–protein interactions, PCA also allows the study of the effects of various regulatory mechanisms on these systems. For example, the use of YFP-based PCA in the detection of a lectin (a carbohydrate binding protein)-mediated interaction between two important cell secretory system proteins has been reported *(86)*. Specifically, complementary fragments of YFP were genetically fused to ERGIC-53 and cathepsin C. A fusion clone of ERGIC-53 with a mutated glycosylation site was also produced. Binding was detected by measuring YFP fluorescence emission. The results of this study were interesting for two reasons. First, an interaction between ERGIC-53 and cathepsin C had never been observed with other standard protein–protein interaction detection methods; however, the high sensitivity of fluorescence-based PCA allowed the detection of the apparently weak interaction between ERGIC-53. Furthermore, this interaction was abrogated by the use of ERGIC-53 with a mutated glycosylation site, indicating that the carbohydrate is intimately involved in the regulation of this novel transient protein–protein interaction (86).

As indicated by the above examples, the ability to detect the disruption of a protein–protein interaction can be just as informative and useful as the ability to detect the occurrence of the interaction in the first place. This is especially true when using pharmacological agents or siRNAs to map large biochemical pathways or in the screening of small molecule libraries against identified intracellular protein–protein interaction targets. PCA has proven to be a highly effective tool in both endeavors (79,87–89) due to its capacity to identify protein binding pairs within a pathway, give information regarding the subcellular localization of protein interactions in cell culture and in vivo, and monitor the response of these interactions to pharmacological probes in a highly specific and quantitative fashion. For example, YFP fragment-fused clones were used to map protein targets downstream of the small GTPase Ras. Specifically, the authors showed that siRNA-mediated knock-down of Ras was sufficient to disrupt the YFP readout from various downstream PCA interactions, including those of Raf with MEK1, MEK1 with ERK2, and Pin1 with Jun. Additionally, the differential cellular localization of these downstream protein complexes was observed in the native cellular environment, representing a great advantage over many traditional studies of protein–protein interactions that require the lysis of cells (89).

Another vitally important application of PCA is its use in drug discovery – both in high throughput screening of small molecule libraries and in the elucidation of the in vivo molecular effects and pharmacokinetics of known therapeutic agents (43). Specifically, the ability of split synthetic renilla luciferase (hRLUC) PCA to monitor the rapamycin-induced heterodimerization of FKBP12 with FRB (mTOR) in living mice was demonstrated by Paulmurugan et al (45). In these studies 293T cells were cotransfected with hRLUC fragment-fused FKBP12 and FRB and injected into living nude mice. The mice were subsequently injected with varying doses of rapamycin at different time intervals. Rapamycin-induced heterodimerization of FKBP12 with FRB was monitored by detection of luminescence with a cooled charged coupled device camera. In this way, the authors were able to monitor the molecular effects of rapamycin administration on living animals in real time and derive dose–response relationships at the molecular level while taking into account all in vivo pharmacokinetic considerations (43).

From the above examples it can be seen that PCA is a highly versatile technique with a wide range of applications from basic science to drug discovery and development. It is a powerful tool that can be used to identify interconnections among critical signaling events, reveal the spatial organization of protein complexes within signaling pathways, identify small molecule modulators of protein complex formation, and elucidate the molecular mechanisms of action of identified therapeutic agents. Because of its simplicity, speed, and high information return, PCA has the potential to rapidly advance our understanding of and ability to wield the vast networks of protein–protein interactions present in healthy and diseased cells.

References

1. Papin JA, et al (2005) Reconstruction of cellular signalling networks and analysis of their properties. Nat Rev Mol Cell Biol 6(2):99–111
2. Pawson T Nash P (2003) Assembly of cell regulatory systems through protein interaction domains. Science 300(5618):445–452
3. Fu H, Subramanian RR, Masters SC (14-3-3) proteins: structure, function, and regulation. Annu Rev Pharmacol Toxicol 40:617–647
4. Raman M Cobb MH (2003) MAP kinase modules: many roads home. Curr Biol,13(22) R886–888
5. Arkin MR Wells JA, (2004) Small-molecule inhibitors of protein–protein interactions: progressing towards the dream. Nat Rev Drug Discov 3(4):301–317
6. Fu H, (2004) Protein–protein interactions: methods and applications Totowa, NJ: Humana Press
7. Golemis E, Adams PD (2005) Protein–protein interactions: a molecular cloning manual Cold Spring Harbor, NY: Cold Spring Harbor Publisher
8. Sarbassov DD, et al (2006) Prolonged rapamycin treatment inhibits mTORC2 assembly and Akt/PKB Mol Cell 22(2):159–168
9. Harlow E, Lane D (eds.) (1996) Antibodies – a laboratory manual. Cold Spring Harbor Laboratory
10. Spector DL, Goldman RD, Leinwand LA (1997) Cells, a laboratory manual Cold Spring Harbor Laboratory Press
11. Ausubel FM, et al (1987) Current protocols in molecular biology New York, NY: Wiley
12. Dudek H et al (1997) Regulation of neuronal survival by the serine-threonine protein kinase Akt. Science 275(5300):661–665
13. Masters SC, Fu H (2001) 14-3-3 proteins mediate an essential anti-apoptotic signal. J Biol Chem 276(48):45193–45200
14. Guan KL, Dixon JE (1991) Eukaryotic proteins expressed in Escherichia coli: an improved thrombin cleavage and purification procedure of fusion proteins with glutathione S-transferase. Anal Biochem 192(2):262–267
15. Rigaut G, Chevchenko A, Rutz B, Wilm M, Mann M, Seraphin B (1999) A generic protein purification method for protein complex characterization and proteome exploration. Nat Biotechnol 17(10):1030–1032
16. Puig O, Caspary F, Rigaut G, Rutz B, Bouveret E, Bragado-Nilsson E, Wilm M, Seraphin B (2001) The tandem affinity purification(TAP) method: a general procedure of protein complex purification. Methods 24(3):218–229
17. Gould KL, Ren L, Feoktistova AS, Jennings JL, Link AJ (2004) Tandem affinity purification and identification of protein complex components. Methods 33(3):239–244
18. Liu X, Constantinescu SN, Sun Y, Bogan JS, Hirsch D, Weinberg RA, Lodish HF (2000) Generation of mammalian cells stably expressing multiple genes at predetermined levels. Anal Biochem 280(1):20–28
19. Benzinger A, Muster N, Koch HB, Yates JR, Hermeking H (2005) Targeted proteomic analysis of 14-3-3 sigma, a p53 effector commonly silenced in cancer. Mol Cell Proteomics 4(6):785–795
20. Burckstummer T, Bennett K, Preradovic A, Schutze G, Hantschel O, Superti-Furga G, Bauch A (2006) An efficient tandem affinity purification procedure for interaction proteomics in mammalian cells. Nat Methods 3(12):1013–1019
21. Knuesel M, Wan Y, Xiao Z, Holinger E, Lowe N, Wang W, Liu X (2003) Identification of novel protein–protein interactions using a versatile mammalian tandem affinity purification expression system. Mol Cell Proteomics 2(11):1225–1233
22. Koch KV, Reinders Y, Ho T-H, Sickmann A, Graf R (2006) Identification and isolation of Dictyostelium microtubule- associated protein interactions by tandem affinity purification. Eur J Cell Biol 85(9–10):1079–1090

23. Hartmann-Petersen R, Gordon C (2005) Quantifying protein–protein interactions in the ubiquitin pathway by surface plasmon resonance. Methods Enzymol 399:164–177

24. Katsamba PS, Park S, Laird-Offringa IA (2002) Kinetic studies of RNA-protein interactions using surface plasmon resonance. Methods 26(2):95–104

25. Raasi S et al (2004) Binding of polyubiquitin chains to ubiquitin-associated (UBA) domains of HHR23A. J Mol Biol 341(5):1367–1379

26. Rich RL, Myszka DG (2000) Advances in surface plasmon resonance biosensor analysis. Curr Opin Biotechnol 11(1):54–61

27. Herman B, Krishnan RV, Centonze VE (2004) Microscopic analysis of fluorescence resonance energy transfer (FRET). Methods Mol Biol 261:351–370

28. Clapp AR, Medintz IL, Mattoussi H (2006) Forster resonance energy transfer investigations using quantum-dot fluorophores. Chemphyschem 7(1):47–57

29. Selvin PR (2000) The renaissance of fluorescence resonance energy transfer. Nat Struct Biol 7(9):730–734

30. Prinz A, Diskar M, Herberg FW (2006) Application of bioluminescence resonance energy transfer (BRET) for biomolecular interaction studies. Chembiochem 7(7):1007–1012

31. Ullman EF et al (1994) Luminescent oxygen channeling immunoassay: measurement of particle binding kinetics by chemiluminescence. Proc Natl Acad Sci U S A 91(12):5426–5430

32. Wilson J et al (2003) A homogeneous 384-well high- throughput binding assay for a TNF receptor using alphascreen technology. J Biomol Screen 8(5):522–532

33. Jameson DM and Croney JC (2003) Fluorescence polarization: past, present and future. Comb Chem High Throughput Screen 6(3):167–173

34. Schade SZ et al (1996) BODIPY-alpha-casein, a pH-independent protein substrate for protease assays using fluorescence polarization. Anal Biochem 243(1):1–7

35. Du Y et al (2006) Monitoring 14-3-3 protein interactions with a homogeneous fluorescence polarization assay. J Biomol Screen 11(3):269–276

36. Fields S, Song O (1989) A novel genetic system to detect protein–protein interactions. Nature 340(6230):245–6

37. Bartel PL, Fields S (1997) The Yeast Two-Hybrid System. Oxford University Press.

38. Gyuris J et al (1993) Cdil, a human G1 and S phase protein phosphatase that associates with Cdk2. Cell 75(4):791–803

39. Zhang L et al (1997) Raf-1 kinase and exoenzyme S interact with 14-3-3zeta through a common site involving lysine 49. J Biol Chem 272(21):13717–13724

40. Johnsson N, Varshavsky A (1994) Split ubiquitin as a sensor of protein interactions in vivo. Proc Natl Acad Sci U S A 91(22):10340–10344

41. Rossi F, Charlton CA, Blau HM (1997) Monitoring protein–protein interactions in intact eukaryotic cells by beta- galactosidase complementation. Proc Natl Acad Sci U S A 94(16):8405–8410

42. Remy I, Michnick SW (1999) Clonal selection and in vivo quantitation of protein interactions with protein-fragment complementation assays. Proc Natl Acad Sci U S A 96(10):5394–5399

43. Galarneau A et al (2002) Beta-lactamase protein fragment complementation assays as in vivo and in vitro sensors of protein protein interactions. Nat Biotechnol 20(6):619–622

44. Hu CD, Chinenoy Y, Kerppola TK (2002) Visualization of interactions among bZIP and Rel family proteins in living cells using bimolecular fluorescence complementation. Mol Cell 9(4):789–798

45. Paulmurugan R, Gambhir SS (2005) Novel fusion protein approach for efficient high-throughput screening of small molecule-mediating protein–protein interactions in cells and living animals. Cancer Res 65(16):7413–7420

46. Ozawa I et al (2001) Split luciferase as an optical probe for detecting protein–protein interactions in mammalian cells based on protein splicing. Anal Chem 73(11):2516–2521

47. Paulmurugan R, Umezawa Y, Gambhir SS (2002) Noninvasive imaging of protein–protein interactions in living subjects by using reporter protein complementation and reconstitution strategies. Proc Natl Acad Sci U S A 99(24):15608–15613

48. Luker KE et al (2004) Kinetics of regulated protein– protein interactions revealed with firefly luciferase complementation imaging in cells and living animals. Proc Natl Acad Sci U S A 101(33):12288–12293

49. Remy I, Michnick SW (2006) A highly sensitive protein–protein interaction assay based on Gaussia luciferase. Nat Methods 3(12):977–979

50. Wehr MC et al (2006) Monitoring regulated protein- protein interactions using split TEV. Nat Methods 3(12):985–993

51. Paulmurugan R, Gambhir SS (2003) Monitoring protein- protein interactions using split synthetic renilla luciferase protein-fragment-assisted complementation. Anal Chem, 75(7):1584–1589

52. Shumway SD, Li Y, Xiong Y (2003) 14-3-3beta Binds to and Negatively Regulates the Tuberous Sclerosis Complex 2 (TSC2) Tumor Suppressor Gene Product, Tuberin. J Biol Chem 278(4):2089–2092

53. Phizicky EM, Fields S (1995) Protein–protein Interactions: Methods for Detection and Analysis. Microbiol Rev 59(1):94–123

54. Zhang L, Chen J, Fu H (1999) Suppression of Apoptosis Signal-Regulating Kinase 1-Induced Cell Death by 14-3-3 Proteins. Proc Natl Acad Sci. USA 96:8511–8515

55. Masters S et al (2002) Survival-Promoting Functions of 14-3-3 Proteins. Biochem Soc Trans 30:360–365

56. Masters SC et al (1999) Interaction of 14-3-3 with a nonphosphorylated protein ligand exoenzyme S of Pseudomonas aeruginosa. Biochemistry 38(16):5216–5221.

57. Wang H et al (1998) Mutations in the hydrophobic surface of an amphipathic groove of 14-3-3zeta disrupt its interaction with Raf-1 kinase. J Biol Chem 273(26):16297–16304

58. Bonnet MC et al (2006) The N-terminus of PKR is Responsible for the Activation of the NF-kappaB Signaling Pathway by Interacting With the IKK Complex. Cell Signal 18(11):1865–1875

59. Meek SE, Lane WS, Piwnica-Worms H (2004) Comprehensive proteomic analysis of interphase and mitotic 14-3-3-binding proteins. J Biol Chem 279(31):32046–32054

60. Blagoev B et al (2003) A proteomics strategy to elucidate functional protein–protein interactions applied to EGF signaling. Nat Biotechnol 21(3):315–318

61. Kung LA, Snyder M (2006) Proteome chips for whole- organism assays. Nat Rev Mol Cell Biol 7(8):617–622

62. Zhu H et al (2001) Global analysis of protein activities using proteome chips. Science 293(5537):2101–2105

63. Jung J W et al (2006) High-throughput analysis of GST- fusion protein expression and activity-dependent protein interactions on GST-fusion protein arrays with a spectral surface plasmon resonance biosensor. Proteomics 6(4):1110–1120

64. Keefe AD, Wilson DS, Seelig B, Szostak JW (2001) One-step purification of recombinant proteins using a nanomolar-affinity streptavidin-binding peptide, the SBP-tag. Protein Expression and Purification 23(3):440–446

65. Gavin AC, Bosche M, Krause R, Grandi P, Marzioch M, Bauer A, Schultz J, Rick JM, Michon AM, Cruciat CM, Remor M, Hofert C, Schelder M, Brajenovic M, Ruffner H, Merino A, Klein K, Hudak M, Dickson D, Rudi T, Gnau V, Bauch A, Bastuck S, Huhse B, Leutwein C, Heurtier MA, Copley RR, Edelmann A, Querfurth E, Rybin V, Drewes G, Raida M, Bouwmeester T, Bork P, Seraphin B, Kuster B, Neubauer G, and Superti-Furga G (2002) Functional organization of the yeast proteome by systematic analysis of protein complexes. Nature 415(6868):141–147

66. Honey S, Schneider B, Schieltz DM, Yates JR, and Futcher B (2001) A novel multiple affinity purification tag and its use in identification of proteins associated with a cyclin-CDK complex. Nucleic Acids Res 29(4). E24

67. Forler D, Kocher T, Rode M, Gentzel M, Izaurralde E, Wilm M (2003) An efficient protein complex purification method for functional proteomics in higher eukaryotes. Nat Biotechnol 21(1):89–92

68. Drakas R, Prisco M, Baserga R (2005) A modified tandem affinity purification tag technique for the purification of protein complexes in mammalian cells. Proteomics 5(1):132–137

69. Schimanski B, Nguyen TN, Gunzl A (2005) Highly efficient tandem affinity purification of trypanosome protein complexes based on a novel epitope combination. Eukaryotic Cell, 4(11):1942–1950

70. Krogan NJ, Cagney G, Yu H, Zhong G, Guo X, Ignatchenko A, Li J, Pu S, Datta N, Tikuisis AP, Punna T, Peregrin-Alvarez JM, Shales M, Zhang X, Davey M, Robinson MD, Paccanaro A, Bray JE, Sheung A, Beattie B, Richards DP, Canadien V, Lalev A, Mena F, Wong P, Starostine A, Canete MM, Vlasblom J, Wu S, Orsi C, Collins SR, Chandran S, Haw R, Rilstone JJ, Gandi K, Thompson NJ, Musso G, St Onge P, Ghanny S, Lam MH, Butland G, Altaf-Ul AM, Kanaya S, Shilatifard A, O'Shea E, Weissman JS, Ingles CJ, Hughes TR, Parkinson J, Gerstein M, Wodak SJ, Emili A, and Greenblatt JF (2006) Global landscape of protein complexes in the yeast Saccharomyces cerevisiae. Nature 440(7084):637–643

71. Rohila JS, CM, Cerny R, Fromm ME, (2004) Improved tandem affinity purification tag and methods for isolation of protein heterocomplexes from plants. Plant Journal 38(1):172–181

72. Raasi S et al (2005) Diverse polyubiquitin interaction properties of ubiquitin-associated domains. Nat Struct Mol Biol 12(8):708–714

73. Hashimoto A, Hirose K, Iino M (2005) BAD detects coincidence of G2/M phase and growth factor deprivation to regulate apoptosis. J Biol Chem 280(28):26225–26232

74. Mathis G (1999) HTRF(R) Technology. J Biomol Screen 4(6):309–314

75. Liu J et al (2003) A homogeneous in vitro functional assay for estrogen receptors: coactivator recruitment. Mol Endocrinol 17(3):346–355

76. Parker GJ et al (2000) Development of high throughput screening assays using fluorescence polarization: nuclear receptor-ligand-binding and kinase/phosphatase assays. J Biomol Screen 5(2):77–88

77. Finley RL, Jr, Brent R (1994) Interaction mating reveals binary and ternary connections between Drosophila cell cycle regulators. Proc Natl Acad Sci U S A 91(26):12980–12984

78. Parrish JR, Gulyas KD, Finley RL, Jr (2006) Yeast two-hybrid contributions to interactome mapping. Curr Opin Biotechnol 17(4):387–393

79. Paulmurugan, R., et al (2004) Molecular imaging of drug-modulated protein–protein interactions in living subjects. Cancer Res 64(6):2113–2119

80. Luker KE, Piwnica-Worms D (2004) Optimizing luciferase protein fragment complementation for bioluminescent imaging of protein–protein interactions in live cells and animals. Methods Enzymol 385:349–360

81. Mossner E, Koch H, Pluckthun A (2001) Fast selection of antibodies without antigen purification: adaptation of the protein fragment complementation assay to select antigen-antibody pairs. J Mol Biol 308(2):115–122

82. Koch H et al (2006) Direct selection of antibodies from complex libraries with the protein fragment complementation assay. J Mol Biol 357(2):427–441

83. Remy I, Wilson IA, Michnick SW (1999) Erythropoietin receptor activation by a ligand-induced conformation change. Science, 283(5404):990–993

84. Korkhov VM et al (2004) Oligomerization of the {gamma}-aminobutyric acid transporter-1 is driven by an interplay of polar and hydrophobic interactions in transmembrane helix II. J Biol Chem 279(53):p. 55728–36

85. Lee HK, Dunzendorfer S, Tobias PS (2004) Cytoplasmic domain-mediated dimerizations of toll-like receptor 4 observed by beta-lactamase enzyme fragment complementation. J Biol Chem 279(11):10564–10574

86. Nyfeler B, Michnick SW, Hauri HP (2005) Capturing protein interactions in the secretory pathway of living cells. Proc Natl Acad Sci U S A 102(18):p. 6350–5

87. Michnick SW (2003) Protein fragment complementation strategies for biochemical network mapping. Curr Opin Biotechnol 14(6):610–617

88. Yu H et al (2003) Measuring drug action in the cellular context using protein-fragment complementation assays. Assay Drug Dev Technol 1(6):811–822

89. Michnick SW, Macdonald ML, Westwick JK (2006) Chemical genetic strategies to delineate MAP kinase signaling pathways using protein-fragment complementation assays (PCA). Methods 40(3):287–293

31

Glycoprotein Analysis

Terry D. Butters and David C. A. Neville

1. Introduction

In eukaryotic cells, one of the most important post-translational modifications of proteins is the covalent addition of carbohydrate. We can consider two major types of modification to amino acid residues: N-glycosylation of asparagine amine side-chain groups and O-glycosylation of serine or threonine hydroxyl side-chain groups (*1*). An additional prerequisite of N-linked glycosylation is that the asparagine is part of the tripeptide sequon asparagine-X-serine/threonine (Asn-X-Ser/Thr) where X can be any amino acid except proline. N-Linked oligosaccharides can be divided into three major classes; the complex type containing N-acetylglucosamine, N-acetylgalactosamine, mannose, galactose, fucose, and sialic acid; the oligomannose type containing N-acetylglucosamine and mannose only, and the hybrid type that has features common to both complex and oligomannose chains (**Fig. 31.1**). All of these structures are synthesized by a common pathway that begins in the endoplasmic reticulum (ER) with the assembly of a lipid-linked donor molecule. The preformed oligosaccharide is transferred to protein co-translationally in the lumen of the ER and by a series of glycosidase (α-glucosidase and α-mannosidase) trimming reactions is modified as the protein progresses through the ER and Golgi apparatus (*2*). The diversity of N-linked oligosaccharide structure is dictated by the accessibility of these partially processed chains to Golgi-resident glycosyltransferases, a group of enzymes able to add monosaccharides to oligosaccharides directly from nucleotide sugar donors. Glycosyltransferases are specific for nucleotide sugar donor, anomericity, glycosidic linkage between sugars and acceptor substrates. Consequently, there are a number of different transferases and each cell, tissue and species has a unique complement of enzymes that control oligosaccharide biosynthesis (*3,4*). O-Linked oligosaccharides contain similar monosaccharide residues to N-glycans but their synthesis has no requirement for *en bloc* addition of carbohydrate to the polypeptide chain. O-glycosylation proceeds by glycosyltransferase catalysed, stepwise addition of monosaccharides to generate, as in the case of mucin glycoproteins, a diverse number of branched oligosaccharides (*5,6*) (see **Fig. 31.2**).

From: *Molecular Biomethods Handbook, 2nd Edition.*
Edited by: J. M. Walker and R. Rapley © Humana Press, Totowa, NJ

Manα1,2Manα1,6
Manα1,6
Manα1,2Manα1,3
Manß1,4GlcNAcß1,4GlcNAcß1,Asn
Manα1,2Manα1,2Manα1,3
Oligomannose type
Manα1,6
Manα1,6
Manα1,3
Manß1,4GlcNAcß1,4GlcNAcß1,Asn
NeuAcα2,6Galß1,4GlcNAcß1,2Manα1,3
Hybrid type
NeuAcα2,6Galß1,4GlcNAcß1,2Manα1,6
Manß1,4GlcNAcß1,4GlcNAcß1,Asn
NeuAcα2,6Galß1,4GlcNAcß1,2Manα1,3
Complex type

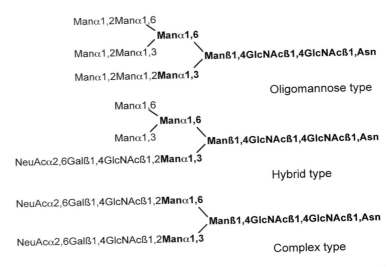

Fig. 31.1. The structure of asparagine(*N*)-linked oligosaccharides. The core unit (in bold) that is found in all three types is derived from a common dolichol lipid donor in the biosynthetic pathway. See **ref. *2***

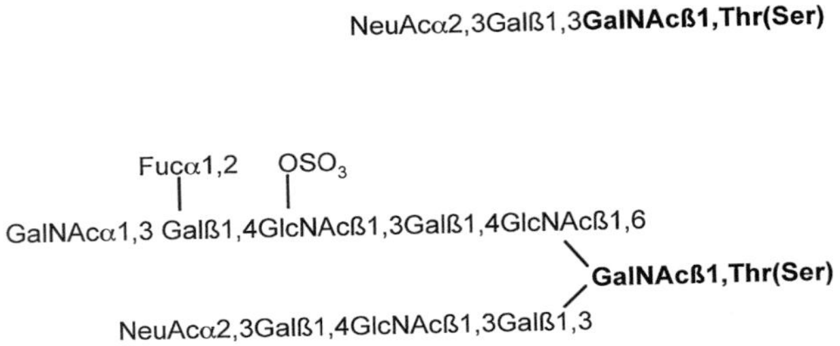

NeuAcα2,3Galß1,3GalNAcß1,Thr(Ser)
Fucα1,2
OSO3
GalNAcα1,3 Galß1,4GlcNAcß1,3Galß1,4GlcNAcß1,6
GalNAcß1,Thr(Ser)
NeuAcα2,3Galß1,4GlcNAcß1,3Galß1,3

Fig. 31.2. Serine or threonine (*O*)-linked oligosaccharide structures found on surface proteins of erythrocytes (top) or in mucin glycoproteins (bottom). The core *N*-acetylgalactosamine residue (in bold) is common to all *O*-linked oligosaccharides. See **ref. *5***

The degree of importance of glycosylation is reflected in the amount of energy and genetic information used by cells in providing the machinery to co-ordinate the correct assembly of protein oligosaccharides. Because many of these processes have been conserved throughout the evolution of eukaryotes there are clearly some vital roles played by the oligosaccharide moieties. These roles are often indirect; in assisting the folding machinery in the ER to ensure the secretion of conformationally correct proteins ***(6)***, or in stabilizing the protein to heat or protease digestion. Functions of the oligosaccharide that have a more direct role include carbohydrate–protein interactions, where the specificity is dictated by the expression of an appropriate sequence of carbohydrate residues. For a more thorough review of oligosaccharide functions see references ***(7,8)***.

A single glycoprotein may be glycosylated with both *N*- and *O*-glycans and several attachment sites may be present in the polypeptide chain. The heterogeneity introduced during oligosaccharide biosynthesis creates a mixture of glycans, termed glycoforms, at the same attachment site on the polypeptide and presents considerable difficulties in analysing structure. To obtain a unique "fingerprint" of a single polypeptide species one needs structural information regarding the oligosaccharide at each attachment point. Attempts to study the sequence of both *N*- and *O*-linked oligosaccharides found on proteins must as a consequence address this enormous diversity of structure (*9*). This information can then be used to manipulate protein oligosaccharides as a means to understand function. For the biologist/biochemist, two questions are posed when proteins from different experimental systems are to be analysed. The first is to ask if the protein is glycosylated. Secondly, if it is a glycoprotein, what is the structural identity, the carbohydrate sequence of the oligosaccharide? An additional question then presents itself: how does the oligosaccharide structure influence the biochemical function of the protein? In this Chapter, a review of some of the current and traditional methodologies used to answer these questions will be presented.

2. Detection of Protein-Linked Oligosaccharide

In many biological systems the target protein may be only available in such small amounts that gross chemical analysis is not a viable option. However, the separation afforded by SDS/PAGE can be used in conjunction with staining methods that detect the presence of carbohydrate. One of the most simple chemical detection methods is the periodate oxidation of adjacent hydroxyl groups of monosaccharides to generate aldehydes. These groups are detected in situ by Schiff's reagent or on Western blots after reaction with more sensitive reporter molecules such as digoxigenin-hydrazide or biotin-hydrazide (*10*). Subsequent reaction of these conjugates with antibody- or streptavidin-labeled enzymes permits colorimetric detection of glycoproteins at the nanogram (fmol) level. Pro-Q® Emerald glycoprotein stains, available from Molecular Probes, (http://probes.invitrogen.com/) can detect specifically the presence of glycoproteins following 1D or 2D gel electrophoresis. This method is also dependent on an initial prior periodate oxidation.

The contribution of carbohydrate to the mass of the polypeptide chain can be assessed after deglycosylation by chemical means using trifluoromethanesulphonic acid. This procedure efficiently cleaves *N*- and *O*-linked oligosaccharide chains leaving the protein reasonably intact (*11*). Selective cleavage of *N*-linked oligosaccharides is provided by endoglycosidase digestion. Endoglycosidases are able to release nondestructively most but not all glycoprotein oligosaccharides. The endoglycosidase isolated from *Flavobacterium meningosepticum*, peptide-N^4-(*N*-acetyl-β-glucosaminyl)asparagine amidase (PNGase F), cleaves between the chitobiose core reducing-terminal GlcNAc residue of oligomannose, hybrid and complex type *N*-glycans and the side chain of the asparagine residue of the protein backbone (**Fig. 31.3**). However, PNGase F is unable to hydrolyse oligosaccharides from plant proteins substituted with core α-1,3-linked fucose and for these structures PNGase A, isolated from sweet almonds, must be used (*12*). Endo-β-*N*-acetylglucosaminidase from *Streptomyces spp.* cleaves the chitobiose core between GlcNAc residues of oligomannose type *N*-glycans but will not hydrolyse small (<3 mannose units) glycans, especially if these are core fucosylated (*13*). Estimates of the

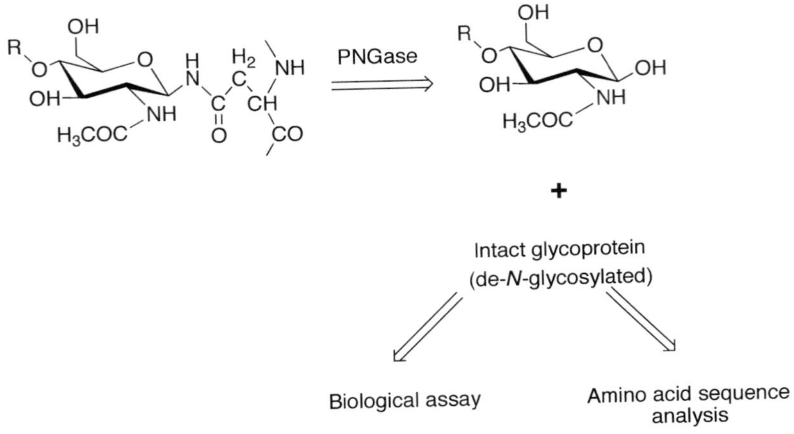

Fig. 31.3. Endoglycosidase release of *N*-linked oligosaccharides. PNGase releases the glycan from the protein without destruction of either oligosaccharide or protein. In addition to glycan composition information, the protein can be evaluated for biological activity or subjected to peptide/amino acid analysis to reveal identity

polypeptide mass by SDS/PAGE before and after deglycosylation may be used to determine the number of *N*-linked oligosaccharide chains.

With this type of information, proteins can be further probed for particular types of oligosaccharide or carbohydrate sequences using a number of lectins. Lectins are plant and animal proteins that are able to bind specifically to sugars that may be either terminal residues or part of an extended sequence *(14)*. Using enzyme-coupled lectins, sensitive visualization of oligosaccharide chains of glycoproteins, after electrophoretic transfer either to nitrocellulose or polyvinylidinefluoride (PVDF) membranes, can identify the type and even portions of the glycan sequence *(15)*. This information aids protein purification or oligosaccharide separation using lectin-affinity chromatography *(16)*. Used in conjunction with specific glycosidase digestion, lectin blot analysis has identified the presence of hybrid-type carbohydrate chains on human monoclonal antibody *(17)*. One important consideration, when using either chemical or lectin staining methods, is the specificity of the reaction. The inclusion of appropriate controls together with the additional use of proteins of known glycosylation type can help confirm identification and reduce errors in interpretation caused by erroneous signals *(18)*.

Direct carbohydrate analysis of glycoproteins blotted onto PVDF membranes has been successfully applied to the examination of *N*-linked oligosaccharides of plant and animal origin. Acid hydrolysis of glycoprotein bands (100 µg protein) followed by monosaccharide compositional analysis by high-performance liquid chromatography (HPLC) was reproducible, and agreed with analyses performed without SDS/PAGE and electroblotting onto PVDF membranes *(19)*. A more sophisticated analysis, using high-pH anion-exchange chromatography (HPAEC) coupled with pulsed amperometric detection (PAD), allows the unequivocal determination of the presence of carbohydrate, by means of a complete monosaccharide composition and oligosaccharide mapping according to size, charge, and isomericity, from 10–50 µg electroblotted glycoprotein bands *(20)*. The derivatization of the released oligosaccharide with the fluorescent molecule 2 aminobenzoic acid (2-AA), followed by HPLC, has allowed both the monosaccharide and oligosaccharide profile of 20 pmol of fetuin (~1 μg protein) to be ascertained *(21)*.

More recently, the in-gel release of *N*-linked oligosaccharides from glycoproteins, separated following SDS-PAGE, has been performed *(22,23)* therefore abrogating the need of protein blotting. The released oligosaccharides may be analysed, with or without subsequent fluorescent derivatization, and subjected to a number of differing analyses including HPLC, mass spectrometry (MS), monosaccharide analysis and exoglycosidase sequencing *(24,25)* as outlined in the following section.

3. Analysis of Oligosaccharides Isolated from Proteins

3.1. Glycan Release and Labeling

Further quantitation of the types of monosaccharide linkage and number of oligosaccharide structures requires release of the oligosaccharide. Chemical methods such as hydrazinolysis involve cleavage of the glycosylamine linkage (*N*-link) or ether linkage (*O*-link) with anhydrous hydrazine (**Fig. 31.4**). Glycosidic bonds between monosaccharides are unaffected and the oligosaccharide (*N*- and/or *O*-linked) is released intact *(26)*. Following re-*N*-acetylation, the terminal *N*-acetylglucosamine (in *N*-linked oligosaccharides) or *N*-acetylgalactosamine (in *O*-linked oligosaccharides) residue can be labeled by

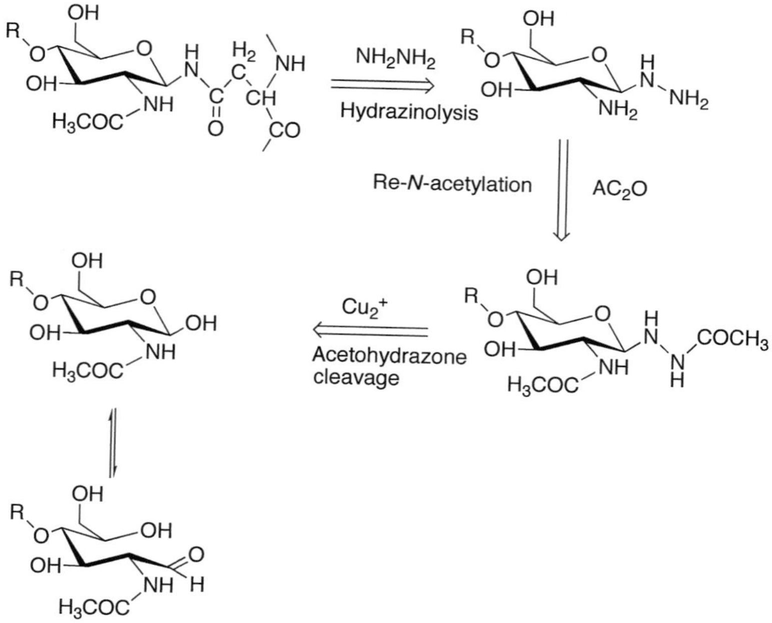

Fig. 31.4. Hydrazinolysis of glycoproteins. Anhydrous hydrazine releases *N*-linked oligosaccharide, as shown, (and *O*-linked oligosaccharides) intact but the protein is destroyed. Any *N*-acetylated sugars are also reduced to amines and re-*N*-acetylation is required. The open and closed ring conformation of the reducing terminal *N*-acetyl-hexosamine residue exists as a tautoisomer in solution

reductive methods using either borotritiide to introduce a radioactive group, or fluorescent molecules that provide a more sensitive reporter group, to aid detection (**Fig. 31.5**). Enzymatic release can be accomplished by endoglycosidases, after first considering the potential lack of hydrolysis noted with certain oligosaccharide types (see previous section). By contrast to hydrazine, endoglycosidase action does not destroy the protein (**Fig. 31.3**) nor change the nature of any sialic acids present, an important advantage when the contribution of oligosaccharide to biological activity is assessed.

O-Linked glycans can be selectively released using anhydrous hydrazine at reduced temperature (27) to minimize any peeling reactions that can occur, or by ß-elimination in the presence of sodium hydroxide. ß-elimination must be directly followed by a reduction step (using NaBH$_4$) to stabilize the glycan to peeling reactions. O-Links can also be removed by other nonreducing conditions using either triethylamine in aqueous hydrazine (28) or aqueous ammonium hydroxide saturated with ammonium carbonate (29). Endoglycosidase catalysed release has been sparingly applied mostly owing to the lack of well-characterized enzymes that allow the release of all O-linked glycans (30). The commercially available enzyme, O-glycanase, has a specificity restricted to the core disaccharide sequence Gal-GalNAc only.

3.2. Fractionation of Oligosaccharides

The physical techniques described later in this chapter require that some preliminary fractionation of oligosaccharides has been achieved, possibly using one or a combination of methods. These include size separation by

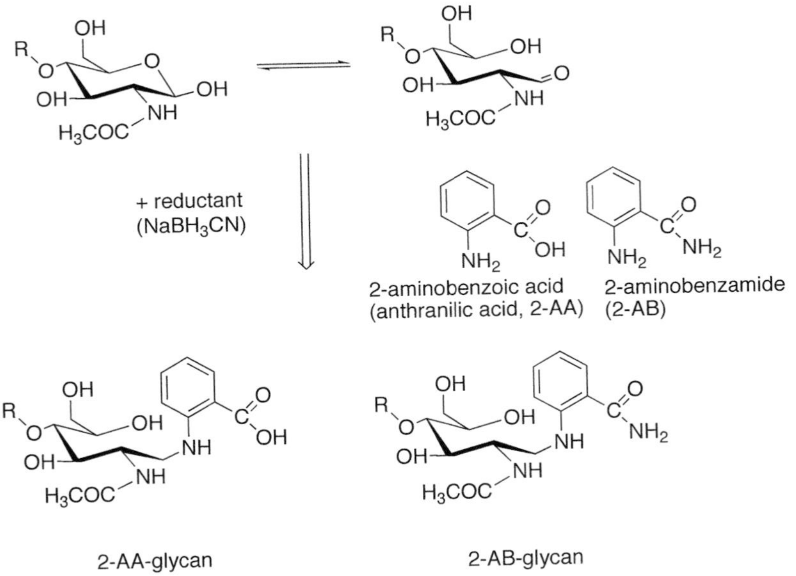

Fig. 31.5. Fluorescence labeling of released oligosaccharides. Following hydrazine or PNGase mediated release of the glycan; the reducing *N*-acetylhexosamine residue can be labeled quantitatively with a fluorescence reporter molecule. The reductive amination scheme using 2-AB and 2-AA is shown here but many other types of fluorescence derivatization can be used. See text for details

low-pressure chromatography using Bio-Gel P-4 *(31)* that can provide some assignment based on the unique hydrodynamic volume of certain uncharged oligosaccharide sequences *(32)*. The application of either strong anion-exchange (SAX), weak anion-exchange (WAX), normal-phase (NP) or reverse-phase (RP) HPLC technology, subsequent to fluorescent derivatization of the released glycans, to carbohydrate analysis provides a greater increase in the resolution and sensitivity of oligosaccharide mixtures *(33,34)*. Chromatography times are far less than low-pressure separations and sensitivity in the femtomolar range can be accomplished. An example of the separating power of HPLC and the level of sensitivity of detection of fluorescently labeled oligosaccharides derived from various glycoproteins is shown in **Fig. 31.6**. HPAEC is able to separate isomeric structures nondestructively, despite the use of basic pH eluants *(35,36)*, and electrochemical detection using pulsed

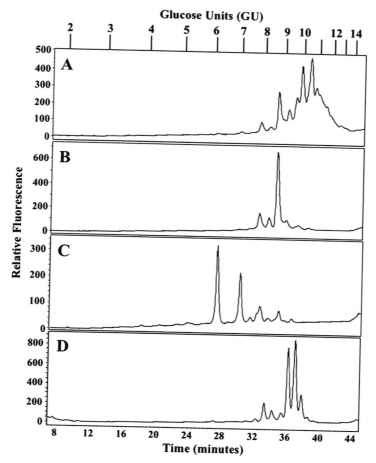

Fig. 31.6. HPLC separation of 2-AA-labeled *N*-linked oligosaccharides. *N*-linked oligosaccharides released from (**A**) ovalbumin and (**B**) transferrin following hydra-zinolysis and from (**C**) ribonuclease B and (**D**) fetuin following PNGase F digestion were labeled with 2-AA and purified. Each chromatogram represents approx 1, 0.3, 2, and 6 pmol of oligosaccharide, respectively. The elution position of each 2-AA-labeled oligosaccharide relative to a 2-AA-labeled dextran hydrolysate external standard, GU values at top, is shown

amperometry allows pmol amounts of carbohydrate to be analysed without the need for derivatization.

The majority of these highly sophisticated technologies have been commercialized but there are alternative techniques that can be performed simply and effectively. The use of immobilized lectins to affinity fractionate oligosaccharides, that comprise a number of quite different structures with similar masses, exploits the exquisite specificities of plant lectins *(37,38)*. Polyacrylamide gel electrophoresis of oligosaccharides labeled with very sensitive fluorophores allows high-resolution separation and detection *(39,40)* and uses equipment that is familiar to most laboratories. Using these methods, coupled with specific glycosidase digestion, oligosaccharide structures have been deduced at the pmol level.

4. Methods for the Structural Analysis of Oligosaccharides

4.1. Oligosaccharide Sequencing Using Glycosidases

The structural characterization of oligosaccharides can be achieved using glycosidases *(41)*, a group of hydrolytic enzymes abundant in nature. Glycosidases have been purified from many sources including plant, vertebrate and invertebrate tissues and microbes. Although most glycosidases are of lysosomal origin or associated with degradative vacuoles involved in the catabolism of glycoconjugates, others, for example α-glucosidases and α-mannosidases, are found in the endomembrane system of eukaryotes where they participate in *N*-glycan biosynthesis. Glycosidases are also found as soluble, secreted enzymes or are located in the outer membrane, for example members of the neuraminidases that are present in bacteria and viruses. Two major groups of enzymes are used in the determination of glycan structure; exoglycosidases that hydrolyse monosaccharides from the nonreducing terminus of glycans and endoglycosidases that cleave between monosaccharide residues located internally to the oligosaccharide.

Structural assignment using sequential exoglycosidase digestion relies on the known specificity and purity of glycosidase-catalysed hydrolysis. Exoglycosidases are usually named after the cleaved monosaccharide and its anomeric configuration. For example, β-galactosidase only hydrolyses glycans containing terminal β-galactose residues and α-fucosidase, terminal α-fucose residues. The strict observance of both glycon and anomericity by exoglycosidases (an exception being the β-hexosaminidases that hydrolyse both *N*-acetylglucosamine and *N*-acetylgalactosamine) is a feature that has considerable predictive value (**Table 31.1**). The selection of enzyme, or even the concentration of enzyme, can be used to determine the anomeric linkage between monosaccharides. The α-fucosidase isolated from *Charonia lampas* cleaves all α-fucosyl residues but at markedly different rates. Consequently, concentrations can be used to remove α1,6-linked fucose, preferentially and predictively, in comparison to α1,3/4-linked fucose. By contrast, almond meal α-fucosidase hydrolyses only α1,3/4-linked fucosyl residues and even at very high concentrations will not cleave α1,6 bonds *(42)*.

In addition to the above substrate specificities, some exoglycosidases have activities that are dependent on the neighboring, or aglycon group. The most complicated example of aglycon specificity is shown by the β-hexosaminidase

Table 31.1. Monosaccharide and linkage specificity for exoglycosidases used in oligosaccharide sequencing.

Enzyme	Source	Monosaccharide hydrolysed	Linkages hydrolysed	Notes
neuraminidase (sialidase)	*Arthrobacter ureafaciens*	neuraminic acid (sialic acid)	$\alpha2,6 > \alpha2,3$ $\alpha2,8$	General purpose sialidase
	Vibrio cholera	neuraminic acid	$\alpha2,3$ $\alpha2,6$ $\alpha2,8$	
	Newcastle disease virus	neuraminic acid	$\alpha2,3$ $\alpha2,8$	
ß-galactosidase	Jack bean	galactose	$\beta1,6 > \beta1,4 > \beta1,3$	General purpose galactosidase
	Streptococcus pneumoniae	galactose	$\beta1,4$	Linkage specific
α-galactosidase	Green coffee bean	galactose	$\alpha1,3$ $\alpha1,4$ $\alpha1,6$	
α-fucosidase	*Charonia lampas*	fucose	$\alpha1,2 > \alpha1,6 > \alpha1,3/4$	General purpose fucosidase
	Almond meal	fucose	$\alpha1,3/4$	Linkage specific
ß-hexosaminidase	Jack bean	*N*-acetylglucosamine	$\beta1,2$ $\beta1,3$ $\beta1,4$ $\beta1,6$	General purpose hexosaminidase
	Streptococcus spneumoniae	*N*-acetylglucosamine	$\beta1,2$	Linkage specific only at certain concentrations
α-mannosidase	Jack bean	mannose	$\alpha1,2$ $\alpha1,6$ $\alpha1,3$	General purpose mannosidase
	Aspergillus saitoi	mannose	$\alpha1,2$	Linkage specific

See ref. *41* for details of preparation and optimal buffer for digestion. Many of these enzymes, either purified or recombinantly expressed, are commercially available from Sigma (http://www.sigmaaldrich.com/), NEB (http://www.neb.uk.com/) Merck (http://www.merckbiosciences.com/), Prozyme (http://www.prozyme.com/).

isolated from *Streptococcus pneumoniae* where hydrolysis of the preferred glycon (GlcNAc linked $\beta1,2$ to mannose) is restricted by further substitutions of the mannose residue, or by the presence of a bisecting GlcNAc (43). Aglycon specificity is also an important property of most endoglycosidases where an extended sequence of carbohydrate several residues away from the site of catalysis determines hydrolytic rates *(44)*. By paying careful attention to the rules for glycosidic cleavage (including enzyme activity, concentration, pH and buffer optima, and ion dependence), oligosaccharide sequences are validly assigned. The use of glycosidases can therefore complement physical and chemical analyses (GC–MS, MS, NMR) and in many cases is sufficient in providing an appropriate level of information.

Any of the techniques described above (usually more than 1) are appropriate to examine enzyme cleavage products. Gel filtration (Bio-Gel P4) relies on the shift in hydrodynamic volume and mass spectrometry relies on the shift in mass after hydrolysis. Usually several rounds of enzyme digestion, recovery of the reaction products, further exoglycosidase digestion and analysis are required to enable full characterization. The covalently attached reporter group at the reducing terminus is retained during exoglycosidase digestion, which proceeds from the nonreducing terminus, allowing the change in mass to be measured or the glycan recovered. Separation using HPLC involves the use of a variety of matrices that exploit the physical/chemical properties of the oligosaccharide. Charged glycans can be resolved using weak anion exchange resins *(45)* and reversed-phase and gel filtration separates carbohydrates according to hydrophilicity or the number of monosaccharide units *(34)*. HPAEC/PAD has the unique advantage that no derivatization or introduction of a reporter group is necessary for detecting separated glycans or monosaccharides and additionally, all the reaction products can be measured. However, the retention times on these columns are not always predictive of structure and identification must rely on the elution times of known oligosaccharide standards. The use of normal-phase HPLC, following fluorescent derivatization, has overcome these difficulties, as the retention time on the column is referenced to an external standard, usually similarly derivatized dextran hydrolysate *(46)*, giving definitive glucose unit (GU) values for each known oligosaccharide. As predictive relative retention time shifts can be assigned to differing monosaccharide linkages, a combination of glycosidase digests and HPLC allows the assignment of oligosaccharide structures. Both neutral and charged oligosaccharides are amenable to this method of analysis. Additionally, similar GU values can be obtained for each oligosaccharide independent of the differing fluorescent molecules used to derivatize the oligosaccharides, either 2-aminopyridine (2-AP) *(34)*, 2-AB *(46)*, 2-AA *(21)* or 2-aminoacridone *(47)*. See Fig. 31-6 for an example of fluorescently labeled oligosaccharides separated by HPLC. The same technique for fluorescence labeling with 2-AA following PNGase treatment of glycoproteins shown here, can also be applied to glycosphingolipids after ceramide glycanase release of the glycan *(48)*.

Enzyme arrays or RAAM, a method where a purified oligosaccharide is subjected to a mixture of glycosidases and the fragmentation or fingerprint obtained is matched to computer databases, allow rapid and reproducible analyses to be made *(49)*. Although this technique had initially only been applied to gel permeation chromatography to separate the fragments, HPLC *(46)*, HPAEC and mass spectrometric methods *(50,51)* can also be used.

4.2. Mass Spectrometry

Mass spectrometry requires relatively little material (low pmol/fmol range) and a number of differing ionization methods and mass spectrometers are used to analyse oligosaccharides. Matrix assisted laser desorption/ionization time-of-flight (MALDI-TOF) techniques involve irradiation of the sample mixed with a UV-absorbing matrix followed by mass separation of the ions. The molecular ions detected give information on the oligosaccharide composition, i.e., number of hexose, deoxyhexose, *N*-acetyl hexosamine and sialic acid residues present, and its ease of use and rapid analysis, used in combination with other separation technologies and/or glycosidase digestion, increases its analytical power. As laser irradiation can impart sufficient energy to cause decomposition of the oligosaccharides, MALDI-TOF instruments that can perform postsource decay (PSD) analysis can give information on oligosaccharide sequence. Fast-atom bombardment (FAB)-MS can give sequence, branching point and linkage information, owing to fragmentation within the ion source of the spectrometer *(52)*. However, without a compound database or other information none of these parameters can be predictively assigned.

To confirm the structure of an unknown glycan, further derivatization techniques such as permethylation of free hydroxyl groups with or without periodate oxidation has to be employed *(53)*.

The above techniques are now largely superseded by the analysis of oligosaccharides in solution using electrospray-ionization mass spectrometry (ESI-MS). This has the advantage that direct coupling to HPLC *(54)*, capillary supercritical fluid chromatography *(55)*, and capillary electrophoresis *(56)* is possible. Initially, molecular ions were separated using a quadrupole (Q) owing to differences in mass and charge. However, advances in electrospray technology, mass spectrometer design and sensitivity have enabled the assignment of oligosaccharide sequence, branching point and linkage information *(57,58)*. This is owing to the fact that current mass spectrometer design allows the use of tandem/hyphenated mass spectrometric techniques in 1 instrument, e.g. Q-Q, Q-TOF, TOF-TOF and others. Molecular ions may be selected using 1 mass analyser, subjected to collision-induced decomposition/dissociation (CID) to fragment the molecule and the fragments analysed by the second mass analyser. However, expert analysis is required to determine both linkage and sequence information from the fragments obtained.

4.3. Nuclear Magnetic Resonance (NMR)

NMR analysis typically requires much larger amounts of free oligosaccharide to confirm the identity of structure and linkage, but can do so unambiguously and nondestructively *(59)*. For high-resolution 2-dimensional studies at high field (500–600 MHz), 1–5 µmol is required. Much less material is needed for a 1D spectrum (50 nmol) but this may be orders of magnitude higher than it is possible to isolate for some biologically active glycoproteins. Therefore, the structural identification depends on reference to databases containing the known chemical shifts of anomeric protons. The quantity of primary biological material required for a single analysis using this technique may be beyond the scope of most studies. The NMR machine provides more than an analytical service and has important applications as a research tool in determining oligosaccharide conformation and molecular dynamics in solution (see Section 5).

4.4. Strategies for Glycosylation Site Analysis

Important biochemical functions of glycoproteins are mediated by the complement of oligosaccharides at particular attachment points on the polypeptide *(60)*. To identify the oligosaccharide composition at specific sites a general strategy is to perform a limited proteolytic digestion of the protein. The peptide mixture can be separated by lectin affinity chromatography to isolate the glycopeptides selectively *(61)* that are further fractionated using reversed-phase HPLC *(62)*. Treatment of each glycopeptide fraction with PNGase F results in cleavage of *N*-linked oligosaccharides and the conversion of the asparagine linked amino acids to aspartic acid. Automated Edman sequencing is used to confirm amino acid composition and reveal amino acid residues substituted by *O*-linked oligosaccharides. The released oligosaccharide can then be analysed for carbohydrate composition, reductively or fluorescently labeled if appropriate, and sequenced using any of the above methods. Lectin micro-columns, permethylation and mass spectrometry methods are now being used to characterize protein glycosylation *(63,64)*. These methods are applicable to the analysis of small amounts of biological material. A method for glycosylation site analysis on in-gel separated glycoproteins has been published (*65*) that can be applied to low pmol amounts of material. This method could also be adapted to purified glycoproteins/glycopeptides. These methodologies highlight the increasing importance of mass spectrometry in the analysis of glycoproteins.

4.5. Monosaccharide Compositional Analysis

Hydrolysis of the glycosidic bonds of isolated oligosaccharides and intact glycoprotein can be achieved using acidic conditions. Trifluoroacetic acid (2*M* TFA) at 100°C for 4–6 h to releases neutral sugars (glucose, galactose, mannose, and fucose) nondestructively, whereas amino sugars (*N*-acetylglucosamine and *N*-acetylglucosamine) are not quantitatively recovered. Amino sugars are quantitatively released by hydrolysis using 6*M* HCl under the same conditions, a treatment that destroys neutral sugars. Separation and detection of the monosaccharides at the pmol level usually require derivatization. Compositional analysis using mass spectrometry of alditol acetates derived from sugars released by acid hydrolysis, and separated by gas chromatography (GC), has been obtained from less than 5 µg of glycoprotein (*66*). A second GC–MS method is analysis of monosaccharides as trimethylsilyl (TMS) derivatives (*67*) following methanolysis and re-*N*-acetylation of the parent glycoprotein-derived glycan, which can, with modifications, routinely be performed on subnanomole amounts of sugar (*68*). Derivatization is unnecessary with HPAEC/PAD (*20*) and analyses using similar amounts of protein can accommodated. HPAEC also has the advantage that acid labile monosaccharides, for example sialic acid, can be quantified after digestion of oligosaccharides or glycoproteins with mild acid conditions (0.1*N* HCl for 1 h at 80°C) or enzymatically using neuraminidases. The availability of specific neuraminidases that discriminate between α2,3- and α2,6-linked sialic acid residues provides additional information about the glycosidic linkage (see **Table 31.1**). Derivatization with 2-AA, followed by C18 RP-HPLC, allows the determination of the monosaccharide composition from sub-microgram quantities of glycoprotein (*69*).

4.6. Glycosidic Linkage Analysis by GC-MS

Information regarding the ways in which monosaccharides are linked to one another in an oligosaccharide can be obtained in the following manner. To begin, permethylation of all the oligosaccharide free hydroxyl groups is performed and then the glycosidic linkages are subsequently hydrolysed. Any free hydroxyl groups are acetylated and the now partially methylated alditol acetates (PMAAs) are separated, subjected to gas collision, and detected following GC-MS. The mass fragments generated are compared to a database of known structures that indicate how the monosaccharides were linked to their neighboring residues (*70*).

5. Glycoprotein Structure and Function

The availability of high resolution methods to sequence the oligosaccharide structure of glycoproteins, together with the acquisition of tools and reagents for glycan manipulation, such as the use of inhibitors (*71*) or knock-out mouse models *(72)*, has been instrumental in ascribing function to glycoproteins *(73)*. A systematic approach to profiling the major oligosaccharide classes found in tissues obtained from transgenic mice has been developed using a "Glycan Isolation Protocol" for the isolation of glycans derived from *N*- and O-linked glycoproteins, proteoglycans, Glycophosphatidylinositol-anchored proteins and glycosphingolipids *(74)*. The field of glycobiology uses these analytical approaches to contribute significantly to our understanding of the oligosaccharide code and allows protein glycan structure to put this into a biologically meaningful context. Although the number of the X-ray crystal structures for proteins has increased dramatically in the last few years, there are few examples of glycoprotein structures where the glycan density is revealed *(75)*. The inherent flexibility of the oligosaccharide is not amenable to the uniform packing that is necessary for obtaining crystals, but high-resolution 2-dimensional NMR methods of analysis can yield important information regarding geometry and conformation. A number of reliable protocols now exist to model oligosaccharide structures *in silico (76)* and to rationalize protein carbohydrate interactions at the cellular level *(77,78)*.

6. Glycoprotein Remodelling

Definition of the role(s) played by the oligosaccharide moiety in glycoprotein function can be made by experimental manipulation either during biosynthesis, or on the mature protein. Glycosylation inhibitors have been used to great effect in changing the normal *N*-glycosylation pattern *(79)*. The uses of inhibitors that block the addition of *N*-linked glycans, for example tunicamycin, have profound effects on protein folding and secretion and consequently many proteins lack biological activity if cells are grown in the presence of such compounds. More selective effects are gained by subtle modification of the N-linked glycan after it has been added to the nascent protein. The deoxynojirimycin and deoxymannojirimycin families, castanospermine, and swainsonine are natural products found in plants that are potent glycosidase inhibitors *(80,81)* and have been used therapeutically to attenuate the infectivity of the HIV and hepatitis B virus *(71,82)*. The addition to tissue-cultured cells of these compounds inhibit α-glucosidase and α-mannosidase processing reactions and prevent or reduce the complement of complex-type oligosaccharides *(83)*. The expression of recombinant glycoproteins in Chinese hamster ovary (CHO) cells in the presence of an α-glucosidase inhibitor generates a uniform population of oligosaccharides that are easily cleaved using endoglycosidases. This protocol efficiently produces a properly folded yet deglycosylated protein that can be used to probe function *(84)* or may be used to obtain X-ray crystal structure where the otherwise heterogeneous nature of the oligosaccharide precludes such analysis *(85)*.

Molecular biology techniques can be applied to glycoprotein remodelling by the substitution of the amino acids (asparagine, serine, and threonine) involved in *N*- and *O*-linked glycosylation, at the genetic level. Site-directed mutagenesis has been successfully applied to the HIV surface glycoprotein, gp 120, to delete *N*-glycosylation attachment points. These experiments provide important information regarding the influence of glycosylation on virus infectivity *(86)*.

Glycoproteins in solution and on the surface of cells can be modified using exoglycosidases, glycosyltransferases, or using chemical probes to aid detection of terminal carbohydrate residues and to investigate function *(87–90)*. Efforts to obtain the genes or cDNAs for glycosidases *(43)* and glycosyltransferases *(72)*, have been successful in providing a range of specific reagents for biologists to manipulate oligosaccharides.

7. Glycoproteomics

The interaction between glycoprotein oligosaccharides and protein ligands is an important process observed in normal and disease biology, including cell migration during embryogenesis, cancer metastasis, inflammation, bacterial and viral infectivity and lymphocyte homing. Initiatives in the glycobiology community to analyse oligosaccharide structure and glycan-binding protein ligands obtained from mouse and human tissue, or cell lines, is generating a valuable knowledge base resource for scientists. The consortium for functional glycomics integrates the core analytical capability with glyco-gene chip arrays to monitor the expression of 2,000 relevant mouse and human transcripts with the creation of new knock-out mouse strains for glycosyltransferases and glycosidases, chemical synthesis of oligosaccharides for ligand binding arrays and bioinformatics (http://www.functionalglycomics. org/static/consortium/main.shtml).

The availability of high resolution, high throughput analytical techniques where protein separation by 2D-electrophoresis, followed by glycan profiling of the individual isoforms and protein sequence identity, is now a possibility to identify some of the pathogenetic mechanisms involved in human disease (http://www.hgpi.jp/).

8. Summary

The many techniques presented here are offered as a guide: the strategy adopted will depend on access to the equipment or analytical techniques described, and the quality of information that is most relevant to the needs of the biologist. If the target protein to be analysed is as complex as the HIV glycoprotein gp120, that contains over 100 glycoforms *(91)*, then only a fully integrated approach will be successful. This includes the release of oligosaccharide, labeling, fractionation and exoglycosidase, NMR, MS sequence, and compositional analysis. For other studies, the separating power of SDS/PAGE used in conjunction with endoglycosidase release to characterize the type of glycan and its contribution to the mass of the protein is an excellent starting point. Enzyme based methods to remove the glycan or modify its structure provides important clues to glycoprotein function and should dictate further strategy. The development of simplified protocols for releasing oligosaccharides and fluorescence labeling followed by conventional high performance chromatography can now be used by most laboratories as an initial platform for obtaining high quality information about glycoprotein structure.

References

1. Allen HJ, Kisailus EC (1992) Glycoconjugates Composition, structure and function Marcel Dekker, New York
2. Kornfeld R, Kornfeld S (1985) Assembly of asparagine-linked oligosaccharides. Annu Rev Biochem 54:631–664
3. Kleene R, Berger EG (1993) The molecular and cell biology of glycosyltransferases. Biochim Biophys Acta 1154:283–325
4. Taniguchi N, Honke K, Fukuda M (2002) Handbook of glycosyltransferases and related genes, Springer, Tokyo
5. Corfield T (1992) Mucus glycoproteins, super glycoforms: how to solve a sticky problem? Glycoconjugate J 9:217–221
6. van den Steen P, Rudd PM, Dwek RA, Opdenakker G (1998) Concepts and principles of O-linked glycosylation. Crit Rev Biochem Mol Biol 33:151–208
7. Gagneux P, Varki A (1999) Evolutionary considerations in relating oligosaccharide diversity to biological function. Glycobiology 9:747–755
8. Varki A (1993) Biological roles of oligosaccharides – all of the theories are correct. Glycobiology 3:97–130
9. Kobata A (1992) Structures and functions of the sugar chains of glycoproteins. Eur J Biochem 209:483–501
10. O'Shannessy DJ, Quarles RH (1987) Labeling of the oligosaccharide moieties of immunoglobulins. J Immunol Meth 99:153–161
11. Edge AS, Faltynek CR, Hof L, Reichert Jr, LE, Weber P (1981) Deglycosylation of glycoproteins by trifluoromethanesulfonic acid. Anal Biochem 118:131–137
12. Tretter V, Altmann F, Marz L (1991) Peptide-N4-(N-acetyl-beta-glucosaminyl) asparagine amidase-F cannot release glycans with fucose attached alpha-1->3 to the asparagine-linked N-acetylglucosamine residue. Eur J Biochem 199:647–652
13. Trimble RB, Tarentino AL (1991) Identification of distinct endoglycosidase (Endo) activities in flavobacterium-meningosepticum – endo-F1, endo-F2, and endo-F3 – endo-F1 and endo-H hydrolyze only high mannose and hybrid glycans. J Biol Chem 266:1646–1651
14. Lis H, Sharon N (1986) Lectins as molecules and as tools. Annu Rev Biochem 55:35–67
15. Kijimoto-Ochiai S, Katagiri YU, Ochiai H (1985) Analysis of N-linked oligosaccharide chains of glycoproteins on nitrocellulose sheets using lectin-peroxidase reagents. Anal Biochem 147:222–229
16. Cummings RD (1994) Use of lectins in analysis of glycoconjugates. Meth Enzymol 230:66–86
17. Tachibana H, Seki K, Murakami H (1993) Identification of hybrid-type carbohydrate chains on the light chain of human monoclonal antibody specific to lung adenocarcinoma. Biochim Biophys Acta 1182:257–263
18. Leonards KS, Kutchai H (1985) Coupling of Ca2+ Transport to ATP Hydrolysis by the Ca2+-ATPase of Sarcoplasmic Reticulum: Potential Role of the 53-Kilodalton Glycoprotein. Biochemistry 24:4876–4884
19. Ogawa H, Ueno M, Uchibori H, Matsumoto I, Seno N (1990) Direct carbohydrate analysis of glycoproteins electroblotted onto polyvinylidene difluoride membrane from sodium dodecyl sulfate-polyacrylamide gel. Anal Biochem 190:165–169
20. Weitzhandler M, Kadlecek D, Avdalovic N, Forte JG, Chow D, Townsend RR (1993) Monosaccharide and oligosaccharide analysis of proteins transferred to polyvinylidene fluoride membranes after sodium dodecyl sulfate-polyacrylamide gel electrophoresis. J Biol Chem 268:5121–5130
21. Anumula KR, Du P (1999) Characterization of carbohydrates using highly fluorescent 2-aminobenzoic acid tag following gel electrophoresis of glycoproteins. Anal Biochem 275:236–242

22. Kuster B, Wheeler SE, Hunter AP, Dwek RA, Harvey DJ (1997) Sequencing of N-linked oligosaccharides directly from protein gels: in-gel deglycosylation followed by matrix-assisted laser desorption/ionization mass spectrometry and normal-phase high-performance liquid chromatography. Anal Biochem 250:82–101

23. Wheeler SF, Harvey DJ (2001) Extension of the in-gel release method for structural analysis of neutral and sialylated N-linked glycans to the analysis of sulfated glycans: application to the glycans from bovine thyroid-stimulating hormone. Anal Biochem 296:92–100

24. Kuster B, Krogh TN, Mortz E, Harvey DJ (2001) Glycosylation analysis of gel-separated proteins. Proteomics 1:350–361

25. Sagi D, Kienz P, Denecke J, Marquardt T, Peter-Katalinic J (2005) Glycoproteomics of N-glycosylation by in-gel deglycosylation and matrix-assisted laser desorption/ionisation-time of flight mass spectrometry mapping: application to congenital disorders of glycosylation. Proteomics 5:2689–2701

26. Takasaki S, Mizuochi T, Kobata A (1982) Hydrazinolysis o asparagine-linked sugar chains to produce free oligosaccharides. Meth Enzymol 83:263–268

27. Merry AH, Neville DC, Royle L, Matthews B, Harvey DJ, Dwek RA, Rudd PM (2002) Recovery of intact 2-aminobenzamide-labeled O-glycans released from glycoproteins by hydrazinolysis. Anal Biochem 304:91–99

28. Cooper CA, Packer NH, Redmond JW (1994) The elimination of O-linked glycans from glycoproteins under non-reducing conditions. Glycoconjugate J 11:163–167

29. Huang Y, Mechref Y, Novotny MV (2001) Microscale nonreductive release of O-linked glycans for subsequent analysis through MALDI mass spectrometry and capillary electrophoresis. Anal Chem 73:6063–6069

30. Takahashi N, Muramatsu T (1992) Handbook of endoglycosidases and glyco-amidases CRC Press, Florida

31. Yamashita K, Mizuochi T, Kobata A (1982) Analysis of oligosaccharides by gel filtration. Methods Enzymol 83:105–126

32. Kobata A, Yamashita K, Takasaki S (1987) BioGel P-4 column chromatography of oligosaccharides: effective size of oligosaccharides expressed in glucose units. Meth Enzymol 138:84–94

33. Anumula KR (2006) Advances in fluorescence derivatization methods for high-performance liquid chromatographic analysis of glycoprotein carbohydrates. Anal Biochem 350:1–23

34. Hase S, Ikenaka K, Mikoshiba K, Ikenaka T (1988) Analysis of tissue glycoprotein sugar chains by two dimensional high-performance liquid chromatographic mapping. J Chromatography 434:51–60

35. Lee YC (1990) High-performance anion-exchange chromatography for carbohydrate analysis. Anal Biochem 189:151–162

36. Townsend RR, Hardy MR (1991) Analysis of glycoprotein oligosaccharides using high-pH anion exchange chromatography. Glycobiology 1:139–147

37. Merkle RK, Cummings RD (1987) Lectin affinity chromatography of glycopeptides. Meth Enzymol 138:232–259

38. Osawa T, Tsuji T (1987) Fractionation and structural assessment of oligosaccharides and glycopeptides by use of immobilised lectins. Annu Rev Biochem 56:21–42

39. Jackson P (1990) The use of polyacrylamide-gel electrophoresis for the high-resolution separation of reducing saccharides labelled with the fluorophore 8-aminonaphthalene-1,3,6-trisulphonic acid. Biochem J 270:705–713

40. Jackson P (1991) Polyacrylamide gel electrophoresis of reducing saccharides labeled with the fluorophore 2-aminoacridone – subpicomolar detection using an imaging system based on a cooled charge-coupled device. Anal Biochem 196:238–244

41. Jacob GS, Scudder P (1994) Glycosidases in structural analysis. Meth Enzymol 230:280–299

42. Butters TD, Scudder P, Rotsaert J, Petursson S, Fleet GW, Willenbrock FW, Jacob GS (1991) Purification to homogeneity of Charonia lampas alpha-fucosidase by using sequential ligand-affinity chromatography. Biochem J 279:189–195

43. Clarke VA, Platt N, Butters TJ (1995) Cloning and expression of the beta-N-acetylglucosaminidase gene from streptococcus pneumoniae – generation of truncated enzymes with modified aglycon specificity. J Biol Chem 270:8805–8814

44. Kobata A (1979) Use of endo- and exoglycosidases for structural studies of glycoconjugates. Anal Biochem 100:1–14

45. Guile GR, Wong SYC, Dwek RA (1994) Analytical and preparative separation of anionic oligosaccharides by weak anion-exchange high-performance liquid chromatography on an inert polymer column. Anal Biochem 222:231–235

46. Guile GR, Rudd PM, Wing DR, Prime SB, Dwek RA (1996) A rapid high-resolution high-performance liquid chromatographic method for separating glycan mixtures and analyzing oligosaccharide profiles. Anal Biochem 240:210–226

47. Camilleri P, Tolson D, Birrell H (1998) Direct structural analysis of 2-aminoacridone derivatized oligosaccharides by high-performance liquid chromatography/mass spectrometric detection. Rapid Commun Mass Spectrom 12:144–148

48. Neville DC, Coquard V, Priestman DA, Te Vruchte DJ, Sillence DJ, Dwek RA, Platt FM, Butters TD (2004) Analysis of fluorescently labeled glycosphingolipid-derived oligosaccharides following ceramide glycanase digestion and anthranilic acid labeling. Anal Biochem 331:275–282

49. Edge CJ, Rademacher TW, Wormald MR, Parekh RB, Butters TD, Wing DR, Dwek RA (1992) Fast sequencing of oligosaccharides: the reagent-array analysis method. Proc Natl Acad of Sci USA 89:6338–6342

50. Tyagarajan K, Forte JG, Townsend RR (1996) Exoglycosidase purity and linkage specificity: assessment using oligosaccharide substrates and high-pH anion-exchange chromatography with pulsed amperometric detection. Glycobiology 6:83–93

51. Tyagarajan K, Townsend RR, Forte JG (1996) The Beta-subunit of the rabbit H,K-ATPase: a glycoprotein with all terminal lactosamine units capped with alpha-linked galactose residues. Biochemistry 35:3238–3246

52. Dell A, Khoo KH, Panico M, McDowell RA, Etienne AT, Reason AJ, Morris HR (1993) FAB-MS and ES-MS of glycoproteins. In: Fukuda M, Kobata A (ed) *Glycobiology: a practical approach.* IRL Press, Oxford, UK

53. Harvey DJ (1992) The role of mass spectrometry in glycobiology. Glycoconjugate J 9:1–12

54. Medzihradszky KF, Maltby DA, Hall SC, Settineri CA, Burlingame AL (1994) Characterisation of protein N-glycosylation by reversed-phase microbore liquid chromatography/electrospray mass spectrometry, complementary mobile phases, and sequential exoglycosidase digestion. J Am Soc Mass Spectrom 5:350–358

55. Leroy Y, Lemoine J, Ricart G, Michalski JC, Montreuil J, Fournet B (1990) Separation of oligosaccharides by capillary supercritical fluid chromatography and analysis by direct coupling to high-resolution mass spectrometer – application to analysis of oligomannosidic N-Glycans. Anal Biochem 184:235–243

56. Kelly JF, Locke SJ, Thibault P (1993) Analysis of protein glycoforms by capillary electrophoresis-electrospray mass spectrometry. Discovery Newsletter (Beckman) 2:1–6

57. Harvey DJ (2005) Proteomic analysis of glycosylation: structural determination of N- and O-linked glycans by mass spectrometry. Expert Rev Proteomics 2:87–101

58. Harvey DJ (2005) Structural determination of N-linked glycans by matrix-assisted laser desorption/ionization and electrospray ionization mass spectrometry. Proteomics 5:1774–1786

59. Dwek RA, Edge CJ, Harvey DJ, Wormald MR, Parekh RB (1993) Analysis of glycoprotein-associated oligosaccharides. Annu Rev Biochem 62:65–100

60. Rademacher TW, Parekh RB, Dwek RA (1988) Glycobiology. Annu Rev Biochem 57:785–838

61. Yeh JC, Seals JR, Murphy CJ, van Halbeek H, Cummings RD (1993) Site-specific N-glycosylation and oligosaccharide structures of recombinant HIV-1 gp120 derived from a baculovirus expression system. Biochemistry 32:11087–11099

62. Rohrer JS, Cooper GA, Townsend RR (1993) Identification, quantification, and characterization of glycopeptides in reversed-phase HPLC separations of glycoprotein proteolytic digests. Anal Biochem 212:7–16

63. Madera M, Mechref Y, Novotny MV (2005) Combining lectin microcolumns with high-resolution separation techniques for enrichment of glycoproteins and glycopeptides. Anal Chem 77:4081–4090

64. Novotny MV, Mechref Y (2005) New hyphenated methodologies in high-sensitivity glycoprotein analysis. J Sep Sci 28:1956–1968

65. Larsen MR, Hojrup P, Roepstorff P (2005) Characterization of gel-separated glycoproteins using two-step proteolytic digestion combined with sequential microcolumns and mass spectrometry. Mol Cell Proteomics 4:107–119

66. Kenne L, Stromberg S (1990) A Method for the microanalysis of hexoses in glyco-proteins. Carb Res 198:173–179

67. Sweeley CC, Bentley R, Makita M, Wells WW (1963) Gas liquid chromatography of trimethylsilyl derivatives of sugars and related subtances. J Am Chem Soc 85:2497–2507

68. Chaplin MF (1982) A rapid and sensitive method for the analysis of carbohydrate components in glycoproteins using gas–liquid chromatography. Anal Biochem 123:336–341

69. Anumula KR (1994) Quantitative determination of monosaccharides in glycoproteins by high-performance liquid chromatography with highly sensitive fluorescence detection. Anal Biochem 220:275–283

70. Montreuil J, Bouquelet S, Debray H, Fournet B, Spik G, Strecker G (1986) Glycoproteins. In: Chaplin MF, Kennedy JF (ed) Carbohydrate analysis: a practical approach, IRL Press, Oxford

71. Dwek RA, Butters TD, Platt FM, Zitzmann N (2002) Targeting glycosylation as a therapeutic approach. Nat Rev Drug Discov 1:65–75

72. Lowe JB, Marth JD (2003) A genetic approach to mammalian glycan function. Annu Rev Biochem 72:643–691

73. Dwek RA, Butters TD (2002) Introduction: glycobiology – understanding the language and meaning of carbohydrates. Chem Rev 102:283–284

74. Manzi AE, Norgard-Sumnicht K, Argade S, Marth JD, van Halbeek H, Varki A (2000) Exploring the glycan repertoire of genetically modified mice by isolation and profiling of the major glycan classes and nano-NMR analysis of glycan mixtures. Glycobiology 10:669–689

75. Petrescu AJ, Butters TD, Reinkensmeier G, Petrescu S, Platt FM, Dwek RA, Wormald MR (1997) The solution NMR structure of glucosylated N-glycans involved in the early stages of glycoprotein biosynthesis and folding. EMBO J 16:4302–4310

76. Wormald MR, Petrescu AJ, Pao YL, Glithero A, Elliott T, Dwek RA (2002) Conformational studies of oligosaccharides and glycopeptides: complementarity of NMR, X-ray crystallography, and molecular modelling. Chem Rev 102:371–386

77. Ritchie GE, Moffatt BE, Sim RB, Morgan BP, Dwek RA, Rudd PM (2002) Glycosylation and the complement system. Chem Rev 102:305–320–319

78. Rudd PM, Elliott T, Cresswell P, Wilson IA, Dwek RA (2001) Glycosylation and the immune system. Science 291:2370–2376

79. Elbein AD (1987) Glycosylation Inhibitors for N-Linked Glycoproteins. Meth Enzymol 138:661–709

80. Fleet GWJ (1988) Amino-sugar derivatives and related compounds as glycosidase inhibitors. Spec Publ -R Soc Chem 65:149–162

81. Watson AA, Fleet GWJ, Asano N, Molyneux RJ, Nash RJ (2001) Polyhydroxylated alkaloids – natural occurrence and therapeutic applications. Phytochemistry 56:265–295

82. Jacob GS, Scudder P, Butters TD, Jones I, Tiemeier DC (1992) Aminosugar attenuation of HIV infection. In: Chu CK, Cutler HG (ed) Natural products as antiviral agents. Plenum Press, New York

83. Karlsson GB, Butters TD, Dwek RA, Platt FM (1993) Effects of the imino sugar N-butyldeoxynojirimycin on the N-glycosylation of recombinant gp120. J Biol Chem 268:570–576

84. Davis SJ, Davies EA, Barclay AN, Daenke S, Bodian DL, Jones EY, Stuart DI, Butters TD, Dwek RA, Van der Merwe PA (1995) Ligand binding by the immunoglobulin superfamily recognition molecule CD2 is glycosylation-independent. J Biol Chem 270:369–375

85. Butters TD, Sparks LM, Harlos K, Ikemizu S, Stuart DI, Jones EY, Davis SJ (1999) Effects of N-butyldeoxynojirimycin and the Lec3.2.8.1 mutant phenotype on N-glycan processing in Chinese hamster ovary cells: application to glycoprotein crystallization. Protein Sci 8:1696–1701

86. Lee WR, Syu WJ, Du B, Matsuda M, Tan S, Wolf A, Essex M, Lee TH (1992) Nonrandom distribution of gp120 N-linked glycosylation sites important for infectivity of human immunodeficiency virus type 1. Proc Natl Acad Sci USA 89:2213–2217

87. Dube DH, Prescher JA, Quang CN, Bertozzi CR (2006) Probing mucin-type O-linked glycosylation in living animals. Proc Natl Acad Sci USA 103:4819–4824

88. Paulson JC, Rogers GN (1987) Resialylated erythrocytes for assessment of the specificity of sialyloligosaccharide binding proteins. Meth Enzymol 138:162–168

89. Prescher JA, Bertozzi CR (2006) Chemical technologies for probing glycans. Cell 126:851–854

90. Whiteheart SW, Passaniti A, Reichner JS, Holt GD, Haltiwanger RS, Hart GW (1989) Glycosyltransferase probes. Meth Enzymol 179:82–95

91. Mizuochi T, Matthews TJ, Kato M, Hamako J, Titani K, Solomon J, Feizi T (1990) Diversity of oligosaccharide structures on the envelope glycoprotein GP 120 of human immunodeficiency virus-1 from the lymphoblastoid cell line H9 – presence of complex-type oligosaccharides with bisecting N-acetylglucosamine residues. J Biol Chem 265:8519–8524

32

Solid-Phase Peptide Synthesis

Mare Cudic and Gregg B. Fields

1. Introduction

Peptides play a central role in numerous biological and physiological processes. They also may be critical for research endeavors in the post-genomic and proteomic era that is characterized by a vast array of new predicted protein sequences. To elucidate the biological function of putative proteins it is important to have facile access to their synthesis. Today we have almost routine technologies for the chemical synthesis of small peptides and proteins, and have made significant progress toward the synthesis of larger proteins via chemoselective ligation (1–5) and expressed protein ligation (6–8). Although these new approaches are impressive and have been employed successfully for the synthesis of many proteins, general protein chemical synthesis is still not routine and there are still many challenges that remain to be confronted.

Methods for synthesizing peptides are divided conveniently into two categories: solution and solid-phase. Classical solution chemistry involves the preparation of fully protected peptide segments and their subsequent condensation in organic solvents for the convergent synthesis of large polypeptides. Solid-phase peptide synthesis (SPPS) uses an insoluble polymeric support for sequential addition of side-chain protected amino acids. The resulting peptide is then cleaved from the resin, typically under acidic conditions. SPPS has numerous advantages over the classical solution procedure, such as automation of the elongation reaction, independence from solubility problems, and minimization of side product formation. On the other hand, in the classical solution procedure, the products can be monitored and purified at each step in the reaction, potentially leading to easier isolation of the desired final peptide. Therefore, solution synthesis retains value in large-scale manufacturing, and for specialized laboratory applications, whereas solid-phase chemistry remains the method of choice in research. In this chapter, an overview of SPPS is presented. For brevity, only commercially available reagents and derivatives utilized for synthesis will be considered here. The reader is referred to a number of comprehensive reviews for further discussion of peptide synthesis techniques (9–22).

From: *Molecular Biomethods Handbook, 2nd Edition.*
Edited by: J. M. Walker and R. Rapley © Humana Press, Totowa, NJ

2. Background

Merrifield introduced SPPS in 1963 (*23*) using acid-labile protecting groups as well as a resin-substrate linker that was cleaved under strongly acidic conditions. The concept of SPPS has been outlined in **Fig. 32.1**. Briefly, an N^α-derivatized amino acid is attached to a commercially available insoluble (solid) support via a linker moiety. The N^α-protecting group is then removed (deprotected) and the amino acid-linker-support is thoroughly washed with solvent. The next amino acid (which is N^α-protected) is then coupled to the amino acid-linker-support as either a preactivated species or directly (in situ) in the presence of an activator. When three functional groups are present in the sequence, the side-chain of the residues also has to be protected. After this reaction is complete, the nascent oligopeptide-linker-support is washed with solvent, thus removing unreacted material. The deprotection and/or coupling

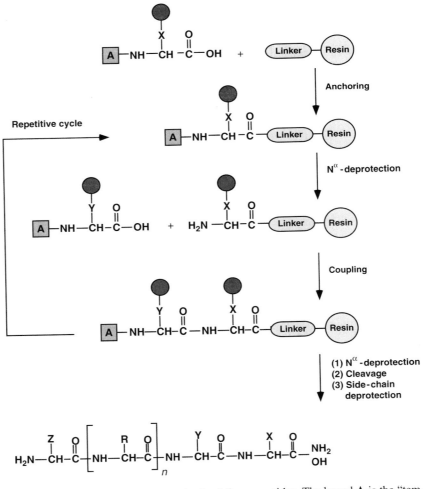

Fig. 32.1. Stepwise solid-phase synthesis of linear peptides. The boxed **A** is the "temporary" N^α-amino protecting group, whereas the red circle is the "permanent" side-chain protecting group. See the text for further details

cycle is repeated until the desired sequence of amino acids is generated. Finally, the peptide-linker-support is cleaved to obtain the peptide as a free acid or an amide, depending on the chemical nature of the linker. Ideally, the cleavage reagent also removes the amino acid side-chain protecting groups, which are stable to the N^α-deprotection conditions.

There are primarily two protocols that have been used for the solid-phase chemical synthesis of peptides and proteins (**Fig. 32.2**). The first protocol (**Fig. 32.2A**) uses the *tertiary*-butyloxycarbonyl (Boc) group for N^α-amino protection. The Boc group is typically removed by trifluoroacetic acid (TFA), and the free amino terminus is neutralized by a tertiary amine. Cleavage of the peptide from the resin is carried out by strong acid, usually hydrogen fluoride (HF). Side-chain protecting groups are suitably "fine-tuned" to be stable to repeated cycles of Boc removal, yet cleanly cleaved by the use of HF or trifluoromethanesulfonic acid (TFMSA). The main drawbacks associated with

A

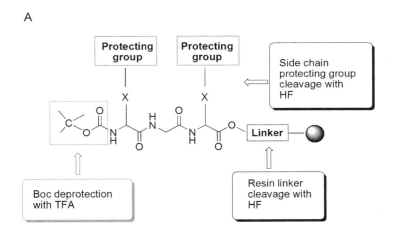

B

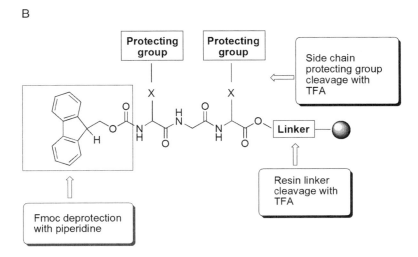

Fig. 32.2. Protection scheme strategy for (**A**) Boc and (**B**) Fmoc chemistries

this strategy is that repetitive TFA acidolysis could lead to acid-catalyzed side reactions, and some peptides containing fragile sequences will not survive the strong acid conditions used to remove side-chain protecting groups and cleave the peptide from the resin. The second protocol (**Fig. 32.2B**) uses the 9-fluore-nylmethyloxycarbonyl (Fmoc) group for N^α-amino protection. Fmoc strategy is based on the orthogonal concept that the two protecting groups belong to independent chemical classes and are removed by different mechanisms. Removal of the Fmoc group is achieved usually with piperidine in N,N-dimethylformamide (DMF) or N-methylpyrrolidone (NMP). Side-chain protection groups that are compatible with N^α-Fmoc protection are removed at the same time as the appropriate anchoring linkages by the use of TFA. The milder conditions of the Fmoc protocol have led to an overall preference for this chemistry (24). However, certain deleterious side reactions are more prevalent in Fmoc-based methodology (25). This review summarizes peptide and protein synthesis using both the Boc and Fmoc solid-phase chemical methods.

3. Polymeric Support (Resin)

The success of solid-phase chemistry is critically dependent on the chemical composition and physical properties of the polymer matrix. In practice, such supports include those that exhibit significant levels of swelling in useful reaction/ wash solvents. Swollen resin beads are reacted and washed batch-wise with agitation, and filtered either with suction or under positive nitrogen pressure. Alternatively, solid-phase synthesis may be carried out in a continuous-flow mode, by pumping reagents and solvents through resins that are packed into columns. The resin support is quite often a polystyrene suspension polymer cross-linked with 1% of 1,3-divinylbenzene. Dry polystyrene beads have an average diameter of about 50 µm, but with the commonly used solvents for peptide synthesis, namely dichloromethane (DCM) and DMF, they swell 2.5 to 6.2-fold in volume (26). Thus, the chemistry of solid-phase synthesis takes place within a well-solvated gel containing mobile and reagent-accessible chains (26,27). This type of resin shows high mechanical stability and acceptable swelling in organic solvents. However, overall reaction rates and yields are limited by the hydrophobic nature and molecular flexibility of the base polymer. Polymer supports have also been developed based on the concept that the insoluble support and peptide backbone should be of comparable polarities (15). A resin of copolymerized dimethylacrylamide, N,N'-bisacry-loylethylenediamine, and acryloylsarcosine methyl ester, commercially known as polyamide or Pepsyn, has been synthesized to satisfy this criteria (28). Increasing popularity has been seen for polyethylene glycol-polystyrene graft supports, which swell in a range of solvents and have excellent physical and mechanical properties for both batch-wise and continuous-flow SPPS (29–33). Meldal and co-workers have developed various PEG-based segmented network resins including poly(ethyleneglycol-acrylamide) (PEGA Versabeads O) (34,35). The hydroxyl groups of Versabeads O can be converted into almost any desired functional group. The intermediate polarity of this resin facilitates compatibility with water as well as organic solvents. The maximum loading values can go up to 1 mmol/g, but lower loadings are easily obtained. The ChemMatrix® resin has loadings between 0.8 and 1.0 mmol/g, which is up to three times the loadings of many other PEG-based resins. ChemMatrix® can be used in a wide array of solvents, including water. Also recently described is a 100% PEG resin that offers an advantage over polystyrene-based resins for long and difficult peptides (36). Owing to a highly crosslinked matrix, the 100% PEG resin has enhanced mechanical and thermal stabilities. Nonstyrene based segmented network resins such as cross-linked poly(oxyethylene-acrylate) resin (CLEAR) was developed and successfully used for peptide synthesis (37). Finally, multiple antigenic peptide (MAP) systems are commercially available that utilize a Lys-branched polystyrene resin core matrix (38). Both Boc- and Fmoc-strategies can be employed with little or no variation of the standard protocols.

Regardless of the structure and nature of the polymeric support chosen, it must contain appropriate functional groups onto which the first amino acid can be anchored. Almost all syntheses by the solid-phase method are carried out in the $C \rightarrow N$ direction, and therefore generally start with the intended C-terminal residue of the desired peptide being linked to the support. This is achieved by the use of a "linker" (see **Fig. 32.1**), which is a bifunctional spacer that on one end incorporates features of a smoothly cleavable protecting group so that eventual cleavage provides either a free acid or amide at the C-terminus, although, in specialized cases, other useful end groups can be obtained (39). The other end of the linker contains a functional group, often a carboxyl that can be activated to allow coupling to functionalized supports. Polymeric supports and linkers had been reviewed in detail by several authors (16,40,41).

4. Protection Schemes

The preceding section outlined the importance of the solid support on the failures and successes of the peptide synthesis. The second key step of the solid-phase procedure is the choice and optimization of protection chemistry. Even when a residue has been incorporated safely into the growing resin-bound polypeptide chain, it may still undergo irreversible structural modification or rearrangement during subsequent synthetic steps. The vulnerability to damage is particularly pronounced at the final deprotection/cleavage step, since these are usually the harshest conditions. So far we dealt only tangentially with combinations of "temporary" and "permanent" protecting groups (**A** and **B**, respectively, in **Fig. 32.1**) and the corresponding methods for their removal. At least 2 levels of protecting group stability are required, insofar as the "permanent" groups used to prevent branching or other problems on the side-chains must withstand repeated applications of the conditions for quantitative removal of the "temporary" N^α-amino protecting group. On the other hand, structures of "permanent" groups must be such that conditions can be found to remove them with minimal levels of side reactions that affect the integrity of the desired product. The necessary stability is often approached by kinetic "fine-tuning," which is a reliance on quantitative rate differences whenever the same chemical mechanism (usually acidolysis) serves to remove both "temporary" and "permanent" protecting groups. An often-limiting consequence of such schemes based on graduated lability is that they force adoption of relatively severe final deprotection conditions. Alternatively, orthogonal protection schemes can be used. These involve two or more classes of groups that are removed by differing chemical mechanisms, and therefore can be removed in any order and in the presence of the other classes. Orthogonal schemes offer the possibility of substantially milder overall conditions, because selectivity can be attained on the basis of differences in chemistry rather than in reaction rates. Quasi-orthogonally protecting schemes had been used in synthesis of complex peptides (i.e., cyclic or branched) and for the construction of peptide libraries. The quasi-orthogonal protecting groups that have become widely accepted will be briefly mentioned below.

4.1. Temporary Protecting Groups

4.1.1. Tertiary-Butyloxycarbonyl (Boc)-Based Chemistry

The so-called "standard Merrifield" system is based on graduated acid lability (**Fig. 32.2A**). The acidolyzable "temporary" Boc group is stable to alkali and nucleophiles, and removed rapidly by inorganic and organic acids (*10*). Boc removal is usually carried out with TFA (20–50%) in DCM for 20–30 min, and, for special situations, HCl (4 N) in 1,4-dioxane for 35 min. Deprotection with neat (100%) TFA, which offers enhanced peptide-resin solvation compared to TFA–DCM mixtures, proceeds in as little as 4 min (*42,43*). Following acidolysis, a rapid diffusion-controlled neutralization step with a tertiary amine, usually 5–10% triethylamine (Et$_3$N) or *N,N*-diisopropylethylamine (DIEA) in DCM for 3–5 min, is interpolated to release the free N^α-amine. Alternatively, Boc-amino acids may be coupled without prior neutralization by using "in situ" neutralization, i.e., coupling in the presence of DIEA or *N*-methylmorpholine (NMM) (*44,45*). "Permanent" side-chain protecting groups are ether, ester, and urethane derivatives based on benzyl alcohol. Alternatively, ether and ester derivatives based on cyclopentyl or cyclohexyl alcohol are sometimes applied, as their use moderates certain side reactions. These "permanent" groups are sufficiently stable to repeated cycles of Boc removal, yet cleanly cleaved in the presence of appropriate scavengers by use of liquid anhydrous HF at 0°C or trimethylsilyl trifluoromethanesulfonate (TMSOTf)/TFA at 25°C. The phenylacetamidomethyl (PAM; for producing peptide acids) or 4-methylbenzhydrylamine (MBHA; for producing peptide amides) anchoring linkages have been designed to be cleaved at the same time (**Fig. 32.3**).

4.1.2. 9-Fluorenylmethoxycarbonyl (Fmoc)-Based Chemistry

The electron withdrawing fluorine ring system of the Fmoc group renders the lone hydrogen on the β-carbon very acidic, and therefore susceptible to removal by weak bases (*46,47*) (**Fig. 32.2B**). Following the abstraction of this acidic proton at the 9-position of the fluorine ring system, β-elimination proceeds to give a highly reactive dibenzofulvene intermediate (*46–50*). Dibenzofulvene can be trapped by excess amine cleavage agents to form stable adducts (*46,47*). The Fmoc group is, in general, rapidly removed by primary (i.e., cyclohexylamine and ethanolamine) and some secondary (i.e., piperidine and piperazine) amines, and slowly removed by tertiary (i.e., Et$_3$N and DIEA) amines. Removal also occurs more rapidly in a relatively polar medium [DMF or *N*-methylpyrrolidone (NMP)] compared to a relatively nonpolar one (DCM). Removal of the Fmoc group is achieved usually with 20–55% piperidine in DMF or NMP for 10–18 min (*51*); piperidine in DCM is not recommended, as

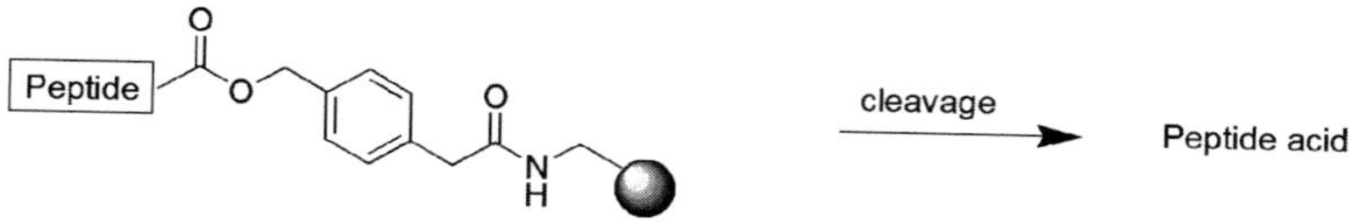

PAM (4-hydroxymethyl-phenylacetamidomethyl)

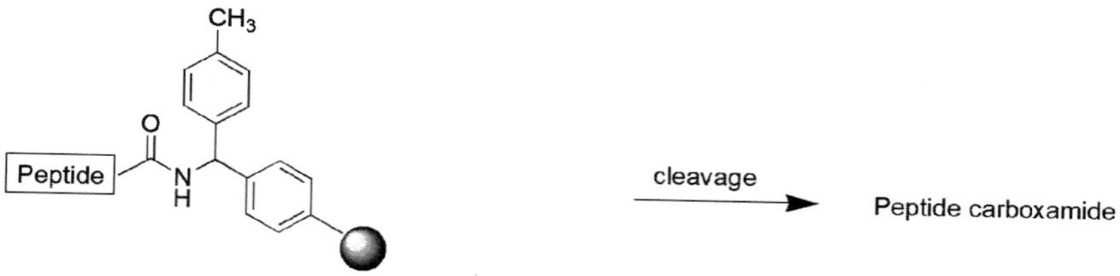

MBHA (4-methylbenzhydrylamine)

Fig. 32.3. Linker-resins for Boc SPPS

an amine salt precipitates after relatively brief standing. Piperidine scavenges the liberated dibenzofulvene to form a fulvene-piperidine adduct. Two percent 1,8-diazabicyclo[5.4.0]undec-7-ene (DBU)–DMF can also be used for Fmoc removal *(52)*. This reagent is recommended for continuous-flow syntheses only, as the dibenzofulvene intermediate does not form an adduct with DBU and thus must be washed rapidly from the peptide-resin to avoid reattachment of dibenzofulvene *(52)*. However, a solution of DBU–piperidine–DMF (1:5:94) is effective for batch syntheses, as the piperidine component scavenges the dibenzofulvene *(53,54)*. After Fmoc removal, the liberated N^{α}-amine of the peptide-resin is free and ready for immediate acylation without an intervening neutralization step. "Permanent" protection compatible with N^{α}-Fmoc protection is provided primarily by ether, ester, and urethane derivatives based on *tert*-butanol. These derivatives are cleaved at the same time as appropriate anchoring linkages, by use of TFA at 25°C. Scavengers must be added to the TFA to trap the reactive carbocations that form under the acidolytic cleavage conditions. The TFA-labile 4-hydroxymethylphenoxy (HMP; for producing peptide acids), 2-chlorotrityl (for producing peptide acids), 5-(4-aminomethyl-3,5-dimethoxyphenoxy)valeric acid (PAL; for producing peptide amides), or 4-(2',4'-dimethoxyphenylaminomethyl)phenoxy (Rink amide) anchoring linkages are used in conjunction with Fmoc chemistry (**Fig. 32.4**).

4.2. Permanent Protecting Groups

Once the means for N^{α}-amino protection has been selected, compatible protection for the side-chains of trifunctional amino acids must be specified. These choices are made in the context of potential side reactions, which should be minimized. Problems may be anticipated either during the coupling steps or at the final deprotection/cleavage. For certain residues (e.g., Cys, Asp, Glu, and Lys), side-chain protection is absolutely essential, whereas for others, an informed decision should be made depending upon the length of the synthetic target and other considerations. Most solid-phase syntheses follow maximal rather than minimal protection strategies. As is clear from the preceding

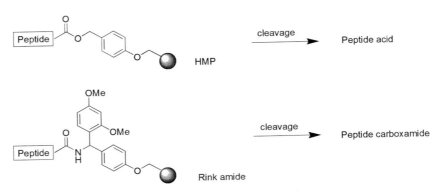

Fig. 32.4. Linker-resins for Fmoc SPPS

Table 32.1. Recommended side-chain protecting groups for Boc and Fmoc SPPS.

Amino acid	Boc chemistry Side-chain protecting group	Fmoc chemistry Side-chain protecting group
Arg	Tos	Pbf
Asn	Xan	Trt
Asp	OBzl, O-2-Ada, OcHx	OtBu, O-1-Ada, OMpe
Cys	Acm, Meb	Acm, Trt
His	Tos, Dnp	Trt
Gln	Xan	Trt
Glu	OBzl	OtBu
Lys	2-ClZ	Boc
Met	Met(O)	
Ser/Thr	Bzl	tBu
Tyr	2,6-Cl₂Bzl, 2-BrZ	tBu
Trp	CHO	Boc

discussion, the Boc and Fmoc groups have risen to the fore as the most widely used. Almost all of the useful N^{α}-Boc and N^{α}-Fmoc protected derivatives can be manufactured in bulk, and are found in the catalogues of the major suppliers of peptide synthesis chemicals. The most widely used "permanent" protecting groups for the trifunctional amino acids for Boc- and Fmoc-strategy have been listed in **Table 32.1**. A plethora of other N^{α}-amino protecting groups, some illustrating remarkably creative organic chemistry, have been proposed over the years *(19,55)*. Chemistries relying on these protecting groups are beyond the scope of the present review.

4.2.1. Asp and Glu

The side-chain carboxyls of Asp and Glu are protected as benzyl (OBzl) esters for Boc chemistry and as *tert*-butyl (OtBu) esters for Fmoc chemistry. To minimize the imide/$\alpha \rightarrow \beta$ rearrangement side reaction, Boc-Asp may be protected with either the 2-adamantyl (O-2-Ada) *(56)* or cyclohexyl (OcHex)

(57) groups. Fmoc-Asp may be protected with the 1-adamantyl (O-1-Ada) group *(56)* or the extremely hindered Mpe (β-3-methylpent-3-yl) protecting group *(58)*. The base-labile 9-fluorenylmethyl (OFm) group offers orthogonal side-chain protection for Boc-Asp/Glu *(59–61)*, whereas the palladium-sensitive allyl (OAl) group *(62,63)* offers orthogonal side-chain protection for both Boc- and Fmoc-Asp/Glu. The *N*-[1-(4,4,-dimethyl-2,6-dioxocyclohexylidene)-3-methylbutyl]aminobenzyl (Dmab) group can be used for quasi-orthogonal protection of Asp during Fmoc chemistry, as Dmab is stable to 20% piperidine and can be removed selectively with 2% hydrazine in DMF *(64)*.

4.2.2. Ser, Thr, and Tyr

The side-chain hydroxyls of Ser, Thr, and Tyr are protected as Bzl and *t*Bu ethers for Boc and Fmoc SPPS, respectively. In strong acid, the Bzl protecting group blocking the Tyr phenol can migrate to the 3-position of the ring *(65)*. This side reaction is decreased greatly when Tyr is protected by the 2,6-dichlorobenzyl (2,6-Cl2Bzl) *(65)* or 2-bromobenzyloxycarbonyl (2-BrZ) *(66)* group; consequently, the latter two derivatives are much preferred for Boc SPPS.

4.2.3. Lys

The ε-amino group of Lys is best protected by the 2-chlorobenzyloxycarbonyl (2-ClZ) or Fmoc group for Boc chemistry, and reciprocally by the Boc group for Fmoc chemistry. Orthogonal side-chain protection for both Boc- and Fmoc-Lys is provided by the palladium-sensitive allyloxycarbonyl (Aloc) group *(63,67)*. In addition, 1-(4,4-dimethyl-2,6-dioxocyclohex-1-ylidene)ethyl (Dde) side-chain protection of Lys during Fmoc chemistry allows for selective deprotection with 2% hydrazine in DMF *(68)*. Lys(Dde) has been successfully employed for the synthesis of branched peptides and peptide templates *(68–71)*. Partial loss of Dde moiety had been noted during the synthesis of long sequences *(72)*, compromising the purity of the final product. Furthermore, Dde has also been reported to undergo intramolecular $N \rightarrow N$ migration, leading to scrambling of its position within the peptide chain. To avoid both side reactions, 1-(4,4-dimethyl-2,6-dioxocyclohexylidene)-3-methylbutyl (ivDde) has been introduced *(72)*. The ivDde group is cleaved under the same conditions as Dde group. Another selectively removable side-chain protecting group for Lys is 4-methyltrityl (Mtt), which is labile to 1% TFA–triisopropylsilane in DCM *(73)*.

4.2.4. Arg

The highly basic trifunctional guanidino side-chain group of Arg may be protected by appropriate benzenesulfonyl derivatives, such as the 4-toluenesulfonyl (Tos) or mesitylene-2-sulfonyl (Mts) groups in conjunction with Boc chemistry, and either 4-methoxy-2,3,6-trimethylbenzenesulfonyl (Mtr), 2,2,5,7,8-pentamethylchroman-6-sulphonyl (Pmc), or 2,2,4,6,7-pentamethyl-dihydro-benzofuran-5-sulfonyl (Pbf) with Fmoc chemistry. These groups most likely block the ω-nitrogen of Arg, and their relative acid lability is Pbf > Pmc > Mtr >> Mts > Tos *(74–76)*.

4.2.5. His

Activated His derivatives are uniquely prone to racemization during stepwise SPPS, owing to an intramolecular abstraction of the proton on the optically active α-carbon by the imidazole π-nitrogen *(77)*. Racemization could be suppressed by either reducing the basicity of the imidazole ring, or by blocking the base directly *(78)*. Consequently, His side-chain protecting groups can be categorized depending on whether the τ- or π-imidazole nitrogen is blocked. The Tos group blocks the N^τ of Boc-His, and is removed by strong acids. However, the Tos group is also lost prematurely during SPPS steps involving 1-hydroxybenzotriazole (HOBt); this allows acylation or acetylation of the imidazole group, followed by chain termination owing to $N^{im} \rightarrow N^\alpha$-amino transfer of the acyl or acetyl group *(79,80)*. Therefore, HOBt should never be used during couplings of amino acids once a His(Tos) residue has been incorporated into the peptide-resin (see Coupling Reactions). Boc-His(Tos) is coupled efficiently using benzotriazol-1-yl-oxy-tris(dimethylamino)phosphonium hexafluorophosphate (BOP) (3 equiv) in the presence of DIEA (3 equiv); these conditions minimize racemization and avoid premature side-chain deprotection by HOBt *(81)*. The 2,4-dinitrophenyl (Dnp) N^τ-protecting group has been used in Boc strategies as well. The advantages of the Dnp group for protection of His are that it is stable to almost all coupling conditions and couples better than Boc-His(Tos) in some difficult sequences. The main drawback of the Dnp group is that is not cleaved by HF and TFMSA, and therefore a separate deprotection step is necessary. Final Dnp deblocking is best carried out at the peptide-resin level before the HF cleavage step, by use of thiophenol in DMF. The τ-nitrogen of Fmoc-His can be protected by the Boc and triphenylmethyl (Trt) groups. It has been shown that the Boc group was very effective at suppressing racemization *(15)*. Unexpectedly, His(Boc) was not completely stable to repetitive base treatment *(82)*. The Trt group is completely stable to repetitive piperidine treatment and is readily removed by 95% TFA. The Trt group reduces the basicity of the imidazole ring significantly (the pK_a decreases from 6.2 to 4.7), although racemization is not eliminated completely when preformed symmetrical anhydride coupling methods are used *(83)*. It is recommended that the appropriate derivatives be coupled as preformed esters or *in situ* with carbodiimide in the presence of HOBt *(78,83)*.

4.2.6. Asn and Gln

Although conditions are available for the safe incorporation of Asn and Gln with free side-chains during SPPS, there are compelling reasons for their protection. Side-chain protecting groups such as 9-xanthenyl (Xan) and Trt minimize the occurrence of dehydration *(84–86)* and pyroglutamate formation *(10)*, and may also inhibit hydrogen bonding that otherwise leads to secondary structures, which substantially reduce coupling rates. In Fmoc synthesis, the Trt protected derivatives Fmoc-Asn(Trt)-OH and Fmoc-Gln(Trt)-OH are the most widely used *(86,87)*. Since intramolecular cyclization of Gln to pyroglutamate is particularly problematic in the Boc strategy, Boc-Gln(Xan)-OH should be used.

4.2.7. Met

The thioether side-chain of Met survives cycles of Fmoc chemistry, but protection during Boc chemistry is often advisable. The reducible sulfoxide function is applied under these circumstances. Smooth deblocking of Met(O) occurs in 20–25% HF in the presence of dimethylsulfide to prevent alkylation of Met.

4.2.8. Trp

There are two main reasons for Trp side-chain protection: oxidation of Trp during peptide synthesis and alkylation of the indole ring by carbonium ions generated during cleavage. The highly sensitive side-chain of Trp is best protected by the N^{in}-formyl (CHO) and N^{in}-Boc groups for Boc and Fmoc chemistry, respectively. Trp(CHO) is deprotected at the peptide-resin level by treatment with piperidine–DMF (9:91), 0°C, 2 h, *before* HF cleavage (*88*). Boc side-chain protection of Trp is partially reduced to a carboxylate function during the TFA cleavage procedure thereby preventing alkylation, peptide re-attachment, or sulfonation. Complete deprotection occurs in aqueous solution (*89,90*). The efficacy of using Trp(Boc) in Fmoc synthesis has now been confirmed by a number of independent studies (*91,92*). The combination of Trp(Boc) and Arg(Pbf) seems to be optimal (*91*).

4.2.9. Cys

The most challenging residue to manage in peptide synthesis is Cys. Compatible with Boc chemistry are the 4-methylbenzyl (Meb), acetamidomethyl (Acm), *tert*-butylsulfenyl (S*t*Bu), and 9-fluorenylmethyl (Fm) β-thiol protecting groups; compatible with Fmoc chemistry are the Acm, S*t*Bu, Trt, and 2,4,6-trimethoxybenzyl (Tmob) groups. The most commonly used group in Fmoc chemistry is Trt because this group generates the free thiol upon deprotection with TFA. Both the Trt and Tmob groups have a tendency to form stable carbonium ions that can realkylate Cys (*93,94*) upon TFA treatment; therefore, effective carbonium ion scavengers are needed. The Meb group is optimized for removal by strong acid (*65*); Cys(Meb) residues may also be directly converted to the oxidized cystine (disulfide) form by thallium (III) trifluoroacetate [Tl(Tfa)$_3$], although some cysteic acid forms at the same time. Cys(Fm) is stable to acid, and cleaved by base. The Acm group is acid- and base-stable and removed by mercuric (II) acetate, followed by treatment with H$_2$S or excess mercaptans to free the β-thiol. Mercuric (II) acetate can modify Trp, and thus should be used in the presence of 50% acetic acid for Trp-containing peptides (*95*). In multiple Cys(Acm)-containing peptides, mercuric (II) acetate may not be a completely effective removal reagent (*96*). Alternatively, Cys(Acm) residues are converted directly to disulfides by treatment with I$_2$ or Tl(Tfa)$_3$ on-resin (*97,98*). Finally, the acid-stable S*t*Bu group is removed by reduction with thiols or phosphines. Cys protecting group strategies have been described in detail (*99*).

5. Coupling Reactions

There are currently four major kinds of coupling techniques that serve well for the *stepwise* introduction of N^α-protected amino acids for solid-phase synthesis. In the solid-phase mode, coupling reagents are used in excess to ensure that reactions reach completion. However the activating group or reaction has to be chosen carefully to achieve a very high coupling efficiency and at the same time avoid potential side reactions (*22,100,101*).

The classical example of an in situ coupling reagent is *N,N*′-dicyclohexylcarbodiimide (DCC) (*102,103*). The related *N,N*-diisopropylcarbodiimide (DIPCDI) is more convenient to use under some circumstances, as the resultant urea co-product is more soluble in DCM. The generality of carbodiimide-mediated couplings is extended significantly by the use of HOBt as an additive, which accelerates carbodiimide-mediated couplings, suppresses racemization, and inhibits dehydration of the carboxamide side-chains of Asn and Gln to the corresponding nitriles (*84,104,105*). More recently, protocols involving phosphonium and aminium/uronium salts of benzotriazole derivatives have been introduced. Benzotriazol-1-yl-oxy-tris(dimethylamino)phosphonium hexafluorophosphate (BOP), 2-(1H-benzotriazol-1-yl)-1,1,3,3-tetramethylaminium hexafluorophosphate (HBTU), 2-(1H-benzotriazol-1-yl)-1,1,3,3-tetramethylaminium tetrafluoroborate (TBTU), and O-(7-azabenzotriazol-1-yl)-1,1,3,3-tetramethylaminium hexafluorophosphate (HATU) have deservedly achieved popularity. Interestingly, X-ray crystallographic analysis has shown that the solid-state structures of HBTU and HATU are not tetramethyluronium salts, but guanidinium N-oxide isomers (106). They all require a tertiary amine such as NMM or DIEA for optimal efficiency (45,107–114). HOBt has been reported to accelerate further the rates of BOP- and HBTU-mediated couplings (112,115). 2-(6-Chloro-1-H-benzotriazole-1-yl)-1,1,3,3-tetramethylaminium hexafluorophosphate (HCTU) is a novel aminium-based coupling reagent that gave superior results compared to TBTU in the synthesis of difficult peptides (100). The superiority of HATU and HCTU had been explained by formation of corresponding 7-azabenzotriazole (OAt) and 6-chloro-1-H-benzotriazole (6-ClOBt) esters that are more reactive than OBt esters (116). The main disadvantage of HATU is its high price, and therefore it is generally recommended for difficult couplings and long sequences. In situ activations by excess HBTU or TBTU can cap free amino groups (117,118); it is not known whether HOBt can suppress this side reaction. Acylations using BOP result in the liberation of the carcinogen hexamethylphosphoramide, which might limit its use in large scale work. The modified BOP reagent benzotriazole-1-yl-oxy-tris-pyrrolidinophosphonium hexafluorophosphate (PyBOP) liberates potentially less toxic by-products (119) and can be used in excess that is especially useful in cyclization steps or for the activation of hindered amino acids. Recently developed is also a new group of coupling reagents that are derived from organophosphorus esters, phosphate, or phosphinyl esters (120). 3-(Diethoxyphosphoryloxy)-3,4-dihydro-4-oxo-1,2,3-benzotriazine (DepODhbt or DEPBT) has been successfully used in the synthesis of linear and cyclic peptides by both solution and solid-phase methods with remarkable resistance to racemization. When DEPBT is used as a coupling reagent, it is not necessary to protect the hydroxyl group of the amino component (such as Tyr, Ser, and Thr) and the imidazole group in the case of His (121,122). Commonly used coupling reagents and additives are presented on **Fig. 32.5**.

A long-known but steadfast coupling method involves the use of active esters, such as pentafluorophenyl (OPfp), HOBt, 6-ClOBt and 3-hydroxy-2,3-dihydro-4-oxo-benzotriazine (ODhbt) esters. Boc- and Fmoc-amino acid OPfp esters are prepared from DCC and pentafluorophenol (123–125) or pentafluorophenyl trifluoroacetate (126). Although OPfp esters alone couple slowly, the addition of HOBt (1–2 equiv) increases the reaction rate (127,128). Fmoc-Asn-OPfp allows for efficient incorporation of Asn with little side-chain dehydration (85). HOBt esters of Fmoc-amino acids are rapidly formed (with DIPCDI) and highly reactive (129,130), as are Boc-amino acid HOBt esters (131). N^{α}-protected amino acid ODhbt esters suppress racemization and are highly reactive, in similar fashion to HOBt esters (120,132).

Preformed symmetrical anhydrides (PSAs) are favored by some workers because of their high reactivity. They are generated in situ from the corresponding

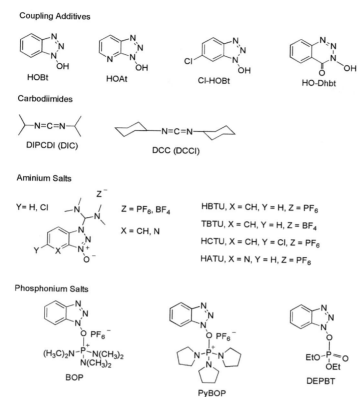

Fig. 32.5. Common coupling reagents and additives for SPPS

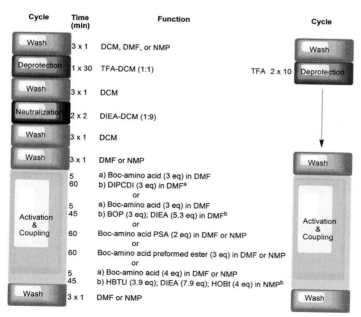

ᵃHOBt (3 eq) is added for Boc-Asn, -Gln, Arg(Tos), and His(Dnp)
ᵇBoc-Asn and -Gln are side-chain protected

Fig. 32.6. General protocol for Boc SPPS

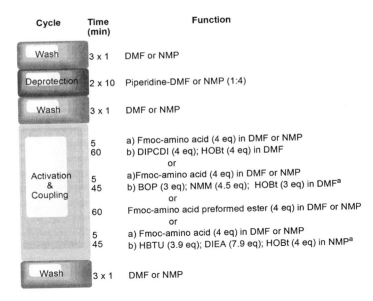

aFmoc-Asn and -Gln are side-chain protected

Fig. 32.7. General protocol for Fmoc SPPS

N^α-protected amino acid (2 or 4 equiv) plus DCC (1 or 2 equiv) in DCM; following removal of the urea by filtration, the solvent is exchanged to DMF for optimal couplings. The solubilities of some Fmoc-amino acids make PSAs a less than optimum activated species.

Fmoc-amino acid fluorides react rapidly under SPPS conditions in the presence of DIEA with very low levels of racemization *(133,134)*. Fmoc-amino acid fluorides are an especially effective method for coupling to *N*-alkyl amino acids *(135,136)*. These fluorides can be prepared and isolated by the reaction of the protected amino acid with cyanuric fluoride or (diethylamino)sulfur trifluoride (DAST), or generated in situ through the aminium reagent tetramethylfluoroformamidinium hexafluorophosphate (TFFH) *(137)*. Furthermore, anionic polyhydrogen fluoride additives such as benzyltriphenylphosphonium dihydrogen trifluoride (PTF) have been used successfully to obtain amino acid fluorides *(138)*. Recommendations for coupling methods are included in **Figs. 32.6** and **32.7**.

6. Chemoselective Ligation

Regardless of the improvements in peptide-synthesis efficiency, stepwise SPPS protocols are most effective in producing up to 50-residue peptides. The recent introduction of chemoselective ligation has dramatically extended the reach of total chemical synthesis of proteins *(2,4,5)*. The initial strategies resulted in the formation of thioester or oxime bonds between peptide fragments. For example, reaction of a peptide bearing a *C*-terminal thioacid with a peptide containing an *N*-terminal bromoacetyl group results in a synthetic protein product containing a thioester bond *(139,140)*. This approach has been used to construct HIV-1 protease *(139)*, a 4 α-helix TASP molecule *(141)*, a folded β-sandwich fibronectin domain model *(142)*, and a tethered dimer of HIV-1 protease *(143)*. A convenient linker that produces *C*-terminal thioacids following Boc chemistry has been described *(144)*. A variation of the thioester approach, in which a peptide *C*-terminal thiol (such as Cys) is reacted with an *N*-terminal bromoacetyl or maleimido peptide to form a thioether bond, has been used to construct linked cytoplasmic domains from the $\alpha_{IIb}\beta_3$ integrin *(145)*, a β-meander TASP molecule *(146)*, and a 129-residue tripod protein *(147)*. Linkers that produce *C*-terminal thiols have been described for both Boc *(148)* and Fmoc *(149)* chemistries. To prevent decomposition of thioester linkers during Fmoc syntheses, an Fmoc deprotection solution containing 1-methylpyrrolidine, hexamethyleneimine, and HOBt in NMP-DMSO (1:1) should be used *(150)*. DBU in the presence of HOBt has been used successfully as well *(151,152)*. Several other approaches have been directed toward stabilization of thioesters *(153)*. More convenient use of chemoselective ligation has been achieved via "safety-catch" type handles *(154–157)*, backbone amide linker (BAL) strategies *(158,159)*, and standard linkers (PAM or HMBA) cleaved by a nucleophile in the presence of an organoaluminum Lewis acid catalyst *(160,161)*. As an alternative to thioester and thioether bonds, peptides containing either aldehyde or *N*-terminal aminooxyacetyl groups can be ligated to form oxime bonds *(162,163)*. An aldehyde containing peptide can also be ligated to a peptide containing a weak nucleophilic base, such as hydrazide, *N*-terminal Cys, or *N*-terminal Thr, to form a hydrazone, thiazolidine, and oxazolidine linkages, respectively *(4,164–167)*.

Chemoselective ligation was made further attractive by "native chemical ligation," in which an amide bond, rather than a thioester, thioether or oxime bond, is generated between fragments *(168)*. A peptide bearing a *C*-terminal thioacid is converted to a 5-thio-2-nitrobenzoic acid ester and then reacted with a peptide bearing an *N*-terminal Cys residue. The initial thioester ligation product undergoes spontaneous rearrangement, leading to an amide bond and the regeneration of the free sulfhydryl on Cys. The ligation strategy was further extended to make use of other thiol additives and their respective reactivities *(169,170)*. The trityl-associated mercaptoproprionic acid-leucine (TAMPAL) resin allows for the convenient generation of any amino acid as a C-terminal thioester *(171)*. Native chemical ligation can proceed intramolecularly to create cyclized proteins *(172,173)*. Conformationally assisted protein ligation, in which the *C*- and *N*-termini to be ligated are brought in close proximity via peptide folding, has been shown to eliminate the absolute need for an *N*-terminal Cys residue *(174)*. Amide bonds can also be generated by chemoselective ligation methods that result in thiazolidine linkages via an $O \rightarrow N$ acyl shift to form hydroxymethyl-thiazolidine *(175)*. Chemoselective ligation can be performed for multiple fragments *(176,177)*, and in either the $N \rightarrow C$ or $C \rightarrow N$ direction in the solid-phase *(178)*. A modular chemoselective ligation strategy was used for the synthesis of a covalently-linked dimer of cMyc and Max transcription factor b/HLH/Z domains *(179)*. The individual cMyc and Max domains were assembled by native chemical ligation, and then linked via oxime bond formation.

Recent advances in the ligation field include use of selenocysteine as a potential Ala surrogate *(180,181)*, thioligation with a removable auxiliary *(182–184)*, and the Staudinger ligation principle *(185–189)*.

7. Cleavage and Side-Chain Deprotection

Boc SPPS is designed primarily for simultaneous cleavage of the peptide anchoring linkage and side-chain protecting groups with strong acid (HF or equivalent), whereas Fmoc SPPS is designed primarily to accomplish the same cleavages with moderate strength acid (TFA or equivalent). In each case, careful attention to cleavage conditions (reagents, scavengers, temperature, and times) is necessary to minimize a variety of side reactions.

Treatment with HF simultaneously cleaves PAM and MBHA linkages and removes the side-chain protecting groups commonly applied in Boc chemistry *(190)*. HF cleavages are always carried out in the presence of a carbonium ion scavenger, usually 10% anisole. For cleavages of Cys-containing peptides, further addition of 1.8% 4-thiocresol is recommended. TMSOTf/TFA has also been used for strong acid cleavage and deprotection reactions, which are accelerated by the presence of thioanisole as a "soft" nucleophile *(191,192)*. TMSOTf (1M)–thioanisole (1M) in TFA (a.k.a. DEPRO™) efficiently cleaves PAM and MBHA linkages *(192,193)*.

The combination of side-chain protecting groups, e.g., *t*Bu (for Asp, Glu, Ser, Thr, and Tyr), Boc (for His and Lys), Tmob (for Cys), and Trt (for Asn, Cys, Gln, and His), and anchoring linkages, e.g., HMP or Rink amide, commonly used in Fmoc chemistry are simultaneously deprotected and cleaved by TFA. Such cleavage of *t*Bu and Boc groups results in *tert*-butyl cations and *tert*-butyl trifluoroacetate formation *(194–198)*. These species are responsible for *tert*-butylation of the indole ring of Trp, the thioether group of Met, and, to a very low degree (0.5–1.0%), the 3'-position of Tyr. Modifications can be minimized during TFA cleavage by utilizing effective *tert*-butyl scavengers. The indole ring of Trp can be alkylated irreversibly by Mtr, Pmc, and Pbf groups from Arg *(91,130,199–201)*, Tmob groups *(85,86)*, and even by some TFA-labile ester and amide linkers *(127,202–205)*. The extent of Pmc modification of Trp is dependent upon the distance between the Arg and Trp residues *(206)*. Cleavage of the Pmc group may also result in *O*-sulfation of Ser, Thr, and Tyr *(201,207)*. Three efficient cleavage "cocktails" for Mtr/Pmc/Pbf/Tmob quenching, and preservation of Trp, Tyr, Ser, Thr, and Met integrity, are TFA–phenol–thioanisole–EDT–H2O (82.5:5:5:2.5:5) (reagent K) *(200)*, TFA–thioanisole–EDT–anisole (90:5:3:2) (reagent R) *(204)*, and TFA–phenol–H$_2$O–triisopropylsilane (88:5:5:2) (reagent B) *(208)*. The use of Boc side-chain protection of Trp also significantly reduces alkylation by Pmc/Pbf groups *(91,92)*.

8. Side Reactions

Side reactions that occur during SPPS have been reviewed extensively *(10,11,14–16,21)*. In general, side reactions can lead to racemized, deletion, truncated, terminated, modified, and/or oxidized peptides. The present discussions focus on new approaches for alleviating well established side reactions.

8.1. Diketopiperazine Formation

The free N^α-amino group of an anchored dipeptide is poised for a base-catalyzed intramolecular attack of the *C*-terminal carbonyl *(10,209,210)*. Base deprotection (Fmoc) or neutralization (Boc) can thus release a cyclic diketo-piperazine while a hydroxymethyl-handle leaving group remains on the resin. With residues that can form *cis* peptide bonds, e.g., Gly, Pro, *N*-methylamino acids, or D-amino acids, in either the first or second position of the $(C \rightarrow N)$ synthesis, diketopiperazine formation can be substantial *(210–212)*. For most other sequences, the problem can be adequately controlled. In Boc SPPS, the level of diketopiperazine formation can be suppressed either by removing the Boc group with HCl and coupling the NMM salt of the third Boc-amino acid without neutralization *(44)*, or else by deprotecting the Boc group with TFA and coupling the third Boc-amino acid *in situ* using BOP, DIEA, and HOBt without neutralization *(212)*. For susceptible sequences being addressed by Fmoc chemistry, the use of piperidine–DMF (1:1) deprotection for 5 min *(210)*, or deprotection for 2 min with a 0.1*M* solution in DMF of tetrabutylam-monium fluoride ("quenched" by MeOH) *(213)* has been recommended to minimize cyclization. Alternatively, the second and third amino acids may be coupled as a preformed N^α-protected-dipeptide, avoiding the diketopi-perazine-inducing deprotection/neutralization at the second amino acid. The stearic hindrance of the 2-chlorotrityl linker may minimize diketopiperazine formation of susceptible sequences during Fmoc chemistry *(214,215)*.

8.2. Aspartimide Formation

A sometimes serious side reaction with protected Asp residues involves an intramolecular elimination to form an aspartimide, which can then partition in water to the desired α-peptide and the undesired by-product with the chain growing from the β-carboxyl *(10,57,216)*. Aspartimide formation is sequence dependent, with Asp(OBzl)-Gly, -Ser, -Thr, -Asn, and -Gln sequences show-ing the greatest tendency to cyclize under basic conditions *(216–218)*; the same sequences are also quite susceptible in strong acid *(10,57,74)*. For mod-els containing Asp(OBzl)-Gly, the rate and extent of aspartimide formation was substantial both in base (50% after 1–3 h treatment with Et_3N or DIEA) and in strong acid (a typical value is 36% after 1-h treatment with HF at 25°C). Aspartimide formation is minimized during Boc chemistry by using the Asp(OcHex) or Asp(O-2-Ada) derivative.

Sequences containing Asp(O*t*Bu)-Gly are somewhat susceptible to base-catalyzed aspartimide formation (11% after 4-h treatment with 20% piperidine in DMF) *(218)*, but do not rearrange at all in acid *(219)*. Piperidine catalysis of aspartimide formation from side-chain protected Asp residues can be rapid, and is dependent upon the side-chain protecting group. Treatment of Asp(OBzl)-Gly, Asp(OcHex)-Gly, and Asp(O*t*Bu)-Gly with 20% piperidine–DMF for 4 h resulted in 100, 67.5, and 11% aspartimide formation, respectively *(218)*, whereas treatment of Asp(OBzl)-Phe with 55% piperidine–DMF for 1 h resulted in 16% aspartimide formation *(220)*. Sequence dependence studies of Asp(O*t*Bu)-X peptides revealed that piperidine could induce aspartimide formation when X = Arg(Pmc), Asn(Trt), Asp(O*t*Bu), Cys(Acm), Gly, Ser, Thr, and Thr(*t*Bu) *(221,222)*. Aspartimide formation can also be conformation dependent *(223)*. This side-reaction can be minimized by including 0.1 M HOBt in the piperidine *(222)* or piperazine *(224)* solution. However, only masking of the Asp-X amide bond via an amide backbone protecting group (i.e., 2-hydroxy-4-methoxybenzyl; Hmb) for the residue in the X position offers complete protection *(225,226)*.

8.3. Racemization of Cys Residues

C-terminal esterified (but not amidated) Cys residues are racemized by repeated piperidine deprotection treatments during Fmoc SPPS. Following 4-h exposure to piperidine–DMF (1:4), the extent of racemization found was 36% D-Cys from Cys(S*t*Bu), 12% D-Cys from Cys(Trt), and 9% D-Cys from Cys(Acm) *(227)*. Racemization of esterified Cys(Trt) was reduced from 11.8% with 20% piperidine–DMF to only 2.6% with 1% DBU–DMF after 4 h treatment *(52,227)*. Several highly hindered bases such as 2,6-dimethyl pyridine, 2,3,5,6-tetramethylpyridine, and 2,6-di-tert-butyl-4-(dimethylamino)pyridine have been successfully used in place of the usual DIEA or NMM to minimize cysteine racemization even with *in situ* coupling protocols and regardless of the thiol protecting group *(228)*. Additionally, the steric hindrance of the 2-chlorotrityl linker has been shown to minimize racemization of *C*-terminal Cys residues *(229)*.

8.4. Interchain Association

Effective solvation of the peptide-resin is perhaps the most crucial condition for efficient chain assembly *(230)*. Under proper solvent conditions, there is no decrease in synthetic efficiency up to 60 amino acid residues in Boc SPPS *(231)*. The ability of the peptide-resin to swell increases with increasing peptide length owing to a net decrease in free energy from solvation of the linear peptide chains *(26)*. Therefore, there is no theoretical upper limit to efficient amino acid couplings, provided that proper solvation conditions exist *(232)*. In practice, obtaining these conditions is not always straightforward. "Difficult couplings" during SPPS have been attributed to poor solvation of the growing chain by DCM. Infrared and NMR spectroscopies have shown that intermolecular β-sheet aggregates are responsible for lowering coupling efficiencies *(233–235)*. A scale of β-sheet structure-stabilizing potential has been developed for Boc-amino acid derivatives *(236)*. Enhanced coupling efficiencies are seen upon the addition of polar solvents, such as DMF, TFE, and NMP *(131,233,237–240)*. Chaotropic salts may be added to organic solvents to disrupt β-sheet aggregates *(241,242)*. Also, using a lower substitution level of the resin to minimize interchain crowding can improve the synthesis *(243)*.

Aggregation also occurs in regions of apolar side-chain protecting groups, sometimes resulting in a collapsed gel structure *(244,245)*. In cases where aggregation occurs owing to apolar side-chain protecting groups, increased solvent polarity may not be sufficient to disrupt the aggregate. A problem of Fmoc chemistry is that the lack of polar side-chain protecting groups could, during the course of an extended peptide synthesis, inhibit proper solvation of the peptide-resin *(240,244,246)*. To alleviate this problem, the use of solvent mixtures containing both a polar and nonpolar component, such as THF–NMP (7:13) or TFE–DCM (1:4), is recommended *(240)*. The addition of DMSO has been demonstrated to inhibit peptide aggregation to an even greater extent than DMF *(247,248)*, or a solvent mixture containing detergents *(249)* can be effective for disrupting such aggregates. The partial substitution or complete replacement of *t*Bu-based side-chain protecting groups for carboxyl, hydroxyl, and amino side-chains by more polar groups would also aid peptide-resin solvation *(240,244,246)*. The incorporation of reversible, amide backbone protecting groups, such as Hmb or 2-hydroxy-6-nitrobenzyl (Hnb), has been demonstrated to be an effective method for disrupting interchain aggregates and thus improving solvation and reaction conditions *(250–252)*. The relative acyl transfer efficiency of the Hnb auxiliary is superior to the Hmb auxiliary, being even more pronounced between more sterically demanding amino acids. On-resin aggregation also has the potential to disrupt the rate of Fmoc deprotection. DBU was shown to be particularly effective in ensuring complete Fmoc-deprotection during difficult peptide syntheses, although caution is required in the presence of Asp-X owing to potential aspartimide formation *(52,253)*.

Microwave energy had been recently used to improve coupling rates of difficult sequences *(254–257)*. A comparison of microwave and conventional heating shows that both provide excellent synthetic results for shorter sequences; however, a clear benefit of microwave irradiation for longer β-peptides has been documented *(257)*.

Even though considerable advances in coupling methods, resin properties, and the choice of coupling solvents have been made, the problem of difficult sequences has not been eliminated. Consequently, the development of new or improved synthetic strategies to overcome this long-standing problem in SPPS remains a continuing goal.

References

1. Borgia JA, Fields GB (2000) Chemical synthesis of proteins. Trends Biotech 18:243–251
2. Dawson PE, Kent SBH (2000) Synthesis of native proteins by chemical ligation. Annu Rev Biochem 69:923–960
3. Miranda IP, Alewood PF (2000) Challenges for protein chemical synthesis in the 21st century: bridging genomics and proteomics. Biopolymers (Peptide Sci) 55:217–226
4. Tam JP, Xu J, Eom KD (2001) Methods and strategies of peptide ligation. Biopolymers (Peptide Sci) 60:194–205
5. Kimmerlin T, Seebach D (2005) "100 years of peptide synthesis": ligation methods for peptide and protein synthesis with applications to β-peptide assemblies. J Peptide Res 65:229–260
6. Muir TW, Sondhi D, Cole PA (1998) Expressed protein ligation: A general method for protein engineering. Proc Natl Acad Sci USA 95:6705–6710
7. Muir TW (2003) Semisynthesis of proteins by expressed protein ligation. Annu Rev Biochem 72:249–289
8. David R, Richter MPO, Beck-Sickinger A (2004) Expressed protein ligation: Method and application. Eur J Biochem 271:663–677
9. Erickson BW, Merrifield RB (1976) Solid-phase peptide synthesis in The Proteins Vol II 3rd Ed (Neurath, H., and Hill, R. L., Eds.) pp 255–527, Academic Press, New York
10. Barany G, and Merrifield RB (1979) Solid-phase peptide synthesis. In: Gross E, Meienhofer J (eds) The Peptides Vol 2. Academic Press, New York, pp 1–284
11. Stewart JM, Young JD (1984) Solid Phase Peptide Synthesis 2nd edn, Pierce Chemical Co., Rockford, IL
12. Merrifield B (1986) Solid phase synthesis. Science 232:341–347
13. Barany G, Kneib-Cordonier N, Mullen DG (1987) Solid-phase peptide synthesis: a silver anniversary report. Int J Peptide Protein Res 30:705–739

14. Kent SBH (1988) Chemical synthesis of peptides and proteins: Annu Rev Biochem 57:957–989

15. Atherton E, Sheppard RC (1989) Solid phase peptide synthesis: a practical approach. IRL Press, Oxford, U.K.

16. Fields GB, Noble RL (1990) Solid phase peptide synthesis utilizing 9-fluorenyl-methoxycarbonyl amino acids. Int J Peptide Protein Res 35:161–214

17. Fields GB (1997) Solid-phase peptide synthesis: methods in enzymology 289. Academic Press, Orlando, FL

18. Sakakibara S (1999) Chemical synthesis of proteins in solution. Biopolymers (Peptide Sci) 51:279–296

19. Albericio F (2000) Orthogonal protecting groups for Nα-amino and C-terminal carboxyl functions in solid-phase peptide synthesis. Biopolymers (Peptide Sci) 55:123–139

20. Anderson L, Blomberg L, Flegel M, Lepsa L, Nilsson B, Verlander M (2000) Large-scale synthesis of peptides. Biopolymers (Peptide Sci) 55:227–250

21. Fields GB, Lauer-Fields JL, Liu R-q, Barany G (2001) Principles and practice of solid-phase peptide synthesis. In: Grant GA (ed) Synthetic peptides: a user's guide, 2nd edn; W.H. Freeman & Co., New York, pp 93–219

22. Albericio F (2004) Developments in peptide and amide synthesis. Curr Opinion Chem Biol 8:211–221

23. Merrifield RB (1963) Solid phase peptide synthesis I: synthesis of a tetrapeptide, J Am Chem Soc 85:2149–2154

24. Angeletti RH, Bonewald LF, Fields GB (1997) Six-year study of peptide synthesis. Meth Enzymol 289:697–717

25. Remmer HA, Fields GB (2000) Chemical synthesis of peptides. In: Reid RE (ed) Peptide and protein drug analysis. Marcel Dekker, Inc., New York, pp 133–169

26. Sarin VK, Kent SBH, Merrifield RB (1980) Properties of swollen polymer networks: solvation and swelling of peptide-containing resins in solid-phase peptide synthesis. J Am Chem Soc 102:5463–5470

27. Live D, Kent SBH (1982) Fundamental aspects of the chemical applications of cross-linked polymers. In: Mark JE (ed) Elastomers and rubber elasticity. American Chemical Society, Washington, DC, pp 501–515

28. Arshady R, Atherton E, Clive DLJ, Sheppard RC (1981) Peptide synthesis, part 1: preparation and use of polar supports based on poly(dimethylac rylamide). J Chem Soc Perkin Trans I: 529–537

29. Hellermann H, Lucas HW, Maul J, Pillai VNR, Mutter M (1983) Poly(ethylene glycol)s grafted onto crosslinked polystyrenes, 2: multidetachably anchored polymer systems for the synthesis of solubilized peptides. Makromol Chem 184:2603–2617

30. Zalipsky S, Albericio F, Barany G (1985) Preparation and use of an aminoethyl polyethylene glycol-crosslinked polystyrene graft resin support for solid-phase peptide synthesis. In: Deber CM, Hruby VJ, Kopple KD (eds) Peptides: structure and function. Pierce Chemical Co., Rockford, IL, pp 257–260

31. Bayer E, Rapp W (1986) New polymer supports for solid–liquid-phase peptide synthesis. In: Voelter W, Bayer E, Ovehinnikov YA, Ivanov VT (eds) Chemistry of peptides and proteins, Vol 3 Walter de Gruyter & Co., Berlin, pp 3–8

32. Bayer E, Albert K, Willisch H, Rapp W, Hemmasi B (1990) 13C NMR relaxation times of a tripeptide methyl ester and its polymer-bound analogues. Macromolecules 23:1937–1940

33. Zalipsky S, Chang JL, Albericio F, Barany G (1994) Preparation and applications of polyethylene glycol-polystyrene graft resin supports for solid-phase peptide synthesis. Reactive Polymers 22:243–258

34. Meldal M (1992) PEGA – a flow stable polyethylene-glycol dimethyl acrylamide copolymer for solid-phase synthesis. Tetrahedron Lett 33:3077–3080

35. Roice M, Johannsen I, Meldal M (2004) High capacity poly(ethylene glycol) based amino polymers for peptide and organic synthesis. QSAR Comb Sci 23:662–673

36. Garcia-Martin F, Quintanar-Audelo M, Garcia-Ramos Y, Cruz LJ, Gravel C, Furic R, Cote S, Tulla-Puche J, Albericio F (2006) ChemMatrix, a poly(ethylene glycol)-based support for the solid-phase synthesis of complex peptides. J Comb Chem 8:213–220

37. Kempe M, Barany G (1996) CLEAR: a novel family of highly cross-linked polymeric supports for solid-phase peptide synthesis. J Am Chem Soc 118:7083–7093

38. Niederhafner P, Sebestik J, Jezek J (2005) Peptide dendrimers. J Peptide Sci 11:757–788

39. Alsina J, Albericio F (2003) Solid-phase synthesis of C-terminal modified peptides. Biopolymers (Peptide Sci) 71:454–477

40. Meldal M (1997) Properties of solid supports. Meth Enzymol 289:83–104

41. Barany G, Kempe M (1997) The context of solid-phase synthesis. In: Czarnik AW, DeWitt SH (eds) A Practical guide to combinatorial chemistry. American Chemical Society, Washington, D.C., pp 51–97

42. Kent SBH, Parker KF (1988) The chemical synthesis of therapeutic peptides and proteins. In: Masshak DR, Liu DT (eds) Banbury report 29: therapeutic peptides and proteins: assessing the new technologies. Cold Spring Harbor, New York, pp 3–16

43. Wallace CJA, Mascagni P, Chait BT, Collawn JF, Paterson Y, Proudfoot AEI, Kent SBH (1989) Substitutions engineered by chemical synthesis at three conserved sites in mitochondrial cytochrome c. J Biol Chem 264:15199–15209

44. Suzuki K, Nitta K, Endo N (1975) Suppression of diketopiperazine formation in solid phase peptide synthesis. Chem Pharm Bull 23:222–224

45. Schnölzer M, Alewood P, Jones A, Alewood D, Kent SBH (1992) In situ neutralization in Boc-chemistry solid phase peptide synthesis: rapid, high yield assembly of difficult sequences. Int J Peptide Protein Res 40:180–193

46. Carpino LA, Han GY (1972) The 9-fluorenylmethoxycarbonyl amino-protecting group. J Org Chem 37:3404–3409

47. Carpino LA (1987) The 9-fluorenylmethyloxycarbonyl family of base-sensitive amino-protecting groups. Acc Chem Res 20:401–407

48. O'Ferrall RAM, Slae S (1970) β-elimination of 9-fluorenylmethanol in aqueous solution: An E1cB mechanism. J Chem Soc (B): 260–268

49. O'Ferrall RAM (1970) β-elimination of 9-fluorenylmethanol in solutions of methanol and t-butyl alcohol. J Chem Soc (B): 268–274

50. O'Ferrall RAM (1970) Relationships between E2 and E1cB mechanisms of β-elimination. J Chem Soc (B): 274–277

51. Fields GB (1994) Methods for removing the Fmoc group. In: Pennington MW, Dunn BM (eds) Methods in molecular biology, Vol. 35: peptide synthesis protocols. Humana Press Inc., Totowa, NJ, pp 17–27

52. Wade JD, Bedford J, Sheppard RC, Tregear GW (1991) DBU as an Nα-deprotecting reagent for the fluorenylmethoxycarbonyl group in continuous flow solid-phase peptide synthesis. Peptide Res 4:194–199

53. Fields CG, Mickelson DJ, Drake SL, McCarthy JB, Fields GB (1993) Melanoma cell adhesion and spreading activities of a synthetic 124-residue triple-helical "mini-collagen". J Biol Chem 268:14,153–14,160

54. Meldal M, Svensen I, Breddam K, Auzanneau FI (1994) Portion-mixing peptide libraries of quenched fluorogenic substrates for complete subsite mapping of endoprotease specificity. Proc Natl Acad Sci USA 91:3314–3318

55. Carreno C, Mendez ME, Kim YD, Kim HJ, Kates SA, Andreu D, Albericio F (2000) Nsc and Fmoc Nα-amino protection for solid-phase peptide synthesis: a parallel study. J Pept Res 56:63–69

56. Okada Y, Iguchi S (1988) Amino acid and peptides, part 19: synthesis of β-1- and β-2-adamantyl aspartates and their evaluation for peptide synthesis. J Chem Soc Perkin Trans I:2129–2136

57. Tam JP, Riemen MW, Merrifield RB (1988) Mechanisms of aspartimide formation: the effects of protecting groups, acid, base, temperature and time. Peptide Res 1:6–18

58. Karlström A, Undén A (1996) A new protecting group for aspartic acid that minimizes piperidine-catalyzed aspartimide formation in Fmoc solid phase peptide synthesis. Tetrahedron Lett 37:4243–4246

59. Bolin DR, Wang CT, Felix AM (1989) Preparation of N-t-butyloxy-carbonyl-Oω-9-fluorenylmethyl esters of asparatic and glutamic acids. Org Prep Proc Int 21:67–74

60. Albericio F, Nicolas E, Rizo J, Ruiz-Gayo M, Pedroso E, Giralt E (1990) Convenient syntheses of fluorenylmethyl-based side chain derivatives of glutamic and aspartic acids, lysine, and cysteine. Synthesis: 119–122

61. Al-Obeidi F, Sanderson DG, Hruby VJ (1990) Synthesis of β- and γ-fluorenylmethyl esters of respectively Nα-Boc-L-aspartic acid and Nα-Boc-L-glutamic acid. Int J Peptide Protein Res 35:215–218

62. Belshaw PJ, Mzengeza S, Lajoie GA (1990) Chlorotrimethylsilane mediated formation of ω-allyl esters of aspartic and glutamic acids. Synth Commun 20:3157–3160

63. Lyttle MH, Hudson D (1992) Allyl based side-chain protection for SPPS. In: Smith JA, Rivier JE (eds) Peptides chemistry and biology Escom, Leiden, The Netherlands, pp 583–584

64. Chan WC, Bycroft BW, Evans DJ, White PD (1995) A novel 4-aminobenzyl ester-based carboxy-protecting group for synthesis of atypical peptides by Fmoc-But solid phase chemistry. J Chem Soc Chem Commun: 2209–2210

65. Erickson BW, Merrifield RB (1973) Acid stability of several benzylic protecting groups used in solid-phase peptide synthesis: rearrangement of O-benzyltyrosine to 3-benzyltyrosine. J Am Chem Soc 95:3750–3756

66. Yamashiro D, Li CH (1973) Protection of tyrosine in solid-phase peptide synthesis. J Org Chem 38:591–592

67. Albericio F, Barany G, Fields GB, Hudson D, Kates SA, Lyttle MH, Solé NA (1993) Allyl-based orthogonal solid-phase peptide synthesis. In: Schneider CH, Eberle AN (eds) Peptides 1992. Escom, Leiden, The Netherlands, pp 191–193

68. Bycroft BW, Chan WC, Chhabra SR, Hone ND (1993) A novel lysine-protecting procedure for continuous flow solid phase synthesis of branched peptides. J Chem Soc Chem Commun: 778–779

69. Fields CG, Lovdahl CM, Miles AJ, Matthias-Hagen VL, Fields GB (1993) Solid-phase synthesis and stability of triple-helical peptides incorporating native collagen sequences. Biopolymers 33:1695–1707

70. Grab B, Miles AJ, Furcht LT, Fields GB (1996) Promotion of fibroblast adhesion by triple-helical peptide models of type I collagen-derived sequences. J Biol Chem 271:12,234–12,240

71. Xu Q, Zheng J, Cowburn D, Barany G (1996) Synthesis and characterization of branched phosphopeptides: prototype consolidated ligands for SH(32) domains. Lett Peptide Sci 3:31–36

72. Chhabra SR, Hothi B, Evans DJ, White PD, Bycroft BW, Chan WC (1998) An appraisal of new variants of Dde amine protecting group for solid phase peptide synthesis. Tetrahedron Lett 39:1603–1606

73. Aletras A, Barlos K, Gatos D, Koutsogianni S, Mamos P (1995) Preparation of the very acid-sensitive Fmoc-Lys(Mtt)-OH. Int J Peptide Protein Res 45:488–500

74. Fujino M, Wakimasu M, Kitada C (1981) Further studies on the use of multi-substituted benzenesulfonyl groups for protection of the guanidino function of arginine. Chem Pharm Bull 29:2825–2831

75. Green J, Ogunjobi OM, Ramage R, Stewart ASJ, McCurdy S, Noble R (1988) Application of the NG-(2,2,5,7,8-pentamethylchroman-6 sulphonyl) derivative of Fmoc-arginine to peptide synthesis. Tetrahedron Lett 29:4341–4344

76. Carpino LA, Shroff H, Triolo SA, Mansour ESME, Wenschuh H, Albericio F (1993) The 2,2,4,6,7-pentamethyldihydrobenzofuran-5-sulfonyl group (Pbf) as arginine side chain protectant. Tetrahedron Lett 34:7829–7832

77. Jones JH, Ramage WI, Witty MJ (1980) Mechanism of racemization of histidine derivatives in peptide synthesis. Int J Peptide Protein Res 15:301–303

78. Riniker B, Sieber P (1988) Problems and progress in the synthesis of histidine-containing peptides. In: Penke B, Torok A (eds) Peptides: chemistry, biology, interactions with proteins. Walter de Gruyter & Co., Berlin, pp 65–74

79. Ishiguro T, Eguchi C (1989) Unexpected chain-terminating side reaction caused by histidine and acetic anhydride in solid-phase peptide synthesis. Chem Pharm Bull 37:506–508

80. Kusunoki M, Nakagawa S, Seo K, Hamana T, Fukuda T (1990) A side reaction in solid phase synthesis: Insertion of glycine residues into peptide chains via Nim -> Nα transfer. Int J Peptide Protein Res 36:381–386

81. Forest M, Fournier A (1990) BOP reagent for the coupling of pGlu and Boc-His(Tos) in solid phase peptide synthesis. Int J Peptide Protein Res 35:89–94

82. Atherton E, Cammish LE, Goddard P, Richards JD, Sheppard RC (1984) The Fmoc-polyamide solid phase method: new procedures for histidine and arginine. In: Ragnarsson U (ed) Peptides 1984 Almqvist & Wiksell Int., Stockholm, pp 153–156

83. Sieber P, Riniker B (1987) Protection of histidine in peptide synthesis: a reassessment of the trityl group. Tetrahedron Lett 28:6031–6034

84. Mojsov S, Mitchell AR, Merrifield RB (1980) A quantitative evaluation of methods for coupling asparagine. J Org Chem 45:555–560

85. Gausepohl H, Kraft M, Frank RW (1989) Asparagine coupling in Fmoc solid phase peptide synthesis. Int J Peptide Protein Res 34:287–294

86. Sieber P, Riniker B (1990) Side-chain protection of asparagine and glutamine by trityl: Application to solid-phase peptide synthesis. In: Epton R (ed) Innovation and perspectives in solid phase synthesis. Solid Phase Conference Coordination, Ltd., Birmingham, U.K, pp 577–583

87. Sieber P, Riniker B (1991) Protection of carboxamide functions by the trityl residue: Application to peptide synthesis. Tetrahedron Lett 32:739–742

88. Fields GB, Carr SA, Marshak DR, Smith AJ, Stults JT, Williams LC, Williams KR, Young JD (1993) Evaluation of peptide synthesis as practiced in 53 different laboratories. In: Angeletti RH (ed) Techniques in protein chemistry IV. Academic Press, San Diego, pp 229–238

89. Franzén H, Grehn L, Ragnarsson U (1984) Synthesis, properties, and use of Nin-Boc-tryptophan derivatives. J Chem Soc Chem Commun: 1699–1700

90. White P (1992) Fmoc-Trp(Boc)-OH: A new derivative for the synthesis of peptides containing tryptophan. In: Smith JA, Rivier JE (eds) Peptides: Chemistry and Biology Escom, Leiden, The Netherlands, pp 537–538

91. Fields CG, Fields GB (1993) Minimization of tryptophan alkylation following 9-fluorenylmethoxycarbonyl solid-phase peptide synthesis. Tetrahedron Lett 34:6661–6664

92. Choi H, Aldrich JV (1993) Comparison of methods for the Fmoc solid-phase synthesis and cleavage of a peptide containing both tryptophan and arginine. Int J Peptide Protein Res 42:58–63

93. Photaki I, Taylor-Papadimitriou J, Sakarellos C, Mazarakis P, Zervas L (1970) On cysteine and cystine peptides, part V: S-trityl- and S-diphenylmethylcysteine and -cysteine peptides. J Chem Soc (C): 2683–2687

94. Munson MC, García-Echeverria C, Albericio F, Barany G (1992) S-2,4,6-Trimethoxybenzyl (Tmob): a novel cysteine protecting group for the Nα-9-fluorenyl-methoxycarbonyl (Fmoc) strategy of peptide synthesis. J Org Chem 57:3013–3018

95. Nishio H, Kimura T, Sakakibara S (1994) Side reaction in peptide synthesis: Modification of tryptophan during treatment with mercury(II) acetate/2-mercaptoethanol in aqueous acetic acid. Tetrahedron Lett 35:1239–1242

96. Kenner GW, Galpin IJ, Ramage R (1979) Synthetic studies directed towards the synthesis of a lysozyme analog. In: Gross E, Meienhofer J (eds) Peptides: structure and biological function. Pierce Chemical Co., Rockford, IL, pp 431–438

97. Albericio F, Hammer RP, García-Echeverría C, Molins MA, Chang JL, Munson MC, Pons M, Giralt E, Barany G (1991) Cyclization of disulfide-containing peptides in solid-phase synthesis. Int J Peptide Protein Res 37:402–413

98. Edwards WB, Fields CG, Anderson CJ, Pajeau TS, Welch MJ, Fields GB (1994) Generally Applicable, Convenient Solid-Phase Synthesis and Receptor Affinities of Octreotide Analogs. J Med Chem 37:3749–3757

99. Albericio Fea, Annis I, Royo M, Barany G (2000) Preparation and handling of peptides containing methionine and cysteine. In: Chan WC, White PD (eds) Fmoc solid phase peptide synthesis. Oxford University Press, Oxford, pp 77–114

100. Marder O, Albericio F (2003) Industrial application of coupling reagents in peptides. Chim Oggi 21:35–40

101. Hachmann J, Lebl M (2006) Search for optimal coupling reagent in multiple peptide synthesizer. Biopolymers (Peptide Sci) 84:340–347

102. Rich DH, Singh J (1979) The carbodiimide method. In: Gross E, Meienhofer J (eds). The peptides, Vol 1 Academic Press, New York, pp 241–314

103. Merrifield RB, Singer J, Chait BT (1988) Mass spectrometric evaluation of synthetic peptides for deletions and insertions. Anal Biochem 174:399–414

104. König W, Geiger R (1970) Eine neue methode zur synthese von peptiden: Aktivierung der carboxylgruppe mit dicyclohexylcarbodiimid unter zusatz von 1-hydroxy-benzotriazolen. Chem Ber 103:788–798

105. König W, Geiger R (1973) N-hydroxyverbindungen als katalysatoren für die aminolyse aktivierter ester. Chem Ber 106:3626–3635

106. Abdelmoty I, Alberici F, Carpino LA, Foxman BM, Kates SA (1994) Structural studies of reagents for peptide bond formation: crystal and molecular structures of HBTU and HATU. Lett Peptide Sci 1:57–67

107. Dourtoglou V, Gross B, Lambropoulou V, Zioudrou C (1984) O-benzotriazolyl-N,N,N′,N′,-tetramethyluronium hexafluorophosphate as coupling reagent for the synthesis of peptides of biological interest. Synthesis: 572–574

108. Fournier A, Wang CT, Felix AM (1988) Applications of BOP reagent in solid phase peptide synthesis: advantages of BOP reagent for difficult couplings exemplified by a synthesis of [Ala15]-GRF(1–29)-NH$_2$. Int J Peptide Protein Res 31:86–97

109. Ambrosius D, Casaretto M, Gerardy-Schahn R, Saunders D, Brandenburg D, Zahn H (1989) Peptide analogues of the anaphylatoxin C3a: synthesis and properties. Biol Chem Hoppe-Seyler 370:217–227

110. Gausepohl H, Kraft M, Frank R (1989) In situ activation of Fmoc-amino acids by BOP in solid phase peptide synthesis. In: Jung G, Bayer E (eds). Peptides 1988 Walter de Gruyter & Co., Berlin, pp 241–243

111. Seyer R, Aumelas A, Caraty A, Rivaille P, Castro B (1990) Repetitive BOP coupling (REBOP) in solid phase peptide synthesis: luliberin synthesis as model. Int J Peptide Protein Res 35:465–472

112. Fields CG, Lloyd DH, Macdonald RL, Otteson KM, Noble RL (1991) HBTU activation for automated Fmoc solid-phase peptide synthesis. Peptide Res 4:95–101

113. Knon R, Trzeciak A, Bannwarth W, Gillessen D (1991) 1,1,3,3-Tetramethyluronium compounds as coupling reagents in peptide and protein chemistry. In: Giratt E, Andreu (eds) Peptides 1990. Escom, Leiden, The Netherlands, pp 62–64

114. Carpino LA, El-Faham A, Minor CA, Albericio F (1994) Advantageous applications of azabenzotriazole (triazolopyridine)-based coupling reagents to solid-phase peptide synthesis. J Chem Soc Chem Commun: 201–203

115. Hudson D (1988) Methodological implications of simultaneous solid-phase peptide synthesis 1: Comparison of different coupling procedures. J Org Chem 53:617–624

116. Sabatino G, Mulinacci B, Alcaro MC, Chelli M, Rovero P, Papini AM (2002) Assessment of new 6-Cl-HOBt based coupling reagents for peptide synthesis. Lett Peptide Sci 9:119–123

117. Gausepohl H, Pieles U, Frank RW (1992) Schiffs base analog formation during in situ activation by HBTU and TBTU. In: Smith JA, Rivier JE (eds) Peptides chemistry and biology Escom, Leiden, The Netherlands, pp 523–524

118. Story SC, Aldrich JV (1992) A resin for the solid phase synthesis of protected peptide amides using the Fmoc chemical protocol. Int J Peptide Protein Res 39:87–92

119. Coste J, Le-Nguyen D, Castro B (1990) PyBOP: a new peptide coupling reagent devoid of toxic by-product. Tetrahedron Lett 31:205–208

120. Carpino LA, Xia J, Zhang C, El-Faham A (2004) Organophosphorus and nitro-substituted sulfonate esters of 1-hydroxy-7-azabenzotriazole as highly efficient fast-acting peptide coupling reagents. J Org Chem 69:62–71

121. Li J, Jiang X, Ye YH, Fan C, Romoff T, Goodman M (1999) 3-(Diethoxyphosphoryloxy)-1,2,3-benzotriazine-4(3H)-one (DEPBT): a new coupling reagent with remarkable resistance to racemization. Org Lett 1:91–93

122. Yo YH, Li H, Jiang X (2004) DEPBT as an efficient coupling reagent for amide bond formation with remarkable resistance to racemization. Biopolymers (Peptide Sci) 80:172–178

123. Kisfaludy L, Löw M, Nyéki O, Szirtes T, Schön I (1973) Die verwendung von pentafluorophenylestern bei peptid-synthesen. Justus Liebigs Ann Chem: 1421–1429

124. Penke B, Baláspiri L, Pallai P, Kovács K (1974) Application of pentafluorophenyl esters of Boc-amino acids in solid phase peptide synthesis. Acta Phys Chem 20:471–476

125. Kisfaludy L, Schön I (1983) Preparation and applications of pentafluorophenyl esters of 9-fluorenylmethyloxycarbonyl amino acids for peptide synthesis. Synthesis: 325–327

126. Green M, Berman J (1990) Preparation of pentafluorophenyl esters of Fmoc protected amino acids with pentafluorophenyl trifluoroacetate. Tetrahedron Lett 31:5851, 5852

127. Atherton E, Cameron LR, Sheppard RC (1988) Peptide synthesis, part 10: Use of pentafluorophenyl esters of fluorenylmethoxycarbonylamino acids in solid phase peptide synthesis. Tetrahedron 44:843–857

128. Hudson D (1990) Methodological implications of simultaneous solid-phase peptide synthesis: A comparison of active esters Peptide Res 3:51–55

129. Fields CG, Fields GB, Noble RL, Cross TA (1989) Solid phase peptide synthesis of [15N]-gramicidins A, B, and C and high performance liquid chromatographic purification. Int J Peptide Protein Res 33:298–303

130. Harrison JL, Petrie GM, Noble RL, Beilan HS, McCurdy SN, Culwell AR (1989) Fmoc chemistry: Synthesis, kinetics, cleavage, and deprotection of arginine-containing peptides. In: Hugli TE (ed) Techniques in Protein Chemistry. Academic Press, San Diego, pp 506–516

131. Geiser T, Beilan H, Bergot BJ, Otteson KM (1988) Automation of solid-phase peptide synthesis. In: Schlesinger DH (ed) Macromolecular sequencing and synthesis: selected methods and applications. Alan R. Liss, Inc., New York, pp 199–218

132. König W, Geiger R (1970) Racemisierung bei peptidsynthesen. Chem Ber 103:2024–2033

133. Carpino LA, Sadat-Aalaee D, Chao HG, DeSelms RH (1990) ((9-Fluorenylmethyl)oxy)carbonyl (Fmoc) amino acid fluorides: convenient new peptide coupling reagents applicable to the Fmoc/tert-butyl strategy for solution and solid-phase syntheses. J Am Chem Soc 112:9651–9652

134. Carpino LA, Mansour ESME (1992) Protected β- and γ-aspartic and -glutamic acid fluorides. J Org Chem 57:6371–6373

135. Wenschuh H, Beyermann M, Krause E, Brudel M, Winter R, Schümann M, Carpino LA, Bienert M (1994) Fmoc amino acid fluorides: convenient reagents for the solid-phase assembly of peptides incorporating sterically hindered residues. J Org Chem 59:3275–3280

136. Wenschuh H, Beyermann M, Haber H, Seydel JK, Krause E, Bienert M, Carpino LA, El-Faham A, Albericio F (1995) Stepwise automated solid phase synthesis of naturally occurring peptaibols using Fmoc amino acid fluorides. J Org Chem 60:405–410

137. Carpino LA, El-Faham A (1995) Tetramethylfluoroformamidinium hexafluorophosphate: a rapid-acting peptide coupling reagent for solution and solid-phase peptide synthesis. J Am Chem Soc 117:5401–5402

138. Carpino LA, Ionescu D, El-Faham A, Beyermann M, Henklein P, Hanay C, Wenschuh H, Bienert M (2003) Complex Polyfluoride Additives in Fmoc-Amino Acid Fluoride Coupling Processes. Enhanced Reactivity and Avoidance of Stereomutation. Org Lett 5:975–977

139. Schnölzer M, Kent SBH (1992) Constructing proteins by dovetailing unprotected synthetic peptides. Science 256:221–225

140. Muir TW, Dawson PE, Kent SBH (1997) Protein synthesis by chemical ligation of unprotected peptides in aqueous solution. Meth Enzymol 289:266–298

141. Dawson PE, Kent SBH (1993) Convenient total synthesis of a 4-helix TASP molecule by chemoselective ligation. J Am Chem Soc 115:7263–7266

142. Williams MJ, Muir TW, Ginsberg MH, Kent SBH (1994) Total chemical synthesis of a folded β-sandwich protein domain: an analog of the tenth fibronectin type 3 module. J Am Chem Soc 116:10,797–10,798

143. Baca M, Muir TW, Schnölzer M, Kent SBH (1995) Chemical ligation of cysteine-containing peptides: synthesis of a 22 kDa tethered dimer of HIV-1 protease. J Am Chem Soc 117:1881–1887

144. Canne LE, Walker SM, Kent SBH (1995) A general method for the synthesis of thioester resin linkers for use in the solid phase synthesis of peptide-a-thioacids. Tetrahedron Lett 36:1217–1220

145. Muir TW, Williams MJ, Ginsberg MH, Kent SBH (1994) Design and chemical synthesis of a neoprotein structural model for the cytoplasmic domain of a multisubunit cell-surface receptor: integrin αIIbβ3 (platelet GPIIb-IIIa). Biochemistry 33:7701–7708

146. Nefzi A, Sun X, Mutter M (1995) Chemoselective ligation of multifunctional peptides to topological templates via thioether formation for TASP synthesis. Tetrahedron Lett 36:229–230

147. McCafferty DG, Slate CA, Nakhle BM, Graham J, HD, Austell TL, Vachet RW, Mullis BH, Erickson BW (1995) Engineering of a 129-residue tripod protein by chemoselective ligation of proline-II helices. Tetrahedron 51:9859–9872

148. Englebretsen DR, Garnham BG, Bergman DA, Alewood PF (1995) A novel thioether linker: chemical synthesis of a HIV-1 protease analogue by thioether ligation. Tetrahedron Lett 36:8871–8874

149. Ramage R, Biggin GW, Brown AR, Comer A, Davison A, Draffan L, Jiang L, Morton G, Robertson N, Shaw KF, Tennant G, Urquhart K, Wilken J (1996) Methodology for chemical synthesis of proteins. In: Epton R (ed) Innovation and perspectives in solid phase synthesis & combinatorial libraries 1996. Mayflower Scientific, Kingswinford, UK, pp 1–10

150. Li X, Kawakami T, Aimoto S (1998) Direct preparation of peptide thioesters using an Fmoc solid-phase method. Tetrahedron Lett 39:8669–8672

151. Clippingdale AB, Barrow CJ, Wade JD (2000) Peptide thioester preparation by Fmoc solid phase peptide synthesis for use in native chemical ligation. J Peptide Sci 6:225–234

152. Bu XZ, Xie GY, Law CW, Guo ZH (2002) An improved deblocking agent for direct Fmoc solid-phase synthesis of peptide thioesters. Tetrahedron Lett 43:2419–2422

153. Gross CM, Lelievre D, Woodward CK, Barany G (2005) Preparation of protected peptidyl thioester intermediates for native chemical ligation by Nα-9-fluorenyl-methoxycarbonyl (Fmoc) chemistry: considerations of side-chain and backbone anchoring strategies, and compatible protection for N-terminal cysteine. J Peptide Res 65:395–410

154. Ingenito R, Bianchi E, Fattori D, Pessi A (1999) Solid-phase synthesis of peptide C-terminal thioesters by Fmoc/t-Bu chemistry. J Am Chem Soc 121:11,369–11,374

155. Shin Y, Winans KA, Backes BJ, Kent SBH, Ellman JA, Bertozzi CR (1999) Fmoc-based synthesis of peptide-thioesters: applications to the total chemical synthesis of a glycoprotein by native chemical ligation. J Am Chem Soc 121:11,684–11,689

156. Quaderer R, Hilvert D (2001) Improved synthesis of C-terminal peptide thioesters on "safety-catch" resins using LiBr/THF. Org Lett 3:3181–3184

157. Camarero JA, Hackel BJ, Yoreo JJD, Mitchell AR (2004) Fmoc-based synthesis of peptide thioesters using an aryl hydrazine support. J Org Chem 69:4145–4151

158. Alasina J, Yokum TS, Albericio F, Barany G (1999) Backbone amide linker (BAL) strategy for Nα-9-fluorenylmethoxycarbonyl solid-phase synthesis of unprotected peptide p-nitroanilide and thioesters. J Org Chem 64:8761–8769

159. Brask J, Albericio F, Jensen KJ (2003) Fmoc solid-phase synthesis of peptide thioesters by masking as trithioorthoesters. Org Lett 5:2951–2953

160. Swwinnen D, Hilvert D (2000) Facile, Fmoc-compatible solid-phase synthesis of peptide C-terminal thioesters. Org Lett 2:2439–2442

161. Sewing A, Hilvert D (2001) Fmoc-compatible solid-phase peptide synthesis of long C-terminal peptide thioesters. Angew Chem Int Ed 40:3395–3396

162. Tuchscherer G (1993) Template assembled synthetic proteins: condensation of a multifunctional peptide to a topological template via chemoselective ligation. Tetrahedron Lett 34:8419–8422

163. Rose K (1994) Facile synthesis of homogeneous artificial proteins. J Am Chem Soc 116:30–33

164. Rao G, Tam JP (1994) Synthesis of peptide dendrimer. J Am Chem Soc 116:6975–6976

165. Spetzler JG, Tam JP (1995) Unprotected peptides as building blocks for branched peptides and peptide dendrimers. Int J Peptide Protein Res 45:78–85

166. Shao J, Tam JP (1995) Unprotected peptides as building blocks for the synthesis of peptide dendrimers with oxime, hydrazone, and thiazolidine linkages. J Am Chem Soc 117:3893–3899

167. Tam JP, Spetzler JC (1997) Multiple antigen peptide system. Meth Enzymol 289:612–637

168. Dawson PE, Muir TW, Clark-Lewis I, Kent SBH (1994) Synthesis of proteins by native chemical ligation. Science 266:776–779

169. Dawson PE, Churchill MJ, Ghadiri MR, Kent SBH (1997) Modulation of reactivity in native chemical ligation through the use of thiol additives. J Am Chem Soc 119:4325–4329

170. Johnson ECB, Kent SBH (2006) Insights into the mechanism and catalysis of the native chemical ligation reaction. J Am Chem Soc 128:6640–6646

171. Hackeng TM, Griffin JH, Dawson PE (1999) Protein synthesis by native chemical ligation: Expanded scope by using straightforward methodology. Proc Natl Acad Sci USA 96:10,068–10,073

172. Camarero JA, Pavel J, Muir TW (1998) Chemical synthesis of a circular protein domain: Evidence for folding-assisted cyclization. Angew Chem Int Ed 37:347–349

173. Camarero JA, Muir TW (1999) Biosynthesis of a head-to-tail cyclized protein with improved biological activity. J Am Chem Soc 121:5597–5598

174. Beligere GS, Dawson PE (1999) Conformationally assisted protein ligation using C-terminal thioester peptides. J Am Chem Soc 121:2633–6333

175. Liu CF, Tam JP (1994) Peptide segment ligation strategy without use of protecting groups. Proc Natl Acad Sci USA 91:6574–6588

176. Tam JP, Yu Q, Miao Z (1999) Orthogonal ligation strategies for peptide and protein. Biopolymers (Peptide Sci) 51:311–332

177. Beligere GS, Dawson PE (1999) Synthesis of a three zinc finger protein, Zif268, by native chemical ligation. Biopolymers (Peptide Sci) 51:363–369

178. Canne LE, Botti P, Simon RJ, Chen Y, Dennis EA, Kent SBH (1999) Chemical protein synthesis by solid phase ligation of unprotected peptide segments. J Am Chem Soc 121:8720–8727

179. Canne LE, Ferré-D'Amaré AR, Burley SK, Kent SBH (1995) Total chemical synthesis of a unique transcription factor-related protein: cMyc-Max. J Am Chem Soc 117:2998–3007

180. Quaderer R, Sewing A, Hilvert D (2001) Selenocysteine-mediated native chemical ligation. Helv Chim Acta 84:1197–1206

181. Gieselman MD, Xie L, van der Donk WA (2001) Synthesis of selenocysteine-containing peptide by native chermical ligation. Org Lett 3:1331–1334

182. Canne LE, Bark SJ, Kent SBH (1996) Extending the applicability of native chemical ligation. J Am Chem Soc 118:5891–5896

183. Offer J, Dawson PE (2000) N-2-mercaptobenzylamine-assisted chemical ligation. Org Lett 2:23–26

184. Offer J, Boddy CNC, Dawson PE (2000) Extending synthetic access to proteins with a removable acyl transfer auxilliary. J Am Chem Soc 124:4642–4646

185. Nilsson BL, Kiessling LL, Raines RT (2000) Staudinger ligation: a peptide from a thioster and azide to form a peptide. Org Lett 2:1939–1941

186. Saxon E, Armstrong JI, Bertozzi CR (2000) A "traceless" Staudinger ligation for chemoselective synthesis of amide bonds. Org Lett 2:2141–2143

187. Nilsson BL, Kiessling LL, Raines RT (2001) High-yielding Staudinger ligation of a phosphothioster and azide to form a peptide. Org Lett 3:9–12

188. Soellner MB, Nilsson BL, Raines RT (2002) Staudinger ligation of alpha-azido acids retains stereochemistry. J Org Chem 67:4993–4996

189. Nilsson BL, Hondal RJ, Soellner MB, Raines RT (2003) Protein assembly by orthogonal chemical ligation methods. J Am Chem Soc 125:5268–5269

190. Tam JP, Merrifield RB (1987) Strong acid deprotection of synthetic peptides: Mechanisms and methods. In: Udenfriend S, Meienhofer J (eds) The peptides, Vol 9. Academic Press, New York, pp 185–248

191. Yajima H, Fujii N, Funakoshi S, Watanabe T, Murayama E, Otaka A (1988) New strategy for the chemical synthesis of proteins. Tetrahedron 44:805–819

192. Nomizu M, Inagaki Y, Yamashita T, Ohkubo A, Otaka A, Fujii N, Roller PP, Yajima H (1991) Two-step hard acid deprotection/cleavage procedure for solid phase peptide synthesis. Int J Peptide Protein Res 37:145–152

193. Akaji K, Fujii N, Tokunaga F, Miyata T, Iwanaga S, Yajima H (1989) Studies on peptides CLXVIII: syntheses of three peptides isolated from horseshoe crab hemocytes, tachyplesin I, tachyplesin II, and polyphemusin I. Chem Pharm Bull 37:2661–2664

194. Jaeger E, Thamm P, Knof S, Wünsch E, Löw M, Kisfaludy L (1978) Nebenreaktionen bei peptidsynthesen III: synthese und charakterisierung von Nin-tert-butylierten tryptophan-derivaten. Hoppe-Seyler's Z Physiol Chem 359:1617–1628

195. Jaeger E, Thamm P, Knof S, Wünsch E (1978) Nebenreaktionen bei peptidsynthesen IV: charakterisierung von C- und C,N-tert-butylierten tryptophan-derivaten. Hoppe-Seyler's Z Physiol Chem 359:1629–1636

196. Löw M, Kisfaludy L, Jaeger E, Thamm P, Knof S, Wünsch E (1978) Direkte tert-butylierung des tryptophans: Herstellung von 2,5,7-tri-tert-butyltryp-tophan. Hoppe-Seyler's Z Physiol Chem 359:1637–1642

197. Löw M, Kisfaludy L, Sohár P (1978) tert-Butylierung des tryptophan-indolringes während der abspaltung der tert-butyloxycarbonyl-gruppe bei peptidsynthesen. Hoppe-Seyler's Z Physiol Chem 359:1643–1651

198. Masui Y, Chino N, Sakakibara S (1980) The modification of tryptophyl residues during the acidolytic cleavage of Boc-groups I: studies with Boc-tryptophan. Bull Chem Soc Jpn 53:464–468

199. Sieber P (1987) Modification of tryptophan residues during acidolysis of 4-methoxy-2,3,6-trimethylbenzenesulfonyl groups: Effects of scavengers. Tetrahedron Lett 28:1637–1640

200. King DS, Fields CC, Fields GB (1990) A cleavage method which minimizes side reactions following Fmoc solid phase peptide synthesis. Int J Peptide Protein Res 36:255–266

201. Riniker B, Hartmann A (1990) Deprotection of peptides containing Arg(Pmc) and tryptophan or tyrosine: elucidation of by-products. In: Rivier JE, Marshall GR (eds) Peptides: chemistry, structure and biology. Escom, Leiden, The Netherlands, pp 950–952

202. Riniker B, Kamber B (1989) Byproducts of Trp-peptides synthesized on a p-benzyloxybenzyl alcohol polystyrene resin. In: Jung G, Bayer E (eds) Peptides 1988. Walter de Gruyter & Co., Berlin, pp 115–117

203. Gesellchen PD, Rothenberger RB, Dorman DE, Paschal JW, Elzey TK, Campbell CS (1990) A new side reaction in solid-phase peptide synthesis: Solid support-dependent alkylation of tryptophan. In: Rivier JE, Marshall GR (eds) Peptides: chemistry structure and biology. Escom, Leiden, The Netherlands, pp 957–959

204. Albericio F, Kneib-Cordonier N, Biancalana S, Gera L, Masada RI, Hudson D, Barany G (1990) Preparation and application of the 5-(4-(9-fluorenylmethyloxy carbonyl)aminomethyl-3,5-dimethoxyphenoxy)valeric acid (PAL) handle for the solid-phase synthesis of *C*-terminal peptide amides under mild conditions. J Org Chem 55:3730–3743

205. Fields CG, VanDrisse VL, Fields GB (1993) Edman degradation sequence analysis of resin-bound peptides synthesized by 9-fluorenylmethoxycarbonyl chemistry. Peptide Res 6:39–47

206. Stierandová A, Sepetov NF, Nikiforovich GV, Lebl M (1994) Sequence-dependent modification of Trp by the Pmc protecting group of Arg during TFA deprotection. Int J Peptide Protein Res 43:31–38

207. Jaeger E, Remmer HA, Jung G, Metzger J, Oberthür W, Rücknagel KP, Schäfer W, Sonnenbichler J, Zetl I (1993) Nebenreaktionen bei peptidsynthesen V: O-sulfonierung von serin und threonin während der abspaltung der Pmc- und Mtr-schutzgruppen von argininresten bei Fmoc-festphasen-synthesen. Biol Chem Hoppe-Seyler 374:349–362

208. Solé NA, Barany G (1992) Optimization of solid-phase synthesis of [Ala8]-dynorphin A. J Org Chem 57:5399–5403

209. Gisin BF, Merrifield RB (1972) Carboxyl-catalyzed intramolecular aminolysis: a side reaction in solid-phase peptide synthesis. J Am Chem Soc 94:3102–3106

210. Pedroso E, Grandas A, de las Heras X, Eritja R, Giralt E (1986) Diketopiperazine formation in solid phase peptide synthesis using p-alkoxybenzyl ester resins and Fmoc-amino acids. Tetrahedron Lett 27:743–746

211. Albericio F, Barany G (1985) Improved approach for anchoring Nα-9-fluorenyl-methyloxycarbonylamino acids as p-alkoxybenzyl esters in solid-phase peptide synthesis. Int J Peptide Protein Res 26:92–97

212. Gairi M, Lloyd-Williams P, Albericio F, Giralt E (1990) Use of BOP reagent for the suppression of diketopiperazine formation in Boc/Bzl solid-phase peptide synthesis. Tetrahedron Lett 31:7363–7366

213. Ueki M, Amemiya M (1987) Removal of 9-fluorenylmethyloxycarbonyl (Fmoc) group with tetrabutylammonium fluoride. Tetrahedron Lett 28:6617–6620

214. Barlos K, Gatos D, Hondrelis J, Matsoukas J, Moore GJ, Schäfer W, Sotiriou P (1989) Darstellung neuer säureempfindlicker harze vom sek.-alkohol-typ und ihre anwendung zur synthese von peptiden. Liebigs Ann Chem: 951–955

215. Barlos K, Gatos D, Kallitsis J, Papaphotiu G, Sotiriu P, Wenqing Y, Schäfer W (1989) Darstellung geschützter peptid-fragmente unter einsatz substituierter triphenylmethyl-harze. Tetrahedron Lett 30:3943–3946

216. Bodanszky M, Kwei JZ (1978) Side reactions in peptide synthesis VII: Sequence dependence in the formation of aminosuccinyl derivatives from β-benzyl-aspartyl peptides. Int J Peptide Protein Res 12:69–74

217. Bodanszky M, Tolle JG, Deshmane SS, Bodanszky A (1978) Side reactions in peptide synthesis VI: A reexamination of the benzyl group in the protection of the side chains of tyrosine and aspartic acid. Int J Peptide Protein Res 12:57–68

218. Nicolás E, Pedroso E, Giralt E (1989) Formation of aspartimide peptides in Asp-Gly sequences. Tetrahedron Lett 30:497–500

219. Kenner GW, Seely JH (1972) Phenyl esters for C-terminal protection in peptide synthesis. J Am Chem Soc 94:3259–3260

220. Schön I, Colombo R, Csehi A (1983) Effect of piperidine on benzylaspartyl peptides in solution and in the solid phase. J Chem Soc Chem Commun: 505–507

221. Yang Y, Sweeney WV, Scheider K, Thörnqvist S, Chait BT, Tam JP (1994) Aspartimide formation in base-driven 9-fluorenylmethoxycarbonyl chemistry. Tetrahedron Lett 35:9689–9692

222. Lauer JL, Fields CG, Fields GB (1995) Sequence dependence of aspartimide formation during 9-fluorenylmethoxycarbonyl solid-phase synthesis. Lett Peptide Sci 1:197–205

223. Dölling R, Beyermann M, Haenel J, Kernchen F, Krause E, Franke P, Brudel M, Bienert M (1994) Piperidine-mediated side product formation for Asp(OBut)-containing peptides. J Chem Soc Chem Commun: 853–854

224. Wade JD, Mathieu MN, Macris M, Tregear GW (2000) Base-induced side reactions in Fmoc-solid phase peptide synthesis: Minimization by use of piperazine as Nα-deprotection reagent. Lett Peptide Sci 7:107–112

225. Quibell M, Owen D, Packman LC, Johnson T (1994) Suppression of piperidine-mediated side product formation for Asp(OBut)-containing peptides by the use of N-(2-hydroxy-4-methoxybenzyl) (Hmb) backbone amide protection. J Chem Soc Chem Commun: 2343–2344

226. Cebrián J, Domingo V, Reig F (2003) Synthesis of peptide sequences related to thrombospondin: Factors affecting aspartimide by-product formation. J Pept Res 62:238–244

227. Atherton E, Hardy PM, Harris DE, Matthews BH (1991) Racemization of C-terminal cysteine during peptide assembly. In: Giralt E, Andreu D (eds) Peptides 1990. Escom, Leiden, The Netherlands, pp 243–244

228. Angell YM, Alsina J, Albericio F, Barany G (2002) Practical protocols for stepwise solid-phase synthesis of cysteine-containing peptides. J Pept Res 60:292–299

229. Fujiwara Y, Akaji K, Kiso Y (1994) Racemization-free synthesis of C-terminal cysteine-peptide using 2-chlorotrityl resin. Chem Pharm Bull 42:724–726

230. Fields CG, Fields GB (1994) Solvents for solid-phase peptide synthesis. In: Pennington MW, Dunn BM (eds) Methods in molecular biology Vol 35: peptide synthesis protocols. Humana Press, Inc., Totowa, NJ, pp 29–40

231. Sarin VK, Kent SBH, Mitchell AR, Merrifield RB (1984) A general approach to the quantitation of synthetic efficiency in solid-phase peptide synthesis as a function of chain length. J Am Chem Soc 106:7845–7850

232. Pickup S, Blum FD, Ford WT (1990) Self-diffusion coefficients of Bocamino acid anhydrides under conditions of solid phase peptide synthesis. J Polym Sci A: Polym Chem 28:931–934

233. Live DH, Kent SBH (1983) Correlation of coupling rates with physico-chemical properties of resin-bound peptides in solid phase synthesis. In: Hruby VJ, Rich DH (eds) Peptides: structure and function. Pierce Chemical Co., Rockford, IL

234. Mutter M, Altmann KH, Bellof D, Flörsheimer A, Herbert J, Huber M, Klein B, Strauch L, Vorherr T, Gremlich HU (1985) The impact of secondary structure formation in peptide synthesis. In: Deber CM, Hruby VJ, Kopple KD (eds) Peptides: structure and function. Pierce Chemical Co., Rockford, IL, pp 397–405

235. Ludwick AG, Jelinski LW, Live D, Kintanar A, Dumais JJ (1986) Association of peptide chains during Merrifield solid-phase peptide synthesis: a deuterium NMR study. J Am Chem Soc 108:6493–6496

236. Narita M, Kojima Y (1989) The β-sheet structure-stabilizing potential of twenty kinds of amino acid residues in protected peptides. Bull Chem Soc Jpn 62:3572–3576

237. Yamashiro D, Blake J, Li CH (1976) The use of trifluoroethanol for improved coupling in solid-phase peptide synthesis. Tetrahedron Lett: 1469–1472

238. Narita M, Umeyama H, Yoshida T (1989) The easy disruption of the β-sheet structure of resin-bound human proinsulin C-peptide fragments by strong electron-donor solvents. Bull Chem Soc Jpn 62:3582–3586

239. Fields GB, Otteson KM, Fields CG, Noble RL (1990) The versatility of solid phase peptide synthesis. In: Epton R (ed) Innovation and perspectives in solid phase synthesis. Solid Phase Conference Coordination, Ltd., Birmingham, UK, pp 241–260

240. Fields GB, Fields CG (1991) Solvation effects in solid-phase peptide synthesis. J Am Chem Soc 113:4202–4207

241. Stewart JM, Klis WA (1990) Polystyrene-based solid phase peptide synthesis: The state of the art. In: Epton R (ed) Innovation and perspectives in solid phase synthesis. Solid Phase Conference Coordination, Ltd., Birmingham, UK, pp 1–9

242. Thaler A, Seebach D, Cardinaux F (1991) Lithium-salt effects in peptide synthesis, part II: improvement of degree of resin swelling and of efficiency of coupling in solid-phase synthesis. Helv Chim Acta 74:628–643

243. Tam JP, Lu YA (1995) Coupling difficulty associated with interchain clustering and phase transition in solid phase peptide synthesis. J Am Chem Soc 117:12,058–12,063

244. Atherton E, Woolley V, Sheppard RC (1980) Internal association in solid phase peptide synthesis: Synthesis of cytochrome C residues 66–104 on polyamide supports. J Chem Soc Chem Commun: 970–971

245. Atherton E, Sheppard RC (1985) Detection of problem sequences in solid phase synthesis. In: Deber CM, Hruby VJ, Kopple KD (eds) Peptides: structure and function. Pierce Chemical Co., Rockford, IL, pp 415–418

246. Bedford J, Hyde C, Johnson T, Jun W, Owen D, Quibell M, Sheppard RC (1992) Amino acid structure and "difficult sequences" in solid phase peptide synthesis. Int J Peptide Protein Res 40:300–307

247. Hyde C, Johnson T, Sheppard RC (1992) Internal aggregation during solid phase peptide synthesis: dimethyl sulfoxide as a powerful dissociating solvent. J Chem Soc Chem Commun:1573–1575

248. Miranda LP, Alewood PF (1999) Accelerated chemical synthesis of peptides and small proteins. Proc Natl Acad Sci USA 96:1181–1186

249. Zhang L, Goldhammer C, Henkel B, Panhaus G, Zuehl F, Jung G, Bayer E (1994) "Magic mixture," a powerful solvent system for solid-phase synthesis of difficult peptides. In: Epton R (ed) Innovation and perspectives in solid phase synthesis 1994. Mayflower Worldwide, Ltd., Birmingham, UK, pp 711–716

250. Johnson T, Quibell M, Owen D, Sheppard RC (1993) A reversible protecting group for the amide bond in peptides: use in the synthesis of 'difficult sequences'. J Chem Soc Chem Commun: 369–372

251. Hyde C, Johnson T, Owen D, Quibell M, Sheppard RC (1994) Some 'difficult sequences' made easy: a study of interchain association in solid-phase peptide synthesis. Int J Peptide Protein Res 43:431–440

252. Miranda LP, Meutermans WDF, Smythe ML, Alewood PF (2000) An activated O -> N acyl transfer auxiliary: Efficient amide-backbone substitution of hindered "difficult" peptides. J Org Chem 65:5460–5468

253. Tickler AK, Clippingdale AB, Wade JD (2004) Amyloid-β as a "difficult sequence" in solid phase peptide synthesis. Protein Pept Lett 11:377–384

254. Yu HM, Chen ST, Wang KT (1992) Enhanced coupling efficiency in solid-phase peptide synthesis by microwave irradiation. J Org Chem 57:4781–4784

255. Erdelyi M, Gogoll A (2002) Rapid microwave-assisted solid phase peptide synthesis. Synthesis: 1592–1596

256. Ferguson JD (2003) Focused microwave instrumentation from CEM corporation. Mol Div 7:281–286.

257. Murray, J. K., and Gellman, S. H. (2005) Application of microwave irradiation to the synthesis of 14-helical β-peptides Org Lett 7:1517–1520

33

Monoclonal Antibodies

Zhong J. Zhang and Maher Albitar

1. Introduction

Activation and clonal expansion of antigen-reactive B cells to mount an immune response is one of our body's most important defenses against foreign materials. Each clone of B cells is able to secrete its own unique antibody, such that an invading pathogen will be countered by millions of antibodies capable of binding to different sites on its surface. Such a polyclonal response is ideal for our body's defense. However, many experimental and clinical situations require access to an unlimited supply of a single antibody with a clearly defined specificity and affinity; i.e., a monoclonal antibody.

In short, monoclonal antibodies are identical antibodies produced by hybridoma cell lines derived from fusion of a B cell with a tumor cell. Kohler and Milstein first described the technique of monoclonal antibody production in 1975, a process that has been put to use in a wide range of laboratory, clinical, and industrial applications (1). The importance of monoclonal antibody production and the theories surrounding it earned them, the 1984 Nobel Prize in Physiology or Medicine. Monoclonal antibodies have since become powerful tools in virtually every field of biological sciences and medicine and are a major driving force in medical diagnostics, from over-the-counter home pregnancy tests to precise laboratory-based immunoassays. More recently, monoclonal antibodies have moved into the medical therapeutic field with products for treatment for various cancers and autoimmune diseases. Therapeutic monoclonal antibodies now represent one of the fastest growing areas of the pharmaceutical industry, with potential market capital of billions of dollars. To date, 19 therapeutic antibodies have been approved for clinical use by the FDA and over 150 antibodies are being tested in clinical trials (**Table 33.1**). The future applications of monoclonal antibodies are limitless. The following is a summary of antibody production and its therapeutic applications.

From: *Molecular Biomethods Handbook, 2nd Edition.*
Edited by: J. M. Walker and R. Rapley © Humana Press, Totowa, NJ

Table 33.1. FDA-approved therapeutic monoclonal antibodies.

Year	Name	Type	Target	Major indication
1986	OKT 3/Muromonab-CD3	Murine	CD3	Transplant rejection
1994	Reopro/Abciximab	Chimeric	GpIIb/gpIIIa	Anticoagulation
1995	Panorex/Edrecolomab	Chimeric	CA17-1A	Colorectal cancer
1997	Rotuxan/Rituximab	Chimeric	CD20	B-cell lymphoma
1997	Zenapax/Daclizumab	Humanized	CD25	Transplant rejection
1998	Remicade/Infliximab	Chimeric	TNF-alpha	Autoimmune disorder
1998	Simulect/Basiliximab	Chimeric	CD25	Transplant rejection
1998	Snagis/Pavilizumab	Humanized	RSV	RSV prophylaxis
1998	Herceptin/Trastuzumab	Humanized	Her2/neu	Breast cancer
2000	Mylotarg/Gemtuzumab	Humanized	CD33	AML
2001	Campath/Alemtuzumab	Humanized	CD52	CLL
2002	Zevalin/Ibritumomab	Murine	CD20	B-cell lymphoma
2002	Humira/Adalimumab	Human	TNF-alpha	Autoimmune disorder
2003	Bexxar/Tositumomab	Murine-I-131	CD20	B-cell lymphoma
2003	Xolair/Omalizumab	Humanized	IgE	Asthma and allergy
2003	Raptva/Efalizumab	Humanized	CD11a	Psoriasis
2004	Erbitux/Cetuximab	Chimeric	EGFR	Colorectal cancer
2004	Avastatin/Bevacizumab	Humanized	VEGF	Solid tumor
2005	Tysabri/Natalizumab	Humanized	CD40	Multiple Sclerosis

TNF, tumor necrosis factor; *RSV*, respiratory syncytial virus; *AML*, acute myeloid leukemia; *CLL*, chronic lymphocytic leukemia; *EGFR*, epidermal growth factor receptor; *VEGF*, vascular endothelial growth factor.

2. Production of Monoclonal Antibodies

Monoclonal antibodies are immunoglobulins secreted by a single clone of B cells with specificity for binding a particular epitope of an antigen. There are five classes of antibodies: IgA, IgD, IgE, IgG, and IgM (*2*). These antibody are heterogeneous molecules but share a common basic structure that determines their unique characteristics. IgG is the most used subtype of antibodies in diagnostics and medical treatment and comprises several distinct structural and functional domains (**Fig. 33.1A**). IgG is made up of two identical heavy chains (50–70 KD) and two identical light chains (25 KD) forming a Y-shaped structure. Each light chain is bound to a heavy chain and the two heavy chains are bound to each other through disulphide bonds. Light chains consist of one variable domain (VL) and a single constant domain (CL), whereas heavy chains comprise one variable domain (VH) and three constant domains (CH). Functionally, immunoglobulin is divided into two antigen-binding fragments (Fabs) and a constant (Fc) region, which are linked via a flexible hinge region. The VL and VH domains of Fabs bind antigens. Each V domain contains three regions with hypervariable sequences, which form loops that are primarily responsible for antigen recognition and are referred to as complementary determining regions (CDRs). The remaining V region is referred to as framework residues (FR). The Fc portion of the antibody mediates effector functions, antibody-dependent cell-mediated cytotoxicity (ADCC),

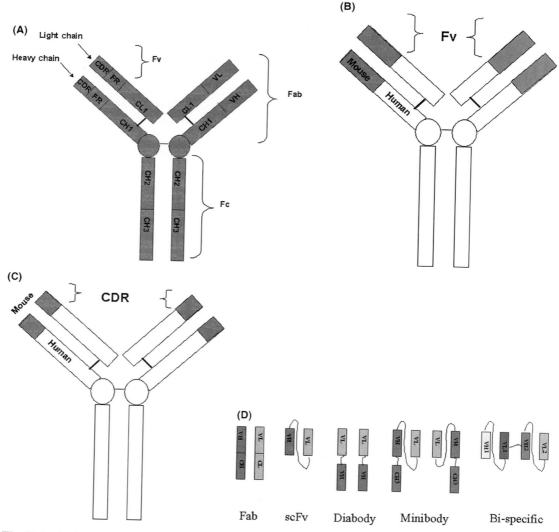

Fig. 33.1. Antibody molecule and its modifications: (**A**) immunoglobulin molecule, (**B**) Recombinant chimeric antibody, (**C**) recombinant humanized antibody, and (**D**) antibody fragments

and complement-dependent cytotoxicity (CDC). In ADCC, antibodies bind to Fc receptors on the surface of effector cells—such as natural killer (NK) cells and macrophages—to trigger phagocytosis or lysis of the targeted cells. In CDC, antibodies kill the targeted cells by triggering the complement cascade.

The features that make antibodies attractive diagnostic and therapeutic tools are their high specificity and distinct structural and functional domains, which have facilitated recombinant protein engineering for the development of antibodies for different uses. Monoclonal antibody production originally employed only murine (rodent) systems, but the focus of development is now shifting to chimeric, humanized, and fully human antibodies. To meet the demand of constantly expanding diagnostic and therapeutic markets, functional antibody fragments and antibodies that conjugate with enzymes, toxins, drugs, and radioactive isotopes have also been developed.

2.1. Murine Monoclonal Antibodies

As mentioned above, monoclonal antibodies are produced by B cells of a single clone and recognize a single epitope. Although these single clone B cells may produce hundreds of antibodies, all are identical in the epitope-binding region. However, B cells are mortal and will eventually die. Kohler and Milstein found that B cells can be immortalized by fusion with myeloma cells, forming hybridoma cells. The cells inherit immortality from their myeloma parent and the ability to secrete large amounts of a specific antibody from their B-cell parent. Hybridoma production involves several steps: 1) selection of the antigen (an entire protein or peptide); 2) selection of an animal for immunization; 3) immunization of the animal; 4) fusion of activated B cells with a myeloma cell line; and 5) screening for and cloning the hybridoma cell line (3). Only animals for which compatible myeloma cell lines are available for fusion may be used. Because most hybridoma cell lines are derived from BALB/C mice, mice are most commonly used as the B-cell donor to avoid histocompatibility problems when B cells are fused with a typical BALB/c myeloma cell line. Animals are injected with the antigen of interest or antigen/adjuvant mixtures to activate B cells, which are then collected from the spleen or lymph nodes. The activated B cells are fused with myeloma cells, and the hybridoma cells are selected by growing cells in medium supplemented with hypoxanthine, aminopterin, and thymidine (HAT). The cloning and selection of the specific hybridoma clone are done by limiting dilution technique and immunoassay. The production of monoclonal antibody using species other than murine follows the same principle.

2.2. Recombinant Monoclonal Antibodies

Because murine antibodies tend to elicit immune responses in humans, and insufficiently activate human effector functions, murine monoclonal antibodies have been relatively unsuccessful as therapeutic reagents (4). These problems have been largely overcome by using recombinant techniques to avoid the human immune response while retaining antibody specificity, as described in the following.

2.2.1. Chimeric Monoclonal Antibodies

The first generation of recombinant monoclonal antibodies consisted of rodent-derived variable domains fused to human constant (C) domains, because the C domains are the most immunogenic areas of antibodies (**Fig. 33.1B**) (5). Because the antigen-binding site of the antibody is localized within the V domain, replacement of murine C domains with human C domains would retain the antibody's binding affinity for an antigen and largely mask the human immune response to a murine antibody. The presence of human C domains also allows more efficient human ADCC and CDC. Several chemotherapeutic agents, including rituximab (anti-CD20) and cetuximab (antiepidermal growth factor receptor [anti-EGFR]), were developed with this technique.

2.2.2. Humanized Monoclonal Antibodies

Procedures have been developed to humanize the variable domains, further reducing the murine content and immunogenicity of monoclonal antibodies. The antigen-binding specificity of an antibody is mainly determined by topography and the characteristics of its CDR surface, such as the conformation of the individual CDR and the nature of its amino acid side chains. Thus, transferring murine CDRs onto the variable domain of a human antibody can markedly decrease the immunogenicity of an antibody (**Fig. 33.1C**) *(6)*. However, CDR grafting may not result in complete retention of antigen-binding properties. Analysis of unique human and murine immunoglobulin heavy- and light-chain variable domains revealed that the precise patterns of exposed residues in the framework differ between human and murine antibodies. Some framework residues from the murine antibody must be preserved in the humanized antibody if significant antigen-binding affinity is to be retained. To achieve the optimal human framework, human variable domains showing the greatest sequence homology to the murine variable domains are chosen from a database. This approach results in humanized monoclonal antibodies that retain the interior and contacting residues that affect their antigen-binding characteristics. This method involves computer modeling, polymerase chain reaction-based techniques, and site-directed mutagenesis. The process of CDR grafting has been successfully used to humanize many antibodies, including trastuzumab (anti-EGFR) and alemtuzumab (anti-CD52).

De-immunization technology targeting murine T-helper cell epitopes is another way to decrease the immunogenicity of the murine-derived monoclonal antibodies. T-helper cell epitopes are antibody sequences that bind to major histocompatibility (MHC) class II molecules and can be recognized by T-helper cells to trigger activation and differentiation of T cells, thereby inducing the human antimurine immune response. The de-immunization procedure involves identifying and removing murine T-helper cell binding epitopes from the antibody, with the assistance of computer prediction of sequence and mutagenesis *(7,8)*.

2.2.3. Fully Human Antibodies

Despite the marked reduction of murine content, the unwanted immunogenicity of humanized antibodies ranges from negligible to intolerable. The development of fully human antibodies is the current trend and can be achieved by using human hybridomas, transgenic animals, and phage display of antibody libraries as described below *(9–11)*.

With the successful cloning of human and murine immunoglobulin genes and the maturation of transgenic techniques, human immunoglobulins can now be produced in animals. Several strains of mice have had their mouse immunoglobulin loci replaced with human immunoglobulin genes *(11,12)*. These transgenic mice produce structurally and functionally normal human antibodies. Cloning and production of these antibodies can be achieved by using usual hybridoma technology.

Production of human antibodies from phage libraries is a field of rapid growth *(13)*. Briefly, human heavy chain and light chain messenger RNAs (mRNAs) are isolated from B cells of different sources, reverse transcribed to cDNA, amplified by PCR, and cloned and expressed on the surface of filamentous bacteriophages. Single colonies expressing antigen-specific antibody can be identified by colony screening techniques with the mixture of antigen and phage libraries. Sources for these mRNAs include individuals who have been immunized with an antigen or exposed to an infectious agent, patients with an autoimmune disease or cancer, and even nonimmune human donors, depending on the desired antibody targets. Adalimumab, a recombinant IgG1 specific for tumor necrosis factor, is the first phage-display-derived human monoclonal antibody approved by the FDA.

2.2.4. Other Recombinant Antibodies

Because intact antibodies are relatively large molecules (about 150 kDa), diffusion through vascular walls and clearance from the blood stream are slow. Rapid development in the field of recombinant DNA technology has also allowed modification of antibodies or antibody fragments for diagnostic and therapeutic applications. Antibody fragments, biospecific antibodies, and antibodies conjugated with enzymes, drugs, and radioactive materials have become available and can be tailored to specific needs (**Fig. 33.1D**).

The Fc fragment of an antibody is not needed for cytokine inactivation, receptor blocking, or viral neutralization, and may cause unwanted effects. Therefore, it is removed from most antibodies used for such purposes. Proteolysis or recombinant engineering is usually used to yield the Fab fragments. The smallest functional fragments of antibodies that bind to an antigen are Fv fragments (VH and LH), which comprise the CDR and FR regions. Joining VH and VL by a flexible peptide linker through recombinant technology produces single-chain variable fragment (scFv) *(14)*. The expression of a scFv is possible and more practical, using a microbial expression system. The pharmacokinetics of such fragments appears to be better, especially in penetrating tissue. Shortening the linker between the VH and LH of an scFv increases intermolecular complexes of VL and VH, resulting in diabodies *(15)*. Triabodies and tetrabodies can also be produced by further reducing the linker length *(16)*. The scFv can be fused to constant domains such as CH3 to form minibodies *(17)*. The generation of bispecific antibodies by fusing two different scFvs is now possible and may provide powerful and more specific therapeutic agents. Indeed, a bispecific antibody (CD30:CD16) has been demonstrated to induce marked regression of xeno-transplanted Hodgkin's lymphoma in mice because of recruitment of CD16-positive NK cells to CD30-positive lymphoma cells *(18)*. Antibodies or antibody fragments tagged with toxin (rituximab/saporin-S6 and Ki-3[scFv]-ETA), drug (gemtuzumab ozogamicin), and radioactive material (131I-tositumomab) have also been developed to effect greater cytotoxicity in the treatment of cancer and have been widely successful *(19,20)*.

3. Therapeutic Application of Monoclonal Antibodies

Next to vaccines, therapeutic monoclonal antibodies are the most significant class of biopharmaceuticals being investigated in recent clinical trials. The FDA has approved 19 monoclonal antibodies for clinical use to date (**Table 33.1**), primarily in the areas of oncologic and autoimmune disorders. Although chemotherapy remains one of the major tools in combating cancers, tumor cell resistance and toxic effects on normal tissues often prevent or limit the use of these cytotoxic chemicals. Thus, the concept of targeted therapy for patients with cancer has intrigued researchers for years. Monoclonal antibody-based immunotherapy has now been used to treat thousands of cancer patients, and its use for treatment of transplant rejection and infectious diseases is also under intensive study.

Two main classes of monoclonal antibodies have been developed for clinical use: unconjugated "naked" antibodies and antibodies conjugated to a drug, a toxin, or a radioisotope. Examples of applications of selected antibodies are described in the following sections.

3.1. Cetuximab (Erbitux) in Colorectal Cancer

The EGFR family consists of four transmembrane receptors, including Her-1 (erbB-1), Her-2 (erbB-2), Her-3 (erbB-3), and Her-4 (erbB-4) *(21,22)*. The EGFR Her-1/erbB-1 comprises three major functional domains: an extracellular ligand-binding domain, a transmembrane domain, and a cytoplasmic tyrosine kinase domain. Binding of ligands activates the cytoplasmic tyrosine kinase of EGFR, causing autophosphorylation of the EGFR tyrosine residue in the cytoplasm. Autophosphorylation initiates a cascade of intracellular signaling transduction, which includes components of the Ras mitogen activated protein kinase (MAPK) and downstream protein kinase C and phospholipase D pathways. Activation of EGFR stimulates tumor growth and progression, including the promotion of proliferation, angiogenesis, invasion, and metastasis, and inhibition of apoptosis *(23,24)*. Overexpression and dysregulation of EGFR have been found in many human malignancies, most notably in the colon/rectum but also in the bladder, brain, breast, cervix, esophagus, lungs, ovaries, pancreas, and kidneys *(25,26)*. Cetuximab, a chimeric monoclonal antibody, binds EGFR and inhibits signal transduction, thereby inhibiting cell growth and inducing apoptosis. Cetuximab is used in association with chemotherapy or as single agent in the treatment of patients with EGFR-expressing colorectal cancer who cannot tolerate chemotherapy *(27)*. The use of cetuximab as a monotherapy produced an overall response rate of approx 10% in these patients, with a disease control rate of 32% *(27, 28)*. It generated even better results when combined with chemotherapy, with a response rate of 23% and disease control in 56% of patients *(28)*. Many clinical trials are also underway to evaluate the effect of cetuximab in other cancers, including head and neck cancer, nonsmall-cell lung cancer, and pancreatic cancer *(29)*.

3.2. Trastuzumab (Herceptin) in Breast Cancer

Her-2 is another tyrosine kinase and belongs to the EGFR family *(21)*. In transgenic mouse models, overexpression of Her-2 in the mammary glands causes breast cancer. Her-2 is overexpressed in 23–30% of breast cancers in humans *(30)*, and tumors that overexpress Her-2 are more aggressive and carry a poor prognosis. Tumor Her-2 status is determined with examination of formalin-fixed paraffin-embedded tumor tissues by immunohistochemistry or fluorescence in situ hybridization (FISH). Tumors with high-level expression (3+ by immunohistochemistry) or shown to be positive by FISH assays are considered Her-2-positive *(31)*. Trastuzumab, a humanized anti-Her-2 monoclonal antibody containing 95% human and 5% murine amino acids *(32)*, binds specifically to the extracellular domain of Her-2. The mechanisms of action are multiple and only partially established. Upon binding its antigen, trastuzumab blocks signal transduction, induces apoptosis, inhibits expression of the vascular endothelial growth factor—a central player of tumor angiogenesis—and induces an immune cytotoxic response *(33,34)*. Trastuzumab alone, as a first-line treatment produces clinical response rates of 26%; the integration of trastuzumab with chemotherapy can increase this rate to 63% to 79% *(35)*. Trastuzumab-containing regimens are first-line therapy for life-threatening disease. Trastuzumab is also indicated as first-line therapy in Her-2-positive and hormone receptor-negative cases. For patients with hormone receptor-positive tumors whose disease is nonlife threatening, hormone therapy is considered as an initial treatment and may be switched to trastuzumab-containing regimens if the disease progresses.

3.3. Bevacizumab (Avastatin) in Colorectal Cancer and Macular Degeneration

The role of vascular endothelial growth factor (VEGF) in angiogenesis has long been established *(36)*. It is also secreted by tumors to stimulate new blood vessel formation and thus facilitates tumor growth. VEGF is overexpressed in many tumors, including colorectal cancers and renal cell carcinoma, which are particularly rich in vessels. This finding led to trials of bevacizumab, an anti-VDGF humanized antibody, in colorectal cancer and eventual approval by the FDA *(37)*. Binding of bevacizumab to its antigen blocks binding of VEGF to its receptor, thus inhibiting endothelial cell proliferation and growth of the new vasculature supplying tumor cells. Anti-VEGF therapy in combination with chemotherapy or radiation has shown greater antitumor effects than either treatment alone *(38,39)*. Bevacizumab in combination with chemotherapy is indicated for first-line treatment of metastatic colorectal carcinoma *(37)*. This antibody is being investigated in clinical trials for other solid tumors such as nonsmall cell lung cancer, renal cell carcinoma, metastatic breast cancer, and hematologic malignancies *(38)*.

Bevacizumab has also proved effective in the treatment of age-related macular degeneration *(40)*. Intravitreal administration of this anti-VEGF antibody demonstrated beneficial morphologic and functional effects, including resolution of macular edema, subretinal fluid, and pigment epithelial detachment. Patients who received treatment had improved visual acuity, decreased retinal thickness, and reduced angiographic leakage, owing to the antineovasculature function of bevacizumab.

3.4. Rituximab (Rituxan) in B-Cell Lymphomas, Leukemias, and Autoimmune Disorders

Patients with hematologic malignancies have benefited most from the advances in cancer treatment over the past several decades. Lymphoma and leukemia are the most common indications for monoclonal antibody-based therapy, owing to the accessibility of tumor cells to this "magic bullet."

Rituxan, a chimeric anti-CD20 antibody, was the first antibody approved for clinical use in hematopoietic tumors *(41,42)*. CD20 is expressed on mature B cells and up to 95% of B cell non-Hodgkin lymphomas, but is generally absent from stem cells and plasma cells. The function of CD20 is still controversial, but it is thought to regulate the cell cycle through calcium channel regulation in the cell membrane. Binding of rituximab by CD20 on cell surfaces triggers cell death directly through apoptosis and also by stimulating an immune reaction against the cells by ADCC and CDC *(43)*.

Rituximab exhibits activity against a range of B cell malignancies, including large-cell lymphoma, follicular lymphoma, mantle cell lymphoma, small lymphocytic lymphoma, and post-transplant lymphoproliferative disorder. It exerts a beneficial effect when used either simultaneously or sequentially with chemotherapy. Combination chemotherapy such as CHOP and rituximab is now the standard of care in cases of diffuse large B cell lymphoma, after a seminal trial showed that this combination leads to better overall survival relative to CHOP alone (44). The use of rituximab has also been demonstrated in indolent lymphomas such as follicular lymphoma and small lymphocytic lymphomas, which are primarily incurable except for some patients treated with bone marrow transplant (45,46). Patients with lymphomas may have an initial response to standard chemotherapy, but most develop resistance. The addition of rituximab has increased the cure rate and improved the survival of such patients. Rituximab is becoming one of the most active single agents in the treatment of indolent B cell lymphomas and can be given as maintenance therapy after clinical remission following chemotherapy (47). It selectively kills malignant cells and normal B cells expressing CD20, without toxicity to any other cells, and lacks dose-limiting toxicity and has not demonstrated overlapping toxicity with chemotherapy. An emerging and promising strategy is the combination of rituximab with immune modulators such as interferons and interleukins (48).

After the success of rituximab, researchers realized that the CD20 antigen is a good target for lymphoid malignancies. Monoclonal antibodies against CD20 can be used as vectors to deliver radioactive substances to kill CD20-positive tumor cells and surrounding tumor cells that do not express CD20. Ibritumomab and tositumomab, two radioactive anti-CD20 conjugates, have been approved by the FDA to treat CD20-positive lymphomas that do not respond adequately to rituximab.

In addition to B-cell malignancies, rituximab has also shown effect in several other disease states. Because of its activity against normal B cells, rituximab has been used effectively in autoimmune disorders such as rheumatoid arthritis and systemic lupus erythematosus (SLE), and even in cases of thrombocytopenic purpura and aplastic anemia.

The important role of B cells in the pathogenesis and development of autoimmune and inflammatory disorders has long been recognized (49). They act as antigen-presenting cells, stimulate autoaggressive T cells, produce inflammatory cytokines and autoantibody (which may initiate inflammatory reactions), and form antigen-antibody immune complex deposits. Addition of rituximab to methotrexate significantly reduces clinical signs and symptoms of rheumatoid arthritis patients and produces better American College of Rheumatology responses than methotrexate alone (50). Treatment of refractory SLE has been difficult and the results are usually poor. Rituximab reduces inflammatory variables and clinical symptoms, and is suggested to be an effective maintenance therapy (51). Anti-CD20 therapy has also been applied to the management of chronic immune thrombocytopenia purpura, aplastic anemia, and refractory polymyositis and dermatomyositis (52–54).

3.5. Alemtuzumab (Campath 1H) in Chronic Lymphocytic Leukemia

CD52 is a glycoprotein present on approximately 95% of all normal human B and T cells, monocytes, and macrophages, as well as most B cell and T cell lymphomas, but not on erythrocytes, neutrophils, platelets, or hematopoietic stem cells (55). The precise function of CD52 is not clear. Alemtuzumab, an anti-CD52 monoclonal antibody, is approved by the FDA for treatment of chronic lymphocytic leukemia (CLL), the most common lymphocytic leukemia (56,57). Alemtuzumab appears to work through ADC and ADCC. As a single agent, it showed response rates between 33% and 57% (58). Rapid elimination of CLL cells in the peripheral blood was seen in 97% of CLL patients, whereas CLL cells in lymph nodes seem more resistant to this treatment. Alemtuzumab has also been used in combination with rituximab in cases of CLL that do not respond to conventional therapy (i.e., refractory cases). This combination led to a 63% response rate in patients with refractory CLL (59). In addition, Alemtuzumab has been used to treat follicular lymphomas, Waldenstrom's macroglobinemia, and mycosis fungoides. Because of its ability to deplete T cells, alemtuzumab has been used successfully to prevent graft-versus-host disease (GVHD) following bone marrow transplantation (60).

3.6. Gemtuzumab Ozogamicin (Myelotarg) in Acute Myeloid Leukemia

Acute myeloid leukemia (AML) is the most common type of acute leukemia in adults. Although most AML patients will achieve remission after chemotherapy, many eventually relapse. Because most patients are seniors and otherwise ill, targeted therapy with limited side effects is desirable.

CD33 is a transmembrane glycoprotein expressed in the maturing myeloid cells and myeloblasts of most AML patients (61). It is not expressed in pluripotent stem cells; therefore, killing of CD33 positive cells would not affect stem cell function. Unconjugated antibodies and antibodies conjugated with radioactive materials, toxins, and synthetic drugs have been used in attempts at targeted killing of CD33-positive cells. The most clinically successful approach so far has been a humanized anti-CD33 antibody conjugated with antibiotic calicheamicin (i.e., gemtuzumab ozogamicin), which has been approved by the FDA for treatment of CD33-positive AML in patients during first relapse who are not candidates for other chemotherapy or who are older than 60 years of age (62). Binding of gemtuzumab ozogamicin to CD33 forms a complex that is internalized; the release of conjugated calicheamicin then leads to cell death. In clinical trials, gemtuzumab ozogamicin therapy led to superior overall response rates relative to combination chemotherapy (63,64).

3.7. Muromonab (OKT-3) in Transplant Rejection

Organ transplantation has become a treatment option for most end-stage diseases of the kidneys, heart, liver, and lungs, but transplant rejection is an ever-present concern. With the discovery that rejection is mainly caused by killing of target cells in the transplanted organ by host cytotoxic T cells, CD3 was identified as a potential target for the treatment of transplant rejection. CD3 is a transmembrane protein that participates in antigen binding by the T cell receptor (TCR) and mediates T cell activation. It is expressed by most T cells, with the exception of T cell precursors.

OKT-3, a murine monoclonal antibody against CD3 antigen, is the first monoclonal antibody approved for clinical use by the FDA (65,66). It appears to interact with CD3/TCR, inducing TCR internalization and reducing interaction with the antigen. OKT-3 coats circulating T cells, facilitating their removal from circulation by the reticuloendothelial system. OKT-3 also induces apoptosis of T cells, thus limiting their ability to cause an alloimmune response. The use of OKT-3 in organ transplantation has increased owing to its ability to reverse allograft rejection. The majority of studies conducted have been in patients with renal transplantation, but promising results have also been demonstrated in liver and heart transplantation. OKT-3 showed a reversal rate of up to 90% when used as the primary rejection treatment for renal transplant, superior to conventional therapy *(66)*. This agent is also useful in acute and resistant rejection after liver transplantation *(67)*. Rejection of heart transplants was also successfully reversed by OKT-3 in several studies *(68)*.

3.8. Adalimumab (Humira) in Rheumatoid Arthritis

Adalimumab, the only fully human monoclonal antibody FDA-approved for treatment of autoimmune diseases such as rheumatoid arthritis, is an antibody against tumor necrosis factor alpha *(69)*. Adalimumab works by binding to TNF-alpha and blocking its reaction with the TNF receptor. Thus, adalimumab downregulates expression of other pro-inflammatory cytokines such as IL-6 and granulocyte-macrophage colony stimulating factor (GM-CSF). This antibody can also lyse target cells in the presence of complement. Because adalimumab is a human antibody, it has a long half-life and low immunogenicity. Patients receiving adalimumab showed significantly less joint damage than those receiving placebo *(70)*. Adalimumab also significantly reduces symptoms and signs of rheumatoid arthritis, improving function and quality of life. Adalimumab has proven efficacy as a monotherapy or in combination with methotrexate or pre-existing therapy.

3.9. Pavilizumab in Respiratory Syncytial Virus Infection

Antibody-containing sera from humans or animals have been widely used for prophylaxis and therapy of viral and bacterial diseases. Respiratory syncytial virus (RSV) infects almost all children by early childhood. During the 1990s, 9000 children each year in the United States will require hospitalization for RSV infection, 2% of whom will die *(71)*. Prematurely born infants and those with congenital diseases have the greatest risk of RSV infection and have more severe consequences than do otherwise healthy infants. Palivizumab, a humanized monoclonal RSV antibody, has been demonstrated to significantly reduce hospital admissions and was recommended as an immunoprophylactic agent. It is the only agent currently approved by the FDA for prevention of RSV infections in high-risk infants *(72)*.

References

1. Kohler G, Milstein C (1975) Continuous cultures of fused cells secreting anti-body of predefined specificity. Nature 256:495–497
2. Franklin EC (1975) Structure and function of immunoglobulins. Acta Endocrinol Suppl (Copenh) 194:77–95
3. Leenaars M, Hendriksen CF (2005) Critical steps in the production of polyclonal and monoclonal antibodies: evaluation and recommendations. ILAR J 46:269–279
4. Schroff RW, Foon KA, Beatty SM, Oldham RK, Morgan AC, Jr (1985) Human anti-murine immunoglobulin responses in patients receiving monoclonal antibody therapy. Cancer Res 45:879–885

5. Morrison SL, Johnson MJ, Herzenberg LA, Oi VT (1984) Chimeric human antibody molecules: mouse antigen-binding domains with human constant region domains. Proc Natl Acad Sci USA 81:6851–6855

6. Jones PT, Dear PH, Foote J, Neuberger MS, Winter G (1986) Replacing the complementarity-determining regions in a human antibody with those from a mouse. Nature 321:522–525

7. Roque-Navarro L, Mateo C, Lombardero J, Mustelier G, Fernandez A, Sosa K, Morrison SL, Perez R (2003) Humanization of predicted T-cell epitopes reduces the immunogenicity of chimeric antibodies: new evidence supporting a simple method. Hybrid Hybridomics 22:245–257

8. Mateo C, Lombardero J, Moreno E, Morales A, Bombino G, Coloma J, Wims L, Morrison SL, Perez R (2000) Removal of amphipathic epitopes from genetically engineered antibodies: production of modified immunoglobulins with reduced immunogenicity. Hybridoma 19:463–471

9. Huls GA, Heijnen IA, Cuomo ME, Koningsberger JC, Wiegman L, Boel E, van der Vuurst de Vries AR, Loyson SA, Helfrich W, van Berge Henegouwen GR, van Meijer M, de Kruif J, Logtenberg T (1999) A recombinant, fully human monoclonal antibody with antitumor activity constructed from phage-displayed antibody fragments. Nat Biotechnol 17:276–281

10. Karpas A, Dremucheva A, Czepulkowski BH (2001) A human myeloma cell line suitable for the generation of human monoclonal antibodies. Proc Natl Acad Sci USA 98:1799–1804

11. Davis CG, Jia XC, Feng X, Haak-Frendscho M (2004) Production of human antibodies from transgenic mice. Methods Mol Biol 248:191–200

12. Ishida I, Tomizuka K, Yoshida H, Tahara T, Takahashi N, Ohguma A, Tanaka S, Umehashi M, Maeda H, Nozaki C, Halk E, Lonberg N (2002) Production of human monoclonal and polyclonal antibodies in TransChromo animals. Cloning Stem Cells 4:91–102

13. McCafferty J, Griffiths AD, Winter G, Chiswell DJ (1990) Phage antibodies: filamentous phage displaying antibody variable domains. Nature 348:552–554

14. Bird RE, Hardman KD, Jacobson JW, Johnson S, Kaufman BM, Lee SM, Lee T, Pope SH, Riordan GS, Whitlow M (1988) Single-chain antigenbinding proteins. Science 242:423–426

15. Holliger P, Prospero T, Winter G (1993) "Diabodies": small bivalent and bispecific antibody fragments. Proc Natl Acad Sci USA 90:6444–6448

16. Iliades P, Kortt AA, Hudson PJ (1997) Triabodies: single chain Fv fragments without a linker form trivalent trimers. FEBS Lett 409:437–441

17. Hu S, Shively L, Raubitschek A, Sherman M, Williams LE, Wong JY, Shively JE, Wu AM (1996) Minibody: a novel engineered anti-carcinoembryonic antigen antibody fragment (single-chain Fv-CH3) which exhibits rapid, high-level targeting of xenografts. Cancer Res 56:3055–3061

18. Arndt MA, Krauss J, Kipriyanov SM, Pfreundschuh M, Little M (1999) A bispecific diabody that mediates natural killer cell cytotoxicity against xenotransplantated human Hodgkin's tumors. Blood 94:2562–2568

19. Polito L, Bolognesi A, Tazzari PL, Farini V, Lubelli C, Zinzani PL, Ricci F, Stirpe F (2004) The conjugate Rituximab/saporin-S6 completely inhibits clonogenic growth of CD20-expressing cells and produces a synergistic toxic effect with Fludarabine. Leukemia 18:1215–1222

20. Matthey B, Borchmann P, Schnell R, Tawadros S, Lange H, Huhn M, Klimka A, Tur MK, Barth S, Engert A, Hansen HP (2004) Metalloproteinase inhibition augments antitumor efficacy of the anti-CD30 immunotoxin Ki-3(scFv)-ETA' against human lymphomas in vivo. Int J Cancer 111:568–574

21. Yarden Y (2001) The EGFR family and its ligands in human cancer: signalling mechanisms and therapeutic opportunities. Eur J Cancer 37 Suppl 4:S3–8

22. Yarden Y, Sliwkowski MX (2001) Untangling the ErbB signalling network. Nat Rev Mol Cell Biol 2:127–137

23. Salomon DS, Brandt R, Ciardiello F, Normanno N (1995) Epidermal growth factor-related peptides and their receptors in human malignancies. Crit Rev Oncol Hematol 19:183–232

24. Nicholson RI, Gee JM, Harper ME (2001) EGFR and cancer prognosis. Eur J Cancer 37 Suppl 4:S9–15

25. Mendelsohn J, Baselga J (2003) Status of epidermal growth factor receptor antagonists in the biology and treatment of cancer. J Clin Oncol 21:2787–2799

26. Ennis BW, Lippman ME, Dickson RB (1991) The EGF receptor system as a target for antitumor therapy. Cancer Invest 9:553–562

27. Cunningham D, Humblet Y, Siena S, Khayat D, Bleiberg H, Santoro A, Bets D, Mueser M, Harstrick A, Verslype C, Chau I, Van Cutsem E (2004) Cetuximab monotherapy and cetuximab plus irinotecan in irinotecan-refractory metastatic colorectal cancer. N Engl J Med 351:337–345

28. Frieze DA, McCune JS (2006) Current status of cetuximab for the treatment of patients with solid tumors. Ann Pharmacother 40:241–250

29. Astsaturov I, Cohen RB, Harari P (2006) Targeting epidermal growth factor receptor signaling in the treatment of head and neck cancer. Expert Rev Anticancer Ther 6:1179–1193

30. Slamon DJ, Clark GM, Wong SG, Levin WJ, Ullrich A, McGuire WL (1987) Human breast cancer: correlation of relapse and survival with amplification of the HER-2/neu oncogene. Science 235:177–182

31. Cell Markers and Cytogenetics Committees College of American Pathologists. (2002) Clinical laboratory assays for HER-2/neu amplification and overexpression: quality assurance, standardization, and proficiency testing. Arch Pathol Lab Med 126:803–808

32. Carter P, Presta L, Gorman CM, Ridgway JB, Henner D, Wong WL, Rowland AM, Kotts C, Carver ME, Shepard HM (1992) Humanization of an anti-p185HER2 antibody for human cancer therapy. Proc Natl Acad Sci USA. 89:4285–4289

33. Petit AM, Rak J, Hung MC, Rockwell P, Goldstein N, Fendly B, Kerbel RS (1997) Neutralizing antibodies against epidermal growth factor and ErbB-2/neu receptor tyrosine kinases down-regulate vascular endothelial growth factor production by tumor cells in vitro and in vivo: angiogenic implications for signal transduction therapy of solid tumors. Am J Pathol 151:1523–1530

34. Clynes RA, Towers TL, Presta LG, Ravetch JV (2000) Inhibitory Fc receptors modulate in vivo cytoxicity against tumor targets. Nat Med 6:443–446

35. Ocana A, Rodriguez CA, Cruz JJ (2005) Integrating trastuzumab in the treatment of breast cancer. Current status and future trends. Clin Transl Oncol 7:99, 100

36. Folkman J (1971) Tumor angiogenesis: therapeutic implications. N Engl J Med 285:1182–1186

37. Ellis LM (2005) Bevacizumab. Nat Rev Drug Discov Suppl: S8, 9

38. Ferrara N, Hillan KJ, Gerber HP, Novotny W (2004) Discovery and development of bevacizumab, an anti-VEGF antibody for treating cancer. Nat Rev Drug Discov 3:391–400

39. Kabbinavar F, Hurwitz HI, Fehrenbacher L, Meropol NJ, Novotny WF, Lieberman G, Griffing S, Bergsland E (2003) Phase II, randomized trial comparing bevacizumab plus fluorouracil (FU)/leucovorin (LV) with FU/LV alone in patients with metastatic colorectal cancer. J Clin Oncol 21:60–65

40. Avery RL, Pieramici DJ, Rabena MD, Castellarin AA, Nasir MA, Giust MJ (2006) Intravitreal bevacizumab (Avastin) for neovascular age-related macular degeneration. Ophthalmology 113:363–372

41. Brekke OH, Sandlie I (2003) Therapeutic antibodies for human diseases at the dawn of the twenty-first century. Nat Rev Drug Discov 2:52–62

42. McLaughlin P, Grillo-Lopez AJ, Link BK, Levy R, Czuczman MS, Williams ME, Heyman MR, Bence-Bruckler I, White CA, Cabanillas F, Jain V, Ho AD, Lister J, Wey K, Shen D, Dallaire BK (1998) Rituximab chimeric anti-CD20 monoclonal antibody therapy for relapsed indolent lymphoma: half of patients respond to a four-dose treatment program. J Clin Oncol 16:2825–2833

43. Smith MR (2003) Rituximab (monoclonal anti-CD20 antibody): mechanisms of action and resistance. Oncogene 22:7359–7368

44. Coiffier B, Lepage E, Briere J, Herbrecht R, Tilly H, Bouabdallah R, Morel P, Van Den Neste E, Salles G, Gaulard P, Reyes F, Lederlin P, Gisselbrecht C (2002) CHOP chemotherapy plus rituximab compared with CHOP alone in elderly patients with diffuse large-B-cell lymphoma. N Engl J Med 346:235–242

45. Buske C, Hiddemann W (2006) Rituximab maintenance therapy in indolent NHL: a clinical review. Leuk Res 30 Suppl 1:S11–15

46. Czuczman MS, Grillo-Lopez AJ, White CA, Saleh M, Gordon L, LoBuglio AF, Jonas C, Klippenstein D, Dallaire B, Varns C (1999) Treatment of patients with low-grade B-cell lymphoma with the combination of chimeric anti-CD20 monoclonal antibody and CHOP chemotherapy. J Clin Oncol 17:268–276

47. Hainsworth JD, Litchy S, Barton JH, Houston GA, Hermann RC, Bradof JE, Greco FA, Minnie Pearl Cancer Research Network (2003) Single-agent rituximab as first-line and maintenance treatment for patients with chronic lymphocytic leukemia or small lymphocytic lymphoma: a phase II trial of the Minnie Pearl Cancer Research Network. J Clin Oncol 21:1746–1751

48. Friedberg JW, Neuberg D, Gribben JG, Fisher DC, Canning C, Koval M, Poor CM, Green LM, Daley J, Soiffer R, Ritz J, Freedman AS (2002) Combination immunotherapy with rituximab and interleukin 2 in patients with relapsed or refractory follicular non-Hodgkin's lymphoma. Br J Haematol 117:828–834

49. Dorner T (2006) Crossroads of B cell activation in autoimmunity: rationale of targeting B cells. J Rheumatol Suppl 77:3–11

50. Looney RJ (2006) B cell-targeted therapy for rheumatoid arthritis: an update on the evidence. Drugs 66:625–639

51. Weide R, Heymanns J, Pandorf A, Koppler H (2003) Successful long-term treatment of systemic lupus erythematosus with rituximab maintenance therapy. Lupus 12:779–782

52. Hansen PB, Lauritzen AM (2005) Aplastic anemia successfully treated with rituximab. Am J Hematol 80:292–294

53. Noss EH, Hausner-Sypek DL, Weinblatt ME (2006) Rituximab as therapy for refractory polymyositis and dermatomyositis. J Rheumatol 33:1021–1026

54. Braendstrup P, Bjerrum OW, Nielsen OJ, Jensen BA, Clausen NT, Hansen PB, Andersen I, Schmidt K, Andersen TM, Peterslund NA, Birgens HS, Plesner T, Pedersen BB, Hasselbalch HC (2005) Rituximab chimeric anti-CD20 monoclonal antibody treatment for adult refractory idiopathic thrombocytopenic purpura. Am J Hematol 78:275–280

55. Salisbury JR, Rapson NF, Codd JD, Rogers MV, Nethersell AB (1994) Immunohistochemical analysis of CDw52 antigen expression in non-Hodgkin's lymphomas. J Clin Pathol 47:313–317

56. Keating MJ, Flinn I, Jain V, Binet JL, Hillmen P, Byrd J, Albitar M, Brettman L, Santabarbara P, Wacker B, Rai KR (2002) Therapeutic role of alemtuzumab (Campath-1 H) in patients who have failed fludarabine: results of a large international study. Blood 99:3554–3561

57. Faderl S, Coutre S, Byrd JC, Dearden C, Denes A, Dyer MJ, Gregory SA, Gribben JG, Hillmen P, Keating M, Rosen S, Venugopal P, Rai K (2005) The evolving role of alemtuzumab in management of patients with CLL. Leukemia 19:2147–2152

58. Osterborg A, Mellstedt H, Keating M (2002) Clinical effects of alemtuzumab (Campath-1H) in B-cell chronic lymphocytic leukemia. Med Oncol 19 Suppl: S21–6

59. Faderl S, Thomas DA, O'Brien S, Garcia-Manero G, Kantarjian HM, Giles FJ, Koller C, Ferrajoli A, Verstovsek S, Pro B, Andreeff M, Beran M, Cortes J, Wierda W, Tran N, Keating MJ (2003) Experience with alemtuzumab plus rituximab in patients with relapsed and refractory lymphoid malignancies. Blood 101:3413–3415

60. Hale G, Waldmann H (1994) CAMPATH-1 monoclonal antibodies in bone marrow transplantation. J Hematother 3:15–31

61. Dinndorf PA, Andrews RG, Benjamin D, Ridgway D, Wolff L, Bernstein LD (1986) Expression of normal myeloid-associated antigens by acute leukemia cells. Blood 67:1048–1053

62. Bross PF, Beitz J, Chen G, Chen XH, Duffy E, Kieffer L, Roy S, Sridhara R, Rahman A, Williams G, Pazdur R (2001) Approval summary: gemtuzumab ozogamicin in relapsed acute myeloid leukemia. Clin Cancer Res 7:1490–1496

63. Sievers EL, Larson RA, Stadtmauer EA, Estey E, Lowenberg B, Dombret H, Karanes C, Theobald M, Bennett JM, Sherman ML, Berger MS, Eten CB, Loken MR, van Dongen JJ, Bernstein LD, Appelbaum FR, Mylotarg Study Group (2001) Efficacy and safety of gemtuzumab ozogamicin in patients with CD33-positive acute myeloid leukemia in first relapse. J Clin Oncol 19:3244–3254

64. Leopold LH, Berger MS, Cheng SC, Cortes-Franco JE, Giles FJ, Estey EH (2003) Comparative efficacy and safety of gemtuzumab ozogamicin monotherapy and high-dose cytarabine combination therapy in patients with acute myeloid leukemia in first relapse. Clin Adv Hematol Oncol 1:220–225

65. Kung P, Goldstein G, Reinherz EL, Schlossman SF (1979) Monoclonal antibodies defining distinctive human T cell surface antigens. Science 206:347–349

66. [Anonymous] (1985) A randomized clinical trial of OKT3 monoclonal antibody for acute rejection of cadaveric renal transplants. Ortho Multicenter Transplant Study Group. N Engl J Med 313:337–342

67. Cosimi AB, Cho SI, Delmonico FL, Kaplan MM, Rohrer RJ, Jenkins RL (1987) A randomized clinical trial comparing OKT3 and steroids for treatment of hepatic allograft rejection. Transplant Proc 19:2431–2433

68. Kremer AB, Barnes L, Hirsch RL, Goldstein G (1987) Orthoclone OKT3 monoclonal antibody reversal of hepatic and cardiac allograft rejection unresponsive to conventional immunosuppressive treatments. Transplant Proc 19:54–57

69. [Anonymous] (2003) Adalimumab (humira) for rheumatoid arthritis. Med Lett Drugs Ther 45:25–27

70. Weinblatt ME, Keystone EC, Furst DE, Moreland LW, Weisman MH, Birbara CA, Teoh LA, Fischkoff SA, Chartash EK (2003) Adalimumab, a fully human anti-tumor necrosis factor alpha monoclonal antibody, for the treatment of rheumatoid arthritis in patients taking concomitant methotrexate: the ARMADA trial. Arthritis Rheum 48:35–45

71. Choy G (1998) A review of respiratory syncytial virus infection in infants and children. Home Care Provid 3:306–311

72. Krilov LR (2002) Palivizumab in the prevention of respiratory syncytial virus disease. Expert Opin Biol Ther 2:763–769

34

Antibody Phage Display

Rob Aitken

1. Introduction

Antibodies now constitute an indispensable tool for research across all areas of biomedicine and the life sciences. Whilst polyclonal antibodies from the serum of an immunized animal remain in widespread use, there is little doubt that monoclonal reagents have significant benefits. Foremost is their recognition of just a single feature (epitope) of the biomolecule of interest (the target or antigen). The conformation of the epitope as recognized by an antibody is of more than academic interest. Linear epitopes—for example, a contiguous stretch of amino acids on a protein antigen—are likely to be bound successfully by an antibody providing they are accessible. These features can be perturbed by chemical modification, but they are more likely to be recognized by the antibody after sample preparation (e.g., denaturation in the preparation of samples for a Western blot, or tissue sample for immunohistochemical analysis) than epitopes that are formed through folding of the target (e.g., conformational epitopes). These considerations may govern whether an antibody will recognize its target in the intended area of application.

1.1. Monoclonal Antibodies from Hybridomas

For around 30 yr, the hybridoma methods of Kohler and Milstein (1) have served as a general method for the production of monoclonal antibodies. The methods are based upon the immortalization of single B lymphocytes taken from a donor and immortalization by fusion with a myeloma cell line. When working with laboratory animals, the B-cell donor must be hyperimmunized with the antigen of interest to ensure that a high proportion of splenic lymphocytes are synthesizing antibody against the intended target. At least in principle, B cells specific for the antigen could be selected before fusion, but in practice this is rarely done. After cell fusion, selection for hybridomas is carried out with drugs that block nucleotide synthesis and salvage; surviving lines are cloned and screened for the synthesis of antibody against the antigen of interest. The system works well but is it labor-intensive and it is difficult to control the precise specificity of antibodies that emerge from screening. More fundamental limitations also exist. Because this method of monoclonal

From: *Molecular Biomethods Handbook, 2nd Edition.*
Edited by: J. M. Walker and R. Rapley © Humana Press, Totowa, NJ

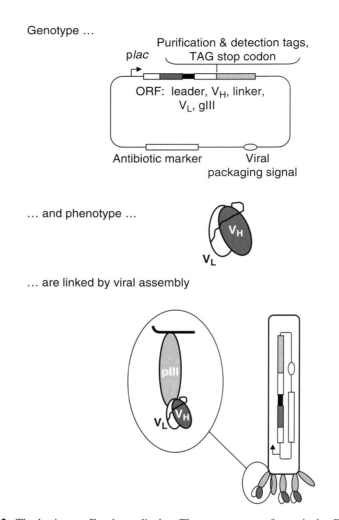

Genotype …

Purification & detection tags,
TAG stop codon

p*lac*

ORF: leader, V$_H$, linker,
V$_L$, gIII

Antibiotic marker   Viral
packaging signal

… and phenotype …

V$_H$

V$_L$

… are linked by viral assembly

pIII

V$_L$ V$_H$

Fig. 34.2. The basis to scFv phage display. The components of a typical scFv phage display vector are shown at the top of the Figure with the organization of the soluble recombinant antibody product shown beneath. The domains of the scFv are labeled, the free-form line indicating the linker peptide extending from the carboxyl terminus of the V$_H$ domain to the amino terminus of the V$_L$ component. The foot of the Figure shows the schematic structure of a phage particle carrying the phagemid vector within the viral capsid (heavy line). The phage particle carries five copies of pIII (light shading) some of which are scFv-pIII fusion proteins (magnified section)

with affinity for the coated surface become immobilized on the surface; others can be washed away. Recoveries are typically low at this stage of selection so the phage are recovered from the surface, infected into bacteria and thereby replicated to much higher numbers. Through repeated rounds of selection, recovery and amplification, target-binding clones are recovered from the library and enriched for those that are favored by the conditions of selection.

At this stage, the antibody fragments are present at the surface of the virus, expressed as fusions to one or other of the components of the viral capsid. This is essential if the antibody is to be displayed at the phage surface. Through simple manipulation, antibody fragment can also be expressed as an independent, freely soluble protein. Guided by a leader peptide (**Fig. 34.2**), the protein is then exported and released into the bacterial periplasm where folding – assembly in the case of Fab fragments – takes place *(9,10)*. Many vectors encode peptide tags to enable purification (e.g., histidine repeats) and detection (e.g., c-myc, Flag) of the translation product (**Fig. 34.2**).

The characterization of viral clones recovered by phage display can take a number of paths. Firstly, immunoassay with either virus ("phage ELISA") or the individual protein ("soluble protein ELISA") can confirm the specificity of an antibody fragment for the target. The natural extension of these experiments is into Western blotting, epitope mapping and the determination of affinity through surface plasmon resonance. By sequencing the reading frame, the antibody fragment can be further characterized to determine the diversity of clones recovered. Purification of soluble antibody enables the biological properties of the protein to be assessed (e.g., seeking the ability of the antibody fragment to inhibit the action of the target molecule or processes in which it is involved). Adaptation of the antibody fragment can take many forms. The natural biological activity of a full length antibody can be restored by recloning the coding sequences into a mammalian expression vector that carries the antibody constant domains *(11,12)*. The capacity of the fragment to bind to target can be harnessed by creating fusions with reporters (e.g., to locate the target molecule in cells *(13)*), enzymes (e.g., for immunoassays for the target molecule *(14)*) or bioactive agents (e.g., toxin fusions enable specific elimination of defined populations of cells in vitro or in vivo *(15)*). With such a range of options, it is little wonder that phage display and recombinant antibody technology has rapidly become a popular experimental technique.

2.2. Library Construction

The flexibility of phage display as a method for the generation of monoclonal reagents becomes apparent even at the earliest stage of a project. Because of this flexibility, it is important for the investigator to be clear about experimental goals and the wider context of the project so that the most appropriate options are exercised. For many projects, a monoclonal reagent is simply required for detection of a biomolecule or for assessment of the function of this target in vitro or in vivo. If this is the case and the format (Fab or scFv) of the monoclonal reagent is not of great importance, then it many be possible to acquire a library from external sources and the time and costs of library construction may be avoided.

If the aim is to use phage display to learn more about the nature of the immune response in a patient or high affinity antibodies are required that have been matured by the response in vivo, the necessity for library generation from that patient, or from a hyperimmunized experimental animal becomes essential.

2.2.1. Source of Material

The construction of a custom library takes as its starting point, cDNA from an appropriate biological source that contains a diverse range of Ig transcripts. Many libraries have been prepared from human donors vaccinated against or infected with particular pathogens or their products. For example, Zwick and colleagues have described the isolation *(16)* and characterization *(17)* of HIV-neutralizing antibodies derived from an HIV seropositive donor. Equally, the immune response active in patients with a range of syndromes and conditions can be sampled if access to lymphoid tissue can be arranged. Fostieri et al. *(18)* reported the isolation from myasthenia gravis patients of Fab antibodies the acetylcholine receptor. Note that samples need to be protected against the degradation of RNA on recovery and during storage so snap-freezing and storage at −80°C, and the use of proprietary protectants (e.g., RNAlater, Ambion) are strongly recommended. Samples from the spleen or lymph nodes are ideal for library construction, but may be hard to obtain from human sources. There may, for example, be ethical, cultural, or legal constraints on access to material from post mortem analysis, or tissues taken during surgery. Informed consent for the sampling of human blood may be easier and there are several reports in the literature of library construction with material sampled in this way *(19–22)*. Before embarking on this approach, it is worth considering that the numbers of B lymphoblasts circulating in the blood are relatively low and the appearance of antigen-specific B cells may be transitory after infection, vaccination etc. These factors can constrain the yield of cDNA and the diversity of Ig transcripts for library construction. It is possible to isolate peripheral blood lymphocytes against a purified antigen *(23,24)* or to expand in vitro small numbers (even single) of B lymphocytes *(25)* to overcome the first of these issues.

To construct large libraries containing antibodies against many, chemically diverse targets, several investigators have deliberately chosen to sample the naïve human repertoire or to use material from normal donors. B lymphocytes bearing IgM at the surface can be selected from blood or lymphoid tissue. Alternatively, transcripts encoding IgM can be specifically recovered by PCR at a later stage driving the construction of the library towards the naive repertoire *(26–29)*.

Sampling material from a vaccinee or an individual who has been exposed to a pathogen *(30–33)* can enrich a display library with high affinity antibodies against targets that may be of immediate relevance (e.g., toxins or other microbial virulence factors *(34,35)*). The library may also represent a snap-shot of the diversity of the humoral response at the time of sampling, aiding analysis of the diversity of the response and its genetic basis (e.g., use of particular families of immunoglobulin genes *(23,36)*). But these features may not be universally beneficial. The library may be overpopulated with clones that are reactive with immunodominant products recognized by the donor's immune system. The library will also be formed from all immunoglobulins expressed by the donor at the time of sampling, but not all antibody sequences express well in the bacterial systems used for propagation of the library, creating gaps in the repertoire of the library *(37)*.

These sorts of limitations have been overcome with the generation of libraries that have been diversified by synthetic methods. Here, scaffolding sequences can be chosen that are known to be expressed successfully in bacteria and then diversified to produce libraries that can be screened for reactivity with a tremendous range of chemically diverse targets *(38–41)*. This is the concept of a "single pot library" – a single resource that contains antibodies to practically any target *(42)*.

2.2.2. Repertoire Recovery

Given a source of cDNA from a lymphoid tissue, the next objective is to recover from it antibody-coding sequences. The use of the polymerase chain reaction with specific primers allows extraction and amplification of antibody-coding sequences from all the other transcripts present in the sample.

Herein lies a paradox: of their nature, antibodies are translated from sequences of enormous diversity. How then can the repertoire be recovered with a manageable number of PCR primers? Fortunately, sequence diversity is concentrated into regions that code for the complementarity-determining regions (CDRs) – those parts of the protein that will contact antigen. The CDRs are supported on sequences (framework regions; FRs) that are more conserved in sequence. In the human and murine immune systems, antibody coding sequences are assembled from gene segments in the developing B lymphocyte that are numerous but which can be grouped into smaller numbers of families because of the conservation of the FR sequences (43). In many other species, the antibody repertoires are founded upon more limited use of Ig gene segments or families (44). Overall, the impact of these features is that huge molecular diversity can be recovered in a representative fashion through a significant but very manageable number of amplification reactions.

A major decision point arises at this point. Is the library to be constructed with Fab or scFv antibody fragments? This governs the actual primer sets that will be used for recovery of the repertoire. If Fab fragments are to be generated, a further question arises: is there to be a preference for antibodies of a particular class? With these considerations in mind, the human antibody heavy chain repertoire can be recovered by PCR with combinations of 8 primers that anneal to the coding sequence for FR1 and 4 that anneal to the coding sequence for IgG constant domain 1. Similar considerations govern the number of reactions and primer sets required for recovery of the light chain repertoires of mice and men (e.g., the de Haard library (28)) although for other species, fewer primer sets are often needed because of more restricted usage of germline segments.

Near identical methods are used if it is decided that a scFv library is to be constructed, the exception being the nature of the primers that are used for amplification: primers specific for the FR1-coding sequence of light and heavy chain cDNA are paired with primers that anneal to FR4-coding sequence (e.g., the Vaughan library (27)). The J segments that are rearranged in B cells to form this part of the Ig reading frame are modest in number in many species – in some animals, only single J segments are utilized – so once again, the repertoire can be recovered with reasonable numbers of PCR reactions using all combinations of heavy chain and light chain primers.

Depending upon the vector to be used for library construction, restriction sites are included in the primers used for PCR. In many cases, the combination of vector-derived sequence and the choice of the restriction site ensures near-native protein sequence in the recombinant product.

2.2.3. Library Construction

In the construction of large libraries from patient material, some investigators have chosen to clone heavy or light chain PCR products into a "holding" vector (e.g., the de Haard library (28)). The purpose of this is 2-fold. First if materials are to be accumulated over a period of time (e.g., from patient material that for logistic reasons cannot be obtained regularly), it enables PCR products to be archived in a stable form pending library construction. Second, when PCR products are digested for transfer into the display vector, thereby generating the library, excision of the inserts can be convincingly demonstrated and there is no ambiguity about their suitability for ligation. Restriction enzymes chosen for cloning are usually able to digest DNA close to the termini of the duplex and where efficiency is an issue of concern, recognition sites can be positioned to ensure efficient digestion. However, excision of the amplicons from a holding vector provides clear confirmation that the antibody sequences are ready for ligation.

Phage display vectors have been extensively adapted by different investigators to match individual needs, but the following properties are typical, irrespective of whether scFv or Fab libraries are to be prepared (**Fig. 34.2**). For display upon filamentous phage, pIII is the preferred anchor *(7)* and phagemid vectors have superseded the use of viral genomic DNA except for specialist purposes (e.g., multivalent display *(45)*). This is largely because shifting from single-stranded DNA carried within the viral capsid to an independently replicating, double-stranded plasmid in bacteria (ideal for purification in high yield, restriction analysis, sequencing, and protein expression studies) is extremely straightforward. Aside from a plasmid origin of replication, a selectable marker and viral sequences to enable packaging into virions, these vectors possess a promoter for expression of the cloned antibody sequence (typically p*lac* for ease of regulation), bacterial leader sequences (e.g., the *pelB* and *ompA* leader sequences) and cloning sites for the Ig inserts (**Fig. 34.2**). Fab display vectors usually carry a simple dicistronic operon for independent expression, translation and export of the heavy and light chain components (e.g., pComb3; *(7)*). In scFv display vectors, the linker sequence that tethers the V_H and V_L components can be included in the vector, or introduced by PCR before ligation into the vector. In order that the antibody fragment will be displayed, the Ig sequence lies in-frame with gIII, the coding sequence for pIII, a minor phage coat protein present in five copies at the tip of the assembled virus (**Fig. 34.2**). The pIII protein mediates infection of the bacterial host by the phage through interaction with the bacterial F pilus and the TolA co-receptor *(46)*. Pioneering work by Smith *(47)* demonstrated that phage infectivity could be retained even when peptides and proteins were fused to pIII. A range of features may be present in the intervening sequence of the display vector. It has become conventional to include an amber stop codon in this part of the vector (**Fig. 34.2**) providing the option of expressing an antibody-pIII fusion protein for display in suppressor strains of *Escherichia coli* (e.g., TG1). Moving the construct into a nonsuppressing bacterial host (e.g., HB2151) then allows expression of the antibody fragment as a soluble protein. The same goal can be achieved with only slightly more effort by excision of the gIII sequence using flanking restriction sites that generate compatible termini, and religation *(7)*. Histidine repeats to facilitate protein purification and tags for immunochemical detection are also common features of this part of the vector (**Fig. 34.2**).

Once the PCR products from repertoire recovery have been cloned into display vectors and transformed into an appropriate strain of *E. coli*, how then is viral assembly initiated? Only two viral sequences are present in the vector: gIII and the packaging signal. By adding helper phage (e.g., VCS M13, Stratagene), the full range of viral proteins can be synthesized in the bacterial host, viral assembly can begin, but it is a single-stranded form of the phagemid rather than the helper phage genome that is packaged into progeny phage. Filamentous bacteriophage are not released from *E. coli* in a catastrophic lytic event (*cf* phage lambda or the T phages) – rather, they are extruded as viral proteins accumulate in the inner membrane and assemble to form the capsid. After DNA is packaged into the virion, the capsid is capped with copies of the minor coat protein pIII. This is a crucial stage as regards the formation of a display library. Low level expression of the antibody-pIII fusion from the phagemid is achieved by growth of the bacteria in low concentrations of glucose thereby allowing some expression from the *lac* promoter. This leads to accumulation of the recombinant protein in the bacterial membrane. As capping takes place, a mixture of pIII proteins – wild-type pIII encoded by the helper phage and antibody-pIII from the phagemid vector – are incorporated into the capsid (**Fig. 34.2**). It is estimated that one or two fusion proteins are most commonly incorporated (*48*), the balance comprising wild-type pIII. Thus progeny phage carry the phagemid, and display at their surface the encoded antibody fragment. When these events take place across the stock of bacteria transformed with the recovered Ig repertoire, a phage display library results.

The properties of helper phage used in this procedure have been extensively refined over recent years. Selection of the library on the target biomolecule can be aided by elimination of phage that only display wild-type pIII and interact with the selecting surface in a nonspecific fashion. Helper phage such as KM13 have been modified to include a trypsin-sensitive site in pIII (*49*). Treatment with the enzyme renders them noninfective. When partnered with a display vector that expresses pIII lacking this susceptibility, proteolysis can be used to inactivate any phage that lack antibody at their surface. An alternative approach is mutation of the helper phage such that it carries a truncated version of gIII that is unable to contribute to the infection process (*50*).

2.2.4. Characterization of the Library

Once the display library has been generated, its size and potential utility can be estimated in a number of ways. The absolute number of virus present can be determined by titration along the simple principle that infection of bacteria with phage will transduce the vector into the bacterial host thereby conferring upon the bacteria resistance to antibiotic. Samples of the library are thus serially diluted and by adding aliquots to cultures of bacteria that express the F pilus, the frequency with which bacteria are converted to antibiotic resistance can be established. Phage stocks of 10^{12} transducing units per ml or more are routinely obtained.

Plasmid DNA can be re-isolated from bacteria infected in this way for further analysis. Restriction analysis of colonies picked at random can determine the frequency of complete Ig inserts within the library. The ligation of amplicons into the display vector is rarely 100% efficient (*48*) and it is useful to know what proportion of the library lacks the heavy or light chain components of a Fab or the V_H or V_L regions of a scFv.

The diversity of Ig sequences carried by the library is also an important parameter. This can be estimated by digesting the Ig inserts with restriction enzymes like *Bst*NI, an enzyme that recognizes a 4 base sequence (5′ CC(A/T)GG 3′) that happens to occur commonly in Ig V region coding sequences. Given the likely occurrence of this sequence in the display vector, it is important that the antibody V region insert is specifically recovered by PCR or restriction digestion before analysis. Failing this, the restriction profile is likely to be obscured by vector-derived fragments.

A more detailed assessment of library diversity can be made by sequencing. For scFv inserts, sequencing primers can be designed against upstream or downstream flanking vector sequences or either strand of the linker region. For Fab inserts, the V region sequences are rather shorter and hence it may be possible to sequence the region of interest using primers against the bacterial leaders upstream of the V_H and V_L inserts. Although more costly and time-consuming, this approach has several significant advantages over restriction analysis. The extent and location of diversity can be thoroughly assessed. If some amplicons from repertoire recovery are disproportionately represented in the library, this can be identified. The degree of diversity present in the library can also be assessed. Perhaps the most important benefit of sequencing is that the reading frames in the library can be checked for integrity. cDNA prepared from lymphoid tissue will include transcripts from B cells undergoing somatic hypermutation, a process with the capacity to introduce stop codons and (more rarely) shifts in the reading frame. Similarly, the use of PCR for repertoire recovery will introduce errors with low frequency. For synthetically diversified libraries, stop codons will be introduced a higher frequency. An alternative method that can be employed to check for the integrity of the reading frame is to pick clones at random from the library and after appropriate manipulation (*see* the following), check for the expression of soluble, recombinant antibody by capture ELISA, dot blotting or Western blotting.

2.3. Screening by Phage Display

2.3.1. Selection Methods

One of the most attractive features of phage display is the speed with which selection from the library can be executed, the flexibility of the method of selection and, most of all, its potential for direct extraction of antibodies directed against the target of interest. It is worth comparing this latter feature with conventional monoclonal methods where the only driving force towards the antibody of interest is the frequency of B cells of the desired specificity amongst the hybridoma population.

In its simplest form, selection can take place upon a convenient surface (often plastic) that has been coated with the target (*8*). This is an application of the "panning" methods originally devised by Smith (*51*). As in most immunochemical procedures, the surface needs to be blocked to minimize nonspecific binding of library phage. To avoid capturing phage that bind to the blocking reagent, the blocker (often skimmed milk, but purified proteins like serum albumin or gelatine are also used) is preincubated with the phage stock. This reduces substantially the chances of interaction with blocking protein present at the selecting surface. The number of phage added to the surface usually ensures that each specificity calculated to exist in the library is represented several thousand-fold, allowing ample opportunity for recovery. After incubation, the surface is washed rigorously and those phage that remain attached are recovered. Recovery can be though change in the pH (*48*), the addition of mild chaotropic agents (*5*) or proteases for those phage systems that are appropriately adapted (*see* description of KM13 above (*49*)). Whilst elution must break the interaction between the displayed antibody and the target-coated surface, it must not be so harsh as to impair the ability of virus to infect bacteria. Fortunately, the infection process is robust.

Recovered phage are then infected into an appropriate strain of bacteria. This serves two important purposes. Firstly, it allows an estimate to be made of the number of virus recovered from selection; as before, this can be done by measuring the frequency with which bacteria are transduced to antibiotic resistance. Secondly, the numbers of phage recovered at the first round of selection are modest (numbers in the range of 10^3 to 10^4 are typical) and represent a very low percentage of the input (10^{10} to 10^{12}). Infection into bacteria, recovery of antibiotic-resistant colonies and reinfection with helper phage allows amplification of the recovered sample to numbers appropriate for a second round of selection. Further rounds often take place on surfaces coated with successively lower concentrations of the target molecule in an effort to refine selection towards those antibodies with the highest affinity of interaction *(48)*. The percentage of phage recovered at each round of selection often climbs sharply from round one to two and further elevation may occur at round 3 *(8,51)*. This can be suggestive of success. Sequencing of clones picked at random through a selection experiment often reveals the emergence of common sequences in the CDRs from collections that initially appear diverse. This indicates that progressive enrichment is taking place during phage selection. It is important to note, however, that this selection is "blind" and that despite careful experimental design, it can drift from the intended direction for a number of reasons. For example, phage that have a low propensity to interact with the selecting surface but are able to replicate quickly will rapidly dominate the output. Similarly, antibodies that react with a contaminant with high affinity rather than the intended target can emerge. Selections that suffer these problems can show all the signs of success as selection proceeds but their failure will only become apparent when tested in immunoassay at a later stage. If these problems arise, again the speed of phage display means that setbacks can be quickly rectified.

The formats for selection are limited only by the ingenuity of the investigators. To avoid conformational change in the target by binding to a plastic surface, solution-based selection methods are popular. Often the target is modified by addition of a small ligand (e.g., biotin). Phage mixed in solution with the target can then be captured to a plastic surface coated with streptavidin or collected by using magnetic beads *(52,53)*. Selection in solution can also be followed by capture to a surface coated with another antibody directed against the target. This selection method is also useful for small target molecules that may not bind efficiently to plastic or when direct binding to a selecting surface may obscure features of potential importance.

Antibodies against small target molecules can also be isolated by phage display through the use of carrier proteins. The target can be coupled to a larger protein carrier either by chemical activation or through genetic fusion and the conjugate then coated to a selecting surface. Naturally, antibodies may be bound during selection via interaction with the carrier. To drive selection towards the molecule of interest, selection in the next round takes place using conjugate employing a different carrier protein *(54)*.

This leads an important principle that can be employed in phage display – the concept of negative selection. Although selection strategies naturally spring to mind in which clones that bind to a coated surface are retained and carried forward to successive rounds, it is equally possible to deplete on a coated surface, leaving behind those antibodies that are captured. This is valuable when seeking antibodies against some feature of the target, one that distinguishes it from other, closely related biomolecules. By applying the library to an irrelevant but similar target, the library can be depleted of antibodies directed towards common or shared motifs (negative selection step). Phage left free in solution can then be taken forward for positive selection against the target. Alternating rounds of negative and positive selection may then drive the process towards the specificities of interest *(55)*.

These examples only serve to illustrate some aspects of selection. Recent reviews *(4,5)* should be consulted to appreciate the enormous variety of selection strategies that have been employed by investigators.

One common feature of selection alluded to earlier is that round-on-round, the diversity of the recovered clones falls as enrichment takes place. When using complex targets or those comprising multiple molecular species, antibodies of potential value are discarded during early rounds of selection. To overcome this wastage, robotic methods have emerged. These are of particular value when deriving antibodies for use in proteomics. Thousands of clones are picked for evaluation at the early stages of selection, and checked by gridding onto membranes coated with the targets of interest *(56,57)*.

2.3.2. Assessing the Output

The assessment of phage numbers can be conveniently determined by titration experiments. This is important in calculating the size of a library, recoveries of virus during selection and amplification when preparing for later rounds of panning. The procedure exploits the ability of phage to infect strains of *E. coli* and transduce them to express the antibiotic marker carried by the phagemid. Hence, serial dilution of the phage stock and infection to *E. coli* TG1 provides a convenient assay.

When selection successfully extracts clones from a library, it is customary to observe low percentage recoveries at the first round of selection that rise by several orders of magnitude in the next round. Further elevation may be seen in later rounds of the selection. This does not necessarily imply that clones against the intended target are emerging but it is a strong indicator of selection on some basis.

The specificity of clones recovered from selection can be conveniently determined by ELISA using various formats. One assay of immediate benefit takes the mixed output of phage from a round of selection and tests its reactivity against the target and a range of irrelevant proteins or other biomolecules. Binding of virus to the immunoassay surface can be detected with reagents against the capsid. Depending upon the supplier, the reagent may be directly conjugated to an enzyme reporter (e.g., horseradish peroxidase) or addition of a secondary antibody–enzyme conjugate may be required. Because the viral input to the assay is mixed in composition, the assay is often termed polyclonal phage ELISA. It can be usefully applied in an initial assessment of the success of a selection protocol. Along with the rising percentage recoveries of virus, increasing ELISA strength in the polyclonal phage ELISA versus the intended target provides signs of specific selection, assuming signals against an irrelevant target remain consistently low. The assay can, for example, confirm that viruses are not emerging through inadvertent selection against blocking materials used in panning.

The natural progression in evaluating the output from selection is to identify individual clones that react with the intended target. Plates used for titrating the output of each round of selection can be used to isolate individual clones for culture, superinfection with helper phage, and the preparation of monoclonal phage stocks. These can then be tested in ELISA as described above.

Some caution has to be exercised with the outcome of monoclonal phage ELISA. Because these assays are typically executed with many clones simultaneously – it is common practice to pick, for example, 96 clones from the output at each round of selection, using microtitre plates for bacterial culture and superinfection – it is rarely possible to titrate the numbers of virus used in the monoclonal phage ELISA. Hence, fluctuations in the ELISA data among clones under test may reflect to some extent variation in the viral input rather than strength of interaction with the target. Another *caveat* is that phage-based ELISA can generate signals of apparent strength but if the affinity of the displayed antibody for the target is moderate or low, the signal may be heavily dependent upon multivalent display (i.e. it benefits from avidity effects rather than affinity). In this instance, expression of the antibody as a monovalent soluble protein fails to generate the signal strength in ELISA that might be expected from initial testing with phage. The final aspect of the technology that needs to be considered is the influence of the bacterial host. Propagation of virus is often carried out in suppressor strains of *E. coli* (e.g., TG1) to ensure translation of the amber stop codon that (depending upon the vector) may be positioned between the antibody and pIII reading frames. This is essential for synthesis of the fusion protein required for display. In this host background, amber stop codons elsewhere in the reading frame (e.g., located in the CDRs where diversification may have been generated synthetically) will also be translated *(56)*. Phage carrying these sequences may be able to bind to the target biomolecule in ELISA. When the construct is transferred to a nonsuppressing bacterial host (e.g., HB2151), a full-length antibody cannot be formed so once more, clones that appear promising from monoclonal phage ELISA are unreactive at a later stage of their characterization. For all these reasons, it is vital that a significant number of clones are chosen from monoclonal phage ELISA for further characterization, and that this choice does not entirely favor clones that generate the strongest signal in phage ELISA.

These issues concern the viral input to ELISA. It is also worth considering the nature of the target at this point in the evaluation process. The outcome of the assay will be used to judge if phage recovered from the screen are of the intended specificity: it is therefore vital that the target used for ELISA is as pure as possible or controls are included in the assay to determine if phage have been isolated that are reactive with a (potentially minor) contaminant, the blocking agent used in selection or another component of the selection system (e.g., naked plastic, biotin, streptavidin etc.). On the assumption that clones recovered from selection are of the intended specificity, it may also be possible to assess at this stage if recognition is taking place of a particular feature of the target biomolecule. For example, competitive ELISA with another monoclonal antibody, a ligand or other biomolecule reactive with the target, or peptides derived from the target sequence can be used to good effect. Finally, the coating of the immunoassay surface with different forms of the target (e.g., the native protein if a recombinant form has been used in selection, close homologues of the target perhaps taken from other species, protein that has been modified at a post-translational stage [phosphorylation, glycosylation, addition of fatty acyl moieties]) or chemical derivatives of small target species (e.g., forms of the target that lack particular molecular features, alternative peptide sequences) can help define antibodies that show particular promise at an early stage of their characterization.

Clones that emerge from this phase of analysis can be sequenced to assess the diversity of the CDRs or (for libraries derived from an immunized source) the range of Ig segments that contribute to the response against the target in vivo. Consensus sequences may appear in the CDRs of antibodies isolated by stringent selection methods, but this step is also worthwhile in identifying whether identical clones are present. Because the DNA of phagemid display vectors is easily isolated for sequencing, this approach has significant benefits over assessing the diversity of recovered clones by restriction analysis with *Bst*NI or other frequently cutting endonucleases. As described above, primers for sequencing may be designed against flanking regions of the antibody reading frame or the coding sequence for the scFv linker.

2.4. Expression of Recombinant Antibodies

Most display vectors have been designed to minimize the degree of manipulation in moving from expression of antibody-pIII fusions to synthesis of soluble, monovalent protein. For some (e.g., the Fab display vector pComb3 *(10)* and its derivatives), the pIII coding sequence is excised by digestion with *Spe*I and *Nhe*I. Because these enzymes generate compatible termini, the vector fragment is then isolated and re-ligated for expression of the Fab in an *E. coli* host. Many scFv display vectors possess an amber stop codon between the reading frames for antibody and the phage coat protein (**Fig. 34.2**). Infection of virus into a nonsuppressing host (e.g., *E. coli* HB2151) therefore leads to expression of the soluble antibody fragment.

In the majority of display vectors, transcription of the recombinant antibody takes place from a *lac* promoter. It is customary to grow the bacteria under glucose repression until adequate biomass has been reached. Removal of the glucose by centrifugation and resuspension in fresh, glucose-free medium containing IPTG inducer then triggers transcription and translation. The choice of growth temperature during the expression phase is important to avoid aggregation of the protein and to minimize toxicity to the bacterial host though some studies suggest that effects on yield can be minimal *(58)*. Expression at 30°C is often chosen as a starting point. Frequently, overexpression of the antibody leads to leakage of the periplasmic contents to the culture medium from which the protein can be purified. Purification is aided significantly by the presence of a histidine repeat sequence at the carboxy-terminus of the protein, a feature that is most conveniently incorporated in the original vector. Material generated in this way can be used in immunoassay or blotting, detection being made with Ig-binding proteins such as Protein A, G or L *(56)* or reagents against the purification and/or other peptide tags (e.g., c-myc, Flag etc.).

Because analysis of the soluble protein differs in many ways from that of the original phage clone, it is prudent to carry forward many different constructs that appear to bind to the target. The movement from a suppressor mutant for expression of a scFv-pIII fusion and propagation of phage to a nonsuppressor host for expression of soluble protein can mean that clones that are positive in phage ELISA react poorly when the soluble antibody is expressed (*see* above). Amber stop codons present in the Ig reading frame will truncate the antibody prematurely in this situation. Some Ig sequences can be expressed more successfully in bacteria than others and whilst some investigations have identified causes for this effect *(59)*, in many cases, they remain unexplained. Clones from custom, immunized libraries may therefore prove difficult to overexpress if they happen to carry problematic framework sequences. It is for this reason that some of the most successful, synthetically diversified libraries are founded upon single frameworks: the framework can be chosen as one that expresses consistently well in a bacterial host *(56)*. The affinity of the antibody-target interaction can also be a relevant consideration *(60)*. Multiple display of an antibody at the phage surface can drive a promising interaction in phage ELISA but when expressed as monovalent soluble protein, constructs with low or modest affinity for the target can give ELISA signals that are close to background.

Some of these potential problems can be foreseen by careful experimental design. For example, Westerns, dot blots or capture ELISA can be used to check for evidence of expression of the protein before target-specific ELISA is undertaken. These data can also be used to normalize extracts or quantities of purified protein that are taken forward to ELISA so that reaction with target can be ranked in the knowledge that roughly equivalent amounts of recombinant antibody have been used in the assay.

Once these issues have been addressed, expression of the antibody can be scaled up and the product purified by nickel chelation chromatography (if a histidine tag is present), or affinity chromatography on Protein A, G, L (according the antibody sequence carried). Determination of the affinity of the purified protein for its target is most commonly assessed by surface plasmon resonance using instruments such as the BiaCore.

2.5. Optimization and Further Modification

Once recombinant antibodies have emerged from selection and characterization, the availability of the coding sequence and the ability to express the protein in bacteria opens up numerous options. The affinity of the antibody for its target can be enhanced by rational or random mutagenesis *(15,61,62)*, manipulations that may further refine the specificity of the antibody for its target. Fusions can be generated, linking the Ig reading frame to enzymes like alkaline phosphatase *(63)* or fluorogens like green fluorescent protein *(64)*. Other manipulations (e.g., the addition of a terminal cysteine residue *(65)* can aid the covalent attachment of other moieties *(66)*. Coupling of the recombinant antibody to other protein domains of modest size (e.g., the human kappa constant domain *(67)*) or other entities (e.g., maltose binding protein *(68)*) may improve yields and / or enable more convenient detection of antibody binding.

Reconstruction of a full-length antibody from a scFv or Fab protein may confer biological activities such as the ability to activate complement upon target recognition but proteins of this size often require expression in eukaryotic systems. The availability of specialized vectors *(11,12)* can assist in achieving this goal.

3. Applications

3.1. Tools for Proteomics

Antibody libraries can be mined for reactivity against a wide range of targets and then to use the recombinant antibodies as reagents for target detection and characterization: this is well-illustrated in the area of proteomics. Ohara and colleagues compared the properties of recombinant Fabs from a library of synthetically diversified human antibodies with polyclonal antisera against the same targets and reported that the Fabs were well-suited to Western blotting and immunohistochemistry (69). Earlier, de Wildt et al. described experiments in which one or two rounds of conventional screening were used to isolate phage from synthetically diversified libraries constructed on single V_H and V_L frameworks. Clones (up to 12,000) were then picked and gridded out using robotics onto membranes coated with the targets to test their specificity (56). The study demonstrated the capacity of large display libraries to yield antibodies against a wide range of targets and the ability to extract antibodies against minor components of complex mixtures, given appropriate (robotic) methods for identification of the recognition of target. Other investigators have described phage selection using blots prepared from 2-dimensional gels – a use of the proteome itself as the target for extraction of specific antibodies from a library.

For naïve or synthetically diversified libraries, the diversity of the resource is such that extraction of antibodies against human protein targets (e.g., tumor necrosis factor (2), human chorionic gonadotropin (28)), molecules that are highly conserved amongst eukaryotes and therefore poorly immunogenic (e.g., ubiquitin (56)) or toxic compounds (e.g., doxorubicin (5)) is possible.

Antibodies isolated through phage display can be developed as diagnostic reagents but a more intriguing prospect is their use in construction of microarrays upon which binding of multiple analytes could be detected (40). Phage display is particularly valuable in this area of application because a single, highly diversified resource (the library) can be conveniently mined for antibodies against very many different targets. Some authors have described the use of stringent selection methods to isolate antibodies of very high affinity *via* phage display (70). These reagents then have the ability to detect very low concentrations of an analyte. For example, Wang and colleagues have reported the formation of a bivalent scFv fusion to alkaline phosphatase that in immunoassay, could detect as few as several hundred *Bacillus anthracis* cells in 2 hours (71). They further showed that replacement of the enzyme reporter with Cy3 dye increased sensitivity of the assay by about 10-fold with no increase in the time taken to conduct the assay.

3.2. Antibody Therapy

When the target is a molecule linked with a disease state, there are numerous reports of the isolation by phage display of antibodies with therapeutic potential. Infectious diseases have proved a productive area for investigation and in one example, antibodies against anthrax toxin have been shown to neutralize the lethal properties of this bacterial virulence factor (72). The pathogenesis of established (e.g., rotavirus (73)) and emergent viral agents (e.g., SARS (74,75)) can also be blocked by recombinant antibodies. Antibodies generated in this way have the potential for treatment of acute infection, blocking the disease process at a key point (e.g., interaction between a receptor and the pathogen *(76)* or its product(s) *(72)*). This provides a therapeutic option when the use of antibiotics or antiviral compounds is undesirable or impossible *(77)*. It also offers prophylaxis when vaccines are unavailable *(78)* or the patient is unable to mount a protective response as a consequence of vaccination *(79)*.

These areas of application deal with infectious agents, but antibody phage display has also been widely applied to the search for antibodies with antitumor activities. Careful design of the selection strategy has enabled, for example, investigators to isolate antibodies that are specific for markers expressed on transformed cells but absent from nontransformed primary cells *(80)*. Therapeutic application need not trigger complement – recruitment of effector cells *(81,82)* can be exploited and in some cases, internalization of the recombinant antibody can have directly antiproliferative effects *(83)*.

3.3. Analysis of Intracellular Processes

Practically all conventional applications of antibody phage display use the recombinant proteins as free, soluble reagents. However in an important exception, intrabodies are deliberately retained in the cytosol *(84)*. This is an important and growing area of application because it provides a natural complement to mutation, gene knockouts and RNAi in the analysis of gene function.

To create an intrabody, the coding sequence of an antibody of some chosen specificity is recloned into a mammalian expression vector – crucially, the insert lacks a leader sequence – and the construct is then transfected into cells. Through this manipulation, the translation product is confined to the cytosol of the transfected cell. If the antibody is successfully folded, it can bind to other molecules present in this location, potentially blocking their normal function. Tagging the antibody with targeting motifs can direct relocalization of the antibody to the nucleus, the mitochondria etc.

Intrabodies find immediate application in the analysis of viral gene function *(85,86)* where interactions between viral proteins and host factors can be disrupted through binding of recombinant antibodies in the cytosol. Other pathogenic processes – inherited conditions like Huntingdon's disease *(87)*, Alzheimer's *(88)* and cancer *(89)* – can similarly be analysed through the application of intrabody techniques.

This approach enables the definition of pathways linked with pathogenesis or the contribution of defined proteins in normal cellular processes. Given the complications of delivering an antibody into the intracellular environment, it perhaps serves more as a route to target discovery and validation than a direct route to therapy.

3.4. Directing Drugs or Other Therapeutic Compounds

Lastly, the specificity of antibodies can be exploited for the specific delivery of drugs and other therapeutics. Obviously, the use of phage display can speed the isolation of antibodies with the desired targeting properties. Genetic fusion has been used to link recombinant antibodies to other proteins that possess toxic activity *(15)* but the introduction of nonnative residues at the terminus of the recombinant antibody has also allowed the application of conjugative chemistry *(66,90)*. By linking enzymes to the antibody, nontoxic prodrugs can be converted to their active form in situ for anticancer therapy *(91)* or thrombolytic agents can be delivered *(92)*. Recombinant antibodies have also been used for the delivery of drugs across the blood brain barrier *(93)*.

3.5. Future Directions

The flexibility of antibody phage display is such that applications are limited only by the imagination of the investigator. Aided by appreciation of the advantages of phage display methods over hybridoma technology, the literature has now expanded enormously. In consequence, this chapter can only provide an overview of how antibodies can be isolated using these methods, and a brief insight to their potential applications. It is inevitable that the use of these methods and their exploitation will continue, driven by the opportunities from "omics" biology and the need for new therapies.

References

1. Kohler G, Milstein C (1975) Continuous cultures of fused cells secreting antibody of predefined specificitiy. Nature 256:495–497
2. Griffiths AD, Malmqvist M, Marks JD, Bye JM, Embleton MJ, McCafferty J, Baier M, Holliger KP, Gorick BD, Hughesjones NC, Hoogenboom HR, Winter G (1993) Human anti-self antibodies with high specificity from phage display libraries. EMBO J 12:725–734
3. Arndt KM, Muller KM, Pluckthun A (1998) Factors influencing the dimer to monomer transition of an antibody single-chain Fv fragment. Biochemistry 37:12,918–12,926
4. Hoogenboom HR (2005) Selecting and screening recombinant antibody libraries. Nat Biotechnol 23:1105–1116
5. Carmen S, Jermutus L (2002) Concepts in antibody phage display. Brief Funct Genomic Proteomic 1:189–203
6. Conrad U, Scheller J (2005) Considerations in antibody phage display methodology. Comb Chem High Throughput Screen 8:117–126
7. Barbas CF, Kang AS, Lerner RA, Benkovic SJ (1991) Assembly of combinatorial antibody libraries on phage surfaces – the gene III site. Proc Natl Acad Sci USA 88:7978–7982
8. McCafferty J, Griffiths AD, Winter G, Chiswell DJ (1990) Phage antibodies – filamentous phage displaying antibody variable domains. Nature 348:552–554
9. Skerra A, Pluckthun A (1988) Assembly of a functional immunoglobulin-Fv fragment in *Escherichia coli*. Science 240:1038–1041
10. Barbas CF, Crowe JE, Cababa D, Jones TM, Zebedee SL, Murphy BR, Chanock RM, Burton DR (1992) Human monoclonal Fab fragments derived from a combinatorial library bind to respiratory syncytial virus-F glyco-protein and neutralize infectivity. Proc Natl Acad Sci USA 89:10,164–10,168
11. Sanna PP, Samson ME, Moon JS, Rozenshteyn R, De Logu A, Williamson RA, Burton DR (1999) pFab-CMV, a single vector system for the rapid conversion of recombinant Fabs into whole IgG1 antibodies. Immunotechnology 4:185–188
12. Boel E, Verlaan S, Poppelier M, Westerdaal NAC, Van Strijp JAG, Logtenberg T (2000) Functional human monoclonal antibodies of all isotypes constructed from phage display library-derived single-chain Fv antibody fragments. J Immunol Meth 239:153–166
13. Casey JL, Coley AM, Tilley LM, Foley M (2000) Green fluorescent antibodies: novel in vitro tools. Protein Eng 13:445–452
14. Mullen BH, Chevrier D, Boulain JC, Guesdon JL (1999) Recombinant single-chain Fv antibody fragment-alkaline phosphatase conjugate for one-step immunodetection in molecular hybridization. J Immunol Methods 227:177–185

15. Chowdhury PS, Vasmatzis G, Lee B, Pastan I (1998) Improved stability and yield of a Fv-toxin fusion protein by computer design and protein engineering of the Fv. J Mol Biol 281:917–928

16. Zwick MB, Kelleher R, Jensen R, Labrijn AF, Wang M, Quinnan GV, Parren P, Burton DR (2003) A novel human antibody against human immunodeficiency virus type 1 gp120 is V1, V2, and V3 loop dependent and helps delimit the epitope of the broadly neutralizing antibody immunoglobulin G1 b12. J Virol 77:6965–6978

17. Cardoso RMF, Zwick MB, Stanfield RL, Kunert R, Binley JM, Katinger H, Burton DR, Wilson IA (2005) Broadly neutralizing anti-HIV antibody 4E10 recognizes a helical conformation of a highly conserved fusion-associated motif in gp41. Immunity 22:163–173

18. Fostieri E, Tzartos SJ, Berrih-Aknin S, Beeson D, Mamalaki A (2005) Isolation of potent human Fab fragments against a novel highly immunogenic region on human muscle acetylcholine receptor which protect the receptor from myasthenic autoantibodies. Eur J Immunol 35:632–643

19. Ando T, Yamashiro T, Takita-Sonoda Y, Mannen K, Nishizono A (2005) Construction of human Fab library and isolation of monoclonal Fabs with rabies virus-neutralizing ability. Microbiol Immunol 49:311–322

20. Edwards BM, Barash SC, Main SH, Choi GH, Minter R, Ullrich S, Williams E, Du Fou L, Wilton J, Albert VR, Ruben SM, Vaughan TJ (2003) The remarkable flexibility of the human antibody repertoire; Isolation of over one thousand different antibodies to a single protein, BLyS. J Mol Biol 334:103–118

21. Coomber DWJ, Hawkins NJ, Clark MA, Ward RL (1999) Generation of anti-p53 Fab fragments from individuals with colorectal cancer using phage display. J Immunol 163:2276–2283

22. Reason DC, Wagner TC, Lucas AH (1997) Human fab fragments specific for the *Haemophilus influenzae* b polysaccharide isolated from a bacteriophage combinatorial library use variable region gene combinations and express an idiotype that mirrors in vivo expression. Inf Immunity 65:261–266

23. Dohmen SE, Mulder A, Verhagen O, Eijsink C, Franke-van Dijk MEI, van der Schoot CE (2005) Production of recombinant Ig molecules from antigen-selected single B cells and restricted usage of Ig-gene segments by anti-D antibodies. J Immunol Methods 298:9–20

24. Koefoed K, Farnaes L, Wang M, Svejgaard A, Burton DR, Ditzel HJ (2005) Molecular characterization of the circulating anti-HIV-1 gp120-specific B cell repertoire using antibody phage display libraries generated from pre-selected HIV-1 gp120 binding PBLs. J Immunol Methods 297:187–201

25. de Wildt RMT, Steenbakkers PG, Pennings AHM, vandenHoogen FHJ, van Venrooij WJ, Hoet RMA (1997) A new method for the analysis and production of monoclonal antibody fragments originating from single human B cells. J Immunol Methods 207:61–67

26. Cardoso DF, Nato F, England P, Ferreira ML, Vaughan TJ, Mota I, Mazie JC, Choumet V, Lafaye P (2000) Neutralizing human anti crotoxin scFv isolated from a nonimmunized phage library. Scand J Immunol 51:337–344

27. Vaughan TJ, Williams AJ, Pritchard K, Osbourn JK, Pope AR, Earnshaw JC, McCafferty J, Hodits RA, Wilton J, Johnson KS (1996) Human antibodies with sub-nanomolar affinities isolated from a large non-immunized phage display library. Nat Biotechnol 14:309–314

28. de Haard HJ, van Neer N, Reurs A, Hufton SE, Roovers RC, Henderikx P, de Bruine AP, Arends JW, Hoogenboom HR (1999) A large non-immunized human Fab fragment phage library that permits rapid isolation and kinetic analysis of high affinity antibodies. J Biol Chem 274:18,218–18,230

29. Gram H, Marconi LA, Barbas CF, Collet TA, Lerner RA, Kang AS (1992) *In vitro* selection and affinity maturation of antibodies from a naive combinatorial immunoglobulin library. Proc Natl Acad Sci USA 89:3576–3580

30. Zhu HP, Wang YC, Jiang M, Ji SD, Bai X, Ruan CG (2005) Generation and characterization of a recombinant single chain Fv antibody to von Willebrand factor A1 domain from phage display library. Thromb Res 116:385–391

31. Cai XH, Garen A (1996) A melanoma-specific V-H antibody cloned from a fusion phage library of a vaccinated melanoma patient. Proc Natl Acad Sci USA 93:6280–6285

32. Manoutcharian K, Acero G, Munguia ME, Montero JA, Govezensky K, Cao C, Ugen K, Gevorkian G (2003) Amyloid-beta peptide-specific single chain Fv antibodies isolated from an immune phage display library. J Neuroimmunol 145:12–17

33. Li Y, Cockburn W, Kilpatrick JB, Whitelam I (2000) High affinity ScFvs from a single rabbit immunized with multiple haptens. Biochem Biophys Res Commun 268:398–404

34. Amersdorfer P, Wong C, Smith T, Chen S, Deshpande S, Sheridan R, Marks JD (2002) Genetic and immunological comparison of anti-botulinum type A antibodies from immune and non-immune human phage libraries. Vaccine 20:1640–1648

35. Hayhurst A, Happe S, Mabry R, Koch Z, Iverson BL, Georgiou G (2003) Isolation and expression of recombinant antibody fragments to the biological warfare pathogen *Brucella melitensis*. J Immunol Methods 276:185–196

36. Rhyner C, Weichel M, Hubner P, Achatz G, Blaser K, Crameri R (2003) Phage display of human antibodies from a patient suffering from coeliac disease and selection of isotype-specific scFv against gliadin. Immunology 110:269–274

37. Duenas M, Ayala M, Vazquez J, Ohlin M, Soderlind E, Borrebaeck CAK, Gavilondo JV (1995) A point mutation in a murine immunoglobulin V region strongly influences the antibody yield in Escherichia coli Gene 158:61–66

38. Lee CV, Liang WC, Dennis MS, Eigenbrot C, Sidhu SS, Fuh G (2004) High-affinity human antibodies from phage-displayed synthetic fab libraries with a single framework scaffold. J Mol Biol 340:1073–1093

39. der Maur AA, Escher D, Barberis A (2001) Anugen-independent selection of stable intracellular single-chain antibodies. Febs Letters 508:407–412

40. Steinhauer C, Wingren C, Hager ACM, Borrebaeck CAK (2002) Single framework recombinant antibody fragments designed for protein chip applications. Biotechniques Suppl., 38–45

41. Desiderio A, Franconi R, Lopez M, Villani ME, Viti F, Chiaraluce R, Consalvi V, Neri D, Benvenuto E (2001) A semi-synthetic repertoire of intrinsically stable antibody fragments derived from a single-framework scaffold. J Mol Biol 310: 603–615

42. Nissim A, Hoogenboom HR, Tomlinson IM, Flynn G, Midgley C, Lane D, Winter G (1994) Antibody fragments from a single pot phage display library as immunochemical reagents. Embo J 13:692–698

43. Cook GP, Tomlinson IM (1995) The human immunoglobulin V_H repertoire. Immunol Today 16:237–242

44. Flajnik MF (2002) Comparative analyses of immunoglobulin genes: surprises and portents. Nat Rev Immunol 2:688–698

45. Little M, Breitling F, Micheel B, Dubel S (1994) Surface display of antibodies. Biotechnol Adv 12:539–555

46. Holliger P, Riechmann L, Williams RL (1999) Crystal structure of the two N-terminal domains of g3p from filamentous phage fd at 1.9 angstrom: evidence for conformational lability. J Mol Biol 288:649–657

47. Smith GP (1985) Filamentous fusion phage – novel expression vectors that display cloned antigens on the virion surface. Science 228:1315–1317

48. de Bruin R, Spelt K, Mol J, Koes R, Quattrocchio F (1999) Selection of high-affinity phage antibodies from phage display libraries. Nat Biotechnol 17:397–399

49. Goletz S, Christensen PA, Kristensen P, Blohm D, Tomlinson I, Winter G, Karsten U (2002) Selection of large diversities of antiidiotypic antibody fragments by phage display. J Mol Biol 315:1087–1097

50. Kramer RA, Cox F, van der Horst M, van den Oudenrijn S, Res PCM, Bia J, Logtenberg T, de Kruif J (2003) A novel helper phage that improves phage display selection efficiency by preventing the amplification of phages without recombinant protein. Nucl Acids Res 31:e59

51. Parmley SF, Smith GP (1988) Antibody-selectable filamentous Fd phage vectors – affinity purification of target genes. Gene 73:305–318

52. Santala V, Saviranta P (2004) Affinity-independent elution of antibody-displaying phages using cleavable DNA linker containing streptavidin beads. J Immunol Methods 284:159–163

53. Chames P, Hufton SE, Coulie PG, Uchanska-Ziegler B, Hoogenboom HR (2000) Direct selection of a human antibody fragment directed against the tumor T-cell epitope HLA-A1-MAGE-A1 from a nonimmunized phage-Fab library. Proc Natl Acad Sci USA 97:7969–7974

54. McElhiney J, Drever M, Lawton LA, Porter AJ (2002) Rapid isolation of a single-chain antibody against the cyanobacterial toxin microcystin-LR by phage display and its use in the immunoaffinity concentration of microcystins from water. Appl Env Microbiol 68:5288–5295

55. Stausbol-Gron B, Jensen KB, Jensen KH, Jensen MO, Clark BFC (2001) De novo identification of cell-type specific antibody-antigen pairs by phage display subtraction – Isolation of a human single chain antibody fragment against human keratin 14. Eur J Biochem 268:3099–3107

56. de Wildt RMT, Mundy CR, Gorick BD, Tomlinson IM (2000) Antibody arrays for high-throughput screening of antibody–antigen interactions. Nat Biotechnol 18:989–994

57. Holt LJ, Enever C, de Wildt RMT, Tomlinson IM (2000) The use of recombinant antibodies in proteomics. Curr Opin Biotechnol 11:445–449

58. Kipriyanov SM, Moldenhauer G, and Little M (1997) High level production of soluble single chain antibodies in small-scale *Escherichia coli* cultures. J Immunol Methods 200:69–77

59. Kipriyanov SM, Moldenhauer G, Martin ACR, Kupriyanova OA, Little M (1997) Two amino acid mutations in an anti-human CD3 single chain Fv antibody fragment that affect the yield on bacterial secretion but not the affinity. Protein Eng 10:445–453

60. Malmborg AC, Duenas M, Ohlin M, Soderlind E, Borrebaeck CAK (1996) Selection of binders from phage displayed antibody libraries using the BIAcore(TM) biosensor. J Immunol Methods 198:51–57

61. Chowdhury PS, Pastan I (1999) Improving antibody affinity by mimicking somatic hypermutation *in vitro*. Nat Biotechnol 17:568–572

62. Daugherty PS, Chen G, Iverson BL, Georgiou G (2000) Quantitative analysis of the effect of the mutation frequency on the affinity maturation of single chain Fv antibodies. Proc Natl Acad Sci USA 97:2029–2034

63. Rau D, Kramer K, Hock B (2002) Single-chain Fv antibody-alkaline phosphatase fusion proteins produced by one-step cloning as rapid detection tools for ELISA. J Immuno Immunochem 23:129–143

64. Hink MA, Griep RA, Borst JW, van Hoek A, Eppink MHM, Schots A, Visser A (2000) Structural dynamics of green fluorescent protein alone and fused with a single chain Fv protein. J Biol Chem 275:17,556–17,560

65. Kipriyanov SM, Dubel S, Breitling F, Kontermann RE, Heymann S, Little M (1995) Bacterial expression and refolding of single chain Fv fragments with C-terminal cysteines. Cell Biophys 26:187–204

66. Albrecht H, Burke PA, Natarajan A, Xiong CY, Kalicinsky M, DeNardo GL, DeNardo SJ (2004) Production of soluble scFvs with C-terminal-free thiol for

site-specific conjugation or stable dimeric scFvs on demand. Bioconjug Chem 15:16–26

67. Hayhurst A, Harris WJ (1999) *Escherichia coli* Skp chaperone coexpression improves solubility and phage display of single-chain antibody fragments. Protein Expr Purif 15:336–343

68. Hayhurst A (2000) Improved expression characteristics of single-chain Fv fragments when fused downstream of the *Escherichia coli* maltose-binding protein or upstream of a single immunoglobulin-constant domain. Protein Expr Purif 18:1–10

69. Ohara R, Knappik A, Shimada K, Frisch C, Ylera F, Koga H (2006) Antibodies for proteomic research: comparison of traditional immunization with recombinant antibody technology. Proteomics 6:2638–2646

70. Harvey BR, Georgiou G, Hayhurst A, Jeong KJ, Iverson BL, Rogers GK (2004) Anchored periplasmic expression, a versatile technology for the isolation of high-affinity antibodies from *Escherichia coli*-expressed libraries. Proc Natl Acad Sci USA 101:9193–9198

71. Wang SH, Zhang JB, Zhang ZP, Zhou YF, Yang RF, Chen J, Guo YC, You F, Zhang XE (2006) Construction of single chain variable fragment (scFv) and BiscFv-alka-line phosphatase fusion protein for detection of *Bacillus anthracis*. Anal Chem 78:997–1004

72. Chen ZC, Moayeri M, Zhou YH, Leppla S, Emerson S, Sebrell A, Yu FJ, Svitel J, Schuck P, St Claire M, Purcell R (2006) Efficient neutralization of anthrax toxin by chimpanzee monoclonal antibodies against protective antigen. J Inf Diseases 193:625–633

73. Higo-Moriguchi K, Akahori Y, Iba Y, Kurosawa Y, Taniguchi K (2004) Isolation of human monoclonal antibodies that neutralize human rotavirus. J Virol 78:3325–3332

74. Duan JZ, Yan XY, Guo XM, Cao WC, Han W, Qi C, Feng J, Yang DL, Gao GX, Jin G (2005) A human SARS-CoV neutralizing antibody against epitope on S2 protein. Biochem Biophys Res Commun 333:186–193

75. Liang MF, Du RL, Liu JZ, Li C, Zhang QF, Han LL, Yu JS, Duan SM, Wang XF, Wu KX, Xiong ZH, Jin Q, Li DX (2005) SARS patients-derived human recom-binant antibodies to S and M proteins efficiently neutralize SARS-coronavirus infectivity. Biomed Envi Sci 18:363–374

76. Chen ZC, Earl P, Americo J, Damon I, Smith SK, Zhou YH, Yu FJ, Sebrell A, Emerson S, Cohen G, Eisenberg RJ, Svitel J, Schuck P, Satterfield W, Moss B, Purcell R (2006) Chimpanzee/human mAbs to vaccinia virus B5 protein neutralize vaccinia and smallpox viruses and protect mice against vaccinia virus. Proc Natl Acad Sci USA 103:1882–1887

77. Schofield DJ, Bartosch B, Shimizu YK, Allander T, Alter HJ, Emerson SU, Cosset FL, Purcell RH (2005) Human monoclonal antibodies that react with the E2 glycoprotein of hepatitis C virus and possess neutralizing activity. Hepatology 42:1055–1062

78. Koch J, Liang MF, Queitsch I, Kraus AA, Bautz EKF (2003) Human recombinant neutralizing antibodies against Hantaan virus G2 protein. Virology 308:64–73

79. Kausmally L, Waalen K, Lobersli I, Hvattum E, Berntsen G, Michaelsen TE, Brekke OH (2004) Neutralizing human antibodies to varicella-zoster virus (VZV) derived from a VZV patient recombinant antibody library. J Gen Virol 85:3493–3500

80. Popkov M, Rader C, Barbas CF (2004) Isolation of human prostate cancer cell reac-tive antibodies using phage display technology. J Immunol Methods 291:137–151

81. Reusch U, Le Gall F, Hensel M, Moldenhauer G, Ho AD, Little M, Kipriyanov SM (2004) Effect of tetravalent bispecific CD19xCD3 recombinant antibody construct and CD28 costimulation on lysis of malignant B cells from patients with chronic lymphocytic leukemia by autologous T cells. Int J Cancer 112:509–518

82. Bruenke J, Fischer B, Barbin K, Schreiter K, Wachter Y, Mahr K, Titgemeyer F, Niederweis M, Peipp M, Zunino SJ, Repp R, Valerius T, Fey GH (2004)

A recombinant bispecific single-chain Fv antibody against HLA class II and Fc gamma RIII (CD16) triggers effective lysis of lymphoma cells. Br J Haematol 125:167–179

83. Belimezi MM, Papanastassiou D, Merkouri E, Baxevanis CN, Mamalaki A (2006) Growth inhibition of breast cancer cell lines overexpressing Her2/neu by a novel internalized fully human Fab antibody fragment. Cancer Immunol Immunother 55:1091–1099

84. Lobato MN, Rabbitts TH (2003) Intracellular antibodies and challenges facing their use as therapeutic agents. Trends Mol Med 9:390–396

85. Accardi L, Dona MG, Di Bonito P, Giorgi C (2005) Intracellular anti-E7 human antibodies in single-chain format inhibit proliferation of HPV16-positive cervical carcinoma cells. Int J Cancer 116:564–570

86. Griffin H, Elston R, Jackson D, Ansell K, Coleman M, Winter G, Doorbar J (2006) Inhibition of papillomavirus protein function in cervical cancer cells by intrabody targeting. J Mol Biol 355:360–378

87. Wolfgang WJ, Miller TW, Webster JM, Huston JS, Thompson LM, Marsh JL, Messer A (2005) Suppression of Huntington's disease pathology in *Drosophila* by human single-chain Fv antibodies. Proc Natl Acad Sci USA 102:11,563–11,568

88. Arbel M, Yacoby I, Solomon B (2004) Inhibition of amyloid precursor protein processing by beta-secretase through site-directed antibodies. Proc Natl Acad Sci USA 102:7718–7723

89. Paz K, Brennan LA, Iacolina M, Doody J, Hadari YR, Zhu ZP (2005) Human single-domain neutralizing intrabodies directed against Etk kinase: a novel approach to impair cellular transformation. Mol Cancer Therap 4:1801–1809

90. Natarajan A, Xiong CY, Albrecht H, DeNardo GL, DeNardo SJ (2005) Characterization of site-specific ScFv PEGylation for tumor-targeting pharmaceuticals. Biocon Chem 16:113–121

91. Alderson RF, Toki BE, Roberge M, Geng W, Basler J, Chin R, Liu A, Ueda R, Hodges D, Escandon E, Chen T, Kanavarioti T, Babe L, Senter PD, Fox JA, Schellenberger V (2006) Characterization of a CC49-based single-chain fragment-beta-lactamase fusion protein for antibody-directed enzyme prodrug therapy (ADEPT). Biocon Chem 17:410–418

92. Ding BS, Gottstein C, Grunow A, Kuo A, Ganguly K, Albelda SM, Cines DB, Muzykantov VR (2005) Endothelial targeting of a recombinant construct fusing a PECAM-1 single-chain variable antibody fragment (scFv) with prourokinase facilitates prophylactic thrombolysis in the pulmonary vasculature. Blood 106:4191–4198

93. Abulrob A, Sprong H, Henegouwen P, Stanimirovic D (2005) The blood-brain barrier transmigrating single domain antibody: mechanisms of transport and antigenic epitopes in human brain endothelial cells. J Neurochem 95:1201–1214

35

Protein Engineering

Thomas Willemsen*, Urs B. Hagemann*, Eva M. Jouaux*, Sabine C. Stebel,
Jody M. Mason, Kristian M. Müller, and Katja M. Arndt

1. Introduction to Protein Engineering

Relating primary sequence to three-dimensional structure has long been the
holy grail of structural biology and appears to be far from achievement. Within
grasp however, is the use of intuitive or unintuitive methodology to modify
existing known protein structures to achieve the desired effect. We use *protein
engineering* as a general term for the design of proteins with useful or valuable
properties. The technique has become possible due to our increasing knowledge
of detailed protein structures, which in turn highlights potential for improving
key facets of protein structure; for example, the mutation of specific residues
with a view to improving binding or catalysis. This *rational design* (Section
2.1) requires the scientist to have a detailed prior knowledge of the protein to
attempt to make specific informed changes to the sequence to exert the desired
effect. The technique is quite straightforward, involving mutation at the genetic
level followed by expression and characterization. This site-directed mutagenesis approach is discussed in Section 2.1.1. However, rational mutations do not
always generate the desired effect. This has invariably led to computer-based
approaches for protein design. These are designed to save time in identifying
mutations that generate the desired effect of low energy structures, and aim for
lower the sequence conformation space that is required in the search. To simplify the procedure, these algorithms are based on approximations that require
less processing time. Unfortunately, approximations can also lead to false
positives which do not yield the predicted desired effect at the protein level.
Computer aided protein engineering strategies are discussed in Section 2.1.2.

The second protein engineering approach, known as *directed evolution*
relies on a selection system to pick from a range of variants. This involves the
construction of protein libraries that contain a wealth of randomized positions.
The generation of libraries is discussed extensively in the chapter "*Directed
Protein Evolution*" in this book. Many of these residues will be intuitively
predicted to have the desired result, while for other residues the outcome of
the change may not be known. By screening these mutations at the protein

---

*TW, UBB and EMJ contributed equally.

From: *Molecular Biomethods Handbook, 2nd Edition.*
Edited by: J. M. Walker and R. Rapley © Humana Press, Totowa, NJ

level for their desired function, sequences conforming to the best molecule for the desired role can be screened. This has the advantage over site-directed mutagenesis or computer-based design that you obtain exactly what you select for. Theory of library-based design strategies is discussed in Section 2.2, and includes a discussion as well as published examples of the phage display (2.2.1.), ribosome display (2.2.2.), and yeast two-hybrid systems (2.2.3) that have been used to screen protein libraries. Also discussed are the advantages and pitfalls of working with any one of these techniques. Protein-fragment complementation assay (PCA) systems are discussed (2.2.4) along with several examples of the screening system in action, as well as methods of cell surface display (2.2.5). Finally, *in vitro* compartmentalization methods are discussed (2.2.6). The chapter closes (Section 3) with a range of examples for each of the techniques highlighted.

2. Methods

2.1. Rational Design Strategies

Rational design is one of the strategies for protein engineering in which a detailed knowledge of the structure and function of the protein is used to predict beneficial changes. These changes are introduced into the protein by site-directed mutagenesis techniques. As an increasing number of high-resolution protein structures is available the creation and application of computational methods to identify amino acid sequences that have low energies for the target structure is used more and more. These two principles can complement each other or be used alone. The major drawback is the need of detailed structural knowledge of a protein, and depending on the design, it can be extremely difficult to predict the effects of various mutations, especially long-range effects.

A variety of strategies have emerged for modulating protein properties, such as stability, specificity, solubility, conformational state, binding affinity, oligomerization state, substrate selectivity for enzymes, protease susceptibility, immunogenicity, and pharmacokinetics (the last three for therapeutical approaches) (see **Fig. 35.1**). Mechanisms for altering these properties include manipulation of the primary structure, incorporation of chemical and post-translational modifications and utilization of fusion-partners *(1)*. There are many rational strategies to change protein characteristics. One simple stabilization strategy is to replace free cysteines, thereby preventing the formation of unwanted intermolecular and intramolecular disulphide bonds. Substituting exposed nonpolar residues with polar residues can enable soluble expression and improve the solubility of the protein. Alteration of the net charge and isoelectric point (pI) of a protein can also affect its solubility. In some cases, increasing the binding affinity for a target protein can produce an increase in biological activity. In other cases, it is possible to reduce undesired biological activities by decreasing the affinity for nontarget molecules. Many proteins undergo conformational changes that are central to their function. In such cases, the conformational equilibrium can be driven towards the desired state.

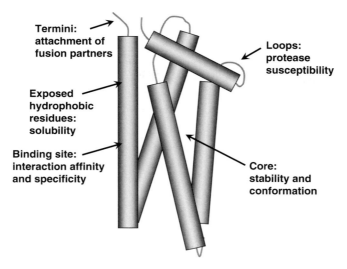

Fig. 35.1. Different strategies for rational protein design

The starting point for rational design is the development of a molecular model, based on the protein structure and function, often in combination with an algorithm. This is followed by experimental construction and analysis of the properties of the designed protein. If the experimental outcome is failure or partial success, then a next round of the design cycle is started *(2)*. Sometimes new mutants based on initial information are developed which leads to a repetition of design steps until a variant is found that meets all the requirements. This iterative process, where theory and experiments alters, is often referred to as a "design cycle."

A possible design strategy procedure is described below, based on the availability of a 3-D structure and sequence of the protein *(3)*.

1. Collect available information from the literature as well as from experimental analysis on the protein of interest, its homologues and other family members.
2. Find as many amino acid sequences as possible of homologues sequences and make a multiple sequence alignment. Take the secondary structure of the protein into account (see, e.g., www.expasy.org for databases and tools).
3. Compare the structures of the protein, homologues and family members by structural alignment to see, whether there is anything remarkable and whether all residues are in an optimal structural environment. Also check whether any of the homologues structures are more stable and if so, why. Examine if the structures possess additional interactions in the form of salt bridges, disulphide bridges, etc. Verify the difference in packing i.e., by looking for any cavities or steric clashes. Take variations in loop length or other conspicuous differences into account. Helpful programs are PyMol and Swiss PDB Viewer.
4. Try and apply the design concepts as described above. Also, apply programs that can predict mutations. You can find a variety of such tools on www.expasy.org/tools/.

5. Simulate the protein under folding conditions and identify the regions that appear to be the least stable. Try to design mutants that counteract the early unfolding processes.

6. Model the mutants you have and check whether the structure has improved and whether the mutation causes other problems, like less favorable torsion angles in the side chain or less optimal packing.

7. Produce the mutants experimentally and analyze their properties.

Nowadays, the first steps of rational design are more and more computer based but historically, site-directed mutagenesis was first. Here, we kept this chronological order.

2.1.1. Site-Directed Mutagenesis

Since the late 1980s protein molecules were altered by site-directed or site-specific mutagenesis of their genes *(4–6)*. In this technique, a mutation is created at a defined site in the DNA leading to a change in the amino acid of the corresponding protein. This method requires the wild-type sequence to be known. The change itself is made by PCR methods where primers containing the desired mutation are used. In the first cycle, there is a priming mismatch for the primers binding the template DNA strand, but after the first cycle, the primer-based strand, containing the mutation, will be at about equal concentration to the original template. After successive cycles, its number will increase exponentially and outnumber the original, unmutated strand, resulting in a nearly homogeneous solution of mutated amplified fragments. For this PCR it is necessary to design primers that are suitable for the desired changes, considering also their annealing temperature.

Two techniques are commonly used to introduce specific amino acid replacements into a target gene. The first of these is termed the overlap extension method (**Fig. 35.2**). In this method, four primers are used in the

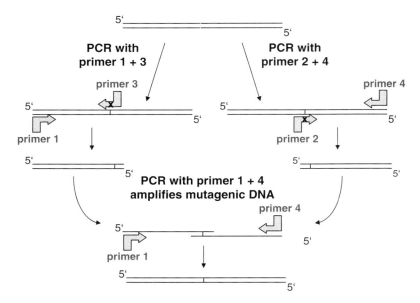

Fig. 35.2. Principle of site-directed mutagenesis by overlap extension. Mutations introduced by primers 2 and 3 are marked with an "x". Further explanations are given in the text

first polymerase chain reaction (PCR) step with two separate PCRs being performed. The primer pairs for these PCRs are 1 and 3 as well as 2 and 4, respectively, with primers 2 and 3 containing the mutant codon with a mismatched sequence. Two double-stranded DNA products containing the desired mutagenic codon are obtained over several PCR cycles. In the second PCR step these two dsDNA products are amplified using primers 1 and 4 resulting in the mutated DNA. A useful variant of the overlap extension method is the megaprimer method (7). In this procedure, two rounds of PCR are performed employing two flanking primers and one internal mutagenic primer that contains the desired base substitutions. A benefit of this method is that mutations can be inserted into the flanking primers so that multiple codons relatively far from each other can be replaced at the once. The second method for performing site-directed mutagenesis is referred to as whole plasmid, single-round PCR (**Fig. 35.3**). In this protocol, two oligonucleotide primers containing the desired mutation(s) are extended with DNA polymerase. In this PCR step, both strands of the template are replicated without displacing the primers to obtain a mutated plasmid containing breaks that do not overlap. As the original wild type plasmid originates from *Eschenichia coli* and is thus methylated on various A and C residues, it may then be selectively digested using DpnI methylase endonuclease resulting in a circular, nicked vector containing the mutant gene. When this nicked vector is transformed into competent cells, the nick in the DNA is repaired by the cell machinery to give a mutated, circular plasmid. The advantages of the whole plasmid, single-round PCR are that only one PCR needs to be performed and only two primers are required. The disadvantages of this technique relative to overlap extension are that it does not work well with large plasmids (>10 kB) and typically only two nucleotides can be replaced at a time (8). Several companies offer kits for performing these methods.

After the PCR step and the cloning and/or transformation, expression and purification of the recombinant protein mutants must be performed for testing and evaluation.

2.1.2. Computational Protein Design

During the past two decades, computer simulations of the dynamics of proteins has become a widely used tool to deepen our understanding of these molecules. Computer simulations can be used to understand the properties of a molecular system in terms of interactions at the atomic level. One of the main challenges is the development of algorithms that can deal directly with structural and

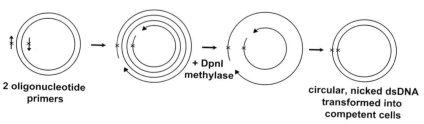

Fig. 35.3. Principle of site-directed mutagenesis by whole plasmid, single-round PCR. Explanations are given in the text

functional specificity. An excellent overview of the strengths and weaknesses of various search algorithms is reported *(9)*, and implementations of these algorithms were quantitatively evaluated *(10)*.

Computational protein design methods seek to identify amino acid sequences that generate low-energy interactions of a specified target protein structure by employing a variety of optimization techniques. These fall into two broad categories: stochastic algorithms, including Monte Carlo, and deterministic algorithms, including dead-end elimination. Stochastic algorithms semi-randomly sample sequence-structure space and move toward lower energy solutions whereas deterministic algorithms perform semi-exhaustive searches.

The advantage of stochastic methods is that they can deal with problems of significant combinatorial complexity because they do not require an exhaustive search. The disadvantage is that there is no guarantee that these methods converge to the global minimum energy solution or even the same solution when run multiple times *(10)*. In contrast, deterministic methods always converge on the same solution.

2.1.2.1. Monte Carlo (MC) Method: These simplest stochastic methods are a widely used class of computational algorithms for simulating the behavior of various physical and mathematical systems. They are distinguished from other simulation methods (such as Molecular Dynamics, see Section 2.1.2.3.) in that they are nondeterministic in some manner, usually by using random numbers. In the context of design, a starting structure is perturbed by a random change in residue type or rotamer at some position. If the change decreases the energy of the structure, it is accepted. Otherwise, the Metropolis criterion, including a Bolzmann weighted probability, is used to accept or reject the change. This permits energetically unfavored uphill moves and escape from local minima. MC methods are especially useful in studying systems with a large number of coupled degrees of freedom, such as liquids, disordered materials, and strongly coupled solids *(11,12)*.

2.1.2.2. Dead-End Elimination (DEE): The DEE algorithm is a method for minimizing a function over a discrete set of independent variables. The basic idea is to identify "dead ends," i.e., "bad" combinations of variables that cannot possibly yield the global minimum and to refrain from searching such combinations further. Hence, good combinations are identified and explored further. The method itself has been developed and applied mainly to the problems of predicting and designing the structures of proteins *(13)*. The basic requirements for DEE are a well-defined finite set of discrete independent variables, a precomputed numerical value, the energy, associated with each element in the set of variables, a criterion or criteria for determining when an element is a "dead end," and an objective function, the energy function, to be minimized. DEE has been used efficiently to predict the structure of side chains on a given protein backbone structure by minimizing an energy function. A large-scale benchmark of DEE compared to alternative methods of protein structure prediction and design is that DEE reliably converges to the optimal solution for a given protein length, and it runs in a reasonable amount of time *(13)*. However, other methods are significantly faster than DEE and thus can be applied to larger and more complex problems. DEE is guaranteed to converge to the global minimum energy solution *(13)*. The effectiveness of DEE for a combinatorial search is due to the systematic elimination or pruning of high-energy rotamers or rotamer-combination. A requirement is that the energy function must be written as the sum of individual and pairwise terms. Additionally, for extremely complex problems, DEE may fail to converge, but due to some large improvements DEE currently seems to be the most powerful method for finding the global minimum energy solution (10).

2.1.2.3. Molecular Dynamics (MD) Simulation: Molecular modeling tools are used in protein engineering studies to indicate which amino acid substitutions or mutations have a high probability of success and should be tested experimentally. Molecular dynamics (MD) are able to correlate the increase in protein stabilization with the conformational and structural changes caused by (single) amino acid replacements. It represents an interface between laboratory experiments and theory. MD also serves as a tool in protein structure determination and refinement using experimental tools such as X-ray crystallography and NMR. Additionally, MD has been applied as a method of redefining protein structure prediction.

The computer simulation method of MD is based on an extremely simple principle: given the coordinates of all atoms in a molecular system and an accurate description of the total potential interaction energy as a function of the atomic coordinates, the force on each atom can be calculated. Describing the interactions accurately in a protein is a key element to protein design and probably the most difficult. The energy functions must be fast and accurate, yet not oversensitive to the fixed backbone approximations and discreteness of the rotamer library (reviewed in **ref. 14**). In chemistry and biophysics, the interaction between the objects can be described by a force field. Molecular mechanics force fields for proteins, such as AMBER, GROMOS, and CHARMM, usually include van der Waals, electrostatics, dihedral angle (torsion), bond angle, and bond stretching (length) terms. These parameters are further adjusted by simulations that attempt to reproduce experimental data, such as small molecular crystal structures. For protein design calculations, considerable modifications are required. Energies must be adjusted to reduce artifacts resulting from the use of discrete rotamers and fixed backbones. Energy terms that describe solvation must be added. Secondary structure propensities have also been used as constraints for sequence design. A reference state needs to be defined, since the relevant value for protein design is the difference in energy between the probed and reference state. Finally, all these terms must be weighted appropriately. For molecular dynamics simulations, the individual energy terms are typically added and must be appropriately parameterized and scaled with respect to one another (15).

Considerations for computational protein design (16):

1. Energy expression or force field used to rank the desirability of each amino acid sequence for a particular backbone.
2. Energy minimization of the target backbone must be determined in order to experimentally test the energy expression. (Published algorithms include MC techniques and DEE).
3. Discrete side chain conformations must be made to restrict the complexity to a reasonable limit. The allowed side chain conformations are typically chosen from a library of discrete possibilities, known as rotamers.
4. Classification of residue position to reduce the size of the design problem. Protein cores are typically composed of hydrophobic amino acids, and

protein surfaces are largely composed of hydrophilic amino acids, but the boundary residues must be selected from the full range of amino acids as these positions are observed to be both.

5. Modeling of backbone flexibility by using a softer van der Waals potential, which means, giving the modeled atoms a fuzzy edge.

Available computer power must be considered when designing MD simulations. Simulation size (number of particles, typically up to 10^5 atoms), time-steps and total time duration must be selected so that the calculation can finish within reasonable time. However, the simulations should be long enough to be relevant to the time scale of the natural processes being studied. Most scientific publications about the dynamics of proteins and DNA use data from simulations spanning nanoseconds to microseconds. To obtain such simulations, several CPU-days to CPU-years are needed. Another factor that impacts total CPU requirement by a simulation is the size of the integration time-step. This is the time length between evaluations of the potential. The time-step must be chosen small enough to avoid discrete errors. Typical time-steps for classical MD are in the order of one femtosecond. Furthermore, a choice should be made between explicit solvent and implicit solvent. Explicit solvent particles (like water) must be calculated extensively by the force field. The impact of explicit solvents on CPU-time can be 10-fold or more. In simulations with explicit solvent molecules, the simulation box must be large enough to avoid boundary condition artifacts.

Limitations must not only be kept in mind when setting up simulations but also when drawing conclusions from such simulations. Consequently, the results of simulations must be critically evaluated and, whenever possible, validated through experiments. When applied in an appropriate way, MD is a tool complementary to experimental methods, which can be used to access atomic details inaccessible to experimental probes *(17)*.

2.2. Library-Based Design Strategies

Library-based design strategies have the advantage that they do not rely on structural information. Various methods for designing libraries exists which are described in detail in the chapter *Directed Protein Evolution*. The success of libraries, however, strongly depends on the selection or screening method. This section introduces the most prominent techniques and discusses advantages and disadvantages of each system.

2.2.1. Phage Display

Phage display is a reliable and widely used selection technique. It enables the rapid screening of peptide libraries or proteins against virtually any desired target both of biological and synthetic origin. This could be either of biological interest or for technical or medical applications. The benefits of phage display rely on the fact that the phenotype is directly linked to the genotype. This is because the peptides to be screened are expressed as fusion proteins of a phage coating protein, and genetic information is packaged into the phage *(18)*.

Typically, phage display as well as ribosome display (see Section 2.2.2) selection rounds are carried out *in vitro* where incubation with the target takes place. Strongest binders remain bound to the target and nonbinders or only weakly interacting binders are removed from the pool upon increasing stringency. The selected pool of binders is amplified, either in *E. coli* for phage display or by RT-PCR in the case of ribosome display. Enriched phages then enter the next round of selection. This procedure is repeated for three to five times and leads to the enrichment of binders dominating the pool. This procedure is called "panning" and without it would be akin to searching for a needle in a haystack.

Phage display was the first display technology shown to physically couple the phenotype with genotype *(19)*. It was originally used to map antibody epitope binding sites by screening peptide-phage libraries against immobilized immunoglobulins. Filamentous phages use its bacterial host to replicate and to assemble the phage particles. For phage display, the phage genome can be modified to incorporate the gene of interest to be displayed in fusion to a surface protein. The most commonly used phage protein for displaying peptides of interest is the minor coat protein 3, which is presented three to five times on the M13 particle (**Fig. 35.4**) *(20)*. The coat protein of gene 3 consists of three domains, a C-terminal constant region which anchors the protein to the phage particle, and two N-terminal domains, N1 and N2, mediating infectivity. N1 binds to the TolA receptor and N2 binds to the F-pilus of *E. coli*. Proteins of interest are usually fused to the N-terminus of the gene 3 protein. During the assembly process, resulting fusion proteins are transported through the inner cell membrane to the bacterial periplasm and incorporated into the phage particle,

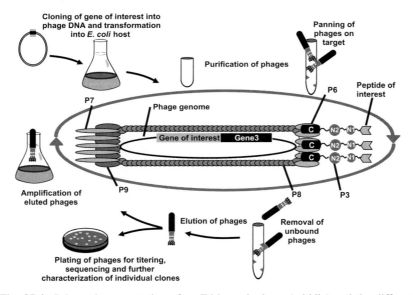

Fig. 35.4. Schematic presentation of an Fd-bacteriophage (middle) and the different steps of a phage panning round. The gene of interest is genetically linked to the N-terminal domain of the phage surface protein 3 and thus is incorporated up to five times in the phage particle (peptide of interest). Another surface protein, which can be used for multivalent display, is the protein P8. After cloning and transformation into the *E. coli* host, phages are purified via polyethylene-glycol precipitation (PEG/NaCl) and incubated with the immobilized target. Unbound phages are removed by increasing washing steps for each selection round. Binders are eluted from the target by acidic pH shift or tryptic digest and amplified upon host *E. coli* infection

while their respective single-stranded DNA (ssDNA) gets packaged in the phage *(20)* thereby coupling phenotype and genotype.

Typically, a selection (or panning) round can be divided into several distinct steps (**Fig. 35.4**) *(21)*. To start, the gene of interest, which can be a library or a single protein, is fused to the gene 3. This modified phage genome is transformed into an *E. coli* host strain (e.g., XL1-blue or ER2738). Upon phage production, the protein of interest is displayed on the phage surface as fusion to protein 3. For the selection, phages are incubated with the target protein, immobilized either in an ELISA well or an immuno test tube. Simple washing steps remove unspecific or weak binding phages. Stringency can be increased from round to round by adding more washing steps and harsher conditions. Phages are well tolerable against heat and denaturing agents *(22)*. Binders are eluted by an acidic pH-shift or by a tryptic digest. These phages are then amplified in an *E. coli* host strain, purified, and enter the next round of selection.

Phage display classically means multivalent display, as the gene 3 protein is modified in the phage genome. This technique is well suited for short peptides that do not influence infectivity of the protein 3. If selection of longer proteins is desired, a trypsin cleavage site should be incorporated between the protein of interest and the protein 3. If phages are eluted by trypsin digest, the protein of interest is cleaved off and the free phages display a wild-type like protein 3. Furthermore, multivalent display is advantageous for low affinity binders. Alternatively, monovalent display can be achieved using a phagemid system *(21)*. In this case, the gene of interest is cloned to a truncated version of gene 3 in a phagemid vector. A phagemid carries in addition to an *E. coli* origin of replication for plasmids and an antibiotic resistance gene an origin of replication for phages, which is only used after cells are super-infected with helper phages. Helper phages provide the full phage genome, including the protein 3. Thus, cells transformed with the phagemid and infected with helper phages express a mixture of wild type and fusion protein 3. Consequently, phages show the same ratio of wild type and fusion protein 3, which ideally is one fusion protein per phage.

Phage display allows for the rapid selection of target-specific binders in three to five panning rounds. Identification of the selected clones occurs via sequencing of the DNA of phage pools and single clones and hence yields directly the primary structure of the selected peptide. Typically, selected peptides harbor affinities in the μM- to the nM-range. Owing to the avidity effect, multivalent display is more sensitive and therefore detects lower-affinity binding.

Beside the protein 3, the major coat protein P8, which is represented up to ~2700 times, can also be used as fusion proteins *(18)*. The high number of displayed peptides in this case was recently shown to have advantages for imaging applications *(23)*. However, the protein 3-based display system is the major method of choice as it enables the screening of large proteins or protein domains. Also, the display efficiency can be increased by choosing different signal sequence domains N-terminally of the protein 3 which are necessary for periplasmic transport during phage assembly *(24)*. Other systems using a split version of the protein 3, so-called "selectively-infective phages" (SIP) have been tested as well but were found to be more susceptible to mutation or recombination events *(25,26)*. The filamentous phage system is limited to proteins which correctly fold in the periplasm of *E. coli*. Other proteins can be screened using lytic phage systems such as T4 *(27)* and T7 *(28)*. The phage assembly and hence incorporation of fusion proteins occurs in the cytoplasm and virions are released upon cell lyses.

2.2.2. Ribosome Display

The first cell-free *in vitro* display described in 1994 was ribosome display *(29)*. The basis of ribosome display is the linkage of the mRNA with the protein of interest. This can be via a stabilized complex on the ribosome (ribosome display) or via a covalent protein-mRNA complex by means of a DNA–puromycin linker (mRNA display).

Typically, a selection round consists of the following steps (**Fig. 35.5**): First, the DNA encoding the gene of interest to be selected needs to be transcribed into mRNA, which is next translated using either a bacterial or a eukaryotic *in vitro* translation system. The stabilization of complexes between the expressed protein, ribosome, and mRNA upon termination of elongation is achieved by a terminator sequence forming a hairpin structure combined with low temperature or chloramphenicol. This is where mRNA-display differs from ribosome display *(30)*. The selected protein is covalently linked to its mRNA via incorporation of puromycin, which has been previously attached to the 3'-end of the mRNA via a short oligonucleotide. Thus, the large complex of ribosome, mRNA and protein in ribosome display is missing in mRNA-display, and unspecific interactions between the selected protein and the ribosomes are circumvented.

Once expressed, the selection rounds itself can be performed. The target of interest is immobilized in an ELISA well or test tube via adsorption, comparable to phage display. Unbound target is removed in washing steps. In mRNA display,

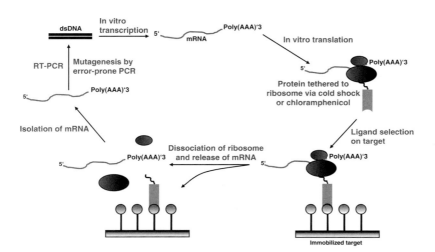

Fig. 35.5. Schematic presentation of a ribosome display round. The gene of interest is transcribed from dsDNA into mRNA and translated into proteins by *in vitro* techniques. The ribosomes remain tethered to the mRNA by either cold shock or chloramphenicol. This step ensures that the genotype remains coupled to the phenotype. The proteins are incubated on the target, and the mRNA of the strongest binding interaction partner is captured after selective washing steps. Using RT-PCR, the mRNA is reverse transcribed into DNA. Using error-prone PCR, defined mutations can be inserted which further increase the binding affinity and specificity

binders are eluted together with their immobilized mRNA, whereas in ribosome display, the mRNA is freed by destroying the protein-ribosome-mRNA complex. In both cases, the mRNA is then amplified by RT-PCR, and the resulting cDNA matrices are transcribed again into mRNA and enter the next round of selection.

One big advantage of ribosome or mRNA display is that it is a cell-free system where expression of toxic proteins or poorly folded proteins can be tolerated. Moreover, the expression and selection of the proteins of interest is not influenced by any growth stress originating from the bacterial host. Importantly, the library size is not limited by transformation efficiencies. Instead, the DNA encoding the library members is directly transcribed into mRNA, and immediately enters the selection process and in this way is only limited by the enzyme reaction. The stringency conditions during the selection rounds are similar to those performed in phage display. However, it is notable that phage particle are very robust. They remain functional even under elevated temperatures or in presence of a chemical denaturant like guanidine. An advantage of mRNA or ribosome display is the potential for affinity maturation through recursive mutagenesis, in which selectants can be further mutated after each round of selection *(31)*. This is faster in comparison to cell-based selection as the encoding DNA does not need to be retransformed into *E. coli* host cells.

2.2.3. Yeast Two-Hybrid System

The "two-hybrid" or "interaction trap" method enables to identify, characterize and even to manipulate protein–protein interactions. It was invented in the early 1990s by Stanke and Fields *(32)*. The yeast-two hybrid system exploits the fact that many eukaryotic transcription factors have at least two distinct functional domains, one that drives DNA-binding to a promoter region and one that activates transcription. It has been shown that DNA-binding and activation domains of one transcription factor can be exchanged from one to another while retaining its function. The basis for this method is the use of the yeast transcription factor GAL4, which is incapable of activating transcription without physical linkage to an activating domain *(33)*. This linkage, which can be mediated by two interacting proteins, is the key to the successful use of the "two-hybrid" method. Only interaction between these proteins connects the DNA-binding domain to the activator domain, resulting in the expression of a reporter gene and thus leading to the identification of interacting partner proteins. The most extensively used vectors are based on GAL4. An alternative system makes use of the DNA-binding domain of the LexA protein and the activator domain of the viral protein 16 (VP16).

In general, in any two-hybrid experiment, a protein of interest is fused to a DNA-binding domain and transfected into a yeast host cell bearing a reporter gene controlled by this DNA-binding domain. This fusion protein, which can not activate transcription on its own, can be used as "bait" or as "target" to screen a library of cDNA clones (prey) that are fused to an activation domain. The cDNA clones capable of forming a protein–protein interaction with the bait protein are identified by their ability to cause activation of the reporter gene (**Fig 35.6A**). The DNA-binding (DBD) domain and the activator domain proteins (AD) can be transformed separately into two different strains, resulting in an AD- and a DBD-strain. In this way, a haploid DBD strain can be mated

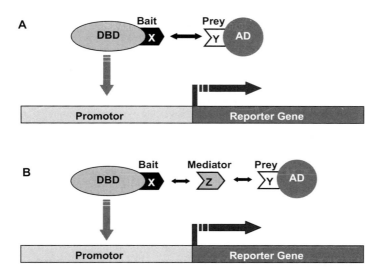

Fig. 35.6. Schematic representation of the yeast two-hybrid (**A**) and yeast three-hybrid system (**B**). (**A**) The bait protein X is genetically fused to a DNA-binding domain (DBD) of a transcription factor, missing the transactivation domain. Upon interaction with the prey protein Y, which is fused to the transactivator domain (AD) of the transcription factor, the transcription of a reporter gene is initiated, and in this manner, an interaction between the bait protein X and the prey protein Y is mapped. (**B**) In the yeast three-hybrid system, the interaction between bait X and prey Y is mediated by a third protein Z

to the haploid AD array to identify individual interacting AD fusions. Another approach would be to mate individual DBD strains with libraries of AD strains (*34*). Reporter gene activation leads to the identification of the selected AD fusion. Thus, this method enables the screening of proteins that interact *in vivo* and is therefore a well-suited method to create a protein–protein interaction map of a cell or an organism.

After transformation and expression of the fusion protein, the first test is to check whether the target protein with the DNA-binding domain exerts autotranscriptional activity. If this should be the case, the experiment needs to be redefined. After testing the autoactivity of the fusion protein, the library of choice in fusion to the activator domain can be transformed. Upon screening on selection marker plates, positive clones are identified via reporter gene assays, e.g., LacZ, and the DNA of the selected clones is prepared and sequenced. After the identification of a selected clone it is necessary to test the specificity again in the two-hybrid system and also in a different system. This can include *in vitro* pull-down assays or co-immunoprecipitations, both evaluating the biological relevance of the interaction.

2.2.3.1. Advantages: One big advantage of the two-hybrid system over classical biochemical and genetic approaches is its use as an *in vivo* assay, with yeast as a live test tube, exhibiting similar conditions to higher eukaryotes. Compared to biochemical approaches that need huge amounts of purified protein or good quality antibodies, the two-hybrid system requires only the cloning of the full-length or even partial cDNA of interest to start the screening.

The genetic reporter gene strategy results in a significant amplification of the read out. This facilitates also detection of weak or transient interactions, which are often the most interesting in signaling cascades. Besides the screening of new interaction partners, the two-hybrid system allows also for mapping of residues crucial for an interaction. The most convincing argument in favor of the two-hybrid is the number and the speed in which many signaling cascades have been resolved in molecular detail.

2.2.3.2. Disadvantages: As mentioned above, the key to the method relies on the fact that the DNA-binding and transcriptional activation are separated. Thus, if the protein of interest exhibits transcriptional function on its own, the use of this protein in a two-hybrid system may not be successful and could be a limiting factor. Furthermore, as the bait and the prey proteins are expressed in fusion to the DNA- and to the activating domains, the resulting chimeras might have different conformations which could result in altered function, resulting in lower activity or even in the inaccessibility of binding sites. If this is the case, it might be worth trying to switch the fusion proteins of bait and prey.

Moreover, the protein of interest needs to be stably expressed and folded in yeast. This can be seen as an advantage rather than a disadvantage, since yeast is closer to higher eukaryotes than *in vitro* experiments or those based on bacterial hosts. Folding problems in yeast can also be accompanied by post-translational modifications that either do not occur or are yeast specific. However, this can possibly be circumvented by co-expressing the enzyme responsible for the posttranslational modification. In addition, it should be noted that the system needs the fusion proteins to be targeted to the nucleus, which could be a limiting factor for, e.g., extracellular proteins. Another problem could be a toxic effect upon expression of the fusion proteins, which has been shown for cyclins and homeobox proteins. Usage of an inducible promoter might circumvent the problem. It has to be noted that after successful identification of two interacting partners, the biological relevance of this interaction remains to be determined to prevent the identification of artificially interacting partners. Even if identified in the assay, it could be possible that these proteins are never in close proximity to each other in the cell. A good representation of the library is necessary to screen successfully. Therefore, it has to be considered that only one out of six fused cDNAs is in the correct frame, which increases the number of clones to be investigated.

2.2.3.3. Reverse Hybrid System: The two-hybrid system does not allow genetic selection of events responsible for dissociation of particular interactions. However, a reverse two-hybrid system makes use of the expression of a counter selectable marker that is toxic and hence leads to a growth arrest. Thus, the dissociation of an interaction provides a selective advantage. One example given here is the "split-hybrid" system, which is based on the *E. coli* TN10-encoded tet repressor/operator system. Upon interaction of the target protein with its prey protein, the transcription of the TetR is initiated. The TetR protein represses then the expression of the HIS3 gene, leading to a growth phenotype on plates without histidine in the growth medium *(35)*. Abrogation of the interaction, either by mutating one of the proteins or by introducing a dissociator protein shuts down the TetR expression and enables again HIS3 expression and thus growth on selective plates. This method can be used in screening large libraries of peptides or compounds that inhibit selectively a protein interaction *(36,37)*.

2.2.3.4. Sos-Recruitment System (SRS): The mammalian GDP-GTP exchange factor hSos (*human son of sevenless*) can only activate Ras when hSos is localized to the plasma membrane in close proximity to Ras. In yeast, functional Ras signaling pathway is required for cell viability. This fact has been exploited in the hSos-recruitment system and similarly in the Ras-recruitment system (RRS). Both systems benefit from the fact that a yeast strain, mutated in the Ras guanyl nucleotide exchange factor cdc25-2, shows temperature sensitive growth. For the screening assay, the target protein is fused to hSos, and the prey protein to be screened is fused to a membrane localization signal. Coexpression of these proteins in a cdc25-2 yeast strain leads to a temperature dependent growth phenotype if the fusion proteins interact and allow hSos recruitment to the membrane *(38–40)*.

2.2.3.5. Yeast Three-Hybrid System: A limitation in the two-hybrid system is the lack of the detection of post-translational modifications, e.g., tyrosine-phosphorylation, which do not occur in *Saccharomyces cerevisiae*. In the so called kinase three-hybrid system, a cytosolic tyrosine kinase has been introduced into the yeast cell, phosphorylating specific substrates *(41)*.

In the yeast three-hybrid system, the target protein activates only transcription via the activating prey protein if a third protein is present. This third protein either mediates the interaction or induces a conformational change thereby promoting interaction (**Fig 35.6B**). In this way it has been shown that the interaction between Sos and the cytoplasmic domain of the EGFR is Grb2-mediated *(42)*. The three-hybrid system can also be extended to the use of a heterodimer of small organic ligands, incorporated into the media plates, which induce dimerization of, e.g., the glucocorticoid receptor and in this way activate the transcription after diffusion into the yeast cell *(43)*. This system is of great interest in pharmacological approaches since small-ligand receptor interactions are the basis for many signaling cascades and misregulation is the cause of many diseases. Hence, the screening of a library of small ligand compounds with the three-hybrid system could identify new drug lead compounds.

Together, these advances have led to a variety of hybrid screening systems each with its own limit and suffering from the fact that each strategy is capable of detecting only a subset of interactions. This argues for the use of multiple systems to maximize coverage.

2.2.4. Protein-Fragment Complementation Assay (PCA)

Protein-Fragment Complementation Assays (PCA) are a powerful tool for studying protein-protein interactions and are used e.g. in protein engineering for selecting tightest binding partners from peptide libraries. For PCA selection, a peptide library and the target protein or a domain thereof are fused to a reporter protein which is dissected into two non-functional fragments, sometimes referred to as $\Delta\alpha$ and $\Delta\omega$ or fragment 1 and 2. Interactions of the studied proteins or domains are demonstrated by restoration of the reporter proteins functionality (**Fig. 35.7**). The reporter protein must monitor the association of the test proteins without promoting it. Interaction must be mediated by the interaction under investigation. A combinatorial approach for generating a reporter protein for PCAs was introduced by Tafelmeyer et al. *(44)*.

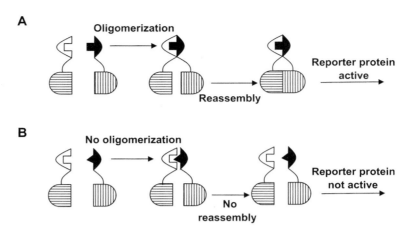

Fig. 35.7. General principle of protein-fragment complementation assays (PCA). Oligomerization domains (black and white) are fused via linkers to the reporter protein fragments (striped). Further explanation are given in the text

In contrast to two-hybrid techniques PCAs are not generally limited to the nucleus, where the proteins lack the appropriate cellular context. Also two-hybrid assays cannot be used to test temporal aspects of protein interactions (*45*).

An interesting point of the PCA system is that, using known interaction domains, it can also be used to study the reporter protein, e.g., mutate residues in the binding interface of the two fragments.

Reporter proteins for PCA have to fulfill several requirements:

- small and monomeric
- overexpression possible in eukaryotic, prokaryotic or both cell types
- the two fragments must be stable and soluble to enable reassembly
- the cleavage site must not be in a functional position
- cleavage site ideally close to the N- or C-terminus to permit different orientation in the fusion protein
- only reassembly of both fragments restores activity to avoid false positives
- miminal auto-reassembly to prevent background (false positive)
- easy discrimination of active and inactive reporters for selection or screening of interacting partners
- no endogenous reporter protein of same activity present in the host or host protein can be efficiently inhibited

Different systems have been developed each with inherent advantages and disadvantages. Here we provide a short overview over the different reporter systems used for PCA.

2.2.4.1. Murine Dihydrofolate Reductase (mDHFR): The dihydrofolate reductase (DHFR) *(46)* is an enzyme in the nucleotide synthesizing pathway, which fulfills the requirements of a reporter protein very well. It is a small (21 kD), monomeric protein of known structure *(47)* and its folding properties and kinetics are well characterized *(48)*. In nucleotide-free media, DHFR is essential for cell growth. The endogeneous DHFR of *E. coli* can be inhibited by the substrate analogue trimethoprim to which it has a 12,000 fold higher affinity compared to mammalian DHFR *(49)*. Consequently, a murine DHFR can be used for simple survival assays in *E. coli*. It has been shown that mDHFR can be disrupted in a loop-region formed by the amino acids 101–108 *(50)* which is the loop between domain two and three, in close proximity to the N-terminus of the enzyme. This permits fusion of either the N-terminus of both fragments to the dimerization domains or alternatively one N- terminal and one C-terminal fusion. Pelletier et al. chose to fragment mDHFR between residue 107 and 108 and fuse interacting proteins N-terminally to the resulting DHFR fragments. The DHFR fragments are stably expressed and reassemble only when fused to a dimerization domains (in this case the leucine zipper of GCN4). After its assisted reassembly mDHFR becomes active and allows *E. coli* to grow on trimethoprim-containing minimal media (**Fig. 35.8**). Without interaction of the dimerization domain no growth will occur. The speed of growth is related to the strength of interaction of the dimerization domain. In addition to cell growth, DHFR activity can be monitored *in vitro* by fluorimetry following the appearance of tetrahydrofolate (THF) (excitation at 310 nm; emission at 360 nm) using the inhibitor methotrexate (MTX) as a control.

The system has two minor disadvantages: As the DHFR needs NADPH as a cofactor, the assay does not function in the periplasm of *E. coli*. Another drawback is the ability of *E. coli* to eventually overcome inhibition of the endogenous DHFR by mutation after some rounds of selection *(51)*. However, this is rare and easily to detect by controls on plates without IPTG. Without induction, no DHFR-fragments are expressed and thus no growth occurs.

The most obvious advantage of the DHFR-PCA is the easy screening of positive interactions by the survival assay, which makes this assay very valuable especially for screening large libraries. The survival assay can be followed by growth competition in liquid culture under selective conditions to enrich the best binding sequence. Another advantage is the control of stringency of the

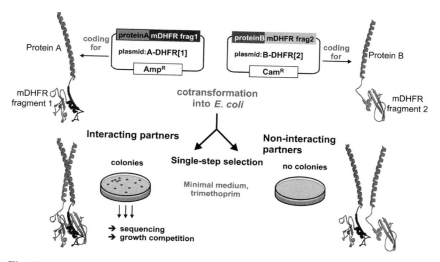

Fig. 35.8. Proteins of interest are genetically fused to mDHFR-fragments and cotransformed in *E. coli* and assayed on minimal medium plates containing trimethoprim. Only interacting proteins enable reassembly of mDHFR, resulting in growths of colonies. Colonies are pooled and best interacting proteins are enriched in growth competitions. Library pools and single clones can be analyzed by sequencing

assay by mutating the binding interface of the two fragments to alter the stability of their reconstituted state, e.g., exchanging wild type isoleucine 114 for alanine or valine *(46)*.

2.2.4.2. Ubiquitin-Based Split-Protein Sensor (USPS): This PCA was developed in 1994 by Johnsson and Varshavsky *(45)*. Ubiquitin acts here as split protein, but for detection of ubiquitin-reassembly an additional protein is needed as reporter. For this, the property of eukaryotic cells is used to cleave ubiquitin-fused proteins by the specific protease UBP. This process is strongly dependent on the correct folding of ub. For USPS ubiquitin is dissected into its two domains and the N-terminal fragment is mutated to inhibit autoreassembly. The reporter protein is fused to the C-terminal fragment. The reporter protein is cleaved on reassembly and correct folding of ubiquitin. Detection depends on the chosen reporter, for example an domain detectable by antibodies or an enzyme which becomes active only after cleavage. The proteins of interest are fused to the ubiquitin fragments which when reassamble permit ubiquitin to fold correctly and the reporter protein is cleaved. However, the signal can be the result of both fragments binding to a common ligand, because USPS detects the proximity of proteins, which does not necessarily means direct interaction. USPS relies on constitutive expression of the host cells ubiquitinase, which had been shown only for cytosol and nucleus.

USPS can also be used *in vitro* with purified fragments and purified proteases such as Ubp1 from yeast.

2.2.4.3. β-Galactosidase: Intracistronic β-galactosidase complementation has long been observed *(52–54)*, and shows that bacterial β-galactosidase activity can be restored when two variants with inactivating mutations in different crucial domains of the enzyme share their intact domains. This is largely efficient but depends on the nature of the mutations *(55)* and holds also true when transferring to mammalian cells *(56)*. Developed in the Blau group, the β-galactosidase-based PCA utilizes this well-known property of β-galactosidase complementation for the first time for time-dependent *in situ* studies of protein–protein interactions in living eukaryotic cells. Rossi et al. *(52)* chose β-gal mutants which have been shown to be unable to complement each other by themselves. The first one lacks only amino acids 11–41 of the wild type and is a naturally occurring mutant described earlier as M15 *(57,58)*. The second contains the first 788 residues of β-gal *(56)*. The proteins of interest are fused to these fragments. Activity of β-gal measured at different time points by either biochemical assays or FACS (summarized in *(53)*) shows the interaction of the fused protein fragments and gives a quantitative readout. As an enzyme, β-gal amplifies the resulting signal allowing monitoring of physiological interaction without overexpression. In contrast to other methods, this PCA can be used to analyze protein–protein interactions in different subcellular compartments of eukaryotic cells. However, because its active form is a large tetramer some interactions might be sterically hindered.

2.2.4.4. β-Lactamase: The bacterial enzyme β-lactamase *(59,60)*, which confers resistance to the antibiotic ampicillin, has long served as a model in protein engineering with well understood properties. Its structure does not suit fragmentation, but this enzyme has significant advantages for use in mammalian cells over other systems. This is because the fragments are small and there is no endogenous β-lactamase activity. In addition in 1998 a cell permeable, fluorescent substrate, called CCF2/AM, was developed *(61)* which detects β-lactamase activity with high sensitivity in eukaryotic cells. A drawback is the high price of these substrates.

The Blau group split β-lactamase after residue 197 *(60,62)*, but found a high background activity in *E. coli*. They were able to reduce the signal-to-noise ratio by stabilizing the α-fragment by adding the empirically found tri-peptide NRG after aa197. The Michnick group established the assay in the cytosol *(59)* using the M182T mutant, which has been reported earlier to stabilize the structure of β-lactamase *(63)*.

2.2.4.5. Luciferase: The enzyme luciferase *(64)* emits light when reacting with a specific substrate in the presence of cofactors. In nature, different types of organisms use this bioluminescence, for example by attracting prey or to scare off predators. In the laboratory, luciferases are used as reporter enzyme for studying the properties of regulatory elements in living organisms *(65)*. Paulmurugan and colleagues used the firefly luciferase to show for the first time a protein-fragment complementation assay that monitors protein interactions in living subjects. The luciferase was split after residue 437 and both fragments ($\Delta\alpha$=437aa, $\Delta\omega$=117aa) were fused to the strongly interacting proteins MyoD and Id. For comparison, the fragments were also fused to inteins, resulting in a reconstituted luciferase by protein splicing. Both approaches, complementation or reconstitution, showed the same high level of luciferase activity after transfection in eukaryotic cells. Best results have been achieved in 293T-cells. In a follow up project Paulmurugan and Gambhir split successfully the synthetic humanized *Renilla* luciferase (hRLUC) for usage in PCA *(66)*. Recently, Remy and Michnick used *Gaussia princeps* luciferase as a PCA reporter protein and found a higher activity compared to the *Renilla* luciferase *(67)*.

Compared to other PCAs the luciferase signal is relatively short living and must be recorded immediately, making the technique somewhat laborious.

2.2.4.6. Green Fluorescent Protein (GFP): A widely used reporter protein for PCA in recent years has been GFP *(68)* and its derivates YFP, CFP and BFP plus the enhanced variants. This method is often referred to as BiFC short for bimolecular fluorescent complementation. Jellyfish *Aequria victoria* GFP is a 238 residue protein that forms an 11-stranded β-barrel with a coaxial helix. The chromophore ρ-hydroxybezylideneimidazolidinon is located with the helix at the center of the barrel *(69)*. Ghosh dissected GFP at a surface loop at residue 157, which has also been shown to accept a 20-residue amino acid insertion *(70)* and fused the resulting fragments with leucine zipper domains for oligomerization. After protein reassembly the fluorophore formes and the protein shows its characteristic fluorescence. In contrast to other PCAs, the complex is stable and does not dissociate, thus allows capturing of transient interactions *(71)*.

2.2.5. Cell-Surface Display

2.2.5.1. Bacterial Display: Bacterial surface display was described in 1986 for the Gram-negative bacteria *E. coli* and *Salmonella* ssp. Short gene fragments were inserted into the genes for the outer membrane proteins LamB, OmpA, and PhoE and were displayed on the cell surface. In 1992 followed the first examples of display techniques using Gram-positive bacteria like *Staphylococcus xylosus* or *S. carnosus* and *Streptococcus gordinii*. The displayed protein mimics a receptor protein like SpaA and M6 respectively and is covalent bound to the outer membrane surface. For staphylococcal display, plasmids are used, while in *S. gordinii* the target genes are incorporated in the genome be homologous recombination. These and other bacterial display systems are reviewed by Lee et al. *(72)*. The main application for bacterial display has been the presentation of antigens, applied to test animals by oral delivery to stimulate the production of specific antibodies by the immune system. Comparison with intracellular expressed or secreted antigens resulted in a more effective immunization using the surface display technique.

Direct comparison with phage display gives better results for the phage-based systems *(73)*, but bacterial display has some advantages. Bacteria are easy to cultivate and can be kept free from contamination by using antibiotic selection markers. Phages in contrast need a host organism, which is susceptible to contamination with wild-type bacteriophages.

2.2.5.2. Yeast Surface Display: *Saccharomyces cerevisae* is generally a good system for expressing heterologous proteins, and transformations are possible both, by plasmid and stable integration of new genes into the genome of yeast cells *(74,75)*. It is generally regarded as safe ("GRAS") and can therefore be used for food and drug production. A big advantage is that yeast as a eukaryotic organism is able to glycosylate and process proteins in its ER, even if it is not fully identical to mammal cells. The first targeting of a heterologous protein to the yeast cell wall was accomplished by Schreuder et al. *(76)*. They fused the protein of interest to the C-terminus of the Aga2p subunit of α-agglutinin. This subunit is connected by two disulfide bonds to the second subunit Aga1p, which is covalently linked to the yeast cell wall (**Fig. 35.9**) The wild-type Aga2p mediates cell-cell contacts during yeast cell mating.

The display of peptide libraries on the surface of yeast was first published by Boder & Wittrup in 1997 *(77)*. In this first attempt to display a fully functional antibody fragment and improve it by random mutation the authors enriched clones with a tenfold higher binding capacity to their target than the wild-type scFv.

Yeast surface display has some advantages over other display techniques. The covalent linkage to the yeast cell wall results in a more stable display of proteins than in other eukaryotic surface expression systems. The displayed proteins can easily be released from the cell surface for further characterization by reduction of the disulfide bonds. The cell wall also gives yeast a higher life time in industrial applications. The culture conditions are well know, thus biomass can be produced in high concentration. Choosing yeast as display system avoids unpredictable bias against expression of some eukaryotic proteins in *E. coli* and of course, this bias also affects phage display. The expression of mammalian proteins in yeast does not work in every case as has been shown for T-cell receptors *(78)*. A limiting factor for library selection by yeast surface display is a smaller achievable library size than in *E. coli*.

Yeast cells can easily be used for quantitative screening by FACS. Alternatively, if it is difficult to obtain a purified ligand or no FACS is available, a ligand can be expressed on mammalian cell surface and binding cells can be selected by density centrifugation *(79)*.

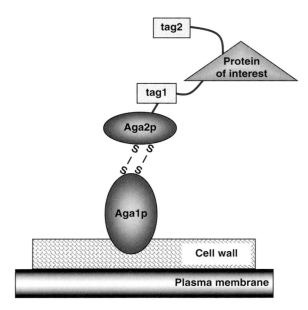

Fig. 35.9. Yeast display. Schematic view of the surface of yeast. The C-terminus of the subunit of the receptor α-agglutinin is covalently anchored in the cell wall, which is located outside the plasma membrane. The second subunit Aga2p is linked via two disulfide bonds. The protein of interest together with several tags, depending on application, is fused to the C-terminus of Aga2p

2.2.5.3. Viral Display: Similar to phage display, proteins can be displayed on the surface of viruses that infect eukaryotic cells. Because the viruses are propagated in the eukaryotic host, the proteins are fully processed by the cellular machinery thus avoiding a main disadvantage of phage display. One widely used host system is the baculovirus *(80)*, which propagates mainly in insect cells, but is transcriptionally silent in mammalian cells, making it relatively safe. It has already been used for expression of recombinant proteins *(81)* and is well established (reviewed *(82)*). Boublik et al. displayed a heterologous protein on the virus surface by fusing it to the surface glycoprotein gp64 *(83)*. Ernst et al. demonstrated the possibility to use a baculovirus system for library selections *(84)*. They expressed HIV-1 glycoprotein gp41 containing a randomized region in Ac-omega and selected for higher affinity to the human antibody 2F5.

Also used for viral display of libraries are retroviruses, originally shown with the murine leukemia virus (MLV) in the human cell line HT 1080 *(85)*. The library was fused to the envelope spike glycoprotein (Env). In contrast to other viruses, retroviruses permit display of large peptides on their surface without reducing infectivity *(86)*. They can be rescued from the target by adding permissive mammalian cells with low loss of high affinity binders. The achievable library size is with 10^6–10^8 *(86)* lower than for phage display but still sufficient for a range of applications.

2.2.5.4. Mammalian Cell Display: In 2005, the first example for library selection in a mammalian cell display system was published. A library with up to 13 residues was displayed on the surface of mammalian cells *(87)*. The library was fused to the chemokine receptor CCR5 and transferred into cells using a retrovirus-based vector. After integration into the genome, the peptide library was constitutively expressed und displayed on the cell surface. As a proof of principle a peptide mimicking the FLAG epitope was successfully enriched after three rounds of selection. Ho et al. fused a small scFV library to the human platelet-derived growth factor receptor PDFGR *(88)*, displayed it on mammalian HEK293 cells, and selected a fully functional scFV against CD22.

2.2.6. In Vitro Compartmentalization (IVC) Methods

In vitro compartmentalization (IVC) uses a water-in-oil (w/o) emulsion with some special surfactants to physically link genotype to phenotype. This is possible because most droplets contain only one gene of a library and the machinery necessary for replication. The surfactants are composed of hydrophilic and lipophilic compounds. Hydrophilic groups associate with the aqueous phase and the lipophilic groups with the oil phase thus forming stable droplets *(89)*. It is thought that such tiny vesicles were part of the primordial soup which enabled the emergence of life *(90)*.

By this emulsification a large reaction volume is divided in many microscopic compartments (up to 10^{10} in 50 µl reaction volume *(89)*) thus increasing the effective concentration of all components used and at the same time reducing diffusion distances *(91)*. These tiny w/o droplets are like the wells of a micro titer plate. If they are re-emulsified in water these w/o droplets are enveloped in water to form w/o/w droplets that can be analyzed by FACS in a much higher efficiency than it would be possible in micro titer or 96 well format if there is a fluorescence-based screening method available *(92)*. The transcription and translation apparatus is provided either by bacterial cell extracts in case of prokaryotic targets and wheat germ or rabbit reticulocyte (RRL) for eukaryotic targets *(89)*.

IVC has several advantages over methods such as phage display, ribosome display or cell surface display in that it can select for properties other than binding, such as sequence specificity, intermolecular catalysis *in trans* (substrate not linked to the catalyst) and regulatory characteristics of proteins and RNA *(92)*. IVC is a highly flexible method with potential for totally new approaches in screening for desired properties.

2.2.6.1. Compartmentalized Self-Replication (CSR): The most simplistic IVC variant is *compartmentalized self-replication (CSR)* (**Fig. 35.10**). CSR was developed for the evolution of enzymes, especially polymerases. PCR is performed in which the individual variants of a polymerase and their respective genes are separated into compartments of an w/o emulsion *(93)*. First the different polymerase variants are cloned into a bacterial host. These bacteria are suspended with appropriate flanking primers and nucleoside triphosphates in a heat stable w/o emulsion. Ideally, each compartment contains only one polymerase variant with its respective gene. During PCR the cells are disrupted and the polymerase is freed. Due to compartmentalization, each polymerase replicates only its own encoding gene and thus only genes that encode for active polymerases are replicated. The more active the variant is the more DNA that is produced. Consequently, there is an increased probability

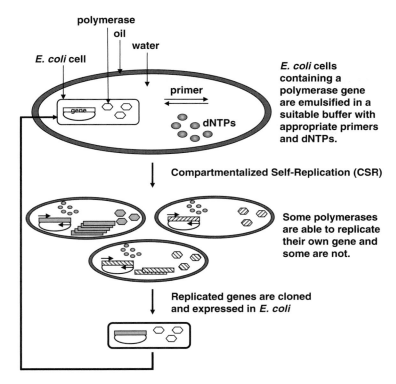

Fig. 35.10. Compartmentalized self-replication

of this variant generating clones for the next round of CSR. Inactive variants fail to amplify their own gene and are thus eliminated from the gene pool. The method bears the potential to select for enzymatic activity under a wide range of conditions.

A modification of this method is short-patch compartmentalized self-replication—spCSR (*94*). SpCSR is based on CSR but in SpCSR only a short region a so-called "patch" of the gene of interest is diversified and replicated. This variation allows for selection of polymerases under conditions where catalytic activity and processivity are compromised resulting in an inefficient full self-replication.

DNA-modifying enzymes like DNA-methyltransferases can be screened in a manner similar to CSR. Instead of amplifying its own DNA the enzyme can modify its own DNA thus cannot be digested after breaking the emulsion (*89*).

Doi et al. (*95*) adjusted IVC to select for endonucleases with altered restriction sites. The DNA coding for the endonuclease is emulsified and translated *in vitro*. An active enzyme cuts its own DNA resulting in sticky ends. In compartments with inactive enzyme, the DNA stays intact. After breaking the emulsion, a biotinylated dNTP is incorporated into the cohesive ends of the cleaved DNA by DNA polymerase, and biotinylated genes are recovered from the mixture using streptavidin coated beads and amplified using PCR. Using this method the coding gene can only be mutated in front of the restriction site of the enzyme as mutations after the restriction site are lost. If a special cleavage site is to be selected, the biotinylated tag could be added to a special oligonucleotide representing the restrictions site to be selected. Thus, only genes coding for enzymes with the correct restriction site will be selected.

2.2.6.2. Microbead Display: The coupling of genotype with phenotype can be achieved by different approaches: In *microbead display* proteins are linked to DNA via microbeads (**Fig. 35.11**). A library of genes coding for a protein with a common tag are labeled with biotin and coupled to streptavidin-coated beads so that every bead carries approximately one gene. These beads additionally carry antibodies against the common tag. The beads are compartmentalized in w/o emulsion and the protein is translated *in vitro*. In each droplet, the transcribed proteins become attached to the antibodies on the bread and thus are linked to the gene encoding them. The emulsion is broken and the beads are incubated with horseradish peroxidase (HRP) coupled ligand or substrate. HRP converts fluorescein tyramide into intermediates that react with the protein which thus becomes labeled with multiple fluorescein molecules. These fluorescent beads can be afterwards sorted by FACS, and the DNA can be amplified and subjected to a new round of selection *(96)*.

If the protein to be screened has enzymatic activity by which a fluorogenic substrate directly is transformed into a fluorescent product, water-oil-water (w/o/w) droplets containing active enzyme can be sorted by FACS *(97)*.

Selection of Diels-Alderase ribozymes can be achieved by coupling a DNA library via a PEG linker to anthracene. These genes are compartmentalized in w/o emulsion and the genes are transcribed to RNA. Mg^{2+} and biotin-maleimide are added to the emulsion and allowed to diffuse into the compartments. If compartments contain active Diels-Alderase ribozymes a cycloadduct of biotin-maleimide is generated, thereby biotinylating the ribozyme coding gene. After

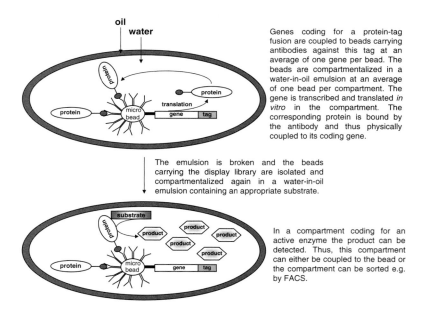

Genes coding for a protein-tag fusion are coupled to beads carrying antibodies against this tag at an average of one gene per bead. The beads are compartmentalized in a water-in-oil emulsion at an average of one bead per compartment. The gene is transcribed and translated *in vitro* in the compartment. The corresponding protein is bound by the antibody and thus physically coupled to its coding gene.

The emulsion is broken and the beads carrying the display library are isolated and compartmentalized again in a water-in-oil emulsion containing an appropriate substrate.

In a compartment coding for an active enzyme the product can be detected. Thus, this compartment can either be coupled to the bead or the compartment can be sorted e.g. by FACS.

Fig. 35.11. Microbead display

breaking the emulsion, genes coding for active Diels-Alderase ribozymes are bound to streptavidin coated magnetic beads and amplified by PCR *(98)*.

3. Applications

3.1. Applications of Rational Design Approaches

Rational design strategies have successfully been used in the field of protein therapeutics by improving existing products and enabling the development of novel therapeutics. Several designed protein therapeutics are currently on the market (**Table 35.1**, from *(1)*).

Some of the most visible and successful applications of rational biotherapeutic engineering methods have occurred in the field of antibodies. Monoclonal antibodies are widely used as a treatment for a variety of conditions from arthritis to cancer. Some antibody products are already available on the market (**Table 35.2** from *(1)*). Antibody variable domains suffer from stability issues like all proteins. However, because antibodies share a common structural scaffold, rational engineering studies have been able to dissect some of the sequential and structural determinants of variable region solubility and stability *(99)*.

For example, the best success for immunogenicity reduction has been the humanization of murine antibodies, which was made possible by the high regularity of antibody sequence and structure and close proximity to the human sequence.

Table 35.1. Engineered protein therapeutics.

Name	Family	Company	Indication	Modification
Proleukin® (aldesleukin)	IL-2	Chiron	Cancer	Mutated free cysteine
Betaseron® (interferon beta-1b)	IFN-β	Berlex/Chiron	Multiple sclerosis	Mutated free cysteine
Humalog® (insulin lispro)	Insulin	Eli Lilly	Diabetes	Monomer not hexamer
NovoLog® (insulin aspart)	Insulin	Novo Nordisk	Diabetes	Monomer not hexamer
Lantus® (insulin glargine)	Insulin	Aventis	Diabetes	Precipitates in dermis
Enbrel® (etanercept)	TNF receptor	Immunex/Amgen/Wyeth	Rheumatoid arthritis	Fc fusion
Ontak® (denileukin diftitox)	Diptheria toxin-IL-2	Seragen/Ligand	Cancer	Fusion
PEG-Intron® (peginterferon alfa-2b)	IFN-a	Schering-Plough	Hepatitis	PEGylation
PEGasys® (peginterferon alfa-2a)	IFN-a	Roche	Hepatitis	PEGylation
Neulasta™ (pegfilgrastim)	G-CSF	Amgen	Leukopenia	PEGylation
Oncaspar® (pegaspargase)	Asparaginase	Enzon	Cancer	PEGylation
Aranesp® (darbepoetin α)	Epo	Amgen	Anemia	Additional glycosylation sites
Somavert® (pegvisomant)	Growth hormone	Genentech/Seragen/Pharmacia	Acromegaly	PEGylation; binding site mutations

Table 35.2. Engineered antibodies.

Name	Company	Target	Indication	Type
Orthoclone OKT3® (muromonab-CD3)	Ortho Biotech/Johnson & Johnson	CD3	Transplant rejection	Murine
ReoPro® (abciximab)	Centocor/Lilly	GPIIb/IIIa	Restenosis	Chimeric
Rituxan® (rituximab)	IDEC/Genentech	CD20	B-cell non-Hodgkins lymphoma	Chimeric
Simulect® (basiliximab)	Novartis	IL-2R	Transplant rejection	Chimeric
Remicade® (infliximab)	Centocor	TNF-a	Crohn's disease, rheumatoid arthritis	Chimeric
Zevalin® (ibritumomab tiuxetan)	IDEC/Schering AG	CD20	B-cell non-Hodgkins lymphoma	Chimeric
Zenapax® (daclizumab)	PDL/Roche	IL-2R	Transplant rejection	Humanized
Synagis® (palivizumab)	MedImmune	RSVF protein	Respiratory syncitial virus	Humanized
Herceptin® (trastuzumab)	Genentech	HER2/neu	Breast cancer	Humanized
Mylotarg® (gemtuzumab ozogamicin)	Celltech/Wyeth	CD33	Acute myeloid leukemia	Humanized
Campath® (alemtuzumab)	Millenium/ILEX	CD52	B-cell chronic lymphocytic leukemia	Humanized

3.1.1. Site-Directed Mutagenesis

To increase protein stability the replacement of free cysteines into serines have been introduced into several therapeutic proteins, including granulocyte colony-stimulating factor (G-CSF) and interferon (IFN) β1b, resulting in a longer half-life *(100,101)*.

The replacement of exposed non-polar for polar residues was applied successfully to the A1 domain of cholera toxin. Of the six variants produced, one retained full biological activity, stability and displayed significant improvement in solubility *(102)*.

A single chain antibody targeting renal cell carcinoma was altered to increase solubility by adding 5 glutamic acid residues to the C-terminus, thus lowering the pI from 7.5 to 6.1 *(103)*.

An example of affinity enhancement is the generation of superagonist variants of human thyrotropin (hTSH) by altering the net charge of the protein. The hTSH receptor has a negative charge, and mutations that introduce positively charged residues or replace negatively charged residues in the peripheral loops of hTSH increase activity *(104,105)*.

4-helix bundle cytokines, including vascular endothelial growth factor (VEGF), hGH and interleukin-6 (IL-6), have been engineered to function as receptor antagonists. Antagonistic VEGF variants were designed as heterodimers, which contain one functional binding site per dimer *(106)*. An IL-6 superantagonist was generated by selecting mutations that disrupt binding to gp130 and incorporated mutations that resulted in increased affinity for the IL-6 coreceptor *(107)*. An especially interesting example of a designed cytokine antagonist is Somavert® (pegvisomant, Genentech/Pharmacia), a hGH variant that has recently successfully completed clinical trials for treatment of acromegaly.

Somavert® contains a point mutation at the second of the two receptor binding sites that blocks receptor dimerization upon binding (108). Eight additional mutations, identified by phage display, that increase the receptor-binding affinity of the first receptor binding site were introduced (109).

A notable example is the design of constitutively active and inactive integrin I domain variants. The integrin I domains can populate two dominant conformations: an "open" conformation, which can bind intracellular adhesion molecule-1 (ICAM-1), and a "closed" conformation, which has very low affinity for ICAM-1. Springer and coworkers introduced pairs of cysteines that form disulfide bonds compatible with either the closed or open conformation (110,111), and they designed mutations in the core of the domain that were computationally selected to stabilize the open conformation and disallow the closed state (112).

Wong and coworkers switched the substrate preference of the 2-deoxyribose-5-phosphate aldolase (DERA) from phosphorylated to nonphosphorylated substrates. The kcat/K_M value for the nonphosphorylated substrate increased 2.5 times for a variant with a single point mutation relative to wild type (113,114).

Lim and coworkers engineered the active site of magnesium-dependent ribonuclease H to form an active metal-independent enzyme. Replacement of an aspartate and a glutamate residue that interact with the metal ion yields an enzyme that is active in the absence of Mg^{2+}. As a result the pH activity profile is dramatically altered (115).

3.1.2. Computational Protein Design

Computation interface design was used to fuse two domains of distantly related homing endonucleases (Dmol and Crel), each carrying a recognition site for a specific DNA target half site (116). The resulting functional chimeric protein combines the two different binding specificities of the parent proteins. The crystal structure of the designed interface confirms the accuracy of the design algorithm. Extending this approach, computational design offers the possibility to create novel interfaces that would go beyond the interaction capabilities of independent modules.

Optimizing the fairly promiscuous calmodulin interface for one of its ligands using a successful computational protein design method, by Shifman and Mayo (117), resulted in a stable interaction in the nanomolar range that is more specific for the selected ligand. This is the first study showing that computational interface redesign is capable of enhancing the specificity of an interaction.

The study of Havranek and Harbury (118) describes the development and experimental verification of a novel computational protocol that automatically selects for sequences that prefer desired cognate interaction over alternative partners and conformations (negative design). The experimental results of the formation of homodimeric or heterodimeric coiled coil interfaces verified the predicted specificities in all instances.

Dwyer and Hellinga used computational design for the enzymatic activity in a protein scaffold of known structure. They demonstrate the feasibility of creating new enzymatic activities by introducing mutations at or near the substrate-binding site (119).

Several authors have compared the behavior of enzymes from thermophilic and mesophilic organisms using MD. The difference in the thermostability was explained by reduced backbone flexibility of the thermostable enzyme for thioredoxin *(120)* and rubredoxin *(121)*.

The automated design of a novel sequence onto a given protein backbone by computational screening of a combinatorial library was achieved by Dahiyat and Mayo *(122)*. NMR spectroscopy showed that the resulting structure, a short zinc-finger protein fold, is in excellent agreement with the designed target structure *(122)*.

Hellinga and coworkers have developed a powerful computational tool DENZYMER to assist in reprogramming the specificities and properties of proteins. This computational technique has been applied to the design of novel variants of *E. coli* periplasmic binding proteins to bind the nonnatural ligands trinitrotoluene, L-lactate, and serotonin with high affinities *(123–126)*.

The success of the computational design process used in these studies strongly suggests that such techniques will play an increasingly important role in protein engineering, especially when paired with experimental data.

3.2. Applications of Library-Based Design Approaches

3.2.1. Phage Display

Phage display is largely used to screen peptide or antibody libraries for ligands using purified and immobilized molecules *in vitro*, with the aim of stabilizing protein–protein interactions or identifying protein–protein interaction domains *(127)*. One example of an FDA approved antibody generated by phage display is Adalimumab (HUMIRA), which is used against rheumatoid arthritis *(128)*. When nonhuman antibodies are used for this approach, immunogenicity can limit application; therefore, the epitope-binding region can be transferred onto the framework of a human IgG antibody. This process is called "humanization."

Another phage display approach is the so called Proside (<u>pro</u>tein <u>s</u>tability <u>i</u>ncreased by <u>d</u>irected <u>e</u>volution) approach which directly links thermodynamic stability of a protein with the infectivity of the filamentous phage *(129)*. In this case, the protein is inserted between two domains of the gene3 protein. Upon incubation of phages with either trypsin or chymotrypsin, only phages harboring well-folded guest-proteins inaccessible to proteolysis remain infective and enter the next round of selection after *E. coli* host amplification. Thus, Proside is independent of interactions with ligands or any specific enzymatic catalysis. Rather, it selects proteins that remain folded upon treatment with proteases, and it is therefore useful for selecting thermodynamic stability.

Moreover, phage display can also be used for *in vivo* screening, so called biopanning. In this approach, phage libraries can be incubated on whole cells targeting a specific receptor or can be used to select for cell-targeting gene therapy vectors *(130)*. Selection remains more specific *in vivo* than *in vitro* as the target protein remains in its "native" conditions and the ligand is challenged by degradation from cellular proteases and competed by native ligands, both improving stability and specificity. This *in vivo* biopanning can be even expanded to select for peptides that are home to receptors differentially expressed on vasculature organs. These selection procedures identify ligands that target specific vascular beds. In this case phages are intravenously injected and circulate in the blood for a certain time period. Nonspecifically bound phages are removed by washing off the tissue cells. Specific clones that bind to selective vascular beds are recovered by host *E. coli* infection and are amplified for further selection rounds *(131)*. Molecular profiles of different diseases can be exploited and lead to the identification of marker genes. Highlighted here are the selection of peptides that "home" to receptors of the lung *(132)* or the breast *(133)*.

3.2.2. Ribosome Display

As for phage display, the list of examples of different approaches is long and applications for ribosome display in biomarker identification, imaging and targeting are likely to evolve further *(134)*. Examples given here include the identification of semi-synthetic factors that have the potential to exhibit transcriptional activity *(135)*; DNA-binding proteins were selected out of a zinc finger protein library which now could be used as novel transcription factors. Another example is the selection of MAP-kinase binders. A combinatorial library of ankyrin repeat proteins (DARPins) displayed with ribosomal display, lead to the isolation of binders displaying nanomolar affinities to JNK1, JNK2, and p38 *(136)*.

3.2.3. Yeast Two-Hybrid System

Aside from the molecular dissection of known interactions and the identification of new potential interacting partners, the evolution of the technique, also mentioned above, enables solving several new problems. The yeast two-hybrid system is the method of choice to study signaling cascades e.g., the Ras/Raf-pathway *(137)*. In the post-genomic era, efforts are now being made to analyze all known genes and proteins and the way they interact in a whole cell/organism with the aim to establish so-called protein linkage maps. These maps consist of all possible protein interactions that occur in a cell and give insight into the overall cell complexity, serving as a starting point for studies at the systems level. The first genome-wide interaction map was generated for the bacteriophage T7 *(138)*. In the same manner, a protein interaction map of the yeast strain *S. cervisiae* was established, comprising 69% of the whole proteome *(139)*. Another screen identified over 5400 interactions of *C. elegans* covering 12% of the genome *(140)*. Other studies have integrated these data with functional genomics data to derive models for genetic pathways. In addition, two-hybrid screens have recently been used to analyze the human proteome, screening ~7200 full-length Open Reading Framess (ORFs) which identified 2754 protein interactions *(141)*.

The identified interaction data from *S. cerevisiae, C. elegans, Drosophila*, and from human permits comparison of these interaction maps and helps to predict additional interactions, missing in one system but found in others. Together with a computer assisted confidence score that relates the interaction to a biological significance, it is also possible to lower the amount of false-positive interactions. Hence, statistical scoring systems facilitate integration of datasets.

3.2.4. Protein-Fragment Complementation Assay

PCAs have been used in many different ways for finding, improving and studying protein–protein interactions. Below are examples given for the presented systems.

3.2.4.1. Murine Dihydrofolate Reductase (mDHFR): Pelletier et al. and Arndt et al. *(51,142,143)* used the DHFR assay to study interactions of coiled coil domains, which are naturally abundant oligomerization domains. The aim was to generate stable heterodimeric artificial coiled coils, which can be used as heterodimerization modules for a variety of protein engineering applications *(144)*. For library design, outer positions were taken from Jun and Fos and core positions from GCN4. The core-flanking residues were randomized with polar and charged residues to create complementary libraries. These libraries were fused to the DHFR fragments and co-transformed in *E. coli* to select for the best heterodimer. In a further study, Amdt and colleagues selected peptides binding natural targets such as C-Jun, C-Fos and C-Myc (*145–148*).

Mossner et al. (*149*) fused a single-chain antibody (scFv) and its antigen to the DHFR-fragments and optimized the linker length and orientation of this system. Replacing the antibody with a library permits use of this assay to select for high affinity antibodies in a robust and easy way.

The DHFR-assay can also be used in mammalian cells when a DHFR-deficient strain is available. Remy et al. studied conformational changes of the erythropoietin receptor upon ligand binding (*150*) and effects of linker length in the assay system. Dimerization was detected by fluorescent-labeled methotrexate, which binds only to the reassembled DHFR. This study demonstrated applicability of the DHFR assay for membrane proteins.

3.2.4.2. Ubiquitin-Based Split-Protein Sensor (USPS): To find new players in the regulation of the galactose pathway in *Saccharomyces cerevisae*, Laser et al. (*151*) partially digested the genome of *S. cerevisae* with the restriction enzyme Sau3A and fused the resulted DNA fragments in all three frames to the gene of the α_{ub}-fragment. The ω-fragment of ubiquitin was fused to Gal4p or Tup1p which are known to bind to the Gal1-operon and were used as bait for the library. Laser successfully identified Nhp6 as new interaction partner to both bait-proteins.

Stagljar et al. used USPS to detect interactions between membrane proteins *in vivo* (*148*). The cleavage of the fusion protein leads to the release of a transcription factor, which activates a reporter gene in the nucleus.

3.2.4.3. β-Lactamase: The developers of the technique SEER (sequence-enabled reassembly) used first GFP but finally the β-lactamase complementation assay (*153,154*) and modules of zinc finger domains to detect specific sequences of DNA. Six or more single zinc fingers were chosen for their combined ability to bind to the DNA sequence of interest. Zinc fingers recognizing the 3′-half of the target were fused to the first fragment of the reporter, and the other fingers to the second fragment. Only if all zinc fingers bind to the DNA in the correct orientation, the β-lactamase can reassemble and become active. β-lactamase proved superior to GFP for this application, because it reassembled and folded much faster than GFP and its enzymatic signal amplification allowed detection of fewer target sites. With this method, the authors were able to specifically detect a target DNA sequence in a complex mixture.

3.2.4.4. Luciferase: Massoud et al. applied the luciferase PCA to study homodimeric protein–protein interactions in mammalian cells and living mice (*155*). They used a split synthetic humanized renilla luciferase (hRLUC) to visualize and quantify the dimerization of herpes simplex virus type 1 thymidine kinase (TK1). Splitting hRLUC resulted in two fragments $\Delta\alpha$ = 229 residues and $\Delta\omega$ = 82 residues (*66*). 293T cells expressing the TK chimeras were implanted in mice and mock-transfected cells as negative controls at another site of the same mice. The luciferase substrate coelenterazine was injected into the mouse tails and the bioluminescence signal recorded by a cooled charged coupled device (CCD) camera. They also tested which order and orientation the luciferase fragments and the TK monomers resulted in the highest bioluminescence. It was possible to locate and quantify luciferase activity with high sensivity in a living subject, which makes this system a valuable tool for studying protein–protein interactions in animals.

3.2.4.5. Green Fluorescent Protein: Hu and Kerppola visualized differential protein interactions in the same cell by multicolored BiFc *(156)*. For this, they performed PCAs with various combininations of four GFP variants (GFP, YFP, CFP, BFP) with two fragmentation sites at aa155 or aa173. The protein fragments were fused to the bZIP domains of Fos and Jun (bFos and bJun) and screened for fluorescence in mammalian cells. The study characterized 12 bimolecular fluorescent complexes with 7 spectral classes, thus providing an impressive set to analyse complex protein interaction networks in living mammalian cells. In the successful complex forming combinations YFP was most prominent.

In 2004, Bracha-Drori et al. and Walter et al. *(157,158)* adapted BiFc for monitoring protein interactions in the nucleus and the cytoplasm of living plants. Using YFP they could visualize protein interactions and show that BiFc occurred in the correct compartement of the plant cells.

3.2.5. Cell-Surface Display

Most examples using cell surface display are from the *de novo* selection and improvement of antibodies.

3.2.5.1. Bacterial Display: Christman et al. applied a bacterial display system for epitope mapping of monospecific antibodies *(159)*. A random library of gene fragments of the classical swine fever virus (CSFV) envelope protein E^{rns} was generated by DNase I digestion. For bacterial surface display, the fragments were fused to a carboxyterminal truncated intimin *(160)*, an E. coli adhesin, which is located far enough from the outer membrane' lipopolysaccharide layer to be sufficiently accessible to the tested antibodies. The epitope-presenting E. coli cells were incubated with specific antibodies produced in mice. A biotinylated anti-mouse antibody was used as a secondary antibody and detected by streptavidin conjugated to the fluorescent dye R-phycoerythrin. Cells were sorted by fluorescence-activated cell sorting (FACS), and FACS-positive clones analyzed for their epitope sequence. Eight of eleven clones presented a carboxy-terminal fragment of E^{rns} on their surface, three displayed other regions.

Metal-binding peptides could become a powerful tool in cleaning the ecosystem from heavy metals and radionuclides. Kjaergaard et al. *(161)* screened a library of approximate 4×10^6 clones for the ability to bind Zn^{2+}. The library was fused to the adhesin FimH, a component of the fimbrial organelle of E. coli. After several rounds of selection of peptide-displaying cells against Zn^{2+}-nitrilotriacetic acid beads, binding clones were analyzed. From those 15 clones, no consensus sequence could be derived but all carried at least one histidine. Data bank research revealed no noteworthy sequence similarities, suggesting that novel Zn^{2+}-binding peptides were selected.

3.2.5.2. Yeast Surface Display: Calmodulin is a highly conserved protein in mammals that is part of a variety of signaling pathways (reviewed in *(162)*). It contains four Ca^{2+}-binding sites and undergoes structural changes upon binding Ca^{2+} ions. There are only few reports about monoclonal antibodies against calmodulin; due to its high conservation it was difficult to deal with the self tolerance mechanism of the immunsystem of the antibody-producing animal system. Yeast display offered an alternative way to the classic method. Feldhaus et al. *(163)* selected from a human nonimmune scFv library displayed on the surface of yeast new antibodies against calmodulin. Sequences were further improved by error-prone PCR to yield specific high affinity binders to the two different conformations of calmodulin. The antibody optained for Ca^{2+}-calmodulin was a scFc with an equilibrium dissociation constant (K_d) of 800 pM and more than 1,000-fold higher specificity for this conformation relative to the Ca^{2+}-free form of the protein. For the latter a single-domain antibody (dAb) was selected with a K_d of 1 nM and more than 300-fold higher specificity relativ to Ca^{2+}-calmodulin.

Red Sea Bream Iridovirus (RSIV) infects, amongst others, cultured and ornamental fishes in Japan *(164)* and can thus lead to severe damage to the economy. Tamaru et al. *(165)* successfully expressed the antigen 380R on the surface of yeast. This may lead to production of an oral vaccine against RSIV.

Finding a binding protein is generally not enough to stimulate the desired cellular response. This response is often the result of multiple amplification events following receptor activation. High valency of receptor interactions are needed, also with complementary molecules on other cells. For example, T-cell activation requires a high number of interactions between T-cell receptors (TCR) and antigen presenting cells. Cho et al. *(166)* presented high levels of a ligand on the surface of yeast to target T cells. This lead to the necessary clustering of TCRs on the surface and to activation of T cells, as demonstrated by increased levels of CD25 and CD69 and a decreased number of TCRs on the surface. The authors also demonstrated the ability to activate T cells in the presence of high concentrations of nonpresenting yeast, suggesting that the system is applicable to library based approaches. More applications for yeast display are reviewed by Kondo and Ueda *(167)*.

3.2.5.3. Viral Display: Buchholz et al. *(85)* applied a viral display system to the selection of protease cleavage sites. They expressed the epidermal growth factor (EGF) on the surface of murine leukemia viruses, linked via a seven-residue linker to the envelope glycoprotein. The virus was propagated on EGF receptor-poor cells without loss of the displayed EGF. In contrast, it did not replicate on EGF receptor-rich cells, because the EGF-displaying viruses were intercepted by the EGF receptors. The authors randomized the seven-residue linker and let the viruses propagate on EGF receptor-rich HT1080 cells. Only viruses whose EGF was proteolytically cleaved from the viral surface were able to infect cells and to replicate. After three passages of selection resulting sequences were all arginine-rich and matched the consensus sequence for furin-like proteases.

To enhance gene delivery to target cells, Raty et al. *(168)* altered the surface of baculo viruses to display avidin, the constructed virus was named Baavi. Avidin is highly positively charged and was therefore expected to improve cell transfection. In this study, Baavi achieved a five-fold increase in transduction efficiency in rat malignant glioma cells and a 26-fold increase in rabbit aortic smooth muscle cells. Even higher transduction efficiency was shown for biotinylated cells.

3.2.5.4. Mammalian Cell Display: Riddle et al. *(169)* mimicked the natural binding of antibodies to tumor cells by displaying the Fc portion of the murine IgG2a heavy chain (IgFc) on the surface of tumor cells in an orientation where its C-terminus pointed away from the surface. In this way they hoped to activate an immune response against the tumor cells equivalent to an antibody-based approach, which showed some inherent problems like poor penetration of the antibody in the tumor and the need for tumor-specific antigens. In a first *in vitro* experiment, they displayed IgFc on the surface of B16 melanoma cells. Indeed, these cells were specifically recognized and rapidly lysed by natural killer cells. Subsequent *in vivo* data demonstrated that tumor formation was severely delayed. Direct intratumoral injection of adenoviral vectors expressing IgFc led to total clearance of the tumor cells but did not prevent metastasis or led to antitumor immunization. For this, an additional immunostimulatory signal was needed, achieved here by coexpression of heat shock protein 70 (hsp70).

For many years, antibodies have been successfully selected and matured by phage display *(170–173)*, bacterial display *(174–176)*, yeast display *(177,178)* and ribosome display *(31,179,180)*, but these techniques are limited by problems with protein folding, posttranslational modification and codon usage. Ho et al. *(88)* for the first time used a mammalian display system for the purpose of antibody maturation. They fused the anti-CD33 scFv and the high-affinity derivative HA22 scFv to the transmembrane domain of human platelet-derived growth factor receptor (PDGFR) and displayed the chimeric protein on human embryonic kidney (HEK) 293T cells. They were able to achieve a 240-fold enrichment of the high-affinity variant relative to the wt scFv. Furthermore, Ho *(88)* selected an antibody with even higher affinity from a scFv library with randomized intrinsic antibody hot spots.

3.2.6. In Vitro Compartmentalization Methods

DNA polymerase from *Thermus aquaticus* (*Taq*) is one of the most important enzymes in modern biotechnology. The various DNA amplification and modification techniques that are used often have requirements that are difficult to achieve with polymerases on the market. Thus, it is important and profitable to adjust polymerases to the conditions needed for special applications till the aim of a "gold standard" polymerase is achieved *(181)*.

Ghadessy et al. *(93)* used three cycles of CSR to select for *Taq* DNA polymerases with 11-fold higher thermostability than wild-type *Taq* and increased resistance to the inhibitor heparin. A few years later Ghadessy et al. *(182)* started from ramdomly mutated *Taq* clones and selected these by CSR for efficient mismatch extension. In three cycles of CSR they enriched *Taq* polymerase with the general ability to extend 3' mispaired termini. This "unfussy" *Taq* promiscuously extended mismatches and was able to incorporate noncanonical substrates with high turnover, processivity, and fidelity.

Bacterial phosphotriesterase (PTE) has the ability to degrade pesticides and nerve agents like soman, sarin, and VX and thus is very interesting for bioremediation or disarmament of chemical weaponry. Griffiths et al. *(183)* used six rounds the microbead display IVC to generate an extremely fast phophotriesterase with 63 times higher k_{cat} than the wild-type enzyme. For selection of active enzymes the substrate was coupled to caged biotin which was afterwards uncaged by UV light. Thus, the product is coupled to the straptavidin coated beads and thus is linked to the coding gene. After breaking the emulsion, the product was detected by an antiproduct antibody which could be detected by a fluorescence labeled secondary antibody. Sorting was done by FACS.

Sequence recognition of enzymes is poorly understood and thus extremely challenging. Methylases as well as endonucleases are valuable tools in biotechnology. M.HaeIII methytransferase methylates the first cytosine after the second guanine of the canonical sequence 5' GGCC 3' but it is known that there is a promiscuous methylation at other sites like AGCC at lower rates *(184)*. Cohen et al. *(184)* altered the sequence preference of HaeIII methyltransferase by use of IVC from GGCC to AGCC and additionally this mutant also methylates at a low rate three other sites (AGCC, CGCC and GGCC) but discriminates as efficiently as the wild type enzyme against other sites. A library of mutated HaeIII genes was translated *in vitro* using IVC. Active enzymes methylated their genes and unmethylated genes were digested with a suitable enzyme NheI. The undigested genes were amplified and subjected to new rounds of IVC.

Ribozymes are catalytically active RNAs which ligate two RNAs which are aligned to a template by a reaction similar to enzymes which synthesize RNA *(138)*. Levy et al. *(184)* selected by microbead display IVC a ligase ribozyme capable to act *trans* on oligonucleotide substrates after two rounds of IVC. The ribozyme coding DNA was coupled to the beads together with an RNA oligonucleotide serving as substrate. DNA coding for functional ribozymes are able to ligate a tagged RNA to the coupled substrate RNA molecule can be selected by antiproduct antibodies. These primary antibodies were likewise detected by fluorescence labeled secondary antibodies, and the beads with DNA coding for active *trans*-acting ligase ribozymes were sorted by FACS.

References

1. Marshall SA, Lazar GA, Chirino AJ, Desjarlais JR (2003) Rational design and engineering of therapeutic proteins. Drug Discov Today 8:212–221
2. Hellinga HW (1997) Rational protein design: combining theory and experiment. Proc Natl Acad Sci USA 94:10015–10017
3. Creveld LD (2001) Molecular dynamics simulations in rational protein design: stabilization of fusarium solani pisi cutinase against anionic surfactants. University of Groningen
4. Balland A, Courtney M, Jallat S, Tessier LH, Sondermeyer P, de la Salle H, Harvey R, Degryse E, Tolstoshev P (1985) Use of synthetic oligonucleotides in gene isolation and manipulation. Biochimie 67:725–736
5. Garvey EP, Matthews CR (1990) Site-directed mutagenesis and its application to protein folding. Biotechnology 14:37–63
6. Wagner CR, Benkovic SJ (1990) Site directed mutagenesis: a tool for enzyme mechanism dissection. Trends Biotechnol 8:263–270
7. Kammann M, Laufs J, Schell J, Gronenborn B (1989) Rapid insertional mutagenesis of DNA by polymerase chain reaction (PCR). Nucleic Acids Res 17:5404
8. Antikainen NM, Martin SF (2005) Altering protein specificity: techniques and applications. Bioorg Med Chem 13:2701–2716
9. Desjarlais JR, Clarke ND (1998) Computer search algorithms in protein modification and design. Curr Opin Struct Biol 8:471–475
10. Voigt CA, Gordon DB, Mayo SL (2000) Trading accuracy for speed: A quantitative comparison of search algorithms in protein sequence design. J Mol Biol 299:789–803
11. Fishman GS (1995) Monte Carlo: concepts, algorithms, and applications. Springer Verlag, New York
12. Metropolis NaU, S (1949) The Monte Carlo method. J Am Stat As 44:335

13. Desmet J, de Maeyer M, Hazes B, Lasters I (1992) The dead-end elimination theorem and its use in protein side-chain positioning. Nature 356:539–542
14. Gordon DB, Marshall SA, Mayo SL (1999) Energy functions for protein design. Curr Opin Struct Biol 9:509–513
15. Pokala N, Handel TM (2001) Review: protein design – where we were, where we are, where we're going. J Struct Biol 134:269–281
16. Street AG, Mayo SL (1999) Computational protein design. Structure 7:R105–109
17. van Gunsteren WF, Mark AE (1992) On the interpretation of biochemical data by molecular dynamics computer simulation. Fur J Biochem 204:947–961
18. Smith GP, Petrenko VA (1997) Phage Display. Chem Rev 97:391–410
19. Smith GP (1985) Filamentous fusion phage: novel expression vectors that display cloned antigens on the virion surface. Science 228:1315–1317
20. Kehoe JW, Kay BK (2005) Filamentous phage display in the new millennium. Chem Rev 105:4056–4072
21. Willats WG (2002) Phage display: practicalities and prospects. Plant Mol Biol 50:837–854
22. Jung S, Honegger A, Plückthun A (1999) Selection for improved protein stability by phage display. J Mol Biol 294:163–180
23. Jaye DL, Geigerman CM, Fuller RE, Akyildiz A, Parkos CA (2004) Direct fluorochrome labeling of phage display library clones for studying binding specificities: applications in flow cytometry and fluorescence microscopy. J Immunol Methods 295:119–127
24. Steiner D, Forrer P, Stumpp MT, Pluckthun A (2006) Signal sequences directing cotranslational translocation expand the range of proteins amenable to phage display. Nat Biotechnol 24:823–831
25. Arndt KM, Jung S, Krebber C, Plückthun A (2000) Selectively infective phage technology. Methods Enzymol 328:364–388
26. Jung S, Arndt KM, Müller KM, Plückthun A (1999) Selectively infective phage (SIP) technology: scope and limitations. J Immunol Methods 231:93–104
27. Jiang J, Abu-Shilbayeh L, Rao VB (1997) Display of a PorA peptide from Neisseria meningitidis on the bacteriophage T4 capsid surface. Infect Immun 65:4770–4777
28. Danner S, Belasco JG (2001) T7 phage display: a novel genetic selection system for cloning RNA-binding proteins from cDNA libraries. Proc Natl Acad Sci USA 98:12954–12959
29. Mattheakis LC, Bhatt RR, Dower WJ (1994) An *in vitro* polysome display system for identifying ligands from very large peptide libraries. Proc Natl Acad Sci USA 91:9022–9026
30. Wilson DS, Keefe AD, Szostak JW (2001) The use of mRNA display to select high-affinity protein-binding peptides. Proc Natl Acad Sci USA 98:3750–3755
31. Hanes J, Jermutus L, Weber-Bornhauser S, Bosshard HR, Plückthun A (1998) Ribosome display efficiently selects and evolves high-affinity antibodies *in vitro* from immune libraries. Proc Natl Acad Sci USA 95:14130–14135
32. Fields S, Song O (1989) A novel genetic system to detect protein-protein interactions. Nature 340:245–246
33. Ma J, Ptashne M (1988) Converting a eukaryotic transcriptional inhibitor into an activator. Cell 55:443–446
34. Walhout AJ, Vidal M (2001) High-throughput yeast two-hybrid assays for large-scale protein interaction mapping. Methods 24:297–306
35. Shih HM, Goldman PS, DeMaggio AJ, Hollenberg SM, Goodman RH, Hoekstra MF (1996) A positive genetic selection for disrupting protein-protein interactions: identification of CREB mutations that prevent association with the coactivator CBP. Proc Natl Acad Sci USA 93:13896–13901
36. Vidal M, Brachmann RK, Fattaey A, Harlow E, Boeke JD (1996) Reverse two-hybrid and one-hybrid systems to detect dissociation of protein-protein and DNA-protein interactions. Proc Natl Acad Sci USA 93:10315–10320

37. Vidal M, Braun P, Chen E, Boeke JD, Harlow E (1996) Genetic characterization of a mammalian protein-protein interaction domain by using a yeast reverse two-hybrid system. Proc Natl Acad Sci USA 93:10321–10326

38. Aronheim A (1997) Improved efficiency sos recruitment system: expression of the mammalian GAP reduces isolation of Ras GTPase false positives. Nucleic Acids Res 25:3373–3374

39. Aronheim A, Zandi E, Hennemann H, Elledge SJ, Karin M (1997) Isolation of an AP-1 repressor by a novel method for detecting protein/protein interactions. Mol Cell Biol 17:3094–3102

40. Köhler F, Müller KM (2003) Adaptation of the Ras-recruitment system to the analysis of interactions between membrane-associated proteins. Nucleic Acids Res 31:e28

41. Osborne MA, Dalton S, Kochan JP (1995) The yeast tribrid system-genetic detection of trans-phosphorylated ITAM-SH2-interactions. Biotechnology (NY) 13:1474–1478

42. Zhang J, Lautar S (1996) A yeast three-hybrid method to clone ternary protein complex components. Anal Biochem 242:68–72

43. Licitra EJ, Liu JO (1996) A three-hybrid system for detecting small lig-and-protein receptor interactions. Proc Natl Acad Sci USA 93:12817–12821

44. Tafelmeyer P, Johnsson N, Johnsson K (2004) Transforming a (beta/alpha)8-barrel enzyme into a split-protein sensor through directed evolution. Chem Biol 11:681–689

45. Johnsson N, Varshavsky A (1994) Split ubiquitin as a sensor of protein interactions *in vivo*. Proc Natl Acad Sci USA 91:10340–10344

46. Pelletier JN, Campbell-Valois FX, Michnick SW (1998) Oligomerization domain-directed reassembly of active dihydrofolate reductase from rationally designed fragments. Proc Natl Acad Sci USA 95:12141–12146

47. Stammers DK, Champness JN, Beddell CR, Dann JG, Eliopoulos E, Geddes AJ, Ogg D, North AC (1987) The structure of mouse L1210 dihydrofolate reductase-drug complexes and the construction of a model of human enzyme. FEBS Lett 218:178–184

48. Blakley RL (1984). Folates and pterins: chemistry and biochemistry of Folates. In: Blakley RL, Cenkovic S (eds), Folates and pterins: chemistry and biochemistry of folates, Vol. 1. John Wiley & Sons, New York, pp 191–253

49. Appleman JR, Prendergast N, Delcamp TJ, Freisheim JH, Blakley RL (1988) Kinetics of the formation and isomerization of methotrexate complexes of recombinant human dihydrofolate reductase. J Biol Chem 263:10304–10313

50. Buchwalder A, Szadkowski H, Kirschner K (1992) A fully active variant of dihydrofolate reductase with a circularly permuted sequence. Biochemistry 31:1621–1630

51. Pelletier JN, Arndt KM, Plückthun A, Michnick SW (1999) An *in vivo* library-versus-library selection of optimized protein–protein interactions. Nat Biotechnol 17:683–690

52. Rossi F, Charlton CA, Blau HM (1997) Monitoring protein–protein interactions in intact eukaryotic cells by beta-galactosidase complementation. Proc Natl Acad Sci USA 94:8405–8410

53. Rossi FM, Blakely BT, Blau HM (2000) Interaction blues: protein interactions monitored in live mammalian cells by beta-galactosidase complementation. Trends Cell Biol 10:119–122

54. Ullmann A, Perrin D, Jacob F, Monod J (1965) [Identification, by *in vitro* complementation and purification, of a peptide fraction of *Escherichia coli* beta-galactosidase]. J Mol Biol 12:918–923

55. Villarejo M, Zamenhof PJ, Zabin I (1972) Beta-galactosidase. *In vivo* - complementation. J Biol Chem 247:2212–2216

56. Mohler WA, Blau HM (1996) Gene expression and cell fusion analyzed by lacZ complementation in mammalian cells. Proc Natl Acad Sci USA 93:12423–12427

57. Beckwith JR (1964) A deletion analysis of the Lac operator region in *Escherichia coli*. J Mol Biol 78:427–430

58. Prentki P (1992) Nucleotide sequence of the classical lacZ deletion delta M15. Gene 122:231–232

59. Galarneau A, Primeau M, Trudeau LE, Michnick SW (2002) Beta-lactamase protein fragment complementation assays as *in vivo* and *in vitro* sensors of protein protein interactions. Nat Biotechnol 20:619–622

60. Wehrman T, Kleaveland B, Her JH, Balint RF, Blau HM (2002) Protein–protein interactions monitored in mammalian cells via complementation of beta - lactamase enzyme fragments. Proc Natl Acad Sci USA 99:3469–3474

61. Zlokarnik G, Negulescu PA, Knapp TE, Mere L, Burres N, Feng L, Whitney M, Roemer K, Tsien RY (1998) Quantitation of transcription and clonal selection of single living cells with beta-lactamase as reporter. Science 279:84–88

62. Ambler RP, Coulson AF, Frere JM, Ghuysen JM, Joris B, Forsman M, Levesque RC, Tiraby G, Waley SG (1991) A standard numbering scheme for the class A beta-lactamases. Biochem J 276 (Pt 1) 269–270

63. Farzaneh S, Chaibi EB, Peduzzi J, Barthelemy M, Labia R, Blazquez J, Baquero F (1996) Implication of lle-69 and Thr-182 residues in kinetic characteristics of IRT-3 (TEM-32) beta-lactamase. Antimicrob Agents Chemother 40:2434–2436

64. Paulmurugan R, Umezawa Y, Gambhir SS (2002) Noninvasive imaging of protein–protein interactions in living subjects by using reporter protein complementation and reconstitution strategies. Proc Natl Acad Sci USA 99:15608–15613

65. Massoud TF, Gambhir SS (2003) Molecular imaging in living subjects: seeing fundamental biological processes in a new light. Genes Dev 17:545–580

66. Paulmurugan R, Gambhir SS (2003) Monitoring protein–protein interactions using split synthetic renilla luciferase protein-fragment-assisted complementation. Anal Chem 75:1584–1589

67. Remy I, Michnick SW (2006) A highly sensitive protein–protein interaction assay based on Gaussia luciferase. Nat Methods 3:977–979

68. Ghosh I, AD, H, Regan L (2000) Antiparallel Leucine zipper-directed protein reassembly: application to the green fluorescent protein. J Am Chem Soc 122:5658–5659

69. Ormo M, Cubitt AB, Kallio K, Gross LA, Tsien RY, Remington SJ (1996) Crystal structure of the Aequorea victoria green fluorescent protein. Science 273:1392–1395

70. Abedi MR, Caponigro G, Kamb A (1998) Green fluorescent protein as a scaffold for intracellular presentation of peptides. Nucleic Acids Res 26:623–630

71. Hu CD, Chinenov Y, Kerppola TK (2002) Visualization of interactions among bZIP and Rel family proteins in living cells using bimolecular fluorescence complementation. Mol Cell 9:789–798

72. Lee SY, Choi JH, Xu Z (2003) Microbial cell-surface display. Trends Biotechnol 21:45–52

73. Lunder M, Bratkovio T, Doljak B, Kreft S, Urleb U, Strukelj B, Plazar N (2005) Comparison of bacterial and phage display peptide libraries in search of target-binding motif. Appl Biochem Biotechnol 127:125–131

74. Romanos MA, Scorer CA, Clare JJ (1992) Foreign gene expression in yeast: a review. Yeast 8:423–488

75. Gellissen G, Melber K, Janowicz ZA, Dahlems UM, Weydemann U, Piontek M, Strasser AW, Hollenberg CP (1992) Heterologous protein production in yeast. Antonie Van Leeuwenhoek, 62:79–93

76. Schreuder MP, Brekelmans S, van den Ende H, Klis FM (1993) Targeting of a heterologous protein to the cell wall of Saccharomyces cerevisiae. Yeast, 9:399–409

77. Boder ET, Wittrup KD (1997) Yeast surface display for screening combinatorial polypeptide libraries. Nat Biotechnol 15:553–557

78. Kieke MC, Shusta EV, Boder ET, Teyton L, Wittrup KD, Kranz DM (1999) Selection of functional T cell receptor mutants from a yeast surface-display library. Proc Natl Acad Sci USA 96:5651–5656

79. Richman SA, Healan SJ, Weber KS, Donermeyer DL, Dossett ML, Greenberg PD, Allen PM, Kranz DM (2006) Development of a novel strategy for engineering high-affinity proteins by yeast display. Protein Eng Des Sel 19:255–264

80. Oker-Blom C, Airenne KJ, Grabherr R (2003) Baculovirus display strategies: Emerging tools for eukaryotic libraries and gene delivery. Brief Funct Genomic Proteomic 2:244–253

81. Smith GE, Summers MD, Fraser MJ (1983) Production of human beta interferon in insect cells infected with a baculovirus expression vector. Mol Cell Biol 3:2156–2165

82. O'Reilly DR, Miller LK, Luckow VA (1992). Baculovirus expression vectors: a laboratory manual 1st ed, W.H. Freeman and Company, New York

83. Boublik Y, Di Bonito P, Jones IM (1995) Eukaryotic virus display: engineering the major surface glycoprotein of the Autographa californica nuclear polyhedrosis virus (AcNPV) for the presentation of foreign proteins on the virus surface. Biotechnology (NY) 13:1079–1084

84. Ernst W, Grabherr R, Wegner D, Borth N, Grassauer A, Katinger H (1998) Baculovirus surface display: construction and screening of a eukaryotic epitope library. Nucleic Acids Res 26:1718–1723

85. Buchholz CJ, Peng KW, Morling FJ, Zhang J, Cosset FL, Russell SJ (1998) *In vivo* selection of protease cleavage sites from retrovirus display libraries. Nat Biotechnol 16:951–954

86. Urban JH, Schneider RM, Compte M, Finger C, Cichutek K, Alvarez-Vallina L, Buchholz CJ (2005) Selection of functional human antibodies from retroviral display libraries. Nucleic Acids Res 33:e35

87. Wolkowicz R, Jager GC, Nolan GR (2005) A random peptide library fused to CCR5 for selection of mimetopes expressed on the mammalian cell surface via retroviral vectors. J Biol Chem 280:15195–15201

88. Ho M, Nagata S, Pastan I (2006) Isolation of anti-CD22 Fv with high affinity by Fv display on human cells. Proc Natl Acad Sci USA 103:9637–9642

89. Rothe A, Surjadi RN, Power BE (2006) Novel proteins in emulsions using *in vitro* compartmentalization. Trends Biotechnol 24:587–592

90. Szostak JW, Bartel DP, Luisi PL (2001) Synthesizing life. Nature 409:387–390

91. Leamon JH, Link DK, Egholm M, Rothberg JM (2006) Overview: methods and applications for droplet compartmentalization of biology. Nat Methods 3:541–543

92. Miller OJ, Bernath K, Agresti JJ, Amitai G, Kelly BT, Mastrobattista E, Taly V, Magdassi S, Tawfik DS, Griffiths AD (2006) Directed evolution by *in vitro* compartmentalization. Nat Methods 3:561–570

93. Ghadessy FJ, Ong JL, Holliger P (2001) Directed evolution of polymerase function by compartmentalized self-replication. Proc Natl Acad Sci USA 98:4552–4557

94. Ong JL, Loakes D, Jaroslawski S, Too K, Holliger P (2006) Directed evolution of DNA polymerase, RNA polymerase and reverse transcriptase activity in a single polypeptide. J Mol Biol 361:537–550

95. Doi N, Kumadaki S, Oishi Y, Matsumura N, Yanagawa H (2004) *In vitro* selection of restriction endonucleases by *in vitro* compartmentalization. Nucleic Acids Res 32:e95

96. Sepp A, Tawfik DS, Griffiths AD (2002) Microbead display by *in vitro* compartmentalisation: selection for binding using flow cytometry. FEBS Lett 532:455–458

97. Bernath K, Hai M, Mastrobattista E, Griffiths AD, Magdassi S, Tawfik DS (2004) *In vitro* compartmentalization by double emulsions: sorting and gene enrichment by fluorescence activated cell sorting. Anal Biochem 325:151–157

98. Agresti JJ, Kelly BT, Jaschke A, Griffiths AD (2005) Selection of ribozymes that catalyse multiple-turnover Diels-Alder cycloadditions by using *in vitro* compartmentalization. Proc Natl Acad Sci USA 102:16170–16175

99. Worn A, Pluckthun A (2001) Stability engineering of antibody single-chain Fv fragments. J Mol Biol 305:989–1010

100. Lin L (1998) Betaseron. Dev Biol Stand 96:97–104

101. Arakawa T, Prestrelski SJ, Narhi LO, Boone TC, Kenney WC (1993) Cysteine 17 of recombinant human granulocyte-colony stimulating factor is partially solvent-exposed. J Protein Chem 12:525–531

102. Culajay JF, Blaber SI, Khurana A, Blaber M (2000) Thermodynamic characterization of mutants of human fibroblast growth factor 1 with an increased physiological half-life. Biochemistry 39:7153–7158

103. Tan PH, Chu V, Stray JE, Hamlin DK, Pettit D, Wilbur DS, Vessella RL, Stayton PS (1998) Engineering the isoelectric point of a renal cell carcinoma targeting antibody greatly enhances scFv solubility. Immunotechnology 4:107–114

104. Weintraub BD, Szkudlinski MW (1999) Development and *in vitro* characterization of human recombinant thyrotropin. Thyroid 9:447–450

105. Grossmann M, Leitolf H, Weintraub BD, Szkudlinski MW (1998) A rational design strategy for protein hormone superagonists. Nat Biotechnol 16:871–875

106. Siemeister G, Schimer M, Reusch P, Barleon B, Marme D, Martiny-Baron G (1998) An antagonistic vascular endothelial growth factor (VEGF) variant inhibits VEGF-stimulated receptor autophosphorylation and proliferation of human endothelial cells. Proc Natl Acad Sci USA 95:4625–4629

107. Savino R, Ciapponi L, Lahm A, Demartis A, Cabibbo A, Toniatti C, Delmastro P, Altamura S, Ciliberto G (1994) Rational design of a receptor super-antagonist of human interleukin-6. Embo J 13:5863–5870

108. Fub G, Cunningham BC, Fukunaga R, Nagata S, Goeddel DV, Wells JA (1992) Rational design of potent antagonists to the human growth hormone receptor. Science 256:1677–1680

109. Cunningham BC, Lowman HB, Wells JA, Clark RG, Olson K, Fuh GG (1988) Human Growth Hormone Variants, USA

110. Lu C, Shimaoka M, Ferzly M, Oxvig C, Takagi J, Springer TA (2001) An isolated, surface-expressed I domain of the integrin alphaLbeta2 is sufficient for strong adhesive function when locked in the open conformation with a disulfide bond. Proc Natl Acad Sci USA 98:2387–2392

111. Shimaoka M, Lu C, Palframan RT, von Andrian UH, McCormack A, Takagi J, Springer TA (2001) Reversibly locking a protein fold in an active conformation with a disulfide bond: integrin alphaL I domains with high affinity and antagonist activity *in vivo*. Proc Natl Acad Sci USA 98:6009–6014

112. Shimaoka M, Shifman JM, Jing H, Takagi J, Mayo SL, Springer TA (2000) Computational design of an integrin I domain stabilized in the open high affinity conformation. Nat Struct Biol 7:674–678

113. DeSantis G, Liu J, Clark DP, Heine A, Wilson IA, Wong CH (2003) Structure-based mutagenesis approaches toward expanding the substrate specificity of D-2-deoxyribose-5-phosphate aldolase. Bioorg Med Chem 11:43–52

114. Heine A, DeSantis G, Luz JG, Mitchell M, Wong CH, Wilson IA (2001) Observation of covalent intermediates in an enzyme mechanism at atomic resolution. Science 294:369–374

115. Babu CS, Dudev T, Casareno R, Cowan JA, Lim C (2003) A combined experimental and theoretical study of divalent metal ion selectivity and function in proteins: application to E. coli ribonuclease H1. J Am Chem Soc 125:9318–9328

116. Chevalier BS, Kortemme T, Chadsey MS, Baker D, Monnat RJ, Stoddard BL (2002) Design, activity, and structure of a highly specific artificial endonuclease. Mol Cell 10:895–905

117. Shifman JM, Mayo SL (2002) Modulating calmodulin binding specificity through computational protein design. J Mol Biol 323:417–423

118. Havranek JJ, Harbury PB (2003) Automated design of specificity in molecular recognition. Nat Struct Biol 10:45–52

119. Dwyer MA, Looger LL, Hellinga HW (2004) Computational design of a biologically active enzyme. Science 304:1967–1971

120. Pedone EM, Bartolucci S, Rossi M, Saviano M (1998) Computational analysis of the thermal stability in thioredoxins: a molecular dynamics approach. J Biomol Struct Dyn 16:437–446

121. Lazaridis T, Lee I, Karplus M (1997) Dynamics and unfolding pathways of a hyperthermophilic and a mesophilic rubredoxin. Protein Sci 6:2589–2605

122. Dahiyat BI, Mayo SL (1997) De novo protein design: fully automated sequence selection. Science 278:82–87

123. Marvin JS, Hellinga HW (2001) Conversion of a maltose receptor into a zinc biosensor by computational design. Proc Natl Acad Sci USA 98:4955–4960

124. de Lorimier RM, Smith JJ, Dwyer MA, Looger LL, Sali KM, Paavola CD, Rizk SS, Sadigov S, Conrad DW, Loew L, Hellinga HW (2002) Construction of a fluorescent biosensor family. Protein Sci 11:2655–2675

125. Yang W, Jones LM, Isley L, Ye Y, Lee HW, Wilkins A, Liu ZR, Hellinga HW, Malchow R, Ghazi M, Yang JJ (2003) Rational design of a calcium-binding protein. J Am Chem Soc 125:6165–6171

126. Looger LL, Dwyer MA, Smith JJ, Hellinga HW (2003) Computational design of receptor and sensor proteins with novel functions. Nature 423:185–190

127. Samoylova TI, Morrison NE, Globa LP, Cox NR (2006) Peptide phage display: opportunities for development of personalized anti-cancer strategies. Anticancer Agents Med Chem 6:9–17

128. Bongartz T, Sutton AJ, Sweeting MJ, Buchan I, Matteson EL, Montori V (2006) Anti-TNF antibody therapy in rheumatoid arthritis and the risk of serious infections and malignancies: systematic review and meta-analysis of rare harmful effects in randomized controlled trials. Jama 295:2275–2285

129. Sieber V, Pluckthun A, Schmid (1998) Selecting proteins with improved stability by a phage-based method. Nat Biotechnol 16:955–960

130. Barry MA, Dower WJ, Johnston SA (1996) Toward cell-targeting gene therapy vectors: selection of cell-binding peptides from random peptide-presenting phage libraries. Nat Med 2:299–305

131. Sergeeva A, Kolonin MG, Molldrem JJ, Pasqualini R, Arap W (2006) Display technologies: application for the discovery of drug and gene delivery agents. Adv Drug Deliv Rev 58:1622–1654

132. Oh Y, Mohiuddin I, Sun Y, Putnam JB, Jr, Hong WK, Arap W, Pasqualini R (2005) Phenotypic diversity of the lung vasculature in experimental models of metastases. Chest 128:596S–600S

133. Essler M, Ruoslahti E (2002) Molecular specialization of breast vasculature: a breast-homing phage-displayed peptide binds to aminopeptidase P in breast vasculature. Proc Natl Acad Sci USA 99:2252–2257

134. Rothe A, Hosse RJ, Power BE (2006) Ribosome display for improved biotherapeutic molecules. Expert Opin Biol Ther 6:177–187

135. Ihara H, Mie M, Funabashi H, Takahashi F, Sawasaki T, Endo Y, Kobatake E (2006) In vitro selection of zinc finger DNA-binding proteins through ribosome display. Biochem Biophys Res Commun 345:1149–1154

136. Amstutz P, Koch H, Binz HK, Deuber SA, Pluckthun A (2006) Rapid selection of specific MAP kinase-binders from designed ankyrin repeat protein libraries. Protein Eng Des Sel 19:219–229

137. Khosravi-Far R, White MA, Westwick JK, Solski PA, Chrzanowska-Wodnicka M, Van Aelst L, Wigler MH, Der CJ (1996) Oncogenic Ras activation of Raf/

mitogen-activated protein kinase-independent pathways is sufficient to cause tumorigenic transformation. Mol Cell Biol 16:3923–3933

138. Bartel DP, Szostak JW (1993) Isolation of new ribozymes from a large pool of random sequences [see comment]. Science 261:1411–1418

139. Uetz P, Giot L, Cagney G, Mansfield TA, Judson RS, Knight JR, Lockshon D, Narayan V, Srinivasan M, Pochart P, Qureshi-Emili A, Li Y, Godwin B, Conover D, Kalbfleisch T, Vijayadamodar G, Yang M, Johnston M, Fields S, Rothberg JM (2000) A comprehensive analysis of protein-protein interactions in Saccharomyces cerevisiae. Nature 403:623–627

140. Li S, Armstrong CM, Bertin N, Ge H, Milstein S, Boxem M, Vidalain PO, Han JD, Chesneau A, Hao T, Goldberg DS, Li N, Martinez M, Rual JF, Lamesch P, Xu L, Tewari M, Wong SL, Zhang LV, Berriz GF, Jacotot L, Vaglio P, Reboul J, Hirozane-Kishikawa T, Li Q, Gabel HW, Elewa A, Baumgartner B, Rose DJ, Yu H, Bosak S, Sequerra R, Fraser A, Mango SE, Saxton WM, Strome S, Van Den Heuvel S, Piano F, Vandenhaute J, Sardet C, Gerstein M, Doucette-Stamm L, Gunsalus KC, Harper JW, Cusick ME, Roth FP, Hill DE, Vidal M (2004) A map of the interactome network of the metazoan C. elegans. Science 303:540–543

141. Rual JF, Venkatesan K, Hao T, Hirozane-Kishikawa T, Dricot A, Li N, Berriz GF, Gibbons FD, Dreze M, Ayivi-Guedehoussou N, Klitgord N, Simon C, Boxem M, Milstein S, Rosenberg J, Goldberg DS, Zhang LV, Wong SL, Franklin G, Li S, Albala JS, Lin J, Fraughton C, Llamosas E, Cevik S, Bex C, Lamesch P, Sikorski RS, Vandenhaute J, Zoghbi HY, Smolyar A, Bosak S, Sequerra R, Doucette-Stamm L, Cusick ME, Hill DE, Roth FP, Vidal M (2005) Towards a proteome-scale map of the human protein–protein interaction network. Nature 437:1173–1178

142. Arndt KM, Pelletier JN, Müller KM, Alber T, Michnick SW, Plückthun A (2000) A heterodimeric coiled-coil peptide pair selected in vivo from a designed library-versus-library ensemble. J Mol Biol 295:627–639

143. Arndt KM, Pelletier JN, Müller KM, Plückthun A, Alber T (2002) Comparison of in vivo selection and rational design of heterodimeric coiled coils. Structure 10:1235–1248

144. Arndt KM, Müller KM, Plückthun A (2001) Helix-stabilized Fv (hsFv) antibody fragments: substituting the constant domains of a Fab fragment for a heterodimeric coiled-coil domain. J Mol Biol 312:221–228

145. Mason JM, Schmitz MA, Müller KM, Arndt KM (2006) Semirational design of Jun-Fos coiled coils with increased affinity: Universal implications for leucine zipper prediction and design. Proc Natl Acad Sci USA 103:8989–8994

146. Mason JM, Müller KM, Arndt KM (2007) Positive Aspects of Negative Design: Simultaneous Selection of Specificity and Interaction Stability. Biochemistry 46:4804–4814

147. Mason JM, Hagemann UB, Arndt KM (2007) Improved Stability of the Jun-Fos Activator Protein-1 Coiled Coil Motif: A Stopped-flow Circluar Dichroism Kinetic Analysis. J Biol Chem 282:23015–23024

148. Jouaux, EM, Schmidkunz K, Müller KM, Arndt KM (2008) Targeting the c-Myc coiled coil with interfering peptides to inhibit DNA binding. J Pept Sci (in press)

149. Mossner E, Koch H, Plückthun A (2001) Fast selection of antibodies without antigen purification: adaptation of the protein fragment complementation assay to select antigen-antibody pairs. J Mol Biol 308:115–122

150. Remy I, Wilson IA, Michnick SW (1999) Erythropoietin receptor activation by a ligand-induced conformation change. Science 283:990–993

151. Laser H, Bongards C, Schuller J, Heck S, Johnsson N, Lehming N (2000) A new screen for protein interactions reveals that the Saccharomyces cerevisiae high mobility group proteins Nhp6A/B are involved in the regulation of the GAL1 promoter. Proc Natl Acad Sci USA 97:13732–13737

152. Stagljar I, Korostensky C, Johnsson N, te Heesen S (1998) A genetic system based on split-ubiquitin for the analysis of interactions between membrane proteins *in vivo*. Proc Natl Acad Sci USA 95:5187–5192

153. Ooi AT, Stains CI, Ghosh I, Segal DJ (2006) Sequence-enabled reassembly of beta-lactamase (SEER-LAC): a sensitive method for the detection of double-stranded DNA. Biochemistry 45:3620–3625

154. Stains CI, Porter JR, Ooi AT, Segal DJ, Ghosh I (2005) DNA sequence-enabled reassembly of the green fluorescent protein. J Am Chem Soc 127:10782–10783

155. Massoud TF, Paulmurugan R, Gambhir SS (2004) Molecular imaging of homodimeric protein–protein interactions in living subjects. Faseb J 18:1105–1107

156. Hu CD, Kerppola TK (2003) Simultaneous visualization of multiple protein interactions in living cells using multicolor fluorescence complementation analysis. Nat Biotechnol 21:539–545

157. Bracha-Drori K, Shichrur K, Katz A, Oliva M, Angelovici R, Yalovsky S, Ohad N (2004) Detection of protein–protein interactions in plants using bimolecular fluorescence complementation. Plant J 40:419–427

158. Walter M, Chaban C, Schutze K, Batistio O, Weckermann K, Nake C, Blazevic D, Grefen C, Schumacher K, Oecking C, Harter K, Kudla J (2004) Visualization of protein interactions in living plant cells using bimolecular fluorescence complementation. Plant J 40:428–438

159. Christmann A, Wentzel A, Meyer C, Meyers G, Kolmar H (2001) Epitope mapping and affinity purification of monospecific antibodies by *Escherichia coli* cell surface display of gene-derived random peptide libraries. J Immunol Methods 257:163–173

160. Wentzel A, Christmann A, Kratzner R, Kolman H (1999) Sequence requirements of the GPNG beta-turn of the *Ecballium elaterium* trypsin inhibitor II explored by combinatorial library screening. J Biol Chem 274:21037–21043

161. Kjaergaard K, Schembri MA, Klemm P (2001) Novel Zn(2+)-chelating peptides selected from a fimbria-displayed random peptide library. Appl Environ Microbiol 67:5467–5473

162. James P, Vorherr T, Carafoli E (1995) Calmodulin-binding domains: just two faced or multi-faceted? Trends Biochem Sci 20:38–42

163. Weaver-Feldhaus JM, Miller KD, Feldhaus MJ, Siegel RW (2005) Directed evolution for the development of conformation-specific affinity reagents using yeast display. Protein Eng Des Sel 18:527–536

164. Williams T (1996) The iridoviruses. Adv Virus Res 46:345–412

165. Tamaru Y, Ohtsuka M, Kato K, Manabe S, Kuroda K, Sanada M, Ueda M (2006) Application of the arming system for the expression of the 380R antigen from red sea bream iridovirus (RSIV) on the surface of yeast cells: a first step for the development of an oral vaccine. Biotechnol Prog 22:949–953

166. Cho BK, Kieke MC, Boder ET, Wittrup KD, Kranz DM (1998) A yeast surface display system for the discovery of ligands that trigger cell activation. J Immunol Methods 220:179–188

167. Kondo A, Ueda M (2004) Yeast cell-surface display–applications of molecular display. Appl Microbiol Biotechnol 64:28–40

168. Raty JK, Airenne KJ, Marttila AT, Marjomaki V, Hytonen VF, Lehtolainen P, Laitinen OH, Mahonen AJ, Kulomaa MS, Yla-Herttuala S (2004) Enhanced gene delivery by avidin-displaying baculovirus. Mol Ther 9:282–291

169. Riddle DS, Sanz L, Chong H, Thompson J, Vile RG (2005) Tumor cell surface display of immunoglobulin heavy chain Fc by gene transfer as a means to mimic antibody therapy. Hum Gene Ther 16:830–844

170. Winter G, Griffiths AD, Hawkins RE, Hoogenboom HR (1994) Making antibodies by phage display technology. Annu Rev Immunol 12:433–455

171. Low NM, Holliger PH, Winter G (1996) Mimicking somatic hypermutation: affinity maturation of antibodies displayed on bacteriophage using a bacterial mutator strain. J Mol Biol 260:359–368

172. de Bruin R, Spelt K, Mol J, Koes R, Quattrocchio F (1999) Selection of high-affinity phage antibodies from phage display libraries. Nat Biotechnol 17:397–399

173. Chowdhury PS, Pastan I (1999) Improving antibody affinity by mimicking somatic hypermutation *in vitro*. Nat Biotechnol 17:568–572

174. Francisco JA, Campbell R, Iverson BL, Georgiou G (1993) Production and fluorescence-activated cell sorting of *Escherichia coli* expressing a functional antibody fragment on the external surface. Proc Natl Acad Sci USA 90:10444–10448

175. Francisco JA, Georgiou G (1994) The expression of recombinant proteins on the external surface of *Escherichia coli*. Biotechnological applications. Ann NY Acad Sci 745:372–382

176. Georgiou G, Stathopoulos C, Daugherty PS, Nayak AR, Iverson BL, Curtiss R, 3rd (1997) Display of heterologous proteins on the surface of microorganisms: from the screening of combinatorial libraries to live recombinant vaccines. Nat Biotechnol 15:29–34

177. Boder ET, Midelfort KS, Wittrup KD (2000) Directed evolution of antibody fragments with monovalent femtomolar antigen-binding affinity. Proc Natl Acad Sci USA 97:10701–10705

178. Feldhaus MJ, Siegel RW, Opresko LK, Coleman JR, Feldhaus JM, Yeung YA, Cochran JR, Heinzelman P, Colby D, Swers J, Graff C, Wiley HS, Wittrup KD (2003) Flow-cytometric isolation of human antibodies from a nonimmune Saccharomyces cerevisiae surface display library. Nat Biotechnol 21:163–170

179. Hanes J, Plückthun A (1997) *In vitro* selection and evolution of functional proteins by using ribosome display. Proc Natl Acad Sci USA 94:4937–4942

180. Gold L (2001) mRNA display: diversity matters during *in vitro* selection. Proc Natl Acad Sci USA 98:4825–4826

181. Pavlov AR, Pavlova NV, Kozyavkin SA, Slesarev AL (2004) Recent developments in the optimization of thermostable DNA polymerases for efficient applications. Trends Biotechnol 22:253–260

182. Ghadessy FJ, Ramsay N, Boudsocq F, Loakes D, Brown A, Iwai S, Vaisman A, Woodgate R, Holliger P (2004) Generic expansion of the substrate spectrum of a DNA polymerase by directed evolution. Nat Biotechnol 22:755–759

183. Griffiths AD, Tawfik DS (2003) Directed evolution of an extremely fast phosphotriesterase by *in vitro* compartmentalization. Embo J 22:24–35

184. Cohen HM, Tawfik DS, Griffiths AD (2004) Altering the sequence specificity of HaeIII methyltransferase by directed evolution using *in vitro* compartmentalization. Protein Eng Des Sel 17:3–11

185. Levy M, Griswold KE, Ellington AL (2005) Direct selection of transacting ligase ribozymes by *in vitro* compartmentalization. Rna 11:1555–1562

36

Directed Protein Evolution

Sabine C. Stebel, Annette Gaida, Katja M. Arndt, and Kristian M. Müller

1. Introduction

Enzymes can dramatically increase the rate of chemical reactions while acting stereoselective and regioselective and are therefore very attractive for industry. However, only few enzymes taken from nature work under the often harsh conditions required by industrial applications. Proteins with desired attributes can be obtained either by searching through the largely unknown naturally occurring species or by improving or altering already characterized proteins. Today, much research effort is devoted to adjusting various enzyme attributes to technical demands and to exploring nonnatural functions of enzymes.

Two basic approaches are used to optimize enzymes to fullfill desired properties: rational design and directed evolution **Fig. 36.1**.

1.1. Rational Design

To optimize a protein by rational design, the structure of the protein or a close homolog should be known. Better results can be obtained, when information about mechanism and function of the protein are available. Scientists planning to redesign an enzyme for the first time should be aware that integration of knowledge into the design process is very time intensive and requires training. Variants are planned based on intuition, sequence alignments and *in silico* modeling. Amino acid exchanges required for optimization are introduced into the gene of the original protein via site-directed mutagenesis. Finally, over-expressed variants require further characterization.

1.2. Directed Evolution

Despite advances in our understanding of protein structure and function this knowledge is by far not sufficient to tailor amino acid exchanges. From this perspective it is very appealing to use random design approaches such as combinatorial strategies to search sequence space for beneficial mutations without prior knowledge of structure or function.

From natural evolution we have learned that organisms and accordingly naturally occurring proteins are constantly changing to adapt to new environmental

From: *Molecular Biomethods Handbook, 2nd Edition.*
Edited by: J. M. Walker and R. Rapley © Humana Press, Totowa, NJ

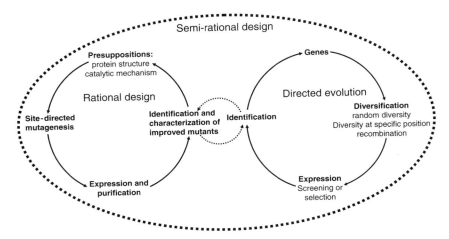

Fig. 36.1. Schema showing how directed evolution and rational design are connected

requirements and microorganisms can even cometabolize xenobiotica they were never adapted to. Directed evolution mimics the Darwinian principles of mutation and selection underlying evolution in nature. In general the term "directed evolution" is used to sum up different techniques for the creation of protein variants by low frequency introduction of point mutations, their selection or screening for the desired properties, and the recombination of beneficial mutations found in different clones. Directed evolution normally consists of repeated cycles of mutagenesis, screening or selection, and recombination **Fig. 36.1**.

1.3. Semi-Rational Design

The experimental combination of rational design and directed evolution is called semi-rational design.

This chapter describes and explains methods used in directed evolution experiments and presents successful applications.

2. Methods for the Creation of Diversity

Crucial to any evolutionary optimization strategy is a suitable library to start with and efficient means of screening or preferably selecting optimized variants from these libraries. A library of mutants is constructed at the genetic level from which the protein library is translated, thus any protein selected can be identified by its DNA sequence. Multiple methods are available to construct such DNA libraries which conceptually can be divided into three groups **Table 36.1**.

2.1. Random Diversity by Disturbed DNA Replication

2.1.1. Chemical and Physical Mutation

The first group comprises methods generating random diversity by disturbed DNA replication.

Physical and chemical mutagens like UV irradiation or alkylating agents were the first employed to purposely damage DNA. UV irradiation generates radicals or is absorbed by the double bond of pyrimidine bases (typically thymidines), which thus excited, can form dimers with neighboring pyrimidine bases. These dimers when not successfully repaired lead to random incorporation of

Table 36.1. Three ways to construct DNA libraries.

Random diversity by disturbed DNA replication	Controlled levels of random diversity at specific positions	Diversity by recombination
• Chemical and physical mutation	• Synthesis of oligonucleotides	**Homologous recombination:**
• Mutator strains	• Whole gene synthesis	• DNA shuffling (DNA shuffling, NExT)
• epPCR		• Staggered extension process (StEP)
• Random insertion / deletion mutagenesis (*PSM, RAISE, RID)*		• Recombination-dependent exponential amplification PCR (RDA-PCR)
• Sequence saturation mutagenesis (SESAM)		• Random chimeragenesis on transient templates (RACHITT)
		• Recombined extension on truncated templates (RETT)
		• Mutagenic and unidirectional reassembly method (MURA)
		• Random-priming in vitro recombination (RPR)
		• Multiplex-PCR-based recombination (MUPREC)
		• In vitro heteroduplex formation and in vivo repair
		Non-homologous recombination:
		• Incremental truncation for the creation of hybrid enzymes (ITCHY, SCRATCHY)
		• Homology-independent protein recombination (SHIPREC)
		• Synthetic shuffling or Assembly of designed oligonucleotides (ADO)
		• Degenerate oligonucleotide gene shuffling (DOGS)
		• Sequence-independent site-directed chimeragenesis (SISDC)
		• Exon shuffling

nucleotides. Alkylation agents like ethylenemethanesulfonat (EMS) alkylate e.g., the oxygens of guanidine at position 6 leading to a transition from GC to AT *(1)*. Hydroxylamine hydroxylates specifically the NH_2 group of cytosine. The resulting hydroxylaminocytosine pairs with adenine leading to a transition from CG to TA *(1)*.

2.1.2. Mutator Strains

Conceptually simple but hard to control regarding the mutation rate are *Escherichia coli* K12 mutator strains like XL1-red from Stratagene, which are deficient in three DNA repair pathways (mutS, mutD, and mutt) increasing the mutation rate up to 5,000 times compared to the wild-type strain.

2.1.3. Error Prone PCR (epPCR)

The most popular method, because it is easy to control and implement, is the generation of random point mutations *by error prone PCR (epPCR) (2)*. *Taq*-DNA-polymerase is prone to errors during polymerase chain reaction. The normal error rate of *Taq*-DNA-Polymerase (1×10^{-4} to 2×10^{-5} errors

Sequence Saturation Mutagenesis (SESAM)

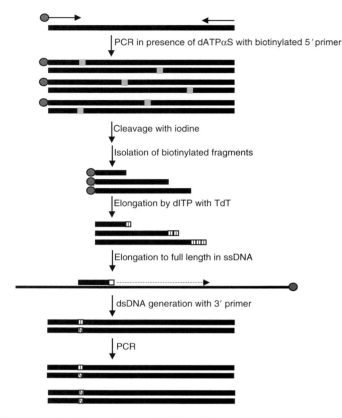

Fig. 36.2. Sequence saturation mutagenesis (SESAM)

per nucleotide) is by far not enough to be used for the construction of a combinatorial library by means of PCR. However it can be easily enhanced by adding small amounts of Mn^{2+} ions, which replace the natural cofactor Mg^{2+}. If necessary, the mutation rate can be further enhanced by using a biased dNTP mixture with unequal representation of nucleotides.

2.1.4. Sequence Saturation Mutagenesis (SESAM)

In the above described methods to mutagenize DNA typically only one nucleotide per codon is changed, thus in average every amino acid can be changed to only about 5 out of 19 possible amino acids. *Sequence saturation mutagenesis (SESAM)* *(3)* overcomes this by substituting nucleotides with a universal base (deoxyinosine, dITP) **Fig. 36.2.** In the first step a PCR is performed with a 5' biotinylated primer and $dATP\alpha S$ in addition to the four natural dNTPs. $dATP\alpha S$ is similar to the natural dATP but carries a sulfur atom instead of an oxygen at the α-phosphate. The resulting phosphate bond is cleaved by iodine and the biotinylated fragments are isolated from the fragment mixture by binding of biotin to immobilized streptavidin. The cleaved and isolated fragments are tailed with dITP by terminal deoxynucleotidyl transferase (TdT), a template-independent DNA polymerase that catalyzes the repetitive random addition of deoxyribonucleotides to the 3' end of single and double stranded

DNA. The resulting elongated strand is extended to full length on long and biotinylated ssDNA templates without amplification of this template. The reverse primer, which can not bind to the long ssDNA template, anneals to the newly synthesized strand and dsDNA is generated that contains a nucleotide analog in one strand and randomly inserted nucleotides at the corresponding position in the complementary strand.

To replace the dITP with standard nucleotides an additional PCR is carried out where the full length genes containing dITP serve as template.

2.1.5. Methods of Random Insertion/Deletion

Random diversity can also be generated by transposons like Tn4430 in *pentapeptide scanning mutagenesis (PSM)* (*4*) **Fig. 36.3**. Tn4430 contains two restriction sites for *Kpn*I 5 bp from both termini. Tn4430 duplicates 5 bp of its target site during transposition. Therefore, if Tn4430 is removed from the target plasmid by digest with *Kpn*I it leaves a 15 bp fingerprint consisting of two times 5 bp from the transposon ends and 5 bp from the duplicated target-site. The gene of interest, which is flanked by two unique restriction sites,

Pentapeptide Scanning Mutagenesis (PSM)

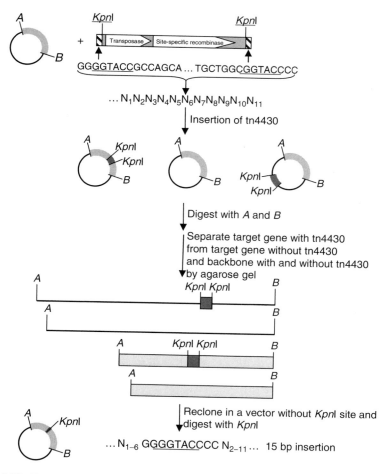

Fig. 36.3. Pentapeptide scanning mutagenesis (PSM)

Random Insertional-deletion Strand Exchange mutagenesis (RAISE)

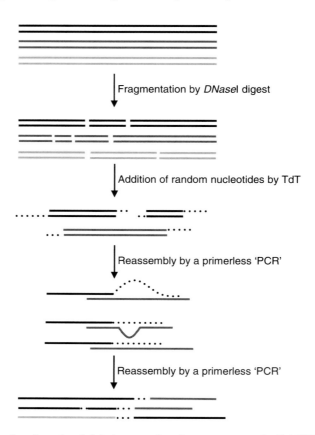

Fig. 36.4. Random insertional-deletion strand exchange mutagenesis (RAISE)

is removed from the plasmid and genes with transposons are separated from those without by agarose gel and cloned into a new vector backbone.

2.1.5.1. Random Insertional-Deletion Strand Exchange Mutagenesis (RAISE): RAISE *(5)* **Fig. 36.4** is a modified version of DNase shuffling (see the following). After DNA digest the generated fragments are incubated with terminal deoxynucleotidyl transferase (TdT), a template-independent DNA polymerase that catalyzes the repetitive random addition of deoxyribonucleotides to the 3' end of single and double stranded DNA. During reassembly of the randomly elongated fragments deletions, insertions, or exchanges are generated dependent of the length of the random insert.

2.1.5.2. Random Insertion and Deletion Mutagenesis (RID): RID *(6)* **Fig. 36.5** can insert randomly up to 16 random bases at random positions along a whole gene. To perform RID the gene of interest is first flanked with two different unique restriction sites and cut by these two enzymes, e.g., *Eco*RI at the 5' end and *Hin*dIII at the 3' end. In the next step a synthetic oligonucleotide linker that has a *Hin*dIII restriction site at the 5' end and a complementary sticky end at the 3' end is ligated to the 5' end of the gene leaving

<u>R</u>andom <u>I</u>nsertion and <u>D</u>eletion (RID)

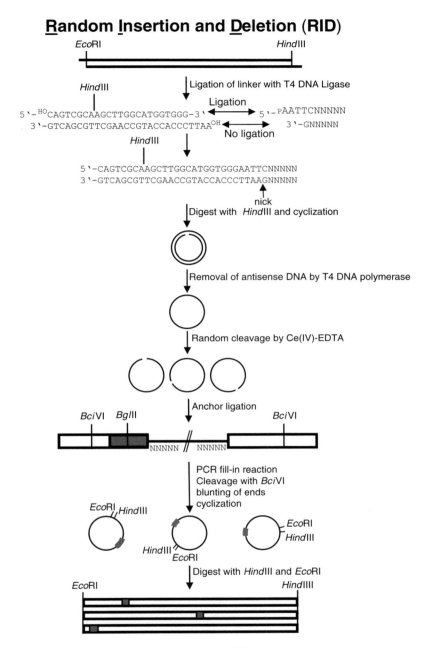

Fig. 36.5. Random insertion and deletion (RID)

a nick as the 3' end does not have a mono-phosphate and thus will not link to the 3' end of dsDNA. The gene is again digested by *Hind*III and cyclized. The DNA strand containing the nick is degraded by T4 DNA polymerase resulting in circular ssDNA that is randomly cut once with ceric ammonium nitrate–EDTA complex (Ce(IV)-EDTA). Random anchors are ligated to both ends. Both anchors contain a unique restriction site e.g., a *Bci*VI site, additional nucleotides to be inserted and a random tail for the hybridization with the unknown 3' end ssDNA and 5' end respectively. The ssDNA is filled in and the ends are blunted if necessary. After renewed cyclization this dsDNA ring is cut with *Eco*RI and *Hind*III thus generating the original gene including a randomly inserted sequence.

2.2. Controlled Levels of Random Diversity at Specific Positions

The techniques described in Section 2.1 randomly generate diversity along the whole gene. The second group of methods encompasses techniques that insert controlled levels of random diversity at specific positions. In principle all the methods of the second group are based on the incorporation of synthetic DNA sequences into the coding gene. The synthesis of oligonucleotides or even whole genes allows the complete control over identity, position, and level of mutation. Most commonly used are degenerate oligonucleotides, which at defined positions contain degenerate codons and can be bought from most suppliers. With such oligonucleotides specific positions in a gene can be completely randomized.

2.3. Diversity by Recombination

2.3.1. Homologous Recombination Methods

2.3.1.1. DNA Shuffling and its Derivates: A big disadvantage of the methods described above is the indiscriminate incorporation of beneficial as well as deleterious mutations. If proteins are to be optimized only by point mutations at some stage the disadvantageous mutations will reduce or completely overlay the beneficial effects of advantageous mutations. In nature this problem is solved by sexual recombination allowing for out crossing of deleterious mutations. The third group of methods comprises approaches mimicking this natural sexual recombination. Unlike in nature where only the genes of two parents are crossed, shuffling can recombine the genes of multiple parents. The first method becoming popular for homologous DNA recombination in the test tube was *DNA shuffling (7)* **Fig. 36.6**. In *DNA shuffling*, the DNA is first digested by DNase I. The digested fragments of the desired size are extracted from an agarose gel and reassembled by a primerless 'PCR' reaction in which the fragments serve each other as primer and template at the same time (recursive PCR). The reconstructed and recombined genes are afterwards amplified using a standard PCR reaction. *Nucleotide exchange and excision technology* (NExT) *(8,9)* **Fig. 36.7** is similar to the DNase digest but much easier to control. NExT uses a statistical fragmentation by incorporation of uridine (dUTP) during PCR, followed by digestion with uracildeglycosylase (UDG) and NaOH instead of DNase I. Additionally NExT uses vent polymerase for the reassembly reaction. Vent is a proofreading polymerase with strand displacement activity. In case of multiple priming events on one strand, vent can remove these oligonucleotides and read on significantly improving yield of reassembled genes.

2.3.1.2. Staggered Extension Process (StEP): STEP *(10)* **Fig. 36.8** is based on fast template switches owing to very short elongation times during a PCR reaction. As a consequence partially elongated strands are generated that can switch the parental template and thus lead to recombination of different parental genes.

A further development of StEP is the *recombination-dependent exponential amplification PCR (RDA-PCR) (11)* **Fig. 36.9**. In RDA-PCR the library is divided into two groups, which are amplified with two different primer pairs adding different overhangs, e.g., group 1 is amplified using primers A and B and group 2 with primer C and D. These two groups are then mixed, divided into two new groups and a StEP reaction is carried out but this time with primer pairs A/D

DNA shuffling

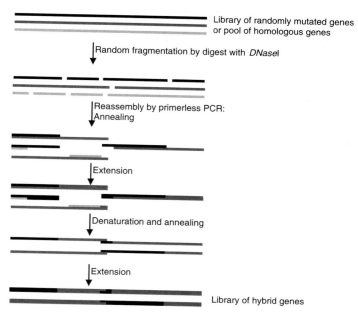

Fig. 36.6. DNA shuffling

<u>N</u>ucleotide <u>Ex</u>change and Excision <u>T</u>echnology (NExT)

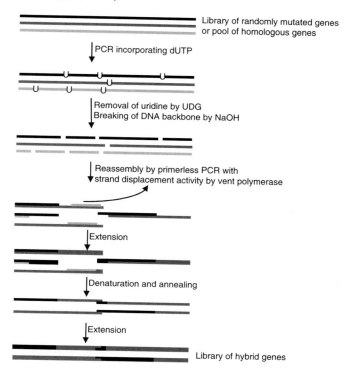

Fig. 36.7. Nucleotide exchange and excision technology (NExT)

Staggered Extension Process (StEP)

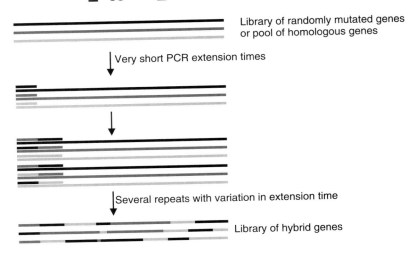

Library of randomly mutated genes
or pool of homologous genes

Very short PCR extension times

Several repeats with variation in extension time

Library of hybrid genes

Fig. 36.8. Staggered extension process (StEP)

Recombination-Dependent Exponential Amplification PCR (RDA-PCR)

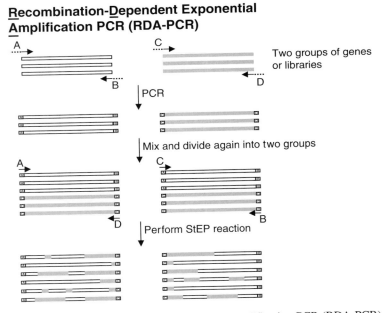

Two groups of genes
or libraries

PCR

Mix and divide again into two groups

Perform StEP reaction

Fig. 36.9. Recombination-dependent exponential amplification PCR (RDA-PCR)

and B/C thus ensuring that only chimeric genes with at least onecross over are amplified. Unfortunately, only chimeric genes with odd numbers of crossovers can be amplified using this method.

2.3.1.3. Random Chimeragenesis on Transient Templates (RACHITT): RACHITT *(12)* **Fig. 36.10** is conceptually similar to StEP. In RACHITT a

<u>R</u>andom <u>C</u>himeragenesis on <u>T</u>ransient <u>T</u>emplates (RACHITT)

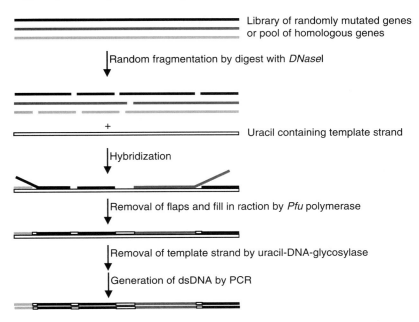

Library of randomly mutated genes or pool of homologous genes

Random fragmentation by digest with *DNaseI*

+   Uracil containing template strand

Hybridization

Removal of flaps and fill in raction by *Pfu* polymerase

Removal of template strand by uracil-DNA-glycosylase

Generation of dsDNA by PCR

Fig. 36.10. Random chimeragenesis on transient templates (RACHITT)

parental DNA strand containing dUTP is generated and fragments of the opposite strand anneal to this parental template. Nonannealed overhangs are digested by the exonuclease activity of *Pfu* DNA polymerase, which also fills in the remaining gaps. The generated fragments are ligated and the uridine containing parental strand is rendered unproductive by digest with endonuclease V. The resulting chimeric strand is amplified by PCR.

2.3.1.4. Recombined Extension on Truncated Templates (RETT): Eukaryotic RNA in contrast to DNA doesn't contain any introns and thus is shorter and more suited for DNA shuffling than eukaryotic DNA. A recombination method more likely useful for eukaryotic genes than the previously described ones is *recombined extension on truncated templates (RETT) (13)* **Fig. 36.11** as it uses RNA. Fragments can be generated by using random primers for reverse transcription or by unidirectional serial truncation of cDNA with exonuclease III. A specific primer is afterwards annealed to complementary ssDNA fragmentation and extended by PCR. Short fragments extended from this specific primer (like in StEP) are annealed to another ssDNA fragment and thus switch templates. This extension is repeated until full length genes are generated, which then are used to generate dsDNA by PCR.

2.3.1.5. Mutagenic and Unidirectional Reassembly Method (MURA): Truncated genes can lead to altered attributes of the enzyme coded by this gene, e.g., specificity and thermal stability. Very similar to RETT is *mutagenic and*

<u>R</u>ecombined <u>E</u>xtensions of <u>T</u>runcated <u>T</u>emplates (RETT)

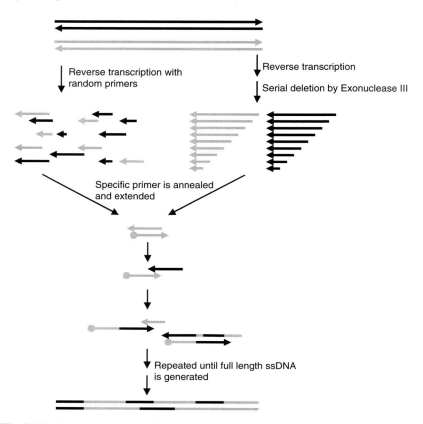

Fig. 36.11. Recombined extension on truncated templates (RETT)

unidirectional reassembly method (MURA) (14) **Fig. 36.12**. In contrast to RETT MURA starts with dsDNA, which is digested by DNaseI like in DNA-shuffling. The resulting fragments however are not reassembled by a primerless PCR but like in RETT the reassembly is achieved using unidirectional primers containing appropriate restriction sites (MURA primer). This unidirectional reassembly additionally to template switches results in N- or C- terminally truncated mutants depending on the location of the primer.

2.3.1.6. Multiplex-PCR-Based Recombination (MUPREC): Only applicable to homologous templates is multiplex-PCR-based recombination (MUPREC) *(15)* **Fig. 36.13**. Multiplex PCR *(16)* is a variant of PCR, which simultaneously amplifies many targets of interest in one reaction by using more than one pair of primers. In this case two different genes are amplified with multiple 5′ and multiple 3′ primers containing point mutations to generate mutated gene fragments of different lengths. These fragments are afterwards mixed and recombined in a reassembly PCR. For this method primers have to be designed

Mutagenic and Unidirectional Reassembly Method (MURA)

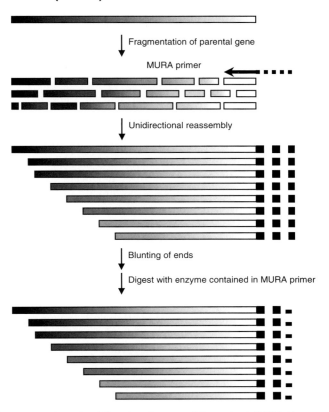

Fig. 36.12. Mutagenic and unidirectional reassembly method (MURA)

Multiplex-PCR-based Recombination (MUPREC)

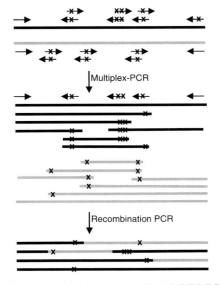

Fig. 36.13. Multiplex-PCR-based recombination (MUPREC)

with comparable melting temperatures. In multiplex-PCR the amount of each primer used influences the frequency of the mutations incorporated.

2.3.1.7. Random-Priming in vitro *Recombination (RPR):* A much earlier published variation of MUPREC is *random-priming* in vitro *recombination (RPR) (17)* that instead of specially designed primers uses random primers of identical length, which results in fragments of many different sizes that can be reassembled by primerless PCR reaction.

2.3.1.8. In vitro *Heteroduplex Formation and* in vivo *Repair:* In vitro heteroduplex formation and in vivo repair *(18)* **Fig. 36.14** is a method that is mainly useful for the recombination of large genes or whole operons as this method has not the size limitations of PCR based methods. If cells are transformed with partially overlapping inserts with included mismatches, each mismatch between the two DNA strands can be repaired independently by combination with homologous regions und this results in chimeric sequences. The *E. coli* mismatch MutHLS repair system consists of three components: MutS for the recognition of mismatches, MuL is a molecular matchmaker that activates the nicking endonuclease MutH. MutH can bind to GATC sequences and nicks the DNA, which is then unwound by helicase II. The mismatch gap is filled in by polymerase III by copying the complementary DNA strand.

In vitro heteroduplex formation and *in vivo* repair

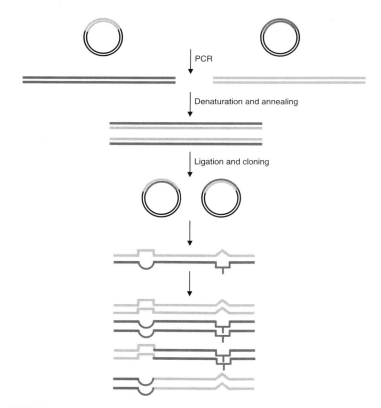

Fig. 36.14. In vitro heteroduplex formation and in vivo repair

2.3.2. Nonhomologous Recombination Methods

2.3.2.1. Incremental Truncation for the Creation of Hybrid Enzymes (ITCHY)/SCRATCHY: It was shown that introns mostly occur at positions with low intermolecular interaction, pointing to proteins being composed of building blocks of domains developed earlier in evolution *(19)*. Nonhomologous recombination or family shuffling explores these largely unknown possibilities.

In contrast to the above mentioned recombination methods, where gene reassembly is based on high homology among the genes to be recombined *incremental truncation for the creation of hybrid enzymes (ITCHY) (20,21)* **Fig. 36.15** allows recombination of nonhomologous templates. Two genes, one incrementally truncated from the 5′ end, the other from the 3′ end are

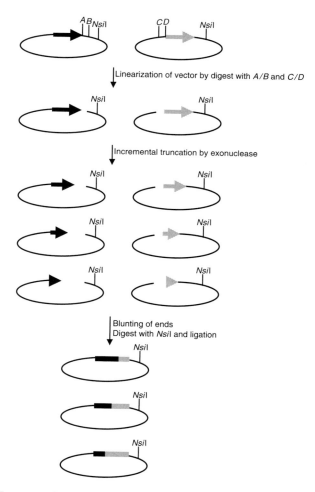

Fig. 36.15. Incremental truncation for the creation of hybrid enzymes (ITCHY)

ligated thus creating chimeras with one cross over. The gene length of the generated chimeras is not conserved and recombination mostly occurs at nonstructurally related sites. The chimeric libraries generated by ITCHY can be afterwards shuffled by the above mentioned methods thus enhancing the cross over rate. This combination of ITCHY technology with DNA shuffling is called SCRATCHY *(22)*.

2.3.2.2. Sequence Homology-Independent Protein Recombination (SHIPREC): A further development of the basic ITCHY idea is *sequence homology-independent protein recombination (SHIPREC) (23)* **Fig. 36.16**. In contrast to ITCHY SHIPCREC generates chimeras that have the cross over at similar structural positions. In SHIPREC two genes are fused together via a linker containing a unique restriction site and digested with *DNase*I. Fragments of the size of the single genes are selected by agarose gel electrophoresis and blunted. The blunted chimeras are afterwards circularized and cut at the linker position thus placing the gene fragment corresponding to the C-terminal part of the protein coded by the first gene behind the gene fragment of the second gene that codes for to the N-terminal part of the second protein. Limiting the size of fragments to the size of the original genes ensures that the chimeras cross at similar parental structures.

2.3.2.3. Synthetic Shuffling or Assembly of Designed Oligonucleotides (ADO): Synthetic shuffling *(24)* **Fig. 36.17** is a combination of the use of degenerate oligonucleotides and DNA shuffling. Instead of fragment-

<u>S</u>equence <u>H</u>omology-<u>I</u>ndependent <u>P</u>rotein <u>R</u>ecombination (SHIPREC)

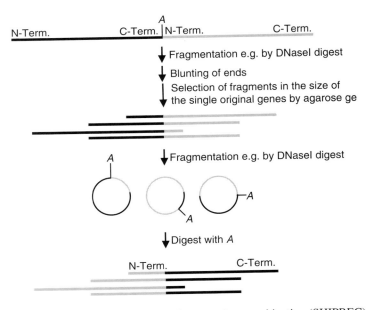

Fig. 36.16. Sequence homology-independent protein recombination (SHIPREC)

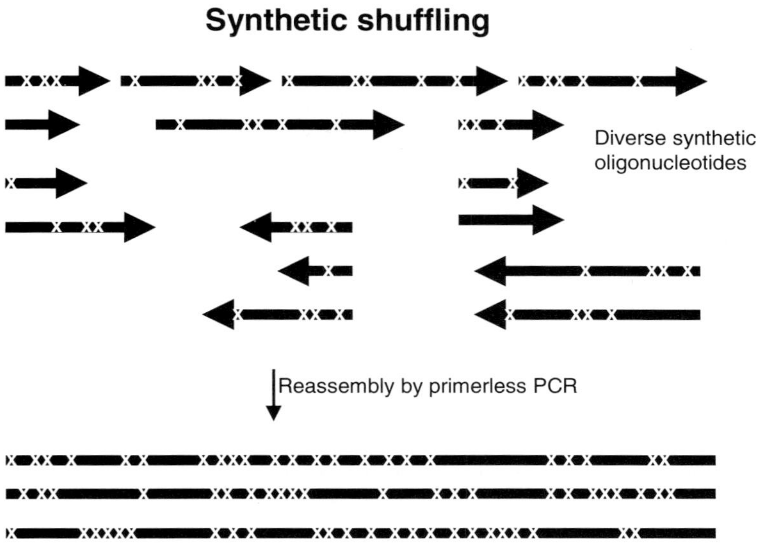

Synthetic shuffling

Fig. 36.17. Synthetic shuffling

ing genes the fragments are designed as degenerate oligonucleotides containing all variations wanted and then reassembled by a primerless PCR reaction. This method unites the benefits of rational design with the statistical approach of shuffling. In principle *Assembly of Designed Oligonucleotides (ADO) (25)* is identical to synthetic shuffling but takes into account conserved regions that can be used as linkers for homologous recombination.

2.3.2.4. Degenerate Oligonucleotide Gene Shuffling (DOGS): DOGS *(26)* **Fig. 36.18** was designed to decrease the amount of parental DNA reassembled from shuffling procedures. For DOGS complementary degenerate primers are designed for conserved motives found in the candidate genes. Each of these segments is flanked by primers and individually amplified. For the reassembly procedure the library of fragments can be put together at different ratios generating many biased libraries containing no parental genes. Conceptually *Structure-based Combinatorial Protein Engeneering (SCOPE) (27)* is identical to DOGS but the fragments generated are not based only on sequence identity but additionally on variable connections among structural elements.

2.3.2.5. Sequence-Independent Site-Directed Chimeragenesis (SISDC): SISDC *(28)* **Fig. 36.19** is additionally to DOGS and SCOPE taking into account the above mentioned assumption that proteins are assembled from earlier developed building blocks. These building blocks are calculated by an algorithm called SCHEMA *(19)*. At the interconnections between these building blocks proteins can be fragmented and exchanged between families. For this specific fragmentation consensus sequences at these points of contact between the building blocks are determined and marker tags are

Degenerate Oligonucleotide Gene Shuffling (DOGS)

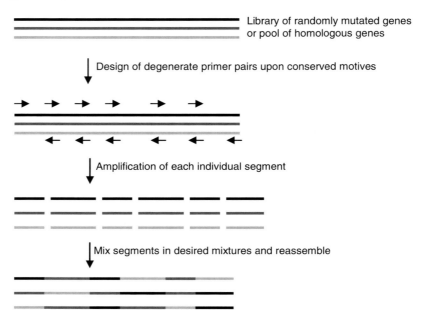

Fig. 36.18. Degenerate oligonucleotide gene shuffling (DOGS)

inserted. These marker tags are inserted by PCR primers into the gene like the DNA fragments are generated in DOGS. Each building block thus is amplified by itself and reassembled again sequentially to the full parental genes. Each tag consists mainly of a recognition site for *Bae*I ([10/15] ACNNNNGTAYC[12/7]), which digests dsDNA at the 5′ end before the tenth random position and at the 3′ end after the twelfth random position thus leaving a five nucleotide overhang at both ends. The custom-made random positions of the *Bae*I recognition are different for each target site. The five nucleotides in front of and after *Bae*I are designed correspond-ing to the consensus sequence of the respective building block ensuring correct order of reassembly of the chimeric genes. To eliminate chimeras with uncut tags, a *Sma*I site is introduced in the downstream part of the *Bae*I site.

2.3.2.6. Exon Shuffling: In eukaryotes crossover reactions often occur in introns creating new combinations of exons. These rearrangements lead to new genes with altered functions during evolution. The natural process of recombining exons from unrelated genes is called exon shuffling. In vitro exon shuffling *(29)* is carried out analog to DOGS or SCOPE but is the best suited method for rearrangement of eukaryotic genes. The exons of multiple related genes are amplified with oligonucleotides that determine the order of reassembly like in SISDC. Each exon is amplified by itself and new genes can be reassembled like using a building set in a reassembly PCR.

Sequence-Independent Site-Directed Chimeragenesis (SISDC)

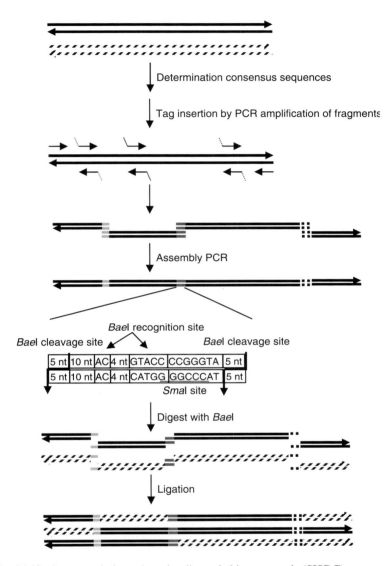

Fig. 36.19. Sequence-independent site-directed chimeragenesis (SISDC)

3. Applications

3.1. Mutator Strain + Selection

E. coli mutator strains belong to the earliest methods used to randomly mutate DNA. In 1985 Liao et al. used a mutD5 *E. coli* mutator strain to generate thermostable enzyme variants of the kanamycin nucleotidyltransferase *(30)*.

Kanamycin nucleotidyltransferase is the enzyme responsible for resistance against the antibiotic kanamycin. Liao cloned the kanamycin resistance first into a shuttle vector and propagated it in an *E. coli* mutD5 mutator strain. Afterwards the gene was transferred into *Bacillus stearothermophilus*. The wild type kanamycin nucleotidyltransferase only confers resistance to kanamycin up to 55°C but Liao was able to identify mutants conferring resistance to *B. stearothermohilus* at 65°C. All these mutants carried the amino acid exchange D80Y and those carrying the additional mutation T130K even conferred resistance up to 70°C.

Esterases can effectively discriminate among stereoisomers and are therefore in use for the production of optical pure compounds. In 1997 Bornscheuer successfully enhanced the enantioselectivity of an esterase from *Pseudomonas fluorescens* by passages of the gene through the mutator strain XL1-Red *(31)*. He was able to increase the enantiomeric excess from 0% up to 25%.

3.1.1. Chemical Mutagenesis

Subtilisin is a mesophilic alkaline serine endo protease of great commercial value. It is used in food and leather processing, and in laundry detergents to remove protein stains from clothing *(24)*. It is highly desirable to enhance wash performance at low temperatures to save energy and reduce the wear on textiles. Thus, cold adapted subtilisins are of high interest. Taguchi et al. used hydroxylamine to chemically mutagenize the gene of subtilisin BPN' from *Bacillus amyloliquefaciens* und engineered a cold adapted protease, which had a 2-fold higher activity at 10°C and only three amino acid substitutions *(32)*. Kano et al. generated with the same methodology applied by Taguchi a subtilisin BPN' mutant active even at 1°C, which only had one amino acid exchange (V84I) *(33)*.

3.1.2. epPCR + Screening

Organic solvents can cause serine proteases to catalyse unusual reactions that are normally not possible in aqueous solutions. Thus serine proteases are promising candidates for the catalysis of unusual chemical reactions. Chen et al. adapted subtilisin E to be active in a dimethylformamide (DMF) solution by sequential rounds of error prone PCR *(34)*. Sequential rounds of error prone PCR generated a mutant enzyme containing 10 amino acid exchanges which was in DMF nearly as active as the wild-type subtilisin E in aqueous solvent. One year later You et al. further enhanced the catalytic activity of subtilisin E, already active in DMF, 16 times by the same strategy *(35)*.

3.1.3. Synthetic Shuffling

Ness et al. succeeded to generate subtilisin variants with 2- to 3-fold higher thermostability and activity at pH 10 *(36)*, but these enzymes could not be produced in useful amounts owing to autoproteolysis. To circumvent this problem they fine tuned these enzymes to be less active at production conditions (pH 7). Based on the library of subtilisin genes from the previous study *(36)* they created synthetic oligonucleotides that were used to assemble a new library of subtilisin genes *(24)*. By this approach the authors found active and highly chimeric enzyme variants that showed the desired attributes they had not been able to obtain by other directed-evolution methods.

3.1.4. DNA Shuffling + Selection

E. coli β-galactosidase encoded by the *lacZ* gene is highly specific for β-D-galactosyl substrates and acts only weakly on ONPG (o-nitrophenyl β-D-fucopyranosides), PNPG (p-nitrophenyl β-D-fucopyranosides) or β-D-fucosyl moieties. Although enzymes are very specific in their choice of substrate Zhang et al. changed the specificity of β-galactosidase from β-D-galactosyl substrates to ONPG by only six amino acid exchanges. The resulting enzyme variant preferred ONPG 1,000-fold and PNPG 66-fold over the former β-D-galactosyl substrate *(37)*.

3.1.5. Rational Design

Recombinant proteins are useful as pharmaceuticals and a multi-billion dollar market. These proteins comprise cytokines, growth factors, enzymes, antibodies and the number of approved pharmaceutical proteins increases every year. Many of these proteins cause serious side-effects and complications, which limit their clinical usefulness. Frequently companies started to modify proteins to either enhance their therapeutic properties or to facilitate their production.

One antibody used in the treatment of metastatic breast cancer is Herceptin (Genentech/Roche) an anti-HER2 monoclonal antibody. Herceptin was developed from the murine monoclonal antibody 4D5 *(38)*, which specifically inhibits the proliferation of human tumor cells that overexpress the human epidermal growth factor receptor 2 oncoprotein p185[Her2]. The application of this antibody was severely limited by a human anti-mouse antibody immune response. Thus, antibody 4D5 was humanized using preassembled oligonucleotides containing the antigen binding loops from Ab 4D5 and the human variable and IgG constant regions.

3.1.6. Shuffling

Dengue fever (DF) and the severe dengue haemorrhagic fever (DHF) are the most important arboviral diseases and they are transmitted by the mosquito *Aedes aegypti*. Up to now no specific treatment for dengue diseases besides supportive intensive care exists. Dengue exists in four serotypes (DEN-1-4) and infection with one serotype only induces resistance against this specific serotype. It is hypothesized that secondary infection with another dengue type can lead to DHF by cross-reaction of antibodies of the dengue type the person is already resistant against. Therefore it is important to have a vaccine that is effective against all four dengue variants *(39)*.

A DNA vaccine consists of a plasmid containing DNA of an infectious organism under a eukaryotic promoter. If such a plasmid is injected into a muscle this leads to the synthesis of the coded protein of the infectious organism. The presence of this protein inside the cell leads to an immune response leading to resistance against this organism. Apt et al. *(40)* developed such a DNA vaccine that confers immunity against all four dengue types by shuffling of codon optimized dengue envelope genes. The DNA vaccine combines epitopes from all four dengue types. This DNA vaccine was successfully tested in mice and rhesus macaques *(41)*.

Further application of directed evolution in vaccine development could be recombination of the antigen-coding genes from different serovars to improve immunogenicity or crossprotective range of vaccines.

Bioremediation is the process of using microorganisms to degrade dangerous chemicals from the environment. Bioremediation is the fastest developing area of environmental restoration. Microorganisms can be used to degrade various chemicals such as hydrocarbons, polychlorated biphenyls, pesticides, metals and much more. By engineering enzymes and metabolic pathways it is possible to enlarge the substrate range that can be metabolized and to accelerate metabolization *(42)*.

Pentachlorophenol (PCP) is a compound that was used and is still used in developing countries as fungicide, wood preservative and as herbicide. PCP is restricted in the US since 1984 as it can affect the endocrine system of vertebrate life forms and may lead to immune system dysfunction.

PCP can be metabolized by *Sphingobium chlorophenolicum*, a gram-negative bacterium isolated from PCP contaminated soil. By employing three rounds of genome shuffling Dai et al. *(43)* developed strains able to grow in presence of $6–8 M$ PCP whereas the wild-type bacterium only grows up to concentrations of $0.6 mM$. These newly developed strains are able to degrade PCP whereas the wild-type does not.

Parathion or diethyl parathion are very potent insecticides and acaricides. Parathion is a cholinesterase inhibitor and can be absorbed through the skin. If incorporated it disrupts neural function by inhibiting the essential enzyme acetylcholinesterase. Cho et al. *(44)* improved by two rounds of directed evolution with DNA shuffling the hydrolysis of methyl parathion by organophosphorus hydrolase (OPH) 25-fold. OPH is a bacterial enzyme that degrades a wide range of neurotoxic organophosphate nerve agents and could be also developed to degrade the chemical weapons sarin and soman.

3.1.7. Family Shuffling

Cytokines are small molecules that are secreted by cells upon immune stimuli. They play important roles in the regulation and mediation of immunity, inflammation, and hematopoiesis. Cytokines possess antiviral and antiproliferating activities and thus could have therapeutic value in the treatment of diseases. Chang et al. *(45)* shuffled a family of over 20 human interferon-a-genes (Hu-IFN-α) and screened for variants with antiviral and antiproliferative properties in murine cells. After two rounds of shuffling and selection they obtained clones that where even more active than the native murine IFNαs. The shuffled clones were up to 250 fold more active than the single IFNαs originally used for shuffling.

3.1.8. ITCHY

Glutathione acetyltransferases (GST) play an important role in many cellular processes e.g., detoxification by conjugating electrophilic compounds to the tripeptide glutathione (GSH). GSTs are ubiquitous in aerobes and form a superfamily of species-independent classes that share a common protein fold.

Griswold et al. *(46)* created an ITCHY-library of chimeric enzymes of human GSTθ-1-1 (hGSTTT1-1) and rat GSTθ-2-2 (rGSTT2-2), that only share 54.3% amino acid identity and exhibit different substrate specificities. The ITCHY library gave rise to variants with improved *kcat* with the substrate used for selection compared to either of the parental enzymes and additionally showed activity on ethacrynic acid, a compound recognized by neither parental enzyme. This combination of a human with nonhuman enzymes to form active chimeras shows that this method could be used for the humanization of proteins with therapeutic values that show no conserved framework allowing for rational grafting.

3.1.9. SHIPREC

Cytochromes are proteins that contain heme groups and are responsible for the transport of electrons. P450 is a family of membrane-bound cytochromes with an absorption maximum of 450 nm when complexed with CO. One of the major roles of the cytochrome P450 system is the detoxification of harmful substances.

Sieber et al. *(23)* produced hybrids of two cytochromes, which share only 16% amino acid sequence identity. They created a library of sequences of the membrane-associated human cytochrome P450 and a soluble bacterial P450 (the heme domain of cytochrome P450 from *Bacillus megaterium*) with single crossovers all along the aligned genes. Two functional P450 hybrids were selected that showed improved solubility in the bacterial cytoplasm.

3.1.10. Enzyme Truncation + Error prone PCR (+Shuffling)

On the first view it seems counterintuitive to truncate an enzyme to enhance its overall stability and activity. Hecky et al. *(47,48)*, however, improved β-lactamase by structural perturbation and compensation. Here, structural perturbation and compensation means that the enzyme is first truncated N- or C-terminally until *in vivo* function is abolished and the truncation is compensated by directed evolution for activity. Afterwards identified mutations are studied in wild-type background. β-lactamase, the enzyme responsible for resistance against β-lactam antibiotics, was N-terminally truncated by five amino acids. After three rounds of error prone PCR, shuffling und selection they found truncated clones that where more active than the wild type protein. Mutations found in the structural perturbed background were inserted into wild type background resulting an overall stabilization of the protein. These mutations increased thermal stability, chemical stability, activity, and shifted the thermal optimum from 35°C to 50°C while maintaining full activity at low temperatures.

The same principle was true for chloramphenicol acetyltransferase (CAT), which is the protein responsible for inactivation of the antibiotic chloramphenicol. An N-terminally 10 amino acids truncated CAT variant could be rescued with seven rounds of directed evolution comprising error prone PCR, NExT shuffling, and selection at 37°C *(8,9)*. After insertion of the mutations found into the wild type background the already high melting temperature of 71°C was further increased by 6°C while activity at room temperature was doubled. Furthermore, solubility and chemical stability in guanidine was enhanced (Stebel et al., in preparation).

References

1. Seyffert W, Ed. (1998) Lehrbuch der Genetik. Gustav Fischer Verlag, Stuttgart, Jena, Lübeck, Ulm
2. Cadwell RC, Joyce GF (1992) Randomization of genes by PCR mutagenesis PCR. Methods Appl 2:28–33
3. Wong TS, Tee KL, Hauer B, Schwaneberg U (2004) Sequence saturation mutagenesis (SeSaM): a novel method for directed evolution. Nucleic Acids Res 32:e26
4. Hayes F, Hallet B (2000) Pentapeptide scanning mutagenesis: encouraging old proteins to execute unusual tricks. Trends Microbiol 8:571–577
5. Fujii R, Kitaoka M, Hayashi K (2006) RAISE: a simple and novel method of generating random insertion and deletion mutations. Nucleic Acids Res 34:e30

6. Murakami H, Hohsaka T, Sisido M (2002) Random insertion and deletion of arbitrary number of bases for codon-based random mutation of DNAs. Nat Biotechnol 20:76–81

7. Stemmer WP (1994) DNA shuffling by random fragmentation and reassembly: in vitro recombination for molecular evolution. Proc Natl Acad Sci USA 91:10,747–10,751

8. Stebel SC, Arndt KM, Müller KM (2006) Versatile DNA fragmentation and directed evolution with nucleotide exchange and excision technology. Methods Mol Biol 352:167–190

9. Müller KM, Stebel SC, Knall S, Zipf G, Bernauer HS, Arndt KM (2005) Nucleotide exchange and excision technology (NExT) DNA shuffling: a robust method for DNA fragmentation and directed evolution. Nucleic Acids Res 33:e117

10. Zhao H, Giver L, Shao Z, Affholter JA, Arnold FH (1998) Molecular evolution by staggered extension process (StEP) in vitro recombination. Nat Biotechnol 16:258–261

11. Ikeuchi A, Kawarasaki Y, Shinbata T, Yamane T (2003) Chimeric gene library construction by a simple and highly versatile method using recombination dependent exponential amplification. Biotechnol Prog 19:1460–1467

12. Coco WM, Levinson WE, Crist MJ, Hektor HJ, Darzins A, Pienkos PT, Squires CH, Monticello DJ (2001) DNA shuffling method for generating highly recombined genes and evolved enzymes. Nat Biotechnol 19:354–359

13. Lee SH, Ryu EJ, Kang MJ, Wang ES, Piao Z, Choi YJ, Jung KH, Jeon JYJ, Shin YC (2003) A new approach to directed gene evolution by recombined extension on truncated templates (RETT). J Mol Catalysis B-Enzymatic 26:119–129

14. Song JK, Chung B, Oh YH, Rhee JS (2002) Construction of DNA-shuffled and incrementally truncated libraries by a mutagenic and unidirectional reassembly method: changing from a substrate specificity of phospholipase to that of lipase. Appl Environ Microbiol 68:6146–6151

15. Eggert T, Funke SA, Rao NM, Acharya P, Krumm H, Reetz MT, Jaeger KE (2005) Multiplex-PCR-based recombination as a novel high-fidelity method for directed evolution. Chembiochem 6:1062–1067

16. Chamberlain JS, Gibbs RA, Ranier JE, Nguyen PN, Caskey CT (1988) Deletion screening of the Duchenne muscular dystrophy locus via multiplex DNA amplification. Nucleic Acids Res 16:11,141–11,156

17. Shao Z, Zhao H, Giver L, Arnold FH (1998) Random-priming in vitro recombination: an effective tool for directed evolution. Nucleic Acids Res 26: 681–683

18. Volkov AA, Shao Z, Arnold FH (1999) Recombination and chimeragenesis by in vitro heteroduplex formation and in vivo repair. Nucleic Acids Res 27:e18

19. Voigt CA, Martinez C, Wang ZG, Mayo SL, Arnold FH (2002) Protein building blocks preserved by recombination. Nat Struct Biol 9:553–558

20. Ostermeier M, Shim JH, Benkovic SJ (1999) A combinatorial approach to hybrid enzymes independent of DNA homology. Nat Biotechnol 17:1205–1209

21. Ostermeier M, Nixon AE, Shim JH, Benkovic SJ (1999) Combinatorial protein engineering by incremental truncation. Proc Natl Acad Sci USA 96:3562–3567

22. Lutz S, Ostermeier M (2003) Preparation of SCRATCHY hybrid protein libraries: size- and in-frame selection of nucleic acid sequences. Methods Mol Biol 231:143–151

23. Sieber V, Martinez CA, Arnold FH (2001) Libraries of hybrid proteins from distantly related sequences. Nat Biotechnol 19:456–460

24. Ness JE, Kim S, Gottman A, Pak R, Krebber A, Borchert TV, Govindarajan S, Mundorff EC, Minshull J (2002) Synthetic shuffling expands functional protein diversity by allowing amino acids to recombine independently. Nat Biotechnol 20:1251–1255

25. Zha D, Eipper A, Reetz MT (2003) Assembly of designed oligonucleotides as an efficient method for gene recombination: a new tool in directed evolution. Chembiochem 4:34–39

26. Gibbs MD, Nevalainen KM, Bergquist PL (2001) Degenerate oligonucleotide gene shuffling (DOGS): a method for enhancing the frequency of recombination with family shuffling. Gene 271:13–20

27. O'Maille PE, Bakhtina M, Tsai MD (2002) Structure-based combinatorial protein engineering (SCOPE). J Mol Biol 321:677–691

28. Hiraga K, Arnold FH (2003) General method for sequence-independent site-directed chimeragenesis. J Mol Biol 330:287–296

29. Kolkman JA, Stemmer WP (2001) Directed evolution of proteins by exon shuffling. Nat Biotechnol 19:423–428

30. Liao H, McKenzie T, Hageman R (1986) Isolation of a thermostable enzyme variant by cloning and selection in a thermophile. Proc Natl Acad Sci USA 83:576–580

31. Bornscheuer UT, Altenbuchner J, Meyer HH (1998) Directed evolution of an esterase for the stereoselective resolution of a key intermediate in the synthesis of epothilones. Biotechnol Bioeng 58:554–559

32. Taguchi S, Ozaki A, Momose H (1998) Engineering of a cold-adapted protease by sequential random mutagenesis and a screening system. Appl Environ Microbiol 64:492–495

33. Kano H, Taguchi S, Momose H (1997) Cold adaptation of a mesophilic serine protease, subtilisin, by in vitro random mutagenesis. Appl Microbiol Biotechnol 47:46–51

34. Chen K, Arnold FH (1993) Tuning the activity of an enzyme for unusual environments: sequential random mutagenesis of subtilisin E for catalysis in dimethylformamide. Proc Natl Acad Sci USA 90:5618–5622

35. You L, Arnold FH (1996) Directed evolution of subtilisin E in *Bacillus subtilis* to enhance total activity in aqueous dimethylformamide. Protein Eng 9:77–83

36. Ness JE, Welch M, Giver L, Bueno M, Cherry JR, Borchert TV, Stemmer WP, Minshull J (1999) DNA shuffling of subgenomic sequences of subtilisin. Nat Biotechnol 17:893–896

37. Zhang JH, Dawes G, Stemmer WP (1997) Directed evolution of a fucosidase from a galactosidase by DNA shuffling and screening. Proc Natl Acad Sci USA 94:4504–4509

38. Carter P, Presta L, Gorman CM, Ridgway JB, Henner D, Wong WL, Rowland AM, Kotts C, Carver ME, Shepard HM (1992) Humanization of an anti-p185HER2 antibody for human cancer therapy. Proc Natl Acad Sci USA 89:4285–4289

39. Locher CP, Heinrichs V, Apt D, Whalen RG (2004) Overcoming antigenic diversity and improving vaccines using DNA shuffling and screening technologies. Expert Opin Biol Ther 4:589–597

40. Apt D, Raviprakash K, Brinkman A, Semyonov A, Yang S, Skinner C, Diehl L, Lyons R, Porter K, Punnonen J (2006) Tetravalent neutralizing antibody response against four dengue serotypes by a single chimeric dengue envelope antigen. Vaccine 24:335–344

41. Raviprakash K, Apt D, Brinkman A, Skinner C, Yang S, Dawes G, Ewing D, Wu SJ, Bass S, Punnonen J, Porter K (2006) A chimeric tetravalent dengue DNA vaccine elicits neutralizing antibody to all four virus serotypes in rhesus macaques. Virology 353:166–173

42. Dua M, Singh A, Sethunathan N, Johri AK (2002) Biotechnology and bioremediation: successes and limitations. Appl Microbiol Biotechnol 59:143–152

43. Dai M, Copley SD (2004) Genome shuffling improves degradation of the anthropogenic pesticide pentachlorophenol by *Sphingobium chlorophenolicum* ATCC 39723. Appl Environ Microbiol 70:2391–2397

44. Cho CM, Mulchandani A, Chen W (2002) Bacterial cell surface display of organophosphorus hydrolase for selective screening of improved hydrolysis of organophosphate nerve agents. Appl Environ Microbiol 68:2026–2030

45. Chang CC, Chen TT, Cox BW, Dawes GN, Stemmer WP, Punnonen J, Patten PA (1999) Evolution of a cytokine using DNA family shuffling. Nat Biotechnol 17:793–797

46. Griswold KE, Kawarasaki Y, Ghoneim N, Benkovic SJ, Iverson BL, Georgiou G (2005) Evolution of highly active enzymes by homology-independent recombination. Proc Natl Acad Sci USA 102:10,082–10,087

47. Hecky J, Mason JM, Arndt KM, Müller KM (2007) A general method of terminal truncation, evolution, and re-elongation to generate enzymes of enhanced stability. Methods Mol Biol 352:275–304

48. Hecky J, Müller KM (2005) Structural perturbation and compensation by directed evolution at physiological temperature leads to thermostabilization of beta-lactamase. Biochemistry 44:12,640–12,654

37

Enzyme Linked Immunosorbent Assay (ELISA)

John Crowther

1. Introduction

There have been very few developments that markedly affect the need to greatly revise the text from the last version of this book. This is testament to the fact that heterogeneous enzyme linked immunosorbent assays (ELISA) provide ideal systems for dealing with a wide range of studies in many biological areas. The main reason for this success is test flexibility, whereby reactants can be used in different combinations, either attached passively to a solid phase support or in the liquid phase. The exploitation of the ELISA has been increased through continued development of specifically produced reagents for example, monoclonal and polyclonal antibodies and peptide antigens coupled with the improvement and expansion of commercial products such as enzyme linked conjugates; substrates and chromogens; plastics technology and design of microwell plates; instrumentation advances and robotics. However, the principles of the ELISA remain the same.

A brief scan of the literature involving ELISA can be used to illustrate the continued success of ELISA. The number of publications with ELISA mentioned in all science areas from 1976 to 2004 is shown in **Table 37.1**. A fairly constant increase in the number of papers using ELISA methods is indicated. A breakdown of publications according to science areas in five yearly periods from 1980 in **Table 37.2** illustrates the versatility in use of the ELISA, as well as highlighting the major areas of use in Medicine and Dentistry; Immunology and Microbiology Molecular biology and Genetics and Biotechnology. It is interesting to note that the earliest exploitation of ELISA was in Immunology and Microbiology and Molecular Biology and Biotechnology, probably reflecting the greatest research areas. Medicine and Dentistry (associated by the search engine) shows the greatest rate of increase in use (probably in the Medical sphere only) from the 1990s.

The search results indicate the continued expansion of ELISA in science and there is no reason to believe that this will change even in the face of modern technologies exploiting molecular methods. The analytical and systematic characteristics of the ELISA are ideally suited to diagnosis at the screening

From: *Molecular Biomethods Handbook, 2nd Edition.*
Edited by: J. M. Walker and R. Rapley © Humana Press, Totowa, NJ

Table 37.1. Literature search in ScienceDirect database for ELISA.

Year	Number	Year	Number
1976	6	1991	743
1977	13	1992	774
1978	14	1993	820
1979	31	1994	870
1980	45	1995	1016
1981	95	1996	1093
1982	125	1997	1119
1983	216	1998	1099
1984	257	1999	1144
1985	367	2000	1118
1986	420	2001	1120
1987	547	2002	1198
1988	565	2003	1253
1989	640	2004	1591
1990	682		

Table 37.2. Breakdown of literature search in science groups.

Subject	1980–1984	1985–1989	1990–1994	1995–1999	2000–2004
Agriculture and biological sciences	87	274	615	804	827
Molecular biology, genetics and biotechnology	374	1,329	1,762	1,845	2,096
Chemistry	8	29	77	208	279
Environmental science	4	13	52	125	162
Immunology and microbiology	514	1,584	2,128	2,450	2,772
Medicine and dentistry	280	971	1,639	2,875	3,372
Neurosciences	21	124	198	380	484
Pharmacology and toxicology	24	108	247	397	497
Veterinary sciences	71	219	522	769	853

level; for surveillance where larger scale sample handling is required and for research. Many of the accepted standard assays in many scientific fields are ELISA based and have replaced other "gold standard" assays. In conjunction with the rapidly evolving use of molecular methods centering on the polymerase chain reaction (PCR) technologies there is the need to use serological confirmatory methods in a dual approach to directly identify and characterise disease agents and to assess disease prevalence through the measurement of specific antibodies or other chemical factors as a result of infection. The use of ELISA methods in testing the environment, and animal, or plant products as safe for human and animal consumption is also a rapidly evolving area for ELISA.

ELISA therefore, has been used in all fields of pure and applied aspects of biology, in particular it forms the backbone of diagnostic techniques. The systems used to perform ELISAs make use of antibodies. These are proteins produced in animals in response to antigenic stimuli. Antibodies are specific chemicals that bind to the antigens used for their production thus they can be used to detect the particular antigens if binding can be demonstrated. Conversely, specific antibodies can be measured by the use of defined antigens, and this forms the basis of many assays in diagnostic biology.

This chapter describes methods involved in ELISAs where one of the reagents, usually an antibody, is linked to an enzyme and where one reagent is attached to a solid phase. The systems allow the examination of reactions

Table 37.3. Brief descriptions of elements common to ELISAs.

Solid phase	This is usually a plastic microtiter plate well. Specially prepared ELISA plates are commercially available. These have 8–12 well formats (even larger possibilities such as 394 well plates), the plates can be used with a wide variety of microtiter equipment, such as multichannel pipets, to allow great convenience to the rapid manipulation of reagents in small volumes.
Adsorption	This is the process of adding an antigen or antibody, diluted in buffer, so that it attaches passively to the solid phase on incubation. This simple way of immobilization of one of the reactants in ELISA is one of the keys to its success.
Washing	Simply flooding and emptying wells with a buffered solution is enough to separate bound and free reagents. Again, this is a key to the simplicity of the ELISA over methods involving complicated separation methods.
Antigen	These are proteins or carbohydrates, which, when injected into animals or as a result of the disease process, elicit the production of antibodies. Such antibodies usually react specifically with the antigen and therefore can be used to detect that antigen.
Antibody	Antibodies are produced in response to antigenic stimuli. These are mainly protein in nature. In turn, antibodies are antigenic.
Antispecies antibody	Antibodies obtained when antibodies from one animal are injected into another species. Thus, guinea pig serum injected into a rabbit would elicit a rabbit anti-guinea pig serum.
Enzyme	A substance that can act at low concentration as a catalyst to promote a specific reaction. Several specific enzymes are commonly used in ELISA.
Enzyme conjugate	An enzyme that is attached irreversibly, by chemical means, to a protein, usually an antibody. Thus, an antispecies enzyme conjugate would be guinea pig antirabbit conjugated to enzyme.
Substrate	The substrate is the chemical compound on which the enzyme reacts specifically. This reaction is used in some way to produce a signal that is read as a color reaction in ELISA.
Chromophore	This is a chemical that alters color as a result of enzyme interacting with substrate, allowing the ELISA to be quantified
Stopping	The process of stopping the action of the enzyme and substrate.
Reading	This implies measurement of the color produced in ELISA. This is quantified using special multichannel spectrophotometers reading at the specific wavelength of the color produced. Tests can be read by eye for crude assessment.

through the simple addition and incubation of reagents. Bound and free reactants are separated by a simple washing procedure. The end product in an ELISA is the development of color that can be quantified using a spectrophotometer. These kinds of ELISA are called heterogeneous assays and should be distinguished from homogeneous assays where all reagents are added simultaneously. The latter assays are most suitable for detecting small molecules such as digoxin or gentamicin.

The development of ELISA stemmed from investigations of enzyme-labeled antibodies *(1–3)*, for use in identifying antigens in tissue. The methods of conjugation were exploited to measure serum components in the first true ELISAs *(4–6)*.

By far the most exploited ELISAs use plastic microtitre plates in an 8 × 12 well format as the solid phase *(7)*. Such systems benefit from a large selection of specialized commercially available equipment including multichannel pipets for the easy simultaneous dispensing of reagents and multichannel spectrophotometers for rapid data capture. There are many books, manuals and reviews of ELISA and associated subjects that should be examined for more detailed practical details *(8–21)*.

The key advantages of ELISA over other assays are summarized in **Table 37.3**.

2. What is ELISA?

Figure 37.1A illustrates a protein that is adsorbed to a plastic surface. The attachment of proteins and hence the majority of all antigens in nature, to plastic, is the key to most ELISAs performed. This process is passive so that protein solutions, in easy to prepare buffer solutions, can be added to plastic surfaces and will attach after a period of incubation at room temperature. The most commonly used plastic surface is that of small wells in microtitre plates. Such plates contain 96 wells measuring approx 5 mm deep by 8 mm diameter in a 12 × 8 format. The main point here is that there has evolved a whole technology of equipment for rapidly handling materials in association with these plates. After the incubation of antigen excess unbound antigen is washed away by flooding the plastic surface, usually in a buffered solution. The plastic can then be shaken free of excess washing solution and is ready for the addition of a detecting system.

The simplest application of the ELISA is illustrated in **Fig. 37.1**. An antibody prepared against the antigen on the plastic is added (**Fig. 37.1B**). The antibody has been chemically linked to an enzyme; this is usually called a conjugate. The antibody is diluted in a buffer (e.g., phosphate buffered saline, pH around 7.2) containing an excess of protein that has no influence on the possible reaction of the antibody and antigen. A very cheap example is that of approx 5% skimmed-milk powder, Marvel, which is mainly the protein from cow milk, casein. The purpose of this excess protein is to prevent any passive attachment of the conjugate (antibody is protein) to any free sites on the plastic not occupied by the antigen. Such sites will be occupied by the excess milk powder proteins by competition with the low concentration of conjugate. These diluting reagents have been called blocking buffers.

Add protein antigen in buffer Wash away non-attached antigen   Antigen coated plate

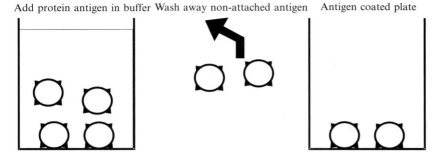

(**A**) Antigen is added in buffer. The protein attaches passively to plastic surface of microtitre plates well. After a period of incubation the non-adsorped protein is washed away.

Add enzyme labelled   Wash away non-bound conjugate   Antigen/conjugate complex
antibodies in blocking buffer   on solid phase

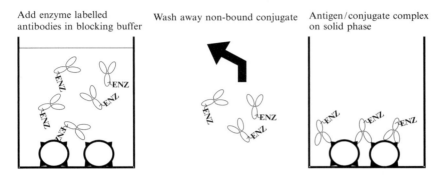

(**B**) Antibodies with enzyme co-valently linked (conjugate) is added in a solution containing iner protein and detergent (to prevent non-specific attachment of the antibodies to plastic wells. The antibody binds to the antigen on well surface. After incubation, non-bound antibodies are washed away.

Add substrate and chromogen,   Colour develops in time
incubate

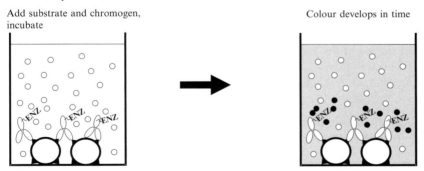

(**C**) Add substrate and chromogenic dye solution. Substrate interacts with enzyme to affect dye solution to give a colour reaction.

Fig. 37.1. Illustration of steps in simple direct ELISA

On addition of the conjugate under these conditions the only reaction that occurs is the specific immunological binding of the antigen and antibody in the conjugate. Thus an antigen-enzyme linked antibody complex is produced and because the antigen is bound to the plastic the enzyme is bound also. Such a process requires incubation (15–60 min) that can be at room temperature. After incubation the plastic surface is washed to remove all unreacted conjugate.

The next stage is illustrated in **Fig. 37.1C**. Here, a substrate for the enzyme is added in solution with a chromogenic chemical that is colorless in the absence of enzyme activity on the substrate. Because there is enzyme linked to the antibody, which is attached specifically to the antigen on the plastic surface, the substrate is catalyzed causing a color change. The rates of such color changes are proportional to the amount of enzyme in the complex. Thus, taking the other extreme, if no antigen were attached to the plastic then no antibody would be bound. Therefore if no enzyme is present to catalyze the substrate so no color change would be observed. The enzyme activity is usually stopped by the addition of a chemical that drastically alters the pH of the reaction or denatures the enzyme e.g., $1 M$ sulfuric acid.

Color can then be assessed by eye or quantified using a multichannel spectrophotometer that is specially designed for use with the microplates and can read a plate (96 samples) in 5 s. Such machines can be interfaced with microcomputers so that a great deal of data can be analyzed in a short time.

There are many systems in ELISA depending on what initial reagent is attached to the solid phase and what order subsequent reagents are added. Thus there is great versatility possible for adaption of ELISAs to solve applied and pure problems in science.

The basic principles of ELISA are summarized below:

1. Passive attachment of proteins to plastics
2. Washing away of unattached protein
3. Addition, at some stage, of a specific antibody linked to an enzyme
4. Use of competing inert proteins to prevent nonspecific reactions with the plastic
5. Washing steps to separate reacted (bound) from unreacted (free) reagents
6. Addition of a specific substrate that changes color on enzyme catalysis or substrate and a colorless chromophore (dye solution) that changes color owing to enzyme catalysis
7. Incubation steps to allow immunological reactions
8. Stopping of enzyme catalysis
9. Reading of the color by spectrophotometer.

Specific details of these stages can be obtained from the references in particular *(8–16)*. The next section illustrates some of the possible variations.

3. Basic Assay Configurations

There are three basic systems used in ELISA: direct ELISA; indirect ELISA; and sandwich ELISA. All these systems can be used to perform competition of inhibition ELISAs.

These systems will be described to illustrate the principles involved with the aid of diagrams. The various stages common to ELISAs will then be described in more detail.

3.1. Direct ELISA

This is the simplest form of ELISA as shown in **Fig. 37.2**. Here an antigen is passively attached to a plastic solid phase by a period of incubation. As indicated

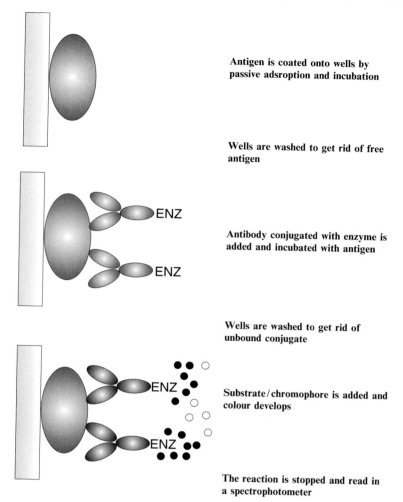

Antigen is coated onto wells by passive adsroption and incubation

Wells are washed to get rid of free antigen

Antibody conjugated with enzyme is added and incubated with antigen

Wells are washed to get rid of unbound conjugate

Substrate/chromophore is added and colour develops

The reaction is stopped and read in a spectrophotometer

Fig. 37.2. Direct ELISA. Antigen is attached to the solid phase by passive adsorption. After washing, enzyme labeled antibodies are added. After an incubation period and washing, a substrate system is added and color allowed to develop

in Subheading 2, the most useful solid phase is a microtiter plate well. After a simple washing step, antigen is detected by the addition of an antibody that is linked covalently to an enzyme. After incubation and washing the test is developed by the addition of a chromogen/substrate whereby enzyme activity produces a color change. The greater the amount of enzyme in the system then the faster the color develops. Usually color development is read after a defined time or after enzyme activity is stopped by chemical means at a defined time. Color is read in a spectrophotometer.

3.2. Indirect ELISA

Antigen is passively attached to wells by incubation. After washing, antibodies specific for the antigen are incubated with the antigen. Wells are washed and any bound antibodies are detected by the addition of antispecies antibodies

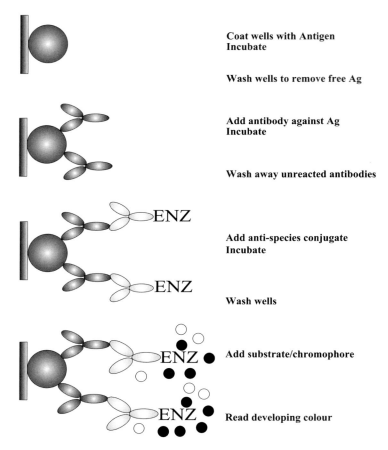

Coat wells with Antigen
Incubate

Wash wells to remove free Ag

Add antibody against Ag
Incubate

Wash away unreacted antibodies

Add anti-species conjugate
Incubate

Wash wells

Add substrate/chromophore

Read developing colour

Fig. 37.3. Indirect ELISA. Antibodies from a particular species react with antigen attached to the solid phase. Any bound antibodies are detected by the addition of an antispecies antiserum labeled with enzyme, this is widely used in diagnosis

covalently linked to an enzyme. Such antibodies are specific for the species in which the first antibody added were produced. After incubation and washing, the test is developed and read as described in Subheading 3.1. The scheme is shown in **Fig. 37.3**.

3.3. Sandwich ELISA

There are two forms of this ELISA depending on the number of antibodies used. The principle is the same for both whereby instead of adding antigen directly to a solid phase, antibody is added to the solid phase, and then acts as to capture antigen. These systems are useful where antigens are in a crude form (contaminated with other proteins) or at low concentration. In these cases the antigen cannot be directly attached to the solid phase at a high enough concentration to allow successful assay based on direct or indirect ELISAs. The sandwich ELISAs depend on antigens having at least two antigenic sites so that at least two antibody populations can bind.

3.3.1. Direct Sandwich ELISA

This is shown in **Fig. 37.4**. Antibodies are protein in nature and can be passively attached to the solid phase. After washing away excess unbound antibody, antigen is added and is specifically captured. The antigen is then detected by a second enzyme labeled antibody directed against the antigen. This antibody can be identical to the capture antibody reacting with a repeating antigenic site or an antibody from a different species directed against the same or a different site. Thus a "sandwich" is created. This type of assay is useful where a single species antiserum is available and where antigen does not attach well to plates.

3.3.2. Indirect Sandwich ELISA

This is similar in principle to the last system but involves three antibodies. **Fig. 37.5** illustrates the scheme. Coating of the solid phase with antibody and capture of antigen are as in Subheading 3.1–3.3, however, here the antigen is detected with a second unlabeled antibody. This antibody is in turn detected using an antispecies enzyme labeled conjugate. It is essential that

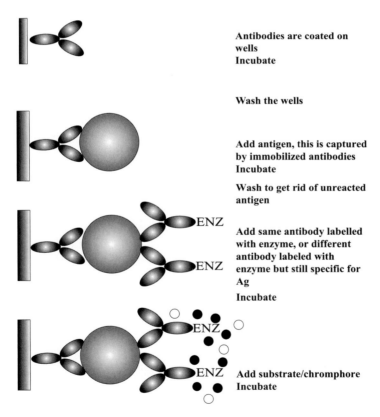

Antibodies are coated on wells
Incubate

Wash the wells

Add antigen, this is captured by immobilized antibodies
Incubate

Wash to get rid of unreacted antigen

Add same antibody labelled with enzyme, or different antibody labeled with enzyme but still specific for Ag
Incubate

Add substrate/chromphore
Incubate

Fig. 37.4. Sandwich ELISA-direct. This system exploits antibodies attached to a solid phase to capture antigen. The antigen is then detected using serum specific for the antigen. The detecting antibody is labeled with enzyme. The capture antibody and the detecting antibody can be the same serum or from different animals of the same species of from different species. The antigen must have at least two different antigenic sites

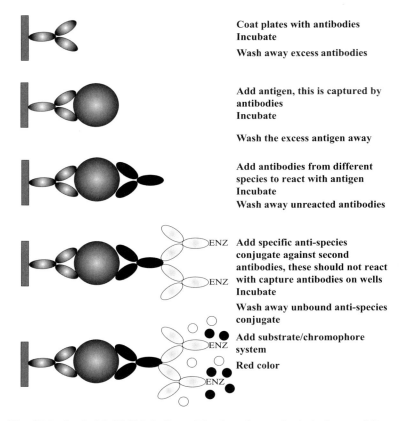

Coat plates with antibodies
Incubate

Wash away excess antibodies

Add antigen, this is captured by
antibodies
Incubate

Wash the excess antigen away

Add antibodies from different
species to react with antigen
Incubate
Wash away unreacted antibodies

Add specific anti-species
conjugate against second
antibodies, these should not react
with capture antibodies on wells
Incubate

Wash away unbound anti-species
conjugate

Add substrate/chromophore
system

Red color

Fig. 37.5. Sandwich ELISA-Indirect. The detecting antibody is from a different species to the capture antibody. The anti-species enzyme-labeled antibody binds to the detecting antibody specifically and not to the capture antibody

the antispecies conjugate does not bind to the capture antibody, therefore the species in which the capture antibody is produced must be different. The same considerations about the need for at least two antigenic sites to allow the "sandwich" are relevant. The advantage of this system is that a single antispecies conjugate can be used to evaluate the binding of antibodies from any number of samples. This is not true of the Direct Sandwich where each serum tested would have to be labeled with enzyme.

4. Competition/Inhibition ELISAs

The systems described in Subheadings 3.1–3.3 are the basic configurations of ELISA. All of these can be adapted to measure antigens or antibodies using competitive or inhibition conditions. Thus each the assays described above require pretitration of reagents to obtain optimal conditions. These optimal conditions are then challenged either by the addition of antigen or antibody. These will be described.

4.1. Direct ELISA Antigen Competition

This is shown in **Fig. 37.6**. The Direct ELISA is optimized whereby a defined amount of antigen coating the plate is bound by an optimal amount of enzyme labeled antibody. Wells coated with the optimal amount of antigen are then set up. This "balanced" situation can then be "challenged" by the addition of samples that could contain the same (or similar) antigen as that attached to the plate. On addition of the enzyme-labeled conjugate the test antigen reacts and prevents that antibody binding to the antigen on the solid phase. Thus the added antigen in the liquid phase and the solid phase antigen, compete for the labeled antibody. The higher the concentration of identical antigen in the test, the greater is the degree of competition. Where the antigen added in the test sample is not the same as the solid phase antigen, then it does not bind to the

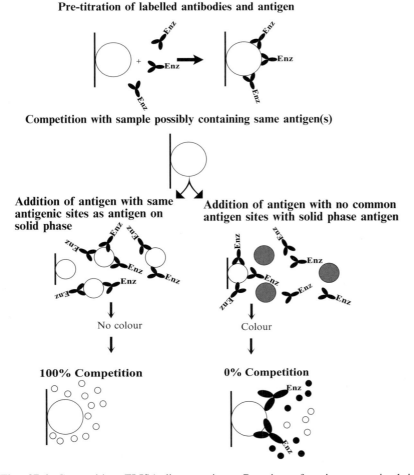

Fig. 37.6. Competition ELISA-direct antigen. Reaction of antigen contained in samples with the enzyme-labeled antibody directed against the antigen on the solid phase blocks the label from binding to the solid phase antigen. If the antigen has no cross-reactivity or is absent, then the labeled antibody binds to the solid phase antigen and a color reaction is observed on developing the test

added conjugate and this can consequently bind without competition to the solid phase antigen.

4.2. Direct ELISA Antibody Competition

This is very similar to the assay in Subheading 4.1, except that test samples are added containing antibodies possibly directed towards the antigen coated on the solid phase. This is shown in **Fig. 37.7**. Thus high concentrations of identical antibody mean that the conjugated pretitrated antibody is inhibited and thus no color reaction is observed (as expected from the pretitration exercise). Such assays are increasing in usefulness with the development of monoclonal antibody (MAb) based tests.

Pre-titration of antigen and labeled antibodies

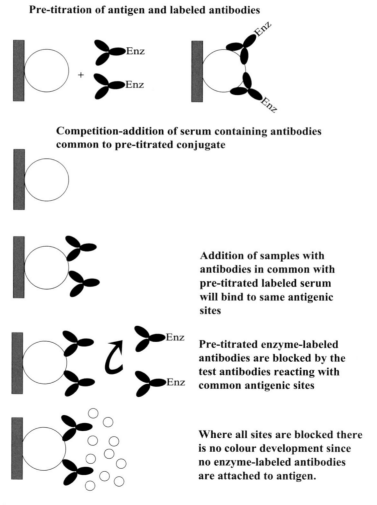

Competition-addition of serum containing antibodies common to pre-titrated conjugate

Addition of samples with antibodies in common with pre-titrated labeled serum will bind to same antigenic sites

Pre-titrated enzyme-labeled antibodies are blocked by the test antibodies reacting with common antigenic sites

Where all sites are blocked there is no colour development since no enzyme-labeled antibodies are attached to antigen.

Fig. 37.7. Competition ELISA-direct antibody. The degree of inhibition by the binding of antibodies in a serum for a pretitrated enzyme-labeled antiserum reaction is determined

4.3. Indirect ELISA Antigen Competition

Figure 37.8 illustrates the principles of this assay. The system relating the antigen, primary antibody and labeled antispecies conjugate is pretitrated. There is inhibition of the binding of primary antibody on addition of test samples containing the same antigen as that coated on the wells. Conversely, where the antigen added does not bind to the primary antibody, then no inhibition occurs and on subsequent addition of the conjugate the expected pretitrated level of color is observed.

4.4. Indirect ELISA Antibody Competition

This is very similar to the assays described in Subheading 2.3. Here test samples containing antibodies that can bind to the solid phase antigen inhibit the pretitrated primary antibody, as shown in **Fig. 37.9**. The key problem with

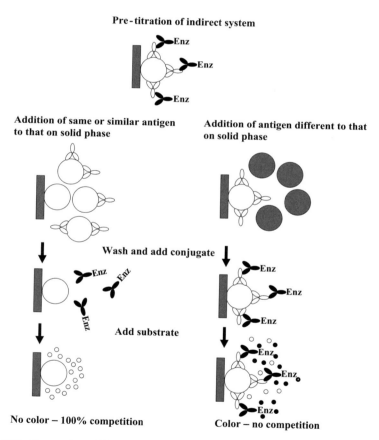

Fig. 37.8. Competition ELISA-indirect antigen. The pretitrated indirect ELISA is competed for by antigen. If the antigen shares antigenic determinants with that of the solid phase antigen, then it binds to the pretitrated antibodies and prevents them binding to the solid phase antigen. If there is no similarity then the antibodies are not bound and can react with the solid phase antigen. Addition of the antispecies enzyme conjugate quantifies the bound antibody

Pre-titration of indirect system

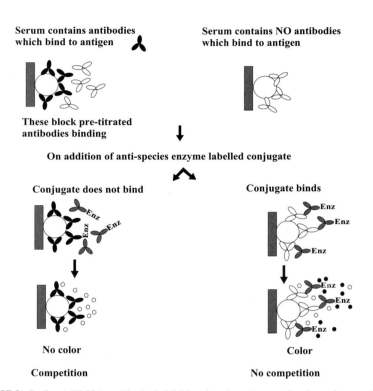

Competition-addition of samples containing antibodies?

Serum contains antibodies which bind to antigen

Serum contains NO antibodies which bind to antigen

These block pre-titrated antibodies binding

On addition of anti-species enzyme labelled conjugate

Conjugate does not bind

Conjugate binds

No color

Color

Competition

No competition

Fig. 37.9. Indirect ELISA-antibody inhibition involves the pretitration of an antigen and antiserum in an indirect ELISA. The addition of a serum containing cross-reactive antibodies will upset the "balance" of the pretitrated system. Because an antispecies conjugate is used, the species from which the sample of serum is taken cannot be the same as that used for the pretitration (the homologous system)

this assay is that the test antibody cannot be from the same species as the primary antibody because this is detected by an antispecies conjugate.

4.5. Sandwich ELISA Direct Antibody Competition

This is shown in **Fig. 37.10**. The situation begins to look a little more complex because more reagents are involved. The figure illustrates two methods where a pretitrated direct sandwich system is competed for by antibody in test samples. The first involves mixing and incubation of the pretitrated antigen with test serum before addition to wells containing the solid phase antibody.

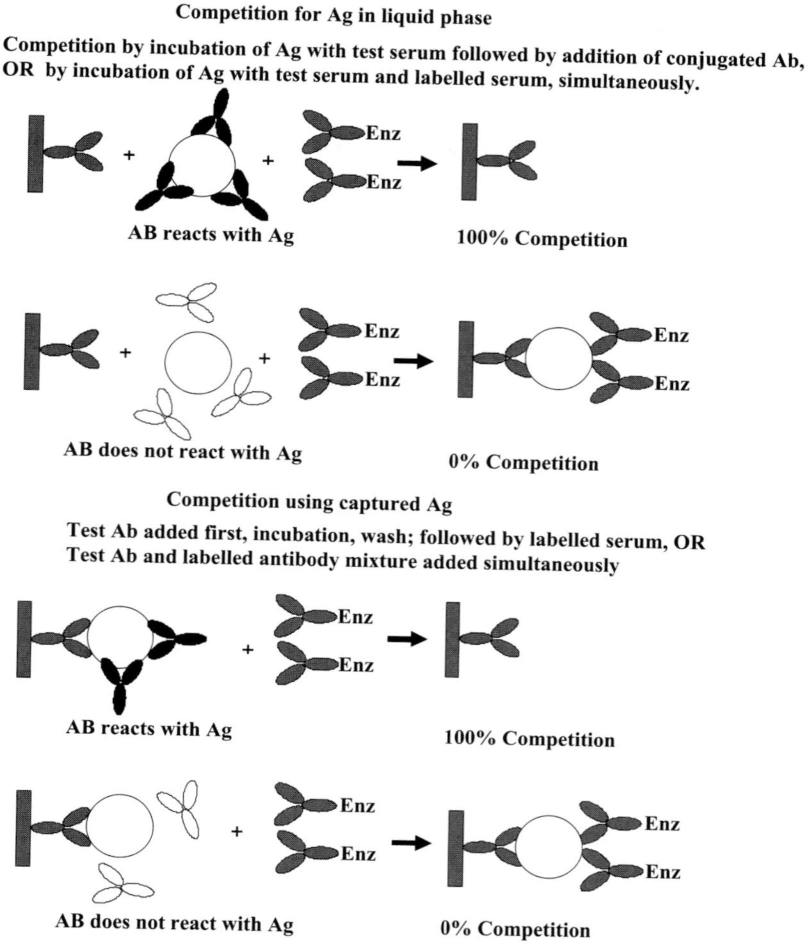

Competition for Ag in liquid phase

Competition by incubation of Ag with test serum followed by addition of conjugated Ab, OR by incubation of Ag with test serum and labelled serum, simultaneously.

AB reacts with Ag   100% Competition

AB does not react with Ag   0% Competition

Competition using captured Ag

Test Ab added first, incubation, wash; followed by labelled serum, OR Test Ab and labelled antibody mixture added simultaneously

AB reacts with Ag   100% Competition

AB does not react with Ag   0% Competition

Fig. 37.10. Competition Sandwich ELISA-direct for antibody

Here, if the antibodies in the test sample bind to the antigen, then they stop the antigen binding to the solid phase antibody. On addition of the pretitrated conjugate there is no color. The second situation involves the use of antigen attached to wells via the capture antibody. After washing the test antibody is added. If this reacts with the captured antigen then it blocks the binding of subsequently added conjugate. In fact both these forms of assay whereby test antibodies are allowed to bind before the addition of detecting second antibody should be termed inhibition or blocking assays because strictly competition refers to the simultaneous addition of two reagents. This can be illustrated in the second situation where the test antibody and second conjugated antibody could be mixed together before addition to the antigen captured on the wells; this is competitive. Note that because we have an enzyme labeled detecting serum then any species serum can be used in the competitive system.

4.6. Sandwich ELISA Indirect Antibody Competition

Figures 37.11 and **37.12** illustrate methods for performing this ELISA. Again we have a more complex situation because five reagents are involved. Basically the Indirect sandwich ELISA is pretitrated. Test antibodies are then added either to the antigen in the liquid phase (**Fig. 37.11**) or to antigen already captured (**Fig. 37.12**). If test antibodies bind to the antigen in either system then the subsequent addition of the second antibody and the antispecies conjugate will be negated. Note here that, as with the Indirect ELISA competition, the species from which the test sera came cannot be the same as that used to optimize the assay i.e., the antispecies conjugate cannot react with the test antibodies.

The assays described are inhibition or blocking assays and can all be further "complicated" with reference to when addition of reagents are made. Thus in **Fig. 37.11**(i) the antigen, test antibodies and detecting antibody could be added together (competition). In **Fig. 37.11**(ii), the test and detecting antibodies could be added together (competition). Similarly for **Fig. 37.12**, the test and detecting antibodies could be premixed to offer competitive conditions.

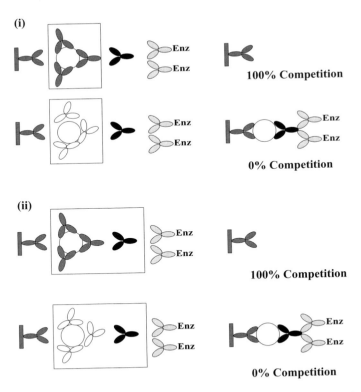

Fig. 37.11. Competition for sandwich ELISA-Indirect (liquid phase antigen) Ag is reacted with competing antibodies followed by addition of second antibody (i) or Ag, competing serum and second antibodies are mixed (ii). Bound second antibody is detected by antispecies against second antibody. This cannot react with species in which test antibody was raised

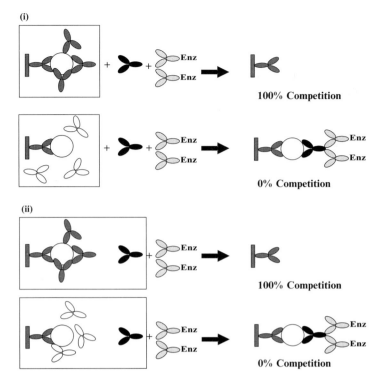

Fig. 37.12. Competition for Sandwich ELISA-Indirect (solid phase antigen)Ag is captured first and then either (i) competing antibodies are added, incubated and then second antibody added, with or without a washing step to remove unbound test antibody and complexes of this antibody and antigen (i) or competing serum and second antibodies are mixed to compete directly (ii). Bound second antibody is detected by antispecies against second antibody. This cannot react with species in which test antibody was raised

4.7. Sandwich ELISAs for Antigen Competition

These have not been illustrated. There is an intrinsic difficulty in that wells are coated with capture antibody. Addition of competing antigens thus serves to increase the concentration of antigen that can be captured resulting in no competition.

5. Summary of Uses of Various Methods Used in ELISA

This section will consider the reasons how and why different systems need to be applied and summarizes the interrelationships of the methods. An overview of the most commonly used systems is shown in **Fig. 37.13**. Although not all applications can be covered here, this will serve to illustrate the versatility of ELISA. Boxes A, B, C and D in the figure cover uses of the systems used in noncompetitive ways.

5.1. A-Direct ELISA

The drawback here is that antibodies from each serum have to be labeled. Antispecies conjugates can be titrated in this method using specific serum proteins from the target species. The Direct ELISA can be used to standardize

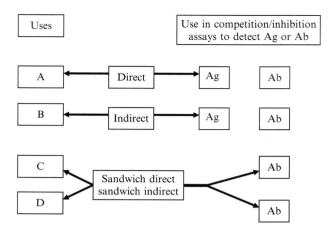

Fig. 37.13. Relationship of methods used in ELISA. Some uses of assays in non competitive ways (A, B and C) are discussed in text. Ag = antigen; Ab = antibody

antispecies conjugates from batch to batch and as a way of estimating the working dilution of conjugate to be used in other ELISA systems.

5.2. B-Indirect ELISA

This is a far more flexible test in that a single antispecies conjugate will detect antibodies. Thus various sera with different specificities can be detected using the same reagent. The Indirect ELISA has been used widely in diagnosis of diseases through the detection of antibodies. The method depends on the availability of enough specific antigen(s) at a suitable concentration for coating plates. Where antigens are at low concentration or in the presence of other contaminating proteins, the test might be impossible to perform. Thus antigens have to be relatively pure and be unaffected by adsorption on to the solid phase.

5.3. C-Sandwich ELISA-Direct

The use of antibodies coated to plates as capture reagents is essential where antigens are at low concentration or are contaminated with other proteins e.g., stool samples. The system also favors presentation of some antigens in a better way than when they are directly coated to plates and also limits changes to conformational epitopes owing to direct coating. The test can be used to detect antibodies via specifically captured antigens, or antigens through the specificity of the capture antibodies. The direct sandwich relies on the conjugation of specific antibodies against the target antigen that causes some problems with variability where new batches are prepared. The antibodies can be identical to the capture antibodies. The test does rely on there being at least two combining sites (epitopes) on the antigen.

5.4. D-Sandwich ELISA-Indirect

This system offers similar advantages as in Subheading 3.3, in that low concentrations of antigen can be specifically captured. This system offers the advantage over the Direct Sandwich ELISA in that a single antispecies conjugate can be used to bind to detecting sera, thus a variety of different species detecting antibodies can be examined. The antispecies conjugate cannot be allowed to react with the initial coating antibodies so that care must be taken to avoid cross-reactions and sera must be prepared in at least two species. If only a single species is available then Fab2 fractions can be prepared from the capture antibodies and a specific anti-Fc conjugate used to develop the test.

5.5. Competition/Inhibition ELISA for all Systems

The advantages examined in the basic ELISAs- in Subheadings 5.1–5.3, all are relevant to the adaptations of the assays in competition/inhibition ELISAs. Thus the affects of coating on antigen, low concentrations of antigen, contaminating proteins, flexibility of using a single conjugate to detect many sera and orientation of antigens are all pertinent to finding the best system for solving problems. Generally competitive methods offer advantages over systems where antibodies or antigens are detected directly. The greatest increase in methods has come through the exploitation of monoclonal antibodies (MAbs) in competition/inhibition systems. **Table 37.4** briefly defines some elements of ELISA.

Table 37.4. shows the most commonly used enzymes and substrate/chromophore systems used in ELISA and the color changes with relevant stopping agents.

A. Commonly used conjugate/substrate systems

Enzyme label	Substrate	Dye	Buffer
Horse radish peroxidase	H_2O_2 (0.004%)	OPD (ortho-phenylene diamine)	Phosphate/ citrate pH 5.0
	H_2O_2 (0.004%)	TMB (tetra methyl benzidine)	Acetate buffer (0.1 M) pH 5.6
	H_2O_2 (0.002%)	ABTS (2,2′-azino di-ethyl	Phosphate/citrate, pH 4.2
	H_2O_2 (0.006%)	5AS (5-aminosalicylic acid) thiazolinesulfonic acid	Phosphate (0.2M), pH 6.8
	H_2O_2 (0.02%)	DAB (diamino benzidine)	Tris or PBS, pH 7.4
Alkaline phosphatase	pnpp	pnpp (paranitrophenyl phosphate)	Diethanolamine (10 mM) plus $MgCl_2$(0.5 mM), pH 9.5.

B. Common enzyme systems, color changes and stopping reactions

Enzyme	System	Color change		Reading wavelength		Stopping solution
		Unstopped	Stopped	Unstopped	Stopped	
Horseradish peroxidase	OPD	Light orange	Orange	450 nm	492 nm	1.25 M H_2SO_4
	TMB	Blue	Yellow	650 nm	450 nm	1% SDS
	ABTS	Green	Green	414 nm	414 nm	No stop
	5AS	Black/brown	Black/brown	450 nm	450 nm	No stop
	DAB	Brown	Brown	N/A	N/A	No stop
Alkaline phosphatase	pnpp	Yellow/green	Yellow/green	405 nm	405 nm	2 M sodium carbonate

6. Uses of ELISA

The purpose of developing ELISAs is to solve problems. These can be divided into pure and applied applications, although the two are interdependent. Thus, a laboratory with a strong research base is essential in providing scientific insight and valuable reagents to allow more routine applications. The methods outlined show the flexibility of the systems. There effective use is up to the ingenuity of scientists. Recent advances in science have given the immunoassayist greater potential for improving the sensitivity and specificity of assays, including ELISA. In particular the development of MAb technology has given us single chemical reagents (antibodies) of defined specificity that can be standardized in terms of activity as a function of their weight. The development of gene expression systems has also given the possibility of expressing single genes as proteins for use in raising antibodies or acting as pure antigens. This technology goes hand-in-hand with developments in the Polymerase Chain Reaction (PCR) technologies, that enables the very rapid identification of genes and their manipulation. In turn improvements in the fields of rapid sequencing and x-ray crystallographic methods has led to a far more intimate understanding of the structure/function relationship of organisms in relation to the immunology of disease. The ELISA fits in rather well in these developments because it is a binding assay requiring defined antibodies and antigens, all of which can be provided. **Table 37.5** illustrates some applications of ELISA with relevant references.

Table 37.5. Applications of ELISA.

General	Specific	References
Confirmation of clinical disease	Titration of specific antibodies.	*21–24,26–28,30,31,41,44,50,53, 54,62–64,69*
	Single dilution assays.	*35,41,53,54,62–64*
	Relationship of titer to protection against disease.	*50,55*
	Kits.	*44,62,63*
Analysis of immune response to whole organisms, purified antigens extracted from whole organisms, expressed proteins (e.g., vaccinia, baculo, yeast, bacteria), measurement. polypeptides, peptides	Antibody quantification.	*30,31,35,38,57,60,62,64*
	Antibody class measurement (IgM, IgG, IgA, IgD, IgE).	*25,33,34,(new 94–old 95)*
	Antibody subclass measurement (IgG1, IgG2b, IgG3).	*33*
	Antibody IG2a, affinity.	*39,49,44*
Antigenic comparison	Relative binding antibodies.	*30,31,60,64,73*
	Affinity differences in binding of antibodies.	*39,43,51,52,60*
	Measurement of weight of antigens.	*29,32,36,37,43,44,48,49,56,64*
	Examination of treatments to antigen (inactivation for vaccine manufacture, heating, enzyme treatments).	*49*

(continued)

Table 37.5. (continued)

General	Specific	References
	Identification of continuous and discontinuous epitopes by examination of binding of poly-clonal and MAbs to denatured and non denatured proteins.	*44,46,48,59*
	Antigenic profiling by MAbs. Comparison of expressed and native problems.	*40,42,44,46,61 47,48,5,92*
	Use of MAbs to identify paratopes in polyclonal sera.	*47,59,79*
Monoclonal antibodies	Screening during production. Competitive assay-antibody assessment.	*40,46 47*
	Comparison of antigens. Use of MAbs to orientate antigens.	*42,44,46,47,59,62 48*
Novel systems	High-sensitivity assays (Amplified-ELISA).	*58*
	Fluorogenic substrates.	*45*
	Biotin/avidin systems.	*68*
More recent references	Food analysis	*70,71,89*
	Fish	*84–87,90*
	AIDS	*78, 82, 90*
	SARS	*93*
	Bird flu	*76,77*
	Allergens	*74,80*
	Emerging diseases	*72*
	Psychiatry	*75*
	Review	*81,(new 95),96*
	Snakes	*91*
	Environment	*83*
	Chemoluminescence	*88*

The ability to develop ELISAs depends on as closer understanding of the immunological/serological/biochemical knowledge of specific biological systems as possible. Such information is already available with reference to literature surveys. Basic skills in immunochemical methods are also a requirement and an excellent manual for this is available (*65*). References (*66,67*) provide excellent text books on immunology. An invaluable source of commercial immunological reagents is available in (*68*). The references from 70 onwards are more recent and reflect newer fields into which ELISA has expanded and also the new problems arising as for example, Avian influenza and SARS. It is difficult to see that there will be a significant reduction in the rate of use of ELISA directly or as part of other molecular systems, but this can only be assessed when the next edition of this book is written. The main danger is methods involving ELISA are now regarded easy to develop. This, as for all tests, is not true and good training in ELISA is even more important today, because there is an incredible spectrum of reagents available for the development of tests. The linking of molecular methods to ELISA and other detection systems based on solid phase assays is exciting and full of potential, but there is a great need to attend to the basic understanding and principles of ELISA.

References

1. Avrameas S, Uriel J (1966) Methode de marquage d'antigenes et d'anticorps avec des enzymes et son application en immunodiffusion. Comptes Rendus Hendomadairesdes Seances de l'Acadamie des Sciences: D: Sciences naturelles (Paris) 262:2543–2545

2. Nakane PK, Pierce GB (1966) Enzyme-labelled antibodies: preparation and application for the localization of antigens. J Histochem Cytochem 14:929–931

3. Avrameas S (1969) Coupling of enzymes to proteins with gluteraldehyde. Use of the conjugates for the detection of antgens and antibodies. Immunochemistry 6:43–52

4. Avrameas S, Guilbert B (1971) Dosage enzymo-immunologique de proteines a l'aide d'immunosadorbants et d'antigenes marques aux enzymes. Comptes Rendus Hendomadaires des Seances de l'Acadamie des Sciences: D: Sciences naturelles (Paris) 273:2705–2707

5. Engvall E, Perlman P (1971) P. Enzyme-linked immunosorbent assay (ELISA). Quantitative assay of immunoglobulin G. Immunochemistry 8:871–874

6. Van Weeman BK, Schuurs AHWM (1971) Immunoassay using antigen enzyme conjugates. FEBS Lett 15:232–236

7. Voller A, Bidwell DE, Huldt G, Engvall E (1974) A microplate method of enzyme linked immunosorbent assay and its application to malaria. Bull Wld Hlth Org 51:209–213

8. Burgess GW (ed) (1988) ELISA technology in diagnosis and research. Graduate School of Tropical Veterinary Science, James Cook University of North Queensland, Townsville, Australia

9. Collins WP (1985) Alternative immunoassays. Wiley, Chichester, UK

10. Collins WP (1985) Complimentary immunoassays. Wiley, Chichester, UK

11. Crowther JR (1995) *ELISA: theory and practice*. Humana, Totowa, NJ

12. Ishikawa E, Kawia T, Miyai K (1981) Enzyme immunoassay. Igaku-Shoin, Tokyo, Japan

13. Kemeny DM, Challacombe SJ (1988) ELISA and other solid-phase immunoassays. Theoretical and practical aspects. Wiley, Chichester, UK

14. Maggio T (1979) *The enzyme immunoassay*. CRC, New York

15. Ngo TT, Leshoff HM (1985) Enzyme-mediated immunoassay. Plenum, New York

16. Voller A, Bidwell DE, Bartlett A (1979) The enzyme-linked immunosorbent assay *(ELISA)*. Dynatech Europe, London, UK

17. Avrameas S, Ternynck T, Guesdon JL (1978) Coupling of enzymes to antibodies and antigens. Scand J Immunol 8 Suppl. 7:7–23

18. Blake C, Gould BJ (1984) Use of enzymes in immunoassay techniques. A review. Analyst 109:533–542

19. Guilbault GG (1968) Use of enzymes in analytical chemistry. Anal Chem 40:459

20. Kemeny DM, Challacombe SJ (1986) Advances in ELISA and other solid-phase immunoassays. Immunol Today 7:67

21. Voller A, Bartlett A, Bidwell DE (1981) Immunoassays for the 80s. MTP, Lancaster, UK

22. Kemeny DM (1987) Immunoglobulin and antibody assays. In: Lessoff MH, Lee TH, Kemeny DM, (eds) Allergy: an international textbook. Wiley, Chichester, UK, p 319

23. Kemeny DM, Chantler S (1988) An introduction to ELISA. In: Kemeny DM, Challacombe SJ (eds) ELISA and other solid phase immunoassays. Theoretical and practical aspects. Wiley, Chichester, UK, p 367

24. Kemeny DM, Challacombe SJ (1988) Micrototitre plates and other solid-phase supports. In: Kemeny DM, Challacombe SJ (eds) ELISA and other solid-phase immunoassays. Theoretical and practical aspects Wiley, Chichester, UK p 367

25. Kemeny DM (1988) The modified sandwich ELISA (SELISA) for detection of IgE anantibody isotypes. In: Kemeny DM, Challacombe SJ (eds) ELISA and other solid-phase immunoassays. Technical and practical aspects. Wiley, Chichester, UK, p

26. Landon J (1977) Enzyme-immunoassay: techniques and uses. Nature 268:483

27. Avrameas S, Nakane PK, Papamichail M, Pesce AJ (eds) (1991) 25 years of immunoenzymatic techniques. J Immunol Methods International Congress, Athens, Greece, Sept 9, p 12

28. Van Weemen BK (1985) ELISA: highlights of the present state of the art. J Virol Methods 10:371

29. Yolken RH (1982) Enzyme immunoassays for the detection of infectious antigens in fluids: current limitations and future prospects. Rev Infect Dis 4:35

30. Abu Elzein EME, Crowther JR (1978) Enzyme-labelled immunosorbent assay technique in FMDV Research. J Hyg Camb 80:391–399

31. Abu Elzein EME, Crowther JR (1979) Serological comparison of a type SAT2 FMDV isolate from Sudan with other type SAT2 strains. Bull Anim Hlth Prod Afr 27:245–248

32. Abu Elzein EME, Crowther JR (1979) The specific detection of FMDV whole particle antigen (140S) by enzyme labelled immunosorbent assay. J Hyg Camb 83:127–134

33. Abu Elzein EME, Crowther JR (1981) Detection and quantification of IgM, IgA, IgG1 and IgG2 antibodies against FMDV from bovine sera using an enzyme-linked immunosorbent assay. J Hyg Camb 86:79–85

34. Anderson J, Rowe LW, Taylor WP, Crowther JR (1982) An enzyme-linked immunosorbent assay for the detection of IgG, IgA and IgM antibodies to rinderpest virus in experimentally infected cattle. Res Vet Sci 32:242–247

35. Armstrong RMA, Crowther JR, Denyer MS (1991) The detection of antibodies against foot-and-mouth disease in filter paper eluates trapping sera or whole blood by ELISA. J Immunol Methods 34:181–192

36. Crowther JR, Abu Elzein EME (1979) Detection and quantification of FMDV by enzyme labelled immunosorbent assay techniques. J Gen Virol 42:597–602

37. Crowther JR, Abu Elzein EME (1979) Application of the enzyme-linked immunosorbent assay to the detection of FMDVs. J Hyg Camb 83:513–519

38. Crowther JR, Abu Elzein EME (1980) Detection of antibodies against FMDV using purified Staphylococcus A protein conjugated with alkaline phosphatase. J Immunol Meth 34:261–267

39. Abu Elzein EME, Crowther JR (1982) Differentiation of FMDV-strains using a competition enzyme-linked immunosorbent assay. J Virol Meth 3:355–365

40. Crowther JR, McCullough KC, Simone EFDE, Brocchi E (1984) Monoclonal antibodies against FMDV: applications and potential use. Rpt Sess Res Gp Stand Tech Comm Eur Comm Cont FMD 7:40–45

41. Crowther JR (1986) Use of enzyme immunoassays in disease diagnosis, with particular reference to rinderpest. In: Nuclear and related techniques for improving productivity of indigenous animals in harsh environments. International Atomic Energy Agency, Vienna, Austria, pp 197–210

42. Crowther JR (1986) ELISA. In: FMD Diagnosis and differentiation and the use of monoclonal antibodies. Paper presented at the 17th Conference of OIE Community FMD, Paris, pp 153–173

43. Crowther JR (1986) FMDV. In: Bergmeyer J, Grassl M (eds) Methods of enzymatic analysis, 3rd edn. VCH Verlagsgesellschaft, Weinheim, Germany, pp 433–447

44. Crowther JR (1996) ELISA. In: (eds) FMD diagnosis and differentiation and the use of monoclonal antibodies. Paper presented at the 17th Conference of OIE Community FMD, Paris, pp 178–195

45. Crowther JR, Anguerita L, Anderson J (1990) Evaluation of the use of chromogenic and fluorigenic substrates in solid phase ELISA. Biologicals 18:331–336
46. Crowther JR, Rowe CA, Butcher R (1993) Characterisation of MAbs against type SAT 2 FMD virus. Epidemiol Infect 111:391–406
47. Crowther JR, Reckziegel PO, Prado JA (1993) The use of MAbs in the molecular typing of animal viruses. Rev Sci Tech Off Int Epiz *12*, 2:369–383
48. Crowther JR (1995) Quantification of whole virus particles (146S) of foot-and-mouth disease viruses in the presence of virus subunits (12S) using monoclonal antibodies in an ELISA. Vaccine 13:1064–1075
49. Curry S, Abrams CC, Fry E, Crowther JR, Belsham G, Stewart D, King AQ (1995) Viral RNA modulates the acid sensitivity of FMDV capsids. J Virol 69:430–438
50. Denyer MS, Crowther JR, Wardley RC, Burrows R (1984) Development of an enzyme-linked immunosorbent assay (ELISA) for the detection of specific antibodies against H7N7 and an H3N3 equine influenza virus. J Hyg Camb 93:609–620
51. Denyer MS, Crowther JR (1986) Use of indirect and competitive ELISAs to compare isolates of equine influenza A virus. J Virol Meth 14:253–265
52. Goldberg ME, Djavadi-Ohaniance L (1993). Methods for measurement of antibody/antigen affinity based on ELISA and RIA. Curr Opin Immunol 5:278–281
53. Hamblin C, Crowther JR (1982) Evaluation and use of the enzyme-linked immunosorbent assay in the serology of swine vesicular disease. In: Wardley RC, and Crowther JR (eds) The ELISA: enzyme-linked immunosorbent assay in veterinary research and diagnosis, Martinus Nijhoff, The Netherlands, pp 232–241
54. Hamblin C, Crowther JR (1982) A rapid enzyme-linked immunosorbent assay for the serological confirmation of SVD. In: Wardley RC, Crowther JR (eds) The ELISA: enzyme-linked immunosorbent assay in veterinary research and diagnosis, Martinus Nijhoff, The Netherlands, pp 232–241
55. Hamblin C, Barnett ITR, Crowther JR (1986) A new enzyme-linked immunosorbent assay (ELISA) for the detection of antibodies against FMDV. II. Appl J Immun Meth 93:123–129
56. Hamblin C, Mellor P, Graham MS, Crowther JR (1990) Detection of african horse sickness antibodies by a sandwich competition ELISA. Epid Infect 104:303–312
57. Hamblin C, Mertens PPC, Mellor PS, Burroughs JN, Crowther JR (1991) A serogroup specific enzyme linked immunosorbent assay (ELISA) for the detection and identification of African Horse Sickness Viruses. J Vir Meth 31:285–292
58. Johannsson A, Ellis DH, Bates DL, Plumb AM, Stanley CJ (1986) Enzyme amplification for immunoasays-detection of one hundredth of an attomole. J Immunol Meth 87:7–11
59. McCullough KC, Crowther JR, Butcher RN (1985) A liquid-phase ELISA and its use in the identification of epitopes on FMDV antigens. J Virol Meth 11:329–338
60. Rossiter PB, Taylor WP, Crowther JR (1988) Antigenic variation between three strains of rinderpest virus detected by kinetic neutralisation and competition ELISA using early rabbit antisera. Vet Microbiol 16:195–200
61. Samuel A, Knowles NJ, Samuel GD, Crowther JR (1991) Evaluation of a trapping ELISA for the differentiation of foot-and-mouth disease virus strains using monoclonal antibodies. Biologicals 19:229–310
62. Sanchez Vizcaino JM, Crowther JR, Wardley RC (1983) A collaborative study on the use of the ELISA in the diagnosis of African swine fever. In: African Swine Fever. (CEC/FAO Research Seminar, Sardinia, Sept. 1981). Wilkinson PJ (ed). Commission of the European Communities Publication EUR 8466 EN, pp. 297–325
63. The sero-monitoring of rinderpest throughout Africa. Phase two. Results for 1993. Proceedings of a research coordination meeting of the FAO/IAEA/SIDA/OAU/IBAR/PARC coordinated research programme organized by the joint FAO/IAEA division of nuclear techniques in food and agriculture, Cairo, Egypt, 7–11, November 1993

64. Wardley RC, Abu Elzein EME, Crowther JR, Wilkinson PJ (1979) A solid-phase enzyme linked immunosorbent assay for the detection of ASFV antigen and antibody. J Hyg Camb 83:363–369

65. Harlow E, Lane D (eds) (1988) Antibodies. A laboratory manual. Cold Spring Harbor Laboratory, Cold Spring Harbor, NY

66. Roitt I (1991) *Essential immunology*. Blackwell Scientific Publications, Oxford, UK

67. Roitt I, Brostoff J, Male D (eds) (1993) *Immunology*. Mosby

68. Linscott's directory of immunological and biological reagents. Linscott's Directory, Santa Rosa, CA

69. Immunogens, Ag/Ab purification, antibodies, avidin–Biotin, protein modification: PIERCE immunotechnology catalogue and handbook, Pierce and Warriner, UK. Published yearly

70. Unusan N (2006) Occurrence of aflatoxin M1 in UHT milk in Turkey. Food Chem Toxicol 44:11 1897–1900

71. Watanabe E et al (2006) Evaluation of performance of a commercial monoclonal antibody - based fenitrothion immunoassay and application to residual analysis in fruit samples. J Food Prot 69:1, (8), 191–198

72. Huestis MA et al (2006) Cannabinoid concentrations in hair from documented cannabis users. Forensic Sci Int September 169:2–3, 129–136

73. Sunwoo HH, Wang WW, Sim JS (2006) Detection of *Escherichia coli* O157: H7 using chicken immunoglobulin Y. Immunol Lett 106:2, 15, 191–193

74. Jennifer M, Maloney MD, Martin D, Chapman P, Scott H, Sicherer MD (2006) Peanut allergen exposure through saliva: assessment and interventions to reduce exposure J Allergy Clin Immunol 118:3, 719–724

75. Huang TL, Lee CT (2006) Associations between serum brain-derived neurotrophic factor levels and clinical phenotypes in schizophrenia patients. J Psychiatr Res 40:7, 664–668

76. Al-Natoura QM, Abo-Shehada MN (2005) Sero-prevalence of avian influenza among broiler-breeder flocks. Jordan Prev Vet Med 70:1–2, 45–50

77. Dundon WG, Milani A, Cattoli G, Capua I (2006) Progressive truncation of the non-structural 1 gene of H7N1 avian influenza viruses following extensive circulation in poultry. Virus Res 119:2, 171–176

78. Neumann J et al (2006) Retroviral vectors for vaccine development: induction of HIV-1-specific humoral and cellular immune responses in rhesus macaques using a novel MLV (HIV-1) pseudotype vector. J Biotechnol 124:3, 615–625

79. Carlos O et al (2006) Evaluation of murine monoclonal antibodies targeting different epitopes of the hepatitis B virus surface antigen by using immunological as well as molecular biology and biochemical approaches. J Immunol Methods 313:1–2, 30, 38–47

80. Dearman RJ et al (2003) Induction of IgE antibody responses by protein allergens: inter-laboratory comparisons. Food Chem Toxicol 41:11, 1509–1516

81. Baker KN et al (2002) Rapid monitoring of recombinant protein products: a comparison of current technologies. Trends Biotechnol 20:4, 1, 149–156

82. Caterino-de-Araujo A et al (1998) Sensitivity of two enzyme-linked immunosorbent assay tests in relation to Western blot in detecting human T-cell lymphotropic virus types I and II infection among HIV-1 infected Patients from São Paulo, Brazil. Diagn Microbiol Infect Dis 30:3, 173–182

83. Speight SE, Hallis BA, Bennett AM, Benbough JE (1997) Enzyme-linked immunosorbent assay for the detection of airborne microorganisms used in biotechnology. J Aerosol Sci 28:3, 483–492

84. Rogers-Lowery CL, Dimock RV, Jr. Kuhn RE (2007) Antibody response of bluegill sunfish during development of acquired resistance against the larvae of the freshwater mussel Utterbackia imbecillis. Dev Comp Immunol 31:2, 143–155

85. Tsutsumi T et al (2006) Application of an ELISA for PCB 118 to the screening of dioxin-like PCBs in retail fish. Chemosphere 65:3, 467–473

86. Liu W et al (2006) Immune response against grouper nervous necrosis virus by vaccination of virus-like particles. Vaccine 24:37–39, 6282–6287

87. Liao T et al (2006) An enzyme-linked immunosorbent assay for rare minnow (*Gobiocypris rarus*) vitellogenin and comparison of vitellogenin responses in rare minnow and zebrafish (*Danio rerio*). Sci Total Environ 364:1–3, 284–294

88. March C et al (2005) Rapid detection and counting of viable beer-spoilage lactic acid bacteria using a monoclonal chemiluminescence enzyme immunoassay and a CCD camera. J Immunol Methods 303:1–2, 92–104

89. Carlin F, Broussolle V, Perelle S, Litman S, Fach P (2004) Prevalence of *Clostridium botulinum* in food raw materials used in REPFEDs manufactured in France. Int J Food Microbiol 91:2, 141–145

90. Pucci B, Coscia MR, Oreste U (2003) Characterization of serum immunoglobulin M of the Antarctic teleost *Trematomus bernacchii*. Comp Biochem Physiol B Biochem Mol Biol 135:2, 349–357

91. Rial A, Morais V, Rossi S, Massaldi H (2006) A new ELISA for determination of potency in snake antivenoms. Toxicon 48:4, 462–466

92. Pullen MA, Laping N, Edwards R, Bray J (2006) Determination of conformational changes in the progesterone receptor using ELISA-like assay. Steroids, 71:9, 792–798

93. Huang J, Ma R, Wu CY (2006) Immunization with SARS-CoV S DNA vaccine generates memory CD4+ and CD8+ T cell immune responses. Vaccine 24:23, 4905–4913

94. Bongertz V (2003) Anti-HIV-1 humoral immune response in Brazilian patients. Clin Appl Immunol Rev 3:6, 307–317

95. Crowther JR (2000) The ELISA guidebook. Methods Mol Biol 149:III–IV, 1–413. Humana, Totowa, NJ

38

Epitope Mapping
Identification of Antibody-Binding Sites on Protein Antigens

Glenn E. Morris

1. What is an Epitope?

An epitope can be simply defined as that part of an antigen involved in its recognition by an antibody. In the case of protein antigens, an epitope would consist of a group of individual amino acid side-chains close together on the protein surface. Epitope mapping, then, becomes the process of locating the epitope, or identifying the individual amino acids involved. Apart from its intrinsic value for understanding protein structure-function relationships, it also has a practical value in generating antibody probes of defined specificity as research tools and in helping to define the immune response to pathogenic proteins and organisms. The epitope concept is becoming increasingly applied to interactions between proteins other than antibodies and antigens *(1,2)*; not every immunologist would be happy about this, but it does make the point that in mapping epitopes, we are studying a biological process of fundamental importance, that of protein–protein interaction. Epitope mapping is usually done with monoclonal antibodies (MAbs), though it can be done with polyclonal antisera in a rather less rigorous way, bearing in mind that antisera behave as mixtures of MAbs. Mapping can be done directly by X-ray crystallography of antibody-antigen complexes, but it can also be done by changing individual amino acids, by using antigen fragments and synthetic peptides or by competition methods in which two or more antibodies compete for the same, or adjacent, epitopes. The term "epitope mapping" has also been used to describe the attempt to determine all the major sites on a protein surface that can elicit an antibody response, at the end of which one might claim to have produced an "epitope map" of the protein immunogen *(3)*. This information might be very useful, for example, to someone wishing to produce antiviral vaccines. However, there is a limit to how far one can go down this road, because the map obtained may be influenced by how MAbs are selected and by the mapping method used. Furthermore, the more strictly correct definition of epitope mapping is based on antigenicity (the ability to recognize a specific antibody), whereas the latter definition is based on immunogenicity (the ability to produce antibodies in a given animal species)

From: *Molecular Biomethods Handbook, 2nd Edition.*
Edited by: J. M. Walker and R. Rapley © Humana Press, Totowa, NJ

and thus depends on the immune system of the recipient animal. Some authors prefer to use the terms "antigenic determinant" and "immunogenic determinant" to make this distinction clear *(4)*. For antigenic determinants, it is possible to think of epitope mapping as a "simple" biochemical problem of finding out how one well-defined protein (a MAb) binds to another (the antigen). Not all antigenic determinants are also immunogenic determinants, however, and Berzofsky *(4)* quotes the example of chicken lysozyme, which is not immunogenic in certain mouse strains although Abs raised against other lysozymes will bind to it. Nevertheless, immunogenicity and antigenicity, although not identical, are sufficiently closely related to make it possible to infer from antibody specificity which regions of a protein are more likely to be immunogenic.

B-lymphocytes display immunoglobulin molecules on their surface and are stimulated to divide when these interact with a suitable antigen. They then undergo somatic mutation in a germinal center of the spleen to refine antibody diversity further and there tends to be selection in favor of B cells that produce higher affinity antibodies *(5)*. The slightly different antibody molecules produced by somatic mutation will generally recognize the same region of protein but with a different affinity or a different tolerance of amino-acid substitutions. These fine specificities can hardly be regarded as defining different epitopes, though it is difficult to decide where exactly to draw the line. A similar problem exists in deciding what point the distinction between two overlapping epitopes should cease to exist. In contrast to the direct stimulation of B cells by immunogen, protein immunogens have to be processed by antigen-presenting cells (APCs) in order to stimulate T cells. APCs digest proteins and display short peptides on their surface in association with products of the major histocompatibility complex (MHC); this displayed complex then stimulates T –cells to divide by interacting with specific T cell receptors (TCRs). Other MHC gene products are involved in proteolytic processing and in transport of peptide fragments to the cell surface *(5,6)*. At least, T cell epitopes are simpler that B-cell epitopes in one respect; they can apparently be treated as simple amino-acid sequences without the problems of protein structure and conformation that pervade all aspects of B-cell epitope mapping. The interested reader is referred to reviews of MHC-peptide interactions *(6)* and prediction of T cell epitopes *(7)*. A simple method for mapping T cell epitopes is to measure the ability of peptide fragments of the protein to stimulate cell division of T lymphocytes *(8)*, but advanced techniques like mass spectrometry *(9)* and ELISPOT assays *(10)* now play a major role. T cell epitope mapping is of vital importance to understanding mechanisms of immunity and an issue of the journal "Methods" was largely devoted to reviews of this rapidly-growing field (volume 29 No. 3 (2003) pp 213–309).

There is also a great deal of interest in mapping epitopes recognized by IgE molecules involved in allergic responses, especially with a view to developing possible vaccines. Many of the methods applicable to IgG and IgM molecules are also applicable to IgE, except that the IgE is likely to derive from patient serum *(11)* or human lymphocyte-derived mAbs *(12)*.

In recent years, a number of literature-derived databases have been developed for B-cell epitopes *(13)*, including conformational epitopes *(14)*.

2. Conformational or Linear Epitopes? Structural or Functional Epitopes?

It is essential to distinguish among conformational ("discontinuous," "assembled") epitopes, in which amino-acids far apart in the protein sequence are brought together by protein folding, and linear ("continuous," "sequential") epitopes, which can often be mimicked by simple peptide sequences. Parts of conformational epitopes can sometimes be mimicked by peptides, but early evidence that most peptide sequences can produce Abs that recognize native proteins *(4)* is no longer accepted *(15)*. The term "mimotope" has been coined to describe peptides that mimic epitopes without corresponding exactly to the antigen sequence; typically, these would be random peptides obtained from random sequence libraries *(16)* or phage-displayed libraries *(17)*.

Most native proteins are formed of highly convoluted peptide chains, so that residues that lie close together on the protein surface are often far apart in the amino-acid sequence *(18)*. Consequently, most epitopes on native, globular proteins are conformation-dependent or "assembled" and they disappear if the protein is denatured or fragmented. Sometimes, by accident or design, antibodies are produced against "local" (linear, sequential) epitopes that survive denaturation, though such antibodies usually fail to recognize the native protein. Conversely, most antibody molecules in polyclonal antisera raised against native proteins do not recognize unfolded antigens or short peptides *(15)*. Historically, there has been something of a culture gap among crystallographers who tend to study assembled epitopes exclusively and people who use MAbs as research tools, for whom assembled epitopes can be something of a nuisance if the MAbs do not work on Western blots. Some authors have even emphasized the distinction between epitopes on native proteins and those on denatured proteins by using such terms as "cryptotopes" or "unfoldons" for the latter *(19)*, but they have never been commonly used. The simplest way to find out whether an epitope is conformational is by Western blotting after sodium dodecyl sulfate-polyacrylamide gel electrophoresis (SDS-PAGE). If the antibody still binds after the protein has been boiled in SDS and 2-mercaptoethanol, the epitope is unlikely to be highly conformational. It must be remembered, however, that few proteins are completely denatured on Western blots and some epitopes identified by Western blotting may still have a conformational element. Similarly, some, though not all, conformational epitopes are also destroyed when the antigen binds to plastic in an ELISA test, which is the commonest primary screen when making monoclonal antibodies *(20)*.

3. Epitope Mapping Methods

A skeleton outline of the approaches that follow is given in **Table 38.1**.

3.1. Structural Approach

At their most elaborate, epitope mapping techniques can provide detailed information on the amino-acid residues in a protein antigen that are in direct contact with the antibody binding site ("contact residues"). X-ray crystallography of antibody-antigen complexes can identify contact residues directly and

Table 38.1. Approaches to epitope mapping.

Structural
　　X-ray diffraction
　　Nuclear magnetic resonance
　　Electron microscopy

Functional
　　Competition
　　　　ELISA
　　　　Ouchterlony plates
　　　　Biosensors

　　Antigen modification
　　　　Chemical modification of side-chains
　　　　Protection by Ab from chemical modification
　　　　Site-directed mutagenesis
　　　　PCR-random mutagenesis
　　　　Homolog scanning
　　　　Viral-escape mutants
　　　　Natural variants and isoforms
　　　　Mass spectrometry

　　Antigen fragmentation
　　　　Chemical fragmentation
　　　　Proteolytic digestion
　　　　Protection by Ab from proteolytic digestion
　　　　Recombinant libraries of random cDNA fragments
　　　　Recombinant subfragments produced by:

　　　　　　PCR
　　　　　　Exonuclease III
　　　　　　Transposon mutagenesis
　　　　　　Early-translation termination

　　Synthetic peptides
　　　　PEPSCAN peptide arrays
　　　　SPOTS synthesis on membranes
　　　　Combinatorial libraries
　　　　Phage-displayed peptide libraries

unequivocally *(21)*, though, not surprisingly in view of the effort required, this method is not in routine use. The method is further restricted by the necessity of obtaining good crystals of Ab–Ag complexes and it has usually been to highly-conformational epitopes on the surface of soluble proteins. Van Regenmortel has made the important distinction between "structural" epitopes as defined by X-ray crystallography and related techniques and "functional" epitopes defined by amino-acid residues, which are important for binding and cannot be replaced *(15)*. The number of contact residues revealed by X-ray crystallography is usually about 15–20, whereas "functional" mapping methods that depend on Ab binding changes generally find about 4–8 important residues. This difference may be more apparent than real, however, partly because there does not seem to be complete agreement on how close amino acids in the Ab and Ag must be to constitute a "contact" and also because some residues in the Ag could be "in contact" with the Ab without contributing significantly to the binding. It is equally true, however, that "functional" mapping methods may give an incomplete picture; fragmentation methods, for example, may detect only the most important continuous part of a discontinuous epitope and additional amino acids may contribute significantly to the binding affinity in the intact antigen. Nuclear magnetic resonance (NMR) of Ab-Ag complexes is another "structural" approach that is in many ways complementary to the crystallographic method (22). NMR methods are performed in solution and thus avoid the need for crystals but they are limited by the size of the antigen that can be studied and are usually applied to peptide antigens (23,24). NMR is therefore unsuitable for direct study of highly assembled protein epitopes. At the other extreme, electron microscopy of Ab-Ag complexes has also been used to identify Ab-binding sites directly, but this is usually applied to very large antigens, such as whole viruses (25,26). When the epitope is known by other methods [e.g., use of anti-peptide antibodies (27) or peptide-mapped mAbs (28)], electron microscopy can provide important data on their disposition on large proteins or viruses.

3.2. Functional Approach

The remaining epitope mapping methods are essentially "functional" in approach, because they involve introducing some additional variable into the basic Ab–Ag interaction and then testing for antigenic function (i.e., does it still bind Ab?). They include protection methods in which the antibody protects the antigen from loss of function and can be usefully divided into four groups:

1. Competition methods
2. Ag-modification methods
3. Ag-fragmentation methods
4. The use of synthetic peptides or peptide libraries

3.2.1. Competition Methods

Competition methods can be very useful when a relatively low degree of mapping resolution is adequate. You may want to establish, for example, that two MAbs recognize different, nonoverlapping epitopes for a 2-site immunoassay, or to find MAbs against several different epitopes on the same Ag so that results from cross reactions with other proteins can be rigorously excluded. The principle behind competition methods is to determine whether two different MAbs can bind to a monovalent Ag at the same time (in which case they must recognize different epitopes) or whether they compete with each other for Ag binding. The traditional approaches to competition mapping involve labeling either Ab or Ag with enzymes or radioactivity and immobilizing the Ag (or one of the competing Abs) on a solid support, such as microtiter plates for ELISA or Sepharose beads (29,30). Abs against the same epitope (or one very close) will clearly displace the labeled Ab from immobilized Ag. An even simpler method based on this principle uses Ouchterlony gel-diffusion plates (31), because single MAbs, or mixtures of MAbs that recognize the same epitope, are unable to form precipitin lines. At a more sophisticated and more expensive level, biosensors that follow Ab-binding in real time can be used to determine directly whether two or more unlabeled MAbs will bind to the same unlabeled Ag (32,33). This BIAcore approach can be used in combination with other methods, such as antigen fragmentation (34).

3.2.2. Antigen Modification Methods

Chemical modification of amino-acid side-chains is a method that is perhaps less widely used today than previously. In principle, addition of modifying groups specifically to amino acids, such as lysine, should prevent antibody binding to epitopes that contain lysine residues and such an approach should be particularly useful for conformational epitopes that are otherwise difficult to map with simple techniques. Unfortunately, such epitopes are also the most sensitive to indirect disruption by chemicals that cause even small conformational changes and great care is needed to avoid false positives. If the Ag can be expressed from recombinant cDNA and the approximate position of the epitope is known, specific mutations can be introduced by site-directed mutagenesis methods (35–37). Alternatively, random mutations can be introduced into part of the antigen by PCR, followed by screening to detect epitope-negative mutants (38). A "site-directed masking" method for proteins of known 3D-structure introduces surface cysteines by mutagenesis and attaches them chemically to a solid phase, thus "masking" different patches of surface around the introduced cysteines (39). An elegant method for conformational epitopes, homolog scanning (40), requires two forms of the Ag (e.g., from different species) to be expressible from recombinant DNA as native proteins, one of them reactive with the Ab and the other not. Functional chimeric proteins can then be constructed by genetic engineering and regions responsible for Ab binding identified. Compared with random mutation methods, this approach is less likely to disrupt the native conformation because protein function is retained. The "escape mutant" approach for viral-surface epitopes that are recognized by neutralizing antibodies involves selection and sequencing of spontaneous mutants whose infectivity is no longer blocked by the antibody (41). Naturally occurring species or isoform differences in amino-acid sequence can also provide very useful information on epitope location, because Abs may or may not cross-react across species or isoforms (42). Protection from chemical modification, as described by Bosshard and coworkers (43), should be more reliable than direct modification because the side-chains in the epitope itself are not altered (protected by Ab) and the modifying groups on the unprotected side-chains are not large (e.g., radioactive acetyl groups). Labeling of individual amino acids is compared in the presence and absence of the protecting Ab. Protection from proteolytic digestion, also known as "protein footprinting" (44), is similar in principle; antigens are exposed to proteases in the presence or absence of antibody (which is fairly protease-resistant) and differences in digestion are detected by gel electrophoresis. For native proteins, that are often resistant to proteases, it does depends on the epitope containing a protease-sensitive site, but assembled epitopes are often found on surface loops that are more likely to be accessible to protease. If the Ab–Ag interaction will survive extensive proteolysis with loss of structure, the Ag fragments remaining attached to the Ab can be identified by mass spectrometry (45); this is really a fragmentation approach rather than a protection or modification method. A recent variant, however, involves protection by antibody against hydrogen-deuterium exchange, with the protected amino acids subsequently identified by mass spectrometry (46,47). Mass spectrometry approaches to epitope mapping, recently and expertly reviewed (48), will increase in importance as the sensitivity and analytical power of these machines continues to develop.

3.2.3. Antigen-Fragmentation Methods

A simpler fragmentation approach for epitopes that survive denaturation is partial protease digestion of the Ag alone, followed either by Western blotting for larger fragments or by HPLC *(49)*. The fragments that bind Ab can be identified by N-terminal microsequencing or by mass spectrometry. Overlapping fragments, produced by different proteases, help to narrow down the epitope location. If the antigen is a recombinant protein, it can be expressed with affinity tags at each end to enable separate affinity purification of fragments after digestion; the epitope can be localized very simply from the overlap between the shortest N-terminal and the shortest C-terminal fragments that bind-antibody *(50)*. Chemical fragmentation is an alternative to proteolysis and has the advantage that cleavage sites are less frequent (e.g., for Cys, Trp, and Met residues) so that fragments can often be identified from their size alone *(51–53)*; for this reason, Ag purity is less important than for proteolytic fragmentation. Conditions for chemical cleavage, however, are usually strongly denaturing, so the method is not useful for assembled epitopes.

Additional methods of generating and identifying antigen fragments are possible if the Ag can be expressed from recombinant cDNA. Random internal digestion of cDNA with DNaseI, followed by cloning and expression of the cDNA fragments to create "epitope libraries," is a popular way of generating overlapping antigenic fragments *(54,55)*. If a MAb recognizes several different fragments, then the epitope must lie within the region of overlap. Epitope expression from the random colonies is screened using the antibody under study and the precise Ag fragment expressed can be identified by DNA sequencing. The power of this approach can be increased by incorporating phage-display methodology in which the antigen fragments are displayed on the surface of filamentous phage. This has the important advantage that Ab-positive clones can be obtained by selection rather than screening *(56,57)*. This approach may be improved by cloning methods that select for in-frame cDNA fragments *(58)*. Another approach is to clone specific, predetermined (rather than random) fragments that have been generated either by using existing restriction enzyme sites in the cDNA or, more flexibly, by using PCR products that have restriction sites in the primers *(59,60)*. The latter approach is especially useful if you want to know whether an epitope is in a specific domain of the antigen or whether it is encoded by a specific exon in the gene, because other methods may give ambiguous answers to these questions. For PCR products, the necessity to clone may be avoided altogether by including a promoter in the forward primer and transcribing/translating the PCR product in vitro *(61)*. Another major advantage of the PCR approach is that it is not always necessary to have your full-length antigen already cloned. Provided the cDNA sequence is known, RT-PCR (reverse transcriptase-PCR) can be used to clone PCR products directly from mRNA or even total RNA *(60)*. Several methods exist for random shortening of the antigens produced from plasmid vectors. Transposon mutagenesis involves the random insertion of stop codons into plasmid DNA using a bacterial transposon *(62,63)*. Unlike previous methods, extensive DNA manipulation is not required and the site of introduction of the stop codon can be identified precisely by DNA sequencing. Another method takes advantage of the spontaneous early termination of translation of mRNA, which occurs in in vitro systems *(64)*. When removal of amino acids abolishes antibody binding, those amino acids may be contact residues, but they may alternatively be needed to maintain the conformation of the real contact residues in the remaining fragment, so care is needed in the interpretation of any results involving loss of antibody binding. A positive binding result, with a synthetic peptide for example, may be needed to confirm the localization. Exonuclease III digests double-stranded DNA nucleotide by nucleotide, but not at 3'-overhangs; because 3' or 5' overhangs can be introduced using restriction enzymes, this method can be used to remove nucleotides progressively from either end *(65)*. This enables production of overlapping recombinant protein fragments that are positive for antibody binding, an approach that determines epitope boundaries reliably.

3.2.4. Peptide Methods

Synthetic peptides have revolutionized our understanding of epitopes to the same extent as X-ray crystallography, though ironically the two approaches are virtually mutually exclusive, because peptides are used for sequential epitopes. In the PEPSCAN method, overlapping peptides (e.g., hexamers) covering the complete Ag sequence are synthesized on pins for repeated screening with different MAbs *(66,67)*. Because the synthesis can be done automatically, this popular approach requires very little work by the end-user. The alternative SPOTS technique performs the multiple-peptide synthesis on a cellulose-membrane support *(68,69)*. Peptides have also been synthesized on micro-arrays for subsequent detection of antibody binding by fluorescein-labeled second antibody and immunofluorescence microscopy *(70,71)*. An alternative approach to the synthesis of peptides based on the Ag sequence is the use of combinatorial libraries of random peptide sequences in solution *(72)*.

The advent of peptide libraries displayed on the surface of phage took this approach a step further by enabling selection of displayed peptides, as opposed to screening *(73,74)*. In this case, random oligonucleotides are cloned into an appropriate part of a phage surface protein and the peptide sequence displayed is identified after selection by sequencing the phage DNA. Selection of random peptides is unique in producing a range of sequences that are related, but not identical, to the Ag sequence; this enables inferences to be made about which amino acids in the epitope are most important for Ab binding. A method has been developed for displaying peptide libraries directly on the surface of *Escherichia coli* in the major flagellum component, flagellin *(75)*, and this may facilitate screening and amplification steps. The great advantage of the Scott and Smith method *(73)* is the use of the fd-tet version of M13 phage, which enables the phage to grow as *E. coli* colonies, rather than the plaques in the E. coli lawn produced by some commercial mapping methods (Ph.D. kit, New England Biolabs: see *76*). Another development displays random-peptide libraries on polyribosomes and the selected mRNA containing the peptide-encoding sequence is amplified by RT-PCR for reselection or sequencing *(77)*. This approach was taken one step further in "mRNA display", in which advantage is taken of the mechanism of puromycin action to make a direct covalent link between a library of expressed RNA sequences and the peptides they encode, enabling co-selection by antibody of antigenic epitope and its corresponding nucleotide sequence *(78,79)*. An advantage shared by all peptide methods is that antigen is not required and this may be important for "rare" Ags that are difficult to purify. Full experimental details of many of these epitope mapping methods, together with background and illustrations of their applications, can be found elsewhere *(80)*.

4. Applications and Epitope Prediction

Epitope mapping is to some degree an end in itself, insofar as it provides fundamental information on the way that proteins recognize each other and recognize ligands in general. In other words, it helps us to understand the protein structure-function relationships that underlie all biological processes. Epitope-mapping studies can also suggest regions of viral proteins that are likely to be immunogenic and thus help in the design of potential vaccines. Antibodies that neutralize infectivity are of particular interest *(22,81–83)*. Epitope mapping of antibodies present in autoimmune disease may throw light on the cause of these diseases, which are often owing to crossreacting antibodies elicited by unrelated proteins or microorganisms *(84–88)*, although T cell epitopes have a major role in autoimmunity. Mapping of antibodies that inhibit protein function (e.g., enzyme activity) can be used to determine which parts of the protein are involved in that function *(89–93)*. Similar use can be made of antibodies that recognize more than one state of the antigen (e.g., native and partly unfolded *(94)*, free or complexed with other proteins *(95)*, and so forth). Antibodies with known binding sites can also be used to determine the topology of trans-membrane proteins by immunoelectron microscopy *(96)*, the domain structure of proteins *(97)*, and the orientation of proteins in relation to intracellular structures *(98)*, or to detect alternative gene products produced by genetic deletion (60) or alternative RNA splicing *(99)*. Finally, this chapter has dealt with experimental epitope mapping methods only, though many attempts have been made to predict epitopes from the amino-acid sequences of antigens *(100–102)*. Epitopes show an obvious correlation with antibody accessibility (i.e., they have to be on the surface of the antigen) and possibly with local mobility of the peptide chain, if the Ab–Ag interaction is of the "induced-fit" variety *(15)*. It is also relatively easy to sequence the variable regions of MAb H and L chains, including the hypervariable regions that recognize the antigen, by performing RT-PCR on hybridoma-cell mRNA *(103)*. Such sequences can be used to create 3-D models of the antigen-combining site, or "paratope" on the antibody *(104)*.

References

1. Wells JA (1995) Structural and functional epitopes in the growth hormone receptor complex. Biotechnology 13:647–651
2. Bialek K, Swistowski A, Frank R (2003) Epitope-targeted proteome analysis: towards a large-scale automated protein protein-interaction mapping utilizing synthetic peptide arrays. Anal Bioanal Chem 376:1006–1013
3. Atassi MZ (1984) Antigenic structure of proteins. Eur J Biochem 145:1–20
4. Berzoksky JA (1985) Intrinsic and extrinsic factors in protein antigenic structure. Science 219:932–940
5. McHeyzer-Williams LJ, McHeyzer-Williams MG (2005) Antigen-specific memory B cell development. Ann Rev Immunol 23:487–513
6. Rudolph MG, Stanfield RL, Wilson IA (2006) How TCRs bind MHCs, peptides, and coreceptors. Ann Rev Immunol 24:419–466
7. Stevanovic S (2005) Antigen processing is predictable: From genes to T cell epitopes. Transpl Immunol 14:171–174
8. Reece JC, Geysen HM, Rodda SJ (1993) Mapping the major human T helper epitopes of tetanus toxin. The emerging picture. J Immunol 151:6175–6184

9. Suri A, Lovitch SB, Unanue ER (2006) The wide diversity and complexity of peptides bound to class II MHC molecules. Curr Opin Immunol 18:70–77

10. Anthony DD, Lehmann PV (2003) T cell epitope mapping using the ELISPOT approach. Methods 29:260–269

11. Hantusch B, Krieger S, Untersmayr E, Scholl I, Knittelfelder R, Flicker S, Spitzauer S, Valenta R, Boltz-Nitulescu G, Scheiner O, Jensen-Jarolim E (2004) Mapping of conformational IgE epitopes on Phl p 5a by using mimotopes from a phage display library. J Allergy Clin Immunol 114:1294–1300

12. Flicker S, Steinberger P, Ball T, Krauth MT, Verdino P, Valent P, Almo S, Valenta R (2006) Spatial clustering of the IgE epitopes on the major timothy grass pollen allergen Phl p 1: importance for allergenic activity. J Allergy Clin Immunol 117:1336–1343

13. Saha S, Bhasin M, Raghava GP (2005) Bcipep: a database of B-cell epitopes. BMC Genomics 6:79

14. Huang J, Honda W (2006) CED: a conformational epitope database. BMC Immunol 7:7

15. van Regenmortel MHV (1989) Structural and functional approaches to the study of protein antigenicity. Immunol Today 10:266–272

16. Lenstra JA, Erkens JH, Langeveld JG, Posthumus WP, Meloen RH, Gebauer F, Correa I, Enjuanes L, Stanley KK (1992) Isolation of sequences from a random-sequence expression library that mimic viral epitopes. J Immunol Methods 152:149–157

17. Mertens P, Walgraffe D, Laurent T, Deschrevel N, Letesson JJ, De Bolle X (2001) Selection of phage-displayed peptides recognised by monoclonal antibodies directed against the lipopolysaccharide of Brucella. Int Rev Immunol 20:181–199

18. Barlow DJ, Edwards MS, Thornton JM (1986) Continuous and discontinuous protein antigenic determinants. Nature 322:747–748

19. Laver WG, Air GM, Webster RG, Smith-Gill SJ (1990) Epitopes on protein antigens: misconceptions and realities. Cell 61:533–556

20. Nguyen Thi Man Morris GE (1996) Production of panels of monoclonal antibodies by the hybridoma method. In: Morris GE (ed) Epitope mapping protocols. Humana Press, Totowa, NJ, pp. 377–389

21. Amit P, Mariuzza R, Phillips S, Poljak R (1986) Three-dimensional structure of an antigen antibody complex. Science 233:747–753

22. Zvi–A, Kustanovich I, Feigelson D, Levy R, Eisenstein M, Matsushita S, Richalet-Secordel P, van Regenmortel MHV, Anglister J (1995) NMR mapping of the antigenic determinant recognised by an anti-gp 120, human immunodeficiency virus neutralizing antibody. Eur J Biochem 229:178–187

23. Morgan WD, Frenkiel TA, Lock MJ, Grainger M, Holder AA (2005) Precise epitope mapping of malaria parasite inhibitory antibodies by TROSY NMR cross-saturation. Biochemistry 18:518–523

24. Megy S, Bertho G, Gharbi-Benarous J, Baleux F, Benarous R, Girault JP (2006) STD and TRNOESY NMR studies for the epitope mapping of the phosphorylation motif of the oncogenic protein beta-catenin recognized by a selective monoclonal antibody. FEBS Lett 580:5411–5422

25. Dore I, Weiss E, Altschuh D, van Regenmortel MHV (1988) Visualization by electron microscopy of the location of tobacco mosaic virus epitopes reacting with monoclonal antibodies. Virology 162:279–289

26. Belnap DM, Watts NR, Conway JF, Cheng N, Stahl SJ, Wingfield PT, Steven AC (2003) Diversity of core antigen epitopes of hepatitis B virus. Proc Natl Acad Sci USA 100:10,884–10,889

27. Benacquista BL, Sharma MR, Samso M, Zorzato F, Treves S, Wagenknecht T (2000) Amino acid residues 4425–4621 localized on the three-dimensional structure of the skeletal muscle ryanodine receptor. Biophys J 78:1349–1358

28. Veliceasa D, Tauscher G, Suranyi G, Kos PB, Liko I, Santore U, Proll E, Ehrig F, Uray K, Hudecz F, Kuhne T, Lukacs N (2005) Characterisation of epitopes on barley mild mosaic virus coat protein recognised by a panel of novel monoclonal antibodies. Arch Virol 150:2501–2512

29. Tzartos SJ, Rand DE, Einarson BL, Lindstrom JM (1981) Mapping of surface structures of Electrophorus acetylcholine receptor using monoclonal antibodies. J Biol Chem 256:8635–8645

30. Le Thiet Thanh, Nguyen thi Man, Buu Mat, Phan Ngoc Tran, Nguyen thi Vinh Ha, Morris, GE (1991) Structural relationships between hepatitis B surface antigen in human plasma and dimers of recombinant vaccine: a monoclonal antibody study. Virus Res 21:141–154

31. Molinaro GA, Eby WC (1984) One antigen may form two precipitin lines and two spurs when tested with two monoclonal antibodies by gel diffusion assays. Mol Immunol 21:181–184

32. Johne B, Gadnell M, Hansen K (1993) Epitope mapping and binding kinetics of monoclonal antibodies studied by real time biospecific interaction analysis using surface plasmon resonance. J Immunol Methods 160:191–198

33. Clement G, Boquet D, Frobert Y, Bernard H, Negroni L, Chate JM, Adel-Patient K, Creminon C, Wal JM, Grassi J (2002) Epitopic characterization of native bovine beta-lactoglobulin. J Immunol Methods 266:67–78

34. Fedosov SN, Orning L, Lovli T, Quadros EV, Thompson K, Berglund L, Petersen TE (2005) Mapping the functional domains of human transcobalamin using mono-clonal antibodies. FEBS J 272:3887–3898

35. Alexander H, Alexander S, Getzoff ED, Tainer JA, Geysen HM, Lerner RA (1992) Altering the antigenicity of proteins. Proc Natl Acad Sci USA 89:3352–3356

36. Vidali M, Hidestrand M, Eliasson E, Mottaran E, Reale E, Rolla R, Occhino G, Albano E, Ingelman-Sundberg M (2004) Use of molecular simulation for mapping conformational CYP2E1 epitopes. J Biol Chem 279:50,949–50,955

37. Mengwasser KE, Bush LA, Shih P, Cantwell AM, Di Cera E (2005) Hirudin binding reveals key determinants of thrombin allostery. J Biol Chem 280:26,997–27,003

38. Ikeda M, Hamano K, Shibata T (1992) Epitope mapping of anti-recA protein IgGs by region specified polymerase chain reaction mutagenesis. J Biol Chem 267:6291–6296

39. Paus D, Winter G (2006) Mapping epitopes and antigenicity by site-directed mask-ing. Proc Natl Acad Sci USA 103:9172–9177

40. Wang LF, Hertzog PJ, Galanis M, Overall ML, Waine GJ, Linnane AW (1994) Structure-function analysis of human IFN-alpha-mapping of a conformational epitope by homologue scanning. J Immunol 152:705–715

41. Ping LH, Lemon SM (1992) Antigenic structure of human hepatitis-A virus defined by analysis of escape mutants selected against murine monoclonal antibod-ies. J Virol 66:208–2216

42. Nguyen thi Man, Cartwright AJ, Osborne M, Morris GE (1991) Structural changes in the C-tenninal region of human brain creatine kinase studied with monoclonal antibodies. Biochim Biophys Acta 1076:245–251

43. Burnens A, Demotz S, Corradin G, Binz H, Bosshard HR (1987) Epitope mappIng by differential chemical modification of free and antibody-bound antigen. Science 235:780–783

44. Jemmerson R, Paterson Y (1986) Mapping antigenic sites on a protein antigen by the proteolysis of antigen-antibody complexes. Science 232:1001–1004

45. Zhao Y, Chait BT (1995) Protein epitope mapping by mass spectrometry. Anal Chem 66:3723–3726

46. Baerga-Ortiz A, Hughes CA, Mandell JG, Komives EA (2002) Epitope mapping of a monoclonal antibody against human thrombin by H/D-exchange mass spectrom-etry reveals selection of a diverse sequence in a highly conserved protein. Protein Sci 11:1300–1308

47. Lu J, Witcher DR, White MA, Wang X, Huang L, Rathnachalam R, Beals JM, Kuhstoss S (2005) IL-1 beta epitope mapping using site-directed mutagenesis and hydrogen-deuterium exchange mass spectrometry analysis. Biochemistry 44:11,106–11,114

48. Hager-Braun C, Tomer KB (2005) Determination of protein-derived epitopes by mass spectrometry. Expert Rev Proteomics 2:745–756

49. Mazzoni MR, Malinski JA, Hamm HE (1991) Structural analysis of rod GTP-binding protein, Gt. Limited proteolytic digestion pattern of Gt with four proteases defines monoclonal antibody epitope. J Biol Chem 266:14,072–14,081

50. Ellgaard L, Holtet TL, Moestrup SK, Etzerodt M, Thogersen HC (1995) Nested sets of protein fragments and their use in epitope mapping-characterization of the epitope for the S4D5 monoclonal antibody binding to receptor-associated protein. J Immunol Meth 180:53–61

51. Morris GE (1989) Monoclonal antibody studies of creatine kinase. The ART epitope: evidence for an intermediate in protein folding. Biochem J 257:461–469

52. Morris GE, Nguyen thi Man (1992) Changes at the N-terminus of human brain creatine kinase during a transition between inactive folding intermediate and active enzyme. Biochim Biophys Acta 1120:233–238

53. Morris GE (2003) Epitope Mapping. In: Pound J (ed) Immunochemical protocols 2nd edn. Humana Press, Totowa, NJ, pp. 161–172

54. Stanley KK (1988) Epitope mapping using pEX. Meth Mol Biol 4:351–361

55. Nguyen thi Man, Morris GE (1993) Use of epitope libraries to identify exon-specific monoclonal antibodies for characterization of altered dystrophins in muscular dystrophy. Amer J Hum Genet 52:1057–1066

56. Wang LF, Du Plessis DH, White JR, Hyatt AR, Eaton BT (1995) Use of a gene-targeted phage display random epitope library to map an antigenic determinant on the bluetongue virus outer capsid protein VP5. J Immunol Methods 178:1–12

57. Pereboeva LA, Pereboev AV, Wangm LF, Morris GE (2000) Hepatitis C epitopes from phage-displayed cDNA libraries and improved diagnosis with a chimeric antigen. J Med Virol 60:144–151

58. Di Niro R, Ferrara F, Not T, Bradbury AR, Chirdo F, Marzari R, Sblattero D (2005) Characterizing monoclonal antibody epitopes by filtered gene fragment phage display. Biochem J 388:889–894

59. Lenstra JA, Kusters JG, van der Zeijst BAM (1990) Mapping of viral epitopes with procaryotic expression systems (review). Arch Virol 110:1–24

60. Thanh LT, Nguyen thi Man Hori S, Sewry CA, Dubowitz V, Morris GE (1995) Characterization of genetic deletions in Becker Muscular Dystrophy using monoclonal antibodies against a deletion-prone region of dystrophin. Amer J Med Genet 58:177–186

61. Burch HB, Nagy FV, Kain KC, Lanar DE, Carr FE, Wartofsky L, Burman KD (1993) Expression polymerase chain reaction for the in vitro synthesis and epitope mapping of autoantigen. Application to the human thyrotropin receptor. J Immunol Methods 158:123–130

62. Sedgwick SG, Nguyen thi Man, Ellis JM, Crowne H, Morris GE (1991) Rapid mapping by transposon mutagenesis of epitopes on the muscular dystrophy protein, dystrophin. Nucleic Acids Res 19:5889–5894

63. Wiens GD, Owen J (2005) Mapping of neutralizing epitopes on *Renibacterium salmoninarum* p57 by use of transposon mutagenesis and synthetic peptides. Appl Environ Microbiol 71:2894–2901

64. Friguet B, Fedorov AN, Djavadi-Ohaniance L (1993) In vitro gene expression for the localization of antigenic determinants-application to the *E. coli* tryptophan synthase beta2 subunit. J Immunol Methods 158:243–249

65. Gross CH, Rohrmann GF (1990) Mapping unprocessed epitopes using deletion mutagenesis of gene fusions. Biotechniques 8:196–202

66. Geysen HM, Meleon RH, Barteling SJ (1984) Use of peptide synthesis to probe viral antigens for epitopes to a resolution of a single amino-acid. Proc Natl Acad Sci USA 81:3998–4002

67. He Y, Zhou Y, Siddiqui P, Niu J, Jiang S (2005) Identification of immunodominant epitopes on the membrane protein of the severe acute respiratory syndrome-associated coronavirus. J Clin Microbiol 43:3718–3726

68. Frank R, Kiess M, Lahmann H, Behn CH, Gausepohl H (1995) Combinatorial synthesis on membrane supports by the SPOT technique. In: Maia HLS (ed) Peptides 1994. ESCOM, Leiden, pp. 479–480

69. Werner A, Rohm KH, Muller HJ (2005) Mapping of B-cell epitopes in E. coli asparaginase II, an enzyme used in leukemia treatment. Biol Chem 386:535–540

70. Holmes CP, Adams CL, Kochersperger LM, Mortensen RB, Aldwin LA (1995) The use of light-directed combinatorial peptide synthesis in epitope mapping. Biopolymers 37:199–211

71. Andresen H, Zarse K, Grotzinger C, Hollidt JM, Ehrentreich-Forster E, Bier FF, Kreuzer OJ (2006) Development of peptide microarrays for epitope mapping of antibodies against the human TSH receptor. J Immunol Methods 315:11–18

72. Houghten RA, Pinilla C, Blondelle SE, Appel JR, Dooley CT, Cuervo JH (1991) Generation and use of synthetic peptide combinatorial libraries for basic research and drug discovery. Nature 354:84–86

73. Scott JK, Smith GP (1990) Searching for peptide ligands with an epitope library. Science 249:386–390

74. Manilal S, Randles KN, Aunao C, Nguyen thi Man, Morris GE (2004) A lamin A/C beta-strand containing the site of lipodystrophy mutations is a major surface epitope for a new panel of monoclonal antibodies. Biochim Biophys Acta 1671:87–92

75. Lu Z, Murray KS, van Cleave V, LaVallie ER, Stahl ML, McCoy JM (1995) Expression of thioredoxin random peptide libraries on the Escherichia coli cell surface as functional fusions to flagellin. Bio/technology 13:366–372

76. Morris GE (2005) Epitope mapping. In: Burns R (ed) "Immunochemical protocols", 3rd edn. Humana Press, Totowa, NJ, pp. 255–268

77. Mattheakis LC, Bhatt RR, Dower WJ (1994) An in vitro display system for identifying ligands from very large peptide libraries. Proc Natl Acad Sci USA 91:9022–9026

78. Wilson DS, Keefe AD, Szostak JW (2001) The use of mRNA display to select high-affinity protein-binding peptides. Proc Natl Acad Sci USA 98:3750–3755

79. Ja WW, Olsen BN, Roberts RW (2005) Epitope mapping using mRNA display and a unidirectional nested deletion library. Protein Eng Des Sel 18:309–319

80. Morris GE (ed.) (1996) Methods in molecular biology vol 66: epitope mapping protocols Humana, Totowa, NJ

81. Wang KS, Strauss JH (1991) Use of a lambda gt11 expression library to localize a neutralizing antibody-binding site in glycoprotein-E2 of Sindbis virus. J Virol 65:7037–7040

82. Hijnen M, Mooi FR, van Gageldonk PG, Hoogerhout P, King AJ, Berbers GA (2004) Epitope structure of the Bordetella pertussis protein P.69 pertactin, a major vaccine component and protective antigen. Infect Immun 72:3716–3723

83. Lynch MP, Kaumaya PT (2006) Advances in HTLV-1 peptide vaccines and therapeutics. Curr Protein Pept Sci 7:137–145

84. Albani S, Roudier J (1992) Molecular basis for the association between hla dr4 and rheumatoid arthritis from the shared epitope hypothesis to a peptidic model of rheumatoid arthritis. Clin Biochem 25:209–212

85. Butler MH, Solimena M, Dirkx R, Hayday A, Decamilli P (1993) Identification of a dominant epitope of glutamic acid decarboxylase (GAD-65) recognized by autoantibodies in Stiff-Man syndrome. J Exp Med 178:2097–2106

86. Carson DA (1994) The value of epitope mapping in autoimmune diseases. J Clin Invest 94:1713

87. Frank MB, Itoh K, McCubbin V (1994) Epitope mapping of the 52-kD Ro/SSA autoantigen. Clin Exp Immunol 95:390–396

88. Palace J, Vincent A, Beeson D, Newsom-Davis J (1994) Immunogenicity of human recombinant acetylcholine receptor alpha subunit: cytoplasmic epitopes dominate the antibody response in four mouse strains. Autoimmunity 18:113–119

89. Liu MS, Ma YH, Hayden MR, Brunzell JD (1992) Mapping of the epitope on lipoprotein lipase recognized by a monoclonal antibody (5D2), which inhibits lipase activity. Biochim Biophys Acta 1128:113–115

90. Pietu G, Ribba AS, Cherel G, Meyer D (1992) Epitope mapping by cDNA expression of a monoclonal antibody which inhibits the binding of von Willebrand factor to platelet glycoprotein-1Ib/IIIa. Biochem J 284:711–715

91. Landis RC, Bennett RI, Hogg N (1993) A novel LFA-1 activation epitope maps to the I-domain. J Cell Biol 120:1519–1527

92. Morris CA, Underwood PA, Bean PA, Sheehan M, Charlesworth JA (1994) Relative topography of biologically active domains of human vitronectin – evidence from monoclonal antibody epitope and denaturation studies. J Bioi Chem 269:23,845–23,852

93. Skirgello OE, Balyasnikova IV, Binevski PV, Sun ZL, Baskin II, Palyulin VA, Nesterovitch AB, Albrecht RF 2nd, Kost OA, Danilov SM (2006) Inhibitory antibodies to human angiotensin-converting enzyme: fine epitope mapping and mechanism of action. Biochemistry 45:4831–4847

94. Morris GE, Frost LC, Newport PA, Hudson N (1987) Monoclonal antibody studies of creatine kinase. Antibody-binding sites in the N-terminal region of creatine kinase and effects of antibody on enzyme refolding. Biochem J 248:53–59

95. Syu WJ, Kahan L (1992) Both ends of Escherichia Coli ribosomal protein-S13 are immunochemically accessible in situ. J Protein Chem 11:225–230

96. Ning G, Maunsbach AB, Leo YJ, Moller JV (1993) Topology of Na,K-ATPase alpha subunit epitopes analyzed with oligopeptide-specific antibodies and double-labeling immunoelectron microscopy. FEBS Lett 336:521–524

97. Morris GE, Cartwright AJ (1990) Monoclonal antibody studies suggest a catalytic site at the interface between domains in creatine kinase. Biochim Biophys Acta 1039:318–322

98. Kruger M, Wright J, Wang K (1991) Nebulin as a length regulator of thin filaments of vertebrate skeletal muscles: correlation of thin filament length, nebulin size, and epitope profile. J Cell Biol 115:97–107

99. Morris GE, Simmons C, Nguyen thi Man (1995) Apo-dystrophins (Dp140 and Dp71) and dystrophin splicing isoforms in developing brain. Biochem Biophys Res Commun 215:361–367

100. Carter JM (1994) Epitope prediction methods. In: Dunn BM, Pennington MW (eds) Peptide analysis protocols. Humana, Totowa, NJ, pp 193–206

101. Flower DR (2003) Towards in silico prediction of immunogenic epitopes. Trends Immunol 24:667–674

102. Haste Andersen P, Nielsen M, Lund O (2006) Prediction of residues in discontinuous B-cell epitopes using protein 3D structures. Protein Sci 15:2558–2567

103. Morris GE, Nguyen C, Nguyen thi Man (1995) Specificity and VH sequence of two monoclonal antibodies against the N-terminus of dystrophin. Biochem J 78:355–359

104. Mandal C, Kingery BD, Anchin JM, Subramaniam S, Linthicum DS (1996) ABGEN: a knowledge-based automated approach for antibody structure modelling. Nature Biotechnol 14:323–328

39

Quantum Dots

Charles Z. Hotz

1. Introduction

Quantum dots are fluorescent probes that are in many respects similar to fluorescent dye molecules. Since their first appearance in biology just a few years ago, many new biological methods using them have since been published. Particularly prevalent are imaging applications that benefit from the brightness and stability inherent to quantum dots (QDs). However, many of the properties of quantum dots differ from other fluorescent biological probes, and these differences are outlined in this chapter. In addition, the various types of QD materials currently available are surveyed, as are the variety of biological applications that have been demonstrated.

1.1. Properties of Quantum Dots

Fluorescence detection is based upon the characteristic of fluorescent probes to absorb light of a given wavelength and emit a fraction of that light at another (longer, lower energy) wavelength. Both QDs and traditional fluorescent dye molecules share this characteristic. However, there are several significant differences between how the two entities interact with light. Fluorescent dyes typically absorb light efficiently in a (absorbance) band that is only slightly shifted in wavelength from the band where light is emitted (see **Fig. 39.1A**). Substantial efforts in instrumentation design have been made to maximally collect as much of the light emitted from the dye, while effectively exciting the absorbance band. This is complicated by the fact that the absorbance and emission bands are spectrally close together for dye molecules. This factor can decrease efficiency, and increase instrument cost, particularly when lasers are required for excitation.

Quantum dots, by comparison, absorb light at all wavelengths shorter than their emission wavelength (**Fig. 39.1B**). This allows multiple colors of QDs to be effectively excited by a single source of light (lamp, laser, LED, etc.) that can be spectrally distant from the emission of any color. The effective "Stokes shift," or wavelength difference between maximum absorbance and maximum emission (typically ~15–30 nm for organic dyes), can be hundreds

From: *Molecular Biomethods Handbook, 2nd Edition.*
Edited by: J. M. Walker and R. Rapley © Humana Press, Totowa, NJ

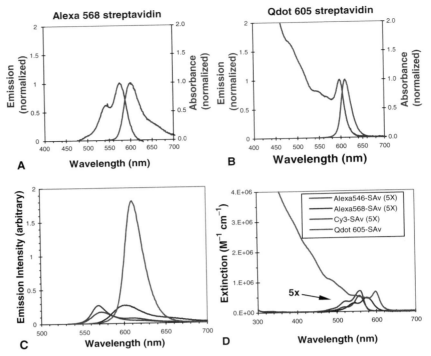

Fig. 39.1. Comparison of the absorbance and emission spectra (normalized) of: (**A**) Alexa® 568 streptavidin conjugate; and (**B**) Qdot®-605 streptavidin conjugate. Note that the quantum dot conjugate can absorb light efficiently far to the blue of the emission. (**C**) Comparison of the emission spectra (nonnormalized) of the streptavidin conjugates of: Qdot® 605 (—), Alexa® 546 (—), Alexa® 568 (—), and Cy3® (—). The spectra were taken under conditions where each fluorophore absorbed the same amount of excitation light. The measured quantum yields of the conjugates were 55%, 8%, 16%, and 11%, respectively. (**D**) Comparison of the absorbance spectra (nonnormalized, each 1 μM of flurophore) of Qdot®-605 streptavidin conjugate (—), Cy3® streptavidin conjugate (—), Alexa® 546 streptavidin conjugate (—), and Alexa® 568 streptavidin conjugate (—). Note that all dye spectra are enhanced 5-fold for clarity. Alexa, Qdot, and Cy3 are registered trademarks of Molecular Probes and GE Biosciences, respectively

of nanometers for a QD, simplifying the design of instrumentation used for detection, and making collection of the emitted light more efficient. In addition, this feature of QDs facilitates multiplexing, the use of more than one fluorescent color simultaneously to generate multiple measurements. Multicolor fluorescence microscopy, for example, which enables the visualization of different cellular structures, particularly benefits from the QDs large separation of absorption and emission wavelengths.

QDs are well-known for their brightness. The primary reason for this feature is that QDs absorb light much more effectively than typical dye molecules. The extinction coefficient (i.e., the measure of light absorbed by a fluorescent material) is much larger for a QD than for typical fluorescent dye (**Fig. 39.1D**). For example, the extinction coefficient for a typical fluorescent dye might be 1 $\times 10^5$, compared to a QD at 2×10^6 – a factor of 20 greater light absorption.

By their nature, QDs exist as polydisperse collections of crystals of slightly different sizes. The emission spectrum of a solution of quantum dots is the average of the spectra of many individual quantum dots that differ slightly in size and emission. Consequently, the width of the observable emission spectrum depends on the uniformity of the quantum dot size distribution. A sample comprised of uniformly sized QDs will have a narrower composite emission spectrum than a sample that is less uniform, although commercially manufactured QDs tend to have consistent and relatively narrow emission spectra from their materials. Typically a QD emission spectrum is nearly Gaussian-shaped, which is in contrast to most fluorescent dyes that display asymmetric emission spectra that tail (sometimes dramatically) to the red (see **Fig. 39.1C**). Typical high-quality quantum dot size distributions result in emission spectrum widths (at half maximum) of 20–3 5 nm, which are noticeably narrower than comparable dyes. These narrow, symmetric, emission spectra make possible detection of multiple colors of QDs together (multiplexing) with low crossover among detection channels.

The quantum yield of a fluorescent material is defined as the ratio of light emitted to light absorbed, and ranges from 0% to 100%. Some organic dyes have quantum yields approaching 100%, but bioconjugates (when coupled to biological affinity molecules) made from these dyes generally have a significantly lower quantum yield. QDs retain their high quantum yield even after conjugation to biological affinity molecules (**Fig. 39.1C**), and are often less effected by environmental conditions than dyes.

A major limitation to dye molecules in many applications is photodestruction. Fluorescent dyes are typically small organic molecules that are steadily bleached (degraded) by the light used to excite them, progressively emitting less light over time. This is owing to chemical modification of the dye molecule, and is irreversible. Although there is a wide range of photostability observed in various fluorescent dye molecules, none approach the stability observed in quantum dots (*1*). Even under conditions of intense illumination (e.g., in a confocal microscope or flow cytometer), little if any degradation is observed. This property makes QDs enabling in applications requiring continuous observation of the probe (cell tracking, some imaging applications, etc.), and potentially more valuable as quantitative reagents.

The length of time required for a fluorescent probe to emit light after absorption is its fluorescence lifetime. Quantum dots have somewhat longer fluorescence lifetimes than typical organic fluorophores (approx 20–40 ns versus <5 ns, respectively) (*2*). This difference can be exploited to reduce autofluorescence background in some measurements, because many sources of background in cellular and other environments are much shorter than QD lifetime. From a practical perspective, a short delay between (short-pulsed) excitation and collection of the emitted light can nearly eliminate autofluorescence of polymeric substrates (or potentially background from other media such as blood) and still allow collection of the majority of the QD emitted light. Additionally, the fluorescence lifetimes of QDs are still much shorter than some long-lived fluorophores, and consequently do not significantly reduce emission at high excitation power owing to saturation.

1.2. Quantum Dot Structure

Quantum dot conjugates are complex, multi-layered structures, and many process steps are required to produce a useful, biological conjugate (**Fig. 39.2**). Some terminology that is used in describing QD structures is:

Core QD – The central QD nanocrystals that determines the optical properties of the final structure. These materials are sensitive to their environment, and not typically fluorescent.

Core/Shell QD – Core nanocrystals that have a crystalline inorganic shell. These materials are brightly fluorescent, and stable.

Water-Soluble QD – Core/Shell QDs that are hydrophilic and are soluble in water and biological buffers. Commercially available water-soluble QDs have a hydrophilic polymer coating.

QD Bioconjugate – A water-soluble QD bound to an affinity molecule.

Quantum dots are not molecules, but rather engineered nanomaterials. Unlike samples of dye molecules where every molecule is in principle identical, each core QD in a sample contains a slightly different number of atoms, and thus can be slightly different in some of the optical properties. Consequently, the methods developed to synthesize QD cores have been optimized to produce quite uniform materials, resulting in narrower emission spectra, as mentioned before *(4,5)*.

Although these "core" QDs determine the optical properties of the conjugate, they are by themselves unsuitable for biological probes owing to their poor stability and quantum yield. It is believed that binding of various molecules to the surface of a core QD results in quenching of the emission. In fact, the quantum yield of QD cores has been reported to be very sensitive to the presence of particular ions in solution *(6)*. Highly luminescent QDs are prepared by coating these core QDs with another material resulting in "core/shell" QDs that are much brighter, and more stable in various chemical and biological environments *(3,7)*. These core-shell QDs are hydrophobic and only organic-soluble as prepared.

A number of methods have been reported to convert these hydrophobic core/shells QDs into aqueous-soluble, biologically useful versions *(4,5,8,9)*.

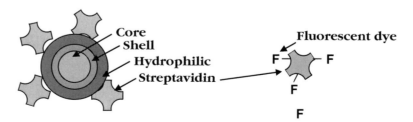

QD Streptavidin Conjugate   **Dye Streptavidin Conjugate**

Fig. 39.2. Schematic of a QD Bioconjugate compared to a typically labeled fluorescent dye protein conjugate (see text for descriptions). Proteins generally carry several fluorescent dye labels (**F**). In contrast, each QD is conjugated to multiple protein molecules

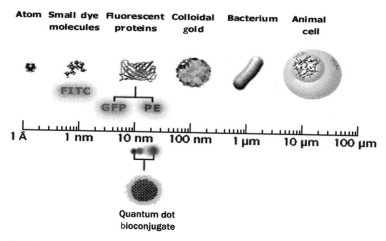

Fig. 39.3. Physical size of quantum dots compared to related entities

Although a comprehensive comparison of these approaches does not exist, significant differences in the stability and brightness, and therefore performance of the resulting aqueous materials do exist. Most commercial preparations of QDs have a hydrophilic polymer coating that confers water-solubility, and provides a functional surface for attachment of biomolecules. High quality, water-soluble quantum dots do not show significant change in peak emission wavelength, or quantum yield, as a function of environment or time.

In addition to the differences in optical properties and size, as outlined above, QDs differ from dye conjugates in another important respect. Quantum dots are polyfunctional with respect to affinity molecules; that is, typically more than one affinity molecule (be it an antibody, protein, oligonucleotide, or small molecule, etc.) can be coupled per single QD, owing to their relatively larger size and greater number of attachment sites. In the case of traditional fluorescent labels, there is generally a one-to-one correspondence of dye to small molecule, and more than one dye molecule per protein or other large molecule (**Fig. 39.2**). In cases where there is an "average" of one affinity molecule to QD, there is typically a distribution of conjugates, some QDs lacking an affinity molecule, and some with more than one.

Quantum dots are described as nanoparticles, and are larger in size than dye molecules. Water-soluble quantum dot conjugates are in the 10–20 nm size range, making them similar in size to large proteins (see **Fig. 39.3**). This size will likely preclude them from certain applications; however, their size does not prevent use in the labeling of cell surfaces, tissue sections, or from accessing intracellular targets in fixed and permeablized cells (see Section 3).

2. Methods

Assuming a laboratory is not equipped or one does not desire preparing quantum dots synthetically, commercial products become the only option for using these materials. Although QD suppliers offer products in a range of colors, the types of available bioconjugates are described below.

2.1. Biotin, Streptavidin, and other Hapten and Hapten-Binding Conjugates

Probably the most general-purpose QD bioconjugate for labeling, streptavidin conjugates are useful when a biotin can be introduced into the system under study. Immunohisto- or cytochemical labeling with biotinylated antibodies allow the use of QD-streptavidin bioconjugates in these applications. Many of the examples in Section 3 of this chapter were carried out with QD-streptavidin bioconjugates. Other hapten-binding antibodies such as anti-DNP, antifluorescein, and anti-GST are also available in various colors. In addition, biotin conjugates are available for instances where one requires a hapten, rather than hapten-binding protein, bound to the QD.

2.2. Antibody Conjugates and Conjugation Kits

A variety of both secondary (antispecies) as well as several primary antibody conjugates are commercially available. These reagents are useful in standard immuno-labeling applications, and are important for multiplex detection; when specific targeting of several antigens is required simultaneously. Also available are antibody conjugation kits, which allow the user to attach their antibodies of interest to any of the available QD colors.

2.3. Transporter-Peptide Bioconjugates

QDs with a short transporter peptide are available for the purpose of live cell labeling. Cells are cultured in the presence of the QD-peptide bioconjugates, which internalize the QDs. The cells continue to grow and divide normally, allowing their use in tracking, motility, proliferation, and related studies. These reagents are available in a number of colors; thus can be used for mixed cell population studies.

2.4. Nontargeted QDs

QDs lacking any attached affinity molecules are also sold. These can be used when it is undesirable to have the QD interact with molecules, surfaces, etc., in its environment. Application examples are diffusion and in vivo circulation studies.

2.5. Reactive QDs

Some users with more experience want the flexibility to make novel bioconjugates from underlying water-soluble QD materials. For these applications, water-soluble QDs in various colors are available with carboxyl- or amine-functional (reactive) surfaces. Using several available conjugation protocols (*10*), one can chemically react materials to these functional groups, forming a covalent bond to the QD. Also available are organic-soluble QDs, however, these find very limited application in biology.

2.6. General Considerations for Selecting QDs for an Application

The discussion in the introduction outlined the considerations for choosing to use QDs as detection reagents: situations requiring photostability, brightness, multiple colors, etc. This section describes the factors that need to be considered when choosing *which* QDs to use for an experiment.

Generally, the first consideration is the detection platform being used. Is a fluorescence microscope being used? If so, one must determine which optical filters are installed, and if they can be used effectively for any colors of available QDs. If not, obtaining appropriate filters may be the first step. Other detection instrumentation may also require optical filters. Assistance in filter selection can be found on any of the optical filter manufacturer websites.

If only one color is being used in the experiment, and sensitivity is required, selection of a redder QD is generally better. This is because the extinction coefficient for QDs is related to the number of atoms in the QD – so the larger the QD (of any given material), the more effectively it will absorb light. Generally redder colors in the 600–660 nm (emission) range are good choices. If particular background issues exist (tissue autofluorescence, etc.), choose colors away from these wavelength ranges.

When multiple colors are being detected together, generally they should be spaced at least 40 nm apart and optical filters need to be selected carefully to avoid cross-talk among detection channels. In certain cases, more than one color can be selected so that they can be viewed simultaneously in a microscope. This involves selection of an excitation filter appropriate for all colors, and a long-pass filter that captures the emission from all colors. Real-time multicolor imaging can be accomplished in this manner.

3. Applications

3.1. Cell and Tissue Imaging

3.1.1. Immunohistochemistry and In-Situ Hybridization

A standard fluorescence microscope is an ideal tool for detection of quantum dot bioconjugates. Lamp-based excitation can be applied through a very wide excitation filter for efficient excitation of the broad QD excitation spectrum. Because the emission spectrum is narrow, a narrow emission filter can be used to maximize signal-to-background. Alternatively, a long pass emission filter can be used to observe several colors simultaneously.

Quantum dots conjugated to immunoglobulin G (IgG) and streptavidin have been used successfully to label the breast cancer marker Her2 on the surface of cancer cells, stain actin and microtubule fibers in the cytoplasm, and detect nuclear antigens (1). Labeling was shown to be specific for intended targets, brighter, and significantly more photostable than comparable organic dyes. A recent study examines formalin-fixed tissue samples using up to 5 QD colors simultaneously, to specifically label targets on the surface, in the cytoplasm, and within the nucleus (11). Osamura and coworkers successfully simultaneously imaged growth hormone protein and its mRNA in a combined IHC/FISH study (12).

3.1.2. Multi-Mode Imaging

The unique combination of properties; that QDs are not only fluorescent, but also electron-dense materials; enables them to be imaged using electron microscopy as well. These attributes allow larger-scale light-microscopic localization of targets, and subsequent high-resolution localization using transmission electron microscopy. Ellisman and coworkers labeled up to three targets in cells or tissues, imaged them using multi-color light microscopy, and subsequently imaged the same samples using electron microscopy. They report the ability to differentiate the various QD labels by size and shape in the electron microscope, effectively multiplexing at this size scale as well *(13)*. It has been reported that QD probes are also "radio-opaque," making them potentially useful to combine with CT scan technology as well *(14)*.

3.1.3. Multiphoton Microscopy

Quantum dots have been shown to be enabling in the area of multiphoton microscopy *(15)*. QD probes are reported to have the largest 2-photon cross-sections (a measure of the ability to absorb light at twice the normal excitation wavelength) of any probe – near the theoretical maximum value. The cross sections are 2–3 orders of magnitude larger than conventional fluorescent probes. Using 2-photon imaging, QDs were intravenously injected into mice and used to dynamically visualize capillaries hundreds of microns deep through scattering media (skin and adipose tissue). The 2-photon technique using QDs has been modeled in the study of receptor-ligand interactions, labeling each with different colors of QDs *(16)*. A recent study uses multicolor 2-photon microscopy to image multiple structures in vascular tissue *(17)*.

3.1.4. Live Cell Imaging

A number of cell lines have been shown to endocytose QDs over a 2–3 h period, and the QDs became localized in endosomes *(18)*. These labeled cells were shown to be stable for as long as 12 d in culture. The investigators also labeled live cells by membrane biotinylation, followed by incubation with QD-avidin conjugate, although this method also resulted in QD endocytosis in the cell lines studied. The authors also used the labeling procedure to study the effect of starvation on aggregation of developing *Dicytostelium discoideum* cells that have been starved for various durations. Cells starved for different durations were labeled with different colored QDs, mixed, and the labeled cells imaged for 2 s intervals, every 2 min for 8 h. They concluded that the cells' propensity to aggregate is an "on-off" phenomenon, not a continuous function of the degree of starvation.

A group has reported the preparation of QDs functionalized with PEG (poly[ethylene glycol]) to study development in *Xenopus* embryos *(19)*. The QDs were microinjected into individual cells of the growing embryo, and because the fluorescence was confined to the progeny of the injected cells, this allowed the embryo development to be studied for many individual cells. The authors further found that the QDs were stable and had no apparent toxicity.

A unique cell motility assay has been reported that involves seeding cells onto a surface that has been previously covered with QDs *(20)*. Upon moving, the cells engulf the QDs, leaving behind a nonfluorescent trail, on an otherwise uniformly fluorescent surface. Using this technique, the investigators were able to quantitate motility, and differentiate between invasive and noninvasive cancer cell lines.

In a powerful demonstration, Jovin and coworkers studied receptor-ligand interactions in real-time by combining EGF-receptor labeling (using visible fluorescent protein) and EGF labeling (using an EGF-QD conjugate) *(21)*. They produced movies demonstrating the binding of EGF to its receptor, the accompanying cell morphological changes, and active trafficking of receptor complex as it is internalized. Through different combinations of receptor labeling (erbB1, erbB2, or erbB3), they were able to determine whether receptor heterodimerization occurred in each case, and also revealed a previously unreported mechanism of retrograde transport.

3.1.5. *Single Molecule Imaging*

The brightness and photostability of QDs make then particularly useful for single-molecule imaging. Few other fluorescent probes can be visualized as single molecules, and none are able to be imaged for sequential images over many minutes. In addition, individual QDs have a "blinking" phenomenon that makes it obvious when a single QD is being imaged. Dahan and coworkers labeled individual glycine receptors on living neuronal cells, and imaged their motion from millisecond to minute time periods *(22)*. The group showed that the receptor diffusion on the cell membrane is influenced by its proximity to a synapse. Capture of the receptor by a synapse was further confirmed by electron microscopic imaging of the QD labeled receptor. The group has compiled their methods for single quantum dot imaging in the cell cytoplasm as well as the membrane *(23)*.

Another group has demonstrated the mechanism of myosin V motion on actin filaments *(24)*. The double-headed protein was differentially labeled with 2 QD colors, and then imaged on surface-bound actin. Successive images revealed that the protein moved in a "hand-over-hand" fashion on the actin filament; each step moving 72 nm.

3.2. Live Animal Imaging

Several reports have appeared using QDs in live animals. Related work is typically accomplished with fluorescent polymers, such as rhodamine green dextran, or with fluorescent proteins (e.g., green fluorescent protein). The lack of photostability and brightness of these reagents limits their utility in longer-duration imaging experiments.

3.2.1. In vivo *Targeting*

Specific targeting of QD-peptide bioconjugates has been carried out in mice *(25)*. Peptides that specifically target lung blood vessel endothelial cells, tumor cell blood vessels, and tumor cell lymphatic vessels were conjugated to QDs and intravenously injected into mice. Specific targeting to the lung and tumor vasculature was observed with the appropriate conjugates, and no acute toxicity was observed after 24 h of circulation. They also observed that the QDs accumulated in the liver and spleen in addition to the targeted tissues, unless the QD was coconjugated with PEG. Although the QD conjugates were specific for the tumor targets, they did not accumulate in the tumor cells, instead remaining in the blood vessel endothelia. The authors speculated as to the possible causes: the size of the QDs, the stability of the particular mercaptoacetic acid-stabilized QD conjugates used, or slow endocytosis into tumor cells.

3.2.2. *Nontargeted* in vivo *Use*

Another group examined the circulation half-lives in vivo of QDs that had various surface modifications *(26)*. They found that the circulation half-life varied from less than 12 min to greater than 70 min depending on the surface modification, which also determined the in vivo localization of the QDs. Long term experiments showed that QDs remain fluorescent after at least 4 mo in vivo.

A collaboration among a group making QDs that emit in the near-infrared (700 nm to greater than 1,000 nm – a wavelength range where light is minimally absorbed by tissue), and a surgical group studying lymph node metastasis has resulted in a new method for mapping lymph nodes *(27)*. Using QDs emitting at over 800 nm along with a real-time overlayed color-near/infrared imaging system, investigators were able to inject QDs at a tumor site, visualize the movement of the QDs within the lymph system until they are trapped owing to their size at the "sentinel" lymph node, making the lymph node location apparent; which is then resected. This technique has been successfully demonstrated in animals as large as pigs. Existing methods for sentinel lymph node identification involve the use of radioactive tracers and colored dyes, which result in poor localization.

3.2.3. In vivo *Toxicity*

The fact that QDs are being used in a number of in vivo studies has raised the question of whether they are toxic to the living organism (or cells) to which they are exposed. Although studies *(28–30)* have attempted to determine the cytotoxicity of QDs in several models, no consistent picture has emerged. One complication is that the studies were carried out on different materials – some (different) commercially available materials, and some laboratory-synthesized. One conclusion is that different surface coatings on QDs have a significant impact on measured toxicity. A recent review of this area points out many of the complications of such studies, as well potential health risks use of these materials could have *(31)*.

3.3. Other Techniques and Applications

3.3.1. *Immunoassays*

The optical properties of quantum dots allow a lower limit of detection than typical fluorescent dyes; as well as assay simplification compared to enzymatic methods of immunoassay detection when used in multiplex format. Immunosorbant assays, where the analyte is present bound to the surface of a plate, are typically detected with enzymatic amplification (ELISA technique). It has been shown that the limit of detection of 605 nm streptavidin conjugate is at least an order of magnitude lower than phycoerythrin-streptavidin conjugate when used in a microplate reader using 250 nm excitation for the QD *(32)*. The use of direct fluorescent detection (as opposed to enzymatic amplification) also allows multiplexed detection without sequential wash and amplification steps.

Several groups have developed immunoassays for pathogens and explosives using QD conjugates *(33–36)* 34 Systematic efforts have resulted in a well-characterized system of producing conjugates as well as measurement of their performance in assays. The sensitivity of these demonstrations is well beyond what can be achieved with dye detection, and up to four simultaneous pathogen determinations have been made. Detection of a single pathogenic bacterium has also been demonstrated *(37)*.

3.3.2. *Western Blotting*

Detection and quantification of proteins is commonly achieved by Western blotting. This is typically accomplished by probing the blot with an antibody to the protein of interest, and detecting the protein via a fluorescent dye linked to the antibody, or more often using a chemiluminescent substrate for increased sensitivity. There are a number of practical complications; fluorescent dyes are not very sensitive, and chemiluminescence makes detecting multiple proteins time-consuming and tedious. When multiple proteins need to be detected and quantified—particularly if the protein bands are overlapping (often this is the case in cell signaling studies where the only difference is the result of protein phosphorylation), the use of quantum dots for detection allows quantifying comigrating bands with the sensitivity of chemiluminescent detection. A study demonstrated multiplex protein detection with QDs and compared the sensitivity to dye-based detection *(38)*.

3.3.3. Flow Cytometry

There have been a number of reports of the use of QDs in flow cytometry *(39–42)*. It would seem that QDs would be the ideal fluorophore for flow cytometry: Narrow emission spectra make the use of many colors possible; one laser excitation is possible owing to the broad QD excitation; as well as their bright emission. Indeed, one group reports the combined use of QDs and dyes to perform T-cell immunophenotyping resolving 17 fluorescence emissions *(43)*.

3.3.4. Fluorescence Resonance Energy Transfer

Fluorescence resonance energy transfer (FRET) is a process that typically involves 1 dye molecule capturing the excited-state energy from another dye molecule, owing to the close proximity of the two molecules. This has been exploited for two purposes: Moving the dye emission further (spectrally) from where it is excited, and using the presence or absence of FRET to determine the proximity of two dye molecules. For the first purpose, QDs already have a very large spectral separation between excitation and emission, and thus transferring the emission to another entity is not particularly beneficial. FRET with QDs is further complicated by the fact that it is difficult to selectively excite one QD in the presence of another, owing to their broad excitation spectra. With regard to using FRET in determining proximity, QDs have been shown to be useful. Coupling an antigen to cadmium telluride QDs and the corresponding antibody to a rhodamine dye, it was shown that formation of the immunocomplex resulted in dye emission upon QD excitation *(44)*. In another report, QD-dye FRET was exploited by creating a complex in which a dye and a QD were coupled via a cleavable linker. In the case of protease detection, the linker was a designed to be cleaved by a particular protease; separating the FRET pair, and allowing the uncoupled dye or QD to be detected *(45)*.

3.3.5. Array Detection

There have been several reports of the use of QDs in array detection. PEGylated QDs were shown to be useful in detection of cell lysates in protein microarrays *(46)*. Additionally, four QD colors were used simultaneously in a DNA microarray, for the purpose of multiplexed genotyping *(47)*.

3.3.6. Neuroscience Applications

A number of reports have emerged demonstrating the utility of quantum dots in a variety of neuroscience applications. Santra and coworkers used TAT-peptide conjugated QDs for imaging rat brain *(48)*. The QDs linked to the cell-penetrating peptide were intra-arterially injected, and were found to efficiently label brain tissue without manipulation of the blood-brain barrier. The QD conjugate was observed to migrate beyond the endothelial cells, and reach the brain parenchyma. Another study has been published that used the observed diffusion of QDs to estimate the dimensions of the extracellular space of the brain, which had not previously been determined in living tissue *(49)*. The authors determined the extracellular space to be at least 2-fold larger than determinations made from fixed tissue. A recent publication emphasizes the importance of QD probes as new tools in neuroscience research *(50)*. Conjugates of neurotransmitters to QDs, including serotonin, have been made and used as probes for their transporters *(51)*. In one investigation, the investigators coupled approx 160 serotonin molecules per QD via a short linker, and characterized these probes by their interaction with serotonin transporters, electrophysiologic measurements, as well as fluorescence imaging. Although results for these initial conjugates show somewhat lower selectivity than high-affinity antagonists, they do show utility in the imaging of membrane proteins in living cells.

References

1. Wu X, Liu H, Liu J, Haley KN, Treadway IA, Larson JP, Ge N, Peale F, Bruchez MP (2003) Immunofluorescent labeling of cancer marker Her2 and other cellular targets with semiconductor quantum dots. Nature Biotech 21:41–46
2. Dahan M, Laurence T, Pinaud F, Chemia DS, Alivasatos AP, Sauer M, Weiss S (2001) Time-Gated Biological Imaging by use of Colloidal Quantum Dots. Opt Lett 26:825–827
3. Quantum Dot Corporation, unpublished results
4. Qu L, Peng ZA, Peng X (2001) Alternative Routes toward High Quality CdSe Nanocrystals. Nano Lett 1:333–337
5. Peng ZA, Peng X (2002) Nearly Monodisperse and shape-controlled CdSe nanocrystals via alternative routes: nucleation and growth. J Amer Chem Soc 124:3343–3353
6. Chen Y, Rosenzweig Z (2002) Luminescent CdS Quantum Dots as Selective Ion Probes. Anal Chem 74:5132–5138
7. Dabboussi BO, Rodriguez-Viejo J, Mikulec FV, Heino JR, Mattoussi H, Ober R, Jensen KF, Bawendi MG (1997) (CdSe)ZnS core-shell quantum dots: synthesis and characterization of a size series of highly luminescent nanocrystallites. J Phys Chem B 101:9463–9475
8. Mattoussi H, Mauro JM, Goldman ER, Anderson GP, Sundar V, Mikulec FV, Bawendi MG (2000) Self-assembly of CdSe-ZnS quantum dot bioconjugates using an engineered recombinant protein. J Amer Chem Soc 122:12,142–12,150
9. Potapova I, Mruk R, Prehl S, Zentel R, Basche T, Mews A (2002) Semiconductor nanocrystals with multifunctional polymer ligands. J Amer Chem Soc 125:320, 321
10. Invitrogen Corp. website. http://probes.invitrogen.com/products/qdot/reactive.html
11. Fountaine TJ, Wincovitch SM, Geho DH, Garfield SH, Pittaluga S (2006) Multispectral imaging of clinically relevant cellular targets in tonsil and lymphoid tissue using semiconductor quantum dots. Mod Pathol 19:1181–1191
12. Matsuno A, Itoh J, Takekoshi S, Nagashima T, Osamura RY (2005) Three-dimensional imaging of the intracellular localization of growth hormone and prolactin and their mRNA using nanocrystal (Quantum dot) and confocal laser scanning microscopy techniques. J Histochem Cytochem 53:833–838
13. Giepmans BN, Deerinck TJ, Smarr BL, Jones YZ, Ellisman MH (2005) Correlated light and electron microscopic imaging of multiple endogenous proteins using Quantum dots. Nat Methods 2:743–749
14. Santra S, Yang H, Holloway PH, Stanley JT, Mericle RA (2005) Synthesis of water-dispersible fluorescent, radio-opaque, and paramagnetic CdS:Mn/ZnS quantum dots: a multifunctional probe for bioimaging. J Amer Chem Soc 127:1656–1657

15. Larson DR, Zipfel WR, Williams RM, Clark SW, Bruchez MP, Wise FW, Webb WW (2003) Water-soluble quantum dots with large two-photon cross-sections for multiphoton fluorescence imaging in vivo. Science 300:1434–1436

16. Swift JL, Heuff R, Cramb DT (2006) A two-photon excitation fluorescence cross-correlation assay for a model ligand-receptor binding system using quantum dots. Biophys J 90:1396–1410

17. Ferrara DE, Weiss D, Carnell PH, Vito RP, Vega D, Gao X, Nie S, Taylor WR (2006) Quantitative 3D fluorescence technique for the analysis of en face preparations of arterial walls using quantum dot nanocrystals and two-photon excitation laser scanning microscopy. Am J Physiol Regul Integr Comp Physiol 290:R114–123

18. Jaiswal JK, Mattoussi H, Mauro JM, Simon SM (2003) Long-term multiple color imaging of live cells using quantum dot bioconjugates. Nature Biotech 21:47–51

19. Dubertret B, Skourides P, Norris DJ, Noireaux V, Brivanlou AH, Libchaber A (2002) Science 298:1759–1762

20. Gu W, Pellegrino T, Parak WJ, Boudreau R, Le Gros MA, Gerion D, Alivisatos AP, Larabell CA (2005) Quantum dot-based cell motility assay. Science STKE:15

21. Lidke DS, Nagy P, Heintzmann R, Arndt-Jovin DJ, Post JN, Grecco HE, Jares-Erijman EA, Jovin TM (2004) Quantum dot ligands provide new insights into erbB/HER receptor-mediated signal transduction. Nat Biotechnol 22:198–203

22. Dahan M, Levi S, Luccardini C, Rostaing P, Riveau B, Triller A (2003) Diffusion dynamics of glycine receptors revealed by single-quantum dot tracking. Science 302:442–445

23. Courty S, Bouzigues C, Luccardini C, Ehrensperger MV, Bonneau S, Dahan M (2006) Tracking individual proteins in living cells using single quantum dot imaging. Methods Enzymol 414:211–228

24. Warshaw DM, Kennedy GG, Work SS, Krementsova EB, Beck S, Trybus KM (2005) Differential labeling of myosin V heads with quantum dots allows direct visualization of hand-over-hand processivity. Biophys J 88:L30–32

25. Akerman ME, Chan WCW, Laakkonen P, Bhatia SN, Ruoslahti E (2002) Nanocrystal targeting in vivo. Proc Nat Acad Sci 99:12,617–12,621

26. Ballou B, Lagerholm BC, Ernst LA, Bruchez MP, Waggoner AS (2004) Noninvasive imaging of quantum dots in mice. Bioconjug Chem 15:79–86

27. Soltesz EG, Kim S, Laurence RG, DeGrand AM, Parungo CP, Dor DM, Cohn LH, Bawendi MG, Frangioni JV, Mihaljevic T (2005) Intraoperative sentinel lymph node mapping of the lung using near-infrared fluorescent quantum dots. Ann Thorac Surg 79:269–277

28. Lovric J, Bazzi HS, Cuie Y, Fortin GR, Winnik FM, Maysinger D (2005) Differences in subcellular distribution and toxicity of green and red emitting CdTe quantum dots. J Mol Med 83:377–385

29. Shiohara A, Hoshino A, Hanaki K, Suzuki K, Yamamoto K (2004) On the cytotoxicity caused by quantum dots. Microbiol Immunol 48:669–675

30. Ryman-Rasmussen, JP, Riviere, JE, Monteiro-Riviere, NA (2007) Surface coatings determine cytotoxicity and irritation potential of quantum dot nanoparticles in epidermal keratinocytes. J Invest Dermatol 127(1):143–153

31. Hardman R (2006) A toxicologic review of quantum dots: toxicity depends on physicochemical and environmental factors. Environ Health Perspect 114:165–172

32. Quantum Dot Corporation, unpublished results

33. Goldman ER, Balighian ED, Mattoussi H, Kuno MK, Mauro JM, Tran PT, Anderson GP (2002) Avidin: a natural bridge for quantum dot-antibody conjugates. J Amer Chem Soc 124:6378–6382

34. Tully E, Hearty S, Leonard P, O'Kennedy R (2006) The development of rapid fluorescence-based immunoassays, using quantum dot-labelled antibodies for the detection of Listeria monocytogenes cell surface proteins. Int J Biol Macromol 39:127–134

35. Goldman ER, Clapp AR, Anderson GP, Uyeda HT, Mauro JM, Medintz IL, Mattoussi H (2004) Multiplexed toxin analysis using four colors of quantum dot fluororeagents. Anal Chem 76:684–688

36. Yang L, Li Y (2006) Simultaneous detection of Escherichia coli O157:H7 and Salmonella Typhimurium using quantum dots as fluorescence labels. Analyst 131(3):394–401

37. Hahn MA, Tabb JS, Krauss TD (2005) Detection of single bacterial pathogens with semiconductor quantum dots. Anal Chem 77:4861–4869

38. Makrides SC, Gasbarro C, Bello JM (2005) Bioconjugation of quantum dot luminescent probes for Western blot analysis. Biotechniques 39:501–506

39. Kahn E, Vejux A, Menetrier F, Maiza C, Hammann A, Sequeira-Le Grand A, Frouin F, Tourneur Y, Brau F, Riedinger JM, Steinmetz E, Todd-Pokropek A, Lizard G (2006) Analysis of CD36 expression on human monocytic cells and atherosclerotic tissue sections with quantum dots: investigation by flow cytometry and spectral imaging microscopy. Anal Quant Cytol Histol 28:14–26

40. Bocsi J, Lenz D, Mittag A, Varga VS, Molnar B, Tulassay Z, Sack U, Tarnok A (2006) Automated four-color analysis of leukocytes by scanning fluorescence microscopy using quantum dots. Cytometry A 69(3):131–134

41. Chattopadhyay PK, Roederer M (2006) Application of quantum dots to multicolor flow cytometry. In: Walker JM (ed) Methods in molecular biology vol 374: quantum dots: applications in biology. Humana, Totowa, NJ, pp. 175–184

42. Abrams B, Dubrovsky T (2006) Quantum dots in flow cytometry. In: Walker JM (ed) Methods in molecular biology vol 374: quantum dots: applications in biology. Humana, Totowa, NJ, pp. 185–204

43. Chattopadhyay PK, Price DA, Harper TF, Betts MR, Yu J, Gostick E, Perfetto SP, Goepfert P, Koup RA, De Rosa SC, Bruchez MP, Roederer M (2006) Quantum dot semiconductor nanocrystals for immunophenotyping by polychromatic flow cytometry. Nat Med 12:972–977

44. Chen Q, Ma Q, Wan Y, Su X, Lin Z, Jin Q (2005) Studies on fluorescence resonance energy transfer between dyes and water-soluble quantum dots. Luminescence 20:251–255

45. Medintz IL, Clapp AR, Brunel FM, Tiefenbrunn T, Uyeda HT, Chang EL, Deschamps JR, Dawson PE, Mattoussi H (2006) Proteolytic activity monitored by fluorescence resonance energy transfer through quantum-dot-peptide conjugates. Nat Mater 5(7):581–589

46. Geho D, Lahar N, Gurnani P, Huebschman M, Herrmann P, Espina V, Shi A, Wulfkuhle J, Garner H, Petricoin E 3rd, Liotta LA, Rosenblatt KP (2005) Pegylated, steptavidin-conjugated quantum dots are effective detection elements for reverse-phase protein microarrays. Bioconjug Chem 16:559–566

47. Karlin-Neumann G, Sedova M, Falkowski M, Wang Z, Lin S, Jain M (2006) Application of Quantum dots to multi-color microarray experiments: four color genotyping. In: Walker JM (ed) Methods in molecular biology vol 374: quantum dots: applications in biology. Humana, Totowa, NJ, pp. 239–252

48. Santra S, Yang H, Stanley JT, Holloway PH, Moudgil BM, Walter G, Mericle RA (2005) Rapid and effective labeling of brain tissue using TAT-conjugated CdS: Mn/ZnS quantum dots. Chem Commun 25:3144–3146

49. Thorne RG, Nicholson G (2006) In vivo diffusion analysis with quantum dots and dextrans predicts the width of brain extracellular space. Proc Natl Acad Sci USA 103:5567–5572

50. Pathak S, Cao E, Davidson MC, Jin S, Silva GA (2006) Quantum dot applications to neuroscience: new tools for probing neurons and glia. J Neurosci 26:1893–1895

51. Rosenthal SJ, Tomlinson I, Adkins EM, Schroeter S, Adams S, Swafford L, McBride J, Wang Y, DeFelice LJ, Blakely RD (2002) Targeting cell surface receptors with ligand-conjugated nanocrystals. J Amer Chem Soc 124:4586–4594

40

Ion-Exchange Chromatography

David Sheehan

1. Introduction

Proteins contain charged groups on their surfaces that enhance their interactions with solvent water and hence their solubility. Charged residues can be cationic (positively charged, e.g., lysine) or anionic (negatively charged, e.g., aspartate) and it is noteworthy that even polar residues can also be charged under certain pH conditions. These charged and polar groups are responsible for maintaining the protein in solution at physiological pH. Because proteins have unique amino acid sequences, the net charge on a protein at physiological pH is determined ultimately by the balance between these charges (i.e., negatively charged proteins possess more negatively charged residues than positively charged groups). This also underlies differing isoelectric points (pIs) of proteins. Ion-exchange chromatography (*1*) separates proteins first on the basis of their charge type and, second, on the basis of relative charge strength (e.g., strongly anionic from weakly anionic).

The basis of ion-exchange chromatography (**Fig. 40.1**) is that charged ions can freely exchange with ions of the same type. In this context, the mass of the ion is irrelevant. Therefore it is possible for a bulky anion like a negatively charged protein to exchange with chloride ions. This process can be later reversed by washing with chloride ions in the form of a NaCl or KCl solution. Such washing removes weakly bound proteins first, followed by more strongly bound proteins with greater net negative charge.

Like most column chromatography techniques, ion-exchange chromatography requires a stationary phase, which is usually composed of insoluble, hydrated polymers, such as cellulose, dextran or Sephadex (*2*). The ion exchange group is immobilized on this stationary phase, and some of the chemical structures of commonly used groups are shown in **Table 40.1**.

In this chapter, the use of microgranular diethylaminoethyl (DEAE) cellulose manufactured by Whatman (Maidstone, UK) is described. As described in Section 3.5, novel formats for ion-exchange chromatography are provided by the immobilization of ion-exchange groups on membrane or filter formats (*3*) and in perfusion chromatography (*4*). The separations can be performed in low pressure or high pressure systems (e.g., FPLC).

From: *Molecular Biomethods Handbook, 2nd Edition.*
Edited by: J. M. Walker and R. Rapley © Humana Press, Totowa, NJ

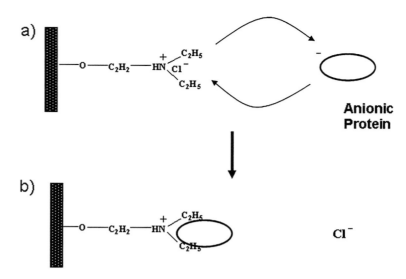

Fig. 40.1. DEAE-cellulose chromatography. a) Anionic (negatively charged) proteins exchange with chloride ions. b) The protein binds electrostatically to the positively charged DEAE group. Washing with a gradient of KCl reverses this process to elute the protein. Proteins generally differ in the precise strength of electrostatic interaction and hence elute at differing chloride ion concentration

Table 40.1. Selected ion exchange groups commonly used in isolation of proteins.

Group	Chemical Structure	pH range
Cation exchangers		
S (methyl sulphonate)	$-\overset{H_2}{C}-SO_3^-$	2–12
SP (sulphopropyl)	$-(CH_2)_2-\overset{H_2}{C}-SO_3^-$	2–12
CM (carboxymethyl)	$-O-\overset{H_2}{C}-COO^-$	6–11
Anion exchangers		
QAE (quaternary aminoethyl)	$-O-(CH_2)_2-\overset{+}{N}-\overset{C_2H_5}{\underset{C_2H_5}{|}}-\overset{}{\underset{H_2}{C}}-CHOH-CH_3$	2–12
Q (quaternary ammonium)	$-\overset{H_2}{C}-\overset{+}{N}\overset{CH_3}{\underset{CH_3}{\overset{|}{<}}}-CH_3$	2–12
DEAE (diethylamino ethyl)	$-O-(CH_2)_2-\overset{+}{N}H\overset{C_2H_5}{\underset{C_2H_5}{<}}$	2–9

2. Methods

2.1. Materials

2.1.1. Buffers

Buffers used will depend on the characteristics of the protein of interest. For proteins not previously purified by DEAE-cellulose chromatography, buffer selection may be helped if the pI of the protein of interest is known. In general, proteins bind to anion exchangers at pH values above their pIs, while binding to cation exchangers, such as CM-cellulose, at pH values below their pIs. Phosphate, Tris, and other common buffers are used in ion-exchange chromatography at concentrations of approx 10–50 mM. Urea (desalted on a mixed bed column of Dowex or else of molecular biology grade) may be included in buffers at concentrations of up to 8 M if separation of denatured samples is required. Care should be taken that the urea does not precipitate in the column during chromatography (especially at lower temperatures). Buffers are prepared fresh before use, and all reagents are of Analar grade. Deionized/distilled water is used.

2.1.2. Resins

Use of microgranular DEAE-cellulose 52 is described in this chapter. Desalting resins, such as sephadex G-25 (Pharmacia), are also useful as it is important that small anions like Cl– do not compete with anionic proteins.

2.1.3. Apparatus

A sintered-glass funnel (no. 1 sinter) is useful for washing resin during equilibration and regeneration. This is usually connected to water suction. For desalting and ion-exchange chromatography, sintered-glass columns are required. Smaller columns could be used for smaller volumes. A gradient-maker (2 × 500 mL) is used to generate salt gradients. A calibrated conductivity meter is also required.

2.2. DEAE Cellulose Chromatography

2.2.1. Sample Preparation

Protein samples require desalting before being applied to the ion-exchange column. This may be achieved by overnight dialysis, by gel filtration on Sephadex G-25 or by desalting of small volumes on PD10 columns (Amersham Biosciences, Uppsala, Sweden) or in centrifugal concentrators (by repeated dilution/filtration) (5).

2.2.2. Resin Equilibration

Before use, resin is washed in water followed by removal of fines achieved by repeatedly stirring the resin with a glass rod, allowing the bulk of the resin to settle, and then aspirating the supernatant. Defined resin is washed 3 times in concentrated buffer (e.g., 200 mM Tris-HCl, pH 8.0) to achieve equilibration. It is gently stirred into slurry, and transferred into a sintered-glass column containing a small volume of water. After settling, the resin is equilibrated with dilute buffer (e.g., 10 mM Tris-HCl, pH 8.0), which is passed through the column until it is completely equilibrated as determined by measuring the pH and conductivity of buffer and column eluate (when these are the same, the column is equilibrated).

2.2.3. Chromatography

Desalted sample is applied to the equilibrated resin, and the effluent is collected. This should be assayed in case the protein of interest has not bound. In cases where a particular protein has not been purified by this method, it may be necessary to develop a new purification procedure for it. The main variables to investigate are choice of ion exchange group, pH, salt concentration, and gradient steepness. In general, approx. 70% of rat-liver cytosolic proteins will bind to DEAE-cellulose at pH 7.5. If the protein of interest has an alkaline pI, then passage through such a column at this pH might be a useful first step in the purification. Conversely, if the protein of interest binds to DEAE-cellulose at pH 7.5, then it is worth repeating the experiment at increasingly higher pH values (e.g., 8.5 and 9.5). Only highly acidic proteins will bind to DEAE-cellulose at pH 10. The column is developed by applying a suitable salt gradient (2 × 500 mL), for example, 0–100 mM NaCl in 10 mM Tris-HCl, pH 8.0 (buffers B and C, aforementioned). Fractions are collected in a fraction collector and assayed for the protein of interest, protein concentration (**6**), and conductivity. The conductivity meter should be carefully calibrated (Note: This property is temperature-dependent), so that conductivity measurements may be expressed as NaCl concentrations, thus facilitating determination of chromatogram reproducibility. These measurements may also be made continuously using on-line UV and conductivity detectors connected to a PC or chart recorder. Appropriate fractions are pooled and concentrated for further study or purification. This is a major factor in the success of the chromatography. In general, fractions should not be pooled in a new purification until sodium dodecyl sulphate-polyacrylamide gel electrophoresis (SDS-PAGE) analysis (**7**) has been carried out on aliquots taken from active fractions. This gives a good indication of fraction purity. It is best to accept some losses of the protein of interest if this means removing significant contaminants. Carrying out the chromatography at different pH values (see previous discussion) usually gives quite different chromatograms, which is often useful for displacing contaminant peaks.

Although shallower gradients (e.g., 0–100, 300–400 mM) generally give better resolution, steeper gradients (e.g., 0–1 M) can be used in initial experiments to identify elution positions of proteins of interest. It is also possible to use stepwise washes (e.g., 100 mM NaCl followed by 200 mM NaCl) rather than continuous gradients. The best approach to developing a new purification procedure, therefore, is to assess the binding (i.e., binding versus nonbinding) of the protein of interest on a small scale on differing ion exchangers at a range of pH values in the alkaline and acidic pH ranges, respectively. Chromatograms where the protein has bound are then developed with a steep gradient. Finally, shallower gradients are assessed at the most promising pH values. It is also possible to use nonlinear gradients for more difficult separations. Lastly, inclusion of "displacer" molecules (i.e., small molecular species that alter the precise retention of individual proteins) can separate proteins that are co-eluting (**1**).

3. Applications

3.1. Separation of Peptides

Because ion-exchange chromatography does not distinguish between large and small ions, it has found uses in separation of peptides in a wide variety of contexts. More usually today, this is performed in a HPLC or capillary electrophoresis format but there are occasions when preparative scale ion exchange is required *(8)*. Naturally occurring bioactive peptides are of major pharmaceutical interest. A thyrotropin-releasing hormone (TRH)-like peptide was successfully isolated from rat thyroid extracts on DEAE-sephadex and shown to be identical to Glu-Glu-Pro, an acidic peptide. Interestingly, a related peptide, Glu-Phe-Pro, did not bind to the anion exchanger because it is neutral and a family of such neutral peptides have now been found to be widespread across mammals based on their behaviour on ion exchange *(9)*. Ion-exchange chromatography is also useful in separating peptides generated by cleavage of purified proteins with agents such as trypsin or CNBr. Separation is performed in the presence of high concentrations of urea (see Section 2.1.1). Urea is a chaotropic agent, which itself has no net charge and thus does not affect the charges on each peptide in the mixture while nonetheless conferring denaturing conditions.

3.2. Separation of Proteins

The overwhelming bulk of ion-exchange chromatography applications involve separation of proteins. This has recently been expertly reviewed *(8)* but some examples of recent applications of DEAE-based anion-exchange purifications are listed in **Table 40.2**. These examples illustrate how DEAE-chromatography is often combined with other ion exchange steps and with affinity chromatography to achieve complete purity in a wide range of biological systems and a wide variety of protein classes. Smilaxin, a protein with anti-HIV properties was essentially purified by DEAE-cellulose chromatography at pH 7.4 but also bound to CM-cellulose at pH 4.6 *(10)*. This illustrates how protein charge characteristics can vary with pH (see Section 2.3.3). A recent purification of a lipase from scorpion showed how DEAE-cellulose can be useful in contributing to purification because the majority of proteins bound to it whereas lipase did not *(11)*. The lipase was further purified by CM-sephadex cation exchange chromatography. A third example is offered by *Leishmania tarentolae* tubulin, which was purified on DEAE-sephadex at pH 6.9 *(12)*. *L. tarentolae* is a non-pathogenic relative of *Leishmania amazonensis* and its tubulin is thought to be suitable for antileishmanial drug screening because its properties are so similar to that of *L. amazonensis*. Lastly, fish (the grass carp, *Ctenopharyngodon idellus*) major histocompatability complex 1 and β-2 microglobulin proteins were purified as recombinant maltose binding protein fusions on DEAE-sepharose *(13)*. After digestion with protease factor Xa, the maltose binding protein moiety was released from the fusions and the proteins of interest were again recovered on DEAE-sephadex.

Table 40.2. Selected examples of use of cation exchange chromatography in isolation of proteins.

Protein	Source	Function	Conditions	Ref.
Smilaxin	*Smilax glabra*	Anti-HIV	pH 7.4	10
Lipase	Scorpion	Enzyme	Protein passed through DEAE	11
Tubulin	*Leishmania tarentolae*	Cytoskeleton	pH 6.7	12
MHC 1	*Ctenopharyngodon idellus*	Immune system	pH 8.0	13

3.3. Applications in Proteomics

Proteomics attempts to study the total complement of proteins expressed in a biological system under any given set of conditions. As such it is a highly dynamic quantity with the potential to offer insights to processes such as the cell cycle, compartmentalization and protein up/down regulation. The most popular proteomics techniques are 2-dimensional electrophoresis (2D SDS PAGE) and various forms of mass spectrometry. However, these techniques can be overcome by the large number of proteins present in even a simple cell. Thus, there is interest in simplifying the proteome by use of procedures to separate sub-proteomes and thus to analyse a smaller number of proteins. Popular approaches include affinity selection based on biospecific recognition and organelle proteomics. Because the mobility of proteins in the isoelectric focusing (IEF) dimension of 2D SDS PAGE is strongly influenced by their net charge, it is possible to select subproteomes by anion or cation exchange based on binding to centrifugal adsorbing units before electrophoresis *(14)*. This has been demonstrated to improve resolution in 2D SDS PAGE. Ion exchange also plays a role in 2-dimensional liquid chromatography where proteins separated by ion-exchange in the first dimension are passed to a second dimension (usually reversed phase or capillary electrophoresis) for further separation. Peaks eluting from the second dimension may be passed on-line to a suitable mass spectrometry analysis *(15)*.

3.4. Downstream Processing of Proteins in Biotechnology

Developments in molecular genetics and genome sequencing have led to increased interest in proteins both as drugs and as targets for drugs. The biological pharmaceutical (BioPharma) sector is now a large and growing aspect of the biotechnology industry *(16)*. A major activity in this sector is purification of valuable proteins by downstream processing of biologically based expression systems in a "good manufacturing environment" (GMP) *(8)*. In comparison with more traditional purification of small molecule pharmaceuticals, the sensitivity of proteins to extremes of pH, temperature, proteolysis and oxidation place particular constraints on the purification protocol used. Many protein purification protocols feature DEAE-cellulose anion exchange chromatography. It is possible to scale up purification from the laboratory scale (e.g., 100 mL resin) to the pilot and production scale by changing the radius of the gel bed. Commercially available arrays of such columns are available where many columns are "stacked" on top of each other allowing gel bed volumes of hundreds of litres and thus industrial-scale binding capacity. Use of a small bed height allows reproduction of laboratory scale separations without undue compression of the gel bed owing to hydrostatic pressure. Another column format is radial flow chromatography where sample is introduced in the centre of the gel bed and flows across rather than down the column. Because of their cheapness, high capacity and desirable flow characteristics, cellulose-based exchange resins continue to be very popular in downstream processing *(8)*.

3.5. Novel Chromatographic Formats

DEAE-cellulose anion exchange chromatography in gel columns has been emphasized in this chapter. However, a variety of other formats for chromatography have been developed, which still depend on ion exchange groups. Membrane-based methods are based on immobilization of anion exchange groups on membranes rather than on hydrated gels thus allowing high flow rates with no loss of resolution *(3)*. Perfusion chromatography uses packings with large "through-pores" or perfusive pores that also allow high flow rates without loss of resolution *(4)*.

Acknowledgements: Work in our laboratory is supported by the Irish Research Council for Science Engineering and Technology, Programme for Research in Third Level Institutions and the Health Research Board of Ireland.

References

1. Ahrer K, Jungbaeur A (2006) Chromatographic and electrophoretic characterization of molecular variants. J Chromatog B 841:110–122
2. Himmelhoch SR (1971) Ion-exchange chromatography. Methods Enzymol 22: 273–290
3. Charcosset C (2006) Membrane processes in biotechnology: an overview. Biotechnology Advances 24:482–492
4. Regnier F (1991) Perfusion chromatography. Nature 350:634, 635
5. Pohl T (1990) Concentration of proteins and removal of solutes. Methods Enzymol 182:68–83
6. Bradford MM (1976) A rapid and sensitive method for the quantitation of microgram quantities of protein utilizing the principle of protein dye binding. Anal Biochem 72:248–254
7. Laemmli UK (1970) Cleavage of structural proteins during the assembly of the head of bacteriophage T4. Nature 227:680–685
8. Levison PR (2003) Large-scale ion exchange column chromatography of proteins: Comparison of different formats. J Chromatog A 790:17–33
9. Ghilchik MW, Tobaruela M, Del Rio-Garcia J, Smyth DG (2000) Characterization of neutral TRH-like peptides in mammary gland, mammary tumours and milk. Biochim Biophys Acta 1475:55–60
10. Chu KT, Ng TB (2006) Smilaxin, a novel protein with immunostimulating, antiproliferative and HIV-1 reverse transcriptase inhibiting activities from fresh *Smilax glabra* rhizomes. Biochem Biophys Res Commun 340:118–124
11. Zouari N, Miled N, Cherif S, Mejdoub H, Gargouri Y (2005) Purification and characterization of a novel lipase from the digestive glands of a primitive animal: the scorpion. Biochim Biophys Acta 1726:67–74
12. Yakovich AJ, Ragone FL, Alfonzo JD, Sackett DL, Werbovetz KA (2006) *Leishmania tarentolae*: Purification and characterization of tubulin and its suitability for antileishmanial drug screening. Exp Parasitol 114:289–296
13. Hao HF, Li XS, Gao FS, Wu WX, Xia C (2006) Secondary structure and 3 dimensional homology modeling of grass carp (*Ctenopharyngodon idellus*) major histocompatibility complex class I molecules. Protein Expression and Purification IN PRESS (doi:10.1016/j.pep.2006.08.003)
14. Doud MK, Schmidt MW, Hines D, Naumann C, Kocourek A, Kashani-Poor N, Zeidler R, Wolf DA (2004) Rapid prefractionation of complex protein lysates with centrifugal membrane adsorber units improves the resolving power of 2D-PAGE-based proteome analysis. BMC Genomics 5:art. No. 25
15. Neverova I, Van Eyk JE (2005) Role of chromatographic techniques in proteomic analysis. J Chromatog B 815:51–63

16. Kraljevic S, Stambrook PJ, Pavelic K (2004) Accelerating drug discovery – Although the evolution of '-omics' methodologies is still in its infancy, both the pharmaceutical industry and patients could benefit from their implementation in the drug development. EMBO Rep 5:837–842

41

Size-Exclusion Chromatography

Paul Cutler

1. Introduction

Size-exclusion chromatography (also known as gel-filtration chromatography) is a technique for separating proteins and other biological macromolecules on the basis of molecular size. Size-exclusion chromatography is a commonly used technique owing to the diversity of the molecular weights of proteins in biological tissues and extracts. It also has the important advantage of being compatible with physiological conditions (1,2).

The solid-phase matrix consists of porous beads packed into a column with a mobile-liquid phase flowing through the column (**Fig. 41.1**). The mobile phase has access to both the volume inside the pores and the volume external to the beads. The high porosity typically leads to a total liquid volume of >95% of the packed column.

Separation can be visualized as reversible partitioning into the two liquid volumes. Large molecules remain in the volume external to the beads because they are unable to enter the pores. The resulting shorter flow path means that they pass through the column relatively rapidly, emerging early. Proteins that are excluded from the pores completely elute in what is designated the void volume, *Vo*. This is often determined experimentally by the use of a high-mol-wt component, such as Blue Dextran 2000 or calf thymus DNA. Small molecules that can access the liquid within the pores of the beads are retained longer and therefore pass more slowly through the column. The elution volume for material included in the pores is designated the total volume, *Vt*. This represents the total liquid volume of the column and is often determined by small molecules, such as vitamin B12.

The elution volume for a given protein will lie between *Vo* and *Vt*. and is designated the elution volume, *Ve*. Intermediate-sized proteins will be fractionally excluded with a characteristic value for *Ve*. A partition coefficient can be determined for each protein as *Kav* (**Fig. 41.1**). In size exclusion, the macromolecules are not physically retained, unlike adsorption techniques; therefore, the protein will elute in a defined volume between *Vo* and *Vt*. If the protein elutes before the void volume *(Ve<Vo)* this suggests channeling

From: *Molecular Biomethods Handbook, 2nd Edition.*
Edited by: J. M. Walker and R. Rapley © Humana Press, Totowa, NJ

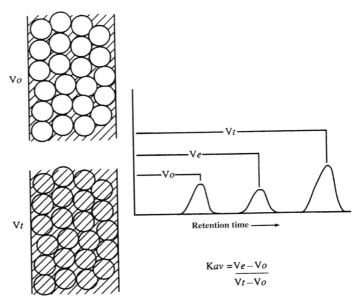

$$K_{av} = \frac{V_e - V_o}{V_t - V_o}$$

Fig. 41.1. The basic principle of size exclusion. Solutes are separated according to their molecular size. Large molecules are eluted in the void volume (V_0) and small molecules are eluted in the total volume (V_t). Solutes within the separation range of the matrix are fractionally excluded with a characteristic elution volume (V_e)

through the column owing to improper packing or operation of the column. If the protein elutes after the total volume *(Ve>Vt)*, then some interaction must have occurred between the matrix and the protein of interest. Size exclusion tends to be used at the end of a purification scheme when impurities are low in number and the target protein has been purified and concentrated by earlier chromatography steps. An exception to this is membrane proteins, where gel filtration may be used first because concentration techniques are not readily used and the material will be progressively diluted during the purification scheme *(3)*.

A range of different preparative and analytical matrices are available commercially. High-performance columns are used analytically for studying protein purity, protein folding, protein–protein interactions, and so forth *(4)*. Preparative separations performed on low-pressure matrices are used to resolve proteins from proteins of different molecular weight, proteins from other biological macromolecules, and for the separation of aggregated proteins from monomers *(5)*. Size exclusion is particularly suited for the resolution of protein aggregates from monomers. Aggregates are often formed as a result of the purification procedures used. Size exclusion is often incorporated as a final polishing step to remove aggregates and act as a buffer-exchange mechanism into the final solution.

Several parameters are important in size-exclusion chromatography. The pore diameter controlling the separation is selected for the relative size of proteins to be separated. Many types of matrix are available. Some are used for desalting techniques where proteins are separated from buffer salts *(6)*. Desalting gels are

Table 41.1. Commonly used preparative size exclusion matrices.

Supplier/matrix	Material type (pH stability)[a]	Separation range[b] kDaltons
Sephadex G10	Dextran	0–0.7
G15	(2–10)[d]	0–1.5
G25		1–5[c]
G50		1.5–3[c]
G75		3–80[c]
Superose 6	Agarose	5–5,000
12	(3–13)	1–300
Superdex Peptide	Agarose/Dextran	0.1–7
75	(3–12)	3–70
200		10–600
Sephacryl S100HR	Dextran/Bisacrylamide	1–100
S200HR	(3–11)	5–250
S300HR		10–1,500
Biogel P-2	Polyacrylamide	0.1–1.8[c]
P-4 gel	(2–10)	0.8–4[c]
P-10 gel		1.5–20[c]
P-60 gel		3–60[c]
P-100gel		5 – 100[c]

[a] In aqueous buffers.
[b] For globular protein.
[c] Different grades are available which effects performance.
[d] pH stability may vary depending on grade and exclusion limit.

used to rapidly remove low-mol-wt material, such as chemical reagents from proteins and for buffer exchange. Because the molecules to be separated are generally very small, typically <1 kDa, gels are generally used with an exclusion limit of approx 2–5 kDa. The protein appears in the void volume *(Vo)* and the reagents and buffer salts are retained. Because of the distinct mol-wt differences, the columns are shorter than other size-exclusion columns and operated at higher flow rates (e.g., 30 cm/h). Some matrices offer a wide range of mol-wt separations and others are high-resolution matrices with a narrow range of operation (**Table 41.1**).

2. Practical Requirements

The preparative separation of proteins by size exclusion is suited to commercially available standard low-pressure chromatography systems. Systems require a column packed with a matrix offering a suitable fractionation range, a method for mobile-phase delivery, a detector to monitor the eluting proteins, a chart recorder for viewing the detector response, and a fraction collector for recovery of eluted proteins (**Fig. 41.2**). The system should be plumbed with capillary tubing with a minimum hold up volume.

Early systems were less sophisticated with a gravimetric feed of the mobile phase from a suspended reservoir, whereas the most modern systems now have computers to control operating parameters and to collect and store data.

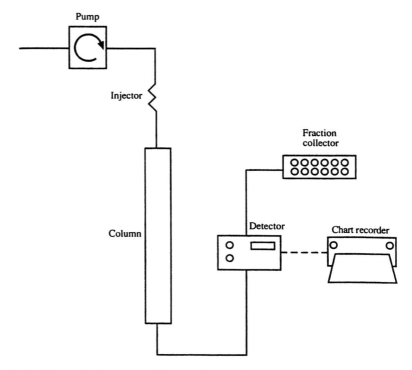

Fig. 41.2. Schematic diagram of the equipment for preparative size-exclusion chromatography

The principle of separation, however, remains the same and high resolution is attainable with relatively simple equipment.

1. Pumps: An important factor in size exclusion is a reproducible and accurate flow rate. The most commonly used pumps are peristaltic pumps, which are relatively effective at low-flow rates, inexpensive, and sanitizable. Peristaltic pumps do, however, create a pulsed flow, and often a bubble trap is incorporated to both prevent air entering the system and to dampen the pulsing effect. More expensive, yet more accurate pumps are those seen on the Äkta systems (GE Healthcare) and BioLogic™ systems (BioRad).

2. Column: Size exclusion, unlike some commonly used adsorption methods of protein separation, is a true chromatography method based on continuous partitioning; hence, resolution is dependent on column length. Columns tend toward being long and thin, typically 70–100 cm long. In some instances, the length of the column required to obtain a satisfactory separation exceeds that which can be packed into a commercially available column (>1 m). In these cases, columns can be packed in series.

The tubing connecting the columns should be as narrow and as short as possible to avoid zone spreading. The column must be able to withstand the moderate pressures generated during operation and be resistant to the mobile phase. The use of columns with flow adapters is recommended to allow the packing volume to be varied and provide a finished support with the required minimum of dead space.

3. Detectors: Protein elution is most often monitored by absorbance in the ultraviolet range, either at 280 nm, which is suitable for proteins with aromatic amino acids, or at 206 nm, which detects the peptide bond. Detection at lower wavelengths may be complicated by the absorbance characteristics of certain mobile phases. The advent of diode-array detectors has enabled continuous detection at multiple wavelengths, enabling characterization of the elutes via analysis of spectral data.

Fluorescence detection either by direct detection of fluorescent tryptophan and tyrosine residues or after chemical derivatization (e.g., by fluorescein) have been used, as have refractive index, radiochemical, electrochemical, and molecular size (by laser-light scattering). In addition to these nonspecific on-line monitoring systems, it is quite common, particularly when purifying enzymes, to make use of specific assays for individual target molecules.

In recent times more advanced detectors have been employed with size exclusion chromatography have included multi-angle laser light scattering *(7)* and mass spectrometry *(8)*.

4. Fraction collectors: A key factor in preparative protein purification is the ability to collect accurate fractions. No matter how efficiently the column may have separated the proteins, the accurate collection of fractions is critical. For the detector to reflect as near as possible in real time the fraction collector, the volume between the detector and the fraction collector should be minimal.

5. Buffers: Size-exclusion matrices tend to be compatible with most aqueous-buffer systems even in the presence of surfactants, reducing agents, or denaturing agents. Size-exclusion matrices are extremely stable, with effective pH ranges of approx 2.0–12.0 (**Table 41.1**). An important exception to this is the silica-based matrices, which offer good mechanical rigidity but low chemical stability at alkaline pHs. Some silica matrices have been coated with dextran, and so forth, to increase the chemical stability and increase hydrophilicity.

The choice of mobile phase is most often dependent on protein stability, necessitating considerations of appropriate pH, and solvent composition as well as the presence or absence of cofactors, protease inhibitors etc. which may be essential to maintain the structural and functional integrity of the target molecule. All buffers used in size exclusion should ideally be filtered through a 0.2-μm filter and degassed by low vacuum or sparging with an inert gas, such as helium.

The majority of protein separations performed using size exclusion are carried out in the presence of aqueous-phase buffers. Size exclusion of proteins in organic phases (sometimes called gel permeation) is not normally undertaken but is sometimes used for membrane-protein separations. The agarose- and dextran-based matrices are not suitable for separations with organic solvents. Synthetic polymers and, to a certain extent, silica are suitable for separations in organic phases. For separation in acidified organic solvents, polyacrylamide matrices are particularly suitable. The separation of the proteins may be influenced by the denatured state of the protein in the organic phase. The equipment must be compatible with the solvent system, e.g., glass or Teflon.

Many matrices retain a residual charge owing to, for example, sulfate groups in agarose or carboxyl residues in dextran. The ionic strength of the buffer should be kept at 0.15–2.0 M to avoid electrostatic or Van Der Waals interactions that can lead to nonideal size exclusion (9,10). Crosslinking agents, such as those used in polyacrylamide, may reduce the hydrophilicity of the matrix, leading to the retention of some small proteins, particularly those rich in aromatic amino-acid residues. These interactions have been exploited effectively to enhance purification in some cases, but are generally best avoided. Interactions with the matrix are commonly seen when charged proteins are being resolved. If low-ionic strength is necessary, then the risk of interaction can be reduced by manipulating the charge on the protein via the pH of the buffer. This is best achieved by keeping the mobile phase above or below the pI of the protein as appropriate. Protein–matrix interaction is a common cause of protein loss during size exclusion. This may be owing to complete retention on the column or retardation sufficient for the material to elute in an extremely broad dilute fraction, thus evading detection above the baseline of the buffer system. Another important consideration is when enzymes are detected off-line by activity assay. The active enzyme may resolve in to inactive subunits. In such cases, a review of the mobile phase is advisable.

6. Selection of matrix: The beads used for size exclusion have a closely controlled pore size, with a high chemical and physical stability. They are hydrophilic and inert to minimize chemical interactions between the solutes (proteins) and the matrix itself. The performance and resolution of the technique has been enhanced by the development of newer matrices with improved properties. Historically, gels were based on starch, although these were superseded by the crosslinked dextran gels (e.g., Sephadex). In addition polystyrene-based matrices were developed for the use of size exclusion in nonaqueous solutions. Polyacrylamide gels (e.g., Bio-Gel® P series) are particularly suited to separation at the lower-mol-wt range owing to their microreticular structure. Composite matrices such as the Superdex® gel (GE Healthcare) have been developed, where dextran chains have been chemically bonded to a highly crosslinked agarose for high speed size exclusion (**Table 41.1**).

3. Practical Procedures

1. Flow rates: In chromatography flow rates should be standardized for columns of different dimensions by quoting linear flow rate (cm/h). This is defined as the volumetric flow rate (cm3/h) per unit cross-sectional area (cm^2) of a given column. Because the principle of size exclusion is based on partitioning, success of the technique is particularly susceptible to variations in flow rates. Conventional low-pressure size exclusion matrices tend to operate at linear flow rates of 5–15 cm/h. Too high a flow rate leads to incomplete partitioning and band spreading. Conversely, very low flow rates may lead to diffusion and band spreading.
2. Preparation of gel matrix: Gel matrices are supplied as either preswollen gels or as dry powder. If the gel is supplied as a dry powder it should be swollen in excess mobile phase as directed by the manufacturers. Swollen gels must be transferred to the appropriate mobile phase. This can be

achieved by washing in a sintered-glass funnel under low vacuum. During preparation, the gel should not be allowed to dry. The equilibrated gel should be decanted into a Buchner flask, allowed to settle, and then fines removed from the top by decanting. The equilibrated gel (an approx 75% slurry) is then degassed under low vacuum.

3. Packing the gel: Good column packing is an essential prerequisite for efficient resolution in size-exclusion chromatography. The column should be held vertically in a retort stand, avoiding adverse drafts, direct sunlight, or changes in temperature. The gel should be equilibrated and packed at the final operating temperature. With the bottom frit or flow adaptor in place degassed buffer (5–10% of the bed volume) is poured down the column side to remove any air from the system. In one manipulation, the degassed-gel slurry is poured into the column using a glass rod to direct the gel down the side of the column, avoiding air entrapment. If available, a packing reservoir should be fitted to columns to facilitate easier packing. The column can be packed under gravity, although a more efficient method is to use a pump to push buffer through the packing matrix. The flow rate during packing should be approx 50% higher than the operating flow rate (e.g., 15 cm/h for a 10 cm/h final flow rate). The bed height can be monitored by careful inspection of the column as it is packing. Once packed, a clear layer of buffer will appear above the bed and the level of the gel will remain constant. The flow should then be stopped and excess buffer removed from the top of the column, leaving approx 2 cm buffer above the gel. The outlet from the column should be closed and the top-flow adaptor carefully placed on top of the gel, avoiding trapped air or disturbing the gel bed.

The packed column should be equilibrated by passing the final buffer through the column at the packing flow rate for at least one column volume. The pump should always be connected to pump the eluent on to the column under positive pressure. Drawing buffer through the column under negative pressure may lead to bubbles forming as a result of the suction. The effluent of the column should be sampled and tested for pH and conductivity to establish equilibration in the desired buffer.

4. Sample application: Several methods exist for sample application. It is critical to deliver the sample to the top of the column as a narrow sample zone. This can be achieved by manually loading via a syringe directly on to the column, although this requires skill and practice. The material may be applied through a peristaltic pump, although this will inevitably lead to band spreading owing to sample dilution. The sample should never be loaded through a pump with a large hold-up volume, such as a syringe pump, or upstream of a bubble trap. Arguably, the best method of applying the sample is via a sample loop in conjunction with a switching valve, allowing the sample to be manually or electronically diverted through the loop and directly on to the top of the column.

5. Evaluation of column packing: The partitioning process occurs as the bulk flow of liquid moves down the column. As the sample is loaded, it forms a sample band on the column. In considering the efficiency of the column partitioning can be perceived as occurring in discrete zones along the axis of the columns length. Each zone is referred to as a theoretical plate and the length of the zone termed the theoretical plate height (H). The value of H is

a function of the physical properties of the column, the exclusion limit, and the operating conditions, such as flow rate, and so forth. Column efficiency is defined by the number of theoretical plates (N) that can be measured experimentally using a suitable sample, e.g., 1% (v/v) acetone (**Fig. 41.3**). Resolution and, hence, the number of theoretical plates, is enhanced by increasing column length.

In addition to determination of the number of theoretical plates (N) described, the performance of the column can be assessed qualitatively by the shape of the eluted peaks (**Fig. 41.4**). The theoretically ideal peak is sharp and triangular with an axis of symmetry around the apex. Deviations from this are seen in practice. Some peak shapes are diagnostic of particular problems that lead to broadening and poor resolution. If the down slope of the peak is significantly shallow, it is possible that the concentration of the load was too high or the material has disturbed the equilibrium between the mobile and stationary phases. If the down slope tends to symmetrical initially, but then becomes shallow, it is common to assume that there is a poorly resolved component; however, it may be suspected that interaction with the matrix is taking place. A shallow upslope may represent insolubility of the loaded material. A valley between 2 closely eluting peaks may suggest poor resolution, but can also be the result of a faulty sample injection.

6. Standards and calibration: Calibration is obtained by use of standard proteins and plotting retention time *(Ve)* against log molecular weight. Successful calibration requires accurate flow rates. The resultant plot gives a sigmoidal curve approaching linearity in the effective separation range of the gel (**Fig. 41.5**).

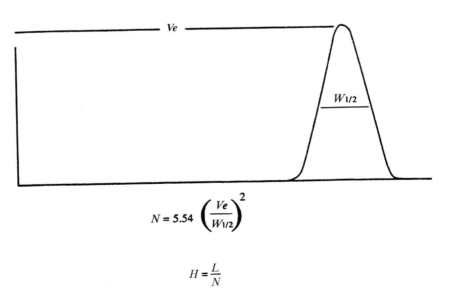

$$N = 5.54 \left(\frac{Ve}{W_{1/2}}\right)^2$$

$$H = \frac{L}{N}$$

Fig. 41.3. Calculation of the theoretical plate height as a measure of column performance. The number of theoretical plates (*N*) is related to the peak width at half-height (W$_{1/2}$) and the elution volume (V$_e$). The height of the theoretical plate (*H*) is related to the column length (*L*)

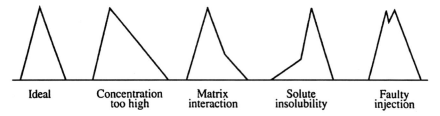

Fig. 41.4. Diagnosis of column performance by consideration of peak shape

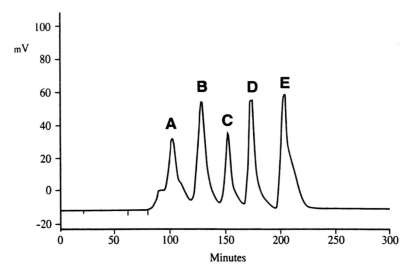

Fig. 41.5. Size exclusion of 5 molecular-weight markers on Superdex 200 (GE Health-care) column (1.6 × 75 cm). Thyroglubin, 670,000 (**A**); γ-globulin, 158,000 (**B**); ovalbumin, 44,000 (**C**); myoglobin, 17,000 (**D**), and vitamin B_{12}, 1350 (**E**)

It should be noted that it is not only the molecular weight that is important in size exclusion, but also the hydrodynamic volume or the Stokes radius of the molecule. Globular proteins appear to have a lower molecular size than proteins with a similar molecular weight, which are in an α-helical form. These, in turn, appear smaller than proteins in random-coil form. It is critical to use the appropriate standards for size exclusion where proteins have a similar shape. This has been useful in some cases for studying protein folding and unfolding. Commonly used mol-wt standards are given in **Table 41.2**.

7. Separation of proteins: The optimum load of size-exclusion columns is restricted to <5% (typically 2%) of the column volume to maximize resolution. Gel-filtration columns are often loaded at relatively high concentrations of protein, such as 2–20 mg/mL. The concentration is limited by solubility of the protein and the potential for increased viscosity, which begins to have a detrimental effect on resolution. This becomes evident

Table 41.2. Molecular weight standards for size exclusion chromatography.

Vitamin B-12	1,350
Ribonuclease A	13,700
Myoglobin	17,000
Chymotrypsinogen A	25,000
Ovalbumin	43,000
Bovine serum albumin	67,000
Bovine gamma globulin	158,000
Catalase	232,000
Ferritin	440,000
Thyroglobulin	670,000
Blue Dextran 2000	~2,000,000

around 50 mg/mL. It is important to remove any insoluble matter before loading by either centrifugation or filtration. Owing to the limitation on loading, it is often wise to consider the ability of the method for scale-up when optimizing the operating parameters (*11*).

8. Column cleaning and storage: Size-exclusion matrices can be cleaned *in situ* or as loose gel in a sintered-glass funnel. Suppliers usually offer specific guidelines for cleaning gels. Common general-cleaning agents include nonionic detergents (e.g., 1% [v/v] Triton X-100) for lipids and 0.2–0.5 *M* NaOH for proteins and pyrogens (not recommended for silica-based matrices). In extreme circumstances, contaminating protein can be removed by use of enzymic digestion (pepsin for proteins and nucleases for RNA and DNA). The gel should be stored in a buffer with antimicrobial activity, such as 20% (v/v) ethanol or 0.02–0.05% (w/v) sodium azide. NaOH is a good storage agent that combines good solubilizing activity with prevention of endotoxin formation. It may, however, lead to chemical breakdown of certain matrices.

References

1. Laurent TC (1993) Chromatography classic: history of a theory. J Chrom 633:1–8
2. Silberring J, Kowalczuk M, Bergquist J, Kraj A, Suder P, Dylag T, Smoulch M, Chervet JP, Ekman R (2004) Size exclusion chromatography. J Chromatogr Libr 69:213–251
3. Findlay JBC (1990) Purification of membrane proteins. In: Harris ELV, Angal S (eds) Protein purification applications. IRL, Oxford, UK, pp. 59–82
4. Irvine GB (2003) High performance size-exclusion chromatography of peptides. J Biochem Biophys Methods 56:233–242
5. Stellwagen E (1990) Gel filtration. *Methods Enzymol.* 182:317–328
6. Pohl T (1990) Concentration of proteins and removal of solutes. Methods Enzymol 182:69–83
7. Oliva A, Llabres M, Farina JB (2004) Applications of multi-angle laser light scattering detection in the analysis of peptides and proteins. Curr Drug Discov Technol 1:229–242

8. Geoghegan KF, Kelly ME (2005) Biochemical applications of mass spectrometry in pharmaceutical drug discovery. Mass Spectrom Rev 24:347–366

9. Gooding KM, Regnier FE (2002) Size exclusion chromatography. Chromatogr Sci Ser 87:49–79

10. Dubin PL, Edwards SL, Mehta MS, Tomalia D (1993) Quantitation of nonideal behavior in protein size exclusion chromatography. *J. Chrom.* 635:51–60

11. Jansen IC, Hedman P (1987) Large scale chromatography of proteins. Adv Biochem Eng 25:43–97

42

Hydrophobic Interaction Chromatography

Paul A. O'Farrell

1. Introduction

The separation of proteins for purification or analysis is carried out by exploiting differences in their biological and/or physiochemical properties. Affinity techniques rely on specific biological properties. Charge and molecular size are the most commonly exploited physiochemical properties, and various methods relying on them are described in other chapters in this volume. Hydrophobicity provides a third general physiochemical property that can also be used for the separation of proteins. Although a soluble protein buries most of its hydrophobic residues within the core of its structure (indeed, this is the major force behind protein folding *(1–3)*), there are generally areas of the surface that are hydrophobic *(4,5)*. Such hydrophobic 'patches' are often very important for the functioning of a particular protein, as many are involved in protein–protein interactions *(6)*. The nature and extent of these patches varies among different proteins, and it is this variation that is exploited in hydrophobic interaction chromatography (HIC). The fact that surface hydrophobicity is a general property of all proteins implies that HIC has the potential to be used in almost any separation protocol. It relies on a property that is orthogonal to both charge and size, and thus it increases the likelihood of achieving significant separation without having to resort to specific affinity methods. Importantly, HIC is a "gentle" method that helps ensure that the protein of interest (POI) retains biological activity.

Although it has become more popular, HIC is still somewhat underused as a separation technique, perhaps because it is poorly understood by many workers. This is not surprising as, despite the existence of a large body of literature on the subject, there is still a lack of consensus as to the exact mechanism of the hydrophobic effect. Although the hydrophobic effect can be described in general terms as the association of nonpolar molecules in a polar medium, many different theories have been posited to explain the association. These incorporate such factors as the entropic advantage gained by the release of ordered water (**Fig. 42.1**), van der Waals and aromatic interactions among nonpolar entities, the masking of protein charges by solvent ions and the

From: *Molecular Biomethods Handbook, 2nd Edition.*
Edited by: J. M. Walker and R. Rapley © Humana Press, Totowa, NJ

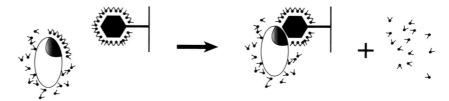

Fig. 42.1. Protein binding to hydrophobic ligand: expulsion of ordered water. The hydrogen bonding structure of liquid water is disturbed by the presence of nonpolar solutes. The water molecules form a shell around the hydrophobic ligand (black hexagon) and the hydrophobic patch on the protein's surface (shaded area) where the hydrogen bonding structure is in fact more ordered that in the bulk solvent. When these two areas associate, some of the ordered water is displaced to the bulk solvent. The resultant increase in entropy represents a thermodynamic advantage that favors the interaction

effect of solvent surface tension. It is clear that a number of different effects are involved in the interaction and it is likely that different effects come into play under different conditions. For example, microcalorimetric studies by Lin et al. *(7)* showed that although adsorption onto an octyl ligand was entropy driven, adsorption onto a less hydrophobic ligand had an increased enthalpic component. Temperature also affects the mechanism of hydrophobic interaction – at room temperature entropic effects dominate, but at higher temperatures, enthalpy becomes more important *(3,8)*. It is clear that the hydrogen bonding structure of water is the major factor that drives the effect, thus modification of this structure can control the strength of hydrophobic interactions. In HIC, this is generally achieved by changing the salt concentration so that, in practice, it is a simple procedure to carry out. The sample is applied to the HIC column in a buffer containing a high concentration of salt and the POI is eluted by decreasing the salt concentration.

Knowledge of a protein's isoelectric point or molecular weight can predict where it will elute in ion-exchange or size-exclusion chromatographies, however there is no comparable parameter for HIC. Asenjo and colleagues have attempted to predict behavior on HIC with some success *(9,10)*. Their method depends on knowing the three-dimensional structure of the protein to assess its surface hydrophobicity. They have noted that it is not simply total surface hydrophobicity that is the main predictor of behavior, rather it is the distribution and size of the surface hydrophobic patches *(11–13)*. As the three-dimensional structure is frequently not available, attempts have also been made to predict surface hydrophobicity using only the protein's amino acid composition *(14)*. Despite these efforts however, the development of a HIC procedure is essentially an empirical process. A number of different parameters must be considered as described in the next section.

2. Experimental Considerations

2.1. Media

Many different absorbant media for HIC are available commercially, and many different combinations of support matrix and ligand are possible (**Table 42.1**). Generally, the choice of support material depends on the mode of

Table 42.1. Commercially available media for HIC.

Supplier	Product	Ligand	Comment
Applied Biosystems www.appliedbiosystems.com	Poros HP2	Phenyl, high density	This has a very porous matrix that supports high flow-rates
Biochrom Labs www.biochrom.com	Hydrocell C3, C4, phenyl	Allyl, butyl, phenyl	Porous polymeric bead matrix, available in different pore sizes
	Hydrocell C3 NP10, C4 NP10, Phenyl NP10	Allyl, butyl, phenyl	Nonporous matrix
Biorad www.bio-rad.com	Macroprep t-butyl HIC, methyl HIC	Butyl, methyl	
GE healthcare/Amersham www.amershambiosciences.com	HiTrap HIC selection kit	Phenyl, butyl, octyl	lit containing different media for method development
Mallinckrodt Baker www.mallbaker.com	Hi-propyl wp-butyl	Propyl butyl	Based on a silica matrix
Millipore www.millipore.com	Prosep thiosorb	proprietary	HCIC medium for antibody purification
Tosoh Bioscience www.tosohbiosep.com	Toyopearl Hexyl-650, SuperButyl-550, butyl-650, PPG-600, phenyl-650, ether-650	Hexyl, butyl, phenyl, polypropylene glycol, ether,	Suitable for HPLC, available in large pore sizes; hexyl is a very hydrophobic ligand
	TSK-GEL butyl-NPR, Phenyl-5PW, Ether-5PW	Butyl, phenyl, ether	Smaller pore size, smaller particles

This table provides only a representative sample of companies offering products for HIC, and only representative products from those companies. It is by no means an exhaustive list.

chromatography to be used. Gravity driven liquid chromatography does not generate high pressures and relatively fragile materials such as agarose can be used. In FPLC and HPLC applications, which run under higher pressures, more robust materials are needed. The manufacturers of a particular chromatography system can provide information about what materials may be suitable for the potential pressures generated. In addition, the support matrix itself should be inert; there should be no functional groups capable of binding protein, as it is preferable to control binding by the choice of ligand. Ligands are available with varying degrees of hydrophobicity, the most common being phenyl groups or alkyl groups of varying chain lengths. The choice of ligand is essentially empirical, but can use prior knowledge about the hydrophobicity of the POI. A weakly hydrophobic protein will require a strongly hydrophobic ligand to ensure binding. With a very hydrophobic protein, a weakly hydrophobic ligand is preferable to avoid harsh and possible denaturing, elution conditions. Method development with an uncharacterized protein should start with a weakly hydrophobic ligand, to avoid loss of material owing to possible irreversible binding. In addition to the hydrophobicity of the ligand, the ligand density also needs to be considered. Increasing ligand density will increase the strength of interaction with the column, owing to increased formation of multivalent interactions *(15,16)*. This effect is dependant on the size of the protein, with larger proteins capable of more interactions with the column. Finally, there may be specific interactions between the ligand and the POI. For example, it has been suggested that phenyl-sepharose in some instances acts more as an affinity matrix rather than as a strictly hydrophobic one *(17)*. A number of kits are commercially available containing small HIC columns with a variety of different matrices. Such kits are a useful place to start when designing a new HIC protocol.

2.2. Binding and Elution

Binding and elution in HIC are achieved by the addition or removal of salts or other solutes. As described above, there is still some controversy as to the exact mechanism of the hydrophobic interaction, but the major effect of solutes is on the molecular interactions among water molecules; in effect, they alter the hydrogen-bonding structure of the solvent. Structure-forming salts increase the strength of hydrophobic interactions, whereas chaotropes have the opposite effect. The Hofmeister, or lyotropic, series *(18)* (**Table 42.2**) arranges ions in the order from those that promote hydrophobic interactions to those that decrease the strength of the interaction. This relates both to a salt's ability to cause a protein to precipitate out of solution (salting-out), as well as to its interactions in HIC. Various aspects of this series as it relates to HIC have been studied *(19,20)*. It should be noted that some salts can have specific interactions with particular proteins, so the series may not be strictly followed by every protein. Any structure-forming salt can be used for HIC, however ammonium sulfate is often used owing to its high solubility and good lyotropic properties. Other factors sometimes come into play in the choice of salt. For example, if the HIC step immediately follows an ion-exchange step, the salt used for elution in that step can be used for binding in HIC. This economy obviates the need for dialysis or other procedures to remove the salt. Indeed, HIC is often placed after ion-exchange chromatography or ammonium sulfate

Table 42.2. The Hofmeister series[a].

Anions	Cations
PO_4^{3-}	NH_4^+
SO_4^{2-}	Rb^+
CH_3COO^-	K^+
Cl^-	Na^+
Br^-	Cs^+
NO_3^-	Li^+
ClO_4^-	Mg^{2+}
I^-	Ca^{2+}
SCN^-	Ba^{2+}

[a]Ions are listed in order from those at the top that promote hydrophobic interaction to those at the bottom that are unfavorable.

precipitation in a multi-step procedure owing to this economy of procedure. The salt concentration used for binding to the column can be determined by a preliminary salting-out experiment – a concentration somewhat below that which causes the POI to precipitate is often suitable. Such an experiment should be carried out with the POI itself at the concentration to be used in HIC, as the salt concentration at which it will precipitate is dependant to a degree on the protein concentration.

In most applications, binding is achieved by loading the column at a high salt concentration. Elution is achieved by reducing the salt concentration, either via a gradient or in a stepwise manner. Although gradient elution should achieve better separation, peaks can sometimes be broad, owing to protein aggregation and slow association/dissociation. This can result in poor resolution and a lower than desirable concentration. A stepwise elution method may be helpful in such circumstances. It has also been reported that sharper peaks can be achieved by including a small amount of solvent (e.g., 0.1–5% ethanol) in the elution buffer.

In some cases simply lowering the salt concentration is not enough to achieve elution and it may be necessary to include a chaotropic agent (e.g., urea), alcohol, or detergent to achieve recovery of the POI. However, these agents can have a deleterious effect on protein structure and are best avoided. If they are found to be necessary, the use of a less hydrophobic adsorption matrix should be considered. It has been reported that the use of a ternary gradient, in which the concentration of a chaotropic agent is increased at the same time as reducing the salt concentration, can result in better resolution (21).

2.3. pH

Although the charged residues of a protein are not directly involved in hydrophobic interactions, HIC is nonetheless affected by the pH of the solvent. It has been observed that there is a general decrease in the strength of binding with increasing pH. This is presumably due to the titration of basic residues, thus increasing the hydrophilicity of the protein (22). The effect of pH is fairly small, and changes in pH are not generally used as a method of effecting binding and elution. However, the effect of pH is different for different proteins, therefore it is possible to modify elution profiles and achieve better resolution by carrying out the procedure at different pH values. Of course, it is important to work in a pH range where the POI is stable, and to bear in mind that proteins may precipitate near their pIs, resulting in reduced recovery.

2.4. Temperature

As entropy plays an important role in the hydrophobic interaction, it may be expected that temperature will have an effect on binding (23). In fact, the strength of binding does generally increase with temperature. These effects are different for different proteins and, as with pH, it is possible to change elution profiles and possibly achieve better resolution by carrying out HIC at different temperatures. However, temperature also affects protein structure and solubility, with the result that its effects on HIC are difficult to predict (17,24,25). Thus, it is often simpler just to work at a temperature where the POI is known to be stable.

3. Applications

HIC can be applied to most proteins and as such, can potentially have a role to play in any protein purification protocol. It is particularly useful in industrial scale applications: it provides an alternative to size-exclusion (which is inefficient to scale up) while being orthogonal to ion-exchange. Affinity chromatography can also be unsuitable for large-scale processes, owing to the high cost of many affinity media. HIC has been investigated as an alternative in this area as well. Husi and Walkinshaw *(26,27)* have demonstrated the utility of HIC in the separation of coagulation proteins from prothrombin concentrate (a common extract of serum). Using phenyl-sepharose as the matrix material and 3 M NaCl in the binding buffer, they were able to separate prothrombin and Factor X, with a significant purification of Factor IX also.

The production of antibodies for therapeutic purposes also provides an opportunity for HIC. Traditionally, antibodies have been purified by affinity chromatography with Protein A or Protein G. However, besides being relatively expensive, leakage of Proteins A or G into the product also causes difficulties owing to their immunotoxicity. Ghosh and Wang *(28)* have purified humanized monoclonal antibody from cell culture using HIC, achieving 97% purity in a single step with high yield. Notably, they were able to achieve significant separation from bovine albumin, a major contaminant in the cell culture. Their method used ammonium sulfate as the salt, and a cassette stack of PVDF membrane sheets, rather than a column filled with a particulate matrix, as the stationary phase. Other workers have used so-called Hydrophobic Charge Induction Chromatography (HCIC) for the purification of antibodies (see *(29)* for a review). Although some would argue that this modality is very different from HIC, hydrophobicity is an important component of the interaction and binding is achieved with a high level of structure-forming salt. What is different is the method of elution. The ligand in this case is uncharged at neutral pH, but charged at lower pH (for example, 4-mercapto-ethyl-pyridine (MEP), with a pKa of 4.8, is commonly used). Thus, by shifting the pH after binding, a positive charge can be induced on the ligand that repels the positively charged antibody.

A different alternative method of elution is used in calcium-dependant HIC. This relies on a property of the protein itself rather than the ligand. Several proteins undergo conformational change on binding or releasing Ca^{2+}, most notably calmodulin. Such conformational change can cause the exposure or sequestration of hydrophobic patches on the protein's surface. Thus, manipulation of the calcium concentration can alter the strength of interaction between the protein and an HIC column. Walsh *et al.* have used this property to isolate protein kinase C *(30)*. The sample was applied to a phenyl-sepharose column in the presence of 2 mM Ca^{2+}. After washing off unbound protein, 1 mM EGTA was applied as a chelating agent. The conformational change induced by the removal of the Ca^{2+} changed the surface hydrophobicity of the protein, causing its release from the column.

As mentioned in the Introduction, proteins maintain their structure by burying hydrophobic residues in the core of the folded molecule. Thus, incorrectly folded molecules generally expose more hydrophobic residues than correctly folded molecules. Because of its sensitivity to protein surface hydrophobicity, HIC can therefore play a role in the area of protein folding.

Foreign proteins expressed in bacteria are often produced as 'inclusion bodies' – aggregates of misfolded protein *(31)*. For the protein to have biological activity, these aggregates must be broken down (by denaturing agents) and the protein induced to refold correctly. However, refolding is generally not 100% successful, and the final preparation will contain both correctly and incorrectly folded protein. These are difficult to separate as they will have the same molecular weight and isoelectric point. However, HIC is capable of separating them owing to the more hydrophobic nature of the misfolded protein. For example, Jing *et al.* *(32)* used phenyl-superose to separate correctly folded recombinant staphylococcal nuclease from a misfolded form that had only 24% of its activity. In fact, HIC can be used in the refolding process itself. Geng and colleagues have successfully used HIC in the refolding of eukaryotic proteins such as interferon and insulin *(33–35)*. In the case of insulin, they were able to achieve correct formation of the disulfide bonds without the addition of reducing agents *(35)*. The method is particularly powerful in that the HIC matrix acts as an artificial chaperone, preventing the misfolded protein molecules from aggregating and giving them the opportunity to refold correctly. It also acts to separate misfolded molecules from correctly folded ones that, being less hydrophobic, are released from the column. For some labile proteins, however, HIC can have the opposite effect *(36,37)*. The hydrophobic ligand can act as a catalyst causing unfolding of the protein. This effect is more pronounced with more hydrophobic ligands and increases with length of exposure to the matrix *(36)*. It has been suggested that the concept of 'critical hydrophobicity', as developed by Jennissen *(16,38)*, can be helpful in such circumstances.

4. Conclusion

HIC has broad applicability in the purification and analysis of proteins. Besides being a general technique that can be used to complement those based on other properties, it can be used to replace some methods such as affinity and size-exclusion that are unsuitable in some circumstances. In addition, it has its own unique applications. Although the exact nature of the hydrophobic interaction is not fully understood, a complete theoretical understanding is not necessary to use it. The extraordinary diversity of protein structure requires that an empirical approach be taken to method development in any particular case. A useful short guide to the steps that can be taken to develop an HIC procedure is presented in reference *(39)*. It has only been possible to give a short summary of HIC here; readers who are interested in a more in depth treatment are directed to other sources *(40–42)*.

References

1. Kauzmann W (1959) Some factors in the interpretation of protein denaturation. Adv Protein Chem 14:1–63
2. Dill KA (1990) Dominant forces in protein folding. Biochemistry 29:7133–7155
3. Makhatadze GI, Privalov PL (1995) Energetics of protein structure. Adv Protein Chem 47:307–425
4. Lee B, Richards FM (1971) The interpretation of protein structures: estimation of static accessibility. J Mol Biol 55:379–400

5. Hofstee B (1975) Accessible hydrophobic groups of native proteins. Biochem Biophys Res Commun 63:618–624
6. Conte LL, Chothia C, Janin J (1999) The atomic structure of protein-protein recognition sites. J Mol Biol 285:2177–2198
7. Lin FY, Chen WY, Ruaan RC, Huang HM (2000) Microcalorimetric studies of interactions between proteins and hydrophobic ligands in hydrophobic interaction chromatography: effects of ligand chain length, density and the amount of bound protein. J Chromatogr A 872:37–47
8. Dill KA (1990) The meaning of hydrophobicity. Science 250:297–298
9. Lienqueo ME, Mahn A, Asenjo JA (2002) Mathematical correlations for predicting protein retention times in hydrophobic interaction chromatography. J Chromatogr A 978:71–79
10. Lienqueo ME, Mahn A, Vasquez L, Asenjo JA (2003) Methodology for predicting the separation of proteins by hydrophobic interaction chromatography and its application to a cell extract. J Chromatogr A 1009:189–196
11. Mahn A, Asenjo J (2005) Prediction of protein retention in hydrophobic interaction chromatography. Biotechnol Adv 23:359–368
12. Salgado JC, Rapaport I, Asenjo JA (2006) Predicting the behaviour of proteins in hydrophobic interaction chromatography. 2: Using a statistical description of their surface amino acid distribution. J Chromatogr A 1107:120–129
13. Salgado JC, Rapaport I, Asenjo JA (2006) Predicting the behaviour of proteins in hydrophobic interaction chromatography. 1: using the hydrophobic imbalance (HI) to describe their surface amino acid distribution. J Chromatogr A 1107:110–119
14. Salgado JC, Rapaport I, Asenjo JA (2005) Is it possible to predict the average surface hydrophobicity of a protein using only its amino acid composition? J Chromatogr A 1075:133–143
15. Fausnaugh J, Kennedy L, Regnier F (1984) Comparison of hydrophobic-interaction and reversed-phase chromatography of proteins. J Chromatography 317:141–155
16. Jennissen H (2005) Hydrophobic interaction chromatography: harnessing multivalent protein-surface interactions for purification procedures. Methods Mol Biol 305:81–99
17. Ibrahim-Granet O, Bertrand O (1996) Separation of proteases: old and new approaches. J Chromatogr B-Biomed Appl 684:239–263
18. Hofmeister F (1888) Zur lohre von der wirkung der salze. Zweite mittheilung. Arch Exp Pathol Pharmakol 24:247–260
19. Melander W (1977) Salt effect on hydrophobic interactions in precipitation and chromatography of proteins: an interpretation of the lyotropic series. Arch Biochem Biophys 183:200–215
20. Arakawa T, Timasheff S (1984) Mechanism of protein salting in and salting out by divalent cation salts: balance between hydration and salt binding. Biochemistry 23:5912–5923
21. El Rassi Z, DeCampo LF, Bacolod MD (1990) Binary and ternary salt gradients in hydrophobic interaction chromatography. J Chromatogr A 499:141–152
22. Fausnaugh JL, Regnier FE (1986) Solute and mobile phase contributions to retention in hydrophobic interaction chromatography of proteins. J Chromatogr 359:31–146
23. Haidacher D, Vailaya A, Horvath C (1996) Temperature effects in hydrophobic interaction chromatography. Proc Natl Acad Sci USA 93:2290–2295
24. Goheen SC, Gibbins BM (2000) Protein losses in ion-exchange and hydrophobic interaction high-performance liquid chromatography. J Chromatogr A 890:73–80
25. Wu SL, Karger BL (1996) Hydrophobic interaction chromatography of proteins. Methods in enzymology 270:27–47

26. Husi H, Walkinshaw M (1999) Separation of human vitamin K-dependent coagulation proteins using hydrophobic interaction chromatography. J Chromatogr B Biomed Sci Appl 736:77–88

27. Husi H, Walkinshaw MD (2001) Purification of factor X by hydrophobic interaction chromatography. J Chromatogr B Biomed Sci Appl 755:367–371

28. Ghosh R, Wang L (2006) Purification of humanized monoclonal antibody by hydrophobic interaction membrane chromatography. J Chromatogr A 1107:104–109

29. Boschetti E (2002) Antibody separation by hydrophobic charge induction chromatography. Trends Biotechnol 20:333–337

30. Walsh M, Valentine K, Ngai P, Carruthers C, Hollenberg M (1984) Ca2+-dependent hydrophobic-interaction chromatography. Isolation of a novel Ca2+-binding protein and protein kinase C from bovine brain. Biochem J 224:117–127

31. Vallejo LF, Rinas U (2004) Strategies for the recovery of active proteins through refolding of bacterial inclusion body proteins. Microbiol Cell Factories 3:11

32. Jing G, Zhou B, Liu L, Zhou J, Liu Z (1994) Resolution of proteins on a phenyl-superose HR5/5 column and its application to examining the conformation homogeneity of refolded recombinant staphylococcal nuclease. J Chromatogr A 685:31–37

33. Geng X, Chang X (1992) High-performance hydrophobic interaction chromatography as a tool for protein refolding. J Chromatogr A 599:189–194

34. Geng X, Bai Q, Zhang Y, Li X, Wu D (2004) Refolding and purification of interferon-gamma in industry by hydrophobic interaction chromatography. J Biotechnol 113:137–149

35. Bai Q, Kong Y, Geng X (2003) Studies on renaturation with simultaneous purification of recombinant human proinsulin from *E. coli* with high performance hydrophobic interaction chromatography. J Liquid Chromatogr Related Technol 26:683–695

36. Jungbauer A, Machold C, Hahn R (2005) Hydrophobic interaction chromatography of proteins. III. Unfolding of proteins upon adsorption. J Chromatogr A 1079:221–228

37. Xiao Y, Jones T, Laurent A, O'Connell J, Przybycien T, Fernandez E (2007) Protein instability during HIC: hydrogen exchange labeling analysis and a framework for describing mobile and stationary phase effects. Biotechnol Bioeng 96:80–93

38. Jennissen H, Demiroglou A (2006) Interaction of fibrinogen with *n*-alkylagaroses and its purification by critical hydrophobicity hydrophobic interaction chromatography. J Chromatogr A 1109:197–213

39. O'Farrell PA (2004) Hydrophobic interaction chromatography. Methods Mol Biol 244:133–138

40. Queiroz JA, Tomaz CT, Cabral JMS (2001) Hydrophobic interaction chromatography of proteins. J Biotechnol 87:143–159

41. Kennedy R (1990) Hydrophobic chromatography. Methods Enzymol 182:339–343

42. Hjerten S (1973) Some general aspects of hydrophobic interaction chromatography. J Chromatogr A 87:325–331

43

Affinity Chromatography

Adam Charlton and Michael Zachariou

1. Introduction

Chromatographic processes allow the separation of small molecules or proteins based on a particular property such as size, polarity, or hydrophobicity. Separation is achieved by differential retardation of the passage of the various constituents of a mixture through a stationary medium. The degree of the retardation of a given entity will be proportional to the magnitude of the selection property for that entity. For example, a more hydrophobic molecule will have a stronger association with the long carbon chain of a reversed phase chromatographic support than will a more hydrophilic entity, thus the hydrophobic molecule will travel through the medium slower, permitting separation of the various species. The ligand-ligate interaction is the cornerstone of chromatographic binding or retardation of macromolecules. Traditionally, a ligand is the small molecule recognized by a ligate, but the more common modern usage, particularly as it applies to chromatography, defines the ligand as the immobilized component of the interaction that binds its ligate.

Rather than relying on a physiochemical property of a molecule or protein, affinity chromatography techniques exploit the specific interactions between certain biomolecules. Such interactions can be exquisitely selective, in many cases allowing for near homogenous recovery of the target protein from extremely complex media.

The predominant contemporary application of affinity chromatography principles is in the production of recombinant proteins, in which an engineered exogenous affinity tag can be translationally fused to the protein product *(1–3)*. This affinity tag can then be exploited for the capture of the protein. The approach has seen almost ubiquitous application in research-scale production of proteins and is making some inroads into biopharmaceutical production. Although affinity chromatography in its most literal guise does not seem to have widespread applicability in the biomedical arena, the core principle underlying affinity chromatography, that of immobilization to a solid support of ligands specific for a particular target, is at the heart of many medically related high-throughput diagnostic technologies. The exquisite selectivity

From: *Molecular Biomethods Handbook, 2nd Edition.*
Edited by: J. M. Walker and R. Rapley © Humana Press, Totowa, NJ

of affinity technologies should lend them to application for the detection of specific disease biomarkers. With increases in the versatility and sensitivity of such high-throughput proteomic technologies their role should only gain prevalence as the pattern of changes to the protein composition of normal and disease state tissues and serum proteins become better understood.

Unlike recombinant protein production, in which the desired affinity can be selected from any natural protein ligand/ligate interaction, diagnostic techniques must display discrimination between naturally occurring protein biomarkers. This discriminating power may be derived from a property of the proteins themselves, or introduced into the system by an antibody of appropriate specificity. As such, there are certain key areas for the application of affinity chromatography in the medical diagnostic field. These include the specific purification of phosphoproteins, glycoproteins and antibodies, each of which will be discussed in this chapter. It must be noted that the basic methods presented in this chapter are intended as a conceptual guide to visualise the technique being discussed; they should not supplant the manufacturer's directions accompanying any materials or reagents.

2. Affinity Chromatography Media

2.1. Affinity Chromatography Interactions

At the heart of all affinity chromatographies is, an affinity interaction. A true affinity interaction is the specific interaction between two biomolecules, the classic example being the antibody–antigen interaction, although countless others exist in nature.

Any binding interaction is always an equilibrium between the formation of the ligand-ligate complex and the free ligand and ligate. The rate at which the ligand-ligate complex is formed is known as the rate of association (k_1) and the rate at which the complex breaks down into free ligand and ligate is the rate of dissociation (k_{-1}). The strength of a binding interaction is given by its dissociation constant, K_d. K_d is measured in molar and is calculated by dividing the rate of dissociation (k_{-1}) by the rate of association (k_1). So for a strong binding interaction, where the interaction is likely to associate quickly (large k_1) and dissociate slowly (small k_{-1}), the dissociation constant ($K_d = k_{-1}/k_1$) will therefore be very small. The smaller the K_d, the tighter the binding interaction, with sub-nanomolar values not uncommon. Examples of binding interactions frequently employed in chromatography, and the K_d range in which they operate, are shown in **Fig. 43.1**.

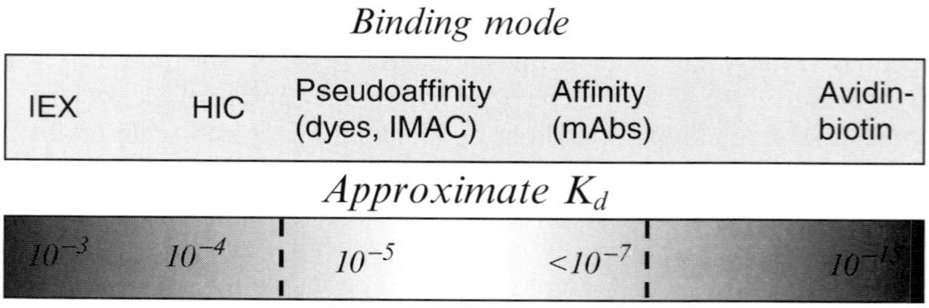

Binding mode

IEX	HIC	Pseudoaffinity (dyes, IMAC)	Affinity (mAbs)	Avidin-biotin

Approximate K_d

| 10^{-3} | 10^{-4} | 10^{-5} | $<10^{-7}$ | 10^{-15} |

Fig. 43.1. Common biological and chromatographic binding interaction and the approximate Kd at which they operate. The typical K_d range for affinity chromatography is shown between the dotted lines

An affinity interaction that can be used for a chromatographic process must be sufficiently strong to enable capture of the ligate, but also sufficiently weak so as to allow the captured biomolecules to be recovered at the completion of the purification process. Broadly speaking, affinity chromatography therefore usually operates in the range of K_d between 10^{-4}–10^{-8}.

2.2. Physical Composition of Affinity Chromatography Supports

2.2.1. Support Structures

A chromatographic support is created by immobilisation of the ligand at the heart of the interaction to a stationary (solid) support or phase matrix. This holds the ligands in one place and allows the mobile (liquid) phase containing the biomolecules of interest to pass over the ligands, sampling them for binding recognition. In this manner the variations in conditions required for the various washes and elution discussed in later sections are readily performed.

The stationary supports for any chromatographic processes fall into two broad categories, being either flat membranes/surfaces or microscopic resins (beads). Resins may be composed of either derivatives of natural substances such as agarose or silica or entirely synthetic. Membranes on the other hand are exclusively synthetic. A schematic representation of this appears as **Fig. 43.2**, and features some of the more common resin matrix compositions.

2.2.2. Spacer Arm Considerations

An important, but often overlooked, aspect in the construction of a chromatographic support is that of the spacer arm. The role of the spacer arm is particularly vital to an affinity chromatography system. A spacer arm provides some physical distance between the stationary support matrix and the ligand. This distance minimizes steric inhibition on the binding interaction that would be imposed by the large support substructure.

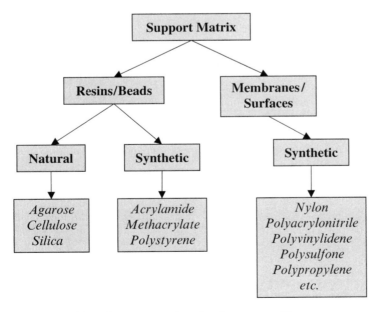

Fig. 43.2. Composition of support matrices for chromatographic processes

Spacer arms are usually a long carbon chain with the general structure $H_2N-(CH_2)_n-X$, where X = -COOH or –NH2 (for subsequent ligand coupling, see Section 2.2.3) and "n," or the length of the carbon chain, is between 2 and 12. As a general rule, the longer the carbon chain the better the reduction in steric hindrance to binding, but a longer carbon chain will also increase the likelihood of nonspecific interactions between it and the biomolecules of the sample. Spacer arms are can be incorporated simultaneously with ligand coupling by the selection of an appropriate activating agent (*4*).

2.2.3. Coupling Chemistries

Coupling of affinity ligands to stationary matrices is achieved via activatable reactive groups that are present in the chemical composition of the matrix itself. For example, the repeating subunit of agarose, shown in **Fig. 43.3**, contains many activatable hydroxyl groups. The choice of the activating agent is limited only to the type of activatable groups that are present on the support matrix of choice and the expected operating parameters of the final

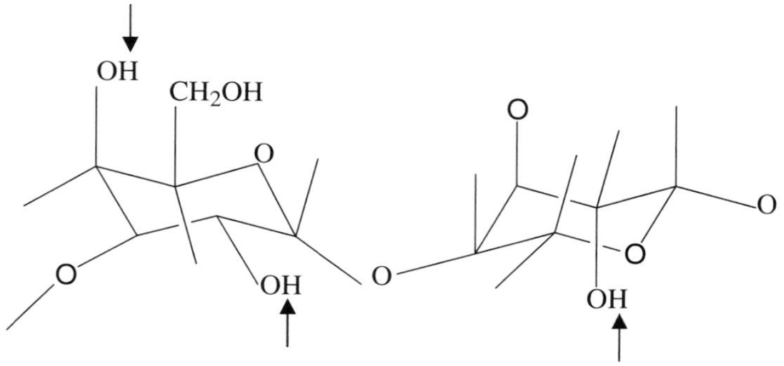

Fig. 43.3. The repeating subunits of Agarose. The activatable hydroxyls are indicated with an arrow

Table 43.1. Properties of common activation chemistries.

Activation reagent	Incubation for activation (h)	Bond type between gel and activator	Activation stability	Suitability for coupling to:			
				Amine	Hydroxyl	Thiol	Phenol
Glutaraldehyde	5–18	Alkylamine	Excellent	Y			
Tosyl chloride	0.5–0.8	Alkylamine or -thiol	Good	Y		Y	
Trichloro-s-triazine	0.5–2	Triazinyl	Good	Y	Y	Y	
carbonyldiimidazole	0.2–0.4	N-substituted carbamate	Stable with <pH 10	Y			
bisepoxirane	5–18	ether	Excellent	Y	Y	Y	
Cyanogen bromide	0.2–0.4	Isourea derivative, carbamate	Stable between pH 5–10	Y			
hydrazine	1–3	Amide	Excellent	Y	Y		
Diazonium	0.5–1.0	Azo	Good	Y			Y
N-hydroxysuccinimide	0.2–1.0	ester	Good	Y			

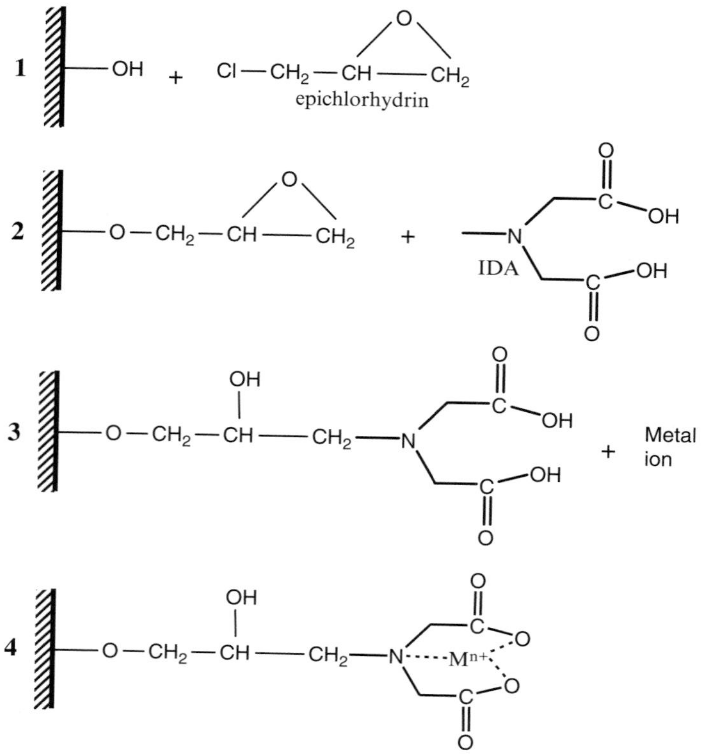

Fig. 43.4. Coupling of an iminodiacetic acid (IDA) chelator to a stationary support via epoxide activation of hydroxyls. (1) At pH10–11 the epichlorhydrin will form an ether bond with the support matrix by reaction with the hydroxyl moiety. (2) pH>9 will cause the ring structure to open, allowing attachment of the IDA group through an amide bond. (3) Charging the chelator with a metal ion creates the completed immobilised metal chelate complex (IMCC) shown in (4) with a three carbon spacer arm *(4)*

process. For example, cyanogen bromide activation, while broadly applicable for a range of biomolecules and relatively mild on both ligand and support, is unstable and prone to breakdown outside of pH 5–10 *(4)*. Some of the more common activating agents are shown in **Table 43.1**.

Consideration of the available activatable groups on the biomolecular ligand is also required. The surface amino acids of proteins display many such potential groups; the amines of lysine residues or N-termini, the hydroxyls of serines or free thiols of unpaired cysteines are some examples. The activation process is exemplified in **Fig. 43.4**, showing the generation of an immobilised metal chelate complex (IMCC), the stationary support for immobilised metal affinity chromatography (IMAC), via epoxy activation of hydroxyl groups.

3. Affinity Chromatography of Phosphoproteins

3.1. Introduction to Phosphoproteins

The post-translational modification of proteins by attachment of a phosphate moiety to specific amino acids, nominally at serine, threonine, or tyrosine in eukaryotes *(5)*, is of particular interest in the postgenomic era. The phosphorylation of proteins is modulated by the activity of the class of enzymes known collectively as kinases and phosphatases for the respective addition and removal of the phosphate groups. Phosphorylation represents the most prevalent of the limited number of reversible post-translational modifications *(5)*. As a potent effector of protein function, phosphorylation can be thought of as a functional "switch" for protein activity, conclusively and reversibly activating or deactivating key proteins in cellular pathways. In fact, it has been asserted that the activity of a phosphorylation regulated protein is far more dependent on its phosphorylation state than even its overall expression level *(6)*. Phosphorylation therefore plays an important part in the regulation of many cellular processes from cell division *(7–8)* and differentiation *(9)* through signal transduction *(10)* and gene expression *(11)* to apoptosis *(12–13)*.

With the pervasiveness of protein phosphorylation events, and their role in the activation of intracellular signalling pathways *(14)*, it is of little surprise that differential protein phosphorylation has been observed in a large number of disease states, either as a causative agent or as an indicator of other dysfunction. Although the transient and largely intracellular nature of phosphorylation events has limited their use as disease biomarkers, proteomic approaches to cellular analyses are beginning to make this approach feasible.

3.2. Phosphoproteins in Pathology

Pathologically relevant, aberrant phosphorylation is unlikely to be isolated to a single protein, but is instead thought of as an alteration in the pattern of phosphorylation to a range of proteins in the disease state. For example, there is direct evidence for an altered, tumor specific, proteome present in certain forms of breast and liver cancer, distinctly altered from that of the equivalent normal cells *(15)*.

With the impact of phosphorylation events in the signalling control of both cellular proliferation and apoptosis it is of very little surprise that defects in phosphorylation are implicated in the pathogenesis of a variety of cancers. It has been postulated that deregulation of kinase activity may be the cause of many cancer progressions, being among the first of the many steps in tumorigenesis *(14)*. Even the action of the classic tumor regulator protein, p53, is thought to be modulated via phosphorylation events *(16–19)*. In fact, over 50% of all known kinases are thought to be involved in at least one form of cancer *(20)*. The impact of differential phosphorylations in various cancers are well documented indeed, with over 18,000 medline citations returned for "phosphorylation and cancer," and have been the subject of a number of recent reviews *(6,20–23)*.

The study of the role of phosphorylation in other disorders is somewhat less mature, but there is increasing evidence for its role in a number of neurodegenerative disorders such as Alzheimer's and Parkinson's diseases, among others *(23)*. Hyperphosphorylation of the microtubule associated *tau* protein is a prerequisite to the formation of the aggregates of the protein. Such aggregates are found in the paired helical filaments, one of the aberrant neuronal structures associated with Alzheimer's disease *(24–25)*. Conversely, a lack of phosphorylation of α-synuclein protein leads to intraneuronal aggregations observed in certain heritable forms of Parkinson's disease *(26–27)*. With advances in proteomic technologies *(28)*, it is likely that altered states of protein phosphorylation will be found to be present in an increasing range of pathological states.

3.3. Purification of Phosphoproteins by Immobilized Metal Affinity Chromatography

In most biological preparations the abundance of phosphoproteins will be comparatively low compared to the total protein content of the sample. As a result, observations of phosphoproteins will be considerably simplified by increasing relative concentration of phosphoproteins in the sample. Selective purification of phosphorylated proteins in a biological sample can be accomplished by a derivation of immobilized metal affinity chromatography (IMAC) technology. IMAC is achieved by using a chelating agent immobilized on a stationary surface to capture a metal ion and form an immobilized metal chelate complex (IMCC). The traditional application of IMAC selects proteins based on their histidine content, exploiting the preference of borderline Lewis metal ions such as Cu^{2+}, Ni^{2+}, Zn^{2+} to accept electrons from borderline Lewis bases such as histidine *(29)*. This results in a co-ordination bond between the imide nitrogen of the histidine side-chain to the free co-ordination sites around the chelated metal ion. Elution of the bound proteins can be enacted by the use of imidazole, the functional moiety of histidine, which will competitively interfere with the IMCC-histidine interaction. Alternatively, the pH may be decreased to <pH 6.5 to prevent histidine, with side-chain pKa of 6.0, from donating electrons thereby inducing elution of the bound protein.

This core IMAC principle was extended to the selective purification of phosphorylated peptides and proteins, by replacing the above borderline Lewis metal ion with a hard Lewis metal ion such as Fe^{3+}, Al^{3+}, or Ga^{3+} *(30–31)*. Instead of displaying affinity for nitrogens, such as in the imide group of histidine, this group of metal ions shows preferential binding of oxygens, such as that in phosphate groups *(32)* or in the side-chains of aspartate and glutamate *(33)*.

3.4. Basic Strategy for the Purification of Phosphoproteins

3.4.1. Media Selection

Select a stationary support appropriate to the application, for example; magnetic beads for plate-screening assay format, agarose/Sepharose beads for preparative columns and macroporous or silica supports for high-pressure analytical application. The support must display a chelating ligand, with iminodiacetic acid (IDA) or nitrilotriacetic acid (NTA) the most common in commercial products. Both chelators have been employed successfully in phosphoprotein enrichments, but lower nonspecific binding has been shown with the NTA ligand *(34)*. This is thought to be due to either the lower metal leaching from the tighter binding tetradentate NTA chelator, with free chelator groups responsible for nonspecific binding *(32)*, or that simply the two remaining co-ordination sites around the metal ion remaining imposes more stringent binding than the three available in the IDA chelator *(34–35)*.

3.4.2. Charging the Medium

Strip any existing metal ions from the stationary support with $0.1M$ EDTA, $0.5M$ NaCl, pH7–8. Wash the support thoroughly with water and equilibrate into $0.1M$ acetic acid (pH<3.5). Charge the support with $0.1M$ $FeCl_3$ in $0.1M$ acetic acid. Wash away unbound metal ions with further washes of $0.1M$ acetic acid.

3.4.3. Sample Preparation and Loading

Follow a preferred tissue/cellular lysis technique to extract the proteins from the desired source. Avoid the carry-over of phosphate containing buffers into the final sample preparation, as these will competitively interfere with phosphoprotein binding to the IMCC. The sample must not contain EDTA or other chelators, as these will strip the metal ions from the support. If buffers containing such compounds are used, perform dialysis to remove them before sample loading. Likewise, avoid the use of phophatase inhibitors that contain sodium orthovanadate, as this will interfere with binding (36); consider sodium fluoride for this purpose instead. The final sample preparation should ideally contain $0.1M$ acetic acid with pH< 3.5. If possible, the total protein concentration should be below 0.1 mg/ml. This will reduce the formation of protein complexes that can result in reduced binding of phosphoproteins as surface phosphates are masked in the complexes. This should also reduce the incidence of copurification of unphosphorylated proteins that may be associated with phosphorylated species in protein aggregates (37).

Apply the prepared sample to the stationary support. Sufficient contact time should be provided for maximum binding; approx 30 min contact time at room temperature should be adequate, although incubations of up to 16 h have been reported (38). Attention should be paid to the stability of the proteins during prolonged incubations, should degradation be observed, conduct the binding at 4°C. For columns, slow linear velocities of between 15 cm/h (31) and 75 cm/h (32) have been used.

3.4.4. Washing

Contamination of the final sample through the nonspecific binding of unphosphorylated proteins can be minimized by washing the column before sample elution. Such nonspecific interactions can be through electrostatic or hydrophobic binding of proteins to the IMCC, free chelator or the spacer arm that separates the chelator from the support. The yield and purity of a particular target protein against the general phosphoprotein background can similarly be enhanced by a carefully selected washing strategy. Removal of hydrophobically bound contaminants has been successfully accomplished by the inclusion of 25–30% acetonitrile in $0.1M$ acetic acid (39–43) although an equivalent concentration of similar organic solvents could conceivably also be effective. Low concentrations, 0.25–2%, of nonionic (e.g., Tween-20) or zwitterionic detergent (e.g., CHAPS) may also be used to achieve this goal (37, 44). Electrostatic binding, particularly of acidic residues to the net positive charge of the metal-chelate complex, is considerably decreased by reducing the pH to less than 3 (45). Also, the inclusion of up to $1M$ NaCl can mitigate the effect of electrostatic binding (46). With detailed prior knowledge of the binding dynamics of a particular protein of interest, stringency washing can be used to improve final purity of that protein. By washing with conditions just outside the elution point of the target protein, the majority of less tightly bound undesired proteins can be excluded.

3.4.5. Elution

The final elution of the enriched phosphoproteins can be achieved by a variety of mechanisms. The most common mechanism is by increased pH, between 7.2 and 10.5, with pH 9.0 most frequently employed. This will disrupt the coordination bond with the metal ion *(31–32)*. Elution can also be effected by competitive interference with binding by the introduction of phosphate ions, akin to imidazole-mediated elution in traditional histidine-selection IMAC. The use of phosphate containing solutions for elution will have the added benefit of providing some buffering capacity at the lower end of the aforementioned elevated pH ranges. Both the increased pH and phosphate ion interference approaches are often used simultaneously for more complete elution in a single step. As a consequence, phosphate buffered saline (PBS) may be an effective eluent under most circumstances.

3.4.6. Media Regeneration

The IMAC supports can be regenerated for reuse by removing the metal ions using the stripping buffer used before the initial charge. The metal ion free support can then be subjected to biological decontamination regimes such as incubation in $1M$ sodium hydroxide for <2 hr or others, depending on the manufacturers recommendations.

4. Affinity Chromatography for Glycoprotein Purification

4.1. Introduction to Glycoproteins

The number of genes identified in the human genome not sufficient to explain diversity of function observed in the human proteome *(47)*. The added level of complexity is, in part, provided by the post-translational modification of proteins. Post-translational modifications are alterations that are made to a protein after it is synthesized, and include some 300 types identified to date *(47)*, a select few of these include; phosphorylation, acylation, methylation, and glycosylation.

One of the most ubiquitous and functionally diverse of the post-translational modifications are the glycosylations, with an estimated 50% of all human proteins bearing such additions *(48)*. The two main classes of glycosylations involve the attachment of a sugar moiety to the amide nitrogen of asparagine or to the hydroxyl oxygen of serine or threonine residues, giving rise to what are termed *N*- or *O*-linked glycosylations, respectively *(49)*. Having extensive intra- and extracellular functions, glycoproteins (also known as glycans) are often involved in mediating cell–cell interactions, in protein folding, targeting and trafficking and in the composition of cell-surface receptors *(50)*, to name a few. A classic example of the pervasiveness of glycosylations, and the impact of their variability are the differences in glycosylations that give rise to the human ABO red blood cell serotype groups *(51)*.

To successfully develop a glycoprotein separation regime, some knowledge of glycoprotein structure is required. Although a comprehensive review of the extremely complex process of protein glycosylation is well beyond the scope of this discussion, some key features are common to all and are summarised below. It should also be noted that the issue is further clouded by the fact that proteins may bear numerous different glycosylations at various sites on the protein and even variable glycosylations at any one given site, either form of heterogeneity give rise to different glycoforms of the one protein *(52)*.

The addition of the sugar moieties of *N*-linked glycosylation begin by attachment of *N*-acetylglucosamine (GlcNAc), which is "preloaded" with a branched structure of 2 GluNAc, 9 mannose and 3 glucose subunits, to an asparagine residue where it is situated in a motif of Asn-Xaa-(Ser/Thr), where

Xaa is any amino acid except Pro. Following attachment of this glycan precursor, further modifications to the sugar structure occurs, including removal of the glucose and some mannose subunits or addition of GlcNAc, galactose, sialic acid, or fucose units *(53–54)*. The additive sugar structures follow three basic designs; high-mannose, complex, or hybrid. High-mannose glycosylations consist of many mannose units added in a branched structure. Complex structures involve the linkages of any of the aforementioned saccharide units in two to four branched systems. These glycosylations often terminate with a sialic acid moiety. As suggested by its name, hybrid glycosylations are a mixture of high-mannose and complex structures. With a very few exceptions (see below) all circulating glycoproteins are of the *N*-linked type. The glycosylation pattern of proteins has a significant impact on their biological efficacy and circulating half-life. It is therefore of major significance to the production and application of therapeutic biopharmaceutical proteins.

O-linked glycosylations are much more complex, with a variety of sugars capable of initiating the glycan chain. Many of these serve primarily intracellular functions and may therefore be of limited applicability as diagnostic biomarkers. One specific type however, those of the *O-N-* acetylgalactosamine (GalNAc) family, often found in the extracellular matrix and the glycoproteins of mucosal secretions *(55)*, with immunoglobulin A and D also glycosylated in this fashion *(56–57)*. This subtype of *O*-linked glycosylations proceed from the initiating GalNAc by attachment of one of eight core polysaccharide motifs *(51,58–59)*, which may then be further extended by the addition of further galactose, GlcNAc, fucose or sialic acid groups *(50)*. *O*-linked glycans as a group are generally less branched than their *N*-linked counterparts, being either linear or diantennic. Another important group of circulating *O*-linked glycosylations are those of the epidermal growth factor-like domain, which occurs in proteins such as tissue-type plasminogen activator *(60)*, Factor VII *(61)*, Factor XII *(62)* and Factor IX *(63)*. These proteins have a (predominantly) single unit *O*-fucosylation *(64)*.

4.2. Glycoproteins in Pathology

Given the widespread impact that glycoproteins have on protein function and molecular recognition, it is of little surprise that variations in the glycosylation patterns of proteins are observed in a number of disease states. Although not commonly the direct causative agent of disorders themselves (except in the obvious case of the some 30 genetic disorders of glycoprotein biosynthetic pathways *(65)* there are a number of instances of differential glycosylation of proteins as a distinct biomarker of the presence of a disease or the extent of its progression, such as the many examples of altered glycosylation and cancer prognosis *(66–68)*. Some selected examples of altered glycosylation detected in disease states appears as **Table 43.2**.

4.3. Purification of Glycoproteins by Lectin Chromatography

The affinity purification of glycoproteins is made possible by exploiting the specific interaction of certain sugar motifs with a class of proteins known collectively as lectins. Individual lectins recognise a particular polysaccharide structure and thus can display quite exceptional specificity for a given type of glycan. For example, lentil lectin (LCA) binds branched mannose *N*-glycans,

Table 43.2. Selected examples of divergent glycosylation in diseases.

Disorder	Protein	Differential glycosylation	Reference
Hepatoma	γ-glutamyl transpeptidase	increased tri- and tetra-antennary branching	*(69)*
Prostate cancer	PSA	Increase in MAA lectin binding	*(70)*
Rheumatoid arthritis	IgG	devoid of galactose	*(71)*
adenocarcinoma (lung, colon, breast)	Normal fecal antigen 2	High-mannose and biantenntic (becomes Carcinoembryonic antigen (CEA), monitoring of prognosis after surgery	*(66)*
Breast carcinoma	various	increase in β1-6 branched N-linked glycoproteins in metastatic lymph nodes associated with poor prognosis	*(72)*
Choriocarcinoma	human chorionic gonadotropin	Devoid of sialic acid, unusual complex-type branching	*(73)*
Myeloma	IgG	change in the ratio of bisected to fucosylated glycans	*(74)*

but only when a fucose group is present on the first GlcNAc unit *(75)*. Lectins are commonly multimeric, with each subunit often providing carbohydrate binding capability, thus lectins are frequently di-to poly-valent *(76)*.

No single lectin can provide complete coverage of the full- range of human glycoproteins (the glycome), and with approximately 1,000 lectins isolated from plants alone, a comprehensive review of all available options is impossible *(77)*. However, some generalizations can be made, such as for serum glycoprotein preparation, which will contain a high proportion of *N*-linked glycans, the broadly specific Concanavalin A of *Canavalia ensiformis* (ConA) and wheat germ agglutinin (WGA) should provide reasonably comprehensive coverage. These lectins recognise either the *N*-linked branched mannoses with terminal mannose or glucose units in the case of ConA *(78)*, or the $(GlnNAc)_2$ core of *N*-glycans in the case of WGA *(79–80)*. See **Table 43.3** for a wider range of lectins *(75,81)*.

The selection of lectins for the majority of *O*- linked glycosylations will be more application specific, as no single lectin or limited subset will display broad enough specificity to cover the large degree of structural diversity in this group. However, the WGA discussed above does also bind sialic acid, a terminal constituent of many glycans, including *O*-linked *(82)*. It is also likely that any given glycoprotein will contain a range of different glycan structures, both *O*- and *N*-linked, so a general approach will often recognize a range of these proteins through one mechanism or another.

As stated above, some lectins are highly specific for particular glycan structures, so if knowledge of the glycan structure of a glycoprotein of interest is available, it is possible to develop strategies to make use of the exquisite selectivity that is offered by some lectins, producing a tailored affinity purification system to suit that glycoprotein. For example, the recognition of the "T-antigen" (sialic acid α2-6Galβ1-3GalNAcα1) on IgA and IgD by

Table 43.3. Selected examples of lectins for glycoprotein purification (Adapted from *76,84*).

Lectin	Abbreviation	Organism	Glycans recognized	Competitive elution with	Notes
Concanavalin A	ConA	*Canavalia ensiformis*	Biantennary and triantennary complex type *N*-glycans	≤0.5*M* methyl-α-D-glucoside	Reload with Mn$_2$ +if pH<5 used
Wheat Germ agglutinin	WGA	*Triticum vulgaris*	(GlnNAc)$_2$ of *N*-glycans, NeuNAc (sialic acid) of *N*- or *O*-glycans	≤0.5*M* GlcNAc	
Lentil	LCH	*Lens culinaris*	As for ConA but with GlcNAc core fucosylation	≤0.5*M* methyl-α-D-glucoside	Mn$_2$ + and Ca$_2$ + cofactors required if pH<5
Snowdrop	GNA (GNL)	*Galanthus nivalis*	α1-3 and α1-6 branched high mannose *N*-glycans	α-methyl mannoside	
Elderberry	SNA	*Sambucus nigra*	NeuNAcα2-6GalNAc of *O*-glycans	lactose	
Maackia amurensis	MAL	*Maackia amurensis*	NeuNAc/Gcα2-3 Galβ1-4GlcNAc of *O*-glycans	lactose	
Jacalin	AIL	*Artocarpus integrifolia*	NeuNAcα2-6Galβ1-3GalNAcα1 (Ser/Thr) of *O*-glycans	0.1*M* galactose	IgA/D binding
Peanut agglutinin	PNA	*Arachis hypogaea*	Galβ1-3 GalNAc (Ser/Thr) *O*-glycans	0.2*M* galactose	

the Jacalin lectin (AIL) of *Artocarpus integrifolia,* can be exploited for the specific purification of these glycoproteins *(83)*.

4.4. Basic Strategy for the Purification of Glycoproteins

4.4.1. Media Selection

This will be the most important step in achieving good enrichment of a specific target glycoprotein, as many individual lectins may have specificity for a relatively narrow range of glycosylation structures. Select either a lectin specific for the target glycoprotein or a broadly specific lectin such as ConA or WGA (see previous section).

4.4.2. Binding

The binding of glycoproteins to lectin-linked supports can occur at near physiological buffer conditions, i.e., 150 m*M* sodium chloride, pH 7.4 with an appropriate buffer such as 20 m*M*, HEPES or Tris-HCl. Avoid the use of phosphate buffers as these may interfere with the specific binding of the glycan with the lectin *(75)*.

4.4.3. Washing

Unbound material can be washed from the support by further application of the binding buffer. Due to the high affinity interaction between the lectin and saccharides, nonspecific binding to the actual ligand should be quite low, but non-specific binding events may take place between elements of the support itself such as the coupling point or spacer group.

4.4.4. Elution

Separation of various glycoproteins is possible by exploiting their differing affinities for a specific lectin. Introduction of an ideal carbohydrate ligate for the specific lectin ligand used (see **Table 43.3**) will compete with the bound glycoprotein for the lectin binding sites. By increasing the concentration of this entity in a step or linear gradient fashion, separation of mixtures of glyco-proteins can be achieved, as the absolute affinity for a single lectin will differ from protein to protein and glycan to glycan. Although bound glycoproteins can dissociated from the lectin by the use of low pH (<5.0), it should be noted that this may result in the loss of the metal cofactor required for some lectins to function (such as ConA, see **Table 43.3**) which will need to be recharged before subsequent use.

4.4.5. Media Regeneration

Being proteins, lectins are sensitive to extremes of conditions so harsh regen-eration regimes are not possible. A decrease in support performance over time may indicate residual protein binding. Tightly bound proteins may be removed by alternate application of 2–3 volumes of high pH (8.5) and low pH (5.5) buffers containing $0.5M$ NaCl **(84)**. The inclusion of low concentrations (0.1%) of nonionic detergent (Tween-20, Triton X-100) may also be useful.

4.4.6. Generation of Novel Lectin-Glycan Affinity Chromatographies

Separation systems to exploit novel lectin-glycoprotein affinities may be developed by directly coupling the specific lectin to a stationary support **(85)**, allowing for selectivity, more specifically tailored to the glycoproteins of one disease state. For example advanced glycation end products (AGEs), commonly associated with predominantly age related degenerations such as macular degeneration, atherosclerosis and Alzheimer's disease, as well as some diabetic complications **(85)**, are known to have affinity for the β-galactoside and galactose binding lectin, galectin-3 **(86)**.

The wide range of lectins available allows exquisite selectivity for specific glycoproteins of known structure. A little insight into the makeup of the par-ticular glycosylations on a protein of interest may yield large rewards in the selectivity of the purification process developed.

5. Affinity Chromatography for Antibody Purification

5.1. Introduction to Antibody-Based Diagnostic Technologies

Applications of antibody technology are the cornerstone of many of the most sensitive and conclusive diagnostic techniques available to modern biomedical science. Delivering quantifiable data and readily amenable to a high-throughput scale, antibody based assay techniques are indispensable in the detection and monitoring of many human disease states.

Antiserum based assay technologies can be applied to any disease state that either has an inflammatory component or to which an antigen can be isolated. In the former case, the immune response itself can be directly queried for dysfunction and in the latter, specific antisera can be raised in another species to detect the human disease biomarker antigen. Antibody based assays are already employed in the diagnosis and quantification of an extremely diverse range of disease biomarkers. Applications exist in the detection of infectious agents *(87–95)*, the diagnosis human disorders and inflammatory processes *(96–100)*, and in the quantification of cytokines *(101–103)* and hormones *(104–107)*, among many others. Antisera is also seeing application in the emerging high-throughput proteomic analyses, with antibody arrays being used in the characterization of the aberrant protein profiles observed in the serum or plasma samples of cancer patients *(108)*. Immunoglobin G (IgG) comprises 75% of plasma antibodies in humans *(109)* and mammalian IgG's form the basis of the majority of the aforementioned diagnostic applications. Humans have four subtypes of IgG *(109)* which, broadly speaking, act best against different types of antigens *(110)*. Of these four subtypes, IgG1 and IgG3 are commonly involved in T-cell mediated immune responses, and are directed against protein antigens such as those of viral or bacterial origin *(111)*. Conversely, IgG2 is associated with T-cell independent immune processes, and is more commonly raised against polysaccharides such as those of bacterial cell membranes *(112)*. IgG4 results from repeated or long-term antigenic exposure and may have a role in allergic sensitization *(113)*.

5.2. Purification of Antibodies by Protein A and Protein G Chromatography

The ability to produce purified IgG from serum is pivotal in the ongoing development of the existing and emerging biomedical applications. It is therefore fortunate that affinity purification of IgG can be achieved through the specific interaction between protein A of *Staphylococcus aureus* *(114,115)* or protein G of *Streptococcus* sp. *(116,117)* and the Fc portion of these antibodies. These two antibody binding proteins display different propensities to bind the antiserum of various mammalian species, and in some cases are even able to discriminate between IgG subtypes of one species (see **Table 43.4**). For example, protein A binds human IgG1, IgG2 and IgG4 equally effectively, but does not bind human IgG3 at all *(118)* so protein A affinity could be used if IgG3 is not implicated in a particular antigen recognition event, or to selectively exclude other IgG subtypes from a IgG3 preparation by their retardation by the protein A ligand. The subtype and species bias between protein A and protein G allow for tailored purification strategies where knowledge of the antibody subclass is available or preference is shown for an antiserum generating host species. Additionally, elution conditions from protein A do also tend to be milder than those required for protein G, maximizing the stability of the target immunoglobin.

The binding of antibodies to protein A or protein G supports can be used as a de facto antibody immobilization for the rapid generation of novel immunoaffinity systems. This can provide a confirmatory proof of concept for an affinity system before the development of direct antibody couplings *(84)*. Such protein A or G mediated couplings have the added advantage that binding is more readily reversible than most antibody–antigen interactions, allowing for the recovery of native protein–antibody complexes. Given that binding of an antibody to protein A or G occurs through the Fc region, which comprises the "stem" of the "Y" shaped antibody molecule, anchorage from this point helps to ensure that the antigen binding Fab regions are presented in the optimum configuration for subsequent binding events.

Table 43.4. IgG and subclasses of various species recognised by Protein A and Protein G (Adapted from *118*).

Species (subclass)	Protein A	Protein G
Human (IgG1)	++++	++++
Human (IgG2)	++++	++++
Human (IgG3)	–	++++
Human (IgG4)	++++	++++
Cow	++	++++
Dog	++	+
Goat	–	++
Guinea pig (IgG1)	++++	++
Guinea pig (IgG2)	++++	++
Hamster	+	++
Horse	++	++++
Rhesus monkey	++++	++++
Mouse (IgG1)	+	++++
Mouse (IgG2a)	++++	++++
Mouse (IgG2b)	+++	+++
Mouse (IgG3)	++	+++
Pig	+++	+++
Rabbit (all subtypes)	++++	+++
Rat (IgG1)	–	+
Rat (IgG2a)	–	++++
Rat (IgG2b)	–	++
Rat (IgG3)	+	++
Sheep	+/–	++

5.3. Basic Strategy for the Purification of Antibodies

5.3.1. Media Selection

Select a stationary support appropriate for the application, such as magnetic beads for high-throughput plate based screening of agarose/sepharose beads for preparative separations. Select either protein A or protein G coupled supports based on the species preference or the expected IgG subclass presented in **Table 43.4**. Given that the two most common circulating IgG subtypes in humans (IgG1 and IgG2, *119*) are recognized equally well by protein A and G; either is a valid choice for preliminary preparation of unknown antiserum.

5.3.2. Sample Preparation and Binding

Binding to Protein A or G supports occurs at physiological pH and ionic strength, so no sample pretreatment other than clarification is necessary. Selective binding may be possible by the addition of higher ionic strength buffers, such as sodium chloride up to 4*M*.

5.3.3. Washing

A buffer homologue of physiological conditions, such as Phosphate-buffered saline (PBS) can be used for the flowthrough of unbound proteins. Improved selectivity of the supports can be achieved for either protein A or G by the inclusion of increased levels of salts such as sodium chloride, with concentrations up to 4M possible (118). As with many chromatographic processes, product purity can be improved by approaching, but not exceeding, the expected elution conditions. Thus in this case a reduction in pH can provide a selective wash step, although care must be taken to avoid premature elution of the target antibody.

5.3.4. Elution

Elution from protein A and G columns are both enacted by decreasing pH (and ionic strength if used in the binding or wash step). Protein G will generally require more extreme conditions than protein A, but the absolute conditions will be application specific. As a rule of thumb, expected elution pH ranges will be 3.5–5 for protein A and 2.5–3.5 for protein G. The exposure of the purified antibodies to pH extremes can be minimized by collection of the eluant into strong buffer solutions such as 1M Tris-HCl, pH8.

5.3.5. Media Regeneration

Protein A and G are quite stable against relatively harsh support regeneration regimes. Hydrophobically bound contaminants can be removed by application of two volumes of low concentrations of nonionic detergent (0.1% Tween-20/Triton X-100) or up to 70% ethanol. Removal of precipitated protein, as implicated by decreased column flow or increased backpressure, may require the use of two volumes of 6M guanidine-HCl, or similar chaotropic denaturant. Any such treatments should be immediately washed from the support with phosphate-buffered saline. The contaminating biological load of the support can be reduced by sanitisation of the support. The support can be sanitised by incubation in 0.1M acetic acid in 20% ethanol for 6 or in 70% ethanol alone for 12 h.

5.3.6. Further Sample Purification Following Protein A or G Chromatography

Leached protein A, protein G or antibodies complexed with either, can be effectively removed from the bulk antiserum preparation by anion exchange chromatography. At pH 8.5, the protein A or G (or antibody complexes) will have much greater affinity for the ion-exchange ligands than will free antibodies. The free antibodies can often be collected in the flowthrough (unbound) of the column, or under quite low eluting salt levels.

6. Immunoaffinity Chromatography

6.1. Introduction to Immunoaffinity Diagnostic Technologies

The application of antibodies in the detection and quantification of many medically relevant molecular species was discussed in Section 5.1; however the use of antibodies is not limited merely to the analysis of samples or the assay of process outcomes. The precise selectivity of antibodies also renders them useful as a versatile platform for the rapid generation of novel affinity interactions. Antibodies, therefore, can function as affinity ligands for chromatographic processes in their own right.

Immunoaffinity chromatography has long been employed in the production of proteins for in vitro research. The introduction of ProteinChip technologies

(Ciphergen, Inc) coupled to the use of surface enhanced laser desorption/ionization (SELDI) mass spectrometry has seen immunoaffinity move rapidly into diagnostic application. ProteinChip technology entails "chips" of aluminium with an activated surface. This surface can contain a range of common traditional chromatographic ligands (ion-exchange, hydrophobic interaction) or affinity ligands such as IMAC. They are also available with activatable surfaces for in-house couplings, as discussed in Section 2. A useful proteomic application for ProteinChips is as a high-density capture substrate for SELDI mass spectrometry systems. This process uses laser activation of the surface (in this case the ProteinChip) to cause thermal ionisation of the biomolecules to make them available for mass spectrometry analysis.

Ideally, an antibody suitable as a ligate for any immunoaffinity chromatography application should have a relatively high K_d, allowing for more gentle elution conditions. Even more desirable is a tightly binding antibody that has a conformational or cofactor requirement, the alteration or exclusion of which can allow for very mild elution from a high-affinity interaction. The classic example of such an ideal interaction is that of the FLAG-tag peptide sequence and the M1 monoclonal antibody designated *(120)*. The recognition of the peptide epitope by the antibody occurs in a calcium-dependent manner *(121)*, thus the exclusion of this cofactor from the system by the addition of EDTA can permit mild elution *(122)*.

6.2. Applications of Immunoaffinity Interaction in Disease Diagnosis

Immunoaffinity chromatography has seen many applications in the monitoring of human health and disease states. A selection of these appears as **Table 43.5**. With novel proteomic approaches such as the aforementioned ProteinChip and SELDI systems already showing significant promise despite being in their relative infancy, the likelihood of the application of immunoaffinity protocols in future medical diagnostic technologies is high.

Table 43.5. Selected examples of immunoaffinity interaction diagnostic technologies.

Purpose	Marker	Notes	Reference
Prostate cancer diagnosis	Serum prostate-specific membrane antigen	ProteinChip capture for SELDI-TOF analysis	*(123)*
Lung cancer diagnosis	Vascular endothelial growth factor (VEGF)	Eight known isoforms, with several post-translational options. Change in isoform abundance profile indicative of disease.	*(124)*
Various, including cancer diagnosis	Ubiquitination state of proteins	Intracellular nature, detection in biological I fluids an indication of tissue damage.	*(125)*
Osteoarthritis diagnosis	Proteolytic fragments of Type-II collagen	Detection in the urine an indicator of pathology	*(126)*
Various liver disease diagnoses	des-gamma-carboxyprothrombin	Different post-translational modification profiles in liver cancer, acute and chronic hepatitis and cirrhosis	*(127)*
Environmental exposure	Polycyclic aromatic hydrocarbons (PAH)	PAH exposure of at risk factory workers detected in the urine	*(128)*

6.3. Basic Strategy for the Immunoaffinity Chromatography of Proteins

The physical conduct of an immunoaffinity separation will be highly dependent on the nature of the particular interaction of the antibody-antigen system being employed. As such, only the most generic highlights likely to be common to all can be presented here.

6.3.1. Media Selection

With a few commercially available exceptions, such as those against recombinant peptide tags like FLAG or hexahistidine, common interfering contaminants like albumin, or commonly separated proteins like cross-species immunoglobulins; the media for immunoaffinity chromatography will be developed in house based upon the chosen antiserum.

6.3.2. Binding

Due to the biological nature of the antibody–antigen interaction, physiological conditions will often prove successful. Some interactions may tolerate more extreme conditions, but this will again be particularly application specific.

6.3.3. Elution

Owing to the very strong binding of most antibody- antigen interactions, disruption of bond will quite often require denaturation of the tertiary structure of both the antibody and the target protein. This can be by the use of ionic detergents such as 1% sodium dodecyl sulphate, or chaotropic agents like $6M$ guanidine-HCL or $8M$ urea. This may not be significant, as in many diagnostic technologies such as mass spectrometry, the biological function of the protein is usually no longer of consequence. In some circumstances elution may be effected by competitive interference of the interaction by the addition of isolated epitope.

6.3.4. Media Regeneration

The reuse of the affinity medium will be quite dependent on the elution conditions employed in Section 5.3.3. For example, the elution of the target protein by denaturation of the antibody–antigen complex will have destroyed the antibody, so reuse will require coupling of fresh antiserum. Even in the case of competitive elution, the peptide mimetic of the target protein will most likely be (effectively) irreversibly bound, requiring stripping and recoupling with fresh antiserum.

References

1. Marston FA (1986) The purification of eukaryotic polypeptides synthesized in *Escherichia coli*. Biochem J 240:1–12
2. Uhlén M, Moks T (1990) Gene fusions for purpose of expression: an introduction. Methods Enzymol 185:129–143
3. Terpe K (2003) Overview of tag protein fusions: from molecular and biochemical fundamentals to commercial systems. Appl Microbiol Biotechnol 60:523–533
4. Hermanson GT, Mallia AK, Smith PK (1992) Immobilized affinity ligand techniques. Academic UK
5. Krebs EG, Beavo JA (1979) Phosphorylation-dephosphorylation of enzymes. Ann Rev Biochem 48:923–959
6. Lim YP (2005) Mining the tumor phosphoproteome for cancer markers. Clin Cancer Res 11:3163–3169

7. Le Breton M, Cormier P, Belle R, Mulner- Lorillon O, Morales J (2005) Translational control during mitosis. Biochimie 87:805–811

8. de Gramont A, Cohen-Fix O (2005) The many phases of anaphase. TIBS 30:559–568

9. Anneren C, Lindholm CK, Kriz V, Welsh M (2003) The FRK/RAKSHB signaling cascade: a versatile signal- transduction pathway that regulates cell survival, differentiation and proliferation. Current Mol Med 3:313–324

10. Hunter T (1995) Protein kinases and phosphatases: the Yin and Yang of protein phosphorylation and signaling. Cell 80:225–236

11. Holcik M, Sonenberg N (2005) Translational control in stress and apoptosis. Nat Rev Mol Cell Biol 6:318–327

12. Burlacu A (2003) Regulation of apoptosis by Bcl-2 family proteins. J Cell Mol Med 7:249–257

13. Amaravadi R, Thompson CB (2005) The survival kinases Akt and Pim as potential pharmacological targets. J Clin Invest 115:2618–2624

14. de Graauw M, Hensbergen P, van de Water B (2006) Phospho-proteomic analysis of cellular signalling. Electrophoresis 27:2676–2686

15. Lim YP, Wong CY, Ooi LL, Druker BJ, Epstein RJ (2004) Selective tyrosine hyperphosphorylation of cytoskeletal and stress proteins in primary human breast cancers: implications for adjuvant use of kinase-inhibitory drugs. Clin Cancer Res 10:3980–3987

16. Fiscella M, Ullrich SJ, Zambrano N, Shields MT, Lin D, Lees-Miller SP, Anderson CW, Mercer WE, Appella E (1993) Mutation of the serine 15 phosphorylation site of human p53 reduces the ability of p53 to inhibit cell cycle progression. Oncogene 8:1519–1528

17. Milne DM, Cambell LE, Cambell DG, Meek DW (1995) p53 is phosphorylated in vitro and in vivo by an ultraviolet radiation-induced protein kinase characteristic of the c-Jun kinase, JNK1. J Biol Chem 270:5511–5518

18. Kobayashi T, Sanbao R, Jabbur JR, Consoli U, Clodi K, Shiku H, Owen-Schaub LB, Andreeff M, Reed JC, Zhang W (1998). Differential p53 phosphorylation and activation of apoptosis-promoting genes Bax and Fas/APO-1 by irradiation and ara-C treatment. Cell Death Diff 5:584–591

19. Blume-Jensen P, Hunter T (2001) Oncogenic kinase signalling. Nature 411:355–365

20. Shimada K, Nakamura M, Ishida E, Konishi N (2006) Molecular roles of MAP kinases and FADD phosphorylation in prostate cancer. Histol Histopathol 21:415–422

21. Bosserhoff AK (2006) Novel biomarkers in malignant melanoma. Clin Chim Acta 367:28–35

22. Ostman A, Hellberg C, Bohmer FD (2006) Protein–tyrosine phosphatases and cancer. Nat Rev Cancer 6:307–320

23. Lee VMY, Goedert M (2001) Neurodegenerative tauopathies. Ann Rev Neurosci 24:1121–1159

24. Grundke-Iqbal I, Iqbal K, Quinlan M, Tung YC, Zaidi MS, Wisniewski HM (1986) Microtubule-associated protein *tau*. A component of Alzheimer paired helical filaments. J Biol Chem 261:6084–6089

25. Montejo de Garcini E, Serrano L, Avila J (1986) Self assembly of microtubule associated protein *tau* into filaments resembling those found in Alzheimer disease. Biochem Biophys Res Commun 141:790–796

26. Fujiwara H, Hasegawa M, Dohmae N, Kawashima A, Masliah E, Goldberg MS, Shen J, Takio K, Iwatsubo T (2002) α-Synuclein is phosphorylated in synuclein-opathy lesions. Nat Cell Biol 4:160–164

27. Wood-Kaczmar A, Gandhi S, Wood NW (2006) Understanding the molecular causes of Parkinson's disease. Trends Mol Med 12:521–528

28. Meri S, Baumann M (2001) Proteomics: posttranslational modifications, immune responses and current analytical tools. Biomol Eng 18:213–220

29. Porath J, Carlsson J, Olsson I, Belfrage G (1975) Metal chelate affinity chromatography a new approach to protein fractionation. Nature 258:598–599

30. Andersson LJ, Porath J (1986) Isolation of phosphoproteins by immobilized metal (Fe3+) affinity chromatography. Anal Biochem 154:250–254

31. Muszynska G, Andersson L, Porath J (1986) Selective adsorption of phosphoproteins on gel-immobilized ferric chelate. Biochemistry 25:6850–6853

32. Scanff P, Yvon M, Pelissier JP (1991) Immobilized Fe^{3+} affinity chromatographic isolation of phosphopeptides. J Chromatogr 539:425–432

33. Zachariou M, Hearn MTW (2000) Adsorption and selectivity characteristics of several human serum proteins with immobilised hard Lewis metal ion–chelate adsorbents. J Chromatogr A 890:95–116

34. Neville DCA, Rozanas CR, Price EM, Gruis DB, Verkman AS, Townsend RR (1997) Evidence for phosphorylation of serine 753 in CFTR using a novel metal-ion affinity resin and matrix-assisted laser desorption mass spectrometry. Protein Sci 6:2436–2445

35. Hochuli E, Dobeli H, Struber A (1987) New metal chelate adsorbents selective for proteins and peptides containing neighbouring histidine residues. J Chromatogr 411:177–184

36. Clontech Laboratories Inc (2006) TALON® PMAC Phosphoprotein Enrichment Kit User Manual

37. QIAgen (2006) PhosphoProtein handbook: for purification and detection of phosphorylated proteins from eukaryotic cells

38. Dubrovska A, Souchelnytskyi S (2005) Efficient enrichment of intact phosphorylated proteins by modified immobilized metal-affinity chromatography. Proteomics 5:4678–4683

39. Posewitz MC, Tempst P (1999) Immobilized gallium(III) affinity chromatography of phosphopeptides. Anal Chem 71:2883–2892

40. Stensballe A, Andersen S, Jensen ON (2001) Characterization of phosphoproteins from electrophoretic gels by nanoscale Fe(III) affinity chromatography with off-line mass spectrometry analysis. Proteomics 1:207–222

41. Ficarro SB, Salomon AR, Brill LM, Mason DE, Stettler-Gill M, Brock A, Peters EC (2005) Automated immobilized metal affinity chromatography/nano-liquid chromatography/electrospray ionization mass spectrometry platform for profiling protein phosphorylation sites. Rapid Commun Mass Spectrom 19:57–71

42. Nuhse TS, Stensballe A, Jensen ON, Peck SC (2003) Large-scale analysis of *in vivo* phosphorylated membrane proteins by immobilized metal ion affinity chromatography and mass spectrometry. Mol Cell Proteomics 2:1234–1243

43. Brill LM, Salomon AR, Ficarro SB, Mukherji M, Stettler-Gill M, Peters EC (2004) Robust phosphoproteomic profiling of tyrosine phosphorylation sites from human T cells using immobilized metal affinity chromatography and tandem mass spectrometry. Anal Chem 76:2763–2772

44. Guerrera IC, Predic-Atkinson J, Kleiner O, Soskic V, Godovac-Zimmermann J (2005) Enrichment of phosphoproteins for proteomic analysis using immobilized Fe(III)-affinity adsorption chromatography. J Proteome Res 4:1545–1553

45. Sigma-Aldrich Inc (2004) PHOS-Select™ Iron affinity gel: technical bulletin

46. Zachariou M, Hearn MTW (1996). Application of immobilized metal ion-chelate complexes as pseudocation exchange adsorbents for protein separation. Biochemistry 35:202–211

47. Jensen ON (2004) Modification-specific proteomics: characterization of post-translational modifications by mass spectrometry. Curr Opin Chem Biol 8:33–41

48. Wong CH (2005) Protein glycosylation: new challenges and opportunities. J Org Chem 70:4219–4225

49. IUPAC-IUB Joint Commission on Biochemical Nomenclature (JCBN). Biochemical nomenclature and related documents, 2nd edn. Portland Press, 1992, pp 84–89

50. Walsh G, Jefferis R (2006) Post-translational modifications in the context of thera-peutic proteins. Nat Biotech 24:1241–1252
51. den Steen PV, Rudd PM, Dwek RA, Opdenakker G (1998) Concepts and principles of O-linked glycosylation. Crit Rev Biochem Mol Biol 33:151–208
52. Rademacher TW, Parekh RB, Dwek RA (1988) Glycobiology. Ann Rev Biochem 57:785–838
53. Kornfeld R, Kornfeld S (1985) Assembly of asparagine-linked oligosaccharides. Annu Rev Biochem 54:631–664
54. Opdenakker G, Rudd PM, Ponting CP, Dwek RA (1993) Concepts and principles of glycobiology. FASEB J 7:1330–1337
55. Strous GJ Dekker J (1992) Mucin-type glycoproteins. Crit Rev Biochem Mol Biol 27:57–92
56. Mellis SJ, Baenziger JU (1983) Structures of the O-glycosidically linked oligosac-charides of human IgD. J Biol Chem 258:11557–11563
57. Mattu TS, Pleass RJ, Willis AC, Kilian M, Wormald MR, Lellouch AC, Rudd PM, Woof JM, Dwek RA (1998) The glycosylation and structure of human serum IgA1, Fab, and Fc regions and the role of N-glycosylation on Fc alpha receptor interac-tions. J Biol Chem 273:2260–2272
58. Hounsell EF, Davies MJ, Renouf DV (1996) O-linked protein glycosylation structure and function. Glycoconj J 13:19–26
59. Peter-Katalinio J (2005) Methods in enzymology: O-glycosylation of proteins. Methods Enzymol 405:139–171
60. Harris RJ, Leonard CK, Guzzetta AW, Spellman MW (1991) Tissue plasminogen activator has an O-linked fucose attached to threonine-61 in the epidermal growth factor domain. Biochemistry 30:2311–2314
61. Bjoern S, Foster DC, Thim L, Wiberg FC, Christensen M, Komiyama Y, Pedersen AH, Kisiel W (1991) Human plasma and recombinant factor VII. Characterization of O-glycosylations at serine residues 52 and 60 and effects of site-directed muta-genesis of serine 52 to alanine. J Biol Chem 266:11051–11057
62. Harris RJ, Ling VT, Spellman MW (1992) O-linked fucose in present in the first epidermal growth factor domain of factor XII but not protein C. J Biol Chem 267:5102–5107
63. Nishimura H, Takao T, Hase S, Shimonishi Y, Iwanaga S (1992) Human factor IX has a tetrasaccharide O-glycosidically linked to serine 61 through the fucose residue. J Biol Chem 267:17520–17525
64. Moloney DJ, Lin AI, Haltiwanger RS (1997) The O-linked fucose glycosylation pathway. Evidende for protein-specific elongation of O-linked fucose in Chinese hamster ovary cells. J Biol Chem 272:19046–19050
65. Freeze HH (2006) Genetic defects in the human glycome. Nat Rev Genetics 7:537–551
66. Fukushima K, Ohkura T, Kanai M, Kuroki M, Matsuoka Y, Kobata A, Yamashita K (1995) Carbohydrate structures of a normal counterpart of the carcinoembryonic antigen produced by colon epithelial cells of normal adults. Glycobiology 5:105–115
67. Hakomori S (1996) Tumor malignancy defined by aberrant glycosylation and sphingo(glyco)lipid metabolism. Cancer Res 56:5309–5318
68. Kobata A (1998) A retrospective and prospective view of glycopathology. Glycoconj J 15:323–331
69. Yamashita K, Totani K, Iwaki Y, Takamisawa I, Tateishi N, Higashi T, Sakamoto Y, Kobata A (1989) Comparative study of the sugar chains of 7-glutamyltranspep-tidases purified from human hepatocellular carcinoma and from human liver. J Biochem 105:728–735
70. Ohyama C, Hosono M, Nitta K, Oh-eda M, Yoshikawa K, Habuchi T, Arai Y, Fukuda M (2004) Carbohydrate structure and differential binding of prostate

specific antigen to *Maackia amurensis* lectin between prostate cancer and benign prostate hypertrophy. Glycobiology 14:671–679

71. Parekh RB, Dwek RA, Sutton BJ, Fernandes DL, Leung A, Stanworth D, Rademacher TW, Mizuochi T, Taniguchi K, Matsuta K, Takeuchi F, Nagano Y, Miyamoto T, Kobata A (1985) Association of rheumatoid arthritis and primary steoarthritis with changes in the glycosylation pattern of total serum IgG. Nature 316:452–457

72. Handerson T, Camp R, Harigopal M, Rimm D, Pawelek J (2005) 1,6-Branched oligosaccharides are increased in lymph node metastases and predict poor outcome in breast carcinoma. Clin Cancer Res 11:2969–2973

73. Mizuochi T, Nishimura R, Derappe C, Taniguchi T, Hamamoto T, Mochizuki M, Kobata A (1983) Structures of the Asparagine-linked Sugar Chains of Human Chorionic Gonadotropin Produced in Choriocarcinoma. J Biol Chem 258:14126–14129

74. Mizuochi T, Taniguchi T, Shimizu A, Kobata A (1982) Structural and numerical variations of the carbohydrate moiety of immunoglobulin G. J Immunol 129:2016–2020

75. QIAgen (2005). Qproteome Glycoprotein Fractionation Handbook

76. Lis H, Sharon N (1998) Lectins: carbohydrate-specific proteins that mediate cellular recognition. Chem Rev 98:637–674

77. Chandra NR, Kumar N, Jeyakani J, Singh DD, Gowda SB, Prathima MN (2006) Lectindb: a plant lectin database. Glycobiology 16:938–946

78. So LL, IJ Goldstein IJ (1968) Protein–carbohydrate interaction. XX. On the number of combining sites on concanavalin A, the phytohemagglutinin of the jackbean. Biochim Biophys Acta 165:398–404

79. Stein MD, Howard IK, Sage HJ (1971) Studies on a phytohemagglutinin from the lentil. IV. Direct binding studies of *Lens culinaris* hemagglutinin with simple saccharides. Arch Biochem Biophys 146:353–355

80. Debray H, Decout D, Strecker G, Spik G, Montreuil J (1981) Specificity of twelve lectins towards oligosaccharides and glycopeptides related to *N*-glycosyl-proteins. Eur J Biochem 117:41–55

81. Rudiger H, Gabius HJ (2002) Plant lectins: Occurrence, biochemistry, functions and applications. Glycoconj J 18:589–613

82. Goldstein IJ (2002) Lectin structure-activity: the story is never over. J Agric Food Chem 50:6583–6585

83. Roque-Barreira MC, Campos-Neto A (1985) Jacalin: an IgA-binding lectin. J Immunology 134:1740–1743

84. Amersham Biosciences (2002). Affinity chromatography: principles and methods. Edition AD

85. Singh R, Barden A, Mori T, Beilin L (2001) Advanced glycation end-products: a review. Diabetologia 44:129–146

86. Vlassara H, Li YM, Imani Y, Wojciechowicz D, Yang A, Liu FT, Cerami A (1995) Identification of galectin-3 as a high-affinity binding protein for advanced glycation end products (AGE): a new member of the AGE-receptor complex. Mol Med 1:634–646

87. Denoyel GA, Gaspar A, Nouyrigat C (1980). Enzyme immunoassay for measurement of antibodies to Herpes Simplex virus infection: comparison with complement fixation, immunofluorescent-antibody, and neutralization techniques. J Clin Microbiol 11:114–119

88. Welch PC, Masur H, Jones TC, Remington JS. Serologic diagnosis of acute lymphadenopathic toxoplasmosis. J Infect Dis 142:256–64

89. Booth JC, Hannington G, Bakir TMF, Stern H, Kangro H, Griffiths PD, Heath RB (1982) Comparison of enzyme-linked immunosorbent assay, radioimmunoassay, complement fixation, anticomplement immunofluorescence and passive haemagglutination techniques for detecting cytomegalovirus IgG antibody. J Clin Pathol 35:1345–1348

90. Steece RS, Talley MS, Skeels MR, Lanier GA (1985) Comparison of enzyme-linked immunosorbent assay, hemagglutination inhibition, and passive latex agglutination for determination of Rubella immune status. J Clin Microbiol 21:140–142

91. Loffeld RJLF, Flendrig JA, Stobberingh E, van Spreeuwel JP, Arends JW (1989) Diagnostic value of an immunoassay to detect anti Campylobacter pylori antibodies in non-ulcer dyspepsia. Lancet 1:1182–1185

92. Bantroch S, Buhler T, Lam JS (1994) Appropriate coating methods and other conditions for ELISA of smooth, rough and neutral LPS of *Pseudomonas aeruginosa*. Clin Diagn Lab Immunol 1:55–62

93. Moser M, Crameri R, Brust E, Suter M, Menz G (1994) Diagnostic value of recombinant Aspergillus fumigatus allergen I/a for skin testing and serology. J Allergy Clin Immunol 93:1–11

94. Verweij PE, Stynen D, Rijs AJMM, de Pauw BE, Hoogkamp-Korstanje JAA, Meis JFGM (1995) Sandwich enzyme-linked immunosorbent assay compared with Pastorex latex agglutination test for diagnosing invasive aspergillosis in immunocompromised patients. J Clin Microbiol 33:1912–1914

95. McHugh TM, Wang YJ, Chong HO, Blackwood LL, Stites DP (1989) Development of a microsphere based fluorescent immunoassay and it comparison to an enzyme immunoassay for the detection of antibodies to three preparations of *Candida albicans*. J Immunol Methods 116:213–219

96. Silver HKB, Gold P, Feder S, Freedman SO, Shuster J (1973) Radioimmunoassay for human alpha$_1$-fetoprotein. Proc Nat Acad Sci USA 70:526–530

97. Pacini F, Fontanelli M, Fugazzola L, Elisei R, Romei C, DiCoscio G, Miccoli P, Pinchera A (1994) Routine measurement of serum calcitonin in nodular thyroid diseases allows the preoperative diagnosis of unsuspected sporadic medullary thyroid carcinoma. J Clin Endocrinol Metab 78:826–829

98. Sulkanen S, Halttunen T, Laurila K, Kolho KL, Korponay-Szabo IR, Sarnesto A, Savilahti E, Collin P, Maki M (1998) Tissue transglutaminase autoantibody enzyme-linked immunosorbent assay in detecting celiac disease. Gastroenterology 115:1332–1328

99. Quinton JF, Sendid B, Reumaux D, Duthilleul P, Cortot A, Grandbastien B, Charrier G, Targan SR, Colombel JF, Poulain D (1998) Anti-*Saccharomyces cerevisiae* mannan antibodies combined with antineutrophil cytoplasmic autoantibodies in inflammatory bowel disease: prevalence and diagnostic role. Gut 42:788–791

100. Vincent C, Nogueira L, Sebbag M, Chapuy- Regaud S, Arnaud M, Letourneur O, Rolland D, Fournie B, Cantagrel A, Jolivet M, Serre G (2000) Detection of antibodies to deiminated recombinant rat filaggrin by enzyme-linked immunosorbent assay. Arthritis Rheum 46:2051–2058

101. Teppo AM, Maury CPJ (1987) Radioimmunoassay of tumor necrosis factor in serum. Clin Chem 33:2024–2027

102. Kahaleh MB, LeRoy EC (1989) Interleukin-2 in scleroderma: correlation of serum level with extent of skin involvement and disease duration. Ann Int Med 110:446–450

103. Sakamoto K, Arakawa H, Mita S, Ishiko T, Ikei S, Egami H, Hisano S, Ogawa M (1994) Elevation of circulating interleukin 6 after surgery: Factors influencing the serum level. Cytokine 6:181–186

104. Starr JI, Mako ME, Juhn D, Rubenstein AH (1978) Measurement of serum proinsulin-like material: cross-reactivity of porcine and human proinsulin in the insulin radioimmunoassay. J Lab Clin Med 91:691–692

105. Bouillon R, Coopmans W, Deqroote DEH, Radoux D, Ellard PH (1990) Immunoradiometric assay of parathyrin with polyclonal and monoclonal region-specific antibodies. Clin Chem 36:271–276

106. Breier M, Gallaher BW, Gluckman PD (1991) Radioimmunoassay for insulin-like growth factor-I: solutions to some potential problems and pitfalls. J Endocrinol 128:347–357

107. Reutens AT, Hoffman DM, Leung KC, Ho KKY (1995) Evaluation and application of a highly sensitive assay for serum growth hormone (GH) in the study of adult GH deficiency. J Clin Endocrinol Metab 80:480–485

108. Haab BB (2005) Antibody arrays in cancer research. Mol Cell Proteomics 4:377–383

109. Spiegelberg HL (1974) Biological activities of Igs of different classes and subclasses. Adv Immunol 19:259–294

110. Burton DR, Woof JM (1992) Human antibody effector function. Adv Immunol 51:1–84

111. Ferrante A, Beard LJ, Feldman RG (1990) IgG subclass distribution of antibodies to bacterial and viral antigens. Pediatr Infect Dis J 9:S16–24

112. Siber GR, Schur PH, Aisenberg AC, Weitzman SA, Schiffman G (1980) Correlation between serum IgG2 concentrations and the antibody response to bacterial polysaccharide antigens. New Engl J Med 303:178–182

113. Aalberse RC, Van der Gaag R, Van Leeuwen J (1983) Serological aspects of IgG4 antibodies I. Prolonged immunisation results in an IgG4-restricted response. J Immunol 130:722–726

114. Bjork I, Petersson BA, Sjoquist J (1972). Some physiochemical properties of protein A from *Staphylococcus aureus*. Eur J Biochem 29:579–584

115. Sjoquist J, Meloun B, Hjelm H (1972). Protein A isolated from *Staphylococcus aureus* after digestion with lysostaphin. Eur J Biochem 29:572–578

116. Bjorck L, Kronvall G (1984). Purification and some properties of streptococcal protein G, a novel IgG-binding reagent. J Immunol 133:969–974

117. Akerstrom B, Brodin T, Reis K, Bjorck L (1985). Protein G: a powerful tool for binding and detection of monoclonal and polyclonal antibodies. J Immunol 135:2589–2592

118. Amersham Biosciences (2002) Antibody Purification Handbook. Edition AC

119. French MAH, Harrison G (1984) Serum IgG subclass concentrations in healthy adults: a study using monoclonal antisera. Clin exp Immunol 56:473–475

120. Hopp TP, Pricket KS, Price VL, Libby RT, March CJ, Ceretti DP, Urda DL, Conlon PJ (1988) A short polypeptide marker sequence useful for recombinant protein identification and purification. Bio/Technology 6:1204–1210

121. Hope TP, Gallis B, Prikett KS (1996) Metal-binding properties of a calcium dependent monoclonal antibody. Mol Immunol 33:601–608

122. Prickett KS, Amberg DC, Hopp TP (1989) A calcium-dependent antibody for identification and purification of recombinant proteins. Biotechniques 7:580–589

123. Xiao Z, Adam BL, Cazares LH, Clements MA, Davis JW, Schellhamme PF, Dalmasso EA, Wright GL Jr (2001) Quantitation of serum prostate-specific membrane antigen by a novel protein biochip immunoassay discriminates benign from malignant prostate disease. Cancer Res 61:6029–6033

124. Landuyta B, Jansenb J, Wildiersa H, Goethalsc L, De Boecka G, Highleya M, van Oosteroma AT, Tjadend U, Guetensa G, de Bruijna EA (2003) Immuno affinity purification combined with mass spectrometry detection for the monitoring of VEGF isoforms in patient tumor tissue. J Sep Sci 26:619–623

125. Vasilescu J, Smith JC, Ethier M, Figeys D (2005) Proteomic analysis of ubiquitinated proteins from human MCF-7 breast cancer cells by immunoaffinity purification and mass spectrometry. J Proteome Res 4:2192–2200

126. Berna M, Schmalz C, Duffin K, Mitchell P, Chambers M, Ackermann B (2006) Online immunoaffinity liquid chromatography/tandem mass spectrometry determination of a type II collagen peptide biomarker in rat urine: Investigation of the impact of collision-induced dissociation fluctuation on peptide quantitation. Anal Biochem 356:235–243

127. Uehara S, Gotoh K, Handa H, Tomita H, Senshuu M (2005) Distribution of the heterogeneity of des-gamma-carboxyprothrombin in patients with hepatocellular carcinoma. J Gastroenterol Hepatol 20:1545–52

128. Bentsen-Farmer RK, Botnen IV, Noto H, Jacob J, Ovrebo S (1999) Detection of polycyclic aromatic hydrocarbon metabolites by high-pressure liquid chromatography after purification on immunoaffinity columns in urine from occupationally exposed workers. Int Arch Occup Environ Health 72:161–8

44

High Performance Liquid Chromatography (HPLC) of Peptides and Proteins

Tzong-Hsien Lee and Marie-Isabel Aguilar

1. Introduction and Theoretical Considerations

The introduction of high performance liquid chromatography (HPLC) to the analysis of peptides and proteins some 25 yr ago revolutionized the biological sciences by enabling the rapid and sensitive analysis of peptide and protein structure in a way that was inconceivable 30 yr ago. Today, HPLC in its various modes has become the pivotal technique in the characterization of peptides and proteins and has therefore played a critical role in the development of peptide and protein-based pharmaceuticals. The extraordinary success of HPLC can be attributed to a number of factors. These include 1) the excellent resolution that can be achieved under a wide range of chromatographic conditions for very closely related molecules as well as structurally quite distinct molecules; 2) the experimental ease with which chromatographic selectivity can be manipulated through changes in mobile phase characteristics; 3) the generally high recoveries and hence high productivity and 4) the excellent reproducibility of repetitive separations carried out over a long period of time, which is due partly to the stability of the sorbent materials under a wide range of mobile phase conditions.

HPLC is extremely versatile for the isolation of peptides and proteins from a wide variety of synthetic or biological sources. The complexity of the mixture to be chromatographed will depend on the nature of the source and the degree of preliminary clean-up that can be performed. In the case of synthetic peptides, RPC is generally employed both for the initial analysis and the final large scale purification. The isolation of proteins from a biological cocktail however, often requires a combination of techniques to produce a homogenous sample. HPLC techniques are then introduced at the later stages following initial precipitation, clarification and preliminary separations using soft gel. Purification protocols therefore need to be tailored to the specific target molecule.

Reversed phase chromatography (RPC) is by far the most commonly used mode of separation for peptides, although ion-exchange (IEC) and size exclusion (SEC) chromatography also find application. The three dimensional structure of proteins can be sensitive to the often harsh conditions employed in

From: *Molecular Biomethods Handbook, 2nd Edition.*
Edited by: J. M. Walker and R. Rapley © Humana Press, Totowa, NJ

RPC, and as a consequence, RPC is employed less for the isolation of proteins where it is important to recover the protein in a biologically active form. IEC, SEC affinity chromatography are therefore the most commonly used modes for proteins, but RPC and hydrophobic interaction (HIC) chromatography are also employed. In addition, each mode of chromatography can be operated at different level of loading from capillary formats to large scale process systems.

An appreciation of the factors that control the resolution of peptides and proteins in interactive modes of chromatography can assist in the development and manipulation of separation protocols to obtain the desired separation. The capacity factor k' of a solute can be expressed in terms of the retention time t_r, through the relationship

$$k' = (t_r - t_o) / t_o \tag{1}$$

where t_0 is the retention time of a nonretained solute. The practical significance of k' can be related to the selectivity parameter α, defined as the ratio of the capacity factors of two adjacent peaks as follows

$$\alpha = k'_i / k'_j \tag{2}$$

which allows the definition of a chromatographic elution window in which retention times can be manipulated to maximize the separation of components within a mixture.

The optimization of high resolution separations of peptides and proteins involves the separation of sample components through manipulation of both retention times and solute peak shape. The second factor that is involved in defining the quality of a separation is therefore the peak width σ_t. The degree of peak broadening is directly related to the efficiency of the column and can be expressed in terms of the number of theoretical plates, N, as follows

$$N = (t_r)^2 / \sigma_r^2 \tag{3}$$

N can also be expressed in terms of the reduced plate height equivalent h, the column length L and the particle diameter of the stationary phase material d_p, as

$$N = hL / d_p \tag{4}$$

The resolution, R_s, between two components of a mixture therefore depends on both selectivity and bandwidth according to

$$R_s = 1/4\sqrt{N}(\alpha - 1)[1/(1 + k')] \tag{5}$$

This equation describes the relationship between the quality of a separation and the relative retention, selectivity and the bandwidth and also provides the formal basis upon which resolution can be manipulated to achieve a particular level of separation. Thus, when faced with an unsatisfactory separation, the aim is to improve resolution by one of three possible strategies: the first is to increase α, the second is to vary k' within a defined range normally $1 < k' < 10$, or third to increase N, for example, by using very small particles in narrow bore columns.

The challenge facing the scientist who wishes to analyze and/or purify their peptide or protein sample is the selection of the initial separation conditions and subsequent optimization of the appropriate experimental parameters. This chapter provides an overview of the different techniques used for the analysis and purification of peptides and proteins and the experimental options available to achieve a high resolution separation of a peptide or protein mixture. The interested reader is also referred to a number of publications that provide a comprehensive theoretical and practical overview of this topic (1–6).

2. Methods

2.1. Reversed Phase Chromatography

Reversed phase high performance liquid chromatography (RPC) involves the separation of molecules on the basis of hydrophobicity. The separation depends on the hydrophobic binding of the solute molecule from the mobile phase to the immobilized hydrophobic ligands attached to the stationary phase, i.e., the sorbent. The solute mixture is initially applied to the sorbent in the presence of aqueous buffers, and the solutes are eluted by the addition of organic solvent to the mobile phase. Elution can proceed either by isocratic conditions where the concentration of organic solvent is constant, or by gradient elution whereby the amount of organic solvent is increased over a period of time. The solutes are therefore eluted in order of increasing molecular hydrophobicity.

The RPC experimental system for the analysis of peptides and proteins usually consists of an n-alkylsilica-based sorbent from which the solutes are eluted with gradients of increasing concentrations of organic solvent such as acetonitrile containing an ionic modifier such as trifluoroacetic acid (TFA) (7,8). Complex mixtures of peptides and proteins can be routinely separated and low picomolar–femtomolar amounts of material can be collected for further characterization. Separations can be easily manipulated by changing the gradient slope, the operating temperature, the ionic modifier or the organic solvent composition.

The extensive use of RPC for the purification of peptides, small polypeptides with molecular weights up to 10,000 Da, and related compounds of pharmaceutical interest has not been replicated to the same extent for larger polypeptides (molecular mass >10,000 Da) and globular proteins. The combination of the traditionally used acidic buffering systems and the hydrophobicity of the n-alkylsilica supports that can result in low mass yields or the loss of biological activity of larger polypeptides and proteins have often discouraged practitioners from using RPC methods for large scale protein separations. The loss of enzymatic activity, the formation of multiple peaks for compositionally pure samples and poor yields of protein can all be attributed to the denaturation of protein solutes during the separation process using RPC (9,10).

2.1.1. Stationary Phases

The most commonly employed experimental procedure for the RPC analysis of peptides and proteins generally involves the use of an octadecylsilica based sorbent and a mobile phase (11). The chromatographic packing materials that are generally used are based on microparticulate porous silica, which allows the use of high linear flow velocities resulting in favorable mass transfer properties and rapid analysis times. The silica is chemically modified by a derivatized silane bearing an n-alkyl hydrophobic ligand. The most commonly used ligand is *n*-octadecyl (C18), while *n*-butyl (C4) and *n*-octyl (C8) also find important application and phenyl and cyanopropyl ligands can provide different selectivity. The process of chemical immobilization of the silica surface results in approximately half of the surface silanol group being modified. The sorbents are therefore generally subjected to further silanization with a small reactive silane to produce an end-capped packing material. The type of *n*-alkyl ligand significantly influences the retention of peptides and proteins and can therefore be used to manipulate the selectivity of peptide and protein separations. While the detailed molecular basis of the effect of ligand structure is not fully understood, a number of factors including the relative hydrophobicity and ligand chain length, flexibility, and the degree of exposure of surface silanols all play a role in the retention process. In addition to effects on peptide selectivity, the choice of ligand type can also influence protein recovery and conformational integrity of protein samples. Generally higher protein recoveries are obtained with the shorter and less hydrophobic *n*-butyl ligands. However, proteins have also been obtained in high yield with *n*-octadecyl silica. Silica-based packings are also susceptible to cleavage at pH values greater than seven. This limitation can severely restrict the use of these materials for separations that require basic pH conditions to effect resolution. In these cases, alternative stationary phases have been developed including cross-linked polystyrene divinylbenzene and porous zirconia, which are all stable to hydrolysis at alkaline pHs.

The geometry of the particle in terms of the particle diameter and pore size, is also an important feature of the packing material. As predicted by Eqn 4, improved resolution can be achieved by decreasing the particle diameter d_p. The most commonly used range of particle diameters for analytical scale RPC is 3–5 μm and nonporous particles of smaller diameter are also available. For preparative scale separations, 10–20 μm particles are utilized. The pore size of RPC sorbents is also an important factor that must be considered. For peptides, the pore size generally ranges between 100 and 300 Å depending on the size of the peptides. Porous materials of ≥300 Å pore size are necessary for the separation of proteins, as the solute molecular diameter must be at least one-tenth the size of the pore diameter to avoid restricted diffusion of the solute and to allow the total surface area of the sorbent material to be accessible. The development of particles with 6,000–8,000 Å pores with a network of smaller pores of 500–1,000 Å can also allow very rapid protein separations to be achieved.

2.1.2. Mobile Phases

One of the most powerful characteristics of RPC is the ability to manipulate solute retention and resolution through changes in the composition of the mobile phase. In RPC, peptide and protein retention is due to multi-site interactions with the ligands. The practical consequence of this is that high resolution isocratic elution of peptides and proteins can rarely be achieved as the experimental window of solvent concentration required for their elution is very narrow. Mixtures of peptides and proteins are therefore routinely eluted by the application of a gradient of increasing organic solvent concentration. RPC is generally carried out with an acidic mobile phase, with trifluoroacetic acid (TFA) the most commonly used additive due to its volatility. Phosphoric acid, perchloric acid, formic acid, hydrochloric acid, acetic acid, and heptaflourobutyric acid can also be used. The effect of ion-pairing reagents on peptide separation is illustrated in **Fig. 44.1** for a series of peptide standards separated on a C18 column. Alternative additives such as nonionic detergents can be used for the isolation of more hydrophobic proteins such as membrane proteins.

The three most commonly employed organic solvents are acetonitrile, methanol, and 2-propanol, which all exhibit high optical transparency in the detection wavelengths used for peptide and protein analysis. Acetonitrile provides the lowest viscosity solvent mixtures and 2-propanol is the strongest eluent. An example of the influence of organic solvent is shown in **Fig. 44.2** where

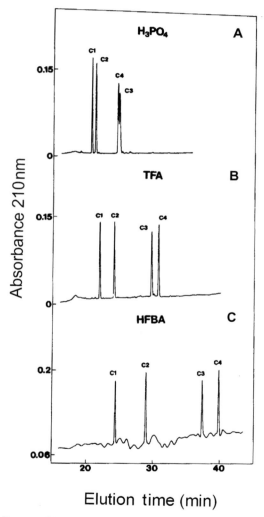

Fig. 44.1. The influence of ion-paring reagent on the separation of a mixture of synthetic peptides in reversed phase chromatography using a SynChropak C18, 25 cm × 4.6 mm ID, 6.5-μm particle size, 30-nm pore size (SynChrom, Linden, IN). Conditions: linear gradient from 0–100% acetonitrile containing A. 0.1% H_3PO_4; B, 0.1% TFA; and C; 0.1% HFBA; flow rate of 1 ml/min, 26°C. Peptide sequences: C1 = Ac-GGGLGGAGGLK-amide, C2 = Ac-KYGLGGAGGLK-amide. C3 = Ac-GGALKALKGLK-amide, C4 = Ac-KYALKALKGLK-amide (reprinted with permission from ref. *3*)

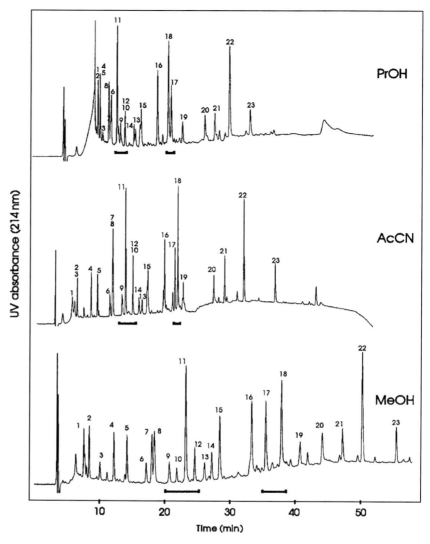

Fig. 44.2. The influence of organic solvent on the reversed phase chromatography of tryptic peptides derived from porcine growth hormone. Column: Bakerbond (J T Baker, Phillipsburg, NJ) RP-C4, 25 cm × 4.6 mm ID, 5-μm particle size, 30-nm pore size. Conditions, linear gradient from 0 to 90% 2-propanol (top), acetonitrile (middle), or methanol (bottom) with 0.1% TFA over 60 min, flow rate of 1 ml/min, 25°C (reprinted with permission from ref. *1*)

changes in selectivity can be observed for a number of peptide peaks in the tryptic map. In addition to the eluotropic effects, the nature of the organic solvent can also influence the conformation of both peptides and proteins and will therefore have an additional effect on selectivity through changes in the structure of the hydrophobic contact region. In the case of proteins, this may also impact on the level of recovery of biologically active material.

2.1.3. Column Geometry

The desired level of efficiency and sample loading size determines the dimension of the column to be used and **Fig. 44.3** summarizes the column dimensions used over the full range of sample scale. For small peptides and proteins, increased resolution is obtained with increases in column length. Thus, for applications such as tryptic mapping, column lengths between 15 and 25 cm and internal diameter (ID) of 4.6 mm are generally employed. However, for larger proteins, low mass recovery and loss of biological activity may result with these columns owing to irreversible binding and/or denaturation. In these cases, shorter columns of between 2 and 20 cm in length can be used. For preparative applications in the 1–500 mg scale, such as the purification of synthetic peptides, so-called semipreparative columns of dimensions 30 cm × 1 cm ID and preparative columns of 30 cm × 2 cm ID can be used.

The selection of the internal diameter of the column is based on the sample capacity and detection sensitivity. While most analytical applications are carried out with columns of internal diameter of 4.6 mm ID, for samples derived from previously unknown proteins where there is a limited supply of material, the task is to maximize the detection sensitivity. In these cases, the use of narrow bore columns of 1 or 2 mm ID can be used, which allow the elution and recovery of samples in much smaller volumes of solvent. Capillary chromatography (see Section 7) is also finding increasing application where capillary columns of internal diameter between 0.2 and 0.4 mm and column length of 15 cm result in the analysis of fmole of sample. The effect of decreasing column internal diameter on detection sensitivity is shown in **Fig. 44.4** for the analysis of lysozyme on a C18 material packed into columns of 4.6 mm, 2.1 mm, and 0.3 mm ID.

		Column diameter (mm)	Typical flow rate	Sample capacity	Maximum pracical sample load
Capillary		0.075	0.25 μL/min	0.05 μg	
		0.15	1.0 μL/min	0.2 μg	
		0.30	5.0 μL/min	1.0 μg	
		0.50	10.0 μL/min	2.0 μg	
Microbore		1.0	20–50 μL/min	0.05–10 μg	
Narrowbore		2.1	100–300 μL/min	0.2–50 μg	
Analytical		4.6	0.5–1.5 mL/min	1–200 μg	10 mg
Semi-preparative		10	2.5–7.5 mL/min	1000 μg	50 mg
Preparative		22	10–30 mL/min	5 mg	200 mg

Fig. 44.3. Summary of the operating conditions associated with the use of HPLC columns for capillary, microbore, narrowbore, analytical, semipreparative, and preparative chromatography

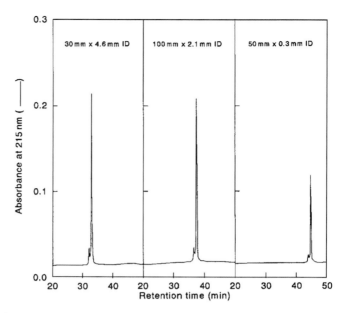

Fig. 44.4. Effect of column internal diameter on detector sensitivity. Column: Brownlee RP-300 C8 (7-μm particle size, 30-nm pore size), 3 cm × 4.6 mm ID and 10 cm × 2.1 mm ID (Applied Biosystems) and 5 cm × 0.32 mm ID. Conditions: linear gradient from 0 to 60% acetonitrile with 0.1% TFA over 60 min, 45°C. Flow rates, 1 ml/min, 200 μl/min, and 4 μl/min for the 4.6, 2.1, and 0.32 mm ID columns respectively. Sample loadings, lysozyme, 10 μg, 4 μg, and 0.04 μg for the 4.6, 2.1, and 0.32 mm ID columns respectively (reprinted from R.L. Moritz, R.J. Simpson 1992, Application of capillary reversed phase high performance liquid chromatography to high sensitivity protein sequence analysis, *J. Chromatogr.*, **599**, 119–130, with kind permission from Elsevier Science – NL, Sara Burgerhartstraat 25, 1055 KV Amsterdam, The Netherlands ref. *22*)

2.1.4. Operating Parameters

There are several operating parameters that can be changed to manipulate the resolution of peptide and protein mixtures in RPC. These parameters include the gradient time, the gradient shape, the mobile phase flow rate, and the operating temperature. The typical experiment with an analytical scale column would utilize a linear gradient from 5% organic solvent up to between 50 and 100% solvent over a time range of 20–120 min while flow rates are between 0.5 and 2.0 ml/min. With microbore columns (1–2 mm ID) flow rates of 50–250 μl/min are used, while for capillary columns of 0.2–0.4 nmm ID, flow rates of 1–4 μl/min are applied. At the preparative end of the scale with columns of 10–20 mm ID, flow rates between 5 and 20 ml/min are required.

The choice of gradient conditions will depend on the nature of the molecules of interest. Generally the use of longer gradient times provides improved separation. However, these conditions also increase the residence time of the peptide or protein solute at the sorbent surface, which may then result in an increase in the degree of denaturation.

The operating temperature can also be used to manipulate resolution. While the separation of peptides and proteins is normally carried out at ambient temperature, solute retention in RPC is influenced by temperature through changes in solvent viscosity. In addition to this, peptide and protein conformation can also be manipulated by temperature. In the case of proteins, where biological recovery is not important, increasing temperature can be used to modulate retention via denaturation of the protein structure. For peptides, secondary structure can actually be enhanced through binding to the hydrophobic sorbent. Changes in temperature can therefore also be used to manipulate the structure and retention of peptide mixtures.

Detection of peptides and proteins in RPC, and in all modes of chromatography, generally involves detection at between 210 and 220 nm, which is specific for the peptide bond, or at 280 nm, which corresponds to the aromatic amino acids tryptophan and tyrosine. The use of photodiode array detectors can enhance the detection capabilities by the on-line accumulation of complete solute spectra. The spectra can then be used to identify peaks specifically on the basis of spectral characteristics and for the assessment of peak purity. In addition, second derivative spectroscopy can provide information on the conformational integrity of proteins following elution.

In summary, RPC is now firmly entrenched as the central tool for the analysis of peptides and proteins and thus plays a pivotal role in the pharmaceutical and biotechnology industries.

2.2. Hydrophobic Interaction Chromatography

Hydrophobic interaction chromatography (HIC) is a valuable technique for the separation of proteins under nondenaturing conditions. HIC involves the use of high salt concentrations to promote hydrophobic interactions between the protein and the hydrophobic stationary phase. Solutes are then eluted in order of increasing hydrophobicity though the application of a descending salt gradient that weakens the hydrophobic interactions between the protein and the sorbent material. The ligands used for HIC materials are less hydrophobic than those in RPC. Thus, in contrast to the denaturing effects of low pH and organic solvent present in RPC systems, the mobile phases used in HIC generally stabilize protein structure.

Both polymeric and silica based HIC supports have been produced and a range of mildly hydrophobic ligands are available to perform HIC. In particular both alkyl and aryl ligands have proven to be successful in obtaining high levels of selectivity. **Figure 44.5** shows the influence of a range of ligands on the retention behavior of a series of globular proteins and demonstrates that protein retention increases in the order hydroxypropyl < methyl < benzyl = propyl < isopropyl < phenyl < pentyl. This figure clearly illustrates the influence of the ligand structure on the retention of proteins in HIC. Other ligand types that can be used include silica-based ether-bonded alkyl phases, neopentylagarose, and phenylagarose.

Selectivity in HIC can be manipulated by changes in the nature of the eluting salt, salt concentration, pH, temperature, and the addition of mobile phase modifiers. Protein retention is strongly dependent on the type of salt employed. Salts defined as being kosmotropic or structure-making are used as they enhance hydrophobic interactions through a salting-out mechanism. An example of the effect of salt on the retention of lysozyme in HIC is shown in **Fig. 44.6**. $(NH_4)_2SO_4$ is the most commonly used salt in HIC, while Na_2SO_4

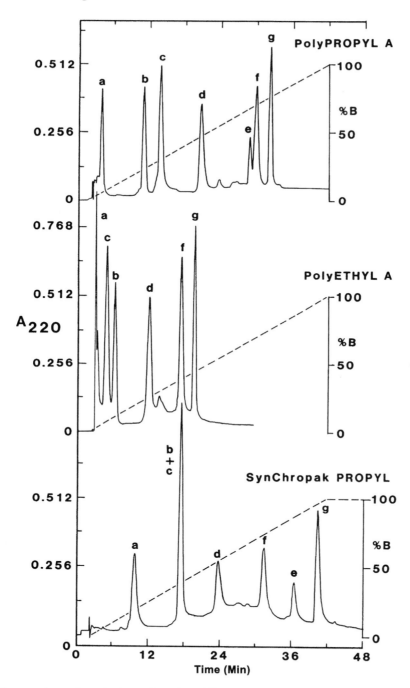

Fig. 44.5. HIC separations of standard proteins using different stationary phases. Stationary phase applied were PolyPROPYL and PolyETHYL Aspartamide and a PROPYL HIC column from other vendor. The elution condition consists of, mobile phase **A**: 1.8 M ammonium sulfate + 0.1 M potassium phosphate, pH 7.0 and mobile phase **B**: 0.1 M potassium phosphate, pH 7.0. A 40 min linear gradient was used from 0 to 100% B at 1 mL/min flow rate. The elution was followed at 220 nm. Peaks: a, cytochrome c; b, ribonuclease A; c, myoglobin; d, conalbumin; e, neochymotrypsin; f, α-chymotrypsin; g, α-chymotrypsinogen. A (reproduced from K Benedek in High Performance Hydrophobic Interaction Chromatography, in HPLC of Peptides and Proteins: Methods and Protocols, Aguilar, MI, Humana Press, 2004, pp 45–53 ref. *23*)

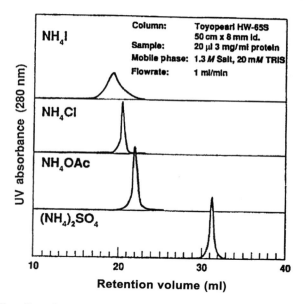

Fig. 44.6. The effect of salt on the elution of lysozyme in HIC. Column; Toyopearl HW-65S (Toyo Soda), 50 cm × 8 mm ID, 30-μm particle size, 100-nm pore size. Conditions; isocratic elution with 20 mM TRIS-HCl, pH 7, containing 1.3 M ammonium iodide, chloride, acetate, or sulphate, at a flow rate of 1 mL/min (reprinted with permission from B.F. Rogetter et al., 1990 in M.R. Ladisch, R.C. Willison, C.C. Painton and S.E. Builder Eds. Protein Purification: From Molecular Mechanisms to Large Scale Processes, Washington DC, American Chemical Society, p. 80–92 ref. *24*)

and NaCl also find application. $(NH_4)_2SO_4$ has a high solubility and low UV absorbance and is readily available in high purity required for HPLC. Initial salt concentrations usually range from 1 to 3 M, and the starting concentration can also influence selectivity of a separation.

The pH of mobile phases used in HIC is typically between five and seven and buffered with sodium or potassium phosphate. The influence of pH on protein retention is dependent on the particular protein as the manipulation of charges located in or near the hydrophobic binding domain will have a profound effect on the affinity of the protein for the sorbent material. Thus, changes in pH represents a useful parameter to modulate selectivity.

The gradient shape is an additional parameter that can be used to manipulate selectivity in HIC. The retention behavior of proteins in HIC generally reveals a linear dependence of retention on salt concentration. The selection of elution conditions to maximize resolution among components therefore follows the same rationale as described for RPC in the previous section.

The addition of other solvent modifiers has also been shown to affect retention in HIC through changes in the surface tension of the mobile phase. These include detergents such as Triton X-100 and CHAPS, organic solvents such as 5–20% methanol, acetonitrile, or even ethylene glycol and urea or guanidine hydrochloride at concentrations of 1–2 M. In all cases, it is possible that these additives may cause denaturation of the target proteins, so care is needed to minimize protein conformational changes when introducing these additives to the mobile phase.

Temperature can also be used to manipulate selectivity in HIC through changes in protein conformation. Depending on the protein solute, chromatography in the range 15–50°C can be used to sharpen individual peaks shapes and hence improve resolution. However, significant band broadening can also be observed as a result of slow conformational interconversions, which results in a decline in resolution.

Overall, HIC is a powerful tool for the purification of proteins in a biologically active form. Moreover, protein structure and conformation play a crucial role in the chromatographic behavior of proteins and subtle changes in selectivity can be achieved through changes in the relative solubility and three-dimensional structure of the protein solute.

2.3. Ion-Exchange Chromatography

High performance ion-exchange chromatography (IEC) is now extensively used in the analysis of proteins, and also to a lesser extent for the analysis of peptides. The early stages of protein purification generally use solubility-based techniques to carry out the initial fractionation. Differences in size and shape of the proteins are then exploited through application of size exclusion or preparative electrophoretic techniques. Adsorptive techniques, including IEC and RPC are then introduced to allow rapid increases in the level of resolution, recovery, and product purity. A significant advantage of IEC over the other adsorptive mods of chromatography is the nondenaturing effects of the solutions used to elute proteins from the ion-exchange sorbents. Thus, while gross conformational changes can be observed in RPC, these are not commonly found in IEC of proteins.

Protein retention in ion-exchange chromatography arises from electrostatic interactions between the peptide or protein and the charged sorbent material and solutes are eluted by increases in the concentration of a displacer salt. As a consequence, the "net charge" concept is widely used to predict the retention characteristics of proteins with both anion and cation-exchange materials. According to this model, and as illustrated in **Fig. 44.7**, a protein will be retained on a cation-exchange column if the solvent pH is lower than the pI of the protein. Conversely, a protein will be retained on an anion-exchange column if the pH is above the pI of the protein. With mobile phases operating at a pH equal to the protein's pI, the surface of the protein is considered to be overall electrostatically neutral and under these conditions, the protein should not be retained on either cation- or anion-exchangers.

While this model can be used to predict the retention behavior of peptides in IEC, this classical model is recognized as a simplistic approach to describing protein retention. The amphoteric nature of proteins results in the existence of localized areas of electrostatic charge at different pHs, which can allow the protein to be retained even under conditions where the protein may be at its isoelectric point.

Overall, the magnitude of electrostatic interactions between proteins and the charged sorbent material in IEC depends on the number and distribution of charged sites on the solute molecule that define the electrostatic contact area of the protein, the charge density of the sorbent and the mobile phase composition. In summary, the magnitude of the electrostatic interactions, and

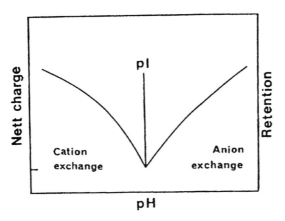

Fig. 44.7. The theoretical relationship between protein net charge and chromatographic retention in ion-exchange chromatography

hence retention, in IEC are dependent on the following structural and chromatographic parameters,

1) The number and distribution of charged sites on the solute molecule that constitute the electrostatic contact area
2) The charge density of the immobilized charged ligand
3) The mobile phase composition

It is these factors that can be used to manipulate peptide and protein surface charge to allow optimization of selectivity in IEC.

The support materials available for high performance ion-exchange chromatography are generally silica-based or polymer-based materials. An ion-exchange material is selected on the basis of the desired particle and pore size, swelling characteristics at the operational pH range. However, the major factor is the capacity of the ion-exchanger, which depends on the nature of the charged functional groups and the charge density as well as the pore size of the material and the charge distribution on the protein solute.

The two classes of ion-exchangers are cation exchangers, which contain negatively charged functional groups, and anion exchangers, which contain positively charged functional groups. The most commonly encountered ligands are listed in **Table 44.1**. Strong cation exchangers normally contain sulphonic acid groups while strong anion exchangers contain quaternary ammonium functional groups. The charged ligands in weak cation exchangers generally contain carboxylic groups while weak anion-exchangers are primary, secondary, or tertiary amines. The terms strong and weak refer to the degree of ionization with pH as strong ion-exchangers are completely ionized over a much wider pH range than weak ion-exchangers.

The selectivity of proteins in IEC can be manipulated by variation in solution pH and ionic strength that alters the electrostatic surface potential of the protein solutes and the charged ligand thereby influencing the strength of the electrostatic interactions. Changes in the nature of the displacer ion and the buffer species represent additional methods by which protein retention can be modified.

Table 44.1. Commonly encountered ligands for ion-exchange chromatography.

Ion exchanger	Functional group	
Strong cation exchanger (SCX)	Methylsulphonate	$-CH_2SO_3^-$
Weak cation exchanger (WCX)	Carboxymethyl	$-OCH_2COO^-$
Strong anion exchanger (SAX)	Methyl trimethyl ammonium	$-CH_2N^+(CH_3)_3$
Weak anion exchanger (WAX)	Diethylaminoethyl	$-OCH_2H_2N^+H(CH_2CH_3)_2$

While NaCl is the most commonly used ionic displacer, a number of other monovalent and multivalent salts can be used. The ions may influence retention through specific interactions with the ion-exchange ligand, thereby changing their ionic properties. In addition, specific salts may alter the conformation of proteins which in turn will influence their retention behavior. At fixed ionic strengths, anions can be ranked in terms of solute retention as follows

$$F^- < CH_3COO^- < Cl^- < HPO_4^{2-} < SO_4^{2+}$$

Similarly, cations are ranked according to the series

$$K^- < Na^+ < NH_4^+ < Ca^{2+} < Mg^{2+}$$

KCl, NaOAc, $MgCl_2$, and $Mg_3(SO_4)_2$ have all been used for the analysis and purification of a wide range of proteins. The effect of different displacer salts on protein retention in weak anion-exchange chromatography is shown in **Fig. 44.8**, which illustrates the profound influence that the nature of the salt can exert on the electrostatic interactions between proteins and ion-exchange materials.

The selection of buffer depends on the pH range required to adsorb the protein to the stationary phase. While selection of a pH can be a straightforward task based on the known pI of the protein, for proteins of unknown pI or closely related proteins such as isoforms or recombinant muteins, a map of retention versus pH can assist in the selection of mobile phase pH. Once the pH range is established, additional changes in selectivity can be obtained through changes in the nature of the buffer species. The most commonly employed buffer species include phosphate and Tris–HCl buffers. A range of buffers, which are commonly used in IEC of proteins, is listed in **Table 44.2**.

While isocratic elution can be used to separate proteins in IEC, gradient elution is generally employed to obtain high resolution separations of proteins in IEC. Linear elution over 16–120 min is generally applied among ionic strengths ranging from 0 to 0.5 M salt. Buffer concentrations usually range between 20 and 50 mM.

A number of additional materials can be added to the mobile phase to further enhance selectivity. For example, hydrophobic interactions may contribute to peptide and protein retention in IEC owing to the nature of the stationary phase material. It has been reported that solutes cannot be eluted with some ion-exchangers without the addition of acetonitrile or methanol to the mobile phase. The percentage organic modifier is usually in the range

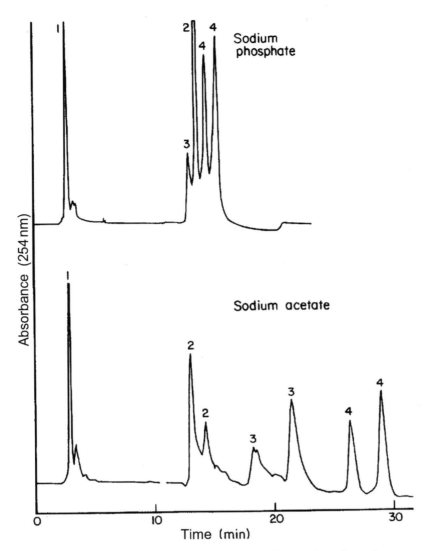

Fig. 44.8. The effect of different displacer salts on the retention of proteins separated by weak anion-exchange chromatography. Column, SynChropak AX-300, 25 cm × 4.1 mm ID, 6.5-μm particle size, 30-nm pore size (SynChrom, Linden, IN). Conditions; Linear gradient from 0 to 1 *M* salt over 30 min at a flow rate of 1 ml/min, detected at 254 nm. Top panel = sodium phosphate, lower panel = sodium acetate. Proteins; 1, myoglobin; 2, conalbumin; 3, ovalbumin; 4, β-lactoglobulins B and A (reprinted with permission from M.P. Nowlan, K.M. Gooding, 1991, in *ref. 3*)

of 10–40%. Higher levels of solvent can cause salt precipitation and may also affect protein conformation.

In summary, high performance ion-exchange chromatography continues to be an important technique for the analysis and purification of proteins under mild nondenaturing conditions and also provides a very useful selectivity alternative for the analysis of peptide samples.

Table 44.2. Buffers commonly used in IEC.

pH range	Buffer
Cation exchange	
1.5–2.5	Maleic acid
2.6–3.6	Citric acid
3.6–4.3	Lactic acid
4.8–5.2	Acetic acid
5.0–6.0	Malonic acid
6.7–7.6	Phosphate
7.6–8.2	HEPES
Anion exchange	
4.5–5.0	*N*-methyl piperazine
5.0–6.0	Piperazine
5.8–6.4	bis-Tris
7.3–7.7	Triethanolamine
7.6–8.0	Tris
8.5–9.0	1,3-diaminopropane
9.5–9.8	Piperazine

2.4. Size Exclusion Chromatography

Size exclusion chromatography (SEC) is frequently used as the first step in the isolation of proteins from complex mixtures where separation is carried out according to molecular size and shape. SEC can also be used for desalting samples through buffer exchange and has also found application in the analysis of peptides. SEC has also been established as a physicochemical tool for estimating molecular size and shape of proteins and has provided insight into protein folding mechanisms by monitoring changes in protein size as a function of changes in the concentration of chemical denaturants.

Separation in SEC is based on differences in molecular size in solution. Porous stationary phases are used with defined pore diameters and elution conditions are used that minimize interaction between the solute molecules and the stationary phase material. The larger the molecule the smaller the amount of accessible pore volume. Molecules that are larger than the largest pore diameter cannot penetrate into the stationary phase pores and pass through the column with the fastest retention time. These molecules are eluted with V_0, while the smallest molecule is eluted in the V_t, the total volume of the column. V_t is the sum of the void volume and the interstitial volume V_i, i.e.,

$$V_t = V_o + V_i \qquad (6)$$

Solute elution volume in SEC is denoted by V_e which should be between V_0 and V_t and can be expressed as follows

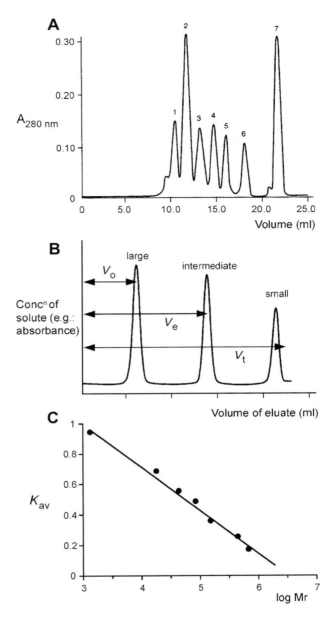

Fig. 44.9. A. Gel filtration chromatography of a series of protein molecular mass standards on a prepacked Superdex 200 HR 10/30 column (Amersham Biosciences). Standards were 1. thyroglobulin (M_r 669,000), 2. ferritin (M_r 440,000), 3. human IgG (M_r 150,000), 4. human transferrin (M_r 81,000), 5. ovalbumin (M_r 43,000), 6. myoglobin (M_r 17,600), 7. vitamin B12 (M_r 1,355). Conditions were: 50 mM sodium phosphate, 150 mM NaCl, pH 7.0, flow rate = 0.25 mL/min (19 mL/cm²/h). Figure reproduced with the kind permission of Amersham Biosciences. **B**. Diagrammatic representation of the measurement of the void volume (V_0), elution volume (V_e) and total volume (V_t) for a gel filtration column. V_0 is the elution volume of molecules too large to enter the pores of the gel media, whereas V_t is the total volume of the column determined with a small molecule. V_e represents the elution volume of a molecule of intermediate molecular mass. Determination of these parameters is best done with standard proteins (see panel **A**) under optimal conditions for flow rate and sample size. From these measurements the coefficient K_{av} can be derived, $K_{av} = (V_e - V_0) / (V_t - V_0)$. **C**. The selectivity curve for a particular gel filtration media is a plot of K_{av} versus log molecular weight, and the data shown here has been derived from Panel **A**. Selectivity curves as provided by the manufacturer are used to choose the gel filtration media that best suits the application, while in the laboratory they are useful for estimation of the molecular mass of an unknown protein (reproduced from P. Stanton in Gel Filtration Chromatography, in HPLC of Peptides and Proteins: Methods and Protocols, Aguilar, MI, Humana Press 2004, pp. 55–74 ref. **25**)

$$V_e = V_o + K_d V_i \qquad (7)$$

where K_d is the distribution coefficient that defines the fraction of internal volume that is accessible to the protein solute as shown in **Fig. 44.9B**.

The packing materials available for high performance SEC are generally silica-based or polymeric. The pore diameter of SEC supports determines the exclusion limits of the material. Columns are characterized in terms of the molecular weight range that can be adequately separated, which is dependent on the pore diameter. Generally pore diameter ranges between 100 and 500 Å. The pore volume is also an important property of an SEC material, which must be sufficiently large to provide a high peak capacity, i.e., the ability to separate seven peaks with a resolution of one. Column efficiency in high performance SEC supports is particularly important as solutes are eluted isocratically and therefore do not exhibit band sharpening, which occurs with gradient elution. SEC supports generally have particle diameters between 5 and 10 μm.

The hydrodynamic shape and volume rather than molecular weight *per se* is the physical property of proteins that causes separation in SEC. To achieve accurate estimations of molecular weight, a column must be calibrated with molecules that have the same overall shape. Under ideal conditions, K_d will be proportional to the logarithm of the molecular weight of the protein as illustrated by a typical calibration curve shown in **Fig. 44.9C** for the protein separation shown in **Fig. 44.9A.** While the majority of applications of SEC have involved the analysis and purification of proteins, SEC has also recently been used in the analysis of peptides. An example of the high level of resolution that can be achieved for peptides is shown in **Fig. 44.10**, which demonstrates excellent separation in the MW range of 75–12,500 Da.

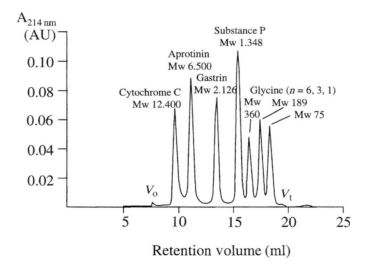

Fig. 44.10. The separation of peptides by size exclusion chromatography. Column; Superdex Peptide HR 10/30 (Pharmacia, Uppsala, Sweden). Conditions; 0.25 *M* NaCl in 0.02 *M* phosphate buffer pH 7.2, flow rate 0.25 mL/min (High performance size exclusion columns Data file No 18-1106-06, 1994, courtesy of Amersham Pharmacia Biotech)

Mobile phase selection is important in SEC to minimize nonspecific interactions between the support and the solutes and also to avoid mobile phase induced changes in solute molecular shape. Both ionic and hydrophobic interactions can also contribute to the elution volume of proteins in SEC as most packings are weakly acidic (owing to residual negative charges) and/or mildly hydrophobic. Ionic interactions can be minimized by increasing the ionic strength of the mobile phase through the addition of up to $0.5\,M$ NaCl. However, increasing ionic strength also results in the enhancement of hydrophobic interactions. Thus a balance is necessary to minimize both undesired interactions. A common mobile phase composition that is employed for SEC of proteins is phosphate buffer at pH 7 with ionic strength of 0.05–0.1 and by optimizing pH and ionic strength, secondary interactions can be almost excluded. However, ionic or hydrophobic interactions can also be used to manipulate selectivity of protein separations.

3. Applications

The application of the four main interactive modes of chromatography to peptide and protein isolation, separation and purification are clearly too broad in nature and number to fully describe here. Examples of these applications include proteolytic mapping, post-translational modifications, neuropeptide processing, glycopeptides, and glycoproteins, MHC-binding peptides, toxins/venoms, membrane proteins, antibodies, combinatorial and proteome analysis, and enzymatic activity. Below is a summary of the some of the key applications to provide a sense of the depth and breadth of impact of HPLC in the life sciences.

3.1. High Resolution Peptide and Protein Separations

RPC is extremely versatile for the isolation of peptides and proteins from a wide variety of synthetic or biological sources and is used for both analytical and preparative applications. Analytical applications range from the assessment of purity of peptides following solid-phase peptide synthesis, to the analysis of tryptic maps of proteins. Preparative RPC is also used for the micropurification of protein fragments for sequencing to large scale purification of synthetic peptides and recombinant proteins *(12–14)*. The complexity of the mixture to be chromatographed will depend on the nature of the source and the degree of preliminary clean-up that can be performed. In the case of synthetic peptides, RPC is generally employed both for the initial analysis and the final large scale purification. The purification of synthetic peptides usually involves an initial separation on an analytical scale to assess the complexity of the mixture followed by large-scale purification and collection of the target product. A sample of the purified material can then be subjected to RPC analysis under the same or different elution conditions to check for purity. The isolation of proteins from a biological cocktail derived from a tissue extract or biological fluid for example, often requires a combination of techniques to produce a homogenous sample. HPLC techniques are then introduced at the later stages following initial precipitation, clarification, and preliminary separations using soft gel.

An example of the high resolution analysis of a tryptic digest of a protein is shown in **Fig. 44.11**. This figure, in which 150 peaks were identified, demonstrates the highly selective separation that can be achieved with enzymatic digests of proteins using RPC as part of the quality control or structure determination of a recombinant or natural protein. The chromatographic separation was obtained with a C2/C18 stationary phase packed in a column of dimensions 10 cm × 4.6 mm internal diameter. Separated components can then be directly subjected to further analysis such as automated Edman N-terminal sequencing or electrospray mass spectrometry.

For peptide applications where incomplete separation is observed in RPC, ion-exchange chromatography represents a very useful alternative separation mode. At neutral pH, basic peptides can be separated by cation-exchange chromatography and acidic peptides can be analyzed by anion-exchange chromatography. However, ion exchange of peptides is more commonly carried out at acidic pH, in the range 2.5–3.0, where most peptides are positively charges and hence cation exchange is applicable. At this pH range, the negative charges associated with aspartate and glutamate residues and the C-terminus are neutralized, while arginine, lysine, histidine residues, and the N-terminus are positively charged.

Commonly used solvents for peptide IEC are usually based on phosphate buffers with NaCl or KCl as the displacer ion. For peptides up to approx 50 residues in length with no significant secondary structure, retention is governed by the number of positive charges. Thus peptides differing by a single charge are generally well-resolved. However peptides with the same charge but different amino acid composition can also be separated owing to differences in overall charge density. In addition, hydrophobic interactions may also contribute to the retention of peptides with ion-exchange resins. In these cases organic

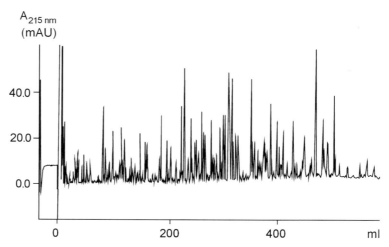

Fig. 44.11. High resolution reversed phase chromatographic separation of a tryptic digest of a 165 kDa protein on a μRPC C2/C18 ST 4.6/100 column, (dimensions 10 cm × 4.6 mm ID, 3-μm particle size, 12-nm pore size). Eluent A: 0.065% trifluoroacetic acid (TFA) in water, eluent B: 0.050%TFA in 84% acetonitrile. Gradient elution was carried out with 0%B for 2 column volumes (CV), 0–50% for 392 CV (650 min); 50–100% B for 55 CV (91 min); 100%B for 10 CV (17 min), flow rate of 1 mL/min and detection was at 215 nm (reprinted with permission from Amersham Bioscience, AKTA™purifier Application Note No. 18-1119-53)

solvent can be added to the mobile phases to further modulate selectivity. Ten to forty percent v/v of either methanol or acetonitrile can be used.

3.2. LC-MS for Peptide/Protein Analysis

One of the most significant recent advances in bioanalytical technology is the advent of mass spectrometry for the analysis and measurement of peptide and protein molecular mass. In particular, the development of on-line electrospray mass spectrometry following RPC (LC-ES-MS) has provided a powerful detection system for the rapid analysis of peptide and proteins *[15,16]*. The identification of proteins, peptide fragments and various modifications is essential for understanding biological processes and the function of proteins for normal healthy and at various disease states. The resulting insights lead to the development of therapies for intervention, and ultimately, the cure of disease. The information and knowledge derived from this type of study are extremely valuable for activities involved with target identification activities during drug discovery.

As described in previous sections, chromatographic analysis of peptide and protein is conventionally detected and quantified by the ultraviolet and/or fluorescence detection. However, quantitative methods combining separation techniques with UV or fluorescence detection are of limited applicability when analysing highly complex biomolecule mixtures. Such samples require high-resolution baseline separations or exceedingly high concentrations of analytes to overcome the impact of the matrix, because of unselective UV/fluorescence detection. Therefore, effective and sensitive peptide/protein detection and quantification from biological samples demands highly selective, robust, and accurate LC-MS methods.

LC-MS is a versatile combination of a commonly used chromatographic technology and mass spectrometry, a powerful identification tool not only for proteins but for all classes of organic molecules. The coupling of LC with MS has had an enormous impact on small molecule and protein profiling, and has proven to be an important alternative method to two-dimensional gel electrophoresis.

Figure 44.12 shows the LC-MS analysis of an Arg-C digest of plasminogen activator separated on a C18 column, with the total ion current in the upper trace and the elution profile detected at 214 nm in the lower trace. The availability of on-line mass spectrometry thus significantly facilitates the identification of the peptide fragments. Other important applications involve the identification of posttranslational modifications of peptides and proteins, assignment of disulphide bonds, and the identification of peptides bound to major histocompatibility complex molecules.

3.3. Capillary Liquid Chromatography

The transfer of analytical HPLC methods from conventional-size columns with typical 3.0–4.6 mm ID to capillary size dimensions of 0.1–0.5 mm ID has been a significant advance in recent years bringing several advantages such as reduction in the consumption and disposal of solvents, working with limited sample amounts and efficient interfacing with electrospray ionization MS. In principle, the various mechanisms utilized in conventional LC separations can be effectively implemented in packed capillary formats. However, most separations utilizing capillary LC are now performed using the reversed phase mode of separations. This is primarily because RPC is highly compatible with MS

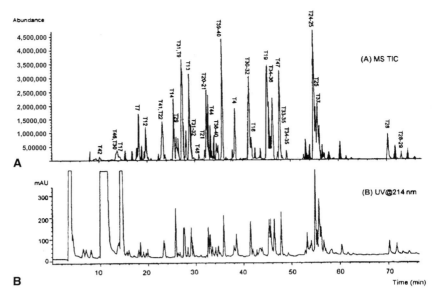

Fig. 44.12. LC-MS of a tryptic digest of single-chain plasminogen activator. Column: Vydac C18, 5-µm particle size, 30-nm pore size. Conditions: linear gradient from 0–60% acetonitrile with 0.1%TFA over 90 min, 45°C, flow rate 0.2 mL/min. (**A**) electrospry mass spectrometry total ion current, (**B**) detection at 214 nm (Reprinted from A. Apffel, J. Chakel, S. Udiavar, WS. Hancock, C. Souders and E. Pungor Jr. Application of capillary electrophoresis, high performance liquid chromatography, on-line electrospray mass spectrometry and matrix-assisted laser desorption ionization-time of flight mass spectrometry to the characterization of single-chain plasminogen activator, 1995, *J. Chromatogr. A* **717**, 41–60, with kind permission from Elsevier Science – NL, Sara Burgerhartstraat 25, 1055 KV Amsterdam, The Netherlands)

detection using ESI and requires only low flow rates to achieve both high separation efficiency and high detection sensitivity. Other modes of LC separation commonly utilized in peptide/protein separations include IEC, SEC, HIC and affinity chromatography. Many of these modes of chromatography are used in sample cleanup, preconcentrations, or fractionation before final analyses.

IEC is primarily used for sample fractionation of either proteomic intact proteins or their proteolytic peptides, and is usually practiced using microcolumns or even conventional columns. However, because of sensitivity requirements for proteomic analysis, the use of capillary IEC is appealing. The sample capacity has been found to be significantly smaller than for capillary RPC using the same dimensions of packed capillary columns. For example, <100 µg of a yeast lysate tryptic digest can be loaded on an 85 cm × 150 µm ID capillary packed with 3 µm SCX particles (300 Å pores), while 500 µg of the same sample can be loaded on the same dimension capillary packed with 3-µm C18 particles (300-Å pores). Desalting of samples can improve the loading capacity to some extent. These properties are important in the selection of capillary column dimensions for two-dimensional separations, particularly considering issues related to detection sensitivity (i.e., with MS). Additionally, IEC elution properties of proteins and peptides potentially provide valuable information for assisting protein identification.

3.4. Multidimensional Peptide and Protein Separations

The design of multidimensional purification schemes to achieve high levels of product purity highlight the power of HPLC techniques in peptide and protein purification *(14,17,18)*. One such example is shown in **Fig. 44.13** where the judicious use of SEC, IEC and RPC resulted in the efficient purification of murine epidermal growth factor *(19)* whereby manipulation of the sample between stages has been minimized and selectivity has been maximized.

Because of the complexity of proteomic samples, two or even multidimensional separations are also being increasingly used to achieve high-resolution separations *(20,21)*. Although comprehensive two-dimensional LC separations have been developed, the fast separation in the second dimension (currently) is generally far from optimal for data-dependent MS/MS peptide identification (e.g., using ion trap MS). Additionally, the interface between the first and the second dimension separation also effectively degrades the detection of low-abundance species. The two-dimensional separations that have been used for proteomic analyses to date achieve their separation efficiencies (combined peak capacities of ~10^3) primarily from the second dimension separation, while the first dimension separation is only used for a limited number of sample fractionations (typically the fraction number is <20). The separation of total human plasma proteins digested with trypsin with high-efficiency capillary SCX/RPC is demonstrated in **Fig. 44.14**. Although used in this way, the first dimension separation efficiency is also important because it determines the number of overlapping (or repeated) components in neighboring fractions.

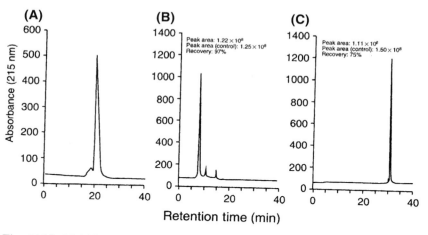

Fig. 44.13. Multidimensional micropreparative HPLC of murine epidermal growth factor (mEGF), using size exclusion, anion-exchange and reversed phase chromatography. (**A**) mEGF (4.5 µg, 750 pmol) was chromatographed on a Superose 12 PC 3.2/30 SEC column (Pharmacia, Uppsala, Sweden), 30 cm × 3.2 mm ID, using a mobile phase of 1%ammonium bicarbonate/0.02%Tween 20 at a flow rate of 0.1 mL/min. (**B**) The major peak in (**A**) was collected and applied to a Mono-Q PC 1.6/5 anion-exchange column (Pharmacia), 30 cm × 3.2 mm ID, using a linear gradient from 0–1 M sodium chloride in 20 mM Tris–HCl, pH 7.5 over 50 min at a flow rate of 0.1 ml/min. (**C**) The major peak from (**B**) was collected and further purified by RPC using a Brownlee RP-300 column, 30 cm × 2.1 mm ID, and a linear gradient from 0–60% acetonitrile in 0.15% TFA over 60 min at a flow rate of 0.1 ml/min. The integrated peak areas and the calculated recovery among stages are indicated in (**B**) and (**C**) (from *19*)

Both CE and capillary LC can also be used as the first separation dimension for sample fractionation; however, the separation sample capacity for the first dimension and the fluid compatibility with MS for the second dimension have to be considered when constructing such two-dimensional separations.

Capillary RPC-MS currently plays a dominant role in proteomic analyses involving peptide mixtures owing to its robustness for a variety of peptide properties (highly acidic/basic and hydrophilic/hydrophobic). Following enzymatic digestion of the global whole-proteome proteins, the resultant extremely complex peptide mixtures can be directly analyzed using capillary RPC-MS or MS/MS. Yates and co-workers have introduced a serial two-dimensional LC for proteomic analysis *(20)*. In this approach, a biphasic microcolumn in which a single capillary with 100 μm ID is first packed with 5 μm C18 for 8 cm and then packed with 5 μm SCX for 4 cm, which is similar to those used in serial column chromatography. The two-dimensional separations are achieved by alternatively eluting with salt step and a 60 min linear aqueous acetonitrile gradients through the whole biphasic column. The system is used for direct analysis of large protein complexes, and this multidimensional protein identification technology (MudPIT), was applied to proteome-wide protein identification. Optimizations included fractionation of a yeast derived proteome sample into three fractions (i.e., soluble, lightly washed, and heavily washed fractions)

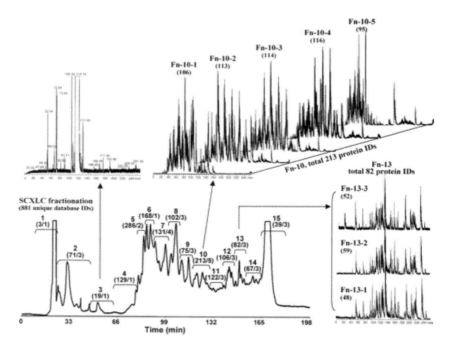

Fig. 44.14. High-efficiency 2D capillary SCX/RPC separation of total human plasma proteins digested with trypsin. The total plasma tryptic digests were first separated in an 80 cm × 320 μm ID fused-silica capillary packed with polysulfoethyl aspartamide-bonded silica particles (3 μm diameter, 300-Å pore size). A linear gradient of 4 m*M* phosphate, pH 2.5 to 0.4 *M* phosphate buffer in 200 min was used to separated the tryptic peptides. The peptides were separated into 15 fractions followed by RPC separation using an 85 cm 30-μm ID capillary (packed with 3 μm C18 particles, 300 Å pore size). The number of proteins identified were given in parentheses (reprinted with permission from *18*)

before the tryptic digestion, extension of C18 packed column length to 10 cm, varying mobile phase composition by adding 0.02% heptafluorobutyric acid (HFBA), using shallow gradient, and using 15 fractionation cycles. In ~84 h required for three runs of the three fractions, a combined 5,540 peptides were assigned, leading to identification of 1,480 proteins. In ~28 h of a single run, 630 soluble proteins from 1,665 assigned peptides were achieved for the soluble protein fraction. By analyzing the data set against the database, 72 out of 231 possible peripheral membrane proteins were detected and identified. The addition of HFBA to the mobile phase has significantly improved the sensitivity and separation resolution in the biphasic column. The separation efficiency of the MudPIT system was evaluated, and a peak capacity of 216 was achieved for the 5-μm C18 packed 10-cm capillary. Combined with 15 cycles (i.e., first stage fractions), a total peak capacity of 3,240 was estimated.

4. Summary

The number of applications of HPLC in peptide and protein purification continue to expand at an extremely rapid rate. Solid phase peptide synthesis and recombinant DNA techniques have allowed the production of large quantities of peptides and proteins that need to be highly purified. The design of multidimensional purification schemes to achieve high levels of product purity highlight the power of HPLC techniques in the production of peptide and proteins-based therapeutics.

Following purification, mass spectrometry can be used to confirm the structural identity of synthetic peptides, while recombinant proteins require further structural analysis by high resolution analytical fingerprinting to confirm the amino acid sequence. RPC will therefore continue to be the central method for the characterization and quality control analysis of synthetic peptides and recombinant proteins. Moreover, the coupling of mass spectrometry to allow on-line identification of samples will become routine and continue to expand the analytical power of HPLC. Other coupled techniques such as LC-CE (capillary electrophoresis) and LC-biosensor will also allow more rapid on-line analysis of sample purity and bioactivity.

Other areas of separation technology in which significant advances are anticipated to emerge are in the areas of miniaturization and high speed analysis to allow the efficient purification of femtomolar to attomolar levels of material. These techniques will have important impact in the discovery of new bioactive peptides and novel proteins as potential candidates for new therapeutics. However, in the postgenomic era, the overwhelming application of HPLC will be in the continuing development of new approaches to proteomic mapping.

References

1. Aguilar M-I (2004) HPLC of peptides and proteins; Methods and protocols, Methods Mol Biol vol 251. Humana Press, NJ
2. Cutler P (2003) Protein purification protocols (2nd edn). Methods Mol. Biol. vol 244. Humana Press, NJ
3. Mant CT, Hodges RS (eds) (1991) High performance liquid chromatography of peptides and proteins: separation, analysis and conformation. CRC Press, Boca Raton, EL
4. Gooding KM, Regnier FE (eds) (1990) HPLC of biological macromolecules: methods and applications. Dekker, NY
5. Hancock WS, Karger BL (eds) (1996) Methods in enzymology, vol 270 (entire volume)
6. Hancock WS, Karger BL (eds) (1996) Methods in enzymology, vol 271 (entire volume)

7. Aguilar MI, Hearn MTW (1996) High resolution reversed phase high performance liquid chromatography of peptides and proteins. Methods Enzymol 270:3–26

8. Mant CT, Hodges RS (1996) Analysis of peptides by high performance liquid chromatography. Methods Enzymol 271:3–50

9. Purcell AW, Aguilar MI, Hearn MTW (1995) Conformational effects in the RP-HPLC of polypeptides. II: the role of insulin A and B chains in the chromatographic behaviour of insulin. J Chromatogr 711:71–79

10. Oroszlan P, Wicar S, Teshima G, Wu S-L, Hancock WS, Karger BL (1992) Conformational effects in the reversed phase chromatographic behaviour of recombinant human growth hormone (rhGH) and N-methionyl recombinant human growth hormone (met-hGH). Anal Chem 64:1623–1631

11. Henry M (1991) Design requirements of silica-based matrices for biopolymer chromatography. J Chromatogr 544:413–443

12. Miller C, Rivier J (1996) Peptide chemistry: development of high performance liquid chromatography and capillary zone electrophoresis. Biopolymers 40:265–318

13. Hoff ER, Chloupek RC (1996) Analytical peptide mapping of recombinant DNA-derived proteins by reversed phase high performance liquid chromatography. Methods Enzymol 271:51–67

14. Nice E (1996) Micropreparative high performance liquid chromatography of proteins and peptides: principles and applications. Biopolymers 40:319–341

15. Link AJ, Eng J, Schietz DM, Carmack E, Mize GJ, Morris DR, Garvik BM, Yates JR III (1999) Direct analysis of protein complexes using mass spectrometry. Nat Biotechnol 17:676–682

16. Fenn JB, Mann M, Meng CK, Wong SF, Whitehouse CM (1989) Electrospray ionization for mass spectrometry of large biomolecules. Science 246:64–71

17. Fujii K, Nakano T, Kawamura T, Usui F, Bando Y, Wang R, Nishimura T (2004) Multidimensional protein profiling technology and its application to human plasma proteome. J Proteome Res 3:712–718

18. Shen Y, Jacobs JM, Camp II DG, Fang R, Moore RJ, Smith RD, Xiao W, Davis RW, Tompkins RG (2004) Ultra-high-efficiency strong cation exchange LC/RPLC/MS/MS for high dynamic range characterization of the human plasma proteome. Anal Chem 76:1134–1144

19. Nice EC, Fabri L, Hammacher A, Andersson K, Hellman U (1993) Micropreparative ion-exchange HPLC. Applications to microsequence analysis. Biomed Chromatogr 7:104–111

20. Washburn MP, Wolters D, Yates JR III (2001) Large-scale analysis of the yeast proteome by multidimensional protein identification technology. Nat Biotechnol 19:242–247

21. Adkins JN, Varnum SM, Auberry KJ, Moore RJ, Angell NH, Smith RD, Springer DL, Pounds JG (2002) Toward a human blood serum proteome: analysis by multidimensional separation coupled with mass spectrometry. Mol Cell Proteomics 1:947–955

22. Moritz RL and Simpson RJ (1992) Application of capillary reversed phase high performance liquid chromotography to high sensitivity protein sequence analysis J Chromatogr 599:119–130

23. Benedek K (2004) High performance hydrophobic interaction chromatography, in HPLC of peptides and proteins: methods and protocols, Aguilar, MI, Humana Press, 45–53

24. Ladisch MR, Willison RC, Painton CC, Builder SE (eds), (1990) Protein purification: from molecular mechanisms to large scale processes, Washington DC, American Chemical Society, 80–92

25. Stanton P (2004) In gel filtration chromatography, in HPLC of peptides and proteins: methods and protocols, Aguilar, MI, Humana Press, pp. 55–74

26. Apffel A, Chakel J, Udiavar S, Hancock WS, Souders C, Pungor Jr. E (1995) Application of capillary electrophosis, high performace liquid chromatography, on-line eletrospray mass spectrometry and matrix-assisted laser desorption ionization-time of flight mass spectrometry to the characterization of single-chain plasminogen activator. J Chromatogr A 717:41–60

45

Amino Acid Analysis

Ian Davidson and Paula O'Connor

1. Introduction

Amino acid analysis is carried out to provide information on the different types and concentrations of amino acids in proteins and peptides from both natural and synthetic sources. It is also an important analysis technique in the determination of levels of free amino acids in foodstuffs and clinical specimens such as physiological fluids and tissues. In addition to the 20 well known amino acids some 700 unusual naturally occurring amino acids have been reported *(1,2)*.

The identification and quantification of amino acids can be divided into five constituent parts, sample purification and preparation, hydrolysis, derivatization, analysis, and data handling.

a) **Sample purification and preparation:** In many types of samples the amino acids can be found in media not compatible with any of the analytical systems available. The presence of buffer salts, urea, detergents etc., can interfere with both the hydrolysis and subsequent derivatization so some purification and sample preparation steps are required before hydrolysis, derivatization and analysis. Methods that utilize postcolumn derivatization of amino acids are generally not affected by buffer component concentrations to the same extent as precolumn derivatization methods.
Sample purification methods are outlined in Section 2.

b) **Hydrolysis of proteins and peptides:** Purified peptides and proteins are subjected to elevated temperatures under acidic conditions to break the peptide bonds to produce free amino acids. Protein and peptide samples are first dried in a hydrolysis tube. In Liquid Phase hydrolysis the acid solution is added to the sample tube and each sample tube is then sealed under vacuum. In vapor phase hydrolysis the individual sample tubes are placed into a hydrolysis vessel and acid solution is added to the vessel before being sealed so only the vapor from the heated acid solution is in contact with the sample. Generally higher sensitivity is achieved with the vapor phase hydrolysis method because any possible contaminants from the acid hydrolysis solution are kept to a minimum.
Hydrolysis methods are outlined in Section 3.

From: *Molecular Biomethods Handbook, 2nd Edition.*
Edited by: J. M. Walker and R. Rapley © Humana Press, Totowa, NJ

c) **Derivatization of free amino acids:** Because amino acids do not have a natural chromophore some form of derivatization is required to aid their detection. In postcolumn derivatization, the derivatization occurs after the liquid chromatography which usually occurs on an ion exchange chromatography column whereas precolumn derivatization is carried out before the chromatography which is typically reverse phase liquid chromatography (RPLC).

It is possible, however, to analyze amino acids without the need for derivatization but specialised detectors such as a mass spectrometer is required.

Derivatization and Underivatized methods are outlined in Sections 4 and 4.8.1, respectively.

d) **Liquid chromatography:** Typically, the derivatized amino acids are separated into the component parts usually by either ion exchange or reverse phase chromatography. The choice of generic chromatography column required is usually determined by the derivatization method.

Capillary electrophoresis (CE) is considered a powerful technique owing to its high separation efficiency, small sample requirement, rapid analysis time and low running costs. It is used as an alternative to HPLC in the separation of free amino acids.

e) **Data Acquisition and Data Handling:** The separated derivatized amino acids are identified by their peak retention times and quantified by measuring the area under the peak or by peak height. Comparison with known amounts of standards run under identical conditions will yield amount of sample. The use of internal standards will improve the accuracy of the method. There are many commercially available acquisition and data handling systems and software packages available.

Basic Calculations are outlined in Section 5.

1.1. Good Laboratory Practice

Amino acid analysis is an accurate analytical technique but success does depend on meticulous work practices. It is extremely important when carrying out amino acid analysis that personal and work area cleanliness is of the highest standard at all stages. Powder free gloves should be worn when handling samples and glassware to avoid contamination. The use of dedicated glassware is recommended and should be kept separate from that used in the general laboratory. Reagents should be of the highest quality available and the water should be of ultra high grade, i.e., HPLC grade or better.

1.2. Internal Standards

Internal Standards are used to monitor physical and chemical losses throughout the analytical process. An accurately known amount of internal standard can be added to a protein or peptide solution before hydrolysis. The recovery of the internal standard reflects the recovery of the amino acids from the protein sample. Calculations, which refer to internal standard recovery allows corrections to be made for losses during analysis and therefore leads to more accurate results. Internal standards can also be added to the mixture of free amino acids, after hydrolysis of peptides and proteins, to correct for differences in sample application and any changes in reagent stability and flow rates.

Ideally, the characteristics of an internal standard are

a) It contains an unnaturally occurring primary amino acid that is commercially available and inexpensive.
b) It should be stable during hydrolysis.
c) Its derivatized response factor should be linear with concentration.
d) It needs to have a unique retention time without coeluting with other amino acids.

Commonly used amino acid standards include norleucine, norvaline, nitrotyrosine and aminobutyric acid.

2. Sample Purification and Preparation Methods

This chapter deals with some of the methods required in purifying samples for amino acid analysis. It is by no means exhaustive and should be used for guidance only. Methods for purifying peptides and proteins such as Gel Filtration, Gel Electro-elution and dialyzing the sample against volatile reagents, have lost popularity in recent years owing to heavy sample losses during the processes leading to poor recovery. None of these techniques are suitable when high sensitivity analysis is required.

2.1. Protein and Peptide purification using HPLC

Reverse Phase Liquid Chromatography (RPLC) should be used to remove significant amounts of buffer salts which could interfere with the hydrolysis and derivatization. The concentration, complexity and size of proteins or peptides present will determine the method of choice (**Tables 45.1–45.3**). Care should be taken when dealing with large or very hydrophobic proteins, as they can remain adsorbed onto the column resulting in poor recovery or even loss of sample. For complex mixtures of peptides and proteins Ion Exchange and/or RPLC can be employed to separate and purify the mixture into its component parts.

2.2. Zip Tips

Zip tips are disposable pipette tips that contain a tiny bed of silica column chromatography media. These tips are available with the following functional groups C_{18}, C_8, C_4, SAX, or SCX. They are similar to RPLC in nature but they use much smaller volumes and can be used to desalt and concentrate femtomole quantities of protein samples. Zip tips are generally not suitable

Table 45.1. HPLC terminology.

LC range	Column ID	Flow rate	Sample capacity	Amount of protein (pmoles)*
Standard	4.6 mm	1 ml/min	1 μg–1 mg	100
Narrowbore	2.1 mm	200 μl/min	2–50 μg	10
Micro	1.0 mm	40 μl/min	0.05–10 μg	1
Capillary	300 μm	4 μl/min	1 ng–1 μg	0.1
Nano	75 μm	200 ηl/min	0.02 ηg–0.05 ηg	0.001

*Please note that the table values are only for initial reference and guidance and should not be taken as absolute values.

Table 45.2. Main types of HPLC column packing.

Type of packing material	Comments
Silica	These are porous silica beads, which have a functional group chemically adsorbed (see **Table 45.1.**) The functional group adsorbed onto the silica will dictate the separation method. As with all these type of columns though there are silanophilic interactions, which are occasionally detected with UV giving rise to ghost peaks. The column packing material is also relatively unstable and therefore has shorter life times compared with polymeric columns.
Perfusion chromatography	These are a polymeric packing material derived from Polystyrene-Divinylbenzene (PS-DVB) and because there is no silica present therefore no silanophilic interactions. These also have larger pore sizes than conventional columns so flow rates can be increased without losing resolution, thus reducing analysis run times. The packing material is available with the equivalent functional groups attached. It is relatively easy to pack columns in-house and so reduce costs.
Monolithic	Solid rods of silica or polymeric material with a porous structure similar to perfusion chromatography. The columns can have the same equivalent functional groups attached. The lack of intraparticular void volume improves mass transfer and separation efficiency, allowing for fast, high-quality separations enabling higher flow rates and therefore reduced analysis run times. One distinct advantage of monolithic columns is when the column blocks usually at the front end, the offending blockage can be cut out and the column can used again albeit a little shorter than before.

Table 45.3. Main types of functional groups found on HPLC Column packing material.

Functional groups	Separation applications
The functional groups listed are available on the packing materials listed above.	The molecular cut offs are only approximate figures.
C18 (Reverse phase)	Peptides (0.1–10 kDa)
C8 (Reverse phase)	Whole proteins (10–70 kDa)
C4 (Reverse phase)	Large proteins (50–150 kDa)
C2 (Reverse phase)	Larger proteins (>200 kDa)
SCX (Strong cation exchange)	Binds negatively charged peptides/proteins
SAX (Strong anion exchange)	Binds positively charged peptides/proteins

for fractionation of even simple protein or peptide mixtures but some degree of fractionation can be achieved by varying the amount of organic solvent in the elution solution. They are commercially available as ZipTip™ from Millipore (Millipore, Bedford, MA) and as Stagetips™ from Proxeon Biosystems (Proxeon Biosystems, Odense, Denmark). These tips can be easily prepared manually in-house by adding the appropriate packing material, for example Poros Media (Applied Biosystems, Foster City, CA) as a slurry to a teased out Gel loader tip (Eppendorf AG, Hamburg, Germany) *(3)*.

2.3. Electrophoresis

1D or 2D gel electrophoresis can be used to separate more complex mixtures of proteins but the samples need to be blotted onto PVDF membrane before hydrolysis *(4,5)*. Sample recoveries are low after blotting and some amino acids such as methionine can be lost altogether.

2.4. Amino Acids in Physiological Fluids and Tissues

Samples including blood, serum, tissue, and cell culture media contain complex mixtures of proteinaceous material, lipids and salts that need to be removed prior to amino acid analysis as they can interfere with derivatization and subsequent analysis. Precipitation of interfering proteins with trichloroacetic acid (TCA), acetone or ethanol followed by centrifugation can reduce the amounts to an acceptable level. The acetone or ethanol, being volatile, can be easily removed by drying in a centrifuge under vacuum. TCA is a little more difficult to get rid of. The supernatant from the TCA-protein precipitate is chilled and the TCA extracted by cold ethyl acetate or ether. This extra extraction process however can lead to losses in amino acid content, which may be significant when high sensitivity is required. The addition of tri-potassium EDTA in the aqueous phase helps reduce the amount of interfering salts. Any lipids present that are not soluble in the aqueous phase, used to re-dissolve the amino acids, are left behind after centrifugation. A final filtration step will separate out any remaining particulate matter. This is a multiple step procedure and losses can occur at each step, the use of suitable internal standards can estimate the extent of these losses *(6–9)*.

2.5. Amino Acids in Foodstuffs

Very little preparation is required for hydrolysis of foodstuff samples other than the removal of high lipid content in some samples. An accurate amount of dried material is weighed into a suitable hydrolysis tube; an acid hydrolysis solution is added and heated to produce the free amino acids, which are then treated according to the preferred derivatization method.

Liquid food samples such as beer, water soluble extracts from cheese or protein hydrolysates are prepared for free amino acid analysis by de-proteinating the samples with TCA. Powder samples are prepared in the same way except that they are first resuspended in water. The de-proteinated samples are then quantified using the chosen derivatization method *(10)*.

2.6. Unusual Amino Acids, Including D-Amino Acids

The purification of these types of amino acids is treated as previously described in Sections 2.1–2.5. Only the derivatization of D-amino acids is different *(11)*.

3. Hydrolysis of Proteins and Peptides

There is no single hydrolysis method that will effectively cleave all proteins to free amino acids completely and quantitatively. This is owing to the varying stability of the peptide bonds between the different amino acids and the amino acid side chains, which are themselves susceptible to the reagents and conditions used to cleave the peptide bonds (**Table 45.4**). The classical hydrolysis conditions, to which all other methods are compared, is liquid phase hydrolysis in which the protein or peptide is heated in $6M$ hydrochloric acid under vacuum at 110°C for 18–24 h *(12)*.

Table 45.4. Stability of amino acid residues and peptide bonds during hydrolysis in $6\,M$ hydrochloric acid at 110°C.

Residue/bond	Stability/modification	Consequence	Remedy
Serine; Threonine	1. Side chain hydroxyl group modified by dehydration, which is increased with increased hydrolysis time and temperature	Serine and Threonine generated in low yield	1. Hydrolyse protein samples for different times between 6 and 72 h. Calculate the yields, extrapolate results to time zero to compensate for losses. *(12,47)*
	2. Ester formation with e.g., glutamic acid can occur at the drying stage *(46)*		2. Dry the hydrolysates rapidly in a rotary evaporator
Tyrosine	The phenolic group ($-C_6H_4OH$) side chain is modified by traces of hypochlorite/chlorine radicals present in the acid *(46)*	Tyrosine generated in low yield.	Incorporate phenol in acid to compete for hypochlorite /chlorine radicals *(12,28,48)*
Methionine	The thioether ($-CH_2-S-CH_3$) side chain is oxidized to the sulphoxide or sulphone *(46)*	Methionine, usually a less common residue anyway is converted to smaller peaks, more difficult to quantify on amino acid analysers.	Add reducing agent (e.g. dodecanthiol or thioglycolic acid) to acid/phenol mixture. *(28,49)*
Cystine; Cysteine	The free sulfhydryl (-SH) and disulphide (-S-S-) side chain groups are oxidized *(46)*	Cystine and Cysteine recovered in low nonquantifiable yields.	Chemically modify before hydrolysis. *(50,51)*
Trytophan	The Indole group side chain is destroyed by oxidation under acid conditions *(46)*	Tryptophan is not quantifiable under these conditions	Add reducing agents (e.g. dodecanthiol or thioglycolic acid to the acid/phenol mixture *(28,47,49)* or hydrolyse under alkaline conditions *(46,52,53)*
Asparagine; Glutamine	Asn and Gln are deaminated to form the respective acids *(46)*	Mixtures of Asp/Asn and Glu/Gln are normally assigned as Asx and Glx respectively in quantification data.	
Bonds between hydrophobic amino acids (e.g., Val-Val or any combination of Ala, Ile, Leu, Val)	Bonds are relatively stable *(46)*	Hydrolyse in poor yield. May be seen as dipeptides or unassigned peaks, on amino acid analyser or not seen at all.	Hydrolyse for longer time or elevated temperature e.g., 165°C *(12,28)*
Phosphorylation	Phosphorylated amino acids are labile	Destroyed under these extreme conditions	Reduce time for hydrolysis to 1–4 h *(54)*
Glycosylation	Amino acid-sugar interactions produces complex secondary reaction products *(46)*	Complex reaction products are difficult to interpret even if they are seen on an analyser.	Deglycosylate before hydrolysis *(55)*

Alternative hydrolysis conditions have been investigated in an effort to reduce total analysis times and increase sensitivity. With the advent of reverse phase HPLC methods, separation times were reduced to less than 20 min, making the long hydrolysis times out of proportion. Elevated temperatures in the acidic vapor phase reduced hydrolysis times to around 30–60 min, which was further reduced to between 10 and 40 min by using microwave irradiation.

Microwave hydrolysis is a relatively new hydrolysis technique that compares well with classical hydrolysis. It has gained popularity in recent years owing to reduced hydrolysis times. Hydrolysis and residue analysis can take place in an autosampler vial thus reducing the risk of sample contamination. This is a step closer towards automation, which may be important in a high throughput laboratory (13,14). It is particularly suited to hydrolysis of microgram quantities of pure proteins and peptides. Samples to be hydrolyzed are aliquoted into vials and freeze dried. These are then hydrolyzed to their amino acid constituents using a CEM MARS 5 microwave (CEM, Mathews, NC.) equipped with a protein hydrolysis kit. After hydrolysis times typically less than 45 min samples are ready for derivatization and analysis (15,16).

To improve recovery of heat labile amino acids various reagents have been added to the $6M$ hydrochloric acid to stabilize the side chains of specific amino acids. For example, free chlorine radicals from the acid can break down the side chain phenolic group of tyrosine; the addition of phenol to the acid competes for these free radicals and thus enhances the recovery of tyrosine. Tryptophan undergoes more stable hydrolysis under alkaline conditions or in the presence of strong reducing agents in the acid (17). Cystine/cysteine is more stable if it is chemically modified before hydrolysis, for example, by reaction with 4-vinylpyridine to form S-pyridylethylated cysteine. Cysteine

Table 45.5. Advantages and disadvantages of various hydrolysis techniques.

Method of hydrolysis	Advantages	Disadvantages
Vapor phase under argon (165°C for 45 min)	High sensitivity. Relatively fast hydrolysis times. Samples can be processed in batches.	Owing to the high pressures the reaction vial and seals require regular inspection. Danger of exploding vials and escaping hot acid can occur with defective vials and seals.
Vapor phase under vacuum (110°C for 18 h)	Conditions not as extreme as in vapor phase under argon. Samples can be processed in batches.	Long duration time for hydrolysis. Most analysers have relatively short derivatization and analysis times. The seals of the reaction vial require regular inspection as above.
Liquid phase (110°C for 18 h)	Conditions not as extreme as in vapor phase under argon.	Long duration time for hydrolysis. Samples are processed individually using a number of manipulations, which is very time consuming.
Microwave irradiation	Rapid hydrolysis times typically less than 1 h. Samples can be processed in batches.	Serine and threonine more susceptible to degradation by microwaves (14)
PVDF blots	Some useful composition data from samples which may not have been pure before SDS gel electrophoresis.	Low recoveries. Methionine may be lost altogether. Samples are difficult to remove successfully from the blot.
Liquid phase under alkaline conditions	Tryptophan is preserved throughout.	Nonvolatile reagents. Relatively high salt content. pH for derivatization difficult to control with such small volumes.

and methionine can also be oxidized to the more stable derivatives cysteic acid and methionine sulphone by reacting with performic acid, which itself is prepared by reacting hydrogen peroxide and formic acid.

The various methods of hydrolysis described here are summarized in **Table 45.5**.

4. Derivatization of Free Amino Acids

The derivatization of amino acids has been well documented since it was first developed in the 1950s *(18)*. The postcolumn derivatization method using ninhydrin remained the predominant method of choice for over 20 yr, this method was usually carried out on dedicated amino acid analyzers and routinely analyzed amino acid concentrations between 10 and 250 picomole/μL. A number of instrument manufacturers still make dedicated analyzers based on the ninhydrin method; these include Jeol (Tokyo, Japan), Hitachi (San Jose, CA) *(19)* and Biochrom (Cambridge, UK).

The development of methods suitable for use with reversed-phase high-performance liquid chromatography (RPLC) resulted in more rapid separation of the amino acid derivatives. Precolumn derivatization became the preferred method of choice, as the resolved peaks did not require dilution and this led to increased sensitivity. Fluorogenic derivatization methodologies were developed such as dansyl chloride *(20)* and *o*-phthaldialdehyde (OPA) *(21)* enabling further increased sensitivity of amino acid detection to less than 1 pmol of an amino acid. However these methods have some disadvantages including derivative instability, reagent interference and lack of reaction with secondary amino acids. 9-fluorenylmethylchloroformate (Fmoc) in conjunction with OPA helped to alleviate some of those problems. Agilent Technologies (Agilent Technologies, Palo Alto, CA) have developed a Zorbax "eclipse amino acid analysis (AAA) column" that uses this method and is suitable to separate the amino acids commonly found in protein hydrolyzates *(22)*.

Derivatization using phenylisothiocyanate (PITC), the first step of the Edman method for determining amino acid sequence of proteins avoids many of the problems described so far. Tarr and coworkers *(23)* first described this method and full details for the application of the method to the analysis of protein hydrolyzates were published in 1984 *(24)*. Because PITC is volatile it is relatively easy to evaporate and therefore does not interfere with the chromatography to any significant degree. This also made it easier for the development of commercial analyzers and employees at Waters Chromatography Division of Millipore Corporation *(25–27)* developed the Waters Pico-Tag System (Millipore, Bedford, MA). Similarly, Applied Biosystems (Foster City, CA) introduced the 420 and 421 Amino Acid Analyzers *(28)*. It should be noted that these Applied Biosystems analyzers are no longer commercially available. Waters also introduced a system *(29,30)* using the fluorescent derivative 6-aminoquinoyl-*N*-hydroxysuccinimidylcarbamate (AQC); they have recently coupled the AQC derivatization with an Acquity Ultra Performance Liquid Chromatography (UPLC) to give analysis times of less than 10 min *(31)*.

4.1. Postcolumn Ninhydrin Derivatization

Ion-exchange chromatography with postcolumn ninhydrin detection is one of the most common methods employed for quantitative amino acid analysis.

The derivatization chemistry is very robust, reliable and reproducible. As a rule, a lithium-based cation-exchange system is employed for the analysis of the more complex physiological samples, and the faster Sodium-based cation-exchange system is used for the more simplistic amino acid mixtures obtained from protein hydrolyzates. Separation of the amino acids on an ion-exchange column is accomplished through a combination of changes in pH and cation strength. A temperature gradient is often employed to enhance separation.

When the amino acid reacts with ninhydrin, the reactant has a characteristic purple color, which absorbs at 590 nm. A yellow coloration indicates an imino acid such as proline, which absorbs at 440 nm. The postcolumn reaction between ninhydrin and amino acid eluted from the column is therefore monitored at both 440 and 590 nm.

The detection limit is considered to be 10 pmol for most amino acid derivatives and 50 pmole for proline and hydroxyproline. Response linearity is obtained in the range of 20–500 pmol with correlation coefficients exceeding 0.999. This method is best suited for protein and peptides that require 0.15 M buffer salts or detergents to aid solubilization.

Good compositional data can be obtained from the analysis of derivatized protein hydrolyzates containing as little as 1 µg of protein/peptide.

4.2. Postcolumn OPA Fluorometric Derivatization

O-Phthaldialdehyde (OPA) reacts with primary amines, in the presence of a thiol compound, to form highly fluorescent isoindole products. This reaction is used with postcolumn derivatization of amino acids by ion-exchange chromatography.

OPA does not react with secondary amines (imino acids such as proline) to form fluorescent substances, however oxidation with sodium hypochlorite does allow this reaction to occur.

The procedure uses a strongly acidic cation-exchange column for the separation of free amino acids using an aqueous gradient of increasing pH and cationic strength followed by postcolumn oxidation with sodium hypochlorite, which is added continuously to the flow from the column. The separated free amino acids are derivatized using OPA and a thiol compound such as N-acetyl-L-cysteine or 2-mercaptoethanol. The derivatization of primary amino acids is not noticeably affected by the continuous supply of sodium hypochlorite.

The OPA-amino acids are detected by the use of a fluorometric detector with an excitation wavelength of 348 nm and an emission wavelength of 450 nm. The detection limit is considered to be at the few tens of picomole level for most of the amino acid derivatives. Response linearity is obtained in the range of a few picomoles to a few tens of nanomoles level.

Good compositional data could be obtained from the analysis of derivatized protein hydrolyzates containing as little as 500 ηg of protein/peptide.

4.3. Precolumn Phenylisothiocyanate (PITC) Derivatization

PITC reacts with the free amino groups of the primary and secondary amino acids to form the corresponding phenylthiocarbamyl (PTC) derivative, which can be detected with high sensitivity at 254 nm.

After the excess PITC is removed under vacuum or dry gas, the derivatized amino acids can be stored dry at −20°C for several weeks with no significant degradation. Once in solution however, there is product degradation after a few days even when the solution is kept cold. It should be noted that glutamine is unstable in a free state (approx 1 wk under acidic conditions at 4°C) and therefore samples containing glutamine should be derivatized and analyzed almost immediately.

The separation of the PTC-amino acids on a reversed-phase HPLC column is accomplished using a gradient change of 50 mM sodium acetate in water and 70% acetonitrile containing 32 mM sodium acetate solution. PTC-amino acids eluted from the column are monitored at 254 nm.

Detection limit is considered to be 1 pmole for most of the amino acid derivatives. Response linearity is obtained in the range of 20–1,000 pmole.

Good compositional data could be obtained from the analysis of derivatized protein hydrolyzates containing as little as 100 ηg of protein/peptide.

4.4. Precolumn AQC Derivatization

6-Aminoquinolyl-N-hydroxysuccinimidyl-carbamate (AQC) reacts with primary and secondary amino acids to form stable, unsymmetrical urea derivatives (AQC-amino acids), which are highly fluorescent and readily amenable to analysis by reversed-phase HPLC.

Separation of the AQC-amino acids on a RPLC column is accomplished through a combination of changes in concentrations of sodium acetate solution and acetonitrile in water. Selective fluorescence detection of the derivatives with excitation wavelength at 248 nm and emission wavelength at 395 nm allows for the direct injection of the reaction mixture with no significant interference from the only major fluorescent reagent by-product, 6-aminoquinoline (AMQ), which has emission maxima of 520 nm. Excess reagent can be rapidly hydrolyzed ($t1/2$ <15 s) to yield AMQ, N-hydroxysuccinimide (NFS) and carbon dioxide.

AQC-amino acids are essentially stable for at least 1 wk at room temperature.

Detection limit is considered to be ranging from 50 to 300 fmol for normal hydrolyzate amino acids, except for cysteine, which has a detection limit of around 800 fmol.

Good compositional data could be obtained from the analysis of derivatized protein hydrolyzates containing as little as 50 ηg of protein/peptide.

4.5. Precolumn OPA Derivatization

As with postcolumn derivatization (see derivatization method 2), OPA in conjunction with a thiol reagent reacts with primary amine groups to form highly fluorescent indole products. The OPA-amino acids are separated by reversed-phase HPLC with fluorometric detection. Instability of the OPA-amino acid derivative requires the HPLC separation and analysis to be performed immediately following derivatization.

This method does not detect secondary amino acids such as proline; to compensate for this the technique may be combined with another technique described in Section 4.7. With the use of photodiode array and fluorescence detection *(32)* this combined method is useful for the analysis of plasma amino acids, which it is claimed is comparable to IEC and could represent an alternative. However two injections per sample are advised and the column must be equilibrated perfectly or co-eluting peaks can occur.

OPA in the presence of 3-mercaptopropionic acid is used to derivatize and quantify amino acids and amines in beer, wine and vinegar samples in a single HPLC run using photodiode array and fluorescence detection *(33)*.

Fluorescence intensity of OPA-amino acids is measured with an excitation wavelength of 348 nm and an emission wavelength of 450 nm.

Detection limits as low as 50 fmol have been reported, although the practical limit of analysis remains at 1 pmol.

Few amino acid analysis methods specialize in the analysis of glutamine and glutamate. Shih et al. *(34)* describe a method that can successfully quantify glutamine, glutamic acid, asparagine , aspartic acid, serine and histidine using precolumn OPA derivatization and fluorescent detection. A modification of this method using UV/VIS detection at 340 nm was used to quantify glutamine levels in glutamine rich hydrolyzates *(35)*. Detection of OPA derivatives from protein biopharmaceuticals has also been successfully validated using UV/VIS detection at 338 nm *(36)*. These methods will be of interest to laboratories that don't have access to a fluorescent detector.

OPA derivatization with *N*-isobutyrylcysteine followed by reverse phase HPLC with fluorogenic detection is used in the determination of amino acid enantiomers. The *N*-isobutyrylcysteine, a chiral thiol compound, forms diastereomeric derivatives, which can be separated by reverse phase chromatography *(37)*.

4.6. Precolumn DABS-Cl Derivatization

Precolumn derivatization of amino acids with Dimethylamino-azobenzenesulphonyl chloride (DABS-Cl) is followed by reversed-phase HPLC separation with visible light detection at 436 nm. This method can analyze imino acids such as proline at the same degree of sensitivity as other amino acids including tryptophan. The other acid-labile residues, asparagine and glutamine, can also be analyzed if they are initially converted into diaminopropionic acid and diaminobutyric acid, respectively.

It should be noted that norleucine might not be appropriate as an internal standard for this method because this compound is eluted in a crowded region of the chromatogram; nitrotyrosine can be used as the internal standard as it elutes in a less crowded region.

The detection limit of DABS-amino acid is about 1 pmol. As little as 2–5 picomoles of an individual DABS-amino acid can be quantitatively analyzed with reliability, and only 10–30 ηg of the dabsylated protein hydrolyzate is required for each analysis.

4.7. Precolumn Fmoc-Cl Derivatization

9-Fluorenylmethylchloroformate (Fmoc-Cl) reacts with both primary and secondary amino acids to form highly fluorescent products. The reaction of Fmoc-Cl with amino acids proceeds under mild conditions in aqueous solution and is completed in 30 s. The derivatives are stable with only the histidine derivative showing any breakdown. Fmoc-Cl is itself fluorescent but the reagent excess and fluorescent side products can be eliminated without loss of Fmoc-amino acids, which are then separated by RPLC. The separation is carried out by gradient elution varied linearly from a mixture of acetonitrile, methanol and acetic acid (10:40:50) to a mixture of acetonitrile and acetic acid (50:50). The 20 amino acid derivatives are separated in around 20 min. Fluorometric detection set at an excitation wavelength of 260 nm and an emission wavelength of 313 nm can be used.

The detection limit is in the fmol range. A linearity range of 0.1–50 pmole is obtained for most of the amino acids.

This method is used for example, to analyze free amino acids in fermented shrimp waste *(38)*.

4.8. Precolumn Dansyl-Cl Derivatization

Precolumn derivatization of amino acids with dansyl chloride (Dans-Cl) followed by RPLC separation with a fluorescence detector set at an excitation wavelength of 340 nm and an emission wavelength of 515 nm. The reaction requires optimal alkaline conditions around pH 9.5 with a reaction time of about 1 h. Dansyl Chloride has to be removed before RPLC because it interferes with the chromatography.

This method, like DABS-Cl, can analyze the imino acids such as proline and hydroxyproline at the same degree of sensitivity as other amino acids including tryptophan.

The detection limit of Dans-amino acid is again in the same order of magnitude as DABS-amino acids at less than 1 pmole.

4.8.1. Detection of Underivatized Amino Acids

A mass spectrometer can be used to detect underivatized amino acids; however problems can arise with the identification of isoleucine and leucine, which have the same mass. The separation of amino acids before detection by mass spectrometry (MS) is achieved either by ion exchange liquid chromatography, RPLC or CE.

Capillary electrophoresis in conjunction with an electrospray ionization tandem mass spectrometry (CE-MS/MS) allows complex mixtures of amino acids as found in physiological fluids to be separated, identified and quantified without derivatization. With this equipment it is possible to detect amino acids at the attomole level (39).

Liquid chromatography electrospray mass spectrometry (LC-MS/MS) has found uses in identification of metabolites from anaerobic protein digestion (40), monitoring the metabolism of amino acids during microbial fermentation (41) and quantification of amino acids on dry blood spots, which represents a quick nonevasive technique for the detection of metabolic disorders (42).

Liquid chromatography coupled to atmospheric pressure chemical ionization mass spectrometry (LC-APCI-MS) can be used to analyze underivatized amino acids in food matrices such as baby foods, juices and honeys (43).

Other techniques that can detect underivatized amino acids include ion exchange chromatography coupled to electrochemical detection (44). This method was assessed in an Association of Biomolecular Resource Facility (ABRF) Amino Acid Research Group (AAARG) collaborative study and found to compare well with pre and post column derivatization techniques for protein determinations using amino acid analysis.

Similarly, Tuma et al. (45) describe a method using CE in conjunction with contactless conductivity detection (CCD).

5. Data Handling and Basic Calculations

From the integrated chromatogram all the amino acids of interest are identified and their peak areas measured but these should be checked for the correct baseline, peak markers and peak absorbance threshold against the relevant integration parameter settings.

Calculations can be carried out manually but it is extremely tedious and time consuming, the use of a spreadsheet can make these tasks more efficient.

Dedicated amino acid analysis systems will have software incorporated, which will carry out all these calculations automatically.

Amino acid identification—by comparing the retention times between the sample chromatogram with that of the standard chromatogram, the amino acids of interest can be identified.

The peak area of the amino acid is found by measuring the width of the peak at half peak height multiplied by the height of the peak.

The amino acid composition of the sample is determined by comparing the peak areas of the amino acid standard with the peak areas of the sample.

The amount of unknown amino acid in the sample can be found from the calculation

A = (peak area of internal standard from the standard x the amount of Internal Standard added to sample)/(peak area of internal standard from the sample)

B = (peak area of amino acid from the sample)/(peak area of amino acid from the standard)

Amount of amino acid in the injection volume (C) = A × B pmoles.
Multiply these values (C) by all dilution factors.

Calculate the amino acid composition expressed as Mole%.

a) Sum the pmoles for each individual amino acid (C) (excluding the Internal Standard). Report the results in pmol/mL

b) Mole% = (pmoles of each amino acid × 100)/(the value of the sum of each amino acid (C))

Calculate the amino acid composition expressed as Weight%

a) Multiply pmoles of each amino acid by the residue weight (molecular weight −18) of an amino acid to convert pmoles to pgrams. Divide by 1,000 to convert to η grams.

b) Sum the η grams for each of the amino acids. Report the results in ηgrams/mL.

c) Divide the weight of each amino acid by the sum of their weights to determine the weight fraction and multiply by 100 to convert to weight%.

Calculate the number of residues in the protein sample
For this the molecular weight of the peptide or protein has to be known.

Number of residues = (η grams of each amino acids/sum of
all amino acids) × molecular weight

6. Relevant Websites

The Association of Biomolecular Resource Facilities (ABRF) www.abrf.org periodically conducts studies into various aspects of amino acid analysis used within its members' laboratories worldwide. It is highly recommended that this website is viewed often as the wealth of information contained is invaluable to both novice and advanced users alike.

http://www.chemie.fu-berlin.de/chemistry/bio/amino-acids_en.html. This website includes information such as molecular formula, molecular mass and 3D structures for individual amino acids.

http://orion1.paisley.ac.uk/Courses/StFunMac/glossary/amino.html gives an introduction to amino acids including structure, ionization and isomers.

http://www.mcb.ucdavis.edu/courses/bis102/AAProp.html features study guides about the properties of amino acid side chains/R groups. It also includes 3D structures of amino acids.

http://micro.magnet.fsu.edu/aminoacids/index.html The amino acid collection contains micrographs of individual amino acids and interesting information on their roles in metabolism.

References

1. Barrett GC, Elmore DT (1998) Amino acids and peptides. Cambridge University Press, UK
2. Anders JC (2002) Advances in amino acid analysis. Biopharm Int 4:32–39
3. Wilm M, Shevchenko A, Houthaeve T, Brit S, Schweigerer L, Fotsis T, Mann M (1996) Femtomole sequencing of proteins from polyacrylamide gels by nano-electrospray mass spectrometery. Nature 370:466–469
4. Tous GI, Fausnaugh JL, Akinyosoye O, Lackland H, Winter-Cash P, Vitorica FJ, Stein S (1989) Amino acid analysis on polyvinylidene difluoride membranes. Anal Biochem 179:50–55
5. Nakagawa S, Fukuda T (1989) Direct amino acid analysis of proteins electroblotted onto polyvinylidene difluoride membrane from sodium dodecyl sulfate-polyacrylamide gel. Anal Biochem 181:75–78
6. Lyndon AR, Davidson I, Houlihan DF (1993) Changes in tissue and plasma free amino acid concentrations after feeding in atlantic cod. Fish Physiol Biochem 10:365–375
7. Amezaga M, Davidson I, McLaggan D, Verhaul A, Abee T, Booth I (1995) The role of peptide metabolism in the growth of *Listeria monocytogenes* ATCC 23074 at high osmolarity. Microbiology 141:41–49
8. Roe AJ, McLaggan D, Davidson I, O'Byrne C, Booth I (1998) Pertubation of anion balance during inhibition of growth of *Escherichia coli* by weak acids. J Bacteriol 180:767–772
9. Menti E, Coutteau P, Houlihan P, Davidson I, Sorgeloos P (2002) Protein turnover, amino acid profile and amino acid flux in juvenile shrimp *Litopenaeus vannamei*: effects of dietary protein source. J Exp Biol 205:3107–3122
10. Fenelon MA, O'Connor P, Guinee TP (2000) The effect of fat content on the microbiology and proteolysis in Cheddar cheese during ripening. J Dairy Sci 83:2173–2183
11. Scaloni A, Simmaco M, Bossa F (2003) D-amino acid analysis. In: Smith BJ (ed) Methods in molecular biology, vol 211, Chapter 15, Protein sequencing protocols, 2nd edn. Humana Press, Totowa, NJ pp 169–180
12. Moore S, Stein WH (1963) Chromatographic determination of amino acids by the use of automatic recording equipment. Methods Enzymol 6:819–831
13. Fountoulakis M, Lahm HW (1998) Hydrolysis and amino acid composition analysis of proteins. J Chromatogr A 826:109–134
14. Weiss M, Manneberg M, Juranville J-F, Lahm H-W, Fountoulakis M (1998) Effect of the hydrolysis method on the determination of the amino acid composition of proteins. J Chromatogr A 795:263–275
15. Jorgensen NOG, Jensen RE (1997) Determination of dissolved combined amino acids using microwave-assisted hydrolysis and HPLC precolumn derivatisation for labelling of primary and secondary amines. Mar Chem 57:287–297
16. Kaiser K, Benner R (2005) Hydrolysis-induced racemization of amino acids. Limnol Oceanogr Methods 3:318–325
17. Ravindran G, Bryden WL (2005) Tryptophan determination in proteins and feedstuffs by ion exchange chromatography. Food Chem 89:309–314
18. Spackman DH, Stein WH, Moore S (1958) Automatic recording apparatus for use in the chromatography of amino acids. Anal Chem 30:1190–1206

19. LCGC North America Advanstar Communications Inc., Iselin, NJ (2006) Product Page 8. Jan 2006

20. Hsu KT, Currie BL (1978) High Performance liquid chromatography of Dns-amino acids and application to peptide hydrolysates. J Chromatogr 166:555–561

21. Lindroth P, Mopper K (1979) High performance liquid chromatographic determination of subpicomole amounts of amino acids by precolumn fluorescence derivatisation with o-phthaldialdehyde. Anal Chem 51:1667–1674

22. Henderson JW, Ricker RD, Bidlingmeyer BA, Woodward C (2000) Rapid, accurate, sensitive and reproducible HPLC analysis of amino acids. Agilent Technologies Technical Note 5980–1193E

23. Knoop DR, Morgan ET, Tarr GE, Coon MJ (1982) Purification and characterization of a unique isoenzyme of cytochrome P-450 from liver microsomes of ethanol-treated rabbits. J Biol Chem 257:8472–8480

24. Hendrickson RL, Meredrith SC (1984) Amino acid analysis by reverse phase high performance liquid chromatography; precolumn derivatisation with phenylisothiocyanate. Anal Biochem 136:65–74

25. Bidlingmeyer BA, Cohen SA, Tarvin TL (1984) Rapid analysis of amino acids using pre-column derivatisation. J Chromatogr 336:93–104

26. Bidlingmeyer BA, Cohen SA, Tarvin TL (1986) Amino acid analysis of submicro-gram hydrolysate samples. In: Walsh K (ed) Methods in protein sequence analysis. Humana Press, Clifton, NJ, 229–245

27. Cohen SA, Strydom DJ (1988) Amino acid analysis utilizing phenylisothiocyanate derivatives. Anal Biochem 174:1–16

28. Dupont D, Keim P, Chui A, Bozzini ML, Wilson KJ (1988) Gas-phase hydrolysis for PTC-amino acids. Applied Biosystems User Bulletin No. 2 1–10

29. Strydom DJ, Cohen SA (1994) Comparison of amino acid analyses by phenyli-sothiocyanate and 6-aminoquinolyl-N-hydroxysuccinimidyl carbamate precolumn derivatisation. Anal Biochem 222:19–28

30. Cohen SA, Michaud DP (1993) Synthesis of a fluorescent derivatising reagent 6-aminoquinoyl-N-hydroxysuccinimydyl carbamate and its application for the analysis of hydrolysate amino acids via high performance liquid chromatography. Anal Biochem 211:279–287

31. LCGC North America Advanstar Communications Inc., Iselin, NJ (2006) The application notebook. Fast and Ultrafast HPLC on Sub-2 Mm Porous Particles. Where do we go from here? by Ronald E. Majors

32. Schwarz EL, Roberts WL, Pasquali M (2005) Analysis of plasma amino acids by HPLC with photodiode array and fluorescence detection. Clinica Chimica Acta 354:83–90

33. Kutlan D, Molnar-Perl I (2003) New aspects of the simultaneous analysis of amino acids and amines as their o-phthaldialdehyde derivatives by high-performance liquid chromatography. analysis of beer, wine and vinegar. J Chromatogr A 987:311–322

34. Shih FF (1985) Analysis of glutamine, glutamic acid and pyroglutamic acid in protein hydrolysates by high performance liquid chromatography. J Chromatogr 322:248–256

35. O'Connor P, FitzGerald RJ (1998) Glutamine enriched peptide products. PCT International Patent Application (PCT/IE98/00068)

36. Bartolomeo MP, Maisano F (2006) Validation of a reversed phase HPLC method for quantitative amino acid analysis. J Biomol Tech 17:131–137

37. Fitznar HP, Loxbbes JM, Kattner G (1999) Determination of enantiomeric amino acids with high performance liquid chromatography and pre-column derivatisation with o-phthaldialdehyde and N-isobutyrylcysteine in seawater and fossil samples (mollusks). J Chromatogr A 832:123–132

38. Lopez-Cervantes J, Sanchez-Machado DI, Rosas-Rodriguez JA (2006) Analysis of free amino acids in fermented shrimp waste by high-performance liquid chromatography. J Chromatogr A 1105:106–110

39. Moini M, Schultz CL, Mahmood H (2003) CE/Electrospray ionisation-MS analysis of underivatised D/L amino acids and several small neurotransmitters at attomole levels through the use of 18-crown-6-tetracarboxylic acid as a complexation reagent/background electrolyte. Anal Chem 75:6282–6287

40. Hecht C, Bieler S, Griehl C (2005). Liquid chromatographic-mass spectrometric-analyses of anaerobe protein degradation products. J Chromatogr A 1088:121–125

41. Dalluge JJ, Smith S, Sanchez-Riera F, McGuire C, Hobson R (2004) Potential of fermentation profiling via rapid measurement of amino acid metabolism by liquid chromatography–tandem mass spectrometry. J Chromatogr A 1043:3–7

42. Zoppa M, Gallo L, Zacchello F, Giordano G (2006) Method for the quantification of underivatized amino acids on dry blood spots from newborn screening by HPLC-ESI-MS/MS. J Chromatogr B 831:267–273

43. Ozcan S, Senyuva HZ (2006) Improved and simplified liquid chromatography/atmospheric pressure ionisation mass spectrometry for the analysis of underivatised free amino acids in various foods. J Chromatogr A 1135(2):179–185

44. Valoren P, Hanko, Rohrer JS (2002) Direct determination of tryptophan using high pressure anion exchange chromatography with integrated pulsed amperometric detection. Anal Biochem 308:204–209

45. Tuma P, Samcova E, Andelova K (2006) Determination of free amino acids and related compounds in amniotic fluid by capillary electrophoresis with contactless conductivity detection. J Chromatogr B 839:12–18

46. Hunt S (1985) Degradation of amino acids accompanying *in vitro* protein hydrolysis. In: Barrett GC (ed) Chemistry and biochemistry of the amino acids. Chapman and Hall, London, pp 376–398

47. Strydom DJ, Anderson TT, Apostal I, Fox WJ, Paxton RJ, Crabb JW (1993) Cysteine and tryptophan amino acid analysis of ABRF92-AAA. In: Angeletti RH (ed) Techniques in protein chemistry IV. Academic Press, San Diego, CA, pp 279–288

48. Bidlingmeyer BA, Tarvin TL, Cohen SA (1986) Amino acid analysis of submicrogram hydrolysate samples. In: Walsh K (ed) Methods in protein sequence analysis. Humana Press, Clifton, NJ, pp 229–244

49. Matsubara H, Sasaki RM (1969) High recovery of tryptophan from acid hydrolysis of proteins. Biochem Biophys Res Commun 35:175–181

50. Amons R (1986) Vapour-phase modifications of sulfhydryl groups in proteins. FEBS Lett 212:68–72

51. Carne AF (1994) Chemical modifications of proteins. In: Walker JM (ed) Methods in molecular biology, basic protein and peptide protocols, vol. 32, Chapter 34. Humana Press, Totowa, NJ, pp 311–320

52. Hugli TE, Moore S (1972) Determination of the tryptophan content of proteins by ion exchange chromatography of alkaline hydrolysis. J Biol Chem 247:2828–2834

53. Simpson RJ, Neuberger MR, Lui T-Y (1976) Complete amino acid analysis of proteins from a single hydrolysate. J Biol Chem 251:1936–1940

54. Capony J-P, Demaille JG (1983) A rapid microdetermination of phosphoserine, phosphothreonine and phosphotyrosine in proteins by automatic cation exchange on a conventional amino acid analyser. Anal Biochem 128:206–212

55. Harvey DJ (2003) Identification of sites of glycosylation In: Smith BJ (ed) Methods in molecular biology, vol 211, Chapter 30, Protein sequencing protocols, 2nd edn. Humana Press Inc., Totowa, NJ, pp 371–383

46

Surface Plasmon Resonance

K. Scott Phillips and Quan Jason Cheng

1. Introduction

SPR is an elegant surface sensitive optical technique most commonly employed for biointeraction analysis on a flat substrate. Although the concept was suggested as early as 1968 (*1,2*), the use of SPR for biosensing in its present capacity started to gain momentum from the mid-1980s (*3*). The most important advantage of SPR is its label-free nature. As explained below, SPR measures changes in the amount of material within about 200 nm of the surface. Because detection is based on refractive index, rather than a reporter molecule such as a fluorophore, there is no need to label the material that will be detected. The downside of this advantage is lack of specificity. Anything that binds or sticks to the surface will be detected, so one must be careful to eliminate this type of interference through careful experimental design, sophisticated surface chemistry, and often the use of a reference channel for comparison. Another advantage of SPR is that it is conducted in real time. Unlike endpoint measurements of binding or surface changes using bulk techniques such as fluorescence, the surface sensitivity of SPR, when used with a properly designed flow cell, allows monitoring of a surface interaction as it occurs. This real-time information can be fit to theoretical models to yield kinetic and thermodynamic parameters. The result is accurate determination of binding constants without waiting for equilibrium to be established, greatly facilitating analysis of large compound libraries. When combined with multiplex instruments, this is especially useful for pharmaceutical screening. SPR is also complementary to other nonlabeled surface sensitive analysis technologies such as QCM or impedance. Assuming complete monolayer coverage, thickness changes as little as several angstroms can be detected. Finally, because SPR is a spectroscopic technique, SPR imaging is also possible. In the applications section, we will discuss the exciting nature of SPR imaging spectroscopy (SPRi). For comprehensive reviews of SPR and SPR imaging, the reader is referred to references (*4–17*).

From: *Molecular Biomethods Handbook, 2nd Edition.*
Edited by: J. M. Walker and R. Rapley © Humana Press, Totowa, NJ

2. How SPR Works

2.1. Instrumentation

A variety of SPR instrumentation is available, ranging from inexpensive (<$10,000 US) to extremely high-end (>$300,000). A review of some instruments was recently published in the Analytical Chemistry A-pages *(18)*. Since then, even more units have become available with powerful new features. **Fig. 46.1** shows an SPR instrument setup with the common *Kretschmann (1)* configuration. The essential parts include a light source, a prism on a rotating stage, and a detector. The substrate sits on top of the prism, usually joined by a thin film of index matching fluid. Substrates are usually glass slides with a refractive index matching the prism. On top of the glass is a ~50 nm layer of gold, sometimes with a thin chromium adhesion layer. The light source (typically a laser) is directed through a series of focusing and polarizing lenses into the prism at an angle normal to the bottom of the gold surface. Snell's law describes the critical angle at which total internal reflection (TIR) occurs. In TIR mode, although no light comes out of the top of the prism at the reflecting gold surface, the photon electrical field extends ~1/4 wavelength beyond it. The decaying em field is *evanescent* because it decays exponentially and is only useful within about ~200 nm of the gold surface. Beyond that, the effects are too small to be experimentally useful in most cases. Near this surface, the light field can interact with a highly delocalized state of weakly bound electrons in gold. When the wavevectors of the incoming light and electron field match, they can resonantly couple. The prism is used to alter the momentum of light to make it ideal for this resonance condition. When the angle of incoming light allows for plasmon resonance, energy is lost, and the amount of reflected light is reduced. This produces a dip shaped curve on an angle vs. reflectivity plot. It is important to understand how this all relates to biointeraction analysis and detection of mass changes on the surface. Basically, an increase in mass near the surface, such as a bound ligand or thin film, changes the refractive index environment near the surface. Because the resonance condition depends on the refractive index near the surface, the minimum angle at which resonance occurs is highly sensitive to small changes.

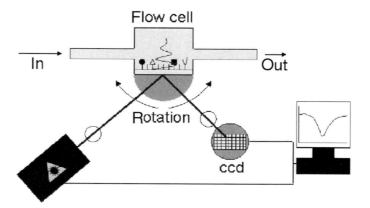

Fig. 46.1. Kretschmann configuration of an SPR setup

2.2. Measurement Modes

SPR measurement is usually performed in one of two ways. In the first, the angle can be scanned while the intensity of reflected light is monitored. As the stage rotates through the minimum angle, this produces a dip-shaped curve like that shown in **Fig. 46.2**. Although suitable for characterization purposes or static measurements, this route is normally too slow for monitoring changes over time. Some instruments include a software routine that can scan through a narrow range of angles around the minimum angle. Because this is much faster, it can be repeated continuously, and the software can adjust the range of angles scanned if the minimum angle changes, such as during a binding event. In this way, a plot of minimum angle versus time can be obtained. The other popular method of measurement is slightly more complex. First a reflectivity plot is obtained by rotating the stage through the minimum angle. Notice in **Fig. 46.2** that the left and right sides of the dip shaped curve have a very steep slope. If the minimum angle condition was to change because of binding, the intensity would rapidly move up or down depending on that slope. In this way, the stage is set before starting an experiment and does not need to be scanned. As shown in **Fig. 46.3**, the change in intensity is plotted vs. time, and it increases (or decreases, depending on which slope is chosen) as binding occurs. A major advantage of this route is speed because data can be collected as fast as the detector can integrate it. The downside is that the data are less useful for theoretical calculations of thickness and must stay within a more narrow linear range. This method is popular for ligand-binding studies and others requiring high sensitivity and fast response.

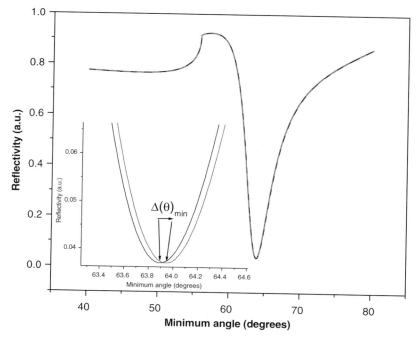

Fig. 46.2. Theoretical reflectivity as a function of minimum angle for a 1 nm (black dashed) and 2 nm (gray) organic film on a gold substrate. The difference in minimum angle can clearly be seen upon zooming in on the dip-shaped curve area (inset)

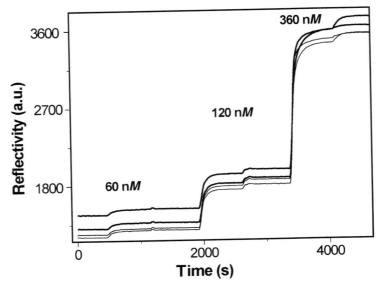

Fig. 46.3. SPR plots of binding versus time for several concentrations of cholera toxin to receptor GM1 in supported membranes on silicate modified gold substrates. From ref. *72*

2.3. Data Analysis

2.3.1. Thickness Evaluation

For thickness determinations, quantitative analysis is performed by comparing the experimental data with theoretically predicted values of an optical multilayer stack. Several free programs are available on the web (Corn Group: http://corninfo.ps.uci.edu/calculations.html, Knoll Group: http://www.mpip-mainz.mpg.de/knoll/soft/index.html) that will calculate thickness. An estimate must be made regarding appropriate input values for the optical parameters of all layers and thickness of individual layers, as well as the substrate thickness and refractive index and the wavelength of light used. To exactly determine the thickness of multiple layers without exact inputs for thickness and refractive index, multiple spectra can be analyzed at different wavelengths or in different media, solving for unknowns in a parallel fashion.

2.3.2. Kinetic Analysis

Kinetic analysis has been made more routine with the aid of software packages specifically designed to work with certain instruments and flow cells. Typically, these set up model differential equations using a background subtracted response-time curve with inputs of analyte concentration, valency of the interaction, and a number of parameters related to mass transfer. A typical equation would involve species X binding to an immobilized species Y to form a complex XY. With a knowledge of surface density and solution concentration of species X and Y, the binding constants for association and dissociation can be solved.

$$d[XY]/dt = k_a [X][Y] - k_d[XY] \qquad (1)$$

The equations are solved numerically and plotted with the original curve to show the closeness of fit. More elaborate models can be used to reduce error resulting from mass transport limitations and better model intermediate binding steps and multivalent binding. Even more accurate values can be obtained by using "global fitting" of sensorgrams at several different concentrations.

3. Applications of SPR

Although the number of publications reporting the use of SPR started out in the dozens, over 2000 were published in 2006 alone. Many investigations using SPR for characterization of biomolecular interactions have extremely high citation rates because with SPR the authors were able to obtain data that was not previously accessible, thereby gaining new understanding of important and previously investigated biological systems. SPR is so versatile because it can be used for many interactions on a flat surface. Generally, larger molecules such as proteins are better for analysis because they have a larger mass and cause greater minimum angle change. However, highly sensitive instruments are pushing the detection limits lower so that SPR can be used with small compounds. Below we group the types of interactions into two main classes, nucleic acids and proteins, although many others have been achieved, such as lipids *(19)*, saccharides *(20)* and gangliosides *(21)*.

3.1. Nucleic Acids

SPR has been used for DNA interactions with many different classes of compounds. Starting with small building blocks, it has been used for sequencing *(22)* and single nucleotide polymorphism analysis *(23)*. SPR imaging has been demonstrated for DNA hybridization *(24)*, DNA/RNA hybridization *(25)*, and DNA/protein interactions *(26)*. DNA/PNA and RNA/PNA interaction have also been investigated *(27)*. DNA interaction with peptide subunits of a larger protein has been monitored to evaluate recognition *(28)*. Chemically induced hairpin formation has been examined in DNA monolayers *(29)*.

3.2. Proteins

Some of the first reports of kinetic analysis were using antibody-antigen interactions *(30)*. However, SPR is so sensitive to nonspecific adsorption that it has been used to screen for nonspecific protein adsorption to help improve biosensor methods *(31)*. The carboxymethyldextran surface developed for gold surface modification was a key selling point of Biacore sensor chip technology and allowed for high immobilization efficiency with reduced hydrophobic nonspecific binding *(32)*. The development of several different commercially available surfaces has also aided in opening up SPR analysis to different areas of biomolecular interaction study. One of the major uses remains the investigation and optimization of antibody antigen interactions *(33–37)*. These are key to many aspects of biology and biochemistry, and are one of the most well-investigated protein interaction systems. Another important area is the interaction of receptors with other proteins and smaller molecules *(38–46)*. It is important to understand how receptors function because they are responsible for many aspects of cell life. Because many membrane-bound receptors rely on changes in conformation and networks of noncovalent interactions, the nonlabeled advantage of SPR is a valuable tool in mechanism elucidation. The planar surface of an SPR substrate is also highly ideal for reconstituation of membrane receptors in "supported lipid membranes" that mimick the real cell membrane. Investigation of multiple protein complexes is also more facile with SPR because of the elimination of interference from fluorophores that are bulky and cause steric hindrance. The major histocompatibility (MHC) and T-cell receptor (TCR) complexes have been frequently studied (47–54). Another area of interest is the investigation of vast and complex protein signaling networks (55–59). Protein kinases are implicated in many disorders and new drugs that target phosphorylation or dephosphorylation by these enzymes are being investigated and found to be very potent with less side-effects. Protein–protein interactions are too numerous, but a few high-impact examples are given as a starting point in the references (60–65). SPR imaging has also been used for protein/protein interaction analysis (see the Following) and even protein–aptamer interactions (66).

4. Recent Advances and Future of SPR

4.1. SPR Imaging

An important area of development is SPR imaging (SPRi), which has similar sensitivity to SPR spectroscopy but allows for spatially resolved measurements. A number of groups have demonstrated working systems (67–72, to name a few) and at least three companies claim to offer SPR imaging instruments. The resolution of the method is limited compared with microscopy, typically to about 50µm, but that is usually enough for quantitative analysis of suitably large arrays on a slide. The use of SPRi for pharmaceutical and genomic/proteomic screening holds out incredible promise for high-throughput analysis without the use and drawbacks of fluorescent labels, reducing costs. This combined with the real-time non-equilibrium analysis might help reduce the time of analysis anywhere that large libraries of compounds are being screened.

4.2. Hyphenated Techniques

Hyphenated techniques are also becoming popular. Many instruments already offer several analysis options in conjunction with SPR. It is often combined with electrochemistry because the gold substrate can be used as a working electrode. It has also been combined with QCM, IR, and even downstream mass spectrometry. An interesting and exciting new technique combines SPR with fluorescence (SPFS) to create a labeled but surface sensitive detection method with ultra-high detection sensitivity (73).

4.3. Materials and Chemistry

As SPR becomes a popular and common technique, many groups are investigating improved surface chemistry for the substrates (74). In general, many binding kinetics experiments are done in pure buffer with only one species of interest present. Thus, linkage chemistry is essential to optimize the accuracy and efficiency of binding constant determinations. The same chemistry that has been used in other methods has also proved useful for SPR. For example, His-NTA linkage used in chromatographic methods *(75)* was found to increase the signal obtained for binding when compared with direct antibody linkages that have higher steric hindrance. The Corn group has also shown the importance of advanced surface chemistry in SPR imaging and gone to great efforts to develop a host of reliable methods using lithography *(76)* or microfluidic patterning *(77)* to pattern surfaces with reactive and nonreactive areas. An interesting recent trend is the use of thin silicate layers (~10 nm) to cover the gold substrate and make the surface more like glass, for which a wide variety of well developed surface chemistry is available *(78–81)*.

When analyzing real samples for clinical or environmental applications, surface chemistry often becomes the limiting factor for accurate and sensitive detection. These solutions have large numbers and concentrations of interfering molecules. Methods that work for fluorescence or other analysis techniques may not be suitable for SPR because any non-specific adsorption on the surface causes an increased signal. A major focus for biosensors proposed for clinical and environmental uses has been the reduction of NS adsorption through better surface chemistry such as biocompatible polymers *(82)*. A new report shows how supported bilayer membranes can be used to "cloak" the surface, followed by removal of the cloak after binding, and measurement of specific signal *(83)*.

4.4. Labels and Amplification

One of the major developments for increasing sensitivity was the use of labeled SPR reagents. Gold nanoparticles labels were found to increase the signal response by >10-fold when compared with unlabeled samples *(84)*. Although this strategy does allow for ultrasensitive detection with SPR, it is no longer a "label-free" method when used in this capacity. Gold nanoparticles may significantly interfere with binding of smaller molecules and the effects on binding constant determination should be carefully considered. For biosensing, however, they provide a means to increase both sensitivity and selectivity through the use of antibody-labeled nanoparticles.

Another exciting new concept is the use of enzymes to provide amplification in SPR imaging of DNA arrays. Two strategies have been developed, one based on the RNase H enzyme *(85)* and another based on ligase T4 *(86)*. The direct detection limit for DNA hybridization is about 1nM, but now genomic samples in the femtomolar range can be achieved. With these techniques added to the repertoire, detection of single-nucleotide polymorphisms also becomes feasible. SPRi looks to be highly competitive with fluorescence-based DNA arrays for high-throughput genomic screening.

5. Conclusions

It should be evident from this brief chapter that SPR has become an indispensable technique for scientific investigation of biomolecular interactions. Although it has some limitations, such as a lower sensitivity than fluorescence, the advantages of being label-free and real-time present a complementary alternative. Moreover, as SPR evolves, researchers are coming up with creative new ways to make it more sensitive, user-friendly, higher-throughput, and versatile for a wide range of investigation topics. A brief survey of the literature above showed that SPR has been applied to crucial high-impact projects in many of the key areas of biology and medicine being investigated today, and that the number of publications using SPR is increasing rapidly. We believe that as the cost of instruments becomes more affordable, it will enjoy widespread use. Further commercialization could make it an indispensable lab instrument just like optical plate readers or fluorescence scanners. The simple and elegant underlying principle of SPR lends to facile modification, such as hyphenated instruments, new materials for substrates, and improved surface chemistry.

References

1. Kretschm E, Raether H (1968) Radiative decay of non radiative surface plasmons excited by light. Zeitschrift Fur Naturforschung Part a-Astrophysik Physik Und Physikalische Chemie A 23:2135–213
2. Otto A (1968) Excitation of nonradiative surface plasma waves in silver by method of frustrated total reflection. Zeitschrift Fur Physik 216:398–&
3. Liedberg B, Nylander C, Lundstrom I (1983) Surface-plasmon resonance for gas-detection and biosensing. Sensors and Actuators 4:299–304
4. Homola J (2003) Present and future of surface plasmon resonance biosensors. Anal Bioanal Chem 377:528–539
5. Calander N (2006) Molecular detection and analysis by using surface plasmon resonances. Current Anal Chem 2:203–211
6. Nedelkov D, Nelson RW (2006) Surface plasmon resonance mass spectrometry for protein analysis. Meth Mol Bio 328:131–139
7. Rich RL, Myszka DG (2005) Survey of the year 2004 commercial optical biosensor literature. J Mol Recognition 18:431–478
8. Homola J, Myszka D, Sinclair S (2002) Surface plasmon biosensors. In: Optical biosensors: present and future: Amsterdam: Newyork: Elsevier, 207, 251
9. McDonnell JM (2001) Surface plasmon resonance: towards an understanding of the mechanisms of biological molecular recognition. Current Opinion Chem Biol 5:572–577
10. Rich RL, Myszka DG (2000) Advances in surface plasmon resonance biosensor analysis. Current Opin Biotechnol 11:54–61
11. Karlsson R, Michaelsson A, Mattsson L (1991) Kinetic-analysis of monoclonal antibody-antigen interactions with a new biosensor based analytical system. J Immunol Methods 145:229–240
12. Phillips KS, Cheng O (2007) Recent advances in surface plasmon resonance based techniques for bioanalysis. Anal Bioanal Chem 387:1831–1840
13. Steiner G (2004) Surface plasmon resonance imaging. Anal Bioanal Chem 379:328–331
14. Cooper MA (2003) Label-free screening of bio- molecular interactions. Anal Bioanal Chem 377:834–842
15. Ince R, Narayanaswamy R (2006) Analysis of the performance of interferometry, surface plasmon resonance and luminescence as biosensors and chemosensors. Analytica Chimica Acta 569:1–20
16. Katsamba PS, Navratilova I, Calderon-Cacia M, Fan L, Thornton K, Zhu MD, Vanden Bos T, Forte C, Friend D, Laird-Offringa I, Tavares G, Whatley J, Shi EG, Widom A, Lindquist KC, Klakamp S, Drake A, Bohmann D, Roell M, Rose L, Dorocke J, Roth B, Luginbuhl B, Myszka DG (2006) Kinetic analysis of a high-affinity antibody/antigen interaction performed by multiple Biacore users. Anal Biochem 352:208–221
17. Besenicar M, Macek P, Lakey JH, Anderluh G (2006) Surface plasmon resonance in protein-membrane interactions. Chem Physics Lipids 141:169–178
18. Mukhyopadyay R (2005) Anal Chem: 313A–317A

19. Salim K, Bottomley MJ, Querfurth E, Zvelebil MJ, Gout I, Scaife R, Margolis RL, Gigg R, Smith CIE, Driscoll PC, Waterfield MD, and Panayotou G (1996) Distinct specificity in the recognition of phosphoinositides by the pleckstrin homology domains of dynamin and Bruton's tyrosine kinase Embo J 15(22):6241–6250

20. Mach H, Volkin DB, Burke CJ, Middaugh CR, Linhardt RJ, Fromm JR, Loganathan D, Mattsson L (1993) Nature of the Interaction of Heparin with Acidic Fibroblast Growth-Factor. Biochemistry 32:5480–5489

21. Kuziemko GM, Stroh M, Stevens RC (1996) Cholera toxin binding affinity and specificity for gangliosides determined by surface plasmon resonance. Biochemistry 35:6375–6384

22. Natsume T, Nakayama H, Jansson O, Isobe T, Takio K, Mikoshiba K (2000) Combination of biomolecular interaction analysis and mass spectrometric amino acid sequencing, Anal Chem 72:4193–4198

23. Caruso F, Jory MJ, Bradberry GW, Sambles JR, Furlong DN (1998) Acousto-optic surface-plasmon resonance measurements of thin films on gold. J App Physics 83:1023–1028

24. Jordan CE, Frutos AG, Thiel AJ, Corn RM (1997) Surface plasmon resonance imaging measurements of DNA hybridization adsorption and streptavidin/DNA multilayer formation at chemically modified gold surfaces. Anal Chem 69:4939–4947

25. Nelson BP, Grimsrud TE, Liles MR, Goodman RM, Corn RM (2001) Surface plasmon resonance imaging measurements of DNA and RNA hybridization adsorption onto DNA microarrays. Anal Chem 73:1–7

26. Wegner GJ, Lee HJ, Marriott G, Corn RM (2003) Fabrication of histidine-tagged fusion protein arrays for surface plasmon resonance imaging studies of protein-protein and protein-DNA interactions. Anal Chem 75:4740–4746

27. Jensen KK, Orum H, Nielsen PE, Norden B (1997) Kinetics for hybridization of peptide nucleic acids (PNA) with DNA and RNA studied with the BIAcore technique. Biochemistry 36:5072–5077

28. Wegner GJ, Lee HJ, Corn RM (2002) Characterization and optimization of peptide arrays for the study of epitope-antibody interactions using surface plasmon resonance imaging. Anal Chem 74:5161–5168

29. Smith EA, Kyo M, Kumasawa H, Nakatani K, Saito I, Corn RM (2002) Chemically induced hairpin formation in DNA monolayers. J Am Chem Soc 124:6810–6811

30. Karlsson R, Michaelsson A, Mattsson L (1991) Kinetic-analysis of monoclonal antibody-antigen interactions with a new biosensor based analytical system. J Immunol Meth 145:229–240

31. Ostuni E, Chapman RG, Holmlin RE et al (2001) A survey of structure-property relationships of surfaces that resist the adsorption of protein. Langmuir 17(18):5605–5620

32. Johnsson B, Lofas S, Lindquist G (1991) Immobilization of proteins to a carboxymethyldextran-modified gold surface for biospecific interaction analysis in surface-plasmon resonance sensors. Anal Biochem 198:268–277

33. Holliger P, Prospero T, Winter G (1993) Diabodies – small bivalent and bispecific antibody fragments. Proc Nat Acad Sci U S A 90:6444–6448

34. Griffiths AD, Malmqvist M, Marks JD, Bye JM, Embleton MJ, McCafferty J, Baier M, Holliger KP, Gorick BD, Hughesjones NC, Hoogenboom HR, Winter G (1993) Human anti-self antibodies with high specificity from phage display libraries. Embo J 12:725–734

35. Marks JD, Griffiths AD, Malmqvist M, Clackson TP, Bye JM, Winter G (1992): Bypassing immunization – building high-affinity human-antibodies by chain shuffling. Bio-Technology 10:779–783

36. Wikstrand CJ, Hale LP, Batra SK, Hill ML, Humphrey PA, Kurpad SN, McLendon RE, Moscatello D, Pegram CN, Reist CJ, Traweek ST, Wong AJ, Zalutsky MR, Bigner DD (1995) Monoclonal antibodies against EGFRvlll are tumor specific and react with breast and lung carcinomas and malignant gliomas. Cancer Res. 55:3140–3148

37. Schier R, McCall A, Adams CP, Marshall KW, Merritt H, Yim M, Crawford RS, Weiner LM, Marks C, Marks JD (1996) Isolation of picomolar affinity Anti-c-erbB-2 single-chain Fv by molecular evolution of the complementarity determining regions in the center of the antibody binding site. J Mol Biol 263:551–567

38. Pevsner J, Hsu SC, Braun JEA, Calakos N, Ting AE, Bennett MK, Scheller RH (1994): Specificity and regulation of a synaptic vesicle docking complex. Neuron 13:353–361

39. Emery JG, McDonnell P, Burke MB, Deen KC, Lyn S, Silverman C, Dul E, Appelbaum ER, Eichman C, DiPrinzio R, Dodds RA, James IE, Rosenberg M, Lee JC, Young PR (1998) Osteoprotegerin is a receptor for the cytotoxic ligand TRAIL. J Biol Chem 273:14363–14367

40. Calakos N, Bennett MK, Peterson KE, Scheller RH (1994) Protein-protein interactions contributing to the specificity of intracellular vesicular trafficking. Science 263:1146–1149

41 Gee SH, Madhavan R, Levinson SR, Caldwell JH, Sealock R, Froehner SC (1998) Interaction of muscle and brain sodium channels with multiple members of the syntrophin family of dystrophin-associated proteins. J Neurosci 18:128–137

42. Alam SM, Travers PJ, Wung JL, Nasholds W, Redpath S, Jameson SC, Gascoigne NRJ (1996) T-cell-receptor affinity and thymocyte positive selection. Nature 381:616–620

43. Greenlund AC, Morales MO, Viviano BL, Yan H, Krolewski J, Schreiber RD (1995) Stat recruitment by tyrosine-phosphorylated cytokine receptors – an ordered reversible affinity-driven process. Immunity 2:677–687

44. Schuster SC, Swanson RV, Alex LA, Bourret RB, Simon MI (1993) Assembly and function of a quaternary signal-transduction complex monitored by surface-plasmon resonance. Nature 365:343–347

45. Donaldson DD, Whitters MJ, Fitz IJ, Neben TY, Finnerty H, Henderson SL, O'Hara RM, Beier DR, Turner KJ, Wood CR, Collins M (1998) The murine IL-13 receptor alpha 2: molecular cloning, characterization, and comparison with marine IL-13 receptor. J Immunol 161:2317–2324

46. Nishikawa J, Saito K, Goto J, Dakeyama F, Matsuo M, Nishihara T (1999) New screening methods for chemicals with hormonal activities using interaction of nuclear hormone receptor with coactivator. Toxicol Appl Pharmacol 154:76–83

47. Lyons DS, Lieberman SA, Hampl J, Boniface JJ, Chien YH, Berg LJ, Davis MM (1996) A TCR binds to antagonist ligands with lower affinities and faster dissociation rates than to agonists. Immunity 5:53–61

48. Corr M, Slanetz AE, Boyd LF, Jelonek MT, Khilko S, Alramadi BK, Kim YS, Maher SE, Bothwell ALM, Margulies DH (1994) T-Cell receptor-Mhc class-I peptide interactions - affinity, kinetics, and specificity. Science 265:946–949

49. Matsui K, Boniface JJ, Steffner P, Reay PA, Davis MM (1994) Kinetics of T-cell receptor-binding to peptide I-E(K) complexes – correlation of the dissociation rate with T-cell responsiveness. Proc Natl Acad Sci USA 91:12862–12866

50. Brown MH, Boles K, van der Merwe PA, Kumar V, Mathew PA, Barclay AN (1998) 2B4, the natural killer and T cell immunoglobulin super-family surface protein, is a ligand for CD48. J Exp Med 188:2083–2090

51. vanderMerwe PA, Bodian DL, Daenke S, Linsley P, Davis SJ (1997) CD80 (B7-1) binds both CD28 and CTLA-4 with a low affinity and very fast kinetics. J Exp Med 185:393–403

52. Corr M, Boyd IF, Frankel SR, Kozlowski S, Padlan EA, Margulies DH (1992) Endogenous peptides of a soluble major histocompatibility complex class-I molecule, H-2I(D)(S) – sequence motif, quantitative binding, and molecular modeling of the complex. J Exp Med 176:1681–1692

53. Kersh GJ, Kersh EN, Fremont DH, Allen PM (1998) High- and low-potency ligands with similar affinities for the TCR: The importance of kinetics in TCR signaling. Immunity 9:817–826

54. Willcox BE, Gao GF, Wyer JR, Ladbury JE, Bell JI, Jakobsen BK, van der Merwe PA (1999) TCR binding to peptide-MHC stabilizes a flexible recognition interface. Immunity 10:357–365

55. Muslin AJ, Tanner JW, Allen PM, Shaw AS (1996) Interaction of 14-3-3 with signaling proteins is mediated by the recognition of phosphoserine. Cell 84:889–897

56. Houseman BT, Huh JH, Kron SJ, Mrksich M (2002) Peptide chips for the quantitative evaluation of protein kinase activity. Nat Biotechnol 20:270–274

57. Bartley TD, Hunt RW, Welcher AA, Boyle WJ, Parker VP, Lindberg RA, Lu HS, Colombero AM, Elliott RL, Guthrie BA, Holst PL, Skrine ID, Toso RJ, Zhang M, Fernandez E, Trail G, Varnum B, Yarden Y, Hunter T, Fox GM (1994) B61 Is a Ligand for the Eck receptor protein-tyrosine kinase. Nature 368:558–560

58. James SR, Downes CI, Gigg R, Grove SJA, Holmes AB, Alessi DR (1996) Specific binding of the Akt-1 protein kinase to phosphatidylinositol 3,4,5-trisphosphate without subsequent activation. Biochem J 315:709–713

59. Ladbury JE, Lemmon MA, Zhou M, Green J, Botfield MC, Schlessinger J (1995) Measurement of the binding of tyrosyl phosphopeptides to Sh2 domains – a reappraisal. Proc Natl Acad Sci U S A 92:3199–3203

60. Floresrozas H, Kelman Z, Dean FB, Pan ZQ, Harper PW, Elledge SJ, Odonnell M, Hurwitz J (1994) Cdk-interacting protein-1 directly binds with proliferating cell nuclear antigen and inhibits DNA-replication catalyzed by the DNA-polymerase-delta holoenzyme. Proc Natl Acad Sci U S A 91:8655–8659

61. Iemura S, Yamamoto TS, Takagi C, Uchiyama H, Natsume T, Shimasaki S, Sugino H, Ueno N (1998) Direct binding of follistatin to a complex of bone-morphogenetic protein and its receptor inhibits ventral and epidermal cell fates in early Xenopus embryo. Proc Natl Acad Sci U S A 95:9337–9342

62. Rickles RJ, Botfield MC, Weng ZG, Taylor JA, Green OM, Brugge JS, Zoller MJ (1994) Identification of Src, Fyn, Lyn, Pi3k and Abl Sh3 domain ligands using phage display libraries. Embo J 13:5598–5604

63. Boll W, Ohno H, Zhou SY, Rapoport I, Cantley LC, Bonifacino JS, Kirchhausen T (1996) Sequence requirements for the recognition of tyrosine-based endocytic signals by clathrin AP-2 complexes. Embo J 15:5789–5795

64. Sapir T, Elbaum M, Reiner O (1997) Reduction of microtubule catastrophe events by LIS1, platelet-activating factor acetylhydrolase subunit. Embo J 16:6977–6984

65. Heiska L, Alfthan K, Gronholm M, Vilja P, Vaheri A, Carpen O (1998) Association of ezrin with intercellular adhesion molecule-1 and -2 (ICAM-1 and ICAM-2) - Regulation by phosphatidylinositol 4,5-bisphosphate. J Biol Chem 273:21893–21900

66. Li Y, Lee HJ, Corn RM (2007) Detection of protein biomarkers using RNA aptamer microarrays and enzymatically amplified surface plasmon resonance imaging. Anal Chem 79:1082–1088

67. Rothenhausler B, Knoll W (1988) Surface-plasmon microscopy. Nature 332:615–617

68. Jordan CE, Corn RM (1997) Surface plasmon resonance imaging measurements of electrostatic biopolymer adsorption onto chemically modified gold surfaces. Anal Chem 69:1449–1456

69. Kanda V, Kariuki JK, Harrison DJ, McDermott MT (2004) Label-free reading of microarray-based immunoassays with surface plasmon resonance imaging. Anal Chem 76:7257–7262

70. Shumaker-Parr JS, Zareie MH, Aebersold R, Campbell CT (2004) Microspotting streptavidin and double-stranded DNA Arrays on gold for high-throughput studies of protein-DNA interactions by surface plasmon resonance microscopy. Anal Chem 76:918–929

71. Lyon IA, Musick MD, Smith PC, Reiss BD, Pena DJ, Natan MJ (1999) Surface plasmon resonance of colloidal Au-modified gold films. Sensors and Actuators B-Chemical 54:118–124

72. Phillips KS, Wilkop T, Wu JJ, Al-Kaysi RO, Cheng Q (2006) Surface plasmon resonance imaging analysis of protein-receptor binding in supported membrane arrays on gold substrates with calcinated silicate films. J Am Chem Soc 128:9590–9591

73. Liebermann T, Knoll W (2000) Surface-plasmon field-enhanced fluorescence spectroscopy. Colloids Surfaces a-Physicochem Eng Aspects 171:115–130

74. Niemeyer CM (2001) Nanoparticles, proteins, and nucleic acids: biotechnology meets materials science. Angewandte Chemie-International Edition 40:4128–4158

75. Sigal GB, Bamdad C, Barberis A, Strominger J, Whitesides GM (1996) A self-assembled monolayer for the binding and study of histidine tagged proteins by surface plasmon resonance. Anal Chem 68:490–497

76. Brockman JM, Frutos AG, Corn RM (1999). A multistep chemical modification procedure to create DNA arrays on gold surfaces for the study of protein-DNA interactions with surface plasmon resonance imaging. J Am Chem Soc 121:8044–8051

77. Lee HJ, Goodrich TT, Corn RM (2001) SPR Imaging measurements of 1-D and 2-D DNA microarrays created from microfluidic channels on gold thin films. Anal Chem 73:5525–5531

78. Phillips KS, Han JH, Martinez M, Wang ZZ, Carter D, Cheng Q (2006) Nanoscale glassification of gold substrates for surface plasmon resonance analysis of protein toxins with supported lipid membranes. Anal Chem 78:596–603

79. Tawa K, Morigaki K (2005) Substrate-supported phospholipid membranes studied by surface plasmon resonance and surface plasmon fluorescence spectroscopy. Biophy J 89:2750–2758

80. Szunerits S, Coffinier Y, Janel S, Boukherrouh R (2006) Stability of the gold/silica thin film interface: Electrochemical and surface plasmon resonance studies. Langmuir 22:10716–10722

81. Reimhult E, Zach M, Hook F, Kasemo B (2006) A multitechnique study of liposome adsorption on Au and lipid bilayer formation on SiO2. Langmuir 22:3313–3319

82. Masson JF, Battaglia TM, Davidson MJ, Kim YC, Prakash AMC, Beaudoin S, Booksh KS (2005) Biocompatible polymers for antibody support on gold surfaces. Talanta 67:918–925

83. Phillips KS, Han JH, Cheng Q (2007) Development of a "membrane cloaking" method for amperometric enzyme immunoassay and surface plasmon resonance analysis of proteins in serum samples. Anal Chem 79:899–907

84. He L, Musick MD, Nicewarner SR, Salinas FG, Benkovic SJ, Natan MJ, Keating CD (2000) Colloidal Au-enhanced surface plasmon resonance for ultrasensitive detection of DNA hybridization. J Am Chem Soc 122:9071–9077

85. Goodrich TT, Lee HJ, Corn RM (2004) Enzymatically amplified surface plasmon resonance imaging method using RNase H and RNA microarrays for the ultrasensitive detection of nucleic acids. Anal Chem 76:6173–6178

86. Lee HJ, Wark AW, Li Y, Corn RM (2005) Fabricating RNA microarrays with RNA-DNA surface ligation chemistry. Anal Chem 77:7832–7837

47

Macromolecular Crystallography

Bernhard Rupp and Katherine A. Kantardjieff

1. Introduction

X-ray-, neutron-, and electron-diffraction are powerful bioanalytical methods delivering information about macromolecular structure at atomic resolution. Diffraction methods have fundamentally influenced our understanding of protein and nucleic acid structure, biochemical reactions and pathways, and macromolecular assembly, as well as aided in the design of pharmaceuticals, enzymes and bio-nanomaterials. The number of therapeutic drugs developed with significant contributions from structure-guided design methods is steadily increasing, and includes well-known examples such as the HIV protease inhibitor saquinovir (Invirase), the anticancer drug imatinib (Gleevec), and the antiviral oseltamivir (Tamiflu), therapeutics against AIDS, leukemia, and influenza respectively *(1)*. Nanomaterials with structurally designed capabilities of controlled release and targeted delivery of bioactive components include bioselective surfaces for manipulation of molecules within cells *(2)*, dendritic polymers as diagnostics for early cancer detection and therapeutic functions *(3,4)*, and nanoparticles for 'smart' delivery of nutrients, DNA and transplanted cells *(5–7)*.

1.1. Basic Challenges in Crystallographic Structure Determination

In structural biology and drug discovery, the most important structure determination technique by far is X-ray crystallography, with its powerful capability of delivering atomic-level detailed models of protein structures. An actual X-ray diffraction experiment is conceptually straightforward: a suitable single crystal of a protein, 50 to a few 100 μm in size, is placed on a goniometer, exposed to brilliant, monochromatic X-rays, and the diffraction pattern is recorded in a frame-by frame fashion. A basic back-transformation formalism applied mathematically to a complete data set – integrated, scaled and merged from the individual diffraction pattern frames – then yields the molecular structure. Yet, despite the conceptual simplicity of such an experiment, a number of formidable tasks are involved in a crystallographic protein structure determination.

From: *Molecular Biomethods Handbook, 2nd Edition.*
Edited by: J. M. Walker and R. Rapley © Humana Press, Totowa, NJ

1.1.1. Protein Crystallization

The first and obvious fact is that without a protein crystal, there is no crystallography experiment. Indeed, a significant portion of time during the course of a structure determination project is spent preparing the protein of interest in a form and purity that is amenable to crystallization. Given that proteins are large, inherently flexible macromolecules, it is easy to understand that screening for and ultimately finding conditions under which the protein molecules self-assemble into a nicely ordered, periodic lattice forming a crystal can be quite challenging.

Despite that X-ray diffraction experiments require crystalline material, they do not require large quantities of material. With an average density for proteins of $1.35 \, g/cm^3$, a typical protein crystal will contain only picograms to micrograms of protein ($\sim 10^9$ to 10^{14} molecules), although more material will be expended during screening for conditions under which diffracting crystals of a protein will form. No principal limitation exists to the size of molecules whose structure is to be determined, and because crystallization is itself a purification technique, we need not worry about impurities being present in the crystals. Crystals generally do not grow well from impure samples.

1.1.2. Phase Determination

A second and critical fact as a principle of any diffraction experiment is that during the recording of the diffraction pattern information is lost, and the back-transform of the data into a molecular model is not possible from diffraction data alone. Although we can readily measure the intensities of the X-rays scattered from our crystal in a diffraction experiment, the phase relations among the X-rays in the diffraction data are lost (we do not have lenses that can focus X-rays). Unfortunately, the phase relations contain substantive information required to reconstruct a protein structure from the diffraction data. This resulting problem is aptly called the "phase problem" in crystallography, and numerous clever strategies to obtain the missing phases (to *solve* the structure) have been devised. The most generally applicable de novo phasing techniques do not require any prior structural information. De novo phasing techniques are based on determining the heavy atom substructure of a labeled protein crystal, from which phase information can be derived. If a model of a structurally similar protein or substantial parts of the structure are already known, *molecular replacement* techniques can be used to obtain starting phases. After either phasing method has succeeded, the resulting models are subsequently *refined* and *rebuilt* until the best correspondence among diffraction data, model, and prior biochemical knowledge is obtained.

1.1.3. Solution Conformation

Because the environment in a protein crystal contains on average 50% aqueous solvent, structures derived from X-ray crystallography generally agree well with solution structures – many enzymes remain active in protein crystals and even facilitate in situ studies. Exceptions are seen, however, in regions of structure that are involved in crystal packing contacts or when crystallization has induced molecules to adopt a nonnative conformation. The latter will affect allosteric conformation changes as well as the conFiguration of multi-domain molecules. In these cases, multiple structures from different crystal forms, as well as in liganded and unliganded (apo) states are determined. Each of the structures provides a different snapshot of the conformational changes during

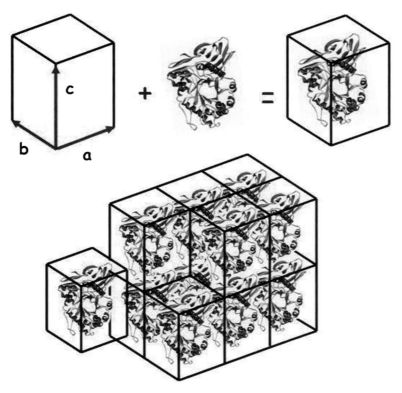

Fig 47.1. A protein crystal is a periodic, ordered self-assembly of protein molecules. The unit lattice (top left, with lattice vectors **a, b** and **c** indicated) contains the molecular motif (top center), and both together form the unit cell (top right). Millions of molecules self-assemble into an ordered macroscopic crystal. Image reproduced with permissions from http://www.ruppweb.org/

catalysis, regulation or receptor binding, enabling a picture of the dynamics of the process to be assembled.

1.2. Structure Models are Archived at the PDB

The international archive for macromolecular structure coordinates, the Protein Data Bank (PDB), was established at Brookhaven National Laboratories in 1971. Two structures were deposited in 1972, but by the late 1970s, researchers had already determined the crystal structures of 132 proteins. With advances in technology, such as high intensity X-ray sources, electronic detectors and high speed computers, as well as advances in experimental methods using low temperature, multiple wavelength anomalous diffraction, and recombinant DNA techniques in protein production, the PDB has grown to more than 50,000 structures in early 2008. Eighty-five percent of these structures have been determined by X-ray diffraction. The protein structures deposited span more than two orders of magnitude in molecular mass, from insulin ($< 10^4$ Da) to ribosomal subunits ($\sim 2.0 \times 10^6$ Da or ~ 2 MDa). However, despite the Protein Structure Initiative (PSI), established in 2000 by the National Institutes of General Medical Sciences and intended to determine the form and function of thousands of proteins over the next decade, membrane proteins – comprising the most important class of receptor molecules for drugs – still represent only approx 1% of the structures deposited in the PDB, and many more new protein folds are expected to be discovered. In the postgenomic era of structural biology and targeted drug design, there is a great deal of work still to be done. Individuals are needed who are adequately familiar with modern diffraction methods, who appreciate the information content of experimentally derived macromolecular structures, and who also understand their limitations.

2. Methods

The fundamental steps in the process of determining a macromolecular crystal structure have not changed from the late 1950s, and still encompass a) sample purification and crystallization; b) data collection and processing; c) structure solution (phase determination); and d) structure building and refinement. What has changed since the late 1950s involves major advances in sample preparation with the advent of recombinant DNA technology. Expression of the cloned gene encoding the protein of interest in a microorganism such as *Escherichia coli* allows the production of large amounts of proteins, even those not very abundant in their native environment. Data collection has benefited from the development of new detectors like phosphor imaging plates and charge coupled devices (CCD detectors). Increasing availability of highly brilliant X-ray radiation from synchrotrons and new crystal flash-cooling techniques have made possible data collection on crystals only few tens of microns (μm) in size and on molecular assemblies as large as virus particles. Because every step following data collection requires a great deal of mathematical manipulation by computer, protein crystallography has also been greatly impacted by the availability of cheap computing power, leading to radical improvements in structure solution, refinement and analysis. More powerful computer-intensive algorithms, such as simulated annealing and maximum likelihood refinement and phasing techniques, can now be applied routinely.

2.1. Principles of Diffraction

All crystallography, not just macromolecular, is explained by the basic theory of X-ray scattering from a crystal, which is a well understood phenomenon.

2.1.1. Diffraction of X-Rays by Electrons

X-ray diffraction is the result of elastic emission (maintaining frequency or wavelength) of radiation owing to the interaction of the electric field vector of the X-rays with the electrons in the atoms. In response to the periodically changing electric field vector of the X-ray, the electrons themselves emit wavelets, which recombine and interfere with one another, producing the phenomenon known as *diffraction*. Because the wavelength of X-rays is of the same order as the diameter of the electron cloud around atoms (1–2 Å), the scattering is pronounced in the forward direction. Diffraction from crystals – comprised of many identically aligned molecules – samples the scattering in discrete directions, which amplifies the signal and leads to discrete diffraction spots. For this reason, it is necessary to use good crystals if the molecules are to be studied with atomic level details, giving rise to the term for this method, *crystallography*. The fact that electrons are the source of X-ray scattering also implies that any reconstruction of a molecular structure from diffraction data will necessarily deliver a detailed image of the scattering molecule in form of the *electron density* of that molecule.

2.1.2. Diffraction by a Periodic Lattice

Consider a crystal to be a periodic array of atoms, described by an array of identical unit cells with unit cell lengths *a, b, c* and angles among the axes denoted as α (between *b* and *c*), β (between *a* and *c*) and γ (between *a* and *b*). We can visualize diffraction as reflection from sets of planes running through such a crystal (**Fig. 47.2**). Only at certain incident angles 2θ are the X-rays diffracted from different planes so that the phase difference among partial waves is a whole number of wavelengths, i.e., they diffract in phase. At other angles the waves reflected from different planes are out of phase and cancel one another out.

The reflecting crystal lattice planes must intersect the cell edges rationally, otherwise the diffraction from the different unit cells interferes destructively. We index the planes by the number of times, *h, k,* and l, that they cut each unit cell vector, **a, b,** and **c**. and these same *h, k, and* 1 values are used to index our diffraction data, the X-ray *reflections* from the planes.

The periodic nature of the lattice as an array of unit cells with regularly spaced lattice planes leads to the *Laue diffraction conditions*

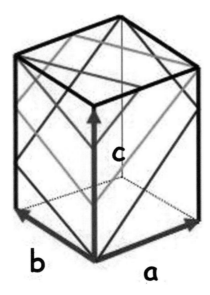

Fig. 47.2. Crystal lattice planoes. The unit cell shown in **Fig. 47.1** contains lattice planes that intersect the cell edges rationally. We index the planes by the number of times, *h, k, l,* that they cut each unit cell edge **a, b,** and **c**, and these same *h, k, l* values are used to index our diffraction data, the X-ray *reflections* from the planes. In the Figure, we see the (2 1 −3) family of planes. Image with permission from http://www.ruppweb.org/

$$\mathbf{a} \cdot \mathbf{S} = h$$

$$\mathbf{b} \cdot \mathbf{S} = k$$

$$\mathbf{c} \cdot \mathbf{S} = l \qquad (1)$$

with $\mathbf{a}$, $\mathbf{b}$, and $\mathbf{c}$ the crystal translation vectors, $\mathbf{S}$ the normal vector (equivalent to the scattering vector $\mathbf{S}_{in} - \mathbf{S}_{out}$ in **Fig. 47.3**) to the reflecting plane with magnitude $2 \sin \theta / \lambda$, and h,k,l integers. Reformulation leads to Bragg's Law

$$2d_{hkl} \sin \theta = n\lambda \qquad (2)$$

where d is the distance among the lattice planes (hkl), θ the reflecting angle, n an integer and λ the wavelength.

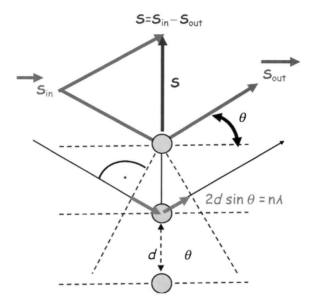

Fig. 47.3. The Bragg equation. The path difference among waves reflected from planes spaced a distance d causes interference, which is constructive when the path difference is $n\lambda$. In this view, diffraction is interpreted as reflection of the X-rays from the (horizontal) lattice planes. The scattering vector $\mathbf{S}$ is then perpendicular to the scattering lattice planes

According to the relations *(1)* and *(2)*, crystals diffract X-rays constructively only in discrete directions hkl. The intensity of a diffracted X-ray in direction hkl, $I(hkl)$, is proportional to the square of the amplitude of the diffracted wave, described as the complex structure factor $\mathbf{F}(hkl)$. $\mathbf{F}(hkl)$ is the summation of all the partial waves scattered from each atom in the crystal in direction hkl, and depends principally on the scattering power of the atoms, f_i (falling off with scattering angle and proportional to the number of electrons each atom has), and the positional coordinates (x, y, z) of each atom:

$$\mathbf{F}_{hkl} = \sum_{i}^{atoms} f_i \cdot e^{2\pi i(hx_i + ky_i + lz_i)} \tag{3}$$

As the atomic scattering factor is a function of the number of electrons present at each position (x, y, z), we can reconstruct the electron density distribution in the unit cell by inverse Fourier transformation of this function, again expressed as a discrete summation over all reflections:

$$\rho(xyz) = \frac{1}{V} \sum_{-h}^{h} \sum_{-k}^{k} \sum_{-l}^{l} \mathbf{F}(hkl) e^{-2\pi i(hx + ky + lz)} \tag{4}$$

The structure factor $\mathbf{F}(hkl)$ used in the electron density reconstruction (4) is expressed in complex form, and can be split into a real magnitude and an imaginary phase part represented by

$$\mathbf{F}_{hkl} = |F_{hkl}| e^{i\varphi(hkl)} \tag{5}$$

The amplitudes $F(hkl)$ can be derived experimentally, and are proportional to the square root of the measured scattered intensities, but the phase angle $\varphi(hkl)$ is not obtained directly from the diffraction pattern, giving rise to the "phase problem" in crystallography.

If we apply Bragg's law to the maximum scattering angle 2θ to which reflections can be measured, we obtain an expression for the maximum resolution (smallest lattice plane spacing) d_{min}:

$$d_{min} = \frac{\lambda}{2\sin(\theta_{max})} \tag{6}$$

As it happens, d_{min} corresponds quite well to the shortest distance apart at which two distinct features such as atoms can be resolved in an electron density map as shown in **Fig. 47.4**.

2.2. Crystallization

Protein crystallization is a special case of phase separation: We must persuade the protein molecules to come out of solution and form a crystalline phase. This is achieved by reducing solubility until a thermodynamically metastable, supersaturated state is reached, from which, upon nucleation, protein crystals may form while the system returns to thermodynamic equilibrium. However, whether crystals form at all, how large they become, and how long it takes, will depend on kinetic phenomena such as the nucleation processes, molecular diffusion, and crystal growth rates.

Crystallographers use several methods to achieve supersaturation in protein solutions from which crystals suitable for X-ray diffraction experiments will grow. These include *vapor diffusion* (hanging, sitting and sandwich drop variations), *microbatch*, *microdialysis* and *free-interface diffusion*. In vapor diffusion, equilibrium is established among a small drop (100 nl–few μl), containing about equal amounts of the purified protein solution and of a precipitant cocktail, and a larger reservoir (100–500 μl) of the same cocktail (**Fig. 47.5**) The precipitant cocktail usually contains a weak organic buffer,

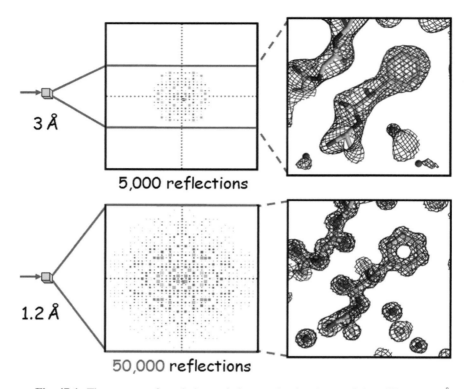

Fig. 47.4. The concept of resolution and electron density. A crystal that diffracts to 3 Å (top panel) generates a limited diffraction pattern with few thousand reflections, and the reconstructed electron density is not as well defined as in case of a well diffracting crystal yielding substantially more data. Note that the 1.2 Å diffracting crystal (bottom panel) gives about 10 times as many reflections, and the electron density is correspondingly well defined and very detailed. The small round spheres of density visible in the high resolution electron density are water molecules filling the solvent channels among the protein molecules in the crystal. Image with permission from http://www.ruppweb.org/

precipitants such as salts, poly-alcohols (poly-ethylene glycols, PEGs), and various additives, detergents or metal ions for example, which are believed to improve crystallization. As the volatile components (generally water unless alcohol or other volatile components are used) evaporate from the crystallization drop and are absorbed into the reservoir, both the precipitant and protein concentrations increase in the protein drop. Once the system reaches the supersaturated state, from which the phase change from solution to crystalline phase is thermodynamically possible, *and* if kinetics are favorable, crystals may form and grow *(8,9)*. Because it is not possible to predict specific crystallization conditions for a protein of unknown structure, many crystallization conditions must be screened (trials), until conditions favorable for crystal growth are found. In high throughput crystallography, thousands of experiments can be set up employing crystallization robots, generally in 96-well crystallization trays. Optimization is a frequently required second step for refining the crystallization conditions, once initial conditions have been

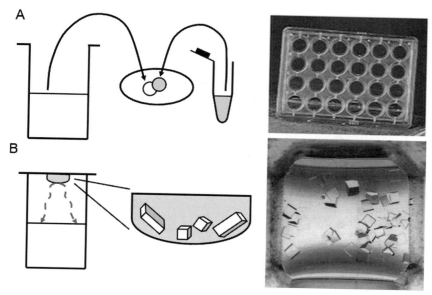

Fig. 47.5. Principle of protein crystallization by vapor diffusion. The left part of the Figure shows the procedure of setting up a hanging drop experiment. A: small (μl) drops of precipitation cocktail from the reservoir and of protein stock are mixed on a siliconized glass slide. The glass slide is turned over and seals the reservoir. With luck, crystals grow within days to months while the solution equilibrates by vapor diffusion. A 24-well Linbro plate for manual hanging drop set-up is shown in the top right panel, and crystals in a sitting drop well in a high throughput, 96-well plate are shown below. Image with permission from http://www.ruppweb.org/

found during screening, to improve crystal quality. Vapor diffusion works well for both screening and optimization.

The microbatch method was originally developed to allow theoretical studies, but it is now generally used for routine crystallization, because it is very rapid, requires no tape sealing, and uses very small amounts of protein (0.2–1 μl) per trial. In microbatch crystallization, the protein solution is simply combined with the crystallization cocktail, and the mixed droplets are dispensed onto and sink to the bottom of small wells covered with paraffin oil to prevent evaporation. The microbatch method is inexpensive and can be quite effective for screening, because it requires very little consumables, setup time, and protein.

In the microdialysis method, the protein of interest is separated from the precipitant solution by a semi-permeable membrane that allows small reagent molecules, but not the protein, to pass (*8–10*). Dialysis buttons, designed for this purpose, range in sample size from 5–350 μl. Microdialysis has the potential advantage that the dialysis buttons can be transferred to different precipitant reservoirs while reusing the same protein solution. Dialysis does generally require more material than vapor diffusion and microbatch methods, but can be useful for growing large crystals for neutron diffraction experiments.

Finally, in free interface diffusion, protein and precipitant solutions are layered such that diffusion can freely occur across the solution interface. Set up in conventional capillary tubes can be tedious and labor intensive, and fairly large amounts of material are needed. Recent developments in microfluidic technology have produced crystallization "chips" for free interface diffusion (*11*).

Fluids are loaded into inlets and dispersed through the fluidic circuitry using pressurized air. Pressure changes automatically open and close flexible polymeric valves to direct the flow of reagents and protein into the various diffusion chambers supporting hundreds of crystallization experiments, each using only about 12 nl of sample. Owing to the small amount of protein they require, the rather expensive crystallization chips are increasingly used for screening purposes. To extract crystals for diffraction experiments, however, the user must dismantle the chip and risk mechanical damage to the crystals. Modified chips, which incorporate thin-walled glass capillaries into the elastomer of the device, allow exposure of crystals to synchrotron radiation while still in the capillaries for direct observation of diffraction patterns with minimal risk *(12)*.

2.3. Laboratory X-Ray Sources

X-rays of a suitable wavelength range for protein crystallography (~0.8–2.3 Å) are generated by three commonly used devices: X-ray *tubes*, *rotating anodes*, and *synchrotrons*. In-house or laboratory sources will produce X-rays using either an evacuated tube or a rotating anode. X-ray tubes consist of a filament that acts as a cathode. Electrons are emitted by the glowing cathode and accelerated by several tens of kVs across the vacuum towards the anode, which consists of a metal target made of a characteristic material, usually copper or chromium, for protein crystallography. As the electron beam impacts the anode, the high kinetic energy of the electrons is converted during deceleration into X-rays producing a) a continuous spectrum consisting of bremsstrahlung (braking radiation) and b) emission lines characteristic of the electronic transitions within the anode material. The characteristic X-ray emission lines, which are important for crystallography, have an intensity that is several orders of magnitude higher than the bremsstrahlung. The $K_{\alpha 1}$ and $K_{\alpha 2}$ components of the X-ray emission are cut out from the bremsstrahlung background and other emission lines by filters, monochromators or X-ray mirrors, and the resulting monochromatic X-rays are collimated and focused onto the crystals. When X-rays are produced by a rotating anode, the cathode and anode are housed under vacuum, in which the anode target rotates at high speed to efficiently distribute and dissipate heat. The wavelength of an in-house source such as a tube or rotating anode generator is fixed by the choice of anode target material and not tunable, as is the case at a synchrotron, and the intensity of the source is less than that of a synchrotron.

2.4. Synchrotrons

At a synchrotron facility, bunches of electrons, several GeV in energy, move in a large, carefully steered, closed electron beam loop containing bending elements and linear segments, collectively called the storage *ring*. In each section, magnetic devices are inserted—bending magnets in the curved sections, insertion devices called wigglers and undulators in the straight sections – to bend, wiggle or undulate the path of the electrons while they pass around the ring (**Fig. 47.6**). Owing to the acceleration experienced in the bending magnets or insertion devices, the electrons emit a narrow fan of intense white (polychromatic) radiation ranging from soft UV to hard X-rays over a very tightly defined angle tangential to the ring. The radiation is "tunable" by cutting out

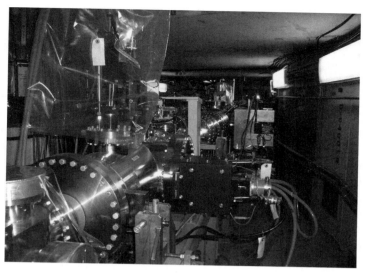

Fig. 47.6. Synchrotron storage ring tunnel. Shown is a straight section of the storage ring, open for maintenance and upgrade, at the Stanford Synchrotron Radiation Laboratory, Menlo Park, CA. Photograph courtesy of K. Kantardjieff

fine bands (few eV or 10^{-5} Å wide) of wavelengths appropriate for particular experiments with monochromator crystals that selectively pass the wavelength of choice. The intensity of X-rays generated by modern third generation synchrotron sources is so high that radiation damage to crystals has become a major concern, and this has given rise to the near-exclusive use of cryo-crystallographic techniques, in which crystals are kept at near-liquid nitrogen temperatures to minimize radiation damage. Synchrotron radiation has additional features that make it attractive for advanced applications. Because it is pulsed, it can be exploited for examining time-dependent phenomena, and because it is highly polarized, it can be used to examine polarization-dependent and angle-dependent effects.

2.5. X-Ray Area Detectors

The detector chosen for a particular experiment must have appropriate design for the energy of the X-rays and the geometry of the experiment. Today, most area detectors for macromolecular crystallography experiments are based either on *image plate* (IP) or *charge coupled device* (CCD) technology.

2.5.1. Image Plates

In an IP X-ray detector, a layer of small crystalline grains consisting of a doped phosphor and organic binders is sandwiched between a support layer and protective layer on a flexible backing. Irradiation excites the crystals in their luminescence centers to a metastable state. Image information formed by X-ray excitation is stable for many hours but decays within days. For readout, the phosphor is photo-stimulated to luminescence by exposure to a visible laser, the light pulses recorded, and the plate finally erased by further exposure to a high intensity halogen lamp. IPs have high quantum efficiency, a wide dynamic range, good linearity of response, a high spatial resolution, a large active area size, a high counting rate capability, and are the least expensive detectors. Their drawback in synchrotron use is the slow readout time, which is generally not an issue for the less intense home-lab X-ray sources.

2.5.2. CCD Detectors

CCDs are comprised of a two-dimensional semiconductor array which directly delivers a digital image of the diffraction pattern. The X-ray photons fall onto a fluorescent screen bonded to an optical taper leading to a photon-sensitive CCD chip. The diffracted X-ray photons are converted into visible light in the fluorescent screen. The light is guided through the taper to the CCD chip, where free electrons in proportion to the number of photons are accumulated. Depending on the specific design of the detector, fast readout electronics generate a raw electronic image of the diffraction pattern, which is further processed by the data collection computer. CCD detectors (**Fig. 47.7**) exhibit high sensitivity, low noise, and excellent linearity of response. However, they can be saturated by very intense X-rays, and multiple passes with suitable exposure times may be necessary to capture data from crystals that diffract strongly. Exposure times for single data frames can be as fast as seconds on synchrotrons, and a whole data set can sometimes be collected within minutes.

2.6. Diffraction Data

Once a suitably sized crystal has been found upon inspection of the crystallization drops, successfully harvested and mounted under cryogenic conditions,

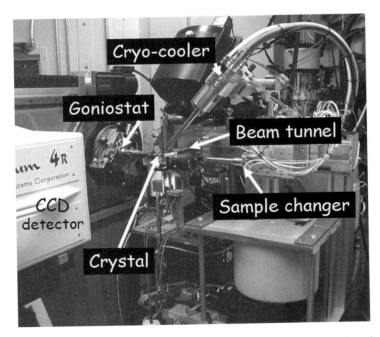

Fig. 47.7. A crystallographic synchrotron beam line end station. The end station of beam line 5.0.2 at the advanced light source (ALS) in Berkley with X-ray beam optics, goniostat, cryo-cooler, sample mounting robot and CCD detector. Image courtesy of G. Snell, ALS

the actual process of structure determination begins. Unlike the sample preparation and crystallization screening stages, which more or less depend on experimentation in the "wet" laboratory, all subsequent steps following data collection – data processing, phase determination and evaluation, electron density reconstruction, model building, structure refinement, validation, and analysis – are conducted in silico with computer programs. Collecting good diffraction data is the final, most important *experimental step* in a crystallographic structure determination. Poor data will invariably result in a poor crystal structure, provided the data can be phased in the first place.

2.6.1. Cryogenic Cooling

Just as any organic or living material, proteins are sensitive to X-ray radiation damage. The energy range of X-rays used for diffraction is in the 6–15 keV range, which is in fact severely ionizing radiation. The ionizing absorption events create radicals, which rapidly destroy any protein crystal, particularly at dose rates experienced at synchrotrons. An efficient way to suppress radiation damage by slowing down the kinetics of the radical reactions is cryogenic cooling. Rapidly quenching or *flash-cooling* crystals to liquid nitrogen temperatures, either in cold nitrogen gas streams or directly into liquid nitrogen, will strongly reduce radiation damage. To prevent the formation of crystalline ice during flash-cooling of the crystals, cryoprotectants, present in the mother liqor or added to the mother liquor, are necessary. Cryoprotection is effectively accomplished during harvesting, when the crystals are scooped up from the drop in cryo-loops and briefly swept though a cryoprotectant before being dipped into liquid nitrogen. Common cryoprotectants are ethylene glycol (the antifreeze in automobile radiators), glycerol, higher alcohols, polyethylene glycols (PEGs), or high concentration solutions of sucrose or salts. Once the protein crystals are flash-cooled and stored in pucks in a liquid nitrogen Dewar (dry shipper), they can be safely sent to a synchrotron for data collection.

2.6.2. Data Collection

The crystal, successfully cryo-mounted in a loop on top of the harvesting pin set in a magnetic base, is placed on a *goniostat* and exposed to intense and collimated X-rays (**Fig. 47.7**). In protein crystallography, the goniostat frequently has only a single axis, φ, which allows the crystal to be rotated in small increments (around one degree of freedom), and during each increment of rotation a diffraction pattern is collected by an electronic IP or CCD detector. From a preliminary sampling of the diffraction pattern, the quality of the diffraction (resolution of the data, cell constants, and sharpness of the reflections) can be determined. If the reflections recorded can be indexed (i.e., a consistent set of directional indices h,k,l, assigned to all reflections) and the crystal is deemed suitable for full data collection, basic data collection parameters such as the rotation increment, the crystal-to-detector distance, and exposure time are optimized.

Depending on the Laue group, which is defined by the symmetry of the crystal, and on the type of diffraction experiment (anomalous data collection or not), a data collection strategy is devised. The symmetry of the crystal is reflected in the diffraction pattern symmetry, the so called Laue symmetry, and a complete data set must contain as many of the unique reflections present in the diffraction pattern as possible. For anomalous data collection, which is extensively used for anomalous phasing techniques, the centro-symmetrically related part of the unique data wedges (containing the so-called Friedel pairs -*h* -*k* -*l* of each reflection *h k l*) of must be also collected.

Once all diffraction pattern images are recorded, they are integrated and scaled into a complete data set. The data set so obtained represents a periodically sampled, reciprocal space transform of the molecules in the crystal. The extent to which the crystal diffracts (well-ordered crystals tend to diffract to a higher resolution than less well-behaved ones) directly determines how detailed or "sharp" the final reconstruction of the electron density will be, and ultimately how accurate and precise the resulting model can be. Although high resolution certainly helps, how accurate the model actually is will depend on the effort the crystallographer puts into the model building and structure refinement. Because crystallography reveals the reconstructed electron density of the atoms that form the protein, there is a keen interplay between the extent of diffraction and amount of detail visible in the electron, as is apparent in **Fig. 47.5**.

2.7. Phase Determination

Although a light microscope can be easily built to create a magnified image of an object using a lens, its resolution is not high enough for us to distinguish atomic detail in a molecular structure. With a microscope, no details of an object can be discerned unless the details of the object are separated by approximately half the wavelength of the radiation used to view them. Although X-rays have the appropriate wavelength to view atoms (in the Å, 10^{-8} cm, or 0.1 nm range), an X-ray microscope to view atoms cannot be built, because the refractive index for X-rays in most matter is practically one. This means, that there is no convenient material we can use to produce a lens that can focus X-rays. Therefore, we need to take the detour of back-transforming X-ray diffraction data mathematically to obtain the desired atomic resolution-level information about the molecular structure.

Our diffraction data, the measured diffraction intensities or reflections that form the data set, return only the magnitude of the diffracted X-rays. The phase relations between the reflections, which unfortunately carry the majority of the information about the molecular structure, are absent. Thus, to complete our X-ray diffraction experiment, and to reconstruct the electron density to obtain an image of our protein in the form of an electron density map, we must obtain the phase information through additional experiments. As noted earlier, this is known as the *crystallographic phase problem*. The strategy of phase determination depends on the molecular system whose structure is being determined, and indeed, can often be quite a time-consuming puzzle. Phasing is also the most critical part of the X-ray structure determination, and as with any other data, poor phases will result only in a poor structure, if it can be solved at all.

2.8. Substructure Methods

Fortunately, there is a generally applicable way to solve macromolecular structures. Instead of determining the position of thousands of atoms at once, it is possible to determine the structure of a few, distinct heavy atoms in a protein structure first, and bootstrap the phase determination from this so called *heavy atom substructure*. Substructure methods require that data sets of isomorphous structures (having the same molecular arrangement, space group, and unit cell dimensions) of the protein and corresponding heavy atom labeled structures are available. The isomorphous data sets are used to generate difference data reflecting the simplified substructure arrangement of the heavy atoms, which can then be determined using the direct methods or Patterson methods described below. Substructure phasing, also called de novo phasing, accounts for about 25% of all structures deposited in the PDB, and the overwhelming majority of new structures are solved by Se-based, *multiple anomalous dispersion (MAD)* phasing discussed in the following sections.

2.8.1. Direct Methods

Molecular structures containing less than 1,000 atoms can be solved by brute force statistical *Direct Methods*, given data to 1.2 Å or better, and most small molecule structures are solved this way. It was shown in the early 1950s that the phases of strongly scattered beams can be estimated from their measured intensities, by investigating the correlation between amplitude and phases of reflections and the electron density distribution in the unit cell. Classical direct methods, as applied to small molecules, assume that the electron density is always positive in the unit cell, that the unit cell consists of discrete atoms, and that the atomic positions are random variables with uniform distribution throughout the unit cell. Classical direct methods calculate phases directly from the amplitudes of the normalized structure factors, and each reflection is involved in multiple probability distributions. The *tangent formula (13)* combines these probability distributions and assigns a most probable phase given the other phase angles. Although there are limits to classical direct methods for complete protein structure solutions, modern, combined reciprocal- and real-space direct methods are extremely powerful in substructure determination *(14)*.

2.8.2. Patterson Function and Synthesis

To locate positions of heavy atoms (large atomic number, many electrons) or anomalous scatterers in the crystallographic unit cell requires the use of mathematics called the *Patterson synthesis*. The marker atoms so located provide phase information, which is deduced from structure factor amplitudes only. In the case of isomorphous replacement, this involves differences between native and derivative structure factor amplitudes, and in the case of anomalous dispersion, it involves anomalous differences between Friedel pairs of reflections and/or dispersive reflections recorded at different wavelengths. The Patterson function is a Fourier synthesis represented as

$$P(uvw) = \frac{1}{V} \sum_{hkl} |F_{hkl}|^2 \cos 2\pi(hu + kv + lw) \tag{7}$$

where $|F_{hkl}|^2$ is proportional to the *intensity* of each reflection we have recorded in our data. Thus, the Patterson function $P(u,v,w)$ can be computed directly from the diffraction data.

$P(u,v,w)$ is a periodic function in Patterson space, whose unit cell vectors **u**, **v**, and **w** are parallel to the unit cell vectors **a**, **b**, and **c** for the crystal. The coordinates u, v, and w are used instead of x, y, and z to emphasize that the *Patterson map* is distinct from the electron density map. In the Patterson map, there will be N^2-1 peaks (excluding the origin), where N is the number of atoms in the structure. But, what exactly do these peaks represent?

The Patterson map is an *interatomic vector map*. Each peak in the map represents a vector whose tail is at the origin and whose head is at the center of the peak. The value of the peak (height) is the sum of the products of the electron density at one end of the vector with the electron density at the other end of the vector. There is a large origin peak at $u = v = w = 0$, because this is where all the self vectors among atoms coincide. A correct interpretation of the Patterson map assigns atomic coordinates to heavy atoms in the structure, thus providing the substructure from which initial phases can be deduced. The Patterson function also lies at the heart of most molecular replacement methods, which will be discussed in a following section.

2.8.3. Isomorphous Replacement

Heavy atoms can be introduced into crystals by soaking techniques, and small changes in the reflection intensities between native crystals and derivatized crystals can be exploited to solve the heavy atom substructure *(15)*. This is called SIR or MIR for *Single* or *Multiple Isomorphous Replacement*. Recall that different atoms contribute to the scattered intensity in proportion to the square of the number of electrons they contain. Consider a mercury atom, which contains ~13 times as many electrons as a carbon atom. The contribution of one Hg atom to the scattered intensity will be equivalent to that of ~170 carbon atoms. Crick and Magdoff *(16)* first estimated the change in scattering intensity (phasing power) resulting from addition of a heavy atom using the following equation:

$$\sqrt{\frac{N_H}{2N_T}} \frac{f_H}{Z_{eff}} \tag{8}$$

where Z_{eff} is the effective atomic number of the atom in the native structure (6.7 for proteins *(17)*), N_T is the total number of atoms in the native structure, and N_H is the number of heavy atoms with scattering power f_H. In our example, then, the change in intensity from the addition of one mercury atom to a protein of ~20 kDa is easily measured. For larger structures such as ribosomal subunits, heavy atom clusters can be exploited for phasing *(18)*.

Soaking the crystals for several hours to days in mother liquor containing a few mill molar heavy atom salts such as Pt, Pb, Hg, and U (Hg for example attaches preferentially to free cysteines) is the classical approach to isomorphous replacement, but osmotic shock, deterioration of the crystals during soaking, and the resulting loss of isomorphism can create problems. As the initial phases are not exact and can have relatively broad probability distributions, it is generally necessary to prepare more than one derivative. Availability of multiple isomorphous derivatives (MIR) also removes the ambiguity in the substructure handedness, which otherwise needs to be overcome in SIR by combination with anomalous phasing or density modification techniques.

2.8.4. Anomalous Phasing Techniques

Heavy atoms (other than C, N, O) often exhibit wavelength-dependent *anomalous scattering*, with the result that a reflection F_{hkl} and its centrosymmetrically related reflection F_{-h-k-l} (also called *Friedel pairs*) are not exactly equal. These small differences can be exploited in SAD and MAD phasing methods (for *Single* and *Multiple Anomalous Diffraction*). Metal atoms such as Fe, already present in the protein, or Se, in selenomethionine (modified methionine that has been incorporated into the protein during expression) are suitable anomalous scatterers. In the case of selenomethionine, one Se-Met residue provides sufficient phasing power for 80–120 residues *(17)*. Heavy atoms soaked into isomorphous crystals can also act as source of anomalous signal, as noted previously.

The elegance of the MAD method *(19)* lies in the fact that anomalous differences exist not only within a data set among the Friedel pairs collected at a wavelength above the absorption edge, but also as dispersive differences among data sets collected at different wavelengths. As all these data sets can be collected at different wavelengths from one single crystal, nonisomorphism among crystals is not an issue. Together, this means that multiple, perfectly isomorphous difference data sets are available, and phases determined from the substructure of anomalous scatterers are of correspondingly high quality. In addition, as the sequence of the protein is normally known, the location of Se atoms in methionine residues provides valuable anchors for the sequence during subsequent model building.

Given very carefully collected and redundant data, even the small anomalous signal resulting from the presence of sulfur atoms of cysteine and methionine residues in native proteins can be exploited for anomalous phasing in combination with density modification techniques. This method is called SSAD (sulfur single wavelength anomalous diffraction). Because the anomalous signal of sulfur is stronger at longer wavelengths (closer to the sulfur absorption edge), characteristic copper (1.54178 Å) or chromium (2.2910 Å) radiation can be used for in-house SSAD phasing *(20)*.

2.8.5. Molecular Replacement

If the atomic coordinates of a previously determined, structurally homologous model are available, these can be used as a search fragment to calculate initial phases for the unknown protein structure in the method known as *Molecular Replacement* (MR). Model phases so derived are then used in the initial construction of the electron density. In MR, we attempt to locate the position of the search molecule in the crystal (hence the name Molecular Replacement, in the sense of repositioning, not substituting, the molecule). To determine the relative orientation of the search molecule in the crystal we first calculate the Patterson map for the search molecule using its atomic coordinates, and then superposition the search map onto the experimental Patterson map for the structure to be solved, which is calculated from the intensity data. Once we have correctly oriented the search molecule (*rotation*), we must locate the search molecule's position in the unit cell with respect to the origin. We step it through the unit cell (*translation*), essentially artificially packing the model into the unit cell of our unknown molecule, now comparing calculated and observed structure factors. When the model is correctly positioned, we will have a good correlation of between calculated and experimental data, and we can use the atomic positions so derived to calculate the structure factors for our unknown molecule. Other, powerful evolutionary algorithms for MR use a direct, six-dimensional search instead of the subsequent 3 + three dimensional (rotation + translation) search to find the correct position of the search model *(21)* or employ additional, sophisticated maximum likelihood search methods *(22)*.

MR does not require high resolution data. It allows a quick determination of initial phases, providing atom positions ready for rebuilding and refinement without the need to completely retrace the chain, and it is very useful for determining the structures of complexes and mutants. However, careless use of model phases will introduce severe *model phase bias*. Model bias is a devious feature: Because phases dominate the reconstruction of the electron density, the initial structure will largely reflect the features of the search model and not necessarily the true structure, although the initial maps can look deceivingly acceptable. Phase bias removal methods such as simulated annealing, omit maps, unrestrained dummy atom refinement, map averaging or a combination thereof must be extensively used to correct the phases and multiple cycles of rebuilding of model may be necessary to obtain a good structure. About 75% of all structures deposited in the protein data bank are solved by molecular replacement techniques exploiting a homologous structure model as a source of initial phases.

2.9. Density Modification and Phase Extension

The initial maps obtained from substructure methods contain noise as a result of measurement errors, imprecision in the heavy atom solutions, and closure errors in the solution of the phasing equations. However, protein molecules pack loosely in a lattice containing substantial solvent channels (about 30–70 % of the crystal volume) filled with nonordered solvent, a fact that can be used to improve the map appearance and improve interpretability. Setting the solvent electron density to a constant value (flattening), in repeated cycles with adjustments in the solvent mask under extension of resolution *(23)*, leads to drastically reduced phase angle errors and, hence, clearer and better interpretable electron density maps. Density modification is also important in permitting phase extension to higher resolution in the frequent case where the derivative or anomalous data used for substructure solution and phasing do not extend to the same high resolution as the native data *(24)*.

A powerful variation of density modification is map averaging, which is applicable in presence of quite frequent non crystallographic symmetry (NCS). The principle of NCS averaging is that if more than one molecule (for example, a dimer) is present in the asymmetric unit of the crystal, the diffraction pattern and hence the back-transformed map, will contain redundant information. The electron density of the different copies of the molecule thus can be averaged (consistent features will amplify whereas noise and ambiguous density will be suppressed), and again, a greatly improved electron density map of the molecule results. Map averaging is also possible among different crystal forms of the same protein *(25)*, and density modification by map averaging is in fact so powerful that virus capsid structures, which are highly symmetric and contain up to 60 copies per molecule, can be phased without additional substructure information.

2.10. Electron Density Map Interpretation

Once an interpretable map is obtained by phase extension methods, a model of the protein, which makes chemical and physical sense, is fitted into the initial electron density map. In the early days of protein crystallography, physical protein models were built by hand *(26)* using metal rods to show chemical bonds. Today, model building is achieved in silico using computer programs that graphically display the electron density and allow placement and manipulation of protein backbone markers and residues, combined with various real space and geometry refinement tools *(27)*. The process of model building is greatly accelerated by automated model building programs *(28)* providing a reasonable starting model, which can then be completed and polished by hand.

Before automatic model building procedures can be used, a set of "guide points" is required, which is essentially a set of Cα backbone atoms placed at recognizable branching points of main and side chain density, at 3.8 Å intervals, and the longest contiguous chain is sought *(29,30)*. This initial set of Cα positions could then be used to query the structural database in search of fragment libraries *(31)*, which along with statistics on use of preferred rotamers *(32)*, can improve the model quality already in the first building cycles. Sequence anchoring on stretches of distinct residues or at marker atom sites then facilitates proper tracing of the chains, as well as recognition and correction of branching errors.

Despite the assisting software available, model building is often perceived as the most dreaded part of a structure determination. Model building certainly constitutes the most intense involvement in the protein structure, and with poor electron density, a large degree of intuition and experience are required. It is here where quality data, good phases, and high resolution deliver substantial pay-offs. Good quality maps at higher resolution reveal much higher detail and allow greater confidence when building the model. At high resolution, electron density shapes of the residues are much less degenerate than at low resolution, aiding proper feature recognition, faster alignment with the known sequence, and less opportunity for tracing errors.

2.11. Model Refinement

Despite meticulous model building, an initial model will still be missing certain parts, and it will have many small errors, such as incorrect bond distances and angles, poor backbone geometry, or improbable torsion angles. These small errors are corrected during the course of *structure refinement*. The refinement program adjusts the atomic position coordinates of the initial model, as well as general scaling parameters, so that the differences between observed and calculated structure amplitudes are minimized *(33)*. The model is usually improved by least-squares minimization of

$$\sum_{hkl} w\left(|F_{obs}| - |F_{cal}|\right)^2 + \sum_{r} w(Y_t - Y)^2 \tag{9}$$

alternately with rebuilding of the model by interactive graphics. Here, w are statistical weights, $|F_{obs}|$ and $|F_{cal}|$ are the observed and calculated structure factor amplitudes and Y and Y_t are the current and target values of *restraints* such as bond lengths and angles. The lower the resolution is, the more important are these restraints. As the model quality is improved, individual atomic temperature factors (a measure for positional displacement either via thermal motion or through disorder) are refined during refinement, and bulk solvent model corrections are applied *(34)*.

The global measure of agreement between calculated and observed structure factor amplitudes is given by the crystallographic *R*-value

$$R = \frac{\sum\limits_{hkl} \left\| F_{\text{obs}} \right| - k \left| F_{\text{cal}} \right\|}{\sum\limits_{hkl} \left| F_{\text{obs}} \right|} \tag{10}$$

In this simple equation $|F_{\text{cal}}|$ and $|F_{\text{obs}}|$ are the calculated and observed structure factor amplitudes, and k is a scaling constant. In the literature, the R-value may be given in percent rather than as a fraction between 0 and 1, e.g., 24.6% instead of 0.246.

The quality of a crystal structure refinement used to be measured with the R-value only. However, R can be reduced artificially by refining more model parameters than justified (called *overfitting*). This fallaciously improves the fit between observed and calculated data, but actually does nothing to improve the model. Common sources of overfitting are the introduction of too many water molecules into the model, or placing various kinds of molecules (solvent or ligands) into spurious density. Today, it is necessary to exclude about 5% of the reflections from refinement, which are used to calculate an index called *Rfree* using the same formula *(10)*. Because the model is never refined against these reflections, they provide an independent assessment of the improvement of the model during refinement/ rebuilding cycles. The refinement is considered complete when it is not possible to reduce *Rfree* further *(35)*, and there is no significant remaining difference electron density or disagreements with the restraint target values. As a crude rule of thumb, R in % is expected to be about 10 times the highest resolution of the data, and the gap between R and R*free* should not be much more than 5%. A valuable final measure of quality, in terms of model stereochemistry, is the Ramachandran *phi/psi* plot *(36)*. Because the backbone torsion angles, φ and ψ, are not restrained during refinement, the Ramachandran plot is a good independent diagnostic. Ideally, 98% of the residues should fall in the allowed core region, and 80% in the most preferred core, as illustrated in **Fig. 47.8**.

2.12. Strategies

2.12.1. Crystallization

Start with pure and monodisperse material. Purity can be ascertained by SDS PAGE, and dispersity can be determined by dynamic light scattering. Commercially available crystallization screening kits, containing as many as 96 different crystallization conditions and based on ionic strength, precipitants, and incomplete factorials, can be purchased for manual or automated screening experiments. Random screening using prior knowledge, such as isoelectric point *(37,38)*, can be utilized for designing specific screening strategies.

2.12.2. Cryo-Crystallography

Radiation damage has been a major concern since the earliest days of macromolecular crystallography, because it limits the information that we can obtain from a single crystal. Symptoms of radiation damage to protein crystals recognizable in the diffraction data include decrease in diffraction intensity and resolution, increase in unit cell volume, and color changes. In refined models, site specific damage, beginning with breakage of disulfide bonds, followed by decarboxylation of aspartates, glutamates, and the C-terminus, and then loss of the hydroxyl group from tyrosines *(39–41)* is molecular evidence of radiation damage. In the late 1980s, flash-cooling techniques for monochromatic macromolecular crystallography, as described earlier, were developed. Because data

Ramachandran plot

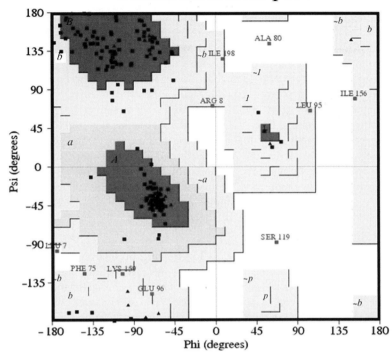

Fig. 47.8. The Ramachandran phi/psi plot. Ramachandran plot showing the distribution of φ/ψ torsion angles pairs for each residue in a protein chain during model building. In this initial structure model, most residues lie in energetically favored core regions (dark shades), while a few highlighted outliers still need further adjustment and rebuilding

collection at ~100 K usually prolongs the crystal lifetime by a factor of ~70 (*42*), the problem of radiation damage had largely been resolved until the advent of third generation synchrotrons in the late 1990s. Ongoing systematic studies on different aspects of radiation damage are continuing to increase our understanding of the underlying physics and chemistry of this process, and software that accounts for the damage effects are actively being developed.

2.12.3. Data Collection
The goal of data collection is to generate data accurate enough to ultimately build a model of sufficient depth of detail to understand your particular protein structure. This entails collecting a complete and accurate set of reflection intensities to as high a resolution as possible. Careful strategies must be used to extract the maximum information from the data within experimental constraints, such as crystal characteristics and properties of the X-ray source. If the crystal diffracts to very high resolution, the detector must be moved off-center to capture those data. Similarly, low resolution data, which are important for phasing, must not be sacrificed at the expense of high resolution data. Two data collections runs at different detector angles and/or exposure times, one for high- and one for low-resolution data coverage are then advisable. If data are collected at two different crystal-to-detector distances, these distances should be optimized to capture enough overlap for proper scal. As data redundancy improves experimental

phases by decreasing the error in merged data and thus in calculated amplitude differences, it is better to collect for phasing fewer intense and well-resolved reflections with high redundancy (several times at different positions in reciprocal space) than to collect many poor reflections at high resolution that simply add to the noise. Exposure times should be adequate to obtain a high signal/noise ratio over the bulk of data set.

In the particular case of data intended for phase determination using anomalous dispersion, synchrotron beamline properties are relevant to determine which and how many wavelengths to use in the experiment. This requires decisions about the data collection sequence and how many data to collect at each wavelength. Although MAD data collected at three wavelengths can provide extremely accurate phases, the probability of radiation damage to the crystal may necessitate the compromise of conducting a two wavelength MAD experiment instead. When single wavelengths are used for anomalous phase determination, complete date sets, including measurements of all anomalous pairs with a very high degree of redundancy in the data, are generally required.

2.12.4. Recombinant DNA Technology

In addition to facilitating overexpression of pure protein, recombinant techniques allow for production of stable mutants, as well as introduction of specific changes into a protein sequence to improve crystallizability *(43)* or provide for site-directed heavy atom labeling *(44–46)*. The most common phasing technique exploits the fact that the amino acid methionine can be replaced with selenomethionine by overexpressing the protein in a suitable, Se-Met auxotroph expression system *(47)*. The incorporated heavy ($z = 34$) Se atoms then act as the source of anomalous signal, and the method, as previously described, is appropriately called multiple anomalous diffraction (MAD) phasing.

2.12.5. Time-Resolved (Laue) Diffraction

The special case of harnessing the full spectrum of synchrotron radiation in Laue crystallography opens up the possibility for time resolved studies, on time scales of seconds to picoseconds, to create molecular movies with high spatial resolution and wide temporal sampling *(48)*. Such analyses are a growing trend in special crystal structure analyses, greatly aided by expanded capabilities such as fast repeated data collection with CCD detectors. To examine the evolution of structural intermediates of reactive protein molecules such as enzymes, for example, one can record a succession of Laue diffraction snapshots with preset lengthening time gaps, while a substrate solution is passed over a crystal of the protein held in a flow cell. Provided that there are no severe conformational changes that alter or destroy the crystal lattice, experimental difference electron density maps produced with Laue data can reveal changes in electron density corresponding to conformational changes and chemical modifications.

3. Applications

3.1. Structure-Guided Drug Discovery

The Philadelphia chromosome arises from translocation between human chromosomes 9 and 22 and fuses two genes, c-ABL and BCR. The fusion protein that results is a constitutively active oncogenic tyrosine kinase that causes cell transformation and chronic myeloid leukemia, and has also been shown to be responsible for malignant transformation in 15–30% of patents with acute lymphoblastic leukemia. Gleevec, or Imatinib, STI-571, is an established first-line treatment for chronic myeloid leukemia. It achieves its effect by binding to the ABL kinase domain and inhibiting its tyrosine kinase activity to produce a normalization of white blood cell counts and reduce the Philadelphia chromosome-positive clones of stem cells in bone marrow. Early treatment elicits high response rates, but acquired resistance to Imatinib, most often a result of point mutations in ABL, is a distinct problem.

In an effort to understand the structural basis of resistance and to design a novel and more potent therapeutic, capable of preventing proliferation of cells including those resistant to Imatinib, scientists at Bristol-Myers Squibb undertook a comparative X-ray crystallographic study. Using molecular replacement techniques, they determined the structures of BCR-ABL in complex with various small molecules that had been shown to be multi-targeted kinase inhibitors (49). As shown in **Fig. 47.9**, they found that, although the central cores of the drugs overlap, the rest of each molecule extends in opposite directions within the enzyme. Mutations imparting Imatinib resistance occur in the activation loop and other regions of the C-terminal lobe of the enzyme. These mutations result in conformational changes unrecognized by Imatinib. One of the molecules screened, Dasatinib, by contrast, is capable of recognizing

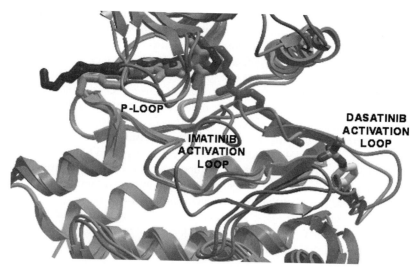

Fig. 47.9. Comparison of the Dasatinib, PD173955 and Imatinib complexes of ABL kinase. A ribbon representation of three complexes, superimposed, with the drugs rendered as sticks. Dasatinib and PD173955 are bound at the upper left of a cleft and shown in dark and light grey, while imatinib (Gleevec) is bound to the right and down, shown in medium grey. The phosphorylated tyrosine is shown at the lower right, rendered by sticks and colored by atom type in tones of grey and white. Ring structures at the ends of the inhibitor molecules overlap, but the rest of the structures extend in opposite directions. The activation loop in the imatinib structure diverges from the conformation found in the Dasatinib structure. All Imatinib-resistant mutations occur in the phosphate-binding loop (P-loop) of ABL kinase, where Dasatinib is capable of binding. Image rendered with ICM Pro v3.4–7h using coordinates from PDB IDs: 1GQG, 1IEP and 1M52

multiple states of the enzyme and still render it inactive. Comparison between structures of Dasatinib and another compound, PD173955, also helped to explain why the latter was not as potent an inhibitor as Dasatinib.

3.2. Elucidating the Transcriptional Molecular Machinery

The human genome consists of approx 3 billion nucleotide pairs organized into 23 chromosomes. If this DNA were to be uncoiled and laid out end to end, it would extend about 3 m. Obviously, this cannot possibly fit into a cell, and extended DNA would be susceptible to breakage during replication and cell division. In eukaryotes, genetic material is thus organized into complexes of DNA with core histones and other chromosomal proteins that together form chromatin. The chromatin repeating unit includes two copies each of four core histones H2A, H2B, H3 and H4 (collective molecular mass 206,000) wrapped by 146 bp of DNA. The fundamental packing unit of chromatin is an 11-nm diameter molecular assembly called the nucleosome. With additional proteins and histone H1, nucleosomes are packaged into 30-nm fibers with six nucleosomes per turn in a spiral or solenoid, and when this 30-nm fiber unwinds, an 11-nm template for transcription is generated. The precise molecular mechanism of transcriptional regulation at the level of the nucleosome was finally elucidated by Tim Richmond et al. in 1997, when they determined the structure of the nucleosome core particle to 2.8 Å resolution (50, 51).

This structure was the culmination of more than 15 yr of work involving a *tour de force* of recombinant DNA technology and protein crystallography. The four core histone proteins were individually expressed in milligram quantities in *E. coli*, purified under denaturing conditions, then refolded into histone octomers and assembled into nucleosome core particles using 146 bp defined-sequence DNA fragment derived from human α-satellite DNA. Crystals were grown by vapor diffusion over the course of one to three weeks and flash cooled in liquid propane at −12°C before data collection on an IP detector on undulator beamline ID13 at the European Synchrotron Radiation Facility (ESRF) in Grenoble. Three heavy atom derivatives were used for MIR phasing, prepared by soaking with mercury nitrate, methyl mercury nitrate and tetrakis(acetoxymercuri)methane (TAMM) *(52)*. The initial MIR electron density map was used to trace 120 bp of DNA and 745 amino acids, and iterative rounds of model building and refinement resulted in a model containing the entire DNA and histone octamer (**Fig. 47.10**).

The structure revealed that the histone amino terminal tails pass over and among the gyres of the DNA superhelix, making contact with neighboring core particles. When the histone tails are *hypoacetylated*, they constrain the wrapping of the DNA on the nucleosome surface by promoting strong nucleosomal interactions. Upon *hyperacetylation*, the nucleosomal interactions are weakened, the histone tails no longer constrain the DNA on the surface of the nucleosome, and the DNA is now accessible to transcription factors. The bending and supercoiling of the DNA on the nucleosome can promote binding of transcription factors and augment interactions among different factors.

3.3. Time Resolved Laue Crystallography

Hydroxymethylbilane synthase (HMBS) is the third enzyme in the heme biosynthetic pathway, catalyzing the polymerization of four molecules of porphobilinogen to form hydroxymethylbilane. All organisms, except viruses, have

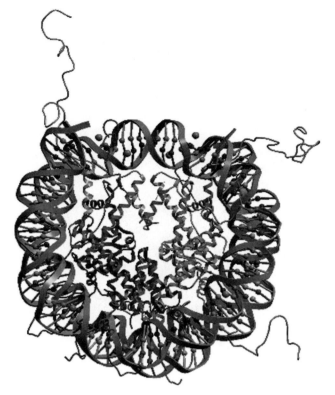

Fig. 47.10. Nucleosome core particle. The nucleosome core particle consists of to copies each of core histone proteins, H2A, H2B, H3 and H4, wrapped by 146 base pairs of DNA. The tails of the histone proteins, which are seen to protrude from among the base pairs, form strong or weak nucleosomal interactions, depending on their state of acetylation. When hyperacetylated, nucleosomal interactions are weakened, the DNA is not constrained on the surface of the nucleosome, and the DNA becomes accessible to transcription factors. Image rendered with ICM Pro v3.4–7h using coordinates from PDB ID: 1AOI

a requirement for one or more of the tetrapyrroles, such as heme, chlorophyll or vitamin B_{12}, for which HMBS activity is vital. Inhibitors of HMBS are believed to be potentially useful as antibiotics and/or herbicides. Furthermore, molecular abnormalities in the gene coding for this enzyme result in half-normal activity of HMBS, which is associated with the autosomal disorder known as acute intermittent porphyria (the madness of King George III).

In a study aimed at understanding the important and highly complex biological chemistry of this molecular system, Helliwell and coworkers conducted a time-resolved experiment at the ESRF Laue beamline ID109 *(53)*. HMBS is suitable for time-resolved studies because it is a slow enzyme ($k_{cat} = 0.1\,s^{-1}$ at 310 K and pH 7.5, compared to $k_{cat} \sim 10^{-7}\,s^{-1}$ for most enzymes), and slower rates can be obtained using mutants, lower pH or lower temperature. The experimental difference maps, produced with the Laue data, revealed an elongated electron density in the putative substrate binding site of the enzyme, located appropriately near the unusual cofactor of HMBS, dipyrromethane.

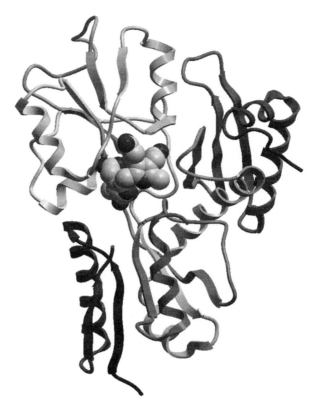

Fig. 47.11. Hydroxymethylbilane synthase. The structure of HMBS as determined by time-resolved and static ensemble X-ray crystallography. The polypeptide backbone is drawn as a ribbon, and the unique dipyrromethane cofactor is rendered as CPK. Because disordered polypeptide backbone, believed to be highly flexible, could not be traced owing to a lack of discernible electron density, the N-terminal domain at the lower left appears disconnected from the remainder of the molecule. Image rendered with ICM Pro v3.4–7 h using coordinates from PDB ID: 1GTK

This density was followed in a structural and functional context over several hours to reveal structural intermediates in the reaction and the change from oxidized (inactive) to reduced (active) form of the cofactor. Although, the role of a disordered loop region containing catalytic residues remains to be elucidated, the structures obtained have provided valuable insights for developing new experiments as well as for designing putative inhibitors (*54*) against pathogens such as *Mycobacterium tuberculosis*.

References

1. Congreve M, Murray CW, Blundell TL (2005) Structural biology and drug discovery. Drug Disc Today 10(13):895–907
2. Curtis A, Wilkinson C (2001) Nanotechniques and approaches in biotechnology. Trends Biotechnol 19:97–101
3. Frechet JM (2002) Dendrimers and supramolecular chemistry. Proc Natl Acad Sci USA 99:4782–4787
4. Patri AK, Majoros IJ, Baker JR (2002) Dendritic polymer macromolecular carriers for drug delivery. Curr Opin Chem Biol 6:466–471

5. Chen H, Scott NR (2002) Nanoscale science and engineering for agriculture and food systems. In: Proc USDA Conference. Washington, DC

6. Quintana A, Raczka E, Piehler L (2002) Design and function of a dendrimer-based therapeutic nanodevice targeted to tumor cells through the folate receptor. Pharm Res 19:1310–1316

7. Zhu SG, Lu HB, Xiang JJ, Tang K, Zhang BC, Zhou M, Tan C, Li GY (2002) A novel nonviral nanoparticles gene vector: poly-L-lysine-silica nanoparticles. Chinese Sci Bull 47:654–658

8. Durcruix A, Giege R (1989) Crystallization of nucleic acids and proteins: A practical approach. Oxford University Press, Oxford, UK, pp 78–82

9. McPherson A (1989) Preparation and analysis of protein crystals Krieger Publishing, Malabar, FL, pp 88–91

10. Zeppezauer M, Eklund H, Zeppezauer ES (1968) Micro diffucion cells for growth of single protein crystals by means of equilibrium dialysis. Arch Biochem Biophys 126(2):564–573

11. Hansen CL, Skordalakes E, Berger JM, Quake SR (2002) A robust and scalable microfluidic metering method that allows protein crystal growth by free interface diffusion. Proc Natl Acad Sci USA 99(26):16531–15536

12. Zheng B, Tice JD, Spencer Roach L, Ismagilov RF (2005) A droplet-based, composit PDMS/glass capillary microfulidic system for evaluating protein crystallization conditions by microbatch and vapor diffusion methods with on-chip x-ray diffraction. Angew Chem Intl Ed Engl 43(19):2508–2511

13. Karle J, Hauptman H (1956) A theory of phase determination for the four types of non-centrosymmetric space groups 1P222, 2P22, 3P12, 3P22. Acta Crystallogr 9:635–651

14. Schneider TR, Sheldrick GM (2002) Substructure solution with SHELXD. Acta Crystallogr D58:1772–1779

15. Carvin D, Islam SA, Sternberg MJE, Blundell TL (2001) The preparation of heavy-atom derivatives of protein crystals for use in multiple isomorphous replacement and anomalous scattering. Int Tables Crystallogr F:247–255

16. Crick FHC, Magdoff BS (1956) The theory of the method of isomorphous replacement for protein crystals. Acta Cryst 9:901–908

17. Hendrickson WA, Ogata CM (1997) Phase determination from multiwavelength anomalous diffraction measurements. Methods Enzymol 276:494–523

18. Schluenzen F, Tocilj A, Zarivach R, Harms J, Glyehmann M, Janell D, Bashan A, Bartels H, Agmon I, Franceschi F, Yonath A (2000) Structure of functionally activated small ribosomal subunit at 3.3 Angstroms resolution. Cell 102:615–623

19. Hendrickson WA (1991) Determination of macromolecular structures from anomalous diffraction of synchrotron radiation. Science 254:51–58

20. Yang C, Pflugrath JW, Courville DA, Stence CN, Ferrara JD (2003) Away from the edge: SAD phasing from the sulfur anomalous signal measured in-house with chromium radiation. Acta Crystallogr D59(11):1943–1957

21. Kissinger CR, Gehlhaar DK, Smith BA, Bouzida D (2001) Molecular replacement by evolutionary search. Acta Crystallogr D57(10):1474–1479

22. Read RJ (2001) Pushing the boundaries of molecular replacement with maximum likelihood. Acta Crystallogr D57:1373–1382

23. Cowtan KD, Main P (1996) Phase combination and cross validation in iterated density-modification calculations. Acta Crystallogr D52:43–48

24. Zhang KYJ, Cowtan KD, Main P (2001) Phase improvement by iterative density modification. Int Tables Crystallog F:311–324

25. Taylor G (2003) The phase problem. Acta Crystallogr D59(11):1881–1890

26. Kendrew JC, Dickerson RE, Strandberg BE, Hart RG, Davies DR, Phillips DC, Shore VC (1960) Structure of myoglobin: a three-dimensional Fourier synthesis at 2A resolution. Nature 185:422–427

27. McRee DE (1999) XtalView/Xfit – a versatile program for manipulating atomic coordinates and electron density. J Struct Biol 125:156–165

28. Cohen SX, Morris RJ, Fernandez FJ, Ben Jelloul M, Kakaris M, Parthasarathy V, Lamzin VS, Kleywegt GJ, Perrakis A (2004) Towards complete validated models in the next generation of ARP/wARP. Acta Crystallogr D60(12):2222–2229

29. Ioerger TR, Sacchettini JC (2002) Automatic modeling of protein backbones in electron density maps via prediction of Ca coordinates. Acta Crystallogr D58:2043–2054

30. Oldfield T (2003) Automated tracing of electron density maps of proteins. Acta Crystallogr D59:483–491

31. Cowtan KD (1998) Modified phased translation functions and their application to molecular-fragment location. Acta Crystallogr D54:750–756

32. Dunbrack RL, Jr (2002) Rotamer libraries in the 21st century. Curr Opin Struct Biol 12:431–440

33. TenEyck LF, Watenpaugh K (2001) Introduction to refinement. Int Tables Crystallogr F:369–374

34. Kostrewa D (1997) Bulk solvent correction: practical application and effects in reciprocal and real space. CCP4. Newsletter Protein Crystallogr 34:9–22

35. Brünger AT (1992) Free R value: a novel statistical quantity for assessing the accuracy of crystal structures. Nature 355:472–475

36. Ramachandran GN, Ramakrishnan C, Sasisekharan V (1963) Stereochemistry of polypeptide chain conFigurations. J Mol Biol 7:95–99

37. Kantardjieff KA, Jamshidian M, Rupp B (2004) Distributions of pI versus pH provide prior information for the design of crystallization screening experiments: response to comment on 'Protein isoelectric point as a predictor for increased crystallization screening efficiency'. Bioinformatics 20(14):2171–2174

38. Kantardjieff KA, Rupp B (2004) Protein isoelectric point as a predictor for increased crystallization screening efficiency. Bioinformatics 20(14):2162–2168

39. Burmeister WP (2000) Structural changes in cryo-cooled protein crystals owing to radiation damage. Acta Cryst D56:328–341

40. Ravelli RBG, McSweeney SM (2000) The 'fingerprint' that X-rays can leave on structures. Structure Fold Des 8:315–328

41. Weik M, Ravelli RBG, Kryger G, McSweeney SM, Raves ML, Harel M, Gros P, DSilman I, Kroon J, Sussman JL (2000) Specific chemical and structural damage to proteins produced by synchrotron radiation. Proc Natl Acad Sci USA 97:623–628

42. Nave C, Garman EF (2005) Towards an understanding of radiation damage in cryocooled macromolecular crystals. J Synchrotron Radiation 12:257–260

43. Dyda F, Hickman AB, Jenkins TM, Engelman A, Craigie R, Davies DR (1994) Crystal structure of the catalytic domain of HIV-integrase: similarity to other polynucleotidyl transferases. Science 266(5193):1981–1986

44. Ebright YW, Chen Y, Ludescher RD, Ebright RH (1993) N-(iodoacetyl)-p-phenylenediamine-EDTA: a reagent for high-efficiency incorporation of an EDTA-metal complex at a rationally selected site within a protein. Bioconjug Chem 4(3):219–225

45. Krebs MP, Behrens W, Mollaaghababa R, Khorana HG, Heyn MP (1993) X-ray diffraction of a cysteine-containing bacteriorhodopsin mutant and its mercury derivative. Localization of an amino acid in the loop of an integral membrane protein Biochemistry 32(47):12830–12834

46. Wallace CJ, Clark-Lewis I (2000) Site-specific independent double labeling of proteins with reporter atoms. Biochem Cell Biol 78(2):79–86

47. Strub MP, Hoh F, Sanchez JF, Strub JM, Bock A, Aumelas A, Dumas C (2003) Selenomethionine and selnocysteine double labeling strategy for crystallographic phasing. Structure 11(11):1359–1367

48. Blakley MP, Cianci M, Helliwell JR, Rizkallah PJ (2004) Synchrotron and neutron techniques in biological crystallography. Chem Soc Rev 33(8):548–557

49. Tokarski JS, Newitt JA, Chang CYJ, Chend JD, Wittekind M, Kiefer SE, Kish K, Lee FYF, Borsillerri R, Lombardo LJ, Xie D, Zhang Y, Klei HE (2006) The structure of dasatinib (BMS-354825) bound to activated ABL kinase domain elucidates its inhibitory activity against imatinib-resistant ABL mutants. Cancer Res 66(11):5790–5797

50. Luger K, Rechsteiner TJ, Flaus AJ, Waye MM, Richmond TJ (1997) Characterization of nucleosome core particles containing histone proteins made in bacteria. J Mol Biol 272(3):301–311

51. Luger K, Mader AW, Richmond RK, Sargent DF, Richmond TJ (1997) Crystal structure of the nucleosome core particle at 2.8A resolution. Nature 389(6648): 251–260

52. O'Halloran TV, Lippard SJ, Richmond TJ, Klug A (1987) Multiple heavy-atom reagents for macromolecular X-ray structure determination. Application to the nucleosome core particle. J Mol Biol 194(4):705–712

53. Helliwell JR, Nieh YP, Habash J, Faulder PF, Raferty J, Cianci M, Wulff M, Hadener A (2003) Time-resolved and static-ensemble structural chemistry of hydroxymethylbilane synthase. Faraday Discuss 122:131–144

54. Kantardjieff K, Rupp B (2004) Structural bioinformatics approaches to the discovery of new antimycobacterial drugs. Curr Pharm Design 10(26):3165–3211

48

Microchip Devices for Bioanalysis

Anna C. Kinsella and Shelley D. Minteer

1. Introduction

Over the last two decades, microchip-based lab analysis systems have become more and more popular. These devices are typically called lab-on-a-chip devices or micro-TAS (micro total analysis systems), because they are designed to integrate an entire analytical instrument onto a small portable device. However, for the benefit of this chapter, we are going to refer to these devices as lab-on-a-chip devices, because this term is broader and includes both the analysis portion of the device, and also any other functions that the device might perform (i.e., microreactors, cell culturing, PCR, separations, etc.). Some of the devices are designed to be disposable and some are designed to be reuseable, but they are typically designed to be small portable, inexpensive devices that complete an entire chemical analysis.

The first lab-on-a-chip device was developed in 1979 when a gas chromatograph was fabricated on a silicon wafer (1). Over the last 25 years, research has continued to decrease the size and increase the functionality of lab-on-a-chip devices. Today, there are lab-on-a-chip devices for gas chromatography (1), liquid chromatography (2), electrophoresis (3–4), immunoassays (5,6), solid phase extraction (7), magnetic separators (8), DNA analysis (9), PCR (10), and cell culturing (11). This chapter will discuss lab-on-a-chip devices for sample preparation, separation, and detection, while also including microreactors and cell culturing.

There are many advantages of lab-on-a-chip devices, but one of the most important is a decreased use of consumable chemicals. Many chemicals and biologicals used in analysis are expensive and others are difficult to dispose of. The lab-on-a-chip device can decrease the use of consumable chemical by several orders of magnitude. This decreases cost, toxicity, and disposal risks. Other advantages include improved performance (sensitivity, detection limits, analysis time, etc.), automation, and design flexibility. However, the main disadvantage of lab-on-a-chip devices has been the ability to integrate them with larger scale systems.

Today, there are more than a dozen commercial lab-on-a-chip products. Most of these products are designed for the life scientist and include products

From: *Molecular Biomethods Handbook, 2nd Edition.*
Edited by: J. M. Walker and R. Rapley © Humana Press, Totowa, NJ

for immunoassays, DNA analysis, protein analysis, enzyme assays, miniaturized replacements for LC systems, and protein crystallization systems. These devices are becoming more and more important to the molecular biologists, clinicians, and biochemists because they can provide more reproducible results and less false results than traditional homogeneous methods, they can analyze smaller sample sizes, which is important in molecular biology where you may only have micro or nanograms of protein, and these devices can decrease analysis time by orders of magnitude.

2. Methods of Microchip Fabrication

Lab-on-a-chip devices are typically fabricated using lithography or laser ablation. Lithography is the process of making three dimensional features on a flat surface, whereas laser ablation is the process of using a laser to engrave features in a surface. There are advantages and disadvantages of both fabrication processes, but typically the choice of fabrication technique is determined by the chip material (glass, polydimethylsiloxane (PDMS), silicon, etc.).

There are two types of lithography that are typically used for producing lab-on-a-chip devices: photolithography and soft lithography. Photolithography is the most widely used type of lithography and brought about the development of the "integrated circuit." Photolithography is the process by which a surface (i.e. silicon wafer, glass slide, etc.) is coated with photoresist. A pattern is transferred to the chip by exposure of the photoresist to a UV light source through an optical mask and subsequent etching of unexposed photoresist. A schematic of the photolithography process is shown in the first three steps of **Fig. 48.1**. Photolithography is commonly used for patterning on silicon wafers, but can also be done on glass or even a polymer like polymethylmethacrylate (PMMA) *(12)*. Photolithography can pattern channels below 50nm, so it is a better technique for producing nanoscale features, then soft lithography.

Soft lithography is the process of using the patterned photoresist from photolithography as a master mold. Although soft lithography can be used on almost all

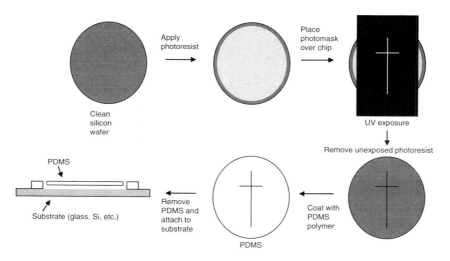

Fig. 48.1. Schematic showing the lithography process

polymers and many other materials, one of the most common methods for using soft lithography for fabricating the microchip devices is replica molding of poly-dimethylsiloxane (PDMS). Replica molding of PDMS is done by using negative photoresist molds on silicon wafers. PDMS is poured over the photoresist mold, cured, and removed to form a PDMS structure containing the negative of the mold, as shown in the last two steps of **Fig. 48.1**. The PDMS can be reversibly or irreversibly bonded to a flat surface to create microchannels or microstructures. Although this technique cannot produce as small of channels as photolithogra-phy, it can produce channels of the micron range with high aspect ratio. Some of the advantages of soft lithography include the low cost of microchip production and the speed of fabrication. Replica microchips can be formed in less than 24 hours from an initial design. However, soft lithography techniques are prone to deformation, defects, and poor reproducibility.

Laser ablation is another popular technique for microchip fabrication. The process involves using laser light to break chemical bonds and eject chemical product from a polymer, glass, ceramic, or metal substrate. It was first devel-oped in 1982 for etching polyethyleneterphthalm (PET) *(13)*. Since then, the technology has been commercialized and is now commercially available from a wide variety of companies. A typical laser ablation system contains a laser light source, optics, and a computer controlled moveable stage. The moveable stage moves the substrate to the area for etching and then the optics focus the laser light on the substrate and can etch channels and structures in a variety of different polymer and nonpolymer substrates.

3. Applications

To develop a micro total analysis system (micro-TAS), an individual chip must include integration of a method for injection of sample, sample preparation, separation, and detection. Very few lab-on-a-chip devices today include the integration of all of these components, but that is the overall goal of miniatur-ized instrumentation. There are a number of methods of sample injection and most methods depend on the type of flow involved in moving the fluid through the chip (microfluidics). For the purpose of this chapter, we will talk about the most popular types of microfluidics: pressure driven flow, electroosmotic flow, centrifugal pumping, and magnetohydrodynamic flow.

The most common pumping mechanism on microchip devices is electroos-motic flow, because it does not require moving components. Electroosmotic flow is flow induced by an electrical voltage being applied across the channel. A common design for microchips using electroosmotic flow is shown in **Fig. 48.2**. The t-shape allows for the electrokinetic injection of the sample. The sample is introduced by applying a high potential (voltage) between the sample reservoir and the sample waste reservoir, while the detection (and possible separation) is performed by applying a potential between the buffer reservoir and the detection reservoir.

Pressure driven flow is popular for flow-injection analysis systems. In a microchip device, pressure drive flow can be introduced by a HPLC pump, syringe pump, micropump, or suction (applying a vacuum to the waste reser-voir.) Centrifugal pumping is not a common type of fluid flow in microchips, but it is used for LabCD type devices (devices that build microchip analysis system for use in a CD drive that will spin the LabCD device and induce a

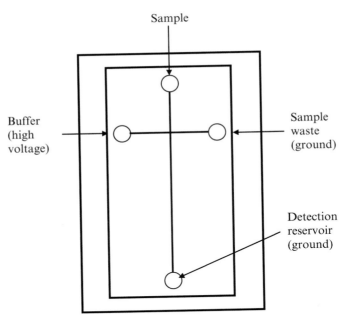

Fig. 48.2. Schematic of a microchip with electrokinetic injection and electroosmotic flow

centrifugal force that will drive the fluid through the analysis channels of the chip). The final flow system is magnetohydrodynamic flow, which is flow that is induced when an AC electrical current is passed across two electrodes in the presence of a magnetic field. This type of flow is rare, but is gaining popularity owing to the fact that it does not require either moving components or a high voltage power supply.

3.1. Electrophoresis

One of the many components that have been miniaturized on lab-on-a-chip devices are separation systems. Early in the development of lab-on-a-chip devices, gas chromatographic columns were miniaturized for lab-on-a-chip devices, but recently there has been more a drive for developing other types of separation systems. One of the most common separation systems to be miniaturized is electrophoresis. Electrophoresis is the separation technique where analytes are separated on the basis of the size and charge, because movement is induced by an electric field gradient. Typically, we consider that there are two types of electrophoresis systems: slab electrophoresis and capillary electrophoresis. However, the capillary electrophoresis system can be mimicked with small microchannels on a glass or polymer chip. Capillary electrophoresis (CE) is easy to tailor to the microchip, because of the easy ability to induce electroosmotic flow in microscale.

Over the last decade, researchers have used microchip-based CE to separate amino acids *(14–16)*, proteins *(17)*, enzyme *(18–20)*, antibodies *(21–23)*, drugs *(24–26)*, neurotransmitters *(27–29)*, DNA *(30–32)*, and many other biomolecules. Some systems require sample preparation depending on the type of sample. This preparation may include filtering or preconcentration.

On-column derivatization is another common component of these microchips, but that depends on the properties of the biomolecule and the detection methods. Frequently, microchip-based CE employs either fluorescence, mass spectrometry (MS) or electrochemical detection. Mass spectrometry is typically done off-chip, so we will not discuss it, but fluorescence detection can be done on-chip. If the analyte is a natural fluorophor, then no derivatization is necessary, otherwise, pre- or postcolumn labeling of the analyte with a fluorophor is needed. The same can be said for electrochemical detection. If the analyte is an electroactive molecule, then no derivatization is necessary, otherwise, pre- or postcolumn derivatization is necessary to produce an electroactive molecule for detection. Electrochemical detection is complicated in an electrophoresis system, because the high separation voltage being applied across the column must be electrically separated from the small amperometric or voltammetric detection voltage being applied to the electrode. Therefore, a decoupler must be used to avoid these electrical interferences. These decouplers can be made of a variety of materials, including polymers, palladium, platinum, etc.

3.2. PCR-on-a-Chip

Polymerase chain reaction is the common technique used today for DNA amplification. It is a thermal cycling three-step process. The three steps include denaturation (30–60 s at 90–96°C) to break the double stranded DNA into single template strands followed by an annealing step (30 s at 55–60°C) that anneals primers to complementary parts of the single template strands, and finally enzyme-catalyzed extension (60 s at 72°C) to synthesis the remainder of the complementary strand. It is a cyclic process, so these steps are repeated over and over until sufficient DNA amplification has occurred. Recently, polymerase chain reaction (PCR) instruments have been miniaturized for lab-on-a-chip devices.

PCR-on-a-chip is becoming a mature technology. PCR microchips have been fabricated from glass and a variety of polymers including: PDMS and polycarbonate. They require much smaller samples than traditional PCR systems. The sample size typically ranges from 1.3 pl to 50 µl. They can also employ traditional polymerase enzymes (like AmpliTaq). Owing to lower thermal mass, faster thermal cycling can be achieved with microchip PCR, so you can actually do 30 cycles in less than 10 min *(33–35)*.

PCR is a common technique in molecular biology to replicate DNA. The amplified DNA can be used for a variety of purposes, but typically is used in lab-on-a-chip devices to increase the concentration of DNA in a sample to increase the sensitivity of the DNA analysis scheme that follows on the chip. Therefore, PCR is typically one of several components on a DNA analysis microchip.

3.3. Sperm Sorter

Portable and disposable microchip devices have been developed to sort motile from nonmotile sperm *(36,37)*. In vitro fertilization is the method commonly used to treat sperm-related infertility, but the sperm must first be sorted to ensure that only high quality are selected to increase the probability of fertilizing oocytes. Macroscale sperm sorting devices include centrifugation, swim-up media techniques, and density gradient separations. Centrifugation has been plagued with problems owing to the fact that the large centrifugal forces can damage the sperm and density gradient separations cause lower DNA integrity after separation *(38)*. Swim-up techniques are less harsh on the sperm, but this bulk technique is not useful for recovering motile sperm from low motility sperm samples or sperm samples that contain large amounts of cellular debris. Therefore, a portable and disposable laminar flow device that separates motile sperm from nonmotile sperm by collecting the sperm that swim from the sperm sample to the media has many advantages, because the gentle procedure ensures the integrity of the sperm while increasing motile sperm purity from 10 to >98% after a single injection into the device *(36,37)*.

3.4. Extraction

Extraction is commonly used for sample preparation to remove contaminants and/or concentrate the analyte. There are two main types of extraction used in microchip devices: liquid phase extraction and solid phase extraction. Liquid phase extraction is done by coating the inside of the transport channel with a species that will interact and concentrate or enrich the sample. This is mostly commonly done by binding organosilanes to glass channels with siloxane chemistry. Solid phase extraction employs the use of solid particles packed in the channel or magnetic particles that can moved to different areas of the microchip. The solid particles could be polymeric or silica, but are typically physically (i.e., with a magnetic field for magnetic particles or with weirs for holding particles in an area of the chip) or chemically (i.e., in a sol-gel matrix) immobilized within the channel and are coated with functional groups to ensure maximum interaction with the analyte. This method is frequently used for DNA purification where a solid support is used for hydrogen bonding-based or electrostatic interaction-based adhesion of DNA to the support structure or by magnetic particles, which are coated with oligonucleotides.

3.5. Cell studies

One of the most interesting areas for microfluidic devices has been for cell culture studies. The microchip devices are ideal for development of small microreactors for monitoring cellular reactions of a single cell to a complete tissue. For instance, mesenchymal stem cells have been cultured on micropatterned PDMS microchip substrates for use in studying cell morphology and alignment in response to substrate surface topography *(39)*. Human connective tissue progenitor cells *(40)*, endothelial cells *(41–43)*, hepatocarcinoma cells *(40)*, cardiac myocytes *(44)*, fungus *(45)*, Escherishia coli *(46)*, and neurons *(11,47)* have also been grown in glass, polydimethylsiloxane, polymethylmethacrylate, and polycarbonate chips. Most microchips require surface coatings before cell culturing. Coatings include collagen, fibernectin, laminin, poly -L-lysine, or gelatin, depending on which coating promotes high cell adhesion for the cell line of interest. Cell culturing on a microchip is primarily performed to allow for the physical or chemical monitoring of the cell or for the study of the effects of surface topography and structure on the growth of the cells.

Researchers have used microchip devices for culturing single cardiac muscle cells to physically monitor contraction of the muscle cell *(48)*. This is a prime example of monitoring of a single cell. However, many researchers have also used cell cultures on microchips to study multiple cells and complete tissues. As examples, researchers have studied the release of neurotransmitters from neurons *(11)*, release of nitric oxide from endothelial cells *(43)*, and uptake of calcium into cells *(49)*.

3.6. Immunoassays and Enzyme Assays

Immunoassays and enzymatic assays have become very popular molecular biology techniques. Immunoassays and enzymatic assays can very easily be performed on a microchip. Many are already performed in a miniaturized environment on a 96-well plate, so it is easy to think about the further miniaturization to a microchip. Most immunoassays and enzymatic assays employ immobilized antibodies and enzymes to simplify the system. Currently, there are immunoassays for a number of proteins (i.e., BSA, Human IgM, ovalbumin, goat IgG, etc.) and enzymatic assays for biomolecules. Competitive immunoassays have been miniaturized to the microchip as well as ELISAs. The same detection schemes typically used for microchip CE are used for immunoassay and enzymatic assay detection (mainly electrochemical and fluorescent detection on-chip and mass spectrometry off-chip).

References

1. Terry SC, Jerman JH, Angell JB (1979) A gas chromatograph air analyzer fabricated on a silicon wafer. IEEE Trans Electron Devices 26:1880–1886
2. Manz A, Miyahara Y, Miura J, Watanabe Y, Miyagi H, Sato K (1990) Sens Actuators. Design of an open-tubular column liquid chromatograph using silicon chip technology. B1:249
3. Zeng Y, Chen H, Pang D, Wang Z, Cheng J (2002) Microchip capillary electrophoresis with electrochemical detection. Anal Chem 74:2441–2445
4. Jacobson SC, Moore AW, Ramsey JM (1995) Fused quartz substrates for microchip electrophoresis. Anal Chem 67:2059–2063
5. Hatch A, Weigl BH, Zebert D, Yager P (1999) Microfluidic approaches to immunoassays. Proc SPIE – Int Soc Opt Eng 3877:169–172
6. Chiem N, Harrison DJ (1997) Microchip-based capillary electrophoresis for immunoassays: analysis of monoclonal antibodies and theophylline. Anal Chem 69:373–378
7. Oleschuk RD, Shultz-Lockyear LL, Ning Y, Harrison DJ (2000) Trapping of bead-based reagents within microfluidic systems: on-chip solid-phase extraction and electrochromatography. Anal Chem 72:585–590
8. Choi JW, Ahn CH, Bhansali S, Henderson HT (2000) A new magnetic bead-based, filterless bioseparator with planar electromagnet surfaces for integrated biodetection systems. Sens Actuators B68:34–39
9. Burns MA, Johnson BM, Brahmasandra SN et al (1998) An integrated nanoliter DNA analysis device. Science 280:1046–1048
10. Kricka LJ, Wilding P (2003) Microchip PCR. Anal Bioanal Chem 277:820–825
11. Li MW, Spence DM, Martin RS (2005) A microchip-based system for immobilizing PC 12 cells and amperometrically detecting catecholamines released after stimulation with calcium. Electroanalysis 17:1171–1180
12. Woodruff GW (2004) Microfluidic channels in polymethylmethacrylate by optimizing aluminum adhesion. Proc Microelect Eng Conf 22:110–113
13. Srinivasan R (1982) Action of far ultraviolet-radiation on poly(ethylene-terphthalate) films – a method for controlled dry etching. Polymer 23:1863, 1864
14. Harrison DJ, Fluri K, Seiler K, Fan Z, Effenhauser CS, Manz A (1993) Micromachining a miniaturized capillary electrophoresis-based chemical analysis system on a chip. Science 261:895–897

15. Jacobson SC, Koutny LB, Hergenroder R, Moore AW, Ramsey JM (1994) Microchip capillary electrophoresis wit an integrated postcolumn reactor. Anal Chem 66:3472–3476

16. Fluri K, Fitzpatrick G, Chiem N, Harrison DJ (1996) Integrated capillary electrophoresis devices with an efficient postcolumn reactor in planar quartz and glass chip. Anal Chem 68:4285–4290

17. Liu Y, Foote RS, Jacobson SC, Ramsey RS, Ramsey JM (2000) Electrophoretic separation of proteins on a microchip with noncovalent, postcolumn labeling. Anal Chem 72:4608–4613

18. Bousse L, Mouradian S, Minalla A, Yee H, Williams K, Dubrow R (2001) Protein sizing on a chip. Anal Chem 73:1207–1212

19. Xue Q, Wainright A, Gangakhedkar S, Gibbons I (2001) Multiplexed enzyme assays in capillary electrophoretic single-use microfluidic devices. Electrophoresis 22:4000–4007

20. Zugal SA, Burke BJ, Regnier FE, Lytle FE (2000) Electrophoretically mediated microanalysis of leucine aminopeptidase using two-photon excited fluorescence detection on a microchip. Anal Chem 72:5731–5735

21. Abad-Villar EM, Tanyanyiwa J, Fernandez-Abedul MT, Costa-Gancia A, Hauser PC (2004) Detection of human immunoglubulin in microchip and conventional capillary electrophoresis with contactless conductivity measurements. Anal Chem 76:1282–1288

22. Cheng SB, Skinner CD, Taylor J, Attiya S, Lee WE, Picelli G, Harrison DJ (2001) Development of a multichannel microfluidic analysis system employing affinity capillary electrophoresis for immunoassays. Anal Chem 73:1472–1479

23. Chiem N, Harrison DJ (1997) Microchip-based capillary electrophoresis for immunoassays: analysis of monoclonal antibodies and theophylline. Anal Chem 69:373–378

24. Wang J, Chatrathi MP, Tian B, Polsky R (2000) Microfabricated electrophoresis chips for simultaneous bioassays of glucose, uric acid, ascorbic acid, and acetominophen. Anal Chem 72:2514–2518

25. Garcia CD, Henry CS (2003) Direct determination of carbohydrates, amino acids, and antibiotics by microchip electrophoresis with pulsed amperometric detection. Anal Chem 75:4778–4783

26. Wicks DA, Li PCH (2004) Separation of fluorescent derivatives of hydroxyl-containing small molecules on a microfluidic chip. Anal Chim Acta 507:107–114

27. Wooley AT, Lao K, Lazer AN, Mathies RA (1998) Capillary electrophoresis chips with integrated electrochemical detection. Anal Chem 70:684–688

28. Lapos JA, Manica DP, Ewing AG (2002) Dual fluorescence and electrochemical detection on an electrophoresis microchip. Anal Chem 74:3348–3353

29. Gawron AJ, Martin RS, Lunte SM (2001) Fabrication and evaluation of a carbon-based dual electrode detector for poly(dimethylsiloxane) electrophoresis chips. Electrophoresis 22:242–248

30. Jacobson SC, Ramsey JM (1996) Integrated microdevice for DNA restriction fragment analysis. Anal Chem 68:720–723

31. Wooley AT, Mathies RA (1994) Ultra-high-speed DNA fragment separations using microfabricated capillary array electrophoresis chips. Proc Natl Acad Sci 91:11,348–11,352

32. Xu F, Jabasini M, Baba Y (2002) DNA separation by microchip electrophoresis using low-viscosity hydroxypropylmethylcellulose-50 solutions enhanced by polyhydroxy compounds. Electrophoresis 23:3608–3614

33. Obeid PJ, Christopoulos TK, Crabtree HJ, Backhouse CJ (2003) Microfabricated device for DNA and RNA amplication by continuous-flow polymerase chain reaction and reverse transcription-polymerase chain reaction with cycle number selection. Anal Chem 75:288–295

34. Rodriguez I, Lesaicherre M, Tie Y (2003) Practical integration of polymerase chain reaction amplification and electrophoretic analysis in microfluidic devices for genetic analysis. Electrophoresis 24:172–178

35. Park N, Kim S, Hahn JH (2003) Cylindrical compact thermal-cycling device for continuous-flow polymerase chain reaction. Anal Chem 75:6029–6033

36. Cho BS, Schuster TG, Zhu X, Chang D, Smith GD, Takayama S (2003) Passively driven integrated microfluidic system for separation of motile sperm. Anal Chem 75:4671–4675

37. Schuster TG, Cho BS, Keller LM, Takayama S, Smith GD (2003) Isolation of motile spermatozoa from semen samples using microfluidics. Reprod Biomed Online 7:75–81

38. Zini A, Finelli A, Phang D (2000) Influence of semen processing technique on human sperm DNA integrity. Urology 6:1081–1084

39. Peterson ETK, Papautsky I (2006) Microtextured polydimethylsiloxane substrates for culturing mesenchymal stem cells. In: Shelley D. Minteer (ed) Methods in molecular biology, Humana Press in Totowa, New Jersey vol. 321, pp 179–197

40. Mata A, Boehm C, Fleischman AJJ, Muschler G, Roy S (2002) Analysis of connective tissue progenitor cell behavior on polydimethylsiloxane smooth and channel microtextures. Biomed Microdevices 4:267–275

41. Borenstein JT, Terai H, King KR, Weinberg EJ, Kaazempur-Mofrad MR, Vacanti JP (2002) Microfabrication technology for vascularized tissue engineering. Biomed Microdevices 4:167–175

42. Gray BL, Lieu DK, Collins SD, Smith RL, Barakat AI (2002) Microchannel platform for the study of endothelial cell shape and function. Biomed Microdevices 4:9–16

43. Spence DM, Torrence NJ, Kovarik ML, Martin RS (2004) Amperometric determination of nitric oxide derived from pulmonary artery endothelial cells immobilized in a microchip channel. Analyst 129:995–1000

44. Kaji H, Nishizawa M, Matsue T (2003) Localized chemical stimulation to micropatterned cells using multiple laminar fluid flows. Labchip 3:208–211

45. Russo AP, Apoga D, Dowell N, Shain W, Turner AMP, Craighead HG, Hoch HC, Turner JN (2002) Microfabricated plastic devices from silicon using soft intermediates. Biomed Microdevices 4:277–283

46. Chang WJ, Akin D, Sedlak M, Ladisch MR, Bashir R (2003) Poly(dimethylsiloxane and silicon hybrid biochip for bacterial culture. Biomed Microdevices 5:281–290

47. Thiebaud P, Lauer L, Knoll W, Offenhausser A (2002) PDMS device for patterned application of microfluids to neuronal cells arranged by microcontact printing. Biosensors and Bioelectronics 17:87–93

48. Li X, Li PCH (2006) Contraction study of a single cardiac muscle cell in a microfluidic chip. In: Shelley D. Minteer (ed) Methods in molecular biology, Humana Press in Totowa, New Jersey vol. 321, pp 199–225

49. Yang M, Li CW, Yang J (2002) Cell docking and on-chip monitoring of cellular reactions with a controlled concentration gradient on a microfluidic device. Anal Chem 74:3991–4001

49

Mammalian Cell Culture

Simon P. Langdon

1. Introduction

Mammalian cell culture is used widely in academic, medical and industrial settings. It has provided a means to study the physiology and biochemistry of the cell and developments in the fields of cell and molecular biology have required the use of reproducible model systems that only cultured cell lines can provide. For medical use, cell culture provides test systems to assess the efficacy and toxicology of potential new drugs. Large-scale mammalian cell culture has allowed production of biologically active proteins, initially production of vaccines and then recombinant proteins and monoclonal antibodies; recent innovative uses of cell culture include tissue engineering to generate tissue substitutes. This chapter will briefly review these areas.

1.1. Developments in Mammalian Cell Culture

The origins of mammalian cell culture began with organ and tissue culture and extend back to 1885 when Wilhelm Roux demonstrated that the medullary plate of a chick embryo could be maintained in saline for several days. For the next few decades, studies focussed on amphibian tissues, as tissue regeneration was feasible. In 1898, the first successful human studies were undertaken with skin being shown to survive in vitro if maintained in ascetic fluid. In 1907, Ross Harrison is credited with being the first to show continued function in vitro and in establishing a general technique of tissue culture *(1)*. His studies demonstrated that not only did tissues from frog embryos survive when explanted into frog lymph clots but also nerve fibres grew from these cells. In 1915, cancer cells were being grown and in 1922, epithelial cells were first cultured. The first continuous rodent cell line was generated in 1943 *(2)* and in 1951 the first human cancer cell line (HeLa) was established *(3)*. This cell line is still widely used today *(4)*.

  In the 1950s, the systematic definition of nutritional components required for cell growth led to the formulation of specialized tissue culture media. The need for vaccine production encouraged rapid progress in the development of

From: *Molecular Biomethods Handbook, 2nd Edition.*
Edited by: J. M. Walker and R. Rapley © Humana Press, Totowa, NJ

mammalian cell culture and the first industrial use arose in the production of a polio vaccine. In the mid 1970's hybridoma technology was developed, as was recombinant DNA technology. Most recently, the derivation of cell culture from organ culture has come full circle with cell culture now being used in tissue engineering to create "neo-organs."

1.2. General Concepts and Terminology

Cell culture refers to the culture of disaggregated cells while organ culture describes the use of nondispersed organs or fragments and both are types of tissue culture. The initial culture removed from the tissue of origin is referred to as the primary culture and when propagated after dilution becomes a secondary culture. The process of dilution and transferring into further containers is termed subculturing or passaging. A culture that continues beyond the primary culture is referred to as a cell line and cell lines may be either continuous and have the ability to undergo indefinite expansion or be finite and generate a limited number of population doublings. The latter undergo senescence unless they undergo transformation.

Cells may grow as adherent cultures or in suspension. Most cell types will adhere to a substrate, e.g., plastic or glass and proliferate as a monolayer whereas suspension cultures do not attach to a substrate and grow within cell culture medium.

2. Methods

2.1. Requirements of Cells in Culture

2.1.1. Substrate

For optimal cell growth and differentiation in culture, most cell types require interaction with a substrate (adherent cultures) but some, e.g., hematopoietic cells do not require this. Traditionally this substrate has been glass (in vitro = in glass) but is now generally a treated plastic. Polystyrene is the most frequently used plastic, though polycarbonate, polytetrafluoroethylene and polyvinyl are also used. The plastics are irradiated or treated with chemicals to produce a charged surface. Cell adhesion can be modified by the use of extracellular components such as collagen, fibronectin, and laminin.

Although monolayer cultures have been the simplest and most convenient mode of culture, more complex models of cells growing in three dimensions within a matrix such as agar can provide improved morphological and biochemical differentiation (5,6).

2.1.2. Media

Many of the synthetic media in use today were developed in the 1950s. The essential components of the basal media are amino acids, carbohydrates, vitamins and salts and to this basal media, serum is generally added. The medium is buffered to produce a stable. pH, ideally pH 7.4 and is maintained at 36–37°C, normally by use of an incubator.

One of the first media to be developed was Eagle's basal medium (BME) (7,8). This contains 13 amino acids, 9 vitamins, 6 inorganic salts, D-glucose, and phenol red (as pH indicator) (see **Table 49.1**). It supports the growth of a wide variety of both normal and cancer cell types. Several variations on this

Table 49.1. Media components.

Amino acids	Inorganic salts	Vitamins	Other
Components in Eagle's basal medium			
Arginine	$CaCl_2$	Biotin	D-Glucose
Cystine	KCl	D-Ca pantothenate	Phenol red
Glutamine	$MgSO_4$	Choline	
Histidine	NaCl	Folic acid	
Isoleucine	$NaHCO_3$	*i*-Inositol	
Leucine	NaH_2PO_4	Nicotinamide	
Lysine		Pyridoxal HCl	
Methionine		Riboflavine	
Phenylalanine		Thiamine HCl	
Threonine			
Tryptophan			
Tyrosine			
Valine			
Additional components added in other media			
Amino acids	Inorganic salts	Vitamins	Other
Alanine	$Fe(NO_3)_3$	Ascorbic acid	HEPES
Asparagine	KH_2PO_4	Biotin	Hypoxanthine
Aspartic acid	$MgCl_2$	Cholesterol	Linoleic acid
Cysteine	Na_2SeO_3	Niacin	Putrescine
Glutamic acid	$CuSO_4$	*p*-aminobenzoic acid	Pyruvate
Glycine	$FeSO_4$	Nicotinic acid	
Hydroxyproline	$ZnSO_4$	Pyridoxine	
Proline	$Ca(NO_3)_2$		
Serine	KNO_3		

medium were then formulated. Increasing the concentrations of individual amino acids gave Eagle's minimum essential medium (MEM) *(8)*. Dulbecco's modified Eagle's medium (DMEM) contained a 4-fold increased concentration of amino acids and vitamins and a 4.5-fold increase in glucose content *(9)*. Iscove's modified Dulbecco medium (IMDM) is a modification of DMEM developed to support hematopoietic precursors and contains additional amino acids and vitamins, sodium pyruvate and HEPES buffer *(10)*.

A medium developed between 1947 and 1949 by Joseph Morgan and Helen Morton, Medium 199, contains many more components than found in Eagle's medium (a total of 60) and was the first synthetic medium produced not requiring animal serum (although long term culture does require serum addition) *(11)*. Although originally developed to study cell nutrition in cancer research it rapidly found use in the early 1950s to help culture the poliovirus in monkey kidney cells. Several other media were initially designed to be used without serum. One of these is CMRL (Connaught Medical Research Institute) 1066, which is a less complex version of Medium 199 *(12)*. Another serum-free medium is Waymouth's medium, initially designed as a total serum-free medium for mouse L929 cells but shown to be useful for other cell lines *(13)*.

Richard Ham designed Ham's nutrient mixtures F10 and F12 for the growth of Chinese Hamster Ovary (CHO) cells, either with or without serum supplementation *(14,15)*. Combination of F12 and DMEM as a 1:1 mix has found broad use in serum-free formulations as this combines the richness of F12 (with its vitamins and trace elements) with the nutrient potency of DMEM. McCoy and colleagues in 1959 described a formulation (McCoy's 5A medium) that supported the growth of many cell types *(16)*. Another medium that is now widely used for many cell types is RPMI (Roswell Park Memorial Institute) 1640 developed by Moore and colleagues *(17)*.

2.1.3. Serum

Although media contain many of the components necessary for growth and differentiation, additional key elements are provided by serum. Important serum components include hormones, growth factors, transport (binding) proteins, enzyme cofactors, lipids, and attachment factors *(18)*. Concentrations of these components will vary from batch to batch and with the age and health status of the animals. Both fetal and newborn calf sera are extensively used but human and equine sera are also occasionally used. The percentage of serum typically added to medium is 5–20%.

2.1.4. Serum-Free Media

There has been a shift towards the use of serum-free media for a number of reasons. Firstly, it is frequently preferable to culture cells with animal-free ingredients to avoid potential contaminants. This has been predominantly to avoid the concerns over animal viruses contaminating cell lines or becoming introduced into recombinant protein or vaccine production. Secondly, because serum varies in its composition between batches and indeed some components are still poorly defined, use of serum-free medium allows for complete definition of the background in which the cells are growing and in which they are being manipulated. Thirdly, certain components of serum are growth-inhibitory.

Although a number of media formulations supported growth for limited periods as described above in some of the complex media, several strategies were undertaken to improve totally defined media. In the 1960s and 1970s, two strategies were successful in producing improved cell growth in defined media. Richard Ham and co-workers increased the concentrations of the components of the basal medium until growth was supported *(14,15)* while Gordon Sato and colleagues identified the key specific supplements required for addition to basal medium *(18,19)*. The essential additives included hormones, binding proteins, lipids, trace elements, and attachment factors.

Ham's studies identified two nutrient mixtures (F10 and F12) that were originally developed to support CHO cells as well as HeLa and murine L-cells. They can be used for both serum-free and serum-containing cultures. The media most frequently selected is then a 1:1 mix of F12 and DMEM although mixes with RPMI 1640 and IMDM are also used. Ham also developed a series of media (MCDB) for the serum-free growth of specific cell types and these were optimized for each cell type, e.g., MCDB 110 for fibroblasts, MCDB 201 for keratinocytes and MCDB 302 for CHO cells *(20)*.

Sato's investigations sought to define the key supplements required to enhance the activity of more basic media. His studies identified insulin, transferrin, and selenium (ITS) and for certain cell types hydrocortisone and epidermal growth factor (HITES). Serum albumin and fibronectin were also key proteins that enhanced growth. Other additives that have been shown to be useful for the growth of certain cell types include estrogen, fibroblast growth factor, glucagons, prostaglandins and triiodothyronine *(18)*.

When cells are transferred from a serum-containing environment to a serum-free medium, it is advisable to reduce the serum percentage gradually to allow adaptation to the new environment. When cells cultures are diluted or transferred to different containers, the trypsin used to detach the cells from plastic is generally inactivated simply by serum addition. In serum-free conditions, trypsin inhibitors can be used. The removal of serum may also cause poorer attachment to the plastic substrate – if this is problematic, then precoating with attachment factors such as collagen or fibronectin can help.

2.2. Primary Cultures

Primary cultures are initial cultures established in vitro from in vivo tissue. The primary tissue may be a tissue explant from which cells can grow or may be broken into single cells or clusters of cells by enzymatic or mechanical procedures. Enzymes routinely used to disaggregate tissue include collagenase and trypsin. Cell suspensions, e.g., blood cell cultures or cultures from peritoneal ascites or pleural effusions are particularly convenient for developing cultures as they already grow as single cells or clusters. Many of the cell types within the initial mix may not readily adhere to the substrate or grow well under the culture conditions and this may lead to the selection of specific cell types within the culture proliferating such that the balance of cells may change with time. The selection process may be advantageous if the desired endpoint is to study the most clonogenic cell type or if cell lines are required. The disadvantage of the selective growth is the loss of heterogeneity and diversity of the culture and the consequent change from the initial cell balance in the tissue of origin to the eventual culture.

Cell cultures should be monitored regularly both macroscopically and microscopically. By eye, the pH indicator color change of the medium provides an indication of the growth of the culture because cell proliferation and metabolism will result in the culture becoming more acidic. Media (plus serum and additives) should be changed regularly to prevent cultures becoming too dense and once they do, they require subculturing.

2.3. Subculture of Cells

When a monolayer culture occupies the complete surface of its container it is said to be confluent and requires subculturing (also referred to as passaging or splitting) to maintain healthy growth. Similarly, a suspension culture that has grown to a point where it has depleted nutrients within the medium requires dilution. The aim is to reduce the cell density to a point where cells will expand optimally again but not so far that they will struggle to survive. Cells are detached from the substrate by proteolytic enzymes such as trypsin that breaks cell–cell and cell–substrate links and allows cells to move into the medium. Once a cell culture is subcultured in this way from a primary to a secondary culture it is referred to as a "cell line."

When cells are subcultured they will generally pass through several well-defined stages of growth. Immediately after trypsinization, monolayer cells will take a period of time to adhere (if a monolayer culture) and repair any damage produced by the proteolytic enzymes. Initial growth is generally relatively slow in this "lag phase." As the culture grows, paracrine interactions will help accelerate growth and an increasing percentage of cells will undergo cell division. This is the most rapid phase – the log phase or exponential phase of growth. As the monolayer fills the substrate area and cells are pushed into close contact with each other (confluency), the growth rate will slow down to a "plateau." In general then, the longer the period of time that cells are in plateau phase, the longer they will stay in the lag phase on subculture.

2.4. Cell Lines

Cell lines provide a renewable source of material for repeat studies. Ideally, cell lines should reflect the properties of their tissue of origin, e.g., reflect genotypic and phenotypic properties and features such as drug sensitivity. Many normal and most cancer cell types can now be cultured. Classic studies in the early 1960s demonstrated that diploid human fibroblasts could undergo only a limited number (circa 50) of divisions in culture before entering crisis and senescence *(21)*. Most cancer cell lines will undergo indefinite numbers of divisions though it is not clear how truly immortal these are. For a cell line to become continuous rather than being finite, either cells must be present at the outset that have the ability to divide indefinitely or cells have to undergo transformation, which can be produced by chemical or viral means. With time in culture, cell lines can become more homogeneous, which is useful with respect to undertaking consistent studies but features such as the ability to differentiate may be lost.

2.5. Cloning

A clone is the population of cells derived from an individual cell and the procedure of isolating this cell and developing its progeny is cloning. The advantage of cloning is to obtain cultures that are genetically homogeneous at the outset. Cells can be cloned on plastic or within a matrix such as agar. The colony forming efficiency (CFE) is a measure of the ability to produce colonies and is the number of colonies produced/number of cells cultured. Although primary cultures have low CFE values (typically <1%), cell lines generally have much higher values typically varying from 10 to 100%.

2.6. Characterization of Cell Lines

With over 3,000 cell lines described in the literature and thousands in regular use, it has become essential to characterize and authenticate cell line models. Characterization is important to relate the cell line model to its tissue of origin and to ensure it appropriately reflects features of the original tissue. Cross-contamination of cell lines has become a major issue and studies conducted through the 1970s and 1980s demonstrated that one in three cell lines were either contaminated or wholly replaced by other cell lines *(22)*. A variety of techniques are now available to characterize cell lines including DNA finger-printing and profiling, cytogenetic analysis, and isoenzyme analysis.

Many cell lines are available through a number of well-recognized banks and collections. These include the American Type Culture Collection (ATCC) (http://www.atcc.org), the European Collection of Animal Cell Cultures (ECACC) (http://www.ecacc.org.uk), the Deutsche Sammlung Von Mikroorganismem Und Zellkulteren GmbH (DSMZ), Corriel Cell Repository (http://locus.umdnj.edu/ccr), Japanese Collection of Research Bioresources (JCRB) (http://cellbank.nibio.go.jp), RIKEN gene bank (www.brc.riken.jp/lab/cell/english/guide.shtml). These are the preferred sources of cell lines because the banks provide guarantees of authentication and freedom from contamination.

2.7. Cryopreservation

Cell stocks can be preserved in long-term storage at temperatures below −130°C for decades if viability is first preserved. This is achieved by the use of cryopreservative agents that prevent ice crystals forming and fragmenting membranes. The most frequently used cryopreservative agent is DMSO (generally at a final concentration of 10%) but glycerol is an alternative. The rates of both freezing and thawing markedly influence viability and a freezing rate of approx 1°C per minute is optimal. Thawing, however, should be rapid and cell ampoules should be warmed at 37°C. It is then vital to wash out the DMSO as quickly as possible. Cells are generally stored in liquid nitrogen tanks at −196°C, but can remain viable for short periods at −80°C.

2.8. Contamination

Two types of cell culture contamination require careful monitoring and continuous vigilance: the contamination of cell cultures with microbial organisms and contamination of one cell line with another. Both types are widely prevalent. The major microbial contaminants are mycoplasma, bacteria, fungi, yeasts, and viruses. In general these are not easy to remove and cultures are best discarded. Unless a laboratory is routinely screening for mycoplasma it is almost inevitable. that all cultures within that laboratory will be infected. Traditionally, mycoplasma has been detected either by Hoescht 33258 (DNA fluorescence) staining or by microbiological culture. PCR methodology now provides a very sensitive, specific, and rapid method. Elimination of mycoplasma from cultures is difficult but possible with certain antibiotics. Bacteria are generally introduced through poor aseptic technique and are frequently first noticed by an increased turbidity or cloudiness in the media, which also becomes rapidly acidic. A number of antibiotics, e.g., penicillin and streptomycin are available to treat cultures though as with most infections the culture is best discarded unless irreplaceable. Fungi are frequent contaminants growing as furry growths in the media. Antimycotics can be used in some instances. Yeast is detected by its small oval appearance budding in short chains and branches. The most difficult infections to detect are viruses and methods of detection include presence of cytopathic effects in susceptible cells, hemadsorption, electron microscopy, and immunofluorescence. More recently, PCR-based techniques have been developed to detect these contaminants.

3. Applications

3.1. Model Systems to Study Cell Biology and Biochemistry

Cell cultures have provided reproducible model systems to study basic features of cell biology and biochemistry and continue to be used extensively in many research laboratories. The main advantage in using cell cultures over the use of intact animals or isolated organs is the ability to control and regulate the cell environment. Functional assays allow study of endpoints such as proliferation, differentiation, and apoptosis and processes such as cell migration and invasion can also be modelled. Cell obtained from many disease types have been cultured and the most extensively studied have been cancer cells. Comparison with normal cells has allowed definition of certain critical features characteristic of cancer cells. Although cell lines can provide often-unlimited quantities of homogeneous populations their limitation can be that they can frequently lose features of differentiation though this can sometimes be modelled by the use of primary cultures.

3.2. Efficacy Testing

Cell lines and primary cultures are used extensively for the testing of novel pharmaceutical agents. For example, the Developmental Therapeutic Program of the US National Cancer Institute (http://dtp.nci.nih.gov/about/irp.html) use a 60 cancer cell line screen for the assessment of novel antitumor agents and this is used to test approx 3,000 new compounds each year (23). The cell line panel encompasses leukemia, melanoma and cancers of the lung, colon, brain, ovary, breast, prostate, and kidney. The screen is used to prioritize for further evaluation, synthetic compounds or natural product samples showing selective growth inhibition or cell killing of particular tumor cell lines. The complexity of a 60-cell line dose response produced by a given compound results in a biological response pattern, which can be analysed in pattern recognition algorithms. Using these algorithms, it is possible to assign a putative mechanism of action to a test compound, or to demonstrate that the response pattern is unique and not similar to that of any of the standard prototype compounds included in the NCI database

3.3. In Vitro Toxicology

In vitro toxicology testing in cell culture is increasingly being used; partially because of high-though put capabilities but also to help reduce in vivo testing. Cell lines, primary cultures and three-D organoid structures are all used.

Primary cultures obtained from human, murine and porcine sources include: epithelial cells (e.g., bladder, cornea, skin, and trachea), endothelial cells (e.g., from aorta, cornea, skin, umbilical cord, and adrenal gland), hematopoietic stem cells, mesenchymal stem cells, hepatocytes, keratinocytes, fibroblasts, and chondrocytes.

Frequently, in vitro systems have been too simple and lacked the necessary complexity required to fully model the intact organism. Other issues have included the problem of de-differentiation in culture. One approach is now to use 3-dimensional systems and even tissue engineering to more appropriately model the in vivo setting. An example of this is the development of a skin model wherein both primary dermal fibroblasts and epidermal keratinocytes are used

(24). These cell types are first isolated from human material and fibroblasts are embedded into a biomatrix to provide a scaffold for the keratinocytes. The keratinocytes then grow over a 3-wk period in a selected growth medium that allows for differentiation into a multiplayer epidermis with stratum basale, spinosum granulosum, and stratum corneum. Applications for the model then include irritation studies, penetration, wound healing studies and biocompatibility tests.

3.4. Industrial Mammalian Cell Culture

Mammalian cell culture has become the primary method for the manufacture of recombinant proteins. The early drive for large-scale mammalian cell culture development was driven by vaccine development in the 1950s. Major epidemics of polio in the 1940s and 1950s spurred on the search to develop a vaccine and when the poliovirus was shown to grow within cultured monkey kidney cells this encouraged development of cell culture systems.

The mid-1970s produced two major technological innovations – recombinant DNA technology and the creation of monoclonal antibodies. The development of recombinant DNA technology in the 1970s led to its use in large-scale production in the 1980s with recombinant insulin being the first true product of modern biotechnology gaining approval in 1982. In parallel, the development of hybridoma technology in 1975 and the ability to produce monoclonal antibodies drove another avenue of biotechnology. Since then, some 165 biopharmaceutical products (recombinant proteins, monoclonal antibodies and nucleic acid-based drugs) have gained approval *(25)* and the market size is estimated at $33 billion and projected to reach $70 billion by the end of the decade *(26–28)*. These products include recombinant hormones and growth factors, blood factors, monoclonal antibody based products, interferons, therapeutic enzymes, and recombinant vaccines. Approximately 100 proteins are licensed in the USA of which 60–70% are produced by mammalian cell culture *(29,30)* (see **Table 49.2**). The mammalian cell lines most widely used to express recombinant proteins include CHO cells, mouse myeloma NSO cells, baby hamster kidney (BHK) cells, human embryo kidney (HEK-293) cells, and C127 cells. Monoclonal antibodies are produced either by hybridoma cells, or as recombinant proteins in cell lines such as CHO cells.

Although mammalian cell culture is more complex, more expensive and slower than *Escherichia coli* or insect or plant cell culture, its ability to produce post-translational protein modifications is frequently an essential requirement for precise cell functionality *(28)*. Microbial cells are easier and cheaper to manipulate than mammalian cells and so have become the method of choice for peptides such as insulin and human growth hormone. However, mammalian cells are uniquely equipped to perform certain processes and have been particularly valuable for the manufacture of large complex proteins where post-translational modifications are required, in particular glycosylation. Both *O*-linked and x-linked glycosylation can influence protein stability, ligand binding, immunogenicity, and serum half-life and these properties are significant for both the efficacy and safety of a wide range of pharmaceuticals including antibodies, blood factors, and some hormones and cytokines.

The productivity of recombinant cell lines has improved dramatically over the last two decades *(29)*. Typically product titres of protein have risen from values of 50 mg/L to 5 g/L. This has been the result of improvements in host

Table 49.2. Examples of biopharmaceuticals produced by mammalian cell culture.

Product type	Product	Cell type	Application
Recombinant blood factors:			
Factor VIII	Helixate Nexgen	BHK	Hemophilia A
	ReFacto	CHO	Hemophilia A
	Kogenate	BHK	Hemophilia A
	Bioclate	CHO	Hemophilia A
Factor VIIa	Novoseven	BHK	Hemophilia
Factor IX	Benefix	CHO	Hemophilia B
Tissue plasminogen	Tenecteplase	CHO	M.I.
Activator	Activase	CHO	Acute M.I.
Recombinant hormones:			
Follicle-stimulating	Follistim	CHO	Infertility
Hormone	Puregon	CHO	Anovulation
	Gonal F	CHO	Anovulation
rHCG	Ovitrelle	CHO	Reproduction
rThyrotrophin-α	Thyrogen	CHO	Thyroid cancer
rLuteinizing hormone	Luveris	CHO	Infertility
Erythropoietin	Aranesp	CHO	Anemia
	Nespo	CHO	Anemia
	Neorecormon	CHO	Anemia
Interferon-β	Rebif	CHO	Multiple sclerosis
	Avonex	CHO	Multiple sclerosis
Monoclonal antibodies:			
Anti-IgE	Xolair	CHO	Asthma
Anti-CD20	Zevalin	CHO	N.H.L.
Others:			
rh α-galactosidase	Fabrazyme	CHO	Fabry disease

M.I. = myocardial infarction, N.H.L. = non Hodgkin lymphoma.

cells, vectors, media and process development. Useful host cell lines require the combination of both rapid growth and high productivity. Both adherent and suspension cultures are used. Adherent cells can either be used in roller bottles that are rotated or can be grown on microcarriers that are cultured in suspension. Use of appropriate media can help adherent cells to grow in suspension. Media have been developed that are free of animal products and have been optimized for the different variants of the CHO cell line

3.5. Cells for Replacement Tissues and Organs

Tissue engineering is a rapidly evolving new discipline that aims to develop biological substitutes to help replace damaged or diseased tissues and organs. Because few prosthetics are as good as the tissue they replace, extensive research effort is evaluating the use of the patient's own cells to generate new tissue. Current examples include: artificial skin, cells for nerve regeneration, bone graft substitutes, cartilage regeneration, and engineered tendons and ligaments. Hepatocytes, pancreatic, and blood cell types are also frequently used

A number of challenges are currently being addressed in this endeavor. Reliable and abundant sources of cells are required and the optimal methods to promote both cell and tissue production are needed. Cell culture is being used to produce the very large number of cells required, e.g., $1\,cm^3$ of bone will contain 150,000,000 cells. Stem cells (both embryonic and adult) offer the most promise to generate the large number of cells required and to have the greatest proliferative potential in vitro. Extensive research effort is currently focussing on the optimization of growth and differentiation conditions for these cultures. Further challenges include how best to regulate cell behavior and function on synthetic scaffolds and then how to maximize the mechanical and functional properties of the resulting tissues.

3.6. Gene Therapy

The development of the ability to genetically engineer cells has led to the ex vivo manipulation of cells in culture and subsequent reintroduction back into patients. Somatic cell therapy is the administration to humans of autologous, allogeneic, or xenogeneic living cells that have been manipulated or processed ex vivo. The genetic manipulation may be designed to have a therapeutic or prophylactic effect or may provide a way of marking cells for later identification. The first approved gene therapy procedure was performed in 1990 on a 4-year old with severe combined immunodeficiency (SCID) and involved removal of white blood cells, insertion of the missing gene within cell culture and infusion of the genetically modified cells back into the bloodstream (Fig. 49.1). This was successful and has led the way to further studies of ex-vivo manipulation of other genes. Some success has now been achieved not only with the treatment of lymphoid diseases but also myeloid immunodeficiencies *(31)*.

As for the development of recombinant proteins and vaccines described above, there is a strong move to the use of serum-free media to prevent the possibility of contamination by animal-derived materials being introduced into the process.

In conclusion, mammalian cell culture is use routinely in both small-scale and large-scale operations and continues to be one of the major tools of the life sciences.

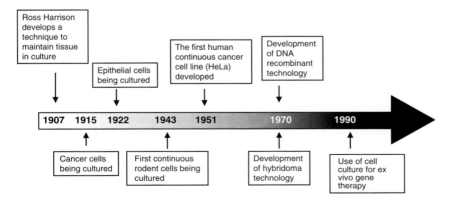

Fig. 49.1. Milestones in mammalian cell culture

References

1. Harrison RG (1907) Observations on the living developing nerve fiber. Proc Soc Exp Biol Med 4:140–143
2. Earle WR, Schilling EL, Stark TH, Straus NP, Brown MF, Shelton E (1943) Production of malignancy in vitro IV. The mouse fibroblast cultures and changes seen in the living cells. J Natl Cancer Inst 4:165–212
3. Gey GO, Coffman WD, Kubicek MT (1952) Tissue culture studies of the proliferative capacity of cervical carcinoma and normal epithelium. Cancer Res 12:364–365
4. Masters JR (2002) HeLa cells 50 years on: the good, the bad and the ugly. Nature Rev 2:315–318
5. Weaver VM, Fischer AH, Peterson OW, Bissel MJ (1996) The importance of the microenvironment in breast cancer progression: recapitulation of mammary tumorigenesis using a unique human mammary epithelial cell model and a three-dimensional culture assay. Biochem Cell Biol 74:833–851
6. Weaver VM, Bissel MJ (1999) Functional culture models to study mechanisms governing apoptosis in normal and malignant mammary epithelial cells. J Mammary Gland Biol Neopl 4:193–201
7. Eagle H (1955) Amino acid metabolism in mammalian cultures. Science 130:432–437
8. Eagle H (1955) Nutrition needs of mammalian cells in culture. Science 122:501
9. Dulbecco R, Freeman G (1959) Plaque formation by polyoma virus Virology 8:396–397
10. Iscove NN, Guilbert LW, Weyman C (1980) Complete replacement of serum in primary culture of erythropoietin-dependent red cell precursors (CFU-E) by albumin, transferring, iron, unsaturated fatty acid, lecithin and cholesterol. Exp Cell Res 126:121–126
11. Morgan JF, Morton HJ, Parker RC (1950) The nutrition of animal cells in tissue culture. Initial studies on a synthetic medium. Proc Soc Exp Biol Med 73:1–8
12. Parker RC (1957) Altered cell strains in continuous culture: a general survey. In: Whitelock O (ed) Special Publications of the New York Academy of Sciences: 5, NY Acad Sci., New York, pp 303–313
13. Waymouth C (1959) Proliferation of sublines of NCTC clone 929 (strain L0 mouse cells in a simple chemically defined medium (MB752/1). J Natl Cancer Inst 22:1003
14. Ham RG (1963) An improved nutrient solution for diploid Chinese hamster and human cell lines. Exp Cell Res 29:515–526
15. Ham RG (1965) Clonal growth of mammalian cells in a chemically defined, synthetic medium. Proc Natl Acad Sci USA 53:288–293
16. McCoy TA, Maxwell M, Kruse PF (1959) Amino acid requirements of the Novikoff hepatoma in vitro. Proc Soc Exp Biol Med 100:115–118
17. Moore GE, Gerner RE, Franklin HA (1967) Culture of normal human leukocytes. JAMA 199:519–524
18. Barnes D, Sato G (1980) Serum-free culture: a unifying approach. Cell 22:649–655
19. Barnes D, Sato G (1980) Methods for growth of cultured cells in serum-free medium. Anal Biochem 102:519–524
20. Ham RG, McKeehan WL (1978) Development of improved media and culture conditions for clonal growth of normal diploid cells. In vitro 14:11–22
21. Hayflick L, Moorhead PS (1961) The serial cultivation of human diploid cell strains. Exp Cell Res 25:585–621
22. Nelson-Rees WA, Daniels DW, Flandermeyer RR (1981) Cross-contamination of cells in culture. Science 212:446–452
23. Boyd MR, Paull KD (1995) Some practical considerations and applications of the National Cancer Institute In Vitro Drug Discovery Screen. Drug Development Research 34:91–109

24. Dieterich C, Schandar M, Noll M, Johannes F, Brunner H, Graeve T, Rupp (2002) In vitro reconstructed human epithelia reveal contributions of *Candida albicans EFG1* and *CPH1* to adhesion and invasion. Microbiology 148:497–506
25. Lawrence S (2005) Biotech drug market steadily expands. Nature Biotechnol 23:1466
26. Pavlou A, Belsy M (2005) The therapeutic antibody market to 2008. Eur J Pharm Biopharm 59:389–396
27. Pavlou A, Reichert J (2004) Recombinant protein therapeutics – success rates, market trends and values to 2010. Nature Biotechnol 22:1513–1519
28. Wurm FW (2004) Production of recombinant protein therapeutics in cultivated mammalian cells. Nature Biotech 22:1393–1398
29. Walsh G (2006) Biopharmaceutical benchmarks 2006. Nature Biotechnol 24:769–776
30. Walsh G (2003) Biopharmaceutical benchmarks 2003. Nature Biotechnol 21:865–870
31. Ott MG, Schmidt M, Schwarzaelder K, Stein S, Siler U, Koehl U (2006) Correction of X-linked chronic granulomatous disease by gene therapy, augmented by insertional activation of MDS1-EVI1, PRDM16 or SETBP1. Nature Med 12:401–409

50

Plant Tissue Culture

Víctor M. Loyola-Vargas, C. De-la-Peña,
R. M. Galaz-Ávalos, and F. R. Quiroz-Figueroa

1. Introduction

Plant tissue culture (PTC) is a set of techniques for the aseptic culture of cells, tissues, organs and their components under defined physical and chemical conditions in vitro and controlled environment (**Fig. 50.1**). PTC technology also explores conditions that promote cell division and genetic re-programming in in vitro conditions and it is considered an important tool in both basic and applied studies, as well as in commercial application *(1)*.

Today, facilities for in vitro cell cultures are found in practically each plant biology laboratory, serving different purposes because tissue culture has turned into a basic asset for modern biotechnology, from the fundamental biochemical aspects to the massive propagation of selected individuals. Today five major areas, where in vitro cell cultures are being currently applied, can be recognized: as a model system for fundamental plant cell physiology aspects, generation of genetic modified fertile individuals, large-scale propagation of elite materials, preservation of endangered species, and metabolic engineering of fine chemicals.

1.1. History of PTC's Development

The theoretical basis for plant tissue culture was proposed by Gottlieb Haberlandt in 1902 *(2,3)*. He predicted that eventually a complete and functional plant could be regenerated from a single cell. Other studies led to the culture of isolated root tips *(4,5)*. The approach of using explants with meristematic cells produce the successful and indefinite culture of tomato root tips *(6)*. The firsts true PTC were obtained by Gautheret *(7)* from cambial tissue of *Acer pseudoplatanus*. Several years later White *(8)* obtained tumor tissue from a *Nicotiana × N. langsdorffii* hybrid and Nobécourt *(9)* and Guatheret *(10)* produced callus from carrot root tips.

During the following years, the culture of young embryos *(11)* and the formation of meristems from callus tissues *(12)* were achieved. The discovery of the first cytokinin (kinetin) *(13)* led to the recognition that the exogenous balance of both auxin and kinetin in the medium influenced the morphogenic

From: *Molecular Biomethods Handbook, 2nd Edition.*
Edited by: J. M. Walker and R. Rapley © Humana Press, Totowa, NJ

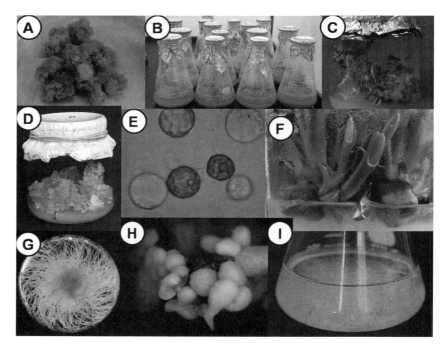

Fig. 50.1. A. Callus from *Catharanthus roseus*. **B.** Suspension culture from *C. roseus*. **C.** Regeneration of plantlets from *C. roseus* callus. **D.** Tumors from *C. roseus*. **E.** Protoplasts from *C. roseus*. **F.** Micropropagation of *Agave tequilana*. **G.** Hairy roots from *C. roseus*. **H.** Somatic embryogenesis of *Coffea canephora*. **I.** Root culture from *C. roseus*. Pictures **A–E, G–I** from the authors' laboratories. Picture **F** from the laboratory of Dr. Manuel Robert all of them at Centro de Investigación Científica de Yucatán

fate of callus *(14)*. A relative high level of auxin to kinetin favored rooting, the reverse led to shoot formation and intermediate levels to the proliferation of callus or wound parenchyma tissue. Several independent groups reported the formation of bipolar somatic embryos *(15–17)*. The first demonstration of the plant cells' totipotency was carried out by Vasil and Hildebrandt using tobacco cells *(18)*. This was followed later by the regeneration of plants from protoplasts *(19)* and the regeneration of the first interspecific hybrid plants (*Nicotiana glauca* × *N. langsdorffii*) *(20)* after Cocking had developed the use of fungal hydrolytic enzymes for the production of protoplasts *(21)*. More recently, the establishment of commercial cultures for the production of secondary metabolites *(22,23)* and the generation of transgenic plants from transformed callus or somatic embryos *(24,25)* has opened the field to major basic and commercial applications *(26–28)*.

1.2. Tissue Culture Media

The nutrition of PTC requires a culture medium. This is formed by both inorganic salts and organic compounds in addition to a carbon source and plant growth regulators *(29)*. Most of our knowledge about the nutrition of plant cultures comes from the solutions done for the hydroponic system of complete plants. In general, the tissue culture medium must contain the essential elements for plant growth *(30)*. The addition of "complexes" such as green tomato extract, coconut milk, orange juice, casein hydrolysate, yeast, and malt extract, to the basic medium frequently resulted in successful growth of the tissues and organs *(30)*.

The success in the application of PTC is profoundly influenced by the nature of the culture medium used. The most important difference among media may be the overall salt level, mainly the amount and quality of the nitrogen source *(31–33)*. It is very important when a medium is chosen, to take into account that some of the culture media's components are not only nutrients, but some of them can have a very deep influence either in the growth of the cultures, or in the differentiation process *(34,35)*. There are several media already published, the choice of one of them will depend on the goal to be reached.

The Murashige and Skoog medium *(31)* is currently the most widely used medium; however, this medium has a high content of nitrogen, as well as a high nitrate/ammonium ratio. Other media reported have less total nitrogen and lower nitrate/ammonium ratio *(32,33,36)*. The Kao and Michayluk medium *(37)* is one of the more complex among all media used in plant tissue culture. It is used mainly for the growth of very low cell density cultures, as well as protoplasts in liquid media.

2. Basic Aspects

2.1. Types of Cell Cultures

PTC includes a set of different techniques to manipulate cells. Among the different PTC that can be obtained are callus, suspension cultures, protoplasts, anther and ovule cultures, somatic embryos, and meristem culture *(30,38–42)*. Depending on particular species employed and the kind of response that is desired, almost every part of a plant can be used as starting material (explant). Among the type of explants frequently used there are leaf portions, isolated meristems, hypocotyls, or root segments among others. For the initiation of the culture three important considerations should be taken into account: a) explant selection, b) election of a suitable culture medium and appropriate environmental conditions for its development, and c) the isolation and maintenance of callus for subsequent experimentation.

2.1.1. Callus

As a first step in many tissue culture experiments, it is necessary to induce callus formation from the primary explant (**Fig. 50.1A**). This explant may be an aseptically germinated seedling of surface-sterilized roots, stem, leaves, or reproductive structures. In the context of PTC, callus is a largely unorganized, proliferating mass of parenchyma cells *(43)* that in a wounded tissue is produced in response to injury *(44)*. Calluses are slow growing, small, and convenient to handle, and hence are a useful means of maintaining and storing germplasm *(45)*. The growth rate and friability of callus produced can vary widely between explants and even within replicates of the same medium *(41)*. This heterogeneity is seen in established calluses as differences in color, morphology, structure, growth, and metabolism. Even an apparently uniform callus may contain cells of different ploidy and metabolic capability *(45)*. Not all cells in an explant contribute to the formation of callus and, more importantly, certain callus cell types are competent to regenerate organized structures. Other callus cell types do not appear to be competent to express totipotency. Early visual selection is usually necessary to select for the cefll type that is regenerable *(44)*. The level of plant growth regulators is a major factor that controls callus formation in the culture medium. Culture conditions (temperature, type of jellification agent, light, etc.) are also important in callus formation and development. A wide variety of media compositions have been used with success to induce calluses. These can be maintained on agar, agarose, gelrite, or any other jellification agent. The formation of callus with an explant marks the beginning of successful PTC, and may be used for a variety of experiments *(43,44)*.

2.1.2. Suspension Cultures

A cell suspension culture could be defined as a rapidly dividing, homogeneous suspension of cells *(46)* (**Fig. 50.1B**). These cultures can be used in biochemical and cell physiology research as well as for the study of growth, metabolism, molecular biology, and genetic engineering experiments. Also cell suspension cultures can be used for medium or large scale secondary metabolites and other fine-chemical production.

There is not a standard method to produce a suitable suspension culture. However, in most of the cases the transference of friable callus to a liquid media, such as Murashige and Skoog *(31)* or Gamborg media *(32)* under agitation during incubation (50–200 rpm), can produce the dispersion of the cells, after several passages. Suspension cultures should ideally consist of single cells, but this is rarely the case and usually small aggregates of 20–100 cells (100–1,000 µm) are found. The suspension cultures grow faster than callus cultures and they are more homogenous; however, the rate of variability also increases producing variability and instability of the cultures. To avoid the problem of instability, the cultures are subcultured when the cells are at the end of the exponential growth phase.

2.1.3. Organ Culture

In addition to callus and suspension cultures, organ culture also has been established. In 1934 Phillip White, one of the pioneers of PTC, developed the first system that allowed indefinite proliferation of roots tips *(6)*. Since then, root cultures became a standard system in studies of inorganic nutrition, nitrogen metabolism, plant growth regulation, and root development *(47)*.

Around 20 years ago, the need for cell organization for the biosynthesis of secondary metabolites in PTC was recognized to be fundamental *(48)*, and encouraged the development of better organ culture systems.

Recent progress on growing roots in isolation has greatly facilitated the study of root-specific metabolism and contributed to our understanding for this remarkable plant organ and showed that they are able to produce the same profiles of natural products as their counterpart in the whole plant *(49–52)*. Root cultures can be established by cultivating roots isolated from aseptic plant cultivate in vitro (**Fig. 50.1I**). One disadvantage of the roots culture is their slow growth under in vitro conditions. To avoid this problem, Flores and Filner *(53,54)* developed a system that involves the generation of fast growing adventitious roots or hairy roots, which are the product of the infection of different tissues with *Agrobacterium rhizogenes* (**Fig. 50.1G**). These hairy root cultures have the same metabolic features as normal root cultures and they produce valuable fine chemicals such as tropane and indole alkaloids among others *(55)*. On the other hand, shoot cultures also have been established. These cultures can be used to produce natural products in which biosynthetic pathway is located in the aerial part of the plant *(56–59)*.

Root and shoot cultures have emerged as powerful tools to study the biochemistry and molecular biology of secondary metabolite biosynthetic pathways. The expression of the metabolic pathway can be regulated manipulating the environmental and nutrimental conditions of the cultures. This manipulation also lets the control of the developmental stage of the cultures. Flores and Filner *(54)* were capable to demonstrate that *Hyosciamus muticus* hairy roots are able to synthesize hyoscyamine at levels equal to or greater than the roots *in planta*. The biosynthetic capacity of hairy root cultures was strictly correlated with a differentiated state; hairy root cultures that were dedifferentiated to callus lost their capability to produce hyoscyamine. When these callus were differentiated back to hairy roots, synthesis of hyoscyamine returned *(54)*. This was the first practical demonstration of the differentiation's role in the expression of secondary metabolic pathways.

2.1.4. Protoplasts

Several of the genetic manipulation techniques, such as the induction of somaclonal variation, somatic hybridization, and transformation, require the use of protoplasts. Protoplasts are a powerful tool to study diverse aspects of development, physiology, and genetics of plant cells *(60)*. Furthermore, protoplasts are basically plant cells without the cell wall (**Fig. 50.1E**). The removal of the cell wall makes it necessary to include osmotic stabilizers into the medium and additional nutritional ingredients to preserve the protoplast and ensure their viability *(41)*. Although almost any explant of most plant species can be used as a source of protoplasts, and procedures are available to isolate and culture protoplasts from monocotyledons and dicotyledons, the ability to isolate protoplasts capable of sustained division and plant regeneration is still restricted to a limited number of species/plant combinations. Among the different parameters that can influence the isolation and culture of protoplasts are the origin of the explant, culture medium, the osmoticum, duration of enzyme incubation, pH of the enzyme solution, and environmental culture conditions. An emphasis must be made on the influence of tissue physiology to the release of viable protoplasts. Embryogenic cell suspensions have been the preferred source of viable protoplasts in some cultivars such as coffee *(61,62)*, sugarcane *(63)*, alfalfa *(64)* mango *(65)*, and wheat *(65,66)*, among others.

The isolation of protoplast using natural plant cell wall enzymatic degradation activity had lead to multiple applications. Recently, Phillip Benfel and his group *(67,68)* used this technique to locate the tissue-specific gene expression in different roots zones. They used five separate transgenic lines expressing the green fluorescent protein (GFP) in stele, endodermis, endodermis plus cortex, epidermal atrichoblast cells, and lateral root cap. After harvesting and protoplasting the root tissue, the protoplasts expressing the GFP were isolated on a fluorescence-activated cell sorter and their mRNA was analyzed with the use of microarrays. This is an elegant method to isolate tissue specific mRNA.

Protoplasts can be fused allowing us to cross natural barriers to produce desirable plant traits that are not possible by sexual means. However, the protoplast fusion is a nonspecific process that can be mediated either by chemicals or by electrical techniques. After the fusion, the heterokaryots (they contain the nuclei of the two parents in a mixed cytoplasm) are isolated and developed into hybrid cells *(69)*. These hybrid cells are characterized and developed into somatic hybrid plants.

2.2. Morphogenesis

Since the first confirmation of Haberlandt's theory *(18)* great effort has been made to understanding the molecular mechanism involved in the stimulation of morphogenesis (from the Greek *morphê* shape and *genesis* creation).

Morphogenesis can be obtained in in vitro plant tissue culture by using synthetic medium supplemented with plant growth regulators among others. However, this "genesis" can also be observed in nature *(70,71)*. The morphogenesis in vitro can go through two different pathways and they are classified as somatic embryogenesis (**Fig. 50.1C**) and organogenesis (**Fig. 50.1H**), the latter can develop organs such as flowers, shoots, and roots. Both somatic embryogenesis and organogenesis can take place either directly or indirectly; direct or adventitious organogenesis often refers when there is not a callus intermediate stage; by contrast when there is a profusely proliferation of callus, before organ formation, it is called indirect or *de novo* organogenesis *(72,73)*.

The main factors involve in the stimulation of both embryogenesis or organogenesis and the kind (direct or indirect) of morphogenesis depend on the nature, concentration, and exposure time of the phytohormones employed, status of endogenous phytohormones, the source and physiological state (the ability to respond) of the explant, the medium of culture, and the culture condition used. The interaction between these factors produces the induction and expression of a specific mode of cell differentiation and development *(74)*.

During morphogenesis' induction three hypothetic phases are recognizable for direct morphogenesis and four for indirect on temporal response caused by the balance of exogenous/endogenous phytohormones (**Fig. 50.2**). In the first phase, the cell can take one of two routes described before. If the cell goes by the direct way, it will change its genetic program to acquire the competence status before it will become a determined cell. In contrast, the cell will pass through a proliferative stage before it gains a competence status. Both routes direct and indirect are a consequence of the response to the physiological status of the explant and hormonal signals. In the second part, the competence cell will get the determined status as a response to influence of phytohormone balance. Afterward, during transition from determined phase into morphogenesis, the cell proceeds independently of the hormonal influence *(75)*. In general, the somatic embryogenesis pathway depends on high concentration of auxin to pass from somatic to determined stage (from 0 to II), whereas organogenesis

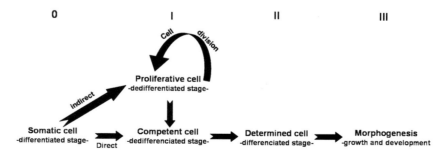

Fig. 50.2. Hypothetic phases of morphogenetic induction from somatic cell to organ or somatic embryo. The numbers represent the morphogetic phases. Adapted from Sugiyama *(75)*

pathway is developed mainly by a high ration of cytokinin:auxin, the species that can be easily regenerated using organogenesis are difficult to regenerate through somatic embryogenesis or vice versa (76). Recently, several genes involved in plant morphogenesis have been discovered (72,76,77).

2.3. Micropropagation

The most widely used commercial application for micropropagation is the vegetative propagation of plants, mainly ornamentals (**Fig. 50.1F**) (30,78–82), and medicinal plants (83). There are three ways by which micropropagation can be achieved; these are enhancing axillary bud breaking, production of adventitious buds directly or indirectly via callus, and somatic embryogenesis directly or indirectly on explants (84,85). The disadvantage of the axillary bud breaking method is that it produces the smallest number of plantlets; however, they are generally genetically true-to-type. On the other hand, somatic embryogenesis is able to produce the greatest number of plantlets, but it is induced in the lowest number of plant species.

Micropropagation protocols are aimed to the rapid multiplication of plantlets true-to-type to the original material. Meristematic tissues, located either on terminal or axillary buds, are induced to proliferate in response to hormonal treatments. Hypocotyls are also frequently used as the original explant. Culture conditions, mainly nitrogen source, light regime, temperature, and the container's atmosphere can play critical roles in favoring bud development into vitroplants (86–90).

Most micropropagation processes are carried out in small culture vessels containing a culture medium solidified with a gelling agent to create a substrate on which the plant tissues are cultured. In spite of its general use, this method has some disadvantages: the culture conditions are heterogeneous because not all the tissues are in contact with the nutrient medium, different media compositions and growth regulator concentrations are required for each stage of the micropropagation process, which implies that tissues or plants need to be continuously transferred to new containers with fresh medium. The multiplication stage also requires frequent transfers as the biomass increases and fills the culture vessels. Consequently, micropropagation is a labor intensive method that greatly increases the production costs of plants produced in vitro and it is only economically viable on a commercial scale in the case of high value-added species (91).

To simplify the whole process, reducing production costs and making micropropagation available to a larger number of species is necessary to develop simpler and cheaper methods, which can decrease the amount of labor. A first step in this direction was the design of semiautomated bioreactors to culture the plants in liquid media (92). A method that combines the advantages of both semisolid and liquid culture media is the temporary immersion system designed by Teisson and collaborators (93). This system alternates short periods of total immersion in liquid medium with longer ones of complete aeration. Satisfactory results for the propagation of various species have been reported using two bioreactors based on this principle (93–97). A new type of bioreactor for micropropagation has been proposed by Robert et al (92). This device has a number of features specifically designed to simplify its operation and reduce production costs.

2.4. Somatic Embryogenesis

Somatic embryogenesis refers to the process by which somatic cells under induction conditions, generate embryogenic cells, which undergo a series of morphological and biochemical changes resulting in the formation of somatic embryos, which could develop into a plant (**Fig. 50.1H**) *(98–100)*. Somatic embryogenesis forms the basis of cellular totipotency that is unique to higher plants. Differing from their zygotic counterpart, somatic embryos are easily tractable, culture conditions can be controlled, and lack of material is not a limiting factor for experimentation *(101)*. These characteristics have made somatic embryogenesis a model for the study of morphological, physiological, molecular, and biochemical events that occur during the onset and development of embryogenesis in higher plants. It also has potentially rich biotechnological applications such as artificial seeds, micropropagation, transgenic plants, etc. *(73)*. Tissue culture systems have been one of the most useful experimental tools used to understand morphogenesis programs.

The somatic embryo resembles the zygotic embryo in various aspects *(102,103)* and it is possible to study diverse subjects related to the embryogenesis process using the somatic embryo system. Nonetheless, other topics cannot be studied, including the moment of fertilization, the differentiation of the endosperm, the absorption of nutrients by the endosperm and its interaction with the embryo, the effect of the mother tissue on embryo's development, the embryo's desiccation, and the embryo's dormancy *(73)*.

Another "type" of embryogenesis can be obtained from diverse sources, different of somatic embryos; e.g., apomictic embryos are derived from an unfertilized egg cell or from maternal tissue *(104)*. It is also possible to obtain in vitro "androgenic" embryos from microspores and pollen grains *(105,106)*. Although somatic embryos are originated from somatic cells *(98,105,107)*, in nature, foliar embryos are observed in several species such as *Bryophyllum calycinum (71)*, or *Camptosorus rhizophyllus (70)*.

The first report to address somatic embryogenesis came in the late 1950s, in cultures of *D. carota (16,17)* and *Oenanthe aquatica (15,108)*. Since then somatic embryos have been obtained in many other plant species *(109)* even though the carrot has been the most widely used model, mainly owing to its feasibility, fast response, and high yields. Somatic embryos from dicots pass through characteristic morphological stages, which are: globular-shaped, oblong-shaped, heart-shaped, enlarged, torpedo-shaped and cotyledonal *(110–113)*.

The basic procedure for producing somatic embryo involves the use of a synthetic medium culture supplemented with plant growth regulators, such as auxin, e.g., 2,4-dichlorophenoxy acetic (2,4-D), cytokinin e.g., kinetin (Kin), abscisic acid (ABA), or combination of two or several growth regulators. In the case of carrot somatic embryogenesis, the tissue initially requires an auxin and later the cells must be transferred into a culture medium with low concentration of auxin or without it.

Components of culture media and growth regulators such as 2,4-D are not the only factors controlling somatic embryogenesis *(80,81)*. It has been demonstrated that other stimuli also induce somatic embryogenesis. For example, stress, including osmotic shock with sucrose or sodium chloride *(114–119)* or the presence of heavy metals—cobalt, nickel, zinc, and cadmium—*(115,120)*, and nutrient starvation *(121,122)*. Other compounds widely used to enhance embryo formation include salicylates (SA) *(123–125)*. It may be happen via inhibition of the ethylene biosynthesis *(123,126–128)*. By contrast, in *Coffea canephora* ethylene is necessary for the induction of somatic embryogenesis *(129)*.

The exogenous application of H_2O_2 enhances its endogenous levels and promotes somatic embryogenesis *(130)* even though Luo et al *(131)* using *Astragalus adsurgens* determined that the endogenous increment in H_2O_2 levels, caused by the exogenous application of SA, was critical to enhancing embryo production.

All data referred above suggest a possible connection or an overlapping between embryogenesis and stress response pathways *(73,103,132,133)*. It has been proposed that the physiological response to stress conditions could depend on two main factors, the physiological state of the cells and the level (time and intensity) of stress condition *(134)*. When the stress level exceeds cellular tolerance, the cells will die, but if there is low levels of stress, the cells could induce mechanisms of adaptation *(134)*. The relationship between different stress conditions and embryogenesis is still not understood, but Lee et al. *(122)* have suggested that undifferentiated cell proliferation could be inhibited and, as a consequence, the embryo production would be stimulated; most likely, the cell is driven into the G_0 stage for its differentiation *(73)*. Indeed, we still do not know the mechanism by which the embryo formation is induced, but the study of such mechanisms may light the understanding of the signalization processes involved in it *(73)*.

Low molecular mass compounds secreted into culture medium can inhibit *(135,136)* or stimulate *(137,138)* somatic embryogenesis. The carrot somatic embryogenesis does not proceed at a high cell density *(139,140)*, it is not due to nutrient uptake or mechanical injury caused by shearing, but factor(s) responsible for the inhibitory effect were found in the culture medium and their molecular masses were estimated under 3.5 kDa *(135)*.

Two factors have been purified and identified, the first was an alcohol, 4-hydroxybenzyl alcohol *(141)* and the other was vanillyl benzyl ether *(136)*. On the contrary to the inhibitors, one peptide growth factor has been identified that is involved on induction of somatic embryogenesis; it is called α-phytosulfokine. The addition of α-phytosulfokine to the somatic embryogenesis induction medium causes an increment in the number of embryos produced *(142,143)*.

Most of proteins secreted into the culture medium are glycoproteins *(144)*. Among them exist a peroxidase that can restore the somatic embryogenesis inhibited by tunicamycin *(145)*. Another protein, an endochitinase, was able to rescue the embryo beyond the globular stage and complete its development under nonpermissible temperature $-32°C$ *(146–149)*. Arabinogalacto proteins (AGPs) are proteoglycans with high carbohydrate content and branched structures. These proteoglycans have been detected in cell culture medium of several plant species. When AGPs from embryogenic culture are added to nonembryogenic cultures, they promote and increase somatic embryogenesis *(150–153)*.

More recently, a number of genes that play specific roles in the initiation of embryogenesis in plants have been identified *(154)*. An increased expression of somatic embryogenesis receptor-like kinase 1 (AtSERK1), which encodes a leu-rich repeat (LRR) transmembrane receptor-like kinase (RLK), is found in cells acquiring embryogenic competence, in embryogenic cells, and in early somatic embryos up to about the 100-celled globular stage *(99)*. Ectopic expression of AtSERK1 confers sustained embryogenic competence to seed-lings under in vitro conditions *(155)*.

LEAFY COTYLEDON (LEC1 and LEC2) genes encode seed-expressed transcription factors. When they were ectopic expressed, both LEC1 and LEC2 promoted somatic embryo formation on the vegetative tissues of the plant *(156,157)*. BABY BOOM (BBM) encodes a transcriptional factor belonging to an AP2/ERF family and it is preferentially expressed in developing embryos and seeds. The ectopic expression of BBM induces spontaneously somatic embryos formation in *Arabidopsis* and *Brassica (158)*. WUSCHEL (WUS) is a gain-of- funtion mutation, which is responsible of transition from vegetative or somatic cellular stage to embryogenic stage, and eventually somatic embryo formation. WUS gen encodes to a homeodomain protein involves in specifying stem fate in shoot and floral meristems *(159)*, also it plays a critical role during embryogenesis *(76)*. Recently, WUS was identified as target of a chromatin-remodeling ATPases -SNF2-class ATPase SPLAYED, known as SYD-through recruiting of SYS by WUS promoter *(160)*.

The loss-of-function of PICKLE (PKL) in roots was enough to express embryogenic characteristics, and somatic embryos were formed when the roots were cut and placed on medium culture. PKL encodes a chromatin remodeling factor and it suggests that PKL is a repressor of embryogenic program *(161)*. AGAMOUS like 15 (AGL15) belongs to family of regulatory factors, which binds specific-sequences to DNA. When it was constitutively expressed, it enhanced production of somatic embryos from zygotic embryos *(162)*.

A higher number of in vitro experimental systems have been developed to elucidate the mechanisms governing the onset and development of morphogenesis; nonetheless, it still remains entirely unknown *(77)*. Mutants with defects in the biosynthetic pathway or perception of a specific growth regulator will be very useful on understanding plant morphogenesis *(77)*.

2.5. Somaclonal Variation

During the massive commercial production of plants, it is important to guarantee their genetic integrity, however after micropropagation, or the plants regeneration from calli or somatic embryos, it has been observed the apparition of phenotypic variation among the produced plants *(163–165)*, such phenomenon has been called somaclonal variation.

Larkin and Scowcroft *(165)* have proposed that the origin of this variation could be from the variability already existed into the original cells or a variation generated during the different step of the in vitro culture. The variation detected between the regenerated plants can be epigenetic *(166,167)* or heritable *(168)*. The epigenetic variation in no heritable through sexual propagation. The heritable variation ranges from gross chromosomal abnormalities *(169)*, changes in the methylation pattern *(170,171)*, to point mutations *(172)*. This variation is stable through out the sexual reproduction *(173)*. The growth regulators, in particular 2,4-D, has been related with the variation produced in tissue cultures *(174)*.

Because, in some cases, the somaclonal variation can occur at higher frequencies than chemical *(175)* or radiation induced mutation *(176)*, it can be used as alternative tool to introduce variation into breeding programs *(172)* and produce commercial varieties with new traits. Among the major traits isolated so far are resistance to pathogens *(177–180)*, tolerance to chilling *(181–183)*, drought tolerance *(184,185)*, altitude *(186)*, and salinity tolerance *(187)*, content of secondary metabolites *(188–191)*, herbicide tolerant genotypes in *Triticum aestivum* L. *(192)*, aluminum resistance *(193,194)* and submergence tolerance and other characters of agronomic importance *(195)*.

2.6. Haploid Cultures

Since the discovery by Blakeslee et al. *(196)*, and Guha and Maheshwari *(197,198)* that embryos with a haploid chromosome number can be obtained, plant scientists are using the production of haploid plants for genetic and mutation studies. Haploids originate from a single gamete, and therefore they are sporophytic plants with the gametophytic chromosome number. Because of this trait recessive characteristics are apparent and the haploid plants can be used to produce homozygous diploid plants useful for plant breeding. This technique has the possibility of shortening the time needed to produce completely homozygous lines compared to conventional breeding. This is particularly important in long reproductive cycle plants such as woody plants and fruit crops *(199)*. Over 200 varieties in 12 species have been developed using doubled haploid methods *(200)*.

This technique also can be used to improve agronomically important cereal crops, such as maize, which are still problematic to be genetically engineered by current techniques *(201,202)*.

3. Applications

3.1. Basic Studies

PTC represents a useful system for the study of the physiological, biochemical, and molecular biology processes in plant cells. The effects of a single factor, on a given process, can be monitoring since the culture conditions can be strictly controlled. One of the best examples of the cell cultures' used for such purposes may be the study of the morphogenetic process. The conditions provided by PTC give us an optimum system for the study of the biochemical and molecular aspects associated with plant differentiation. Also, the response of PTC in response to elicitation is an excellent system to study the plant cells' response to the pathogens attack. A number of genes involved in different aspects of such response, including those in perception of the stimulus as well as in the signalling pathway, have been isolated and characterized in cell cultures from different species *(203)*.

The changes in the membrane's fluidity and the cellular mechanisms for resistance to metals, salinity, or drought among others, can be analyzed without having the interference of tissue organization *(204,205)*. The mechanism of the plant cell wall biosynthesis has been widely studied using protoplast as the main tool *(206–208)*.

One of the fields where PTC has been most useful is the study of secondary metabolism; the use of elicitors in cell cultures has led to the identification of enzymes involved in the biosynthesis of different compounds *(209–212)*. PTC has been the model for the study and elucidation of the purine salvage pathway in higher plants *(213,214)* as well as for the study of different aspects of nutrition of plant cells *(215)*.

3.2. Massive Plant Production

Considerable progress has been achieved to scale up the culture vessel to propagate thousands of uniform plantlets under in vitro conditions of plants of agricultural, horticultural, medicinal, and forestry importance *(89)*. Micropropagation has several advantages over conventional methods of vegetative propagation. Among the advantages offered by micropropagation are: 1) with few resources large number of plants can be produced, 2) micropropagation of species may be carried out throughout the year, and 3) micropropagated plants are generally pathogen-free material *(83)*. Therefore, large-scale plant production through cell tissue and embryo cultures using bioreactors is promising for industrial plant propagation *(216)*.

Automation of micropropagation in a bioreactor has been advanced as a possible way for reducing costs. Bioreactors provide a rapid and efficient plant propagation system for many species, using liquid media to avoid intensive manual handling. These bioreactor-cultures have several advantages compared with agar- based cultures, with a better control of the plant tissue's contact with the culture medium, and optimal nutrient and growth regulator supply as well as aeration and medium circulation, the filtration of the medium and the scaling-up of the cultures *(217)*. Since the first use of bioreactor for micropropagation *(218)*, it has been used for the propagation of several species and plant organs including shoots, bulbs, microtubers, corms, and somatic embryos *(219)*.

To fully achieve the potential to scale-up of propagation in bioreactors for commercial micropropagation, the understanding of the signals and molecular mechanisms that control morphogenesis in liquid media will be reached. Further basic and applied researches will provide the information necessary for an efficient and economic use of bioreactors for massive plant propagation *(217)*.

3.3. Production of Virus-Free Plants

Plant diseases are caused by fungi, bacteria, viruses, mycoplasma-like organisms, and nematodes *(220)*. In crop species that are routinely propagated vegetatively there is usually a severe risk of passing on systemic viral infections during the propagation process *(221)*. Other pathogens can be transmitted during micropropagation but because of the intimate, intracellular association of viruses with plant tissue, viruses constitute by far the largest threat to vegetative propagated crops.

To carry plants through borders, the international trades require that plants be healthy and pathogen-free. In addition, to avoid losses, the production of plants must begin with healthy plants. However, most of the cultivars of different species are contaminated with different pathogenic agents, such as bacteria, fungi and virus. PTC provides a set of techniques to produce plant pathogen-free.

Virus-free plants of many species and/or cultivars have been produced by culture of meristematic tissue *(220,222)*, somatic embryogenesis *(223)*, and grafting *(224)*. The use either one technique or another will depend on several factors, mainly of the specie's regeneration capacity. The widely used technique to produce virus-free plants is the in vitro meristem-tip culture. This protocol can be used either alone or combined with chemo or thermotherapy *(225)* from a wide range of plants *(220)*.

When chemotherapy is used, the chemicals are applied to plants or tip-meristem cultures for several days. Also it is possible, at the same time, to apply thermotherapy for several weeks. In general, combinations of both treatments give good results. The amount of the chemicals and the duration of the thermotherapy treatments will depend on the infection's severity, the virus present and the plant specie.

In the grafting technique, the shoots tips are excised from virus-infected plants and grafted onto decapitated rootstock seedlings in a green house. By this method, virus-free plants are produced from the mother plants infected by viruses (224).

In all the cases, regenerated plants (treated with chemo- and thermotherapy) from tip-cultures, somatic embryogenesis or grafted must be indexed for the viruses. Actually, there is a set of assay to test the presence of virus in plant tissues (226), such as the double antibody sandwich-enzyme linked immuno-sorbent assay (DAS-ELISA), and the reverse transcription polymerase chain reaction (RT-PCR) protocols.

3.4. Embryo Rescue and Dangerous Extinction Plants

Plant breeding takes place through hybridization and selection of new plants. The primary objective in plant breeding is to increase the genetic variability and desirable characteristics in crops. It is done by crossing plants to join together traits in offspring from two different plants. However, in many cases the hybridization is not entirely successful because embryo development is arrested in its development or matureness, producing a weak embryo, which will not germinate; in other cases, the endosperm is not properly formed. Under these conditions embryos die (abortion). When embryos are from a desirable genotype, they can be rescued from being aborted by culturing them under suitable conditions on an artificial nutrient medium (227–229).

The term of embryo rescue is confinable only to those circumstances where embryos need to be saved, otherwise they are endangered and neither germinate nor form seedlings. When embryos are not getting aborted but they are excise and culture, it is named embryo culture (227). The aim of embryo rescue technique is to promote the development of an immature or weak embryo into a viable plant; the plant embryo could be isolated by excising from maternal tissue, with ovaries or with ovules. The last two cases are done when embryos can not be removed. The application of embryo rescue culture technique is used to produce interspecific and intergeneric hybrids, recover maternal haploids, obtain plants with genes for disease and insect resistance, for earliness and number of flowers per plant, salt tolerance, herbicide-resistance or tolerance, and other favorable agronomic traits. Additionally, general factors should be considered when embryo rescue technique are used. Among them are genotype and developmental stage of the embryo, culture media, temperature and light, time of culture, plant growth regulators and supplements to the culture medium such as different nitrogen or carbon sources (227,229,230).

The protocols for embryo rescue are simple and carry out an enormous potential in salvage embryo with advantageous characteristics from cross-breeding. On the other hand, embryo culture technique can also be used to save plant species from extinction. Embryo culture is useful when endangered plant produces a few seeds, seeds can be eaten by insect, birds, or any animal, depredation of its inhabit and plant itself. Many techniques have been employed to propagate for example culture axillary buds (231), organogenesis (232), and somatic embryogenesis (233).

3.5. Germplasm Collections and Seed Conservation

Every year, an important number of plant species disappear, partly owing to the loss of natural habitat. Plants with a complex reproductive biology are particularly endangered given the reduction of their natural habitats, along with the small sizes of their populations and their prolonged life cycle. Furthermore, endangered, asexually propagated plants have to deal with the reduction of their genetic variability, which increases their susceptibility to an abrupt environmental change or to the introduction of new elements into their ecosystem. In vitro culture represents an alternative to preserve and regenerate endangered species' populations through micropropagation techniques.

Not only tropical, but also exotic species are endangered. The use of improved plant varieties have resulted in the diminished use of traditional varieties of several crops, such as maize, potato, tomato, etc. Quite often, these traditional varieties, which may have been bred for hundreds of years, are adapted to very specific environments or conditions, and are still cultivated by farmers of small communities, isolated by distance or geographical conditions. Besides their cultural value, they may represent an unexplored source for resistance genes to pathogens, insects, drought, etc. In vitro culture provides the technology for preservation of such phytogenetic resources, which may not be adapted to flourish either in nurseries or under greenhouse conditions. In vitro cultures may also be used to preserve extended collections of germplasm in reduced areas under strictly controlled environments. This approach is particularly valuable in the case of plants that are vegetatively propagated. Terminal or axillary buds cultured in vitro may also be preserved by cryogenic techniques, thus minimizing the excessive tissue manipulation required. The preservation of valuable tropical genetic resources, deposited in germplasm banks and maintained by means of in vitro techniques, represents a growing trend in tissue culture applications.

3.6. Secondary Metabolites

Higher plants produce a large number of diverse organic chemicals, some of which are of pharmaceutical and industrial interest. Once the technology for culturing plant cells, in the same way as fungal and bacterial cells was available, the production of natural products were among the first applications to be pursued. The first attempt of the use of plant cells for the production of secondary metabolites took place in the 1950s *(234–236)*. Later, in Germany and Japan in particular, the development of scale-up techniques for suspension cultures led to development of the industrial application of cell cultures commercially *(22,237,238)*. However, differing from fungi and bacteria, the pattern of natural products yield by plant cells in culture frequently showed variations from those of organized tissues *(239)*. Despite numerous attempts by several laboratories around the world, in vitro cell cultures have not turned out to be efficient factories of natural products, because since many of the economically important plant products are neither formed in sufficiently large quantities nor at all by plant cell cultures. However, the culture of organs, such as roots or shoots, lead to the production of complex chemicals in amounts equals or higher than those of the mother plant *(210)*. In addition, cell cultures have proved to be an invaluable source for enzymes and genes involved in the synthesis of these natural products, as well as for establishing the relationship between cell differentiation and secondary metabolism *(54)*.

Different approaches to enhance yields of secondary metabolites included the induction of cell lines from highly productive tissues or individuals, the cloning and systematic screening of heterogeneous cell populations for strains with a high biosynthetic potential (240), and the formulation of culture media composition (241). Another approach involves selection of mutant cell lines that overproduce the desired product (242). The use of abiotic factors, such as heat or cold, salts of heavy metals, and UV radiation, and the use of biotic elicitors of plant and microbial origin, such as fungi cell walls, methyl jasmonate, salicylic acid, and nitric oxide, has been shown to enhance secondary product formation (243–247). The use of immobilized cell technology has also been applied successfully (248,249).

The better understanding of the tight regulation governing secondary metabolism pathways and also, of its close relationship with branches of the primary metabolism, can now be applied through metabolic engineering strategies to promote the accumulation of valuable natural products in in vitro cultures (250–252). Metabolic engineering is aimed to improve cell processes, by means of recombinant DNA technology, for commercial purposes. Genes coding for enzymes involved in limiting steps in a pathway may be overexpressed in cell cultures favoring carbon flux through it. Alternatively, new enzymatic activities can be introduced, resulting in the formation of new compounds. Recently, the identification of regulatory genes, controlling the coordinated activation of a set of enzymes involved in secondary metabolism, has opened new possibilities for the genetic manipulation of the whole pathway, by means of a single gene.

3.7. Transgenic Plants

The Green Revolution in the mid-1960s saved hundreds of millions of human lives. However, in the last 10–15 years cereal productivity has declined. Among the different factors for this decrease are the salinization of the soil, the quality and amount of water, and the possibility that crops may have reached the physiological limits of their productivity (27). On the other hand, plants are known for their wide diversity, which allows them to survive in an ever-changing and often stressful environment. A multiplicity of traits encompasses features that are required for optimal growth and reproduction, and includes aspects of stress tolerance, nutrient use, plant morphology, resistance to pathogens, and the production of secondary metabolites (253). For crops other quality traits are required, such as improved postharvest storage, flavor, nutritional content and color (254). However, in the case of crops most of these traits need to be transferred to them. Agriculture techniques allow the transferred of some of these characteristics between plants of the same specie but not among members of different species. The chemically induced fusion of plant protoplasts brought a solution to this problem and opened a new research field (255). This technique established the possibility of the genetic manipulation of plants by bypassing problems of sexual incompatibility (256).

The first report of the genetic transformation of plant cells was also published by the Cocking group in the United Kingdom (257) by the direct delivery of DNA into protoplasts of petunia. Only a few years later, the Ti (tumor- inducing) plasmid was used as a vector for gene transference and production of the first transgenic plant (258).

Actually, transgenic organisms allow scientists to cross the physical and genetic barriers that separate pools of genes among organisms and produce plants with new traits. At the same time transgenic plants are used as an important research tool *(259)*. Today, all transformation systems for creating transgenic plants require separate processes for introducing cloned DNA into plant cells, for identifying or selecting those transformed cells and for regenerating and recovering fully developed and fertile plants from the transformed cell *(259)*. Different techniques to introduce foreign genes into plant genomes have been used; these include the *Agrobacterium* system and the bombardment of DNA-covered microprojectiles. Selective markers, such as antibiotic resistance, chromophores, or fluorochromes, are incorporated to distinguish the transformed tissues from those untransformed. The first generation of genetically modified plants suitable for agriculture was largely produced using antibiotic resistance markers for the preparation of plant transformation vectors or for the plant transformation process itself *(260)*.

Genetically modified plants would rise from individual cells and, because DNA insertion is a random process, an efficient regeneration procedure could increase the probability of recovering a transgenic plant. For this reason, the use of tissues with a high morphogenetic or embryogenic potential is recommended. Protoplasts can also be used; however, they may require a considerable amount of labor before regenerating a new plant, although with better odds of obtaining actual transformants.

In addition to the traits already mentioned genetically modified crops could also manufacture industrial and pharmaceutical compounds as renewable resources with a production system based on solar energy *(254)*.

4. Future Progress

Plant cell cultures have become an invaluable tool to plant scientists, cell cultures have remained an important tool in the study of plant biology, and today in vitro culture techniques are standard procedures in most of the plant biology's laboratories. Cell cultures will remain as an important tool in the study of morphogenesis. Molecular, physiological, and biochemical studies on somatic embryogenesis and plant regeneration processes will continue lightening the way cells choose any morphogenetic pathway. In addition to *Arabidopsis* model, the isolation of new mutants from PTC will help in this task.

Cell cultures have remained, and will continue, an extremely important tool in the study of primary metabolism, e.g., the use of protoplasts and vacuoles for the study of the mechanisms of toxicity of heavy metals *(261)*, as well as the production of resistant plants based in PTC technology *(262)*.

The development of medicinal plant cell culture techniques has led to the identification of complete pathways of alkaloid biosynthesis *(263)*. Similar information arising from the use of cell cultures for molecular and biochemical studies is generating research activity on metabolic engineering of plant secondary metabolite production *(264)*.

The helpfulness of this knowledge goes beyond basic research. Massive propagation of plants represents today an economically rewarding enterprise and this will increase in the following years by incorporating new plants into the market, mainly exotic plants with new flower colors and fragrances. Thanks to the development of genomics, proteomics, and metabolomics, plant biotechnology is experimenting new and exciting advances. These "omics" approaches, with no doubt, will accelerate the discovery, isolation and characterization of genes conferring new agronomic traits to crops.

Successful genetic engineering programs will focused in the development of new plant varieties with traits that increase the quality of the crops to fight undernourishment and in this way the increase in the yields without the use of chemicals in the field will remain an important task. The new plant varieties must also let an increase in the use of the land for agricultural aim by overcoming problems such as salinity, drought and desertification. PTC technique will also allow the production of roots for food in bioreactors (265), under controlled conditions. Technologies for cell culture in large volumes for the production of fine chemicals in genetically modified cells cultured should be established. This technique presents advantages over their production in field grown plants that normally occupy considerable extensions of land.

The use of in vitro techniques in embryo rescue during plant breeding, to save dangerous extinction plants, and the construction of germplasm banks to preserve plants with valuable traits will help the continuous necessity of genetic improvement programs.

In summary, the advancements made with this technology have gone well beyond what the pioneers lead by Gottlieb Haberlandt could have imagined.

Acknowledgments: We are grateful to Emily Wortman–Wunder for editorial assistance. The work of the laboratory of V.M.L.-V. is partially funded by CONACYT (Grant No. 61415). V.M.L-V. is a recipient of scholarship from CONACYT, Mexico.

References

1. Thorpe TA (1990) The current status of plant tissue culture. In: Developments in crop science 19. Plant tissue culture: applications and limitations, Bhojwani SS (ed) Elsevier, Amsterdam, pp 1–33
2. Haberlandt G (1902) Kulturversuche mit isolierten pflanzenzellen. Sber Akad Wiss Wein 111:69–92
3. Krikorian AD, Berquam DL (1969) Plant cell and tissue cultures: the role of Haberlandt. Bot Rev 35:59–87
4. Kotté W (1922) Kulturversuch isolierten wulzelspitzen. Beitr Allg Bot 2:413–434
5. Robbins WJ (1922) Cultivation of excised root tips and stem under sterile conditions. Bot Gaz 73:376–390
6. White PR (1934) Potentially unlimited growth of excised tomato root tips in a liquid medium. Plant Physiol 9:585–600
7. Gautheret RJ (1934) Culture du tissue cambial. C R Acad Sci (Paris) Sér III 198:2195–2196
8. White PR (1939) Potentially unlimited growth of excised plant callus in an artificial nutrient. Am J Bot 26:59–64
9. Nobécourt P (1939) Sur la perennite et l'augmentation de volume des cultures de tissus vegétaux. C R Séanc Soc Biol Paris 130:1270–1271
10. Guatheret RJ (1939) Sur la possibilité de réaliser la culture indéfinie des tissue de tubersules de carotte. C R Acad Sci (Paris) Sér III 208:118–121
11. van Overbeek J, Conklin ME, Blakeslee AF (1941) Factors in coconut milk essential for growth and development of very young *Datura* embryos. Science 94:350–351
12. Skoog F, Tsui C (1948) Chemical control of growth and bud formation in tobacco stem segments and callus cultured *in vitro*. Am J Bot 35:782–787

13. Miller CO, Skoog F, Von Saltza MH, Strong FM (1955) Kinetin, a cell division factor from deoxyribonucleic acid. J Am Chem Soc 77:1392

14. Skoog F, Miller CO (1957) Chemical regulation of growth and organ formation in plant tissues cultured *in vitro*. Symp Soc Exp Bot 11:118–130

15. Krikorian AD, Simola LK (1999) Totipotency, somatic embryogenesis, and Harry Waris (1893–1973). Physiol Plant 105:348–355

16. Steward FC, Mapes MO, Mears K (1958) Growth and organized development of cultured cells. II.Organization in cultures grown from freely suspended cells. Am J Bot 45:705–708

17. Reinert J (1959) Uber die kontrolle der morphogenese und die induktion von adventivembryonen an gewebekulturen aus karotten. Planta 53:318–333

18. Vasil V, Hildebrand AC (1965) Differentiation of tobacco plants from single, isolated cells in micro cultures. Science 150:889–892

19. Takebe I, Labib G, Melchers G (1971) Regeneration of whole plants fron isolated mesophyll protoplasts of tobacco. Naturwissenschaften 58:318–320

20. Carlson PS, Smith HH, Dearing PD (1972) Parasexual interspecific plant hybridisation. Proc Natl Acad Sci (USA) 69:2292–2294

21. Cocking EC (1960) A method for the isolation of plant protoplasts and vacuoles. Nature 187:962–963

22. Tabata M, Mizukami H, Hiraoka N, Konoshima M (1974) Pigment formation in callus cultures of *Lithospermum erythrorhizon*. Phytochemistry 13:927

23. Fujita Y, Takahashi S, Yamada Y (1984) Selection of cell lines with high productivity of shikonin derivatives through protoplast of *Lithospermum erythrorhizon*, in Third european congress on biotechnology Vol. I, 9/10/1983, Verlag Chemie, Weinheim, pp 161–166

24. Caplan A, Herrera-Estrella L, Inze D, Van Haute E, Van Montagu M, Zambryski JSP (1983) Introduction of genetic material into plant cells. Science 222:815–821

25. Herrera-Estrella L, Depicker A, Van Montagu M, Schell J (1983) Expression of chimaeric genes transferred into plant cells using a Ti-plasmid-derived vector. Nature 303:209–213

26. Trigiano RN, Gray DJ (2005) Plant development and biotechnology, CRC Press, Boca Raton, Florida

27. Vasil IK (2005) The story of transgenic cereals: the challenge, the debate, and the solution – A historical perspective. In Vitro Cell Dev Biol Plant 41:577–583

28. Loyola-Vargas VM, Vázquez–Flota FA (2006) Plant cell culture protocols, Humana Press, Totowa, New Jersey

29. George EF (1993) Plant propagation by tissue culture. Part 1. The technology, Exegetics Limited, Great Britain

30. Conger BV (1980) Cloning Agricultural Plants Via *in vitro* Techniques, CRC Press, Boca Raton, Florida

31. Murashige T, Skoog F (1962) A revised medium for rapid growth and bio-assays with tobacco tissue cultures. Physiol Plant 15:473–497

32. Gamborg OL, Miller RA, Ojima K (1968) Nutrient requirements of suspension cultures of soybean root cells. Exp Cell Res 50:151–158

33. Phillips GC, Collins GB (1979) *In vitro* tissue culture of selected legumes and plant regeneration from callus cultures of red clover. Crop Sci 19:59–64

34. Halperin W, Wetherell DF (1965) Ammonium requirement for embryogenesis *in vitro*. Nature 205:519–520

35. Wetherell DF, Dougall DK (1976) Sources of nitrogen supporting growth and embryogenesis in cultured wild carrot tissue. Physiol Plant 37:97–103

36. Nitsch JP, Nitsch C (1969) Haploid plants from pollen grains. Science 163:85–87

37. Kao KN, Michayluk R (1975) Nutritional requeriments for growth of *Vicia hajastana* cells and protoplasts at a very low population density in liquid media. Planta 126:1095–1100

38. Dodds JH, Roberts LW (1995) Experiments in plant tissue culture, Cambridge University Press, Cambridge

39. Gamborg OL, Phillips GC (1995) Plant cell, tissue and organ culture. Fundamental methods, Springer-Verlag, Germany

40. Street HE (1977) Plant tissue and cell culture, University of California Press, Oxford

41. Thorpe TA (1981) Plant tissue culture. Methods and applications in agriculture, Academic Press, New York

42. Vasil IK (1985) Cell culture and somatic cell genetics of plants. Vol. 2. Cell growth, nutrition, cytodifferentiation, and cryopreservation, Academic Press, Orlando

43. Constabel F (1984) Callus culture: induction and maintenance. In: Cell culture and somatic cell genetics of plants, Vasil IK (ed) Vol. 1, Academic Press, Orlando, pp. 27–35

44. Smith RH (1992) Plant tissue culture. Techniques and experiments, Academic Press, Inc., San Diego

45. Allan E (1991) Plant cell culture. In: Plant cell and tissue culture, Stafford A, Warren G (eds) Open University Press, London, pp 1–24

46. King PJ (1984) Induction and maintenance of cell suspension cultures. In: Cell culture and somatic cell genetics of plants, Vasil IK (ed) Vol. 1, Academic Press, Orlando, pp 130–138

47. Butcher DN, Street HE (1964) Excised root culture. Bot Rev 30:513–586

48. Lindsey K, Yeoman MM (1983) The relationship between growth rate, differentiation and alkaloid accumulation in cell cultures. J Exp Bot 34:1055–1065

49. Loyola-Vargas VM, Miranda-Ham ML (1995) Root culture as a source of secondary metabolites of economic importance. Rec Advan Phytochem 29:217–248

50. Canto-Canché B, Loyola-Vargas VM (1999) Chemical from roots, hairy roots, and their application. Adv Exp Med Biol 464:235–275

51. Flores HE, Vivanco JM, Loyola-Vargas VM (1999) "Radicle" biochemistry: the biology of root-specific metabolism. Trends Plant Sci 4:220–226

52. Bais HP, Loyola-Vargas VM, Flores HE, Vivanco JM (2001) Root-specific metabolism: the biology and biochemistry of underground organs. In Vitro Cell Dev Biol Plant 37:730–741

53. Flores HE, Filner P (1985) Hairy roots of Solanaceae as a source of alkaloids. Plant Physiol 77:12s

54. Flores HE, Filner P (1985) Metabolic relationships of putrescine, GABA and alkaloids in cell and root cultures of Solanaceae. In: Primary and secondary metabolism in plant cell cultures, Neumann KH, Barz W, Reinhard E (eds) Springer-Verlag, Heidelberg, pp 174–186

55. Guillon S, Tremouillaux-Guiller J, Pati PK, Rideau M, Gantet P (2006) Hairy root research: recent scenario and exciting prospects. Curr Opi Plant Biol 9:341–346

56. Jordan M, Humam M, Bieri S, Christen P, Poblete E, Munoz O (2006) *In vitro* shoot and root organogenesis, plant regeneration and production of tropane alkaloids in some species of *Schizanthus*. Phytochemistry 67:570–578

57. Hernández-Domínguez E, Campos F, Vázquez-Flota FA (2004) Vindoline synthesis in *in vitro* shoot cultures of *Catharanthus roseus*. Biotechnol Lett 26:671–674

58. Ekiert H, Choloniewska M, Gomólka E (2001) Accumulation of furanocoumarins in *Ruta graveolens* L. shoot culture. Biotechnol Lett 23:543–545

59. Kirakosyan A, Hayashi H, Inoue K, Charchoglyan A, Vardapetyan H (2000) Stimulation of the production of hypericins by mannan in *Hypericum perforatum* shoot cultures. Phytochemistry 53:345–348

60. Davey MR, Anthony P, Power JB, Lowe KC (2005) Plant protoplast technology: status and applications. In Vitro Cell Dev Biol Plant 41:202–212

61. Acuña JR, de Pena M (1991) Plant regeneration from protoplasts of embryogenic cell suspensions of *Coffea arabica* L. cv. caturra. Plant Cell Rep 10:345–348

62. Toruan-Mathius N (1992) Isolation and protoplasts culture of *Coffea arabica* L. Biotechnol Forest Tree Improvement 49:89–98
63. Aftab F, Iqbal J (1999) Plant regeneration from protoplasts derived from cell suspension of adventive somatic embryos in sugarcane (*Saccharum* spp. *hybrid* cv. CoL-54 and cv. CP-43/33). Plant Cell Tiss Org Cult 56:155–162
64. Arcioni S, Davey MR, Dos Santos AVP, Cocking EC (1982) Somatic embryogenesis in tissues from mesophyll and cell suspension protoplasts of *Medicago coerulea* and *M. glutinosa*. Z Pflanzenphysiol 106:105–110
65. Ara H, Jaiswal U, Jaiswal VS (2000) Plant regeneration from protoplasts of mango (*Mangifera indica* L.) through somatic embryogenesis. Plant Cell Rep 19:622–627
66. Vasil IK, Vasil V, Redway F (1990) Plant regeneration from embryogenic calli, cell suspension cultures and protoplasts of *Triticum aestivum* L. (Wheat). In: Progress in plant cellular and molecular biology., Nijkamp HJJ, Van der Plas LHW, Van Aartrijk J (eds) Kluwer Academic Publishers, Dordrecht, pp 33–37
67. Birnbaum K, Shasha DE, Wang JY, Jung JW, Lambert GM, Galbraith DW, Benfey PN (2003) A gene expression map of the Arabidopsis root. Science 302:1956–1960
68. Birnbaum K, Jung JW, Wang JY, Lambert GM, Hirst JA, Galbraith DW, Benfey PN (2005) Cell type-specific expression profiling in plants via cell sorting of protoplasts from fluorescent reporter lines. Nat Meth 2:615–619
69. Hammatt N, Lister A, Blackhall NW, Gartland J, Ghose TK, Gilmour DM, Power JB, Davey MR, Cocking EC (1990) Selection of plant heterokaryons from diverse origins by flow cytometry. Protoplasma 154:34–44
70. Yarbrough JA (1936) The foliar embryos of *Tolmiea menziesii*. Am J Bot 123:16–20
71. Yarbrough JA (1932) Anatomical and developmental studies of the foliar embryos of *Bryophyllum calycinum*. Am J Bot 19:443–453
72. Phillips GC (2004) *In vitro* morphogenesis in plants – Recent advances. In Vitro Cell Dev Biol Plant 40:342–345
73. Quiroz-Figueroa FR, Rojas-Herrera R, Galaz-Avalos RM, Loyola-Vargas VM (2006) Embryo production through somatic embryogenesis can be used to study cell differentiation in plants. Plant Cell Tiss Org Cult 86:285–301
74. Gaj MD (2004) Factors influencing somatic embryogenesis induction and plant regeneration with particular reference to *Arabidopsis thaliana* (L.) Heynh. Plant Growth Regul 43:27–47
75. Sugiyama M (1999) Organogenesis *in vitro*. Curr Opi Plant Biol 2:61–64
76. Zuo J, Niu QW, Frugis G, Chua NH (2002) The WUSCHEL gene promotes vegetative-to-embryonic transition in *Arabidopsis*. Plant J 30:349–359
77. Sugiyama M (2000) Genetic analysis of plant morphogenesis *in vitro*. Int Rev Cytol 196:67–84
78. George EF (1996) Plant propagation by tissue culture. Part 2, Exegetics Limited, England
79. Debergh PC, Zimmerman RH (1993) Micropropagation. Technology and application, Kluer Academic Publishers, Netherlands
80. Herman EB (1991) Recent Advances in Plant Tissue Culture. Regeneration, Micropropagation and Media 1988–1991, Agritech Consultants, Inc., USA
81. Herman EB (1995) Recent advances in plant tissue culture III. Regeneration and micropropagation: techniques, systems and media 1991–1995, Agritech Consultants, USA
82. Kyte L, Kleyn J (1996) Plant from test tubes. An introduction to micropropagation, Timber Press, Portland
83. Debnath M, Malik CP, Bisen PS (2006) Micropropagation: a tool for the production of high quality plant-based medicines. Current Pharmaceutical Biotechnology 7:33–49

84. Murashige T (1974) Plant propagation through tissue cultures. Annu Rev Plant Physiol 25:135–166

85. George EF (1993) Plant propagation and micropropagation. In: Plant propagation by tissue culture. Part 1, George EF (ed) Exegetics Limited, England, pp 37–66

86. Hazarika BN (2006) Morpho–physiological disorders in *in vitro* culture of plants. Sci Hortic 108:105–120

87. Huang C, Chen C (2005) Physical properties of culture vessels for plant tissue culture. Biosys Eng 91:501–511

88. Chen C (2004) Humidity in plant tissue culture vessels. Biosys Eng 88:231–241

89. Zobayed SMA, Afreen F, Xiao Y, Kozai T (2004) Recent advancement in research on photoautotrophic micropropagation using large culture vessels with forced ventilation. In Vitro Cell Dev Biol Plant 40:450–458

90. Lowe KC, Anthony P, Power JB, Davey MR (2003) Novel approaches for regulating gas supply to plant systems *in vitro*: application and benefits of artificial gas carriers. In Vitro Cell Dev Biol Plant 39:557–566

91. Pierik RLM, Ruibing MA (1997) Developments in the micropropagation industry in the Netherlands. Plant Tiss Cult Biotechnol 3:152–156

92. Robert ML, Herrera-Herrera JL, Herrera-Herrera G, Herrera-Alamillo MA, Fuentes-Carrillo P (2006) A new temporary immersion bioreactor system for micropropagation. In: Plant cell culture protocols, Loyola-Vargas VM, Vázquez-Flota F (eds) Humana Press, Totowa, New Jersey, pp 121–129

93. Etienne H, Berthouly M (2002) Temporary immersion systems in plant micropropagation. Plant Cell Tiss Org Cult 69:215–231

94. Berthouly M, Dufour M, Alvard D, Carasco C, Alemanno L, Teisson C (1995) Coffee micropropagaction in a liquid medium using the temporary immersion technique, in 16ᵉ Colloque Scientifique International sur le Café, Association Scientifique Internationale du Café, Paris, pp 514–519

95. Cabasson C, Alvard D, Dambier D, Ollitrault P, Teisson C (1997) Improvement of *Citrus* somatic embryo development by temporary immersion. Plant Cell Tiss Org Cult 50:33–37

96. Etienne H, Lartaud M, Michaux-Ferrière N, Carron MP, Berthouly M, Teisson C (1997) Improvement of somatic embryogenesis in *Hevea brasiliensis* (mull. arg.) using the temporary immersion technique. In Vitro Cell Dev Biol Plant 33:81–87

97. Lorenzo JC, González BL, Escalona M, Teisson C, Espinosa P, Borroto C (1998) Sugarcane shoot formation in an improved temporary immersion system. Plant Cell Tiss Org Cult 54:197–200

98. Zimmerman JL (1993) Somatic embryogenesis: A model for early development in higher plants. Plant Cell 5:1411–1423

99. Schmidt EDL, Guzzo F, Toonen MAJ, De Vries SC (1997) A leucinerich repeat containing receptor-like kinase marks somatic plant cells competent to form embryos. Development 124:2049–2062

100. Komamine A, Murata N, Nomura K (2005) Mechanisms of somatic embryogenesis in carrot suspension cultures – morphology, physiology, biochemistry, and molecular biology. In Vitro Cell Dev Biol Plant 41:6–10

101. Kawahara R, Komamine A (1995) Molecular basis of somatic embryogenesis, In: Biotechnology in agriculture and forestry. Vol. 30. Somatic embryogenesis and synthetic seed I, Bajaj YPS (ed) Springer-Verlag, Berlin, pp 30–40

102. Dodeman VL, Ducreux G, Kreis M (1997) Zygotic embryogenesis *versus* somatic embryogenesis. J Exp Bot 48:1493–1509

103. Fehér A, Pasternak TP, Dudits D (2003) Transition of somatic plant cells to an embryogenic state. Plant Cell Tiss Org Cult 74:201–228

104. Nogler GA (1984) Gametophytic Apomixis. In: Embryology of Angiosperms, Johri BM (ed) Springer-Verlag, Berlin, pp 475–518

105. Raghavan V (2000) Developmental biology of flowering plants, Springer-Verlag, NY

106. Maraschin SF, de Priester W, Spaink HP, Wang M (2005) Androgenic switch: an example of plant embryogenesis from the male gametophyte perspective. J Exp Bot 56:1711–1726

107. Bhojwani SS, Razdan MK (1983) Plant Tissue Culture: Theory and Practice, Elsevier, Amsterdam

108. Waris H (1957) A striking morphogenetic effect of amino acid in seed plant. Suom Kemistil 36B:121

109. Rojas-Herrera R, Quiroz-Figueroa FR, Sánchez-Teyer F, Loyola-Vargas VM (2002) Molecular analysis of somatic embryogenesis: An overview. Physiol Mol Biol Plants 8:171–184

110. Kato H, Takeuchi M (1963) Morphogenesis *in vitro* starting from single cells of carrot root. Plant Cell Physiol 4:243–245

111. Halperin W (1966) Alternative morphogenetic events in cell suspensions. Am J Bot 53:443–453

112. Schiavone FM, Cooke TJ (1985) A geometric analysis of somatic embryo formation in carrot cell culture. Can J Bot 63:1573–1578

113. Nakamura T, Taniguchi T, Maeda E (1992) Studies on somatic embryogenesis of coffee by scanning electron microscope. Jpn J Crop Sci 61:476–486

114. Wetherell DF (1984) Enhanced adventive embryogenesis resulting from plasmolysis of cultured wild carrot cells. Plant Cell Tiss Org Cult 5:221–227

115. Kamada H, Kobayashi K, Kiyosue T, Harada H (1989) Stress induced somatic embryogenesis in carrot and its application to synthetic seed production. In Vitro Cell Dev Biol Plant 25:1163–1166

116. Litz RE (1986) Effect of osmotic stress on somatic embryogenesis in *Carica* suspension cultures. J Am Soc Hortic Sci 111:969–972

117. Galiba G, Yamada Y (1988) A novel method increasing the frequency of somatic embryogenesis in wheat tissue culture by NaCl and KCl supplementation. Plant Cell Rep 7:55–58

118. Ikeda-Iwai M, Umehara M, Satoh S, Kamada H (2003) Stress-induced somatic embryogenesis in vegetative tissues of *Arabidopsis thaliana*. Plant J 34:107–114

119. Pasternak TP, Prinsen E, Ayaydin F, Miskolczi P, Potters G, Asard H, Van Onckelen HA, Dudits D, Fehér A (2002) The role of auxin, pH, and stress in the activation of embryogenic cell division in leaf protoplast–derived cells of alfalfa. Plant Physiol 129:1807–1819

120. Kiyosue T, Takano K, Kamada H, Harada H (1990) Induction of somatic embryogenesis in carrot by heavy metal ions. Can J Bot 68:2301–2303

121. Smith DL, Krikorian AD (1989) Release of somatic embryogenic potential from excised zygotic embryos of carrot and maintenance of proembryonic cultures in hormone-free medium. Am J Bot 76:1832–1843

122. Lee EK, Cho DY, Soh WY (2001) Enhanced production and germination of somatic embryos by temporary starvation in tissue cultures of *Daucus carota*. Plant Cell Rep 20:408–415

123. Roustan J-P, Latche A, Fallot J (1989) Effet de l'acide salicylique et de l'acide acétylsalicylique sur la production d'éthylène et l'embryogenèse somatique de suspensions cellulaires de carotte (*Daucus carota* L.). C R Acad Sci (Paris) Sér III 308:395–399

124. Hutchinson MJ, Saxena PK (1996) Acetylsalicylic acid enhances and synchronizes thidiazuron-induced somatic embryogenesis in geranium (*Pelargonium x hortorum* Bailey) tissue cultures. Plant Cell Rep 15:512–515

125. Quiroz-Figueroa FR, Méndez-Zeel M, Larqué-Saavedra A, Loyola-Vargas VM (2001) Picomolar concentrations of salicylates induce cellular growth and enhance somatic embryogenesis in *Coffea arabica* tissue culture. Plant Cell Rep 20:679–684

126. Leslie CA, Romani RJ (1986) Salicylic acid: a new inhibitor of ethylene biosynthesis. Plant Cell Rep 5:144–146

127. Roustan JP, Latche A, Fallot J (1989) Stimulation of *Daucus carota* somatic embryogenesis by inhibitors of ethylene synthesis: cobalt and nickel. Plant Cell Rep 8:182–185

128. Hutchinson MJ, Murr D, Krishnaraj S, Senaratna T, Saxena PK (1997) Does ethylene play a role in thidiazuron–regulated somatic embryogenesis of geranium (*Pelargonium* x *Hortorum* bailey) hypocotyl cultures? In Vitro Cell Dev Biol Plant 33:136–141

129. Hatanaka T, Sawabe E, Azuma T, Uchida N, Yasuda T (1995) The role of ethylene in somatic embryogenesis from leaf disks of *Coffea canephora*. Plant Sci 107:199–204

130. Kairong KR, Xing GS, Liu XM, Xing GM, Wang YF (1999) Effect of hydrogen peroxide on somatic embryogenesis of *Lycium barbarum* L. Plant Sci 146:9–16

131. Luo JP, Jiang ST, Pan LJ (2001) Enhanced somatic embryogenesis by salicylic acid of *Astragalus adsurgens* Pall.: relationship with H_2O_2 production and H_2O_2–metabolizing enzyme activities. Plant Sci 161:125–132

132. Dudits D, Bögre L, Györgyey J (1991) Molecular and cellular approaches to the analysis of plant embryo development from somatic cells *in vitro*. J Cell Sci 99:473–482

133. Dudits D, Györgyey J, Bögre L, Bakó L (1995) Molecular biology of somatic embryogenesis. In: *In vitro* embryogenesis in plants, Thorpe TA (ed) Kluwer Academic Publishers, Dordrecht 267–308

134. Lichtenthaler HK (1998) The stress concept in plants: an introduction. Ann NY Acad Sci 851:187–198

135. Higashi K, Daita M, Kobayashi T, Sasaki K, Harada H, Kamada H (1998) Inhibitory conditioning for carrot somatic embryogenesis in high-cell-density cultures. Plant Cell Rep 18:2–6

136. Umehara M, Ogita S, Sasamoto H, Koshino H, Asami T, Fujioka S, Yoshida S, Kamada H (2005) Identification of a novel factor, vanillyl benzyl ether, which inhibits somatic embryogenesis of Japanese larch (*Larix leptolepis* Gordon). Plant Cell Physiol 46:445–453

137. Yang H, Matsubayashi Y, Hanai H, Sakagami Y (2000) Phytosulfokine-α, a peptide growth factor found in higher plants: its structure, functions, precursor and receptors. Plant Cell Physiol 41:825–830

138. Igasaki T, Akashi N, Ujino-Ihara T, Matsubayashi Y, Sakagami Y, Shinohara K (2003) Phytosulfokine stimulates somatic embryogenesis in *Cryptomeria japonica*. Plant Cell Physiol 44:1412–1416

139. Fridborg E (1978) The effect of activated charcoal on tissue cultures; adsorption of metabolites inhibiting morphogenesis. Physiol Plant 43:104–106

140. Osuga K, Kamada H, Komamine A (1993) Cell density is an important factor for synchronization of the late stage of somatic embryogenesis at high frequency. Plant Tiss Cult Lett 10:180–183

141. Kobayashi T, Higashi K, Sasaki K, Asami T, Yoshida S, Kamada H (2000) Purification from conditioned medium and chemical identification of a factor that inhibits somatic embryogenesis in carrot. Plant Cell Physiol 41:268–273

142. Kobayashi T, Eun CH, Hanai H, Matsubayashi Y, Sakagami Y, Kamada H (1999) Phytosulphokine-α, a peptidyl plant growth factor, stimulates somatic embryogenesis in carrot. J Exp Bot 50:1123–1128

143. Igasaki T, Akashi N, Shinohara K (2006) Somatic embryogenesis in *Cryptomeria japonica* D. Don: gene for phytosulfokine (PSK) precursor. In: Somatic embryogenesis, Mujib A, Samaj J (eds) Springer, Berlin, Heidelberg, pp 201–213

144. Satoh S, Kamada H, Harada H, Fujii T (1986) Auxin–controlled glycoprotein release into the medium of embryogenic carrot cells. Plant Physiol 81:931–933

145. Cordewener J, Booij H, Van der Zandt H, Van Engelen FA, Van Kammen A, De Vries SC (1991) Tunicamycin-inhibited carrot somatic embryogenesis can be restored by secreted cationic peroxidase isoenzymes. Planta 184:478–486

146. Lo Schiavo F, Giuliano G, De Vries SC, Genga A, Bollini R, Pitto L, Cozzani F, Nuti-Ronchi V, Terzi M (1990) A carrot cell variant temperature sensitive for somatic embryogenesis reveals a defect in the glycosylation of extracellular proteins. Mol Gen Genet 223:385–393

147. De Jong AJ, Cordewener J, Lo Schiavo F, Terzi M, Vandekerckhove J, Van Kammen A, De Vries SC (1992) A carrot somatic embryo mutant is rescued by chitinase. Plant Cell 4:425–433

148. Baldan B, Guzzo F, Filippini F, Gasparian M, LoSchiavo F, Vitale A, De Vries SC, Mariani P, Terzi M (1997) The secretory nature of the lesion of carrot cell variant ts11, rescuable by endochitinase. Planta 203:381–389

149. De Jong AJ, Hendriks T, Meijer EA, Penning M, Lo Schiavo F, Terzi M, Van Kammen A, De Vries SC (1995) Transient reduction in secreted 32 kD chitinase prevents somatic embryogenesis in the carrot (*Daucus carota* L.) variant ts11. Devel Genet 16:332–343

150. Van Hengel AJ, Tadesse Z, Immerzeel P, Schols H, Van Kammen A, De Vries SC (2001) *N*-acetylglucosamine and glucosamine-containing arabinogalactan proteins control somatic embryogenesis. Plant Physiol 125:1880–1890

151. Egertsdotter U, Mo LH, Von Arnold S (1993) Extracellular proteins in embryogenic suspension cultures of Norway spruce (*Picea abies*). Physiol Plant 88: 315–321

152. Egertsdotter U, Von Arnold S (1995) Importance of arabinogalactan proteins for the development of somatic embryos of Norway spruce (*Picea abies*). Physiol Plant 93:334–345

153. Letarte J, Simion E, Miner M, Kasha K (2006) Arabinogalactans and arabinogalactan-proteins induce embryogenesis in wheat (*Triticum aestivum* L.) microspore culture. Plant Cell Rep 24:691–698

154. Ikeda M, Umehara M, Kamada H (2006) Embryogenesis-related genes; Its expression and roles during somatic and zygotic embryogenesis in carrot and Arabidopsis. Plant Biotechnol J 23:153–161

155. Hecht V, Vielle-Calzada JP, Hartog MV, Schmidt EDL, Boutilier K, Grossniklaus U, De Vries SC (2001) The Arabidopsis *somatic embryogenesis receptor kinase 1* gene is expressed in developing ovules and embryos and enhances embryogenic competence in culture. Plant Physiol 127:803–816

156. Lotan T, Ohto M, Matsudaira YK, West MAL, Lo R, Kwong RW, Yamagishi K, Fischer RL, Goldberg RB, Harada JJ (1998) Arabidopsis leafy cotyledon1 is sufficient to induce embryo development in vegetative cells. Cell 93:1195–1205

157. Stone SL, Kwong LW, Yee KM, Pelletier J, Lepiniec L, Fischer RL, Goldberg RB, Harada JJ (2001) Leafy cotyledon encodes a B3 domain transcription factor that induces embryo development. Proc Natl Acad Sci (USA) 98:11806–11811

158. Boutilier K, Offringa R, Sharma VK, Kieft H, Ouellet T, Zhang L, Hattori J, Liu C-M, Van Lammeren AAM, Miki BLA, Custers JBM, Van Lookeren-Campagne MM (2002) Ectopic expression of BABY BOOM triggers a conversion from vegetative to embryonic growth. Plant Cell 14:1737–1749

159. Laux T, Mayer KF, Berger J, Jurgens G (1996) The WUSCHEL gene is required for shoot and floral meristem integrity in Arabidopsis. Development 122:87–96

160. Kwon CS, Chen C, Wagner D (2005) Arabidopsis SPLAYED in dynamic control of stem cell fate in is a primary target for transcriptional regulation by WUSCHEL. Genes Dev 19:992–1003

161. Ogas J, Chen J-C, Sung ZR, Somerville C (1997) Cellular Differentiation Regulated by Gibberellin in the Arabidopsis thaliana pickleMutant. Science 277:91–94

162. Harding EW, Tang W, Nichols KW, Fernandez DE, Perry SE (2003) Expression and maintenance of embryogenic potential is enhanced through constitutive expression of AGAMOUS-like 15. Plant Physiol 133:653–663

163. Bayliss MW (1973) Origin of chromosome number variation in cultured plant cells. Nature 246:529–530

164. Gengenbach BG, Connelly JA, Pring DR, Conde MF (1981) Mitochondrial DNA variation in maize plants regenerated during tissue culture selection. Theor Appl Genet 59:161–167

165. Larkin PJ, Scowcroft WR (1981) Somaclonal variation –a novel source of variability from cell cultures for plant improvement. Theor Appl Genet 60:197–214

166. Kaeppler SM, Kaeppler HF, Rhee Y (2000) Epigenetic aspects of somaclonal variation in plants. Plant Mol Biol 43:179–188

167. Monk M (1990) Variation in epigenetic inheritance. Trends Genet 6:110–114

168. Larkin PJ, Ryan SA, Brettell RIS, Scrowcroft WR (1984) Heritable somaclonal variation in wheat. Theor Appl Genet 67:443–456

169. Lee M, Phillips RL (1988) The chromosomal basis of somaclonal variation. Annu Rev Plant Physiol Plant Mol Biol 39:413–437

170. Kaeppler SM, Phillips RL (1993) Tissue culture-induced DNA methylation variation in maize. Proc Natl Acad Sci (USA) 90:8773–8776

171. Bebeli PJ, Karp A, Kaltsikes PJ (1990) Somaclonal variation from cultured immature embryos of sister lines of rye differing in heterochromatic content. Genome 33:177–183

172. Skirvin RM, Coyner M, Norton MA, Motoike S, Gorvin D (2000) Somaclonal variation: do we know what causes it? AgBiotechNet 2:1–4

173. Orton TJ (1984) Case histories of genetic variability *in vitro*: celery. In: Cell culture and somatic cell genetics of plants. Vol. 3. Plant regeneration and genetic variability, Vasil IK (ed) Academic Press, Inc., Orlando, pp 245–366

174. Evans DA (1988) Applications of somaclonal variation. In: Biotechnology in Agriculture, Mizrahi A (ed) Alan R. Liss, Inc., New York 203–223

175. Van den Bulk RW, Löfer HJM, Lindhout WH, Koornneef M (1990) Somaclonal variation in tomato: effect of explant source and comparison with chemical mutagenesis. Theor Appl Genet 80:817–825

176. Novak FJ, Daskalov S, Brunner H, Nesticky M, Afza R, Dolezelova M, Lucretti S, Herichova A, Hermelin T (1988) Somatic embryogenesis in maize and comparison of genetic variability induced by gamma radiation and tissue culture techniques. J Plant Breed 101:66–79

177. Yang ZP, Yang XY, Huang DC (1998) Studies on somaclonal variants for resistance to scab in bread wheat (*Triticum aestivum* L.) through *in vitro* selection for tolerance to deoxynivalenol. Euphytica 101:213–219

178. Claxton JR, Arnold DL, Clarkson JM, Blakesley D (1998) The regeneration and screening of watercress somaclones for resistance to *Spongospora subterranea* f. sp. *nasturtii* and measurement of somaclonal variation. Plant Cell Tiss Org Cult 52:155–164

179. Ahmed KZ, Mesterhazy A, Bartok T, Sagi F (1996) *In vitro* techniques for selecting wheat (*Triticum aestivum* L) for *Fusarium*–resistance .2. Culture filtrate technique and inheritance of *Fusarium*–resistance in the somaclones. Euphytica 91:341–349

180. Muhammad AJ, Othman RY (2005) Charactherization of Fusarium wiltresistant and Fusarium wilt-susceptible somaclones of banana cultivar Rastali (Musa AAB) by random amplified polymorphic DNA and retrotransposon markers. Plant Molecular Biology Reporter 23:241–249

181. Bertin P, Kinet JM, Bouharmont J (1996) Heritable chilling tolerance improvement in rice through somaclonal variation and cell line selection. Aust J Bot 44:91–105

182. Bertin P, Bouharmont J, Kinet JM (1997) Somaclonal variation and improvement of chilling tolerance in rice: Changes in chilling–induced chlorophyll fluorescence. Crop Sci 37:1727–1735

183. Bertin P, Bouharmont J (1997) Use of somaclonal variation and *in vitro* selection for chilling tolerance improvement in rice. Euphytica 96:135–142

184. Mohamed MA, Harris PJC, Henderson J (2000) *In vitro* selection and characterisation of a drought tolerant clone of *Tagetes minuta*. Plant Sci 159:213–222

185. Bajji M, Bertin P, Lutts S, Kinet JM (2004) Evaluation of drought resistance-related traits in durum wheat somaclonal lines selected *in vitro*. Aust J Exp Agricul 44:27–35

186. Bertin P, Busogoro JP, Tilquin JP, Kinet JM, Bouharmont J (1996) Field evaluation and selection of rice somaclonal variants at different altitudes. Plant Breed 115:183–188

187. Lutts S, Kinet JM, Bouharmont J (1998) NaCl impact on somaclonal variation exhibited by tissue culture– derived fertile plants of rice (*Oryza sativa* L.). J Plant Physiol 152:92–103

188. Bariaud-Fontanel A, Tabata M (1988) Somaclonal variation in the berberine-producing capability of a culture strain of *Thalictrum minus*. Plant Cell Rep 7:206–209

189. Berlin J (1990) Screening and selection for variant cell lines with increased levels of secondary metabolites. In: Secondary Products from Plant Tissue Culture, Charlwood BV, Rhodes MJC (eds) Oxford University Press, Oxford 119–137

190. Dougall DK (1990) Somaclonal variation as a tool for the isolation of elite cell lines to produce secondary metabolites. In: Production of Secondary Metabolites from Plant Tissue Cultures and its Biotechnological Perspectives, Loyola-Vargas VM (ed) CICY, Merida, Yucatan, pp 122–137

191. Ravindra NS, Kulkarni RN, Gayathri MC, Ramesh S (2004) Somaclonal variation for some morphological traits, herb yield, essential oil contentand essential oil composition in an Indian cultivar of rose–scented geranium. Plant Breed 123:84–86

192. Bozorgipour R, Snape JW (1997) An assessment of somaclonal variation as a breeding tool for generating herbicide tolerant genotypes in wheat (*Triticum aestivum* L.). Euphytica 94:335–340

193. Jan VV, De Macedo CC, Kinet JM, Bouharmont J (1997) Selection of Al-resistant plants from a sensitive rice cultivar using somaclonal variation, *in vitro* and hydroponic cultures. Euphytica 97:303–310

194. Bidhan R, Asit BM (2005) Towards development of Al-toxicity tolerant lines in indica rice by exploiting somaclonal variation. Euphytica 145:221–227

195. Adkins SW, Shiraishi T, McComb JA, Ratanopol S, Kupkanchanakul T, Armstrong LJ, Schultz AL (1990) Somaclonal variation in rice-submergence tolerance and other agronomic characters. Physiol Plant 80:647–654

196. Blakeslee AF, Belling J, Farnham ME, Bergner AD (1922) A haploid mutant in the Jimson weed, "*Datura stramonium*". Science 55:646–647

197. Guha S, Maheshwari SC (1964) *In vitro* production of embryos from anthers of *Datura*. Nature 204:497

198. Guha S, Maheshwari SC (1966) Cell division and differentiation of embryos in the pollen grain of *Datura in vitro*. Nature 212:97–98

199. Germaná MA (2006) Doubled haploid production in fruit crops. Plant Cell Tiss Org Cult 86:131–146

200. Thomas WTB, Forster BP, Gertsson B (2003) Doubled haploids in breeding. In: Doubled haploid production in crop plants, a manual, Maluszynski M, Kasha KJ, Forster BP, Szarejko I (eds) Kluwer Academic Publishers, Dordrecht 337–349

201. Feiyu T, Yazhong T, Tianyong Z, Guoying W (2006) *In vitro* production of haploid and doubled haploid plants from pollinated ovaries of maize (*Zea mays*). Plant Cell Tiss Org Cult 84:100210–100214

202. Guangyuan H, Jinrui Z, Kexiu L, Zhiyong X, Mingjie C, Junli C, Yuesheng W, Guangxiao Y, Beáta B (2006) An improved system to establish highly embryo-

genic haploid cell and protoplast cultures from pollen calluses of maize (*Zea mays* L.). Plant Cell Tiss Org Cult 86:15–25

203. Loyola-Vargas VM, Vázquez-Flota FA (2006) An introduction to plant cell culture: Back to the future. In: Plant cell culture protocols, Loyola-Vargas VM, Vázquez-Flota FA (eds) Humana Press, Totowa, New Jersey, pp 1–8

204. Leckie F, Scragg AH, Cliffe KC (1990) The effect of continuous high shear stress on plant cell suspension cultures. In: Progress in plant cellular and molecular biology, Nijkamp HJJ, Van der Plas LHW, Van Aartrijk J (eds) Kluwer Academic Publishers, The Netherlands, pp 689–693

205. Dracup M (1991) Increasing salt tolerance of plants through cell culture requires greater understanding of tolerance mechanisms. Aust J Plant Physiol 18:1–15

206. Takeuchi Y, Komamine A (1982) Effects of culture conditions on cell division and composition of regenerated cell walls in *Vinca rosea* protoplasts. Plant Cell Physiol 23:249–255

207. Takeuchi Y, Komamine A (1981) Glucans in the cell walls regenerated from *Vinca rosea* protoplasts. Plant Cell Physiol 22:1585–1594

208. Takeuchi Y, Komamine A (1978) Composition of the cell wall formed protoplasts isolated from cell suspension cultures of *Vinca rosea*. Planta 140:227–232

209. Zenk MH (1991) Chasing the enzymes of secondary metabolism: Plant cell cultures as a pot of gold. Phytochemistry 30:3861–3863

210. Loyola-Vargas VM, Hernández-Sotomayor SMT (2003) Hairy root cultures of *Catharanthus roseus*: A model for primary and secondary metabolic studies. In: Plant Genetic Engineering Vol. 1: Applications and limitations, Singh RP, Jaiwal PK (eds) Sci Tech Publishing LLC, Houston, pp 297–315

211. Collin HA (2001) Secondary product formation in plant tissue cultures. Plant Growth Regul 34:119–134

212. Verpoorte R, Van der Heijden R, Memelink J (2000) Engineering the plant cell factory for secondary metabolite production. Transg Res 9:323–343

213. Shimazaki A, Ashihara H (1982) Adenine and guanine salvage in suspension cultured cells of *Catharanthus roseus*. Ann Bot 50:531–534

214. Hirose F, Ashihara H (1983) Comparison of purine metabolism in suspension cultured cells of different growth phases and stem tissue of *Catharanthus roseus*. Z Naturforsch [C] 38:375–381

215. Kartosentono S, Indrayanto G, Zaini NC (2002) The uptake of copper ions by cell suspension cultures of *Agave amaniensis*, and its effect on the growth, amino acids and hecogenin content. Plant Cell Tiss Org Cult 68:287–292

216. Paek KY, Chakrabarty D, Hahn EJ (2005) Application of bioreactor systems for large scale production of horticultural and medicinal plants. Plant Cell Tiss Org Cult 81:287–300

217. Ziv M (2005) Simple bioreactors for mass propagation of plants. Plant Cell Tiss Org Cult 81:277–285

218. Takayama S, Misawa M (1981) Mass propagation of Begoniahiemalis plantlet by shake culture. Plant Cell Physiol 22:461–467

219. Paek KY, Hahn E-J, Son SH (2001) Application of biorreactors for large-scale micropropagation systems of plants. In Vitro Cell Dev Biol -Plant 37:149–157

220. Kartha KK (1984) Elimination of viruses. In: Cell culture and somatic cell genetics of plants. Vol. 1. Laboratory procedures and their applications, Vasil IK (ed) Academic Press Inc., Orlando, pp 577–585

221. Warren G (1996) The regeneration of plants from cultured cells and tissues. In: Plant cell and tissue culture, Stafford A, Warren G (eds) John Wiley & Sons, England, pp 82–100

222. Verma N, Ram R, Hallan V, Kumar K, Zaidi AA (2004) Production of cucumber mosaic virus-free chrysanthemums by meristem tip culture. Crop Protection 23:469–473

223. Eisa S, Koyro HW, Kogel KH, Imani J (2005) Induction of somatic embryogenesis in cultured cells of *Chenopodium quinoa*. Plant Cell Tiss Org Cult 81:243–246

224. Katoh N, Yui M, Sato S, Shirai T, Yuasa H, Hagimori M (2004) Production of virus-free plants from virus-infected sweet pepper by *in vitro* grafting. Sci Hortic 100:1–6

225. Verma N, Ram R, Zaidi AA (2005) *In vitro* production of *Prunus* necrotic ringspot virus-free begonias through chemo- and thermotherapy. Sci Hortic 103:239–247

226. Torrance L (1998) Developments in serological methods to detect and identify plant viruses. Plant Cell Tiss Org Cult 52:27–32

227. Sharma DR, Kaur R, Kumar K (1996) Embryo rescue in plants – a review. Euphytica 89:325–337

228. Reed SM (2005) Embryo rescue. In: Plant development and biotechnology, Trigiano RN, Gray DJ (eds) CRC Press, Boca Raton, Florida 235–239

229. Stewart JM (1981) *In vitro* fertilization and embryo rescue. Env Exp Bot 21:301–315

230. Alan LM, Henning MJ (2003) Production of haploid and doubled haploid plants of melon (*Cucumis melo* L.) for use in breeding for multiple virus resistance. Plant Cell Rep 21:1121–1128

231. Martínez-Palacios A, Ortega-Larrocea MP, Chávez VM, Bye R (2003) Somatic embryogenesis and organogenesis of *Agave victoriae -reginae*: Considerations for its conservation. Plant Cell Tiss Org Cult 74:135–142

232. Manjkhola S, Dhar U, Joshi M (2006) Organogenesis, embryogenesis, and synthetic seed production in *Arnebia euchroma* - A critically endangered medicinal plant of the Himalaya. In Vitro Cell Dev Biol Plant 41:244–248

233. Moebius-Goldammer KG, Mata-Rosas M, Chávez-Avila VM (2003) Organogenesis and somatic embryogenesis in *Ariocarpus kotschoubeyanus* (Lem.) K. Schum. (Cactaceae), an endemic and endangered Mexican species. In Vitro Cell Dev Biol Plant 39:388–393

234. West FR Jr, Mika ES (1957) Synthesis of atropine by isolated roots and root–callus cultures of belladonna. Bot Gaz 119:50–54

235. Straus J (1959) Anthocyanin synthesis in corn endosperm tissue cultures 1. Identity of the pigments and general factors. Plant Physiol 34:536–541

236. Tulecke W, Nickell LG (1959) Production of large amounts of plant tissue by submerged culture. Science 130:863–864

237. Tabata M, Ogino T, Yoshioka K, Yoshikawa N, Hiraoka N (1978) Selection of cell lines with higher yield of secondary products. In: Frontiers of Plant Tissue Culture, Thorpe TA (ed) The International Association for Plant Tissue Culture, Calgary, Canada, pp 213–221

238. Fujita Y, Hara Y, Suga C, Marimoto T (1981) Production of shikonin derivatives by cell suspension cultures of *Lithospermum erythrorhizon*. II. A new medium for the production of shikonin derivatives. Plant Cell Rep 1:61–63

239. Hara Y, Morimoto T, Fujita Y (1987) Production of shikonin derivatives by cell suspension cultures of *Lithospermum erythrorhizon* V. Differences in the production between callus and suspension cultures. Plant Cell Rep 6:8–11

240. Fujita Y, Takahashi S, Yamada Y (1985) Selection of cell lines with high productivity of shikonin derivatives by protoplast culture of *Lithospermum erythrorhizon* cells. Agric Biol Chem 49:1755–1759

241. Mizukami H, Konoshima M, Tabata M (1977) Effect od nutritional factors on shikonin derivative formation in *Lithospermum* callus cultures. Phytochemistry 16:1183–1186

242. Widholm JM (1977) Selection and characterization of biochemical mutants. In: Plant tissue culture and its bio-technological application, Barz W, Reinhard E, Zenk MH (eds) Springer-Verlag, Berlin, pp 112–122

243. Eilert U (1998) Induction of alkaloid biosynthesis and accumulation in plants and *in vitro* cultures in response to elicitation. In: Alkaloids. Biochemistry, ecology,

and medicinal applications, Roberts MF, Wink M (eds) Plenum Press, New York, pp 219–238

244. Kurz WGW, Constabel F, Eilert U, Tyler RT (1988) Elicitor treatment: a method for metabolite production by plant cell cultures *in vitro*. In: Topics in Pharmaceutical Sciences 1987, Breimer DD, Speiser P (eds) Elsevier Science Publishers B. V., Amsterdam, pp 283–290

245. Ketchum REB, Gibson DM, Croteau RB, Shuler ML (1999) The kinetics of taxoid accumulation in cell suspension cultures of *Taxus* following elicitation with methyl jasmonate. Biotechnol Bioeng 62:97–105

246. Lee-Parsons CWT, Ertük S, Tengtrakool J (2004) Enhancement of ajmalicine production in *Catharanthus roseus* cell cultures with methyl jasmonate is dependent on timing and dosage of elicitation. Biotechnol Lett 26:1595–1599

247. Xu MJ, Dong JF, Zhu MY (2005) Nitric oxide mediates the fungal elicitor-induced hypericin production of *Hypericum perforatum* cell suspension cultures through a jasmonic-acid-dependent signal pathway. Plant Physiol 139:991–998

248. Brodelius P (1985) The potential role of immobilization in plant cell biotechnology. Trends Biotechnol 3:280–285

249. Yeoman MM (1987) Techniques, characteristics, properties, and commercial potential of immobilized plant cells. In: Cell culture and somatic cell genetics of plants. Vol. 4. Cell culture in phytochemistry, Constabel F, Vasil IK (eds) Academic Press, Co., San Diego, pp 197–215

250. Hughes EH, Hong SB, Gibson SI, Shanks JV, San KY (2004) Metabolic engineering of the indole pathway in *Catharanthus roseus* hairy roots and increased accumulation of tryptamine and serpentine. Metabolic Engineering 6:268–276

251. Verpoorte R, Memelink J (2002) Engineering secondary metabolite production in plants. Curr Opi Biotechnol 13:181–187

252. Ayora-Talavera T, Chappell J, Lozoya-Gloria E, Loyola-Vargas VM (2002) Overexpression in *Catharanthus roseus* hairy roots of a trucated hamster 3-hydroxy-3-methylglutaryl-CoA reductase gene. Appl Biochem Biotechnol 97:135–145

253. Rommens CM (2006) Kanamycin resistance in plants: an unexpected trait controlled by a potentially multifaceted gene. Trends Plant Sci 11:317–319

254. Nap JP, Metz PLJ, Escaler M, Conner AJ (2003) The release of genetically modified crops into the environment. Part I. Overview of current status and regulations. Plant J 33:1–18

255. Power JB, Cummind SE, Cocking EC (1970) Fusion of isolated protoplasts. Nature 225:1016–1018

256. Cocking EC (2000) Turning point article plant protoplasts. In Vitro Cell Dev Biol Plant 36:77–82

257. Davey MR, Cocking EC, Freeman J, Pearce N, Tudor I (1980) Transformation of petunia protoplasts by isolated *Agrobacterium* plasmids. Plant Sci Lett 18:307–313

258. Schell J, Van Montagu M, Holsters M, Zambryski P, Joos H, Inzé D, Herrera-Estrella L, Depicker A, De Block M, Caplan A, Dhaese P, Van Haute E, Hernalsteens JP, De Greve H, Leemans J, Deblaere R, Willmitzer L, Schröder J, Otten L (1983) Ti plasmids as experimental gene vectors for plants. In: Advances in gene technology: molecular genetics of plants and animals, Downey K, Voellmy RW, Ahmad F, Schultz J (eds) Academic Press, New York/London, pp 191–209

259. Miki B, McHugh S (2004) Selectable marker genes in transgenic plants: applications, alternatives and biosafety. J Biotechnol 107:193–232

260. Goldstein DA, Tinland B, Gilbertson LA, Staub JM, Bannon GA, Goodman RE, McCoy RL, Silvanovich A (2005) Human safety and genetically modified plants: a review of antibiotic resistance markers and future transformation selection technologies. Journal of Applied Microbiology 99:7–23

261. Lee M, Lee K, Lee J, Noh EW, Lee Y (2005) AtPDR12 contributes to lead resistance in *Arabidopsis*. Plant Physiol 138:827–836
262. Song W-Y, Soh EJ, Martinoia E, Lee YJ, Yang YY, Jasinski M, Forestier C, Hwang I, Lee Y (2003) Engineering tolerance and accumulation of lead and cadmium in transgenic plants. Nat Biotechnol 21:914–919
263. Zenk MH (1995) Chasing the enzymes of alkaloid biosytnhesis. In: Organic reactivity: Physical and biological aspects, Golding BT, Maskill H (eds) The Royal Society of Chemistry, Cambridge, pp 89–109
264. Verpoorte R, Van der Heijden R Memelink J (1998) Plant biotechnology and the production of alkaloids. Prospects of metabolic engineering. In: The Alkaloids. Vol. 50, Cordell GA (ed) Academic Press, San Diego, pp 453–508
265. Choi SM, Son SH, Yun SR, Kwon OW, Seon JH, Paek KY (2000) Pilot–scale culture of adventitious roots of ginseng in a bioreactor system. Plant Cell Tiss Org Cult 62:187–193

51

Stem Cells and Regenerative Medicine

Mohan C. Vemuri and Chellu S. Chetty

1. Introduction

Stem cells and regenerative medicine is a rapidly progressing science that addresses the use of stem cells via cell therapy for human diseases. Successful use of stem cells in regenerative medicine depends on two important features of stem cells; a) stem cells can proliferate and self renew almost indefinitely, and b) they can differentiate into specialized cell types that make up tissues such as pancreas, heart, liver, blood, and others. Further, stem cells can be engineered to replace worn-out cells and to regenerate damaged tissue. These advances open up new ways of stem cell based treatment through regenerative medicine and tissue engineering.

2. Types of Stem Cells

There are two types of stem cells, embryonic stem cells and adult stem cells. Embryonic stem cells (ESC), derived from an early stage embryo such as blastocyst are the most primitive, unspecialized, and pluripotent cells. Pluripotent stem cells can become any type of cell in the epidermal, endodermal, and mesodermal cell lineages, including germ cells but they can not grow into a whole organism. Adult stem cells are isolated from the tissues of aborted fetuses, umbilical cord blood, or living children and adults. Because they are isolated from tissues of an organism, they are termed tissue specific adult stem cells (ASC) or nonembryonic stem cells. Unlike ESCs, adult stem cells are only multipotent and turn into fewer cell types. Multipotent stem cells can form multiple lineages that constitute an entire tissue or tissues, such as hematopoietic stem cells.

The self renewal capacity of ESCs is relatively high compared to tissue specific adult stem cells. Stem cell numbers decline and the multilineage potential gets restricted as the embryo grows into an offspring and further into an adult. This is a limitation in harvesting the full potential of stem cells. Another hurdle is to identify the stem cells and grow them in large numbers with out altering their stem cell properties and capabilities for clinical transplantation. This particular aspect has been the main focus of current research and has tremendous developments, enabling stem cells to enter the next stage of clinical trials.

From: *Molecular Biomethods Handbook, 2nd Edition.*
Edited by: J. M. Walker and R. Rapley © Humana Press, Totowa, NJ

3. Human Embryonic Stem Cells (hESCs)

Embryonic stem cells are derived from the inner cell mass of a blastocyst, when the human embryo consists of about 150 cells and are generally cultured on a layer of mitotically inactive mouse embryonic fibroblast cells to inhibit spontaneous differentiation. The first human ESC lines were derived by a group of scientists at the University of Wisconsin at Madison led by James Thomson (1). Human ESCs at this early developmental stage are pluripotent and contain the versatile potential to turn into any of the 200 cell types of human body. Further, hESCs can remain in an undifferentiated state and divide indefinitely if they are grown in the presence of appropriate chemokines and cytokines (2,3). This combination of unlimited "self-renewal" and ability to differentiate into mature cell types of the three primary germ layers makes hESCs an attractive source for identical, well-defined and genomically characterized cells for regenerative cell therapy.

3.1. Human ESC Culture Expansion

The basic composition of culture media used in the derivation methodology and maintenance of hESCs, comprises a mix of Dulbecco's Modified Eagle's Media (DMEM) or Knock-Out™ DMEM (KO-DMEM), or Dulbecco's Modified Eagle's Media/F12 (DME/F12) with nonessential amino acids, β-mercaptoethanol and L-glutamine in the presence of bovine sera. The choice of serum includes either 10–15% fetal bovine serum (FBS), ES cell-tested FBS, or Knock-Out™ Serum Replacement (KO-SR). Some recent studies suggest the addition of FGF2 to basal media to facilitate hESC maintenance (4,5) in serum free culture media. This step is a major advance in developing simplified hESC culture systems.

3.2. Human ESC Phenotype

Human ESCs tend to grow as compact colonies with high nucleus to cytoplasm ratios. Expression of stem cell specific markers such as the transcription factors oct-4, nanog, TRA-1-60, TRA-1-81, and the cell surface markers SSEA-3 and SSEA-4 in humans is correlated with pluripotency (6). These markers are important for monitoring and assessing pluripotency of hESCs when testing different culture conditions (**Fig. 51.1**). The loss of pluripotency

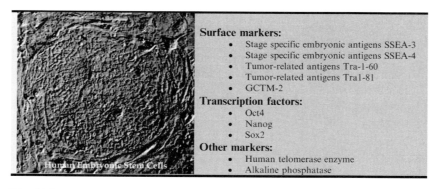

Fig. 51.1. Human embryonic stem cell markers

markers warrants a greater consideration towards possible differentiation of stem cells into tissue specific lineages.

4. Human Adult Stem Cells

Adult stem cells are harvested from aborted fetuses, umbilical cord blood, or adult tissues. During development, stem cells progress towards cell specific lineages through progenitors, mature into differentiated cell types, and assemble to form tissues. Current studies show that tissue specific stem cells are isolated from bone marrow, specific regions in brain, blood vessels, skin, cornea and retina of the eye, mammary gland, endocrine gland, prostate, lung, intestine lining, and other adult tissues *(7)*. These adult stem cell populations exhibit self renewal, proliferation, differentiation properties in defined culture conditions. They can also be mobilized from stem cell "niches" through injury or wounding and in disease conditions. A major limitation of adult stem cells is their inability to self renew indefinitely. In addition, their potential for proliferation and differentiation diminishes with age and differs significantly among tissue specific adult stem cell types. Despite such limitations, continuing studies on hematopoietic, mesenchymal and neural adult stem cells provide valuable insights into the use of stem cell based therapies through transplantation.

5. Hematopoietic Stem Cells

Hematopoietic stem cells (HSC) are isolated from bone marrow and are the primary adult stem cell candidates currently used to treat various hematological diseases including malignancies. HSCs give rise to all the blood lineages, including myeloid, lymphoid, and erythroid cell types *(8)*. Repopulation of the hematopoietic compartment following myelo-ablative chemotherapy and radiation uses HSCs derived either directly from bone marrow or from mobilized peripheral blood *(9)*. Depending on their transplantational efficiency to repopulate the bone marrow, they are also categorized into long-term (LT-HSCs) or short-term (ST-HSCs) self renewing hematopoietic stem cells. LT-HSCs are considered most primitive, while ST-HSCs are in transition to progenitor cell state. LT-HSCs have been shown to be effective in whole bone marrow and immune reconstitution in animal models and in human bone marrow transplantation studies *(10–12)*. ST-HSCs are also effective in transplantation, but the response could be transient and might need recurring regimens of transplantation. Currently, culture conditions that allow HSCs to grow in large numbers and remain as primitive stem cells without differentiation are considerable challenges for the clinical potential of HSCs *(13–15)*.

5.1. HSC Culture Expansion

Efficient methods to expand HSCs in culture can significantly enhance the therapeutic application of this cell type and reduce the burden of bone marrow transplants. Combination of growth factors utilized for ex vivo expansion include Flt-3 Ligand/TPO/IL-6 /IL-11, IL-3/TPO/SCF/Flt-3 Ligand2, IL-3/GCSF/SCF3, and SCF/G-CSF/MGDF. Recent

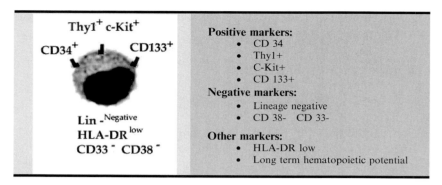

Fig. 51.2. Human hematopoietic stem cell markers

studies suggest that the cytokine leukemia inhibitory factor (LIF) plays an important role in the development of ex vivo expansion systems for murine and human HSCs.

5.2. HSC Phenotype

Presence of cell surface glycoprotein CD34 and further fractionation of CD34+ population into lineage committed progenitors and primitive HSCs is the most widely accepted criteria for the prospective isolation of human HSCs. Lineage-committed cells are depleted using a combination of markers (Lineage negative or Lin-). More recently, it has been proposed that a distinct panel of species specific markers (**Fig. 51.2**) may improve the accuracy of HSC identification and isolation from human tissues (*16,17*).

6. Multipotent Mesenchymal Stromal Cells (MSC)

Bone marrow, in addition to HSCs that form blood and immune cells, also contains stromal stem cells, referred as MSCs (*18*). Although stroma was originally considered to be structural supportive frame work for hematopoietic system, ongoing studies show that the MSCs derived from stroma are distinctly different from the HSC fraction. MSCs can give rise to a wide array of lineages necessary for connective tissue formation including bone, fat, and vascular tissue (*19,20*). In addition, they are currently evaluated in combination with HSCs to overcome allogenic barriers of immune rejection in bone marrow transplantation (*21*). Human MSCs, in a xenogeneic fetal transplant model (*22*) engraft and survive in the developing sheep fetus. Further, the human MSCs are not rejected when implanted into immunocompetent fetal sheep. These and other studies have established that MSCs possess important therapeutic potential for stromal reconstitution, gene therapy, and bone and cartilage repair (*19*).

6.1. Culture Expansion of Human Bone Marrow Derived MSCs

MSCs comprise a mere 0.01–0.0001% of total bone marrow nucleated cells and need in vitro cell culture expansion to get sufficient numbers for clinical applications. Standard culture expansion protocols for MSCs involve attachment of the cells to the plastic surface of a culture flask (*23*). The attached cells following an initial lag phase expand through rapid divisions and turn confluent before they enter into stationary phase. Morphologically they are spindle shaped and resemble fibroblasts in culture, but when confluent they acquire a flattened morphology. MSC-culture media comprises a basal medium, qualified fetal calf serum (FCS), and addition of different growth factors like TGF β, hydrocortisone, and FGF-2 *(24)*. A recent study compared the composition of different media and how they enable optimal growth of human MSCs in a culture. The study suggests that Modified Eagle Medium alpha (a-MEM) is the optimal type of basal medium and that stable glutamine and low glucose concentration favor MSC-isolation and in vitro expansion *(25)*.

6.2. MSC Phenotype

MSCs are increasingly utilized in a wide variety of biomedical applications *(25,26)*. However among groups of investigators, there is a lack of common consensus on the criteria of a MSC. MSC identification relies on a combination of positively and negatively expressed markers that facilitates their characterization among other cellular subsets (**Fig. 51.3**). A recent publication from the International Society of Cellular Therapy has come out with three minimal criteria for defining human "multipotent mesenchymal stromal cells" (MSC). First, MSC must be plastic-adherent when maintained in standard culture conditions. Second, MSC must express CD105, CD73, and CD90, and lack CD45, CD34, CD14 (or CD11b), CD79a (or CD19), and HLA-DR surface molecules. Lastly, MSC must differentiate to osteoblasts, adipocytes, and chondroblasts in vitro *(27)*.

7. Neural Stem Cells (NSC)

NSCs are defined an undifferentiated population of cells that self renew continuously with an ability to differentiate into multipotential mature cell lineages of both neuronal and glial subpopulations. As undifferentiated NSCs progress towards mature cell types, they turn into lineage specific neural precursor cells (NPC) that are restricted to one of many distinct lineages such as neurons or astrocytes *(28,29)*. NSCs and NPCs are a potential cell source for cell based therapies in neurodegenerative disorders such as Parkinson's disease or multiple sclerosis *(30)*. However,

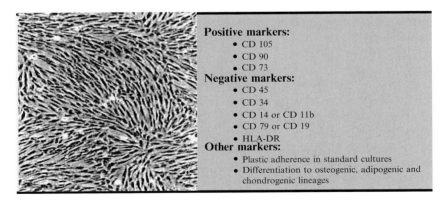

Positive markers:
- CD 105
- CD 90
- CD 73

Negative markers:
- CD 45
- CD 34
- CD 14 or CD 11b
- CD 79 or CD 19
- HLA-DR

Other markers:
- Plastic adherence in standard cultures
- Differentiation to osteogenic, adipogenic and chondrogenic lineages

Fig. 51.3. Human multipotent mesenchymal stromal cell markers

their limited number in the developing fetus and lack of proper methods to isolate subpopulations from more differentiated cell types in CNS are major challenges that are currently investigated by researchers *(31)*. Culture expansion strategies to overcome their limited number and cell markers appropriate for selective isolation of NSC/NPC subtypes is the key for generating clinical grade NSCs *(32)*.

7.1. NSC Culture Expansion

Current methods allow extended human NSC culture periods of up to 2 yr and if the cultures are derived from embryonic or fetal tissues, they are expanded a million fold in vitro *(33)*. Although these developments help push forward cell therapy based clinical trials, the limited life span of these cells in a culture dish poses a restraint *(34)*. Methods are developed to culture hNSCs, but usually the critical ingredients of a good culture medium involve the use of epidermal growth factor (EGF), fibroblast growth factor (FGF)-2, and the NSCs are cultured as floating aggregates termed neurospheres *(35)*. Cell line, hNS1 (formerly called HNSC.100, a model cell line of hNSCs) is a human embryonic forebrain-derived, multipotent, clonal cell line can grow in a chemically defined HSC medium supplemented with 20 ng/ml each of EGF and FGF-2 *(32)*.

7.2. NSC Phenotype

Undifferentiated NSCs express high levels of the intermediate filament proteins vimentin and nestin. Additionally, proliferating NSCs usually show little or no expression of mature neural or glial markers. Several subtypes of NSCs exist, depending on when and where these cells are isolated *(36)*. Neuroepithelial stem cells are the earliest form and can be directed to different neural fates with signaling molecules *(37,38)*. Neuroepithelial stem cells, unlike neurosphere-forming stem cells, are harvested as a relatively pure homogenous population and can serve as useful control for studies on stem cell markers. In addition to the neurosphere forming assays, expression of Sox2, Sox3, musashi, MCM-2, bmi1, prominin-1, and nestin without the expression of neuronal and glial markers is generally accepted as NSC phenotype *(39)*. In addition, integrin subunits α6 and β1 are highly expressed on human neural precursors. NSC and NPC subtypes can selectively be identified and prospectively isolated using cell specific markers (**Fig. 51.4**).

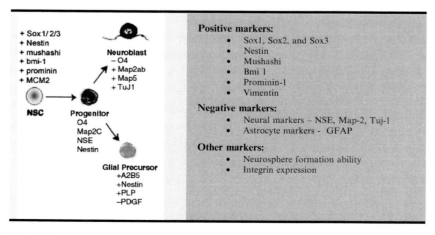

Fig. 51.4. Human Neural Stem Cell Markers

Table 51.1. Some gene therapy applications for stem cells.

Stem cell	Gene	Stem cell therapy application
HSC	Phox	Chronic granulomatous disease
	MGMT	Bone marrow protection-chemoprotection
	Globins	Thallesemias, Sickle Cell Anemia
MSC	Collagen	Osteogenesis Imperfecta
	Erythropoietin	Anemia
	Insulin	Diabetes
	several	Secreted therapeutic proteins
	Dystrophin?	Muscular Dystrophy
NSC	Unknown	Parkinson's disease, other neurodegenerative
hESC	Fetal genes	Theoretical / unlimited possibilities in review

8. Stem Cell Therapy Applications in Human Diseases

Some concerns exist, although advances in research in animal models demonstrate positive potential of stem cell therapies for human diseases *(40,41)*. If the disease can be identified early during development, interventional stem cell therapy can correct at fetal stages *(42)*. It offers a distinct advantage when coupled with fetal disease screening and genetic counseling. Selective gene therapy applications for stem cells are being studied (**Table 51.1**). However, the only human stem cell used in gene therapy trials so far is the hematopoietic stem cell.

9. Hematological Malignancies and Blood Diseases

Successful stem cell therapy is achieved with adult bone marrow transplantation for leukemia and lymphoma. It is now believed that treatment of selective inherited blood disorders such as hemophilia, anemia, inborn errors of metabolism, and autoimmune diseases can greatly benefit from stem cell therapy *(43,44)*. Bone marrow transplantation is done now as a transplant of HSCs collected from the peripheral blood of matched donor, usually a sister or a brother *(45)*. One of the major limitations in this type of therapy is the low number of stem cells that could be harvested from a single donor. Cord blood stem cells and hESCs are proving to be alternative resources. Establishment of cord blood banks and refinement of methods in cord blood stem cell isolation is expected to considerably increase the use of even allogenic HSCs for transplantation.

10. Neurological Diseases and Spinal Cord Lesions

Parkinson's disease is one of the major neurological ailments in which dopamine neurons are lost in a specific area of the brain called, the substantia nigra. Depending on the number of neurons lost and the extent of the disease development owing to the slow death of dopaminergic neurons, the disease intensity could vary from moderate shaking of head, hands, and legs to severe uncontrollable movement disorder, called as dyskinesia. Stem cells injected into the brains of mice with disease similar to Parkinson's disease resulted in the improvement of their symptoms. Current advances in stem cell research also have developed methods to turn hESCs or NSCs into dopamine neurons. These culture methods can generate large number of dopamine precursor cells for replacement therapy in Parkinson's disease patients (46). Dopamine neurons derived in vitro from hESCs (47) show molecular and functional properties comparable to dopamine neurons, in vivo, including the secretion of dopamine and elicit a neurophysiological signal that is critical for functional restorative therapy (48). Fetal tissue transplants in patients with Parkinson's disease showed encouraging and consistent results, suggesting the clinical utility of embryonic/fetal stem cells, but still need refinements as human clinical trials resulted in increased dyskinesia in small number of human patients (49,50). Preclinical studies with autologous olfactory ensheathing stem cells show increased functional recovery in the treatment of spinal cord lesions. Promising stem cell treatments are on the horizon with human fetal NPCs in Huntington disease clinical trials (51), neuroblastoma and glioma in children, oligodendrocyte precursors for myelin based diseases (52). The risks associated with stem cell transplantation trials are difficult to assess, but have not become overtly apparent throughout preclinical investigations. Other conditions in which stem cell therapy is being explored include corneal, retinal lesions, motor neuron disease, cerebrovascular disease, Alzheimer disease, and muscular dystrophy.

11. Ischemic Heart Disease

Researchers are working toward using stem cells to replace damaged heart cells and restore cardiac function (53). Both adult and ESCs are used in these studies. The cells that were transplanted include CD34+ cells from peripheral blood, and MSCs from bone marrow (54). In patients with heart failure, myoblast transplantation is emerging as a therapeutical option to speed up the function of remaining myocytes (55). Both skeletal myoblasts and autologous bone marrow transplantation have entered into Phase 1 safety studies in humans and are backed by extensive studies in animals. These studies show that the procedure is safe in humans and that it leads to improved myocardial function. Phase 1 trials indicate relative safety while phase II/III are currently underway to determine the extended clinical benefit. An extensive review on clinical trials to improve myocyte function in human heart failure patients confirms the great potential of stem cell therapy for ischemic heart disease (56,57). The stem cell therapies are timely and appropriate as the incidence of heart failure cases is reaching to an alarming epidemic proportion.

12. Stem Cells to Treat Diabetes

Diabetes is caused by the destruction of insulin producing β-islet cells of the pancreas (type I) or owing to insulin receptor resistance (type II). Current approaches using stem cells are focused on generating β-islet cells ex vivo suitable for transplantation and to stimulate the endogenous production of β-islet cells in the pancreas (58). Culture methods are currently available to differentiate hESCs into insulin-producing beta-cells (59). The insulin content of one million stem cell derived insulin positive cells is about 200 ng, whereas the insulin content of normal islets is about 10 μg per million cells. Stem cell derived insulin positive cells have 50 times less insulin per cell than normal cells. Therefore, it is necessary to conduct further studies that will enhance insulin production and regulate its response to physiological glucose concentration, before stem cells are used for treating diabetes.

13. The Future with Stem Cells

Stem cells are at the frontier in therapeutics as part of a multidisciplinary approach of cell therapy, gene therapy and regenerative medicine *(60,61)*. The extraordinary research done with stem cells has come a long way, and practical utility of stem cells in clinical settings can only be realized through intensive and additional studies on all types of stem cells. It is important to be able to direct the differentiation of pure cell populations in large quantities and safety concerns must be met, as well. The hESCs should not cause teratomas or carcinomas when transplanted in vivo or immunologically rejected. To have ESCs available for research or clinical purposes, moral and bioethical aspects should be taken into consideration. A great deal of basic research needs to be continued to explore the full potential of stem cells in regenerative medicine for efficient and effective ways to treat diseases.

Acknowledgments: The authors thank Divya Vemuri for reading and editing the manuscript.

References

1. Thomson JA, Itskovitz-Eldor J, Shapiro SS et al (1998) Embryonic stem cell lines derived from human blastocysts. Science 282:1145–1147
2. Vallier L, Alexander M, Pedersen RA (2005) Activin/Nodal and FGF pathways cooperate to maintain pluripotency of human embryonic stem cells. J Cell Sci 118:4495–4509
3. Levenstein ME, Ludwig TE, Xu RH et al (2006) Basic fibroblast growth factor support of human embryonic stem cell self-renewal. Stem Cells 24:568–574
4. Wang G, Zhang H, Zhao Y et al (2005) Noggin and bFGF cooperate to maintain the pluripotency of human embryonic stem cells in the absence of feeder layers. Biochem Biophys Res Commun 330:934–42
5. Xu C, Rosler E, Jiang J et al (2005) Basic fibroblast growth factor supports undifferentiated human embryonic stem cell growth without conditioned medium. Stem Cells 23:315–323
6. Hoffman LM, Carpenter MK (2005) Characterization and culture of human embryonic stem cells. Nat Biotechnol 23:699–708
7. Terskikh AV, Bryant PJ, Schwartz PH (2006) Mammalian stem cells. Pediatr Res 59:13R–20R
8. Bryder D, Rossi DJ, Weissman IL (2006) Hematopoietic stem cells: the paradigmatic tissue-specific stem cell. Am J Pathol 169:338–346
9. Bhattacharya D, Rossi DJ, Bryder D et al (2006) Purified hematopoietic stem cell engraftment of rare niches corrects severe lymphoid deficiencies without host conditioning. J Exp Med 203:73–85
10. Bhattacharya D, Bryder D, Rossi DJ et al (2006) Rapid lymphocyte reconstitution of unconditioned immunodeficient mice with non-self-renewing multipotent hematopoietic progenitors. Cell Cycle 5:1135–1139

11. Parkman R, Cohen G, Carter SL et al (2006) Successful immune reconstitution decreases leukemic relapse and improves survival in recipients of unrelated cord blood transplantation. Biol Blood Marrow Transplant 12:919–927

12. Crooks GM, Weinberg K, Mackall C (2006) Immune reconstitution: from stem cells to lymphocytes. Biol Blood Marrow Transplant 12:42–46

13. Kirouac DC, Zandstra PW (2006) Understanding cellular networks to improve hematopoietic stem cell expansion cultures. Curr Opin Biotechnol 17:538–547

14. Suzuki T, Yokoyama Y, Kumano K et al (2006) Highly efficient ex vivo expansion of human hematopoietic stem cells using Delta11-Fc chimeric protein. Stem Cells 24:2456–2465

15. Madlambayan GJ, Rogers I, Purpura KA et al (2006) Clinically relevant expansion of hematopoietic stem cells with conserved function in a single-use, closed-system bioprocess. Biol Blood Marrow Transplant 12:1020–1030

16. Yao CL, Feng YH, Lin XZ et al (2006) Characterization of serum-free ex vivo-expanded hematopoietic stem cells derived from human umbilical cord blood CD133(+) cells. Stem Cells Dev 15:70–78

17. Gordon MY, Levicar N, Pai M et al (2006) Characterization and clinical application of human CD34+ stem/progenitor cell populations mobilized into the blood by granulocyte colony-stimulating factor. Stem Cells 24:1822–1830

18. Majumdar MK, Keane-Moore M, Buyaner D et al (2003) Characterization and functionality of cell surface molecules on human mesenchymal stem cells. J Biomed Sci 10:228–241

19. Magne D, Vinatier C, Julien M et al (2005) Mesenchymal stem cell therapy to rebuild cartilage. Trends Mol Med 11:519–526

20. Tocci A, Forte L (2003) Mesenchymal stem cell: use and perspectives. Hematol J 4:92–6

21. Aggarwal S, Pittenger MF (2005) Human mesenchymal stem cells modulate allogeneic immune cell responses. Blood 105:1815–1822

22. Liechty KW, Mackenzie TC, Shaaban AF et al (2000) Human mesenchymal stem cells engraft and demonstrate site-specific differentiation after in utero transplantation in sheep. Nat Med 6:1282–1286

23. Meuleman N, Tondreau T, Delforge A et al (2006) Human marrow mesenchymal stem cell culture: serum-free medium allows better expansion than classical alpha-MEM medium. Eur J Haematol 76:309–316

24. Muller I, Kordowich S, Holzwarth C et al (2006) Animal serum-free culture conditions for isolation and expansion of multipotent mesenchymal stromal cells from human BM. Cytotherapy 8:437–444

25. Sotiropoulou PA, Perez SA, Salagianni M et al (2006) Characterization of the optimal culture conditions for clinical scale production of human mesenchymal stem cells. Stem Cells 24:462–471

26. Dominici M, Hofmann TJ, Horwitz EM (2001) Bone marrow mesenchymal cells: biological properties and clinical applications. J Biol Regul Homeost Agents 15:28–37

27. Dominici M, Le Blanc K, Mueller I et al (2006) Minimal criteria for defining multipotent mesenchymal stromal cells. The International Society for Cellular Therapy position statement. Cytotherapy 8:315–317

28. Martinez-Serrano A, Rubio FJ, Navarro B et al (2001) Human neural stem and progenitor cells: in vitro and in vivo properties, and potential for gene therapy and cell replacement in the CNS. Curr Gene Ther 1:279–299

29. Merkle FT, Alvarez-Buylla A (2006) Neural stem cells in mammalian development. Curr Opin Cell Biol 18:704–709

30. Galvin KA, Jones DG (2002) Adult human neural stem cells for cell-replacement therapies in the central nervous system. Med J Aust 177:316–318

31. Vescovi AL, Parati EA, Gritti A et al (1999) Isolation and cloning of multipotential stem cells from the embryonic human CNS and establishment of transplantable human neural stem cell lines by epigenetic stimulation. Exp Neurol 156:71–83

32. Villa A, Snyder EY, Vescovi A et al (2000) Establishment and properties of a growth factor-dependent, perpetual neural stem cell line from the human CNS. Exp Neurol 161:67–84

33. Svendsen CN, Ter Borg MG, Armstrong RJ et al (1998) A new method for the rapid and long term growth of human neural precursor cells. J Neurosci Methods 85:141–152

34. Cai J, Limke TL, Ginis I et al (2003) Identifying and tracking neural stem cells. Blood Cells Mol Dis 31:18–27

35. Mori H, Ninomiya K, Kino-Oka M et al (2006) Effect of neurosphere size on the growth rate of human neural stem/progenitor cells. J Neurosci Res 84:1682–1691

36. Ellis P, Fagan BM, Magness ST et al (2004) SOX2, a persistent marker for multipotential neural stem cells derived from embryonic stem cells, the embryo or the adult. Dev Neurosci 26:148–165

37. Dupin E, Real C, Ledouarin N. (2001) The neural crest stem cells: control of neural crest cell fate and plasticity by endothelin-3. An Acad Bras Cienc 73:533–545

38. Moody SA, Je HS (2002) Neural induction, neural fate stabilization, and neural stem cells. Scientific WorldJournal 2:1147–1166

39. Cai J, Shin S, Wright L et al (2006) Massively parallel signature sequencing profiling of fetal human neural precursor cells. Stem Cells Dev 15:232–244

40. Kassem M (2006) Stem cells: potential therapy for age-related diseases. Ann N Y Acad Sci 1067:436–442

41. Yates F, Daley GQ (2006) Progress and prospects: gene transfer into embryonic stem cells. Gene Ther 13:1431–1439

42. Peranteau WH, Endo M, Adibe OO et al (2006) CD26 inhibition enhances allogeneic donor cell homing and engraftment after in utero hematopoietic cell transplantation. Blood 108:4268–4274

43. Tuch BE (2006) Stem cells – a clinical update. Aust Fam Physician 35:719–721

44. Van Laar JM, Tyndall A (2006) Adult stem cells in the treatment of autoimmune diseases. Rheumatology (Oxford) 45:1187–1193

45. Eapen M, Rubinstein P, Zhang MJ et al (2007) Comparable long-term survival after unrelated and HLA-matched sibling donor hematopoietic stem cell transplantations for acute leukemia in children younger than 18 months. J Clin Oncol 24:145–151

46. Paul G, Ahn YH, Li JY et al (2006) Transplantation in Parkinson's disease: the future looks bright. Adv Exp Med Biol 557:221–248

47. Iacovitti L, Donaldson AE, Marshall CE et al (2007) A protocol for the differentiation of human embryonic stem cells into dopaminergic neurons using only chemically defined human additives: studies in vitro and in vivo. Brain Res 112:19–25

48. Goldman SA, Windrem MS (2006) Cell replacement therapy in neurological disease. Philos Trans R Soc Lond B Biol Sci 361:1463–1475

49. Snyder BJ, Olanow CW (2005) Stem cell treatment for Parkinson's disease: an update for 2005 Curr Opin Neurol 18:376–385

50. Correia AS, Anisimov SV, Li JY et al (2005) Stem cell-based therapy for Parkinson's disease. Ann Med 37:487–498

51. Pineda JR, Rubio N, Akerud P et al (2007) Neuroprotection by GDNF-secreting stem cells in a Huntington's disease model: optical neuroimage tracking of brain-grafted cells. Gene Ther 14:118–128

52. Okano H (2006) Adult neural stem cells and central nervous system repair. Ernst Schering Res Found Workshop 215–228

53. Torella D, Ellison GM, Mendez-Ferrer S et al (2006) Resident human cardiac stem cells: role in cardiac cellular homeostasis and potential for myocardial regeneration. Nat Clin Pract Cardiovasc Med 3 Suppl 1:S8–13

54. Boyle AJ, Whitbourn R, Schlicht S et al (2006) Intra-coronary high-dose CD34+ stem cells in patients with chronic ischemic heart disease: a 12-month follow-up. Int J Cardiol 109:21–27

55. Gallo P, Peschle C, Condorelli G (2006) Sources of cardiomyocytes for stem cell therapy: an update. Pediatr Res 59:79R–83R

56. Saha M, Ferro A (2006) Cardiac stem cell therapy: present and future. Br J Clin Pharmacol 61:727–729
57. Puceat M (2006) Stem cell therapy in heart failure: where do we stand and where are we heading? Heart Fail Monit 5:44–49
58. Miszta-Lane H, Mirbolooki M, James Shapiro AM et al (2006) Stem cell sources for clinical islet transplantation in type 1 diabetes: embryonic and adult stem cells. Med Hypotheses 67:909–913
59. Schroeder IS, Kania G, Blyszczuk P et al (2006) Insulin-producing cells. Methods Enzymol 418:315–333
60. Sanchez PL, San Roman JA, Villa A et al (2006) Contemplating the bright future of stem cell therapy for cardiovascular disease. Nat Clin Pract Cardiovasc Med 3 Suppl 1:S138–151
61. Caplice NM (2006) The future of cell therapy for acute myocardial infarction. Nat Clin Pract Cardiovasc Med 3 Suppl 1:S129–132

52

Cryopreservation

Conservation of Bioresources at Ultra Low Temperatures

John G. Day, Keith C. Harding, Jayanthi Nadarajan, and Erica E. Benson

Summary Cryopreservation is the ultra-low temperature storage (usually in liquid nitrogen at ca. −135 to −196°C) of living cells, tissues and organs capable of resuming normal functions after retrieval from a cryobank. This chapter explains the basic principles of cryopreservation with respect to strategies currently used to cryoprotect the diverse biological materials held in cryogenic storage. Approaches used to minimize or obviate the lethal and sublethal effects of cryoinjury are particularly highlighted. Examples of how cryopreservation has been universally applied to safeguard and preserve the wide spectrum of biological resources used in agriculture, biotechnology, healthcare, and biodiversity conservation are summarized and general guidance is offered for the management of bioresources in cryobanks.

Keywords Biological resource center; cryoinjury; cryopreservation; vitrification.

1. Introduction

Survival at low temperatures is found in nature amongst diverse organisms *(1,2)*. The recent sequencing *(3)* of the Arctic marine psychrophile, *Colwellia psychrerythraea* suggests tolerance to cold may be conferred by complex and synergistic molecular adaptations rather than specific genes *per se*. Understanding survival mechanisms in both natural (e.g., permafrost) and man-made cryobanks is important for environmental security and the sustainable use of biological resources that benefit mankind. Low temperatures slow metabolism and under appropriate conditions enhance longevity and confer stability on living cells. These attributes have been widely exploited by cryoconservationists and medical practitioners who have a requirement to secure viable biological resources in a stable condition. *In vitro* fertilization (IVF) and transplant organ surgery are examples of applications in which cells and tissues are preserved for short to extended periods in liquid nitrogen (LN) or low temperature refrigerators. Alternatives to cryogenic storage such as the serial subculture of actively growing cells in culture collections do not bestow the same level of stability and security as they risk genetic selection, instability,

From: *Molecular Biomethods Handbook, 2nd Edition.*
Edited by: J. M. Walker and R. Rapley © Humana Press, Totowa, NJ

loss of totipotency, and contamination. Moreover, maintenance of active cultures is costly, time consuming and resources inefficient for many types of biological samples. In these cases, there are no practicable alternatives to cryopreservation. This is true for human and animal gametes and embryos, recalcitrant tropical forest tree seeds and vegetatively propagated crop plant germplasm. Thus, cryopreservation in the liquid and vapor state of liquid nitrogen is the main focus of this chapter. Successful cryogenic storage in LN cryobanks is dependent upon the use of cryoprotective strategies and understanding the basic principles of cryobiology is fundamental in their development.

1.1. Historical Perspectives of Cryopreservation

Advances in cryopreservation have been driven by discoveries and technological inventions arising from the convergence of disparate disciplines. Current progress in contemporary cryobiological research would not have been possible without knowledge of the biophysical phenomena pertaining to the behavior of water, nature's solvent. The complex transitional changes of H_2O at low temperatures is a major determinant of survival and the efficacy of cryoprotection is largely determined by its unique chemical, thermal, colligative, and osmotic properties. Charting the historical progress of cryopreservation highlights developments across many research disciplines (**Table 52.1** and associated bibliography) and it is beyond the scope of this chapter to comprehensively cover them. Newcomers to cryobiology are advised to explore historical progress in an interdisciplinary context and will find that many of the field's most significant early advances remain relevant today.

1.2. Cryopreservation Theory and Practice

The development of robust cryopreservation protocols for a wide range of biological diversity is a major challenge best approached by applying fundamental theory to a practical framework, with due consideration of the physiological complexity of the taxa concerned (**Tables 52.2 and 52.3**) and the cryoprotective parameters to ensure their survival. Despite the vast diversity of the biological materials that have been successfully cryopreserved (**Table 52.2**) all storage protocols are underpinned by a generic knowledge of: (I) water behavior; (II) cryoinjury and (III) cryoprotection. Water exists in four states as a liquid, glass, solid and vapor, the formation of which is greatly influenced by temperature. Manipulation of the liquid, glassy and solid (ice) states of water is the main goal of cryoconservationists whose aim it is to devise protocols that avoid the formation of lethal intracellular ice. There are two main approaches to cryopreservation; the first is variously termed "traditional," controlled rate, two-step, or equilibrium freezing. This requires the control of extracellular ice crystallization, a process described as nucleation or "seeding" which is the point at which ice crystals are initiated. It is a common misconception that water freezes at 0°C, but this is rarely the case and in the absence of conditions that permit H_2O molecules to aggregate, water can supercool to temperatures well below zero. The lowest temperature being at, or around, −40°C (the point of homogeneous ice nucleation). This is a thermodynamic process, concomitant with ice formation, exothermic energy is released (**Fig. 52.1**) as the latent heat of fusion, conversely ice melting is accompanied by an endothermic event.

Table 52.1. Selected historical advances, bibliographic and information sources in cryopreservation.

Year	Principal investigator(s)	Advance/bibliography	Citation/information source
1665	Boyle	Published monograph 'New Experiments & Observations Touching Cold'	(4)
1776	Spallanzani	Recovery of spermatozoa cooled in snow	(5)
1901	van't Hoff	Awarded 1st Nobel Prize for Chemistry: laws of solution dynamics and osmotic pressure	http://nobelprize.org
1907	Lidforss	Proposal that sugars act as in vivo protectants in acclimated plants exposed to freezing	(6)
1912	Maximov	Discovery of the cryoprotective effects of glycerol and sugars in plant cell freezing	(7)
1940	Luyet & Gehenio	Publication of 'Life and Death at Low Temperatures'	(8)
1949	Polge et al.	Discovery of the cryoprotective effects of glycerol in avian spermatozoa	(9)
1950	Smith	Cryoprotection of red blood cells	(10)
1951	Smith & Polge	Birth of first calf (Frosty) from AI using cryopreserved semen	(11)
1953	Lovelock	Demonstration of osmotically induced colligative cryoinjury in red blood cells	(12)
1956	Sakai	Demonstration of survival of winter-hardy mulberry twigs exposed to LN	(13)
1957	Lovelock & Bishop	Successful application of DMSO as a cryoprotectant	(14)
1961	Smith	Comprehensive review of the biological effects of freezing and supercooling	(15)
1964	Cryobiology Society	Founding of the Society for Cryobiology	www.societyforcryobiology.org
1964	SLTB	Founding of the Society for Low Temperature Biology	www.sltb.info
1965	Mazur	Proposed the '2-factor hypothesis of cryoinjury' dehydration and intracellular ice	(16)
1966	Meryman	Milestone Reviews in 'Cryobiology'	(17)
1966	Parkes	Documentation of early experiments exploring the biological effects of low temperatures	(18)
1966	Sakai	Successful cryopreservation of plant tissues	(19)
1968	Meryman	Proposal of the minimum volume hypothesis of cryoinjury	(20)
1970	Smith	Publication of 'Current Trends in Cryobiology'	(21)
1972	Whittingham et al.	Successful cryopreservation of mouse embryos	(22)
1975	Franks	Publication of 'Water: A Comprehensive Treatise'	(23)

(continued)

Table 52.1. (continued).

Year	Principal investigator(s)	Advance/bibliography	Citation/information source
1980	Withers & King	Development of a routine controlled rate freezing protocol for plant cell preservation	(24)
1982	Kartha et al.	First development of droplet freezing technique applied to Cassava meristems	(25)
1983	Trounson & Mohr	First Human pregnancy following cryopreservation of the embryo	(26)
1984	Zeilmaker et al.	Birth of children following transfer of intact frozen–thawed embryos	(27)
1984	Fahy et al.	Proposal of vitrification as an approach to cryopreservation	(28)
1985	Rall & Fahy	Successful vitrification of mouse embryos	(29)
1985	Kartha	Publication of 'Cryopreservation of Plant Cells & Organs'	(30)
1990	Fabre & Dereuddre	Development of the encapsulation/dehydration cryopreservation method for plant germ-plasm	(31)
1990	Sakai et al.	Development, application and thermal analysis of plant vitrification solution PVS2	(32)
1990	Watson	Comprehensive review of domestic animal AI and the cryopreservation of spermatozoa	(33)
1994	Leibo et al.	Fertilization of oocytes by 37-year-old cryopreserved bovine spermatozoa	(34)
1995	Day & McLellan	Publication of the first comprehensive cryopreservation protocols manual	(35)
1995	Grout	Publication of 'Genetic Preservation of Plant Cells in Vitro'	(36)
1995	Bajaj	Publication of 'Cryopreservation of Plant Germplasm I'	(37)
1991	Watson & Holt	Publication of 'Cryobanking the Genetic Resource'	(38)
1999	Benson	Publication of 'Plant Conservation Biotechnology'	(39)
2000	Engelmann et al.	Publication of 'Cryopreservation of Tropical Plant Germplasm'	(40)
2004	Fuller et al.	Publication of 'Life in the Frozen State'	(>2)
2004	Leibo	Review of the early history of gamete cryobiology	(41)
2004	Benson	Review of the history of cryo-conserving algal and plant cells	(42)
2004	Mazur	Review of the principles of cryobiology	(43)
2005	Panis et al.	Development of a widely applicable droplet-vitrification protocol for plant germplasm	(44)
2007	Day & Stacey	Publication of Cryopreservation and Freeze-drying protocols.	(45)

Table 52.2. Examples of cryobanking protocols for diverse biological resources.

Biological resource	Taxa[1]	Germplasm-tissue type[2]	Cryogenic modality[3]	Cryoprotection regime[4]	Cryogenic approaches[5]	Cooling-rewarming regime[6]	Cryo store[7]	Ref
Viruses		Viral suspension	URF	none	Plunge (CV)	Direct plunge in LN. Rewarm at ca. 37°C until all ice has melted.	−70°C (F)	(71)
Eubacteria	Bacteria	Cell suspension	CRF	C (15% v/v glycerol)	PF (CV)	Mix glass beads with bacterial suspension in cryoprotectant, placed in −80°C freezer. Rewarm at ambient temperatures ca. 25°C.	−80°C (F)	(72)
		Cell suspension	CRF	C (5% v/v DMSO)	PF (CS)	1 step, place in LN_{vapor}. Rewarm at ambient temperatures ca. 25°C.	−196°C LN_{vapor}	(72)
	Cyanobacteria	Unicellular, filamentous	CRF	C (5–10% v/v DMSO; or 10% v/v MeOH)	CF or PF (CV)	2-step, −1°C/min to −40°C, hold 30min, direct plunge in LN. Rewarm at ca. 40°C until all ice is melted.	−196°C LN_{liquid}	(73)
Protista	Protozoa	Axenic, naked amoeba	CRF	C (5% v/v DMSO)	PF (CV)	3-step, place samples for 1h at −20°C, transfer to −70°C, incubate 1h then plunge in LN. Rewarm at 37°C until all ice is melted.	−196°C LN_{liquid}	(74)
	Plasmodium falciparum in host cell suspension		CRF	C (10% v/v DMSO)	CF or PF (CV)	2-step, −1°C/min to −40°C, hold 30min, direct plunge in LN. Rewarm at 37°C until all ice is melted.	−196°C LN_{vapor}	(75)
	Microalgae (general method)	Unicellular, short filaments or small clumps of cells	CRF	C (5–10% v/v DMSO; or 10% v/v MeOH)	CF or PF (CV)	2-step, −1°C/min to −40°C, hold 30min direct plunge in LN. Rewarm at ca. 40°C until all ice is melted.	−196°C LN_{liquid}	(73)
Fungi	Yeast (general method)	Unicellular, short filaments or small clumps	CRF	C (5% v/v glycerol)	PF (CV)	2 step, incubate for 2h in −30°C alcohol bath then plunge in LN. Rewarm at ca. 40°C until all ice is melted.	−196°C LN_{vapor}	(76)

(continued)

Table 52.2. (continued).

Biological resource	Taxa[1]	Germplasm-tissue type[2]	Cryogenic modality[3]	Cryoprotection regime[4]	Cryogenic approaches[5]	Cooling-rewarming regime[6]	Cryo store[7]	Ref
	Filamentous taxa (general method)	Filamentous/ hyphae and spores	CRF	C (10% v/v glycerol)	CF (CV)	2-step, −1°C/min to −40°C, hold briefly at −35°C, directly plunge in LN. Rewarm at 37°C until all ice is melted.	−196°C LN$_{vapor}$	(77)
	Basidiomycete (new "Perlite" method)	Mycelia	CRF	C (5% v/v glycerol)	CF (CV)	Fungal cultures grown in directly in cryovials moistened with glycerol. Controlled cooling at −1°C/min to −70°C and transfer to LN. Rewarm at 37°C in a water bath.	−196°C LN$_{liquid}$	(78)
Plants	Bryophytes	Protonemata	E-D	SA, D (Pre-treatments of sucrose, ABA, tissue embedded in 3% w/v calcium alginate dispensed onto filter paper strips. Evaporative desiccation in a sterile air flow)	UR (CV)	Direct plunge of cryovials in LN and transfer to cryostorage boxes. Rewarm at 40°C in a water bath.	−196°C LN$_{vapor}$	(79)
Higher Plant Germplasm		Cell Suspensions	CRF	SA, C, O (6% w/v mannitol or 10% w/v Proline → either 1M DMSO + 1M glycerol + 2M + 1M proline or 1M DMSO + 1M glycerol + 2M sucrose and added in equal volume to cell suspension diluting CPA by 50%)	CF(CV)	Cryovials, 2-step, 0°C, −1°C/min to −35°C, hold 30 min, transfer to LN. Rewarm at 40°C in a water bath.	−196°C LN$_{vapor}$	(24)
		Shoot meristems	CRF	A, C, O (Cold acclimation 1 wk 16h (22°C) light-8h (−1°C) dark cycles. PGD Cryoprotectant comprising 10% w/v each of polyethylene glycol$_{800}$ + glucose + DMSO)	CR(CV)	2-step, 4°C 30 min. −0.5°C/min to −40°C, then LN, with optional seeding cryovials directly plunged in LN. Rewarmed for 1 min. at 45°C transfer to a water bath at 45°C for 2 min, rinsed in culture medium.	−196°C LN$_{liquid}$	(80)

Shoot meristems and embryos	E-D	O, D (0.75 M sucrose loaded in 3% w/v calcium alginate, evaporatively desiccated in a sterile air flow)	UR germplasm encased in calcium alginate beads (CV)	Cryovials containing the beads directly plunge in LN. Rewarm by transferring cryovials to ambient temperatures (ca. 25°C).	−196°C LN$_{liquid}$	(31)
Shoot meristems and embryos	VPVS2	PVS2 (30% u/v glycerol + 15% v/v ethylene glycol +15% v/v DMSO +0.4M sucrose)	UR (CV)	Cryovials containing the beads directly plunge in LN. Rewarm by transferring cryovials to ambient temperatures (ca. 25°C) and unload with 1.2M sucrose.	−196°C LN$_{liquid}$	(57)
Shoot meristems and embryos	E-V PVS2 UR	V(3% w/v calcium alginate beads loaded with PVS2)	UR (CV)	Cryovials containing the beads directly plunge in LN. Rewarm by transferring cryovials to ambient temperatures (ca. 25°C) and unload with 1.2M sucrose.	−196°C LN$_{liquid}$	(57)
Shoot meristems	DF URF	C, V (10% v/v DMSO)	DF (2.5 μl cryoprotectant droplets on aluminium foil)	Droplets supported on foils directly plunge in LN contained in cryovials. Rewarm by transferring droplets-foils to liquid culture medium at ambient temperatures (ca. 25°C).	−196°C LN$_{liquid}$	(70)
Shoot meristems	D-V PVS2 UR	V(2M glycerol + 0.4M sucrose w/v of 30% u/v glycerol + 15% ethylene glycol+15% w/v DMSO +0.4M sucrose)	D-V (15 μl PVS2 droplets on aluminium foil)	Droplets supported on foils directly plunge in LN contained in cryovials. Rewarm by transferring droplets-foils to 1.2M sucrose unloading solution at ambient temperatures (ca. 25°C).	−196°C LN$_{liquid}$	(44)
Temperate Forest tree germplasm — Embryogenic suspension cultures	CRF	SA, C, (0.4M sorbitol → 5 % v/v DMSO)	CF (CV)	0°C, −0.5°C/min −15°C hold 15 min then −0.5°C/min to −50°C, hold 10 min, transfer to LN. Rewarmed at 40°C in a water bath.	−196°C LN$_{liquid}$	(81)

(continued)

Table 52.2. (continued).

Biological resource	Taxa[1]	Germplasm-tissue type[2]	Cryogenic modality[3]	Cryoprotection regime[4]	Cryogenic approaches[5]	Cooling-rewarming regime[6]	Cryo store[7]	Ref
	Tropical Rain Forest tree germplasm	Zygotic embryos	URF	D (Evaporatively desiccated, laminar airflow, up to 6h at 23°C and 55% RH)	Embryos desiccated to critical moisture contents (CV)	Directly plunge in LN, Rewarm in a water bath at 40°.	−196°C LN$_{liquid}$	(82)
Animals	Nematodes	*Bursaphelenchus* spp.	URF	O (Transfer from 10 to 25% v/v ethylene glycol).	50 µl drops of nematode suspension transferred to strips of chromatography paper (Roche nylon membranes)	Strips in cryovials directly plunged in LN and held for several minutes and then transferred to a mechanical freezer.	−140°C	(83)
	Insects	Mediterranean Fruit Fly (*Ceratitis capitata*) embryos	URV	SA, D, V Transfer from Ispropyl alcohol to hexane to 10% v/v ethylene glycol in culture medium to 40% v/v ethylene glycol or + 0.5 M trehalose + 5% w/v polyethylene glycol.	Transfer to 25 mm d 8.0µm pore size polycarbonate membrane (Nucleopore® Whatman)	Annealed over LN$_{vapor}$ for 1 min then plunged in LN. Rewarm in LN$_{vapor}$ for1 min then plunged into culture medium containing 0.5 M trehalose for 2 min. At ambient temperature.	−196°C LN$_{liquid}$	(84)
	Mollusk *Crassostrea gigas*	Spermatozoa	CRF	O, C (1 M trehalose + 10% v/v DMSO)	CF (CS)	3 step, 100°C/min from 25°C to −120°C, from −120°C cool at 15°C/min to a chamber temperature of −150°C, hold at −150°C for 1 min, then plunge in LN. Thaw in a 25°C waterbath.	−196°C LN$_{liquid}$	(85)
	Fish	Spermatozoa	CRF	C (1–5% v/v DMSO, ethylene glycol, methanol, or ethanol)	PF (CV or CS)	3 step, 2.5 min at −20°C, 2.5 min at −40°C, then plunge in LN. Rewarm at 37°C until all ice is melted.	−196°C LN$_{vapor}$	(86)

Taxonomic group[1]	Material type[2]	Cooling system[3]	Special additives[4]	Cooling system / vessel[5]	Protocol[6]	Storage temperature[7]	Ref
Avian (wild, endangered and domesticated)	Spermatozoa	URF	SA (6% v/v dimethyl-acetamide)	DF (CV)	Using a 1 ml automatic pipette, take up around 0.5 ml and allow individual droplets fall into the LN. Transfer droplets to CV. Hold vial and gently agitate in a 60°C (bath) until the pellets liqufy, when this happens, remove them quickly from the water bath.	−196°C LN$_{liquid}$	(87)
Mammals	Spermatozoa	CRF	C (5% v/v glycerol)	PF (CS)	Suspend the straws horizontally 5 cm above the surface of the LN for 7 min and then plunge in LN. Thawing: remove straws from LN and thaw in air for 2–3 s then plunge into a water bath at 35°C for 15 s.	−196°C LN$_{liquid}$	(88)
	embryos	CRF	O, C (1.5 mol/L PrOH plus 0.2 mol/L sucrose)	CF (CS)	Straws are cooled at −1°C/min to −7°C, ice nucleation or "seeding" is initiated, samples are held for 10 min at −7°C then cooled −0.3°C/min to −35°C, then cooled at −50°C/min to −150°C before storage. To thaw, straws are held in air for 10 s, then warmed in a 20°C water bath until the ice melts (approx 20 s). The contents of the straws are then expelled into diluent.	−196°C LN$_{vapor}$	(63)

[1] Taxonomic group.
[2] Material type; e.g. naked DNA, single cell, cell suspension, spore, gamete, zygotic embryo, somatic embryo, callus, colonial type, coenocytic, tissue, organ, whole organism or symbiotic association.
[3] Controlled rate freezing (CRF); ultra rapid freezing (URF); ultra rapid UR; vitrification (V); plant vitrification solution number 2 (PVS2); encapsulation/dehydration (E-D); (E-V) encapsulation-vitrification; droplet freezing (DF); droplet-vitrification (D-V).
[4] Acclimation (A); desiccation (D); osmotic (O); colligative (C); vitrification (V); special additives (SA).
[5] Cooling system: programmable controlled rate freezer (CF); passive freezer (PF); droplet freezer (DF); vessel used: cryovial (CV); cryostraw (CS).
[6] Cooling and warming protocols employed.
[7] Storage temperature and refrigerator used: ultra freezer (F); storage in vapor phase LN (LN$_{vapor}$); storage in liquid phase LN; (LN$_{liquid}$).

Table 52.3. Examples of cryobanking protocols applied to biomedical resources.

Biological resource / application	Taxa[1]	Germplasm-tissue type[2]	Cryogenic modality[3]	Cryoprotection regime[4]	Cryogenic approach[5]	Cooling-rewarming regime[6]	Cryo store[7]	Ref
Articular cartilage	Human	Isolated chondrocytes	CRF, C	C (10% v/v DMSO)	CR (CV)	Two-step, −1°C/min to −60°C, transfer to LN$_{vapor}$, rewarm at 22°C	−180°C. LN$_{vapor}$	(89)
Stem cells	Human and other mammals	Umbilical cord blood (CD34) cells	Various, derived by testing different modalities, using volumetric responses, cooling rate optima determination and modeling of CPA parameters	Various	Various	Various		(90,91)
Haematopoietic progenitor cells		Autologous grafts						
Hepatocytes for transplantation in acute liver failure	Human	Isolated hepatytocytes purifed from liver tissue	Various CRF	C (10% v/v DMSO)	CR(CV)	Various options of multistep protocols: e.g. 4°C to −70 or −80°C usually at −1°C/min^{-1} transferred to LN$_{vapor}$, rapid rewarming at 37°C, addition of high levels of glucose to the rewarming medium	−140°C LN$_{vapor}$	(92)
Research and metabolite production	Human & other mammals	Cell suspension	CRF	C (10 v/v DMSO or glycerol)	CF (CV)	2 step, cooling at 1–5°C/min to <−60°C, then plunge in LN. Rewarm at 37°C until all ice is melted.	−196°C LN$_{vapor}$	(93)
Transplantation	Human	Bone marrow cell suspension	CRF	C (10 v/v DMSO)	CF (CB)	4 step, 6°C hold for 12 min, cool at −2°C/min to −5°C, then cool at −1°C/min to −40°C, then cool at −5°C/min to −160°C.	−196°C LN$_{vapor}$	(94)
Transfusion	Human	Red blood cells	CRF	C (40% w/v glycerol)	PF (CB)	Maintain the sample at 25–32°C, then place in a cardboard or metal canister and place in a freezer at −65°C or below. Thawing in either a 37°C water-bath, or 37°C dry warmer.	<−65°C	(95)

IVF	Human	Spermatozoa	See Table 5.2.2					(88)
		oocytes	CRF	O, C (1.5 mol/l PrOH plus 0.2 mol/l sucrose)	CF (CV)	Cool from room temp to −7°C at −2°C/min, hold at −7°C for 10 min, initiate ice nucleation, then resume cooling to −150°C for storage. To thaw, hold in air for 30 s, then place in a 30°C waterbath for 30 s or until the ice has just melted.	−196°C LN$_{vapor}$	(96)
		Embryos	See Table 5.2.2.	For example method	CF (CV)	For example method		(63)
Fertility preservation for patients undergoing chemotherapy	Rat/ Human	Ovarian Tissue	CRF	C (1.5 mol/l ethylene glycol + 0.1 mol/l sucrose)	CF (CV)	Use an open freezing system that changes temperature by moving samples above the surface of LN. −2-step, −2°C/min to 1°C, 0.5°C/min to −5°C, −0.3°C/min to −9.3°C, 10 min hold, soak time (nucleation) cool at −0.3°C/min to −40°C, then −10°C/min to −140°C, plunged to LN.	−196°C LN$_{vapor/liquid}$	(97,98)
Skin grafts	Human	Skin and keratinocytes	CRF	SA, C, O (Trehalose and various combinations DMSO, glycerol)	CF (CV)	Cryovials and various controlled cooling rates using passive and programmable freezing units. Rapid rewarming in a 37°C water-bath.	−196°C LN$_{vapor/liquid}$	(99–101)

[1] Taxonomic group.
[2] Material type; e.g naked DNA, single cell, cell suspension, spore, gamete, zygotic embryo, somatic embryo, callus, colonial type, coenocytic, tissue, organ, whole organism or symbiotic association.
[3] Controlled rate freezing (CRF); ultra rapid freezing (URF); vitrification (V); droplet freezing (DF).
[4] Acclimation (A); desiccation (D); osmotic (O); colligative (C); vitrification (V); special additives (SA), cryoprotective additive (CPA).
[5] Cooling system: programmable controlled rate freezer (CF); passive freezer (PF); droplet freezer (DF). vessel used: cryovial (CV); cryostraw (CS); cryocyte bag (CB).
[6] Cooling and warming protocols employed
[7] Storage temperature and refrigerator used: ultra freezer (F); storage in vapor phase LN (LN$_{vapor}$); storage in liquid phase LN (LN$_{liquid}$).

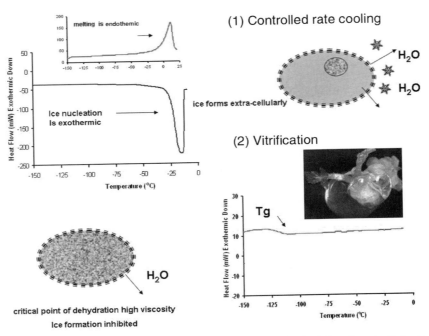

Fig. 52.1. Schematic comparing the physical and thermal principles of controlled rate cooling and vitrification. DSC thermograms demonstrating: ice nucleation, melting and vitrification (Tg). On controlled slow cooling: (*I*) ice forms extracellularly and a vapor deficit created across the cell membrane cause the movement of water to the outside of the cell. Colligative cryoprotectants protect against the deleterious effects of solute concentration. Vitrification (*II*) requires the concentration of solutes (e.g., by encapsulation-dehydration) through evaporative and/or osmotic dehydration and/or the loading of high concentrations of penetrating cryoprotectants. The cell viscosity reaches a critical high, such that on exposure to freezing temperatures water is unable to nucleate and the cells vitrify

The second approach to cryoprotection requires the cell to achieve a critically high viscosity such that on exposure to freezing temperatures water forms a vitrified state. Glasses are highly viscous solidified liquids they are amorphous, metastable and non-crystalline and, because of their lack of organized structure are far less damaging to cells compared to ice.

Glass formation also involves thermal changes of which the most significant is the glass transition temperature or Tg, the temperature at which a glass is initiated (**Fig. 52.1**). Glasses are metastable and their behavior in biological tissues is highly complex as water can devitrify and convert back to ice. Knowledge of the thermal events associated with ice nucleation, melting and the Tg is very useful in developing cryopreservation protocols. Specialist thermal analysis using a differential scanning calorimeter (DSC) may be employed to study and optimize vitrification procedures (**Fig. 52.1**).

Tolerance to cryopreservation depends upon the ability to overcome or avoid cryoinjury, for which Mazur (*16*) proposed that two factors were involved; colligative damage and ice. Ice promotes structural and osmotic damage and causes mechanical injury to fragile cell structures (*46*). Colligative injury is the excessive concentration of solutes, which is detrimental to cellular function.

When slow to moderate cooling rates (**Tables 52.2** and **52.3**) are applied ice usually nucleates extracellularly causing a vapor pressure deficit between the outside and inside of the cell and to retain osmotic equilibrium H_2O passes to the outside. Rates of water loss are determined by cooling rate, the dynamics of extracellular ice nucleation and cryoprotection. Lovelock (*12*) demonstrated that salt concentration was the primary cause of freezing injury and Meryman (*20*) proposed a minimal volume hypothesis for cryoinjury (**Table 52.1**). As cryopreserved cells shrink their rate of water loss can be expressed as a function of cell size and knowledge of cell permeability and the kinetics of water loss may be used to help predict their freezing profiles (*16*). Mathematical equations and theoretical models of thermodynamic behavior and membrane permeability (*47–49*) have very important applications in optimizing controlled rate cooling and cryoprotective protocols for animal and human cells (*50*). However, their application in plant, algal, and microbial cells can be confounded by the presence of cell walls, extracellular mucilage etc.

Successful cryopreservation protocols are dependent upon optimizing cooling rate in conjunction with cryoprotective strategies. There are two main types of chemical cryoprotectants: (I) penetrating/colligative and (II) non-penetrating/osmotic and they are frequently used in combination. Traditional controlled rate cooling protocols use penetrating cryoprotectants such as dimethyl sulphoxide (DMSO) or glycerol, although their permeabilities vary among cell types. As cells are exposed to controlled cooling (e.g., −1°C/min) ice forms extracellularly causing the withdrawal of intracellular water. This is desirable as it reduces the amount of H_2O molecules available for initiating lethal ice crystals. In many systems it is essential to induce extracellular ice nucleation (**Tables 52.2** and **52.3**) as from this point onwards the operator has some control over the excursion of water. Moreover, as water is removed, the freezing point becomes increasingly depressed allowing more time for water to exit the cell. Often a "hold" is programed into controlled cooling protocols allowing additional H_2O molecules to move across the cell membrane. However, a balance must be achieved such that dehydration does not result in excessive, deleterious concentration of solutes and this is where colligative cryoprotectants come into play. These chemicals penetrate cells and act as cellular solvents as they protect against the damaging concentration of solutes that occurs as water is lost from the cell and obviates the deleterious and potentially lethal reduction in cell volume. Following these treatments and when cells are finally exposed to terminal freezing temperatures and LN it is possible that the intracellular solution is so concentrated that it becomes vitrified (**Fig. 52.1**). Alternatively, if some H_2O molecules remain available for nucleation, the ice crystals formed are so small they are innocuous. Non-penetrating cryoprotectants have multiple protective roles, they depress the freezing point, cause osmotic dehydration and reduce the amount of water available for freezing, they may also impair ice nucleation by restricting the molecular mobility of H_2O molecules (*51–54*).

Cryopreservation using ultra rapid rates of cooling usually involves a cryoprotective strategy, which allows cells and tissues to be directly plunged into LN. This approach normally requires the formation and stabilization of a vitrified state, which is achieved by attaining a critically high cell viscosity, by evaporative and/or osmotic removal of water, or the loading of high concentrations of penetrating cryoprotectants, or both. Cryopreservation by this method is quite different to controlled rate cooling that, as part of the protective strategy, necessitates the formation of extracellular ice to initiate the process of freeze-dehydration (**Fig. 52.1**). Vitrified systems comprise of two types: (I) partially vitrified in which the solution external to the cell forms ice while the intracellular component remains ice free, or, (II) totally vitrified in which both the external and intracellular compartments become vitrified and in effect this is cryopreservation in the absence of ice. As well as their physical protective properties cryoprotectants also impart additional defences against cryoinjury *(53,55)* as they can stabilize proteins and membranes and act as antioxidants.

Rewarming of cryopreserved samples also requires stringent optimization as small innocous ice crystals are capable of growing to a size that may cause injury. Similarly, relaxation of glasses on rewarming can fracture fragile and particularly rigid cell structures or, they can devitrify and form ice if they are rewarmed too slowly. By applying these general principles of cryobiological theory it is now possible to consider the different types of protocols used to preserve biological resources.

2. Cryopreservation Methodology

Cryoprotection is pivotal to successful cryogenic storage, although some robust organisms, such as the unicellular alga *Chlorella protothecoides* *(56)*, survive without the need for cryoprotective additives or controlled cooling. Naturally cold hardened *(19,57)* and/or evaporatively desiccated *(58)* higher plant germplasm can also survive LN without chemical protection. However, the capacity to recover from cryopreservation without the need for chemical additives is not normally the case for animal and human cells. Cryopreservation is usually undertaken using two main approaches, controlled rate cooling coupled with colligative cryoprotection or vitrification, the generic methodologies of which may be described as follows.

2.1. Controlled Rate Cooling

Protocols based on regulating cooling rates usually apply single or combined colligative cryoprotectants that are often used in conjunction with osmotic additives (see Section 1.2) followed by cooling steps intercepted by the manual, automatic or passive induction of ice nucleation (see Section 1.2). Survival can be improved by pre-culture and cold hardening treatments applied before cryopreservation, these usually simulate natural acclimation responses. For example, culturing algal cells at lower than normal growth temperatures *(59)*, or applying biochemical additives to enhance stress tolerance in plants *(60)*. Post-storage survival in mammalian and human cells can be improved by adding antioxidant supplements to the freezing media *(53,61)*. Modifications to post-storage culture can also significantly enhance the level and rate of recovery *(62)*. Factors critical to controlled cooling methods are cryoprotectant composition in which a penetrating colligative additive must be included as well as cooling regime. Different cell types have specific optimal cooling rates (**Fig. 52.2**) that are largely determined by balancing the two components of cryoinjury *(16)*. If cooling is too rapid, intracellular ice occurs; conversely at suboptimally slow rates of cooling colligative dehydration damage is enhanced. Complex cooling regimes, capable of more effectively dissipating the latent heat of fusion on ice formation can also be beneficial

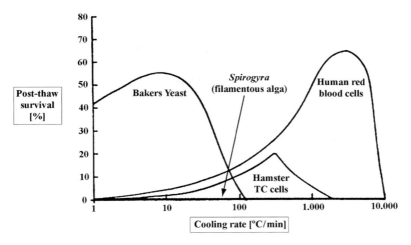

Fig. 52.2. The effects of cooling rate on survival following the cryopreservation of four different cell types

(62,63). Computerized, controlled rate programmable freezers (CRFs) (e.g., Planer Products, Sunbury, UK; Cryomed, Waltham, MA,USA; CryoLogic, Musgrave, Victoria, Australia) provide the most reliable means of controlling cooling parameters, which in sequence are:

a. Loading temperature (ambient/subzero X°C).
b. The 1st cooling ramp (−Y°/min).
c. Temperature of initiating ice nucleation (−Z°C) with an optional hold.
d. A 2nd or 3rd optional cooling ramp (−Y°/min).
e. An intermediate terminal transfer temperature at, or near the point of homogeneous ice nucleation (ca. −40°C).
f. A hold (X minutes).
g. Transfer to liquid nitrogen.
h. Storage in liquid or vapor phase LN.
i. Optimized rewarming using rapid (30–45°C), 2-step, or ambient conditions.

   Computerized programmable freezers have the advantage of providing data outputs allowing each run to be documented for protocol development and quality control purposes. Programmable freezers accurately regulate cooling rates over a broad range of temperatures by feeding pressurized vapor-phase LN into a sample chamber controlled by an electronic-solenoid feedback system. Where it is necessary to manipulate cryodehydration, for example, following extracellular ice nucleation some machines can be fitted with an automatic seeding facility. Furthermore, "soak times" or "dwell periods" may be built into the program to allow for freeze-dehydration and transfers to LN. It is important to transfer the cryogenic vial quickly from the cooling chamber to the storage vessel to prevent sample rewarming. Substitutes for LN-cooled electronically programed freezers may also be applied and these include passive coolers that rely on the thermal conductivity of an insulated containment vessel placed in an electrical deep freeze or refrigerator and/or a solvent bath. Simple cooling ramps can be devised by placing cryovials in a polystyrene box (~10 × 10 × 10 cm internal dimensions with walls and lid ~3.5 cm thick) placed in a −80°C freezer. The insulated container retards heat transfer allowing the contents of the cryogenic vial to cool relatively slowly (−1°C/min). Undisturbed, the sample reaches the ambient temperature, at a specific rate of cooling that is dependent on the insulation properties of the container. These systems can be calibrated over a time course using thermometers, thermocouples and simple data logging devices. Over a narrow range of temperatures passive cooling systems have a near-linear cooling rate. It is also possible to modulate the cooling properties of the cooling vessel or refrigerated chamber by adding a solvent such as isopropyl alcohol. This is the basis for commercial systems that use solvent-containing units to passively cool at ca. −1°C/min over the temperature range 0°C to −40°C (e.g., Mr. Frosty, Nalgene Nunc, Rochester, NY, USA). Alternatively, samples can be cooled using direct immersion in an industrial methylated spirit (denatured ethanol) bath *(62)*. When the sample reaches a sufficiently low temperature (e.g., −30 to −80°C), it is removed and plunged into LN. The conventional approach to controlled rate cooling cryopreservation creates an approximately linear change of temperature with time during the first of cooling ramp. Morris et al. *(64)* demonstrated that human spermatozoa can be successfully cryopreserved by manipulating the cooling regime to provide non-linear changes in temperature with time over critical temperatures. Recently an alternative freezer, which allows controlled rate cooling without the need for LN or a permanent electrical supply, also manufactured by Asymptote, UK, has been successfully tested on horse semen *(65)*.

2.2. Vitrification

At the glass transition temperature (Tg) molecular motion ceases and a liquid becomes a glassy solid (**Fig. 52.1**). In controlled rate cooling it is possible that on exposure to freezing temperatures the intracellular viscosity of the cell is sufficiently high that cells become vitrified inside, while remaining frozen extracellularly. This is a partially vitrified system and although the glassy state may account in part for survival, ice nucleation is still required to evoke osmotic, freeze-induced dehydration. Ice-free cryopreservation, initially pioneered for animal cells *(28)* and applied to plants *(57)* and algae *(66)* involves a very different cryoprotective strategy; such that ice formation is inhibited both inside and outside the cell, resulting in total vitrification. The glassy state offers great benefits for larger and/or structurally complex, heterogeneous tissues for which it is difficult to optimize colligative cryoprotection and cooling rates. Vitrification does not require controlled cooling and the need for programmable freezing apparatus is circumvented making cryopreservation more amenable to researchers from non-specialist laboratories. However, as glass formation usually requires the excessive concentration of solutes, and cells must be able to tolerate dehydration. Pathways to achieve vitrified and frozen states are frequently interdependent and increasingly "hybrid" protocols are being developed that incorporate components of colligative cryoprotection/cooling and vitrification procedures, albeit their final end point is usually the glassy state *(51)*.

The "conventional approach" to vitrification developed for human and animal systems uses mixtures of traditional liquid cryoprotectants (DMSO, glycerol, ethylene glycol, polyols, and sugars) at high concentrations (**Tables 52.2** and **52.3**). Those that penetrate the cell cumulatively increase solute concentration while non-penetrating additives act synergistically by withdrawing water osmotically, their combined effect enhances the overall viscosity of the cell. Exposing cells to high concentrations of cryoprotective additives can be injurious and strategies have been devised to reduce their toxicity. These include their sequential "loading" and "unloading" to avoid osmotic shock, and application at chilling temperatures.

Vitrification solutions, of which plant vitrification solution number 2 (PVS2) is the most widely used, have been applied to many different types of plant genetic resources (57); however, alternative approaches exist. Fabre and Dreuddre (31) developed the encapsulation/dehydration method in which tissues are entrapped in calcium-alginate beads, osmotically dehydrated in high molarity sucrose solutions, then evaporatively desiccated in a sterile air flow, or over silica gel. This approach can be applied even to the most complex of genetic resources systems, as exemplified by the simultaneous preservation of orchid seed with its fungal symbiont (67). The sugar-loaded alginate matrix supports very stable glasses, so long as the system is sufficiently desiccated to a critical moisture content that inhibits devitrification on rewarming as well as cooling (68). For cells sensitive to desiccation a hybrid of chemical vitrification and encapsulation/dehydration was developed (57) in which alginate beads are loaded with vitrification cocktails such as PVS2.

The capacity of water molecules to come together and nucleate to initiate ice can also be influenced by the critical mass/volume of a liquid solution. For very small (μl) volumes the probability of neighboring H_2O molecules existing in sufficient numbers to aggregate and nucleate ice is more limited as compared to larger volumes. Moreover, if cells and tissues are contained in micro droplets of cryoprotective additives and cooled ultra rapidly by direct plunging into LN the capacity to form ice is increasingly restricted and the system becomes predisposed to vitrification. This approach, termed "droplet freezing" was first devised by Kartha (30) for cassava shoot-tips (69) and has latterly been applied to potato (70) using DMSO. A modification of the technique using PVS2 microdroplets as the cryoprotectant system has recently (44) achieved considerable success in cryopreserving a wide range of plant germplasm. Glass formation and stabilization in these different vitrification systems is highly complex (51) and their efficacies cannot solely be assigned to enhanced viscosity. Thermal analysis studies linked to the thermodynamic modelling of molecular mobility are yielding evidence (52–54) suggesting that mixtures of highly concentrated additives restrict the mobility and energetic behavior of H_2O molecules and impact their potential for ice formation and growth.

3. Applications of Cryopreservation

Cryopreservation is applied in a multitude of scientific sectors and has resulted in the development of a cryoengineering industry (69), capable of manufacturing precision instruments that measure and control ultra-low temperatures and supplying containment vessels that safely withstand extreme low temperatures and high pressures of coolant gases. Storage protocols must be robust and reproducible and support good levels of survival whilst retaining fitness-for-purpose on retrieval from the cryobank. In the case of reproductive cells, maintenance of genetic stability and totipotency is also essential *(101,102)*. Similarly, molecular, metabolic and functional competencies must be assured for cryobanked resources used in validation and testing in biotechnology, healthcare and pharmaceutical sectors. Stringent safety, security and validation measures are also crucial for assuring confidence in the use of cryopreserved bioresources by custodians, donors and beneficiaries *(103)*.

3.1. Cryopreserving Biological Resources

Biological resources are living assets selected from the spectrum of biodiversity used for the benefit of mankind. In addition germplasm from endangered species also requires human intervention to facilitate *in situ* and *ex situ* conservation projects that use assisted breeding and reintroduction practices. Cryo-conservation ensures the long-term security, stability, and sustainable use of biodiversity and storage protocols must support survival in vastly different levels of biological complexity (**Table 52.1**). In 1999 the total world market for products of biodiversity was estimated as between US$ 500 billion and 800 billion *(104)* a fact that goes a long way to justifying the long-term cryopreservation of biological resources. The diversity of currently cryopreserved living resources is mirrored by the many different approaches used for their cryogenic storage (**Tables 52.2** and **52.3**). However, it is cautioned that the information provided in the above tables only summarizes key cryogenic components, and for full methodological procedures the reader is directed to the primary bibliographic source.

3.1.1. Microorganisms and Biotechnology

Cryopreservation is the method of choice for conserving many microorganisms *(105)* as their storage in LN circumvents the need for repeated subculturing and mitigates against the destabilizing changes associated with the long-term culture of actively growing organisms *(62)*. Cryogenic storage ensures the safe, long-term security of microorganisms of both present and potential economic value. It supports their continued capacity to generate active products and participate in processes used, for example, by the brewing industry and in the manufacture of industrial enzymes. There is therefore a major financial incentive to cryopreserve high-value microorganisms having global annual sales of US$30–60 billion *(104)*. This is particularly the case for those used by the pharmaceutical sector for the production of drugs and natural healthcare products. Cryogenic storage of microorganisms exploited by biotechnology industries underpins the stringent requirement for phenotypic and genotypic stability in master stock-cultures used for patenting, commercialization and sustainable exploitation. Moreover, modern biotechnological approaches to drug discovery, such as bioprospecting *(106)*, genetic manipulation, genomics, and proteomics have increased the need to develop robust cryopreservation protocols that safeguard elite genetic combinations and cell lines. Although lyophilization is an alternative option to cryogenic storage, preservation in LN is increasingly viewed as the preferred approach. This is because the stability of production of primary and secondary metabolites *(107)* is confirmed at ultra-low temperatures, whereas, production losses of secondary metabolites can occur in suboptimally lyophilized fungi *(108)*.

3.1.2. Agriculture and Aquaculture

One of the earliest and most significant contributions that cryopreservation has made is in artifical insemination (AI) assisted livestock breeding and animal husbandry. Thus, over the last 50 years cryogenic storage has been routinely applied for the preservation of the spermatozoa, ova, oocytes, and embryos of a wide range of domesticated fowl and mammals (**Table 52.2**). Cryopreserved bull semen has facilitated world-wide bovine breeding programs resulting in a doubling of milk production in dairy cows from 26,000 to 52,000 litres of milk per cow per year between 1950 and 1980. Only semen from bulls with the greatest genetic potential for milk production was used and although this genetic improvement could have been achieved without the use of cryopreservation, the time required to achieve the same level of genetic improvement would have been greatly extended. Furthermore, the use of cryopreserved bovine germplasm is far more cost effective than can be achieved by using non-cryopreserved AI procedures. It has been estimated that the cost for one AI using fresh semen is about three times more than for cryopreserved semen and transportation costs per insemination are more than double, and for each live calf, costs are more than triple *(109)*.

The Aquaculture sector is now considered one of fastest growing areas of "agriculture" with growth-rates at 26% per annum being quoted by some experts *(110)*. A key challenge to the sector is improvement of the genetic quality of fish, shrimp, and mollusk breeding stocks to increase productivity. This is because traditional approaches to genetic improvement can take a long time, in catfish; for instance, a male typically spawns with only one female each season. Even if genetically superior males and females can be identified, the process of developing breeding stock and improved lines can take a decade or more. Cryopreservation of fish germplasm accelerates this process as it improves the efficiency and capacity of hatchery operations by providing sperm on demand and simplifying the timing of induced spawning by permitting out of season breeding. Furthermore, it can significantly reduce operational costs by allowing hatcheries to eliminate the need to maintain live males. Cryopreservation also secures valuable genetic lineages, such as endangered species, "model" strains used in research, or improved farmed strains. This could be critical for marine species including shellfish, where valuable brood stocks must normally be stored in natural waters. It is projected that cryopreserved sperm of aquatic species will become a new and economically significant industry within the coming decade.

3.1.3. Cryopreservation for Crops, Forestry, and Phyto-Pharming

Cryopreservation is extensively used for the *ex situ* conservation of plant germplasm *(39,111)* and is the method of choice for preserving genetic resources that cannot be conserved by traditional seed banking. These include vegetatively propagated crops and forestry species that either do not produce seeds or, that must be produced by clonal proliferation to maintain their desired traits. Examples include tuber crops and *Alliums (112)*, horticultural species such as soft and top fruits *(80)* maintained through grafting on rootstocks, or by vegetatively proliferating cuttings. Cryopreservation is essential to modern commercial conifer forestry industries as it is used to maintain totipotent somatic cell lines and embryos of elite "plus" trees that have desired timber traits *(113)*. Many tropical plants produce seeds recalcitrant to traditional seed storage and cryogenic storage provides an alternative approach to their conservation *(40)*. Plant germplasm cryopreservation has significant indirect benefits for the sustainable exploitation and security of economically important phytodiversity *(114)*. *Ex situ* conservation in field genebanks, arboreta and plantations risk potentially catastrophic losses through pathogen attack, pest infestation, natural disasters, conflict and increasingly, climate change. The establishment of global genetic resources networks *(111)* capable of maintaining large cryopreserved holdings *(115)* of precious plant germplasm provides assurance against the risk of loss from conservation in the field. Moreover, as plant germplasm cryopreservation is usually integrated with *in vitro* manipulations, sterile tissue culture practices can be linked to virus eradication procedures. Cryopreserved disease-indexed germplasm can be transported with phytosanitary passports across international boundaries reducing the risk transferring phytopathological diseases. The biotechnological production of plants and products used in pharmaceutical, food and bioengineering industries also has a requirement for cryopreservation *(116, 117)*. These programs apply genetic manipulations, recombinant DNA technologies, genomics, and proteomics to cultures that use LN-storage for culture stabilization, patent deposition, and licensing.

3.1.4. Cryopreservation for Endangered Species and Environmental Protection

Cryopreservation has the potential to assist the *ex situ* and *in situ* conservation of endangered species and their habitats by: (I) protecting germplasm collected from individuals residing in at risk native habitats *(118)* or, from *ex situ* wild life sanctuaries, reserves, zoos and botanical gardens *(119–121)*; (II) using cryogenically stored gametes, oocytes and embryos in IVF and AI assisted reproduction programs; (III) providing a stable and safe means of transferring and exchanging at risk reproductive materials across international borders; (IV) facilitating cooperative breeding projects of rare species undertaken by geographically dispersed wildlife protection agencies; (V) holding at risk germplasm under low maintenance and cost effective storage regimes until the time is appropriate to use them in assisted breeding projects and/or reintroduction programs *(122)*; (VI) securing germplasm under stable conditions for DNA fingerprinting and genomic analysis used to plan back-from-the-brink breeding strategies for species represented by narrow genepools and (VII) sequentially cryo-conserving biodiversity unique to extreme habitats, (e.g., Antarctica) over time courses such that the preserved samples may be used in environmental impact monitoring.

Practical logistics is a major problem for cryopreserving germplasm acquired from endangered and at risk species. Donor scarcity coupled with the fact that endangered species are often located in remote, inaccessible or high risk regions which make it difficult and costly to procure precious samples and transfer them with the rapidity required to ensure their safe deposition in cryogenic storage. Lack of materials available for storage protocol work up is a significant limitation as the development of cryoprotective strategies necessitates the sacrifice of a certain amount of material *(123)*. Also, germplasm from at risk and endangered donors may be more sensitive to cryopreservation owing to compromised health, physiological status, age and a narrowed genepool. Genotype variation in semen cryopreservation is also a limiting factor in the conservation of rare animals. Included in this category are the genetic breeding stocks of domesticated breeds placed at risk by disease epidemics such as foot and mouth and Bovine Spongiform Encephalopathy (BSE). Thus, understanding the molecular genetic reasons as to why the germplasm of certain at risk species or individuals are particularly sensitive to cryogenic manipulations is essential *(124)*.

3.1.5. Cryopreserving Biological Resources Limited by Access and Supply

Conserving the genetic resources of endangered species is particularly prone to logistical problems, however availability issues are also relevant to other types of living materials. Thus, this section highlights some practical solutions that may help overcome the difficulties associated with cryopreserving biological resources that are rare, or in limited supply or for which rapid protocol work up is desirable because of their rapid deterioration. Simplified cooling units (e.g., Mr Frosty^R) and vitrification protocols offset the need for controlled rate freezers in remote laboratories. Furthermore, instruments that operate without LN and use battery-supplied electricity may assist field-based cryo-conservation *(65)*. Planning experiments for cryopreservation protocol work-up when germplasm is limited has been greatly assisted by Taguchi experimental designs as initially developed for tropical rain forest tree germplasm *(82,123)*. In the Taguchi method, fractional factorial experiments are designed using orthogonal arrays and as such they require a far smaller number of observations than for traditional full factorial experiments *(125)*. Taguchi experiments use signal to noise ratios (SNR) as the statistical variable, which reduces variation and define the consistency of performance. This is achieved by moving mean performance to a nominal or target value (e.g., a critical moisture content required for glass formation) as well as reducing variation around this target. Taguchi designed experiments and analyses can thus predict the optimal treatments required in developing a cryopreservation protocol using a minimal number of observations *(123,126)*. This approach is recommended when germplasm is scarce and method work up needs to be undertaken rapidly. Similarly, probabilistic approaches have been developed to help predict the amount of germplasm required to be cryopreserved to ensure an appropriate level of survival after cryogenic storage *(127)*. In combination these approaches will assist the future application of cryopreservation for the conservation of some our most valuable and vulnerable living resources.

3.2. Cryopreservation of Biomedical Resources

Cryogenic storage of biomedical resources (see **Table 52.3**) comprises two main applications: (I) donor and autologous materials used in the direct healthcare of a recipient patient (e.g., blood transfusion products, transplant and graft cells, tissues and organs, vascular and bone tissues, reproductive cells/tissues for IVF) and (II) biotechnologically altered, procured or manufactured cell lines and engineered tissue products used in therapeutic treatments, diagnostics, pharmaceutics, clinical research, and translational medicine. The main tissues and organs used for human transplant purposes are: blood products, stem cells, bone, tendon, amniotic membranes, corneas, vascular graft tissues and heart valves, articular cartilage, osteochondral allografts, skin grafts, keratinocytes, and pancreatic islet cells *(128)*. The cryopreservation of these systems is highly desirable although not all are as yet, fully amenable to clinically optimal cryogenic storage at ultra-low temperatures.

Most of the cryopreserved materials used in healthcare have a crucial underpinning role in supporting multi-component treatment strategies and an effective operational interface among cryobiologists, the users of cryopreserved medical resources and their custodians is therefore essential. A case in point is the human heart valve allograft that, although it can be cryopreserved successfully, requires a technically critical and time consuming post-storage preparative procedure before being transplanted. The frozen valves used for surgery are usually recovered in the operating theatre while the patient is on cardiopulmonary bypass. Thus, improved post-storage manipulations that assist in the efficacy of thawing and cryoprotectant dilution are being progressed *(129)* providing an excellent example as to the importance of pursuing concomitant applied and basic low temperature research to advance the practical use of transplant tissues *(128)*. Similar examples include the cryogenic storage of reproductive cells from patients undergoing chemotherapy for which preservation advances are particularly significant *(130,131)* for ovarian tissues. Furthermore patients with liver failure can be treated with cryopreserved hepatocyte grafts, cell transplants, and constructed bioengineered products (**Table 52.3**). Recently, cryopreservation has been evaluated for the storage of human teeth with a view to developing dental cryobanks for transplantation *(132)*. Autologous transplantations, particularly of haematopoietic stem cells for the treatment of malignancies are particularly increasing. This is because harvesting during the early stages of treatment is a safety measure as even though there may be no immediate requirement to perform stem cell transplants this possibility may arise in the future. It is crucial to store these materials in long-term cryogenic as they are "living insurance policies" should transplantations be required in the future *(91)*.

The stringency of recovery requirements for medical bioresources is highly variable; some tissue grafts, such as bones, are required to provide mechanical support only and it is not necessary for their component cells to remain viable. This contrasts with transplants and grafts that must retain high levels of functionality and integrity after cryopreservation, as is the case for corneas *(133)*. Importantly, the effective use of revived tissues must be considered not only in terms of the direct impacts of cryogenic storage, but also as to how the process may affect their reintegration with recipient systems and particular vascular tissues. This capability has been highlighted by Pegg *(134)* who defined "cryopreservation" in a clinical context as a storage procedure that preserves functional and viable cells, including their entire and intact extracellular structure. Meeting this target is difficult and the efficacy of the various cryoprotection regimes (see **Table 52.3**) resides particularly in limiting the damage caused by the direct and indirect effects of ice, which is highly injurious to physiological, mechanical, and structural stability. For this reason vitrification in the absence of ice is considered a powerful tool in cryo-conserving complex structures and engineered tissue constructs. Improving the interface between post-cryopreservation recovery and the clinical and therapeutic uses of cryobanked transplant tissues is thus crucial.

As the safety and security of biomedical resources is paramount storage protocols must stringently comply with procedures that protect against, the risks associated with biomedical resources as well as complying with ethical standards *(135,136)*. Risks include: donor, operator, and recipient safety; premature or accidental rewarming; mistaken identity, transmission of infection;

and including within cryotanks, stringent equipment quality assurance (e.g., cryovials, dewars, and controlled rate freezers) and the use of safety warning and alarm systems *(137)*. Critical to these practices is the need for cryogenic containers that are used to store human tissues to be sealed using means that prevents exchange of material between the specimen and LN *(138,139)*. Alternatives *(140)* to cryopreservation in LN liquid and vapor offer a different long-term storage approach, although the benefits of these must be balanced with the need to confirm long-term impacts on stability and risks of operating in the event of power failure.

Clearly the applications of cryopreservation in medical and healthcare sectors are becoming increasingly diverse, complex and pervasive and this trend will continue as a result of advances in bioengineering, transplant surgery, reproductive technologies, and translational medicine. How cryopreserved resources are managed will therefore play an increasingly important role in developing improved cryogenic storage methods. Biological resource centers are thus particularly well placed to facilitate the cohesion among cryobiologists, tissue and cell bank curators, and medical practitioners.

4. Management of Cryopreserved Resources: Biological Resource Centers (BRCs)

Cryopreserved materials are held in formal, or informal, collections located in medical, academic, public service, private, government, or commercial organizations. Cryopreserved "collections" usually form the basis of Biological Resource Centres (BRCs), as they perform a key role in delivering documented, characterized cultures/cell-lines, semen, plant material etc. as "seed" stocks for: (I) use in medicine, agriculture or bioindustry; (II) as reference strains for biological assays and published scientific literature; (III) as type strains for taxonomical studies, and (IV) as centers for conservation of biodiversity.

As indicated (Section 3) in the case of cryopreserved biomedical resources culture collections must conform to three fundamental responsibilities to establish, sustain, and maintain the value of their stored materials: (I) purity (freedom from contaminant organisms; (II) authenticity (correct identity of each sample) and (III) stability, including correct functional characteristics. BRCs maintain practices, including the application of optimized cryopreservation protocols, to ensure that the samples of organisms they hold and distribute sustain these important attributes. In addition, for those organizations dealing with microorganisms and biomedical materials, master and distribution banks for each organism and robust quality control systems are normally established *(141)*. It is particularly important that high standards are maintained in IVF facilities, those handling therapeutic materials, genetically manipulated organisms, and patent depositories where the preserved cells must remain viable for at least 30 years *(96,141,142)*. Security and stability of stored material is assured through adoption of appropriate management systems to restrict access to authorized personnel, appropriate alarms for nitrogen storage vessels, and documented procedures for filling and maintenance of nitrogen storage. Monitoring using temperature alarm systems and auditing to ensure correct maintenance and documentation are also important activities for BRC operation.

The provision of specimens from BRCs is of little value unless they are accompanied by passport information on their identity, provenance, and characteristics. Accurate records are vital to enable retrieval of the stored ampules or straws efficiently. There may also be a legal requirement for cryogenically stored genetically modified, infectious, or other hazardous materials. Numerous commercial database systems are specially designed for this purpose, but it is important to select a system that is flexible to the full range of user requirements. It is also sensible to have an up to date hard-copy version or back-up electronic copies to ensure that amendments to storage records for additions or withdrawals can be made at the storage site to avoid transcript errors.

In conclusion, there are clear commercial and scientific drivers for the implementation of storage of biological resources for reference or future exploitation. Cryopreservation provides the most appropriate and widely applicable approach to the long-term conservation of biological materials. There remain some constraints on the type of material that can be successfully held; however, new cryoprotective approaches have considerably extended the range and diversity of materials that can be preserved. On going challenges include the preservation of complex tissues and organs, improving the preservation of recalcitrant plant germplasm and freeze-sensitive medical bioresources and expanding the use of cryo-conservation for endangered and at risk species.

Acknowledgements: The authors acknowledge the European Union's 5th Framework Programme, Quality of Life and Management of Living Resources, Research Infrastructures Biological Collections, COBRA Project QLRT-2000-01645 and CRYMCEPT Project (QLK5-CT-2002-01279). J Nadarajan acknowledges the European Social Fund, The Forest Research Institute of Malaysia and the University of Abertay Dundee for the support of her postgraduate studies.

References

1. Fox D (2006) Sub-zero survivors. New Scientist, 12th August, pp 34–38
2. Fuller B, Lane N, Benson EE (2004) Life in the frozen state CRC Press, London UK
3. Methé BA, Nelson KE, Deming JW, Momen B, Melamud E, Zhang X, Moult J, Madupu R, Nelson WC, Dodson RJ, Brinkac LM, Daugherty SC, Durkin AS, DeBoy RT, Kolonay JF, Sullivan SA, Zhou L, Davidsen TM, Wu M, Huston AL, Lewis M, Weaver B, Weidman JF, Khouri H, Utterback TR, Feldblyum TV, Fraser CM (2005) The psychrophilic lifestyle as revealed by the genome sequence of *Colwellia psychrerythraea* 34H through genomic and proteomic analyses. PNAS 102:10913–10918
4. Boyle R (1665) New experiments and observations touching cold. Royal Society of London
5. Spallanzani L (1776) Opuscoli di Fisca Animale E Vegetabile. Socia della Academie Di Londra De' Currosi della Natura di Germania Di Berlino Stockolm Gottinga Bologna Siena etc. Modena, Italy
6. Lidforrs B (1907) Die Wintergrune Flora. Lunds Universitets Arsskrift 2:1–76
7. Maximov N (1912) Chemical protective agents of plants against freezing injury. Berichte Deutschen Bot Gesellschaft 30:52–65
8. Luyet BJ, Gehenio PM (1940) Life and death at low temperatures. Biodynamica, Normandy Missouri

9. Polge C, Smith AU, Parkes AS (1949) Revival of spermatozoa after vitrification and dehydration at low temperatures. Nature 164:666

10. Smith AU (1950) Prevention of hemolysis during freezing and thawing of red blood cells. Lancet 2:910–911

11. Smith AU, Polge C (1950) Survival of spermatozoa at low temperatures. Nature 166:668

12. Lovelock JE (1953) The haemolysis of human red blood cells by freezing and thawing. Biochim Biophys Acta 10:414–426

13. Sakai A (1956) Survival of plant tissue at superlow temperatures. Low Temp Sci Ser B 14:17–23

14. Lovelock JE, Bishop MWH (1959) Prevention of freezing damage to living cells by dimethylsulphoxide. Nature 183:1394–1395

15. Smith AU (1961) Biological effects of freezing and supercooling. Williams and Wilkins, Baltimore, MD

16. Mazur P (1965) Causes of injury and frozen and thawed cells. Fed Proc 24: S175–S182

17. Meryman HT (1966) Cryobiology. Academic, London

18. Parkes AS (1966) Sex science and society. Oriel, Newcastle on Tyne, UK

19. Sakai A (1960) Survival of a twig of woody plants at −196°C. Nature 185:393–394

20. Meryman HT (1968) A modified model for the mechanisms of freezing injury in erythrocytes. Nature 218:333–336

21. Smith AU (1970) Current trends in cryobiology. Plenum, New York

22. Whittingham DG, Leibo SP, Mazur P (1972) Survival of mouse embryos frozen to −196°C and −269°C. Science 178:411–414

23. Franks F (1975) Water: a comprehensive treatise. Plenum, New York

24. Withers LA, King P (1980) A simple freezing unit and routine cryopreservation method for plant cell cultures. CryoLetters 1:213–220

25. Kartha KK, Leung NL, Moroginski LA (1982) *In vitro* growth and plant regeneration from cryopreserved meristems of cassava (*Manihot esculenta* Crantz). Zeitschrift Pflanzenphysiol Bd 107:S 133–140

26. Trounson A, Mohr L (1983) Human pregnancy following cryopreservation thawing and transfer of an eight-cell embryo. Nature 305:707–709

27. Zeilmaker GH, Alberta AT, Van Gent, Imprinetta, Rijkmans, Camilla MPM, Drogendijk, A at C (1984) Two pregnancies following transfer of intact frozen–thawed embryos. Fertil Steril 42:293–296

28. Fahy GM, MacFarlane DR, Angell CA, Meryman HT (1984) Vitrification as an approach to cryopreservation. Cryobiology 21:407–426

29. Rall WF, Fahy G (1985) Ice-free cryopreservation of mouse embryos at −196°C by vitrification. Nature 313:573–575

30. Kartha KK (1985) Cryopreservation of plant cells and organs. CRC, Boca Raton, FL

31. Fabre J, Dereuddre J (1990) Encapsulation-dehydration an new approach to cryopreservation of *Solanum* shoot-tips. CryoLetters 11:413–426

32. Sakai A, Kobayashi S, Oiyama I (1990) Survival by vitrification of nucellar cells of navel orange *Citrus sinensis* Osb var brasiliensis Tanaka cooled to −196°C. J Plant Physiol 137:465–470

33. Watson PF (1995) Artificial insemination and the preservation of semen. In: Lamming GE (ed) Marshall's physiology of reproduction. Churchill Livingstone, Edinburgh, Scotland, pp 747–869

34. Leibo SP (2004) The early history of gamete cryobiology. In: Fuller B, Lane N, Benson EE (eds) Life in the frozen state. CRC, Boca Raton, FL, pp 347–370

35. Day JG, McLellan MR (1995) Cryopreservation and freeze-drying protocols. Humana, Totowa, NJ

36. Grout B (1995) Genetic preservation of plant cells *in vitro,* Springer lab manual. Springer-Verlag, Berlin, Germany

37. Bajaj YPS (1995) Cryopreservation of plant germplasm I biotechnology in agriculture and forestry. vol 32. Springer-Verlag, Berlin, Germany

38. Watson PF, Holt WV (2001) Cryobanking. The Genetic Resource Taylor and Francis, London

39. Benson EE (1999) Plant conservation biotechnology. Taylor and Francis, London

40. Engelmann F, Takagi H (2000) Cryopreservation of tropical plant germplasm; Current research progress and application. Japanese International Research Center for Agricultural Sciences, Tskuba, Japan, International Plant Genetic Resources Institute, Rome, Italy

41. Leibo SP, Semple ME, Kroetsch TG (1994) *In-vitro* fertilization of oocytes by 37-year-old cryopreserved bovine spermatozoa. Theriogenology 42:1257–1262

42. Benson EE (2004) Cryoconserving algal and plant diversity: historical perspectives and future challenges. In: Fuller B, Lane N, Benson EE (eds) Life in the frozen state. CRC, Boca Raton, FL, pp 299–328

43. Mazur P (2004) Principles of cryobiology. In: Fuller B, Lane N, Benson EE (eds) Life in the frozen state. CRC, Boca Raton, FL, pp 299–328

44. Panis B, Piette B, Swennen R (2005) Droplet vitrification of apical meristems: a cryopreservation protocol applicable to all Musaceae. Plant Science 168:45–55

45. Day JG, Stacey GN (2007) Cryopreservation and freeze-drying protocols. Methods in molecular biology, Humana, Totowa, NJ

46. Fleck RA, Pickup RW, Day JG, Benson EE (2006) Characterisation of cryoinjury in *Euglena gracilis* using flow-cytometry and cryomicroscopy. Cryobiology 52:261–268

47. Kedem O, Katchalsky A (1958) Membrane permeability modelling: Thermodynamic analysis of the permeability of biological membranes to non-electrolytes. Biochim Biophys Acta 27:229–246

48. Rubinsky B, Pegg DE (1988) A mathematical model for the freezing process in biological tissues. Proc R Soc Lond 234:343–358

49. Chuenkhum S, Cui Z (2006) The parameter conversion from the Kedem-Katchalsky model into the two-parameter model. CryoLetters 27:185–199

50. Gilmore JA, McGann LE, Gao DY, Peter AT, Kleinhans FW, Crister JK (1995) Effect of cryoprotectant solutes on water permeability of human spermatozoa. Biology of Reproduction 53:985–995

51. Benson EE (2008) Cryopreservation theory. In: Reed BM (ed) Plant cryopreservation: a practical guide. Springer, Germany, pp 15–32

52. Fahy GM, Wowk B, Wu J, Paynter S (2004) Improved vitrification solutions based on the predictability of vitrification solution toxicity. Cryobiology 48:22–35

53. Fuller BJ (2004) Cryoprotectants: the essential antifreezes to protect life in the frozen state. CryoLetters 25:375–388

54. Volk GM, Walters C (2006) Plant vitrification solution 2 lowers water content and alters freezing behaviour in shoot tips during cryoprotection. Cryobiology 52:48–61

55. Benson EE, Bremner DH (2004) Oxidative stress in the frozen plant: a free radical point of view. In: Fuller B, Lane N, and Benson EE (eds) Life in the frozen state. CRC, FL, pp 205–242

56. Morris GJ, Clarke KJ, Clarke A (1977) The cryopreservation of *Chlorella* 3 Effect of heterotrophic nutrition on freezing tolerance. Arch Microbiol 114:249–254

57. Sakai A (2004) Plant cryopreservation. In: Fuller B, Lane N, Benson EE (eds) Life in the frozen state. CRC, FL, pp 329–346

58. Da Costa Nunes E, Benson EE, Oltramari AC, Araujo PS, Moser JR, Viana AM (2003) *In vitro* conservation of *Cedrela fissilis* (Meliaceae) a native tree of the Brazilian Atlantic Forest. Biodiversity and Conservation 12:837–848

59. Morris GJ (1976) The cryopreservation of *Chlorella* 2 effect of growth temperature on freezing tolerance. Arch Microbiol 107:309–312

60. Luo J, Reed BM (1997) Abscisic acid-responsive protein bovine serum albumin and proline pretreatments improve recovery of *in vitro* currant shoot tips and callus cryopreserved by vitrification. Cryobiology 34:240–250

61. Marco-Jiménez F, Lavara R, Vicente JS, Viudes-de-Castro MP (2006) Cryopreservation of rabbit spermatozoa with freezing media supplemented with reduced and oxidised glutathione. CryoLetters 27:261–268

62. Day JG, Brand JJ (2005) Cryopreservation methods for maintaining cultures. In: Andersen RA (ed) Algal culturing techniques. Academic, NY, pp 165–187

63. Fuller BJ, Paynter SJ (2007) Cryopreservation of mammalian embryos. In: Day JG, Stacey GN (eds) Cryopreservation and freeze-drying protocols. Humana, Totowa, NJ, pp 323–337

64. Morris GJ, Acton E, Avery S (1999) A novel approach to sperm cryopreservation. Human Reproduction 14:1013–1021

65. Faszer K, Draper D, Green JE, Morris GJ, Grout BWW (2006) Cryopreservation of horse semen under laboratory and field conditions using a Stirling cycle freezer. CryoLetters 27:179–184

66. Harding K, Day JG, Lorenz M, Timmerman H, Friedl T, Bremner DH, Benson EE (2004) Introducing the concept and application of vitrification for the cryo-conservation of algae – a min-review. Nova Hedwigia 79:207–226

67. Wood CB, Pritchard HW, Miller AP (2000) Simultaneous preservation of orchid seed and its fungal symbiont using encapsulation-dehydration is dependent upon moisture content and storage temperature. CryoLetters 21:125–136

68. Benson EE, Reed BM, Brennan R, Clacher KA, Ross DA (1996) Use of thermal analysis in the evaluation of cryopreservation protocols for *Ribes nigrum* L germplasm. CryoLetters 17:347–362

69. Benson EE, Johnston J, Muthusamy J, Harding K (2005) Physical and engineering perspectives of *in vitro* plant cryopreservation. In: Dutta Gupta S, Ibaraki Y(eds) Plant tissue culture engineering. Springer, Netherlands, pp 441–473

70. Mix-Wagner G, Schumacher HM, Cross RJ (2002) Recovery of potato apices after several years of storage in liquid nitrogen. CryoLetters 24:33–41

71. Gould EA (1995) Virus cryopreservation and storage In: Day JG, McLellan MR (eds) Cryopreservation and freeze-drying protocols. Humana, Totowa, NJ, pp 7–20

72. Tindall BJ (2007) Vacuum-drying and cryopreservation of prokaryotes. In: Day JG, Stacey GN (eds) Cryopreservation and freeze-drying protocols. Humana, Totowa, NJ, pp 73–97

73. Day JG (2007) Cryopreservation of microalgae and cyanobacteria. In: Day JG, Stacey GN (eds) Cryopreservation and freeze-drying protocols. Humana, Totowa, NJ, pp 139–149

74. Kilvington S (1995) Cryopreservation of pathogenic and non-pathogenic free-living amoebae. In: Day JG, McLellan MR (eds) Cryopreservation and freeze-drying protocols. Humana, Totowa, NJ, pp 63–69

75. Christofinis GJ, Miller H (1983) A simplified method for cryopreservation of *Plasmodium falciparum* from continuous *in vitro* cultures. Ann Trop Med Parisitol 77:123–126

76. Bond C (2007) Cryopreservation of yeast cultures. In: Day JG, Stacey GN (eds) Cryopreservation and freeze-drying protocols. Humana, Totowa, NJ, pp 107–115

77. Ryan MJ, Smith D (2007) Cryopreservation and freeze-drying of fungi employing centrifugal and shelf freeze-drying. In: Day JG, Stacey GN (eds) Cryopreservation and freeze-drying protocols. Humana, Totowa, NJ, pp 125–138

78. Homolka L, Ludmilla L, Nerud F (2006) Basidiomycete cryopreservation on perlite: Evaluation of a new method. Cryobiology 52:446–453

79. Burch J, Wilkinson T (2002) Cryopreservation of protonemata of *Ditrichum cornubicum* (Paton) comparing the effectiveness of four cryoprotectant pretreatments. CryoLetters 23:197–208

80. Reed BA, Dumet DJ, DeNoma JM, Benson EE (2001) Validation of cryopreservation protocols for plant germplasm conservation: a pilot study using. *Ribes* L Biodiversity & Conservation 10:939–949

81. Find JI, Krogstrup P, Moller JD, Noergaard JV, Kristensen MMH (1993) Cryopreservation of embryogenic suspension cultures of *Picea sitchensis* and subsequent plant regeneration. Scan J Forest Res 8:156–162

82. Nadarajan J, Staines HJ, Benson EE, Mansor M, Krishnapillay B, Harding K. (2006) Optimization of cryopreservation protocol for *Stericulia cordata* Blume Zygotic embryos using Taguchi experiments. J Tropical Forest Sci 18:166–172

83. Irdani T, Carletti B, Ambrogioni L, Roversi PF (2006) Rapid-cooling and storage of plant nematodes at −140°C. Cryobiology 52:319–322

84. Rajamohan A, Leopold RA, Wang WB, Harris M, McCombs SD, Peabody NC, Fisher K (2003) Cryopreservation of the Mediterranean fruit fly. CryoLetters 24:125–132

85. MacFadzen IRB (1995) Cryopreservation of *Crassostrea gigas*. In: Day JG, McLellan MR (eds) Cryopreservation and freeze-drying protocols. Humana, Totowa, NJ, pp 145–149

86. Kopeika E, Kopeika J, Zhang T (2007) Cryopreservation of fish sperm. In: Day JG, Stacey GN (eds) Cryopreservation and freeze-drying protocols, Humana, Totowa, NJ, pp 201–215

87. Wishart G (2007) Cryopreservation of avian spermatozoa. In: Day JG, Stacey GN (eds) Cryopreservation and freeze-drying protocols. Humana, Totowa, NJ, pp 217–223

88. Curry MR (2007) Cryopreservation of mammalian semen. In: Day JG, Stacey GN (eds) Cryopreservation and freeze-drying protocols. Humana, Totowa, NJ, pp 301–310

89. Pegg DE, Wusteman MC, Wang L (2006) Cryopreservation of articular cartilage Part 1: Conventional cryopreservation methods. Cryobiology 52:335–346

90. Hunt CJ, Pegg DE, Armitage SE (2006) Optimising cryopreservation protocols for haematopoietic progenitor cells: a methodological approach for umbilical blood cord. CryoLetters 27:73–85

91. Spurr EE, Wiggins NE, Marsden KA, Lowenthal RM, Ragg SJ (2002) Cryopreserved human haematopoietic stem cells retain engraftment potential after extended (5–14) years of cryostorage. Cryobiology 44:210–217

92. Terry C, Dhawan A, Mitry RR, Hughes RD (2006) Cryopreservation of isolated human hepatocytes for transplantation: state of the art. Cryobiology 53:149–159

93. Morris CB (2007) Cryopreservation of animal and human cell lines. In: Day JG and Stacey GN (eds) Cryopreservation and freeze-drying protocols. Humana, Totowa, NJ, pp 225–234

94. Watt SM, Austin E, Armitage S (2007) Cryopreservation of haematopoietic stem/ progenitor cells for therapeutic use. In: Day JG, Stacey GN (eds) Cryopreservation and freeze-drying protocols. Humana, Totowa, NJ, pp 235–257

95. Sputtek A (2007) Cryopreservation of red blood cells and platelets. In: Day JG, Stacey GN (eds) Cryopreservation and freeze-drying protocols. Humana, Totowa, NJ, pp 281–299

96. Paynter SJ, Fuller BJ (2007) Cryopreservation of mammalian oocytes. In: Day JG, Stacey GN (eds) Cryopreservation and freeze-drying protocols. Humana, Totowa, NJ, pp 311–322

97. Dittrich R, Maltaris T (2006) A simple freezing protocol for the use of an open freezing system for cryopreservation of ovarian tissue. Cryobiology 52:166

98. Newton H, Aubard Y, Rutherford A, Sharma V, Gosden R (1996) Low temperature storage and grafting of human ovarian tissue. Human Reprod 11:1487–1491

99. Strumia MM, Hodge CC (1945) Frozen human skin grafts. Ann Surg 121:860–865

100. Konstantinow A, Muhlbauer W, Hartinger AG, von Donnersmarck G (1991) Skin banking: a simple method for cryopreservation of split thickness skin and cultures epidermal keratinocytes. Ann Plast Surg 26:89–97

101. Donelly ET, Steele EK, McClure N, Lewis SEM (2001) Assessment of DNA integrity and morphology of ejaculated spermatozoa from fertile and infertile men before and after cryopreservation. Human Reproduction 16:1191–1199

102. Harding K (2004) Genetic integrity of cryopreserved plant cells: a review. CryoLetters 25:3–22

103. Stacey G (2004) Fundamental issues for cell-line banks in biotechnology and regulatory affairs. In: Fuller B, Lane N, Benson EE (eds) Life in the frozen state. CRC, London, pp. 437–452

104. Kate KT, Laird SA (1999) The commercial use of biodiversity–access to genetic resources and benefit sharing. Earthscan Publications, London

105. Kirsop B, Doyle A (1991) Maintenance of microorganisms and cultured cells. Academic, London

106. Haefner B (2003) Drugs from the deep: marine natural products as drug candidates. Discovery Today 8:536–544

107. Hédoin H, Pearson J, Day JG, Philip D, Young AJ, Hall TJ (2006) *Porphyridium cruentum* A-408 and *Planktothrix* A-404 retain their capacity to produce biotechnologically exploitable metabolites after cryopreservation. J Appl Phycol 18:1–7

108. Ryan MJ, Smith D, Bridge PD, Jeffries P (2003) The relationship between fungal preservation method and secondary metabolite production in *Metarhizium anisopliae* and *Fusarium oxysporum*. W J Microbiol Biotechnol 19:839–844

109. Radhakrishna TG, Ramanatha CL, Gupta C, Reddy NC (1983) Economics of artificial insemination and calves born from liquid semen and frozen semen. Ind J Anim Reprod 3:44–45

110. Ludvigsen S (2003) Speech by the Norwegian Minister of Fisheries – seminar hosted by the Brazilian Ministry of Fisheries – Brasilia – 7 October 2003

111. Ashmore SE (1997) Status report on the development and application of *in vitro* techniques for the conservation and use of plant genetic resources IPGRI Rome Italy

112. Keller ER, Senula A, Leunufna S, Grube M (2006) Slow growth storage and cryopreservation-tools to facilitate germplasm maintenance of vegetatively propagate crops and living plant collections. Int J Refrigeration 29:411–417

113. Park YS, Barrett JD, Bonga JM (1998) Application of somatic embryogenesis in high-value clonal forestry: deployment genetic control and stability of cryopreserved clones. In Vitro Cell Dev Biol-Plant 34:231–239

114. Benson EE, Harding K, Johnston J, Day JG (2005) From ecosystems to cryobanks: the role of cryo-conservation. In: Benett IJ, Bunn E, Clarke H, McComb JA (eds) The preservation and sustainable utilization of global plant diversity. Contributing to a sustainable future. Australian Branch of the International Association for Plant Tissue Culture & Biotechnology, Perth Western, Australia, pp 30–44

115. Panis B, Tien Thinh N (2001) Cryopreservation of Musa germplasm International Network for the Improvement of Banana and Plantains Technical Guidelines INIBAP Montpellier France

116. Schumacher HM (1999) Cryo-conservation of industrially important plant cell cultures. In: Benson EE (ed) Plant conservation biotechnology. Taylor and Francis, London, pp 125–138

117. Touno K, Yoshimatsu K, Shimomura K (2006) Characteristics of *Atropa belladonna* hairy roots cryopreserved by vitrification method. CryoLetters 27:65–72

118. Crosier A, Pukashenthi BS, Henghali JN, Howard J, Dickman AJ, Marker L, Wildt DE (2006) Cryopreservation of spermatozoa from wild-born Namibian cheetahs (*Acinonyx jubatus*) influence of glycerol on cryosurvival. Cryobiology 52:169–181

119. Pickard A, Holt WV (2004) Cryopreservation as a supporting measure in species conservation: not the frozen zoo! In: Fuller B, Lane N, Benson EE (eds) Life in the frozen state. CRC, FL, pp 393–414

120. Pence VC (1999) The application of biotechnology for the conservation of endangered plants. In: Benson EE (ed) Plant conservation biotechnology. Taylor and Francis, London, pp 227–250

121. González-Benito ME, Martin C, Iriondo JM, Pérez C (1999) Conservation of the rare and endangered plants endemic to Spain. In: Benson EE (ed) Plant conservation biotechnology. Taylor and Francis, London, pp 251–264

122. Touchell DH, Dixon KW (1993) Cryopreservation of seed of Western Australian native species. Biodiversity and conservation 2:594–602

123. Muthusamy J, Staines HJ, Benson EE, Mansor M, Krishnapillay B (2005) Investigating the use of fractional replication and Taguchi techniques in cryopreservation: a case study using orthodox seeds of a tropical rainforest tree species. Biodiversity and conservation 14:3169–3185

124. Thurston LM, Watson PF, Holt WV (2002) Semen cryopreservation: a genetic explanation for species and individual variation. CryoLetters 23:255–262

125. Nadarajan J (2005) Development of efficient experimental strategies for the cryopreservation of problematic tropical rainforest tree germplasm. PhD Thesis University of Abertay Dundee and The Forest Research Institute of Malaysia

126. Nadarajan J, Staines HJ, Benson EE, Mansor M, Krishnapillay B, Harding K (2006) Optimization of cryopreservation protocol for *Sterculia cordata* Blume Zygotic embryos using Taguchi experiments. J Tropical Forest Sci 18:166–172

127. Dussert S, Engelmann F, Noirot M (2003) Development of probabilistic tools to assist in the establishment and management of cryopreserved plant germplasm collections. CryoLetters 24:149–160

128. Wusteman M, Hunt CJ (2004) The scientific basis for tissue banking. In: Fuller B, Benson EE, Lane N (eds) Life in the frozen state. CRC, Boca Raton, FL, pp 541–562

129. Armitage WJ, Dale W, Alexander EA (2005) Protocols for thawing and cryoprotectant dilution of heart valves. Cryobiology 50:17–20

130. Donnez J, Dolmans MM, Demylle D, Jadoul P, Pirard C, Squifflet J, Martinez-Madrid B, van Langendonckt A (2004) Livebirth after ortotopic transplantation of cryopreserved ovarian tissue. Lancet 16:1405–1410

131. Meirow D, Levron J, Eldar-Geva T, Hardan I, Fridman Y, Zalel E, Schiff J, Dor J (2005) Pregnancy after transplantation of cryopreserved ovarian tissues in a patient with ovarian failure after chemotherapy. N Engl J Med 353:318–321

132. Oh HY, Che ZM, Hong JC, Lee EJ, Lee SJ, Kin J (2005) Cryopreservation of human teeth for future organization of a tooth bank – A preliminary study. CryoLetters 51:322–329

133. Routledge C, Armitage WJ (2003) Cryopreservation of cornea: a low cooling rate improves functional survival of endothelium after freezing and thawing. Cryobiology 46:277–283

134. Pegg DE (2001) The current status of tissue cryopreservation. CryoLetters 2:105–114

135. Human Fertilisation and Embryology Authority (1998) Consultation on the safe cryopreservation of gametes and embryos HFEA London UK

136. Bielanski A, Bergeron H, Lau PCK, Devenish J (2003) Microbial contamination of embryos and semen during long term banking in liquid nitrogen. Cryobiology 46:146–152

137. Tomlinson M (2005) Managing risks associated with cryopreservation. Human Reprod 20:1751–1756

138. Tedder RS, Zuckerman MA, Goldstone AH, Hawkins AE, Fielding A, Briggs EM, Irwin D, Blair S, Gorman AM, Patterson KG, Linch DC, Heptonstall J, Brink NS (1995) Hepatitis B transmission from a contaminated cryopreservation tank. Lancet 346:137–140

139. Morris GJ (2005) The origin ultrastructure and microbiology of the sediment accumulating in liquid nitrogen storage vessels. Cryobiology 50:231–238

140. Medrano A, Cabrera C, González F, Batista M, Gracia A (2002) Is sperm cryopreservation at −150°C a feasible alternative? CryoLetters 23:167–172
141. Stacey GN, Day JG (2007) Long-term *ex situ* conservation of Biological Resources and the role of Biological Resource Centres. In: Day JG, Stacey GN (eds) Cryopreservation and freeze-drying protocols. Humana, Totowa, NJ, pp 1–14
142. Budapest Treaty Regulations (1977) Budapest treaty on the international recognition of the deposit of microorganisms for the purposes of patent procedure. World Intellectual Property Organisation Geneva

53

Magnetic Resonance Imaging

Pottumarthi V. Prasad and Pippa Storey

1. Introduction

Magnetic resonance imaging (MRI) evolved in the early 1970s and has undergone tremendous growth over the last two decades, primarily as a diagnostic tool. The 2003 Nobel Prize in Physiology or Medicine was awarded to two scientists responsible for the development of nuclear magnetic resonance as an imaging technique. The versatility of the technique has led to increasing interest from the basic science community in recent years. This chapter is a condensed summary of the book that was recently published *(1)*. It provides the reader with a concise outline of the fundamental concepts behind MRI and an introduction to a few biological applications. Interested readers can find more detailed information and other relevant bibliography in the book *(1)*.

2. Principles of Magnetic Resonance

Magnetic resonance imaging exploits the phenomenon of nuclear magnetic resonance (NMR), whereby atomic nuclei exposed to a strong magnetic field absorb and reemit electromagnetic waves at a characteristic or "resonant" frequency, which falls in the radiofrequency (RF) range. Because there are no known adverse effects from either the strong magnetic fields or the radio waves, MRI is considered safe for human studies and suitable for longitudinal animal experiments.

Because the resonant frequency of the nuclei is an extremely precise measure of the local magnetic field, it provides a very sensitive probe of their molecular environment. In this capacity, magnetic resonance has long been used in chemistry for the analysis of molecular structure and interactions, and for the identification of chemical compounds. Only recently (since the early 1970s) has it been applied to in vivo spectroscopy and imaging. For a more detailed description, please refer to the introductory chapter of the book *(2)*.

From: *Molecular Biomethods Handbook, 2nd Edition.*
Edited by: J. M. Walker and R. Rapley © Humana Press, Totowa, NJ

2.1. Behavior of Nuclei in a Magnetic Field

The phenomenon of nuclear magnetic resonance derives from the fact that certain nuclei possess tiny magnetic moments, similar to that of a common bar magnet (**Fig. 53.1**). In the presence of an applied magnetic field, the magnetic moments undergo a rotational motion known as "precession," which is analogous to the slow wobble exhibited by a spinning top or gyroscope. The explanation of nuclear precession lies in the relationship between the magnetic moment of the nucleus and its intrinsic spin.

2.1.1. Larmor Precession

Because the magnetic moment of the nucleus is derived from its spin, the orientation of the magnetic moment is locked to the spin axis. This is expressed through the equation

$$\mu = \gamma \mathbf{I}, \tag{1}$$

where μ is the magnetic moment of the nucleus and $\mathbf{I}$ is its spin. Note that each is a vector quantity (as indicated by the bold script), and thus has both magnitude and direction. The direction of $\mathbf{I}$ is given by the spin axis, whereas that of μ determines the orientation of the nucleus' intrinsic magnetic field (**Fig. 53.1**). The factor γ is known as the gyromagnetic ratio, and is a property of the nucleus.

Because the magnetic moment of the nucleus is parallel to its spin, any change in the direction of the magnetic moment requires a corresponding reorientation of the spin axis. A similar situation exists with a gyroscope; any reorientation of the gyroscope is necessarily accompanied by a change in the direction of its spin axis. The result is that when a gyroscope is subjected to a gravitational field it does not immediately fall over, but instead remains upright, albeit with a slow wobble about the vertical known as precession. Similarly, when a nucleus is subjected to a magnetic field, its magnetic moment does not simply swing into alignment with the field, but instead precesses about the direction of the field, as depicted in **Fig. 53.2**.

2.1.2. Larmor Frequency

The frequency at which the nucleus precesses about the magnetic field is known as the Larmor frequency ω_L. It can be shown from classical mechanics

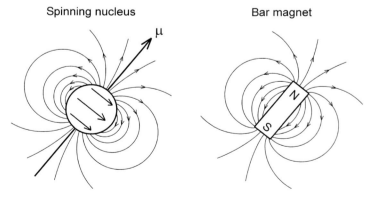

Spinning nucleus   Bar magnet

Fig. 53.1. Nuclei with nonzero spin possess a magnetic moment μ, and produce a tiny magnetic field analogous to that of a bar magnet. The curves indicate lines of magnetic flux

Precession

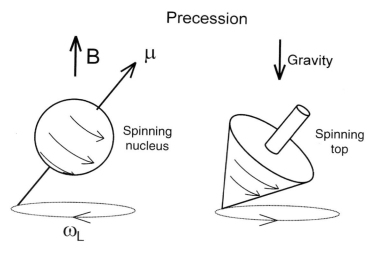

Fig. 53.2. In the presence of an external magnetic field B_0, a nucleus with nonzero spin precesses about the direction of the field, just as a spinning top precesses about the direction of gravity **g**

that the value of the Larmor frequency is proportional to the strength of the magnetic field B_0 and the gyromagnetic ratio of the nucleus,

$$\omega_L = \gamma B_0. \tag{2}$$

The values of γ for some of the nuclei commonly used in biological studies are shown in **Table 53.1**. The most important of these for magnetic resonance imaging (MRI) is hydrogen, because it is present throughout the body in water and fat. Many of the other nuclei that are prevalent in the body, such as carbon-12 and oxygen-16, do not exhibit magnetic resonance because they have no net spin.

2.2. Excitation and Signal Detection

2.2.1. Nuclear Magnetization

The magnetic field of a nucleus is a complicated function of space (**Fig. 53.1**), but is uniquely specified by its magnetic moment μ. The net magnetic field of all the nuclei in a given volume of tissue can similarly be specified by the vector sum of their magnetic moments. The sum is known as the nuclear magnetization, and denoted **M**. The component of **M** that lies in the transverse plane (perpendicular to the static field **B**$_0$) rotates at the Larmor frequency ω_L as the nuclei precess. This produces an oscillating magnetic field that can be detected with an RF receiver coil. The receiver coil consists essentially of one or more loops of wire, through which lines of magnetic flux may pass. As the transverse magnetization rotates, the magnetic flux through the loop oscillates, inducing a small alternating voltage in the coil. The MR signal is thus proportional to the transverse component of **M**.

At equilibrium, the nuclei precess with random phases, as shown in **Fig. 53.3**. The transverse components of their magnetic moments therefore cancel out, and produce no detectable signal. There is however a small net magnetization

Table 53.1. Some of the nuclear isotopes used for *in vivo* magnetic resonance imaging and spectroscopy, listed with their natural abundance, nuclear spin, and gyromagnetic ratio γ.

Nuclear isotope	Natural abundance [%]	Net spin	$\gamma/2\pi$ [MHz/T]
^{1}H	99.98	1/2	42.58
^{2}H	0.015	1	6.53
^{3}He	0.00014[§]	1/2	−32.44
^{7}Li	92.6	3/2	16.5
^{13}C	1.11	1/2	10.71
^{14}N	99.6	1	3.1
^{15}N	0.36	1/2	−4.3
^{19}F	100	1/2	40.05
^{23}Na	100	3/2	11.26
^{31}P	100	1/2	17.23
^{39}K	93.1	3/2	2.0
^{129}Xe	26.44	1/2	−11.84

[§] The helium-3 used in magnetic resonance studies is derived from the decay of tritium (^{3}H).

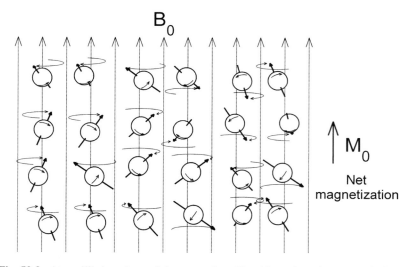

Fig. 53.3. At equilibrium the nuclei precess about $\mathbf{B}_0$ with random phases, producing no net transverse magnetization. However, slightly more of the nuclei are oriented towards the field than away from it, giving rise to a small net longitudinal magnetization $\mathbf{M}_0$

$\mathbf{M}_0$ in the longitudinal direction (parallel to $\mathbf{B}_0$). It cannot be detected directly, because it does not oscillate. It is necessary for producing the signal, however, as we will soon show.

Excitation of nuclear magnetization

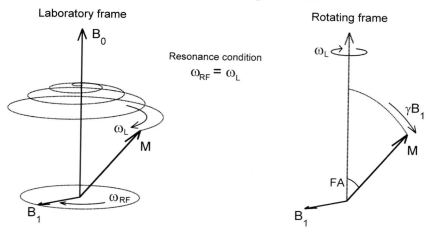

Fig. 53.4. When an RF field B$_1$ is applied at the Larmor frequency, the net magnetization is tipped away from the longitudinal direction. In a frame rotating at the Larmor frequency, the B$_1$ field appears stationary, and the tipping can be interpreted as a secondary precession of the nuclei about B$_1$

The equilibrium magnetization arises because the nuclei exhibit a slight preference for being aligned along the direction of the external magnetic field, because that lowers their energy. The small excess of nuclei pointing along the field (upwards) gives rise to the equilibrium magnetization **M**$_0$ (**Fig. 53.3**).

2.2.2. RF Excitation

By applying a transverse oscillating magnetic field to the tissue at exactly the Larmor frequency ω_L, the nuclear magnetization can be tipped away from the longitudinal axis, producing a finite component in the transverse plane. The excess nuclei that had been pointing upwards at equilibrium then precess in synchrony, emitting a detectable signal. The process is one of resonant excitation, and is similar to the mechanism involved in pushing a child's swing.

Just as the swing can be made to oscillate by applying a periodic force, the nuclei in a sample of tissue can be made to precess in synchrony by applying a rotating magnetic field in the transverse plane. The applied field is denoted **B**$_1$(t), and its frequency of rotation must exactly match the Larmor frequency of the nuclei to satisfy the resonance condition. Because the Larmor frequency falls in the radiofrequency regime, the process is described as RF excitation, and the resonance condition is written $\omega_{RF} = \omega_L$. As the **B**$_1$(t) field transfers energy to the nuclei, the amplitude of their transverse magnetization gradually increases (**Fig. 53.4**).

When the **B**$_1$(t) field is switched off, the transverse magnetization continues to rotate at the Larmor frequency, producing an oscillating magnetic field that can be detected by the RF receiver coil

2.3. Spin Relaxation

The signal following an RF pulse will not persist indefinitely, however, owing to internuclear and intermolecular forces, which cause a loss of phase coherence among the spins and a corresponding attenuation of the transverse magnetization. The nuclei simultaneously lose energy to their surroundings, resulting in a recovery of the longitudinal magnetization to its equilibrium value. These processes are termed transverse and longitudinal relaxation respectively.

2.3.1. Longitudinal Relaxation (Loss of Energy)

The timescale on which longitudinal relaxation occurs is denoted T_1, and defined as the reciprocal of the rate of energy loss. Because longitudinal relaxation is caused by interactions between the nuclei and their environment, the value of T_1 varies according to the molecule in which the nucleus is bound and the type of tissue in which it is present. For example, the T_1 of tissue water tends to be longer in body fluids such as blood and cerebrospinal fluid than in "solid" tissues such as the white matter of the brain. Intensity differences among these tissues can be achieved on an MR image by tailoring the acquisition so that it is sensitive to T_1.

The recovery of the longitudinal magnetization follows an exponential curve

$$M_{\parallel}(t) = M_0 + [M_{\parallel}(0) - M_0]\, e^{-t/T1} \tag{3}$$

where $M_{\parallel}$ denotes the longitudinal magnetization and t is the time following the RF excitation. The value of the longitudinal magnetization immediately after the excitation $M_{\parallel}(0)$ is determined by its value before the excitation and by the flip angle of the RF pulse.

2.3.2. Transverse Relaxation (Loss of Phase Coherence)

Transverse relaxation occurs more rapidly than longitudinal relaxation as a result of additional processes that cause dephasing among the spins. Dephasing occurs because of local variations in the magnetic field, which arise in part from the influence of neighboring nuclei and molecules. The timescale, T_2, associated with these microscopic dephasing processes depends on the tumbling rate of the molecules, because rapid motion tends to average out the effects of the interactions over time. Free water in body fluids, for example, relaxes relatively slowly (on the order of 1 s), because its molecules are in constant rotation. By comparison, molecules that are very large or bound to cell membranes have very short T_2 values (on the order of microseconds). Dephasing can also result from larger-scale variations in magnetic field strength, which arise from inhomogeneities in the applied field and differences in magnetic susceptibility among the tissues themselves. Susceptibility differences occur around air-filled cavities, such as the sinuses and petrous bones in the head, and in tissue containing deoxygenated blood or byproducts of hemorrhage. The resulting mesoscopic field variations further shorten the transverse relaxation time, to a value denoted by T_2^*.

2.3.3. The Fid and The Spin Echo

The attenuation of the transverse magnetization following RF excitation is known as the "free induction decay" or "FID" (**Fig. 53.5**). It is described by an exponential decay with timescale T_2^*

$$M_{\perp}(t) = M_{\perp}(0)\, e^{-t/T_2^*} \tag{4}$$

Here $M_{\perp}$ is the amplitude of the transverse magnetization and t is the time following the RF excitation. The value of $M_{\perp}(0)$ is determined by the longitudinal magnetization available before the excitation and by the flip angle of the RF pulse.

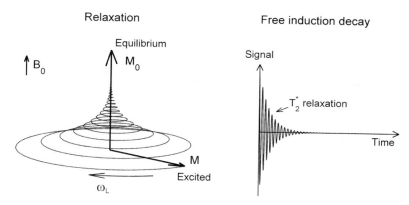

Relaxation   Free induction decay

Fig. 53.5. When the excitation field B_1 is turned off, the net magnetization **M** continues to rotate about B_0 at the Larmor frequency, producing a signal that can be detected with an RF coil. However it undergoes transverse relaxation, producing a gradual attenuation of the signal known as a free induction decay (FID). The nuclei simultaneously lose energy to the environment, resulting in longitudinal relaxation, and a return of the magnetization to its equilibrium value $\mathbf{M}_0$

The dephasing owing to mesoscopic field inhomogeneities is considered reversible, because its effect can be undone using a simple refocusing procedure. The procedure relies on the use of a 180° RF pulse (the refocusing pulse) to reverse the phase differences that have accumulated among the spins. The echo registered under these conditions is called a spin echo and follows the same exponential decay as in Eq. 4, except that the decay constant is T_2 rather than T_2^*.

2.4. Common Abbreviations and Symbols

γ: gyromagnetic ratio; B_0: static magnetic field; B_1: radiofrequency field; BOLD: blood oxygenation level dependent; FID: free induction decay; FA: flip angle; FOV: field of view; M_0: equilibrium magnetization; MRI: magnetic resonance imaging; MRS: magnetic resonance spectroscopy; NMR: nuclear magnetic resonance; RF: radiofrequency; SAR: specific absorption rate; SNR: signal-to-noise ratio; T: tesla (1 T = 10,000 gauss); T_1: time constant for longitudinal relaxation; T_2: time constant for irreversible transverse relaxation (describing the attenuation of the spin echo); T_2^*: time constant for total transverse relaxation (describing the decay of the FID); TE: echo time; TR: repetition time; voxel: volume element

3. Methods

3.1. Instrumentation

The central component of an MR scanner is the primary magnet, which produces the $\mathbf{B}_0$ field. The scanner also includes gradient coils and higher-order shim coils to adjust the spatial variations in $\mathbf{B}_0$. RF coils and related circuitry are required for spin excitation and signal reception, and a computer system is used to control the acquisition and process the results.

The most important specification of the primary magnet is its field strength, because that determines the available signal. Magnetic field strength is measured in gauss (G) or tesla (T), where $1\,T = 10,000\,G$. Gauss is the more natural unit for the magnetic fields encountered in everyday situations; the earth's own magnetic field for example is about $0.5\,G$ ($5 \times 10^{-5}\,T$). The fields used in MR scanners however are of the order of 10,000–100,000 times stronger, and are quoted in tesla. Clinical MR scanners typically have field strengths of 1.5 T or 3.0 T, whereas the high-field systems used for animal studies have strengths of up to around 14 T. The fields must not only be strong, but also very stable, and this is achieved with the use of electromagnets made from coils of superconducting wire, which must be maintained at liquid helium temperature (4 K).

To optimize the spatial homogeneity of the magnetic field, the scanner is equipped with gradient and higher-order shim coils, which are used to adjust the linear and quadratic variations in the field. The gradient coils serve a second purpose, because they are also used for encoding the spatial information that is required to produce an image. An MR system typically includes three gradient coils that produce linearly varying magnetic fields along the three principal X, Y, and Z directions. On human whole body scanners, the maximum gradient field strength is typically on the order of 40 mT/m, whereas on small bore scanners it can be up to 3000 mT/m. Higher gradient fields can support finer spatial resolution.

The next essential element of the MRI scanner is the radio-frequency coil, used both for spin excitation and signal reception. Coils are typically classified as surface coils, which are placed over the region of interest, or volume coils, which enclose the region of interest. Surface coils may consist of a single loop or an array of multiple elements. A given coil may be used to transmit or receive or both. A typical scanner system is usually equipped with multiple coils designed specifically for each application (**Fig. 53.6**). The coil must be tuned to the resonant frequency of the nucleus of interest (e.g., hydrogen, sodium or phosphorus).

Multiple computer systems are required to control the various components of the scanner, to acquire and postprocess the data, to interface with the operator and to provide options for data archival and display.

3.2. Image Formation

Imaging can be performed using 2D or 3D acquisitions, which involve the excitation of nuclei in a specified slice or slab of tissue respectively. Once excited, all the tissue within the slice or slab emits signal simultaneously. To produce an image, therefore, additional mechanisms are needed to determine how much signal originated from each point. This is achieved by "encoding" spatial information into the phase and frequency of the signal. Both slice-selective excitation and spatial encoding involve the use of magnetic field gradients.

3.2.1. Slice-Selective Excitation

Slice-selective excitation is achieved by applying the RF field in the presence of a magnetic field gradient. The gradient introduces a small spatial variation into the strength of the $\mathbf{B}_0$ field, producing a corresponding variation in the Larmor frequency (**Fig. 53.7**). Only those nuclei whose Larmor frequency ω_L equals the frequency of the applied RF field ω_{RF} will then be excited. The condition $\omega_L = \omega_{RF}$ is satisfied for nuclei lying in a particular slice of tissue oriented

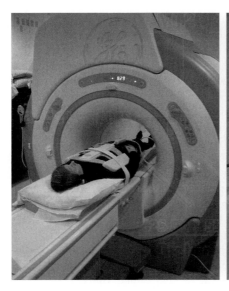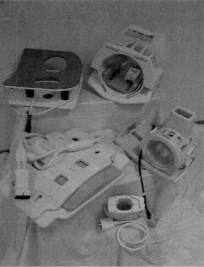

Fig. 53.6. (**A**) A 1.5 T whole body clinical MRI scanner (GE Healthcare, Milwaukee, WI). A torso phased array coil has been placed over the subject's chest for localized signal reception. (**B**) Examples of other coils used in clinical MRI. Clockwise from top left: a breast coil, head coil, extremity coil (for knee, ankle and foot imaging), wrist coil, and torso coil

Slice-selective excitation

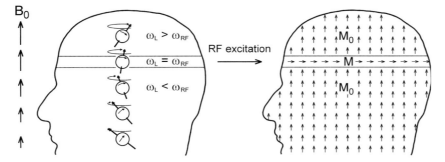

Fig. 53.7. To acquire an image of a particular slice of tissue, the scanner must excite the nuclear magnetization only within that slice. Slice-selective excitation is achieved by applying a magnetic field gradient in the direction perpendicular to the plane of the slice (in this case the superior/inferior direction). The gradient produces a linear variation in the strength of the static field, which gives rise to a spatial variation in the value of the Larmor frequency. Only those spins whose Larmor frequency matches the frequency of the applied RF field will be excited

perpendicular to the magnetic field gradient. The thickness of the slice is determined by the bandwidth of the RF pulse and the amplitude of the gradient, each of which can be chosen independently. The orientation of the slice can be controlled by adjusting the direction of the magnetic field gradient. The gradient coils can be used singly or in combination to excite a slice in any oblique plane.

3.2.2. Spatial Encoding

By applying a magnetic field gradient during data acquisition, position information is encoded into the frequency of the signal (**Fig. 53.8**). Because the detected signal comes from the entire slice, it will contain a range of different frequencies, corresponding to contributions from tissue at different points along the direction of the gradient. The origin of each contribution can be identified by its frequency. This technique, known as frequency encoding, is not sufficient by itself to reconstruct an image, however, because it provides position information in only one direction.

Position information along the perpendicular direction is obtained through a mechanism known as phase encoding, which is used in combination with frequency encoding to produce an image in two dimensions. A gradient pulse is applied in the phase-encoding direction before signal acquisition. The gradient alters the Larmor frequency of the spins, but only for a brief period, resulting in a relative phase shift among them (**Fig. 53.8**). The detected signal therefore contains components with different phases, which originate from different positions along the direction of the gradient. To extract the amplitude of each component, the entire process of excitation and signal acquisition must be repeated many times, with gradient pulses of incrementally different strengths. The phase change among successive acquisitions uniquely identifies the position of the tissue along the direction of the gradient. Phase encoding is in fact mathematically equivalent to frequency encoding, except that the data are acquired in a discrete rather than continuous manner.

3.2.3. Image Reconstruction

Image reconstruction is summarized in **Fig. 53.9**. The MRI data are recorded as a series of lines in a two-dimensional array known as "k-space." By applying a 2D Fourier transform to the k-space data, the spatial distribution of the signal is recovered. The phase information is usually discarded, leaving a map of the signal amplitude, which constitutes the image.

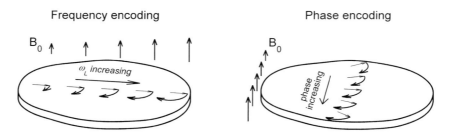

Fig. 53.8. Having excited the nuclear magnetization within a desired slice of tissue, spatial information regarding the position of the spins within the imaging plane must be encoded into their signal. This is achieved using frequency encoding in one direction and phase encoding in the perpendicular direction. In frequency encoding, a magnetic field gradient is applied during the signal acquisition. The position of the spins along the direction of the gradient can therefore be deduced from the frequency of the signal. In phase encoding, a magnetic field gradient is applied briefly before data acquisition. This introduces a phase variation among the spins, which is imprinted on their signal. To extract position information from the phase of the signal, the process must be repeated many times with phase-encoding gradients of incrementally different amplitudes

Image reconstruction

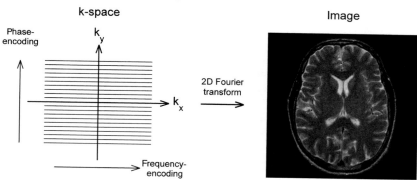

k-space

Image

Phase-encoding

k_y

2D Fourier transform

k_x

Frequency-encoding

Fig. 53.9. Following each excitation, signal is acquired as a function of time and recorded as a line of data along the frequency-encoding direction of "k-space," the Fourier reciprocal of the image domain. The process is repeated with phase-encoding gradients of incrementally different amplitudes, and the signals recorded as adjacent lines in k-space. After all the k-space data is acquired, the image can be extracted by means of a 2D fast Fourier transform. (Note that, in accordance with convention, the image is rotated so that the anterior of the head is at the top)

The resolution of the image in the phase-encoding direction is determined by the number of k-space lines collected. An image with a resolution of 256 pixels in the phase-encoding direction for example requires the acquisition of 256 k-space lines. Resolution in the frequency-encoding direction is determined by the amplitude of the frequency-encoding gradient and the duration of the acquisition period.

It is useful to note that data in k-space can be interpreted as "spatial-frequency components" of the image. Data near the center of k-space ($\mathbf{k} = 0$) correspond to low spatial-frequency components, and represent the large-scale or "coarse" spatial structure in the image. Data near the outer edges of k-space correspond to high spatial-frequency components, and represent the fine structure in the image.

3.2.4. Pulse Sequences

The acquisition of an MR image requires repeated RF pulses and signal acquisitions, each of which must be synchronized with magnetic field gradients. The entire process is known as a pulse sequence, and can be tailored to provide optimal signal contrast for each application. Among the simplest and most commonly used pulse sequences is the so-called "gradient-echo" sequence.

In a gradient-echo sequence, a single RF excitation pulse is applied during each TR period, and data are acquired during the subsequent free induction decay. The term gradient echo refers to the resurgence of signal that occurs at the center of the acquisition period (**Fig. 53.10**). It arises because the frequency-encoding gradient itself produces dephasing among the spins, and the center of the acquisition period is the moment at which that component of the dephasing is zero. The fact that the gradient echo occurs at the center of the acquisition period rather than the beginning results from the application of a negative preparatory gradient pulse, which "prewinds" the spins.

Gradient-echo pulse sequence

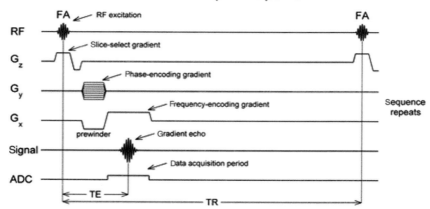

Fig. 53.10. A simple pulse sequence illustrating the implementation of slice selection and spatial encoding. The presentation of a pulse sequence is analogous to an orchestral score, with time increasing from left to right, and the parts played by each component of the scanner displayed one above the other. The top line illustrates the RF pulses produced by the transmitter, whereas the lines marked G_z, G_y, and G_x indicate the magnetic field gradients in the slice-select, phase-encoding and frequency-encoding directions respectively. The label ADC denotes the analog-to-digital converter, which is turned on during signal acquisition

The term "echo time" (TE) is used in the context of gradient echo sequences to denote the interval between RF excitation and the center of the gradient echo. The value of TE is important in determining the signal contrast of the image. Because the transverse magnetization is subject to T_2^* dephasing during the FID, regions of tissue where T_2^* is short compared to TE will exhibit greatly attenuated signal. By comparison, regions with longer T_2^* will have relatively higher signal. Gradient-echo images are therefore described as T_2^*-weighted. The degree of T_2^*-weighting depends on the value of TE, which for gradient-echo sequences ranges from about 1 ms upwards.

Gradient-echo sequences often employ very short TR values (of the order of a few milliseconds), with the result that the images also exhibit T_1 weighting. Tissues with shorter T_1 appear brighter than those with longer T_1 because their longitudinal magnetization will have more fully recovered before each excitation. The degree of T_1 weighting is also influenced by the value of the flip angle, because a higher FA causes greater saturation of the longitudinal magnetization. The FAs typically used in gradient echo sequences range from about 10° to about 40°.

There exists a vast array of other pulse sequences that employ alternative means of spatial encoding and which impart different contrast properties to the acquired image. For more specific details readers should refer to the book chapter *(3)* and the references therein.

3.3. Contrast Preparation

Images are most useful when they can distinguish different tissue types and this is achieved by proper choice of contrast properties. In MRI there are a number of endogenous mechanisms that allow for adjusting the contrast properties of the image. In addition, exogenous contrast material can be used to further enhance contrast.

The most common form of contrast is based on differences in relaxation parameters, T_1, T_2, and T_2^*. Other mechanisms responsible for contrast are flow and diffusion. A more rigorous discussion on this topic is beyond the scope of this review. However **Fig. 53.11** provides a sampling of some of the different types of signal contrast that can be achieved.

3.4. Exogenous Contrast Agents

Further scope for modifying signal contrast in MR imaging is provided by the use of exogenous contrast materials. MR contrast agents do not contribute to the signal directly, but rather alter the signal of surrounding water protons via their effect on relaxation rates.

3.4.1. Types of Contrast Agents

The contrast agents currently in clinical or laboratory use can be roughly divided into two types: those incorporating paramagnetic ions such as gadolinium or manganese *(4,5)*, and those containing superparamagnetic iron oxide (SPIO) particles *(6)*. Paramagnetic ions are typically chelated to organic ligands or bound to macromolecules such as albumin. This minimizes their toxicity, and also reduces their tumbling rates, thereby increasing their effectiveness or "relaxivity." When water molecules bind to the agent and tumble with it in solution, they experience randomly oscillating magnetic fields that stimulate

Types of signal contrast in MRI

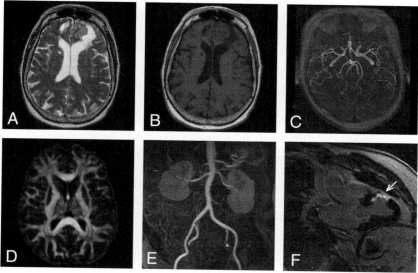

Fig. 53.11. Example images demonstrating a few of the many different sources of signal contrast available in MRI. (**A**) A T_2-weighted image of a patient with an inferior frontal meningioma. (**B**) A T_1-weighted image of the same patient. (**C**) A maximum intensity projection (MIP) of a 3D time-of-flight MR angiogram. (**D**) A diffusion anisotropy map showing myelinated white matter tracts. (**E**) A MIP of a 3D contrast-enhanced MR angiogram. (**F**) A delayed enhancement image of a patient with a myocardial infarct (arrow)

longitudinal relaxation, thereby shortening T_1. Although only a small fraction of the water can bind to the agent at any one time, the bound fraction is in continual exchange with the free water, so that the T_1-shortening effect is distributed throughout the bulk fluid. The result is an enhancement of signal on T_1-weighted images.

Superparamagnetic iron oxide particles have much stronger magnetic moments than individual paramagnetic ions, and therefore alter the magnetic field over a much longer range. The resulting magnetic field gradients induce rapid dephasing of water protons, causing strong signal attenuation on T_2- and T_2^*-weighted images. Although SPIO particles are primarily "T_2 agents," they also shorten T_1 relaxation times, and can be used to produce enhancement on T_1-weighted images. In such applications, the concentration of the agent and the echo time of the sequence must be chosen to minimize T_2 and T_2^* effects, so that they do not counteract the T_1-related signal enhancement.

3.4.2. Biodistribution

The range of applications of exogenous contrast agents is determined largely by their biodistribution and pharmacokinetics. The standard gadolinium chelates are useful for first-pass angiography (**Fig. 53.11e**) *(7)*, but gradually diffuse into the extracellular space over time. This property has however proven useful for imaging infarcts, which exhibit delayed enhancement relative to viable tissue owing to their slower distribution kinetics (**Fig. 53.11f**) *(8,9)*. Macromolecules and small particles are confined to the vascular space, and show promise for quantitative imaging of perfusion and vascular volume *(10)*.

Currently one of the most exciting avenues of research in MR imaging is the development of so-called "targeted" and "smart" contrast agents. Targeted agents *(11)* incorporate ligands such as antibodies that bind to specific molecular markers in the tissue, whereas smart agents *(12)* are activated by the presence of specific ions or enzymes. These agents open the way to visualization of gene expression in vivo, an emerging field known as "molecular imaging."

4. Representative Biological Applications

This section provides representative examples that highlight the utility of MRI for biological applications. It is divided under three subcategories: *(1)* to highlight the exquisite anatomical detail available, *(2)* to illustrate the types of functional information that can be derived using either endogenous mechanisms or exogenous agents both in health and disease, and *(3)* to introduce some cutting edge applications that are evolving to elucidate molecular processes such as gene expression and to monitor the migration of implanted stem cells.

4.1. Structural

4.1.1. Mouse Phenotyping

Upon creation of a new genetic disease model, it is usually characterized by looking for changes in anatomy, physiology, behavior and function. Many of these tests can be done in vivo, but the final step is to perform histopathology to look for organ and biochemical abnormalities. This is not a desirable endpoint if there is only one mouse, and it is required for reproduction. Additionally, given the enormous numbers of mouse mutants produced, it is difficult for mouse pathologists to characterize each mouse in depth. By adapting the techniques and tools of MRI, which is inherently noninvasive, it is possible to take detailed images of the inside of a mouse without conventional "slicing and dicing." This way, it is possible to make anatomic, physiologic and functional measurements in the same living mouse. The field of mouse phenotyping with MRI is rapidly growing.

Recently, there has been interest in preserving and imaging the entire mouse for phenotyping purposes *(13)*. Whole body perfusion and fixing can be achieved by an ultrasound-guided ventricular puncture via the beating heart *(14)*. **Fig. 53.12** shows representative examples of perfusion-fixed whole body MR images.

4.2. Functional

4.2.1. MEMRI

The manganese ion (Mn^{2+}) has long been used in biomedical research as an indicator of calcium (Ca^{2+}) influx in conjunction with fluorescent microscopy, as it is well established that Mn^{2+} enters cells through voltage-gated Ca^{2+} channels. Mn^{2+} is also paramagnetic, resulting in a shortening of the spin-lattice relaxation time constant, T_1, which yields positive contrast enhancement on T_1-weighted MR images, specific to tissues where the ion has accumulated. Manganese-Enhanced MRI (MEMRI) utilizes a combination of these properties of Mn^{2+} to elucidate anatomical information as well as identify regions of cellular activity.

The following three features of Mn^{2+} allow MRI to trace neuronal tracts in an activity dependent manner in the olfactory system of the mouse:

1. Mn^{2+} can be used to measure Ca^{2+} influx.
2. Mn^{2+} can be transported along axons and traverse synapses.
3. Mn^{2+} is paramagnetic and hence MRI detectable.

The initial study involved exposing mice to a nasal lavage of a concentrated Mn^{2+} solution and imaging at multiple time points following exposure *(15)*. Similar to what Tjälve et al. observed with radioactive Mn^{2+} in the pike and later the rat, the olfactory pathway in the mouse exhibited contrast enhancement on T_1-weighted MRI images (**Fig. 53.13**) *(15–17)*. The peak signal intensity in the olfactory bulbs occurred at 29 hours post Mn^{2+} exposure; after 72–96 hours, the signal intensity returned to baseline *(15)*. The return to baseline signal intensity, indicating the "wash-out" of the ion from tissue, allows for longitudinal studies to be performed in the same animal *(15)*.

4.2.2. Oxygenation in Kidneys

Blood oxygenation level dependent (BOLD) MRI exploits the fact that deoxygenated hemoglobin is slightly paramagnetic and hence behaves as an endogenous intravascular contrast agent *(18,19)*. In principle, one can monitor changes in tissue oxygenation using this technique by assuming that the regional blood oxygenation levels are in dynamic equilibrium with the surrounding tissue. The BOLD signal changes are influenced by both changes in regional blood flow (perfusion) and regional oxygen consumption (or extraction). Hence, in principle, BOLD MRI measurements are not very specific, i.e., one cannot differentiate changes in perfusion from changes in oxygen extraction.

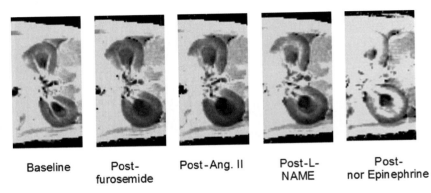

| Baseline | Post-furosemide | Post-Ang. II | Post-L-NAME | Post-nor Epinephrine |

Fig. 53.14. A set of pre- and post pharmaceutical R_2^* (=$1/T_2^*$) maps in rat kidneys in the axial plane. Although this was not performed to address any specific scientific question, it is a very nice demonstration of the advantage and efficacy of the technique. These images were all acquired within about an hour, with about 10 min between administrations of different agents. There is no other known technique that would allow such dynamic information. This is possible mainly because the technique does not rely on administering any exogenous agents. Of course the observed effects would still depend on the pharmacokinetics of the agents used that is not necessarily a limitation of the technique itself. Furosemide stops the reabsorptive function along the medullary thick ascending limbs and thereby reduces the oxygen consumption in the medullary segments. So one can observe reduction in the brightness of R_2^* maps in the medulla (lower R_2^* implied better oxygenation). Angiotensin II is a vasoconstrictor that is commonly used and we observed little effect on the R_2^* maps. However, following subsequent administration of L-NAME and norepinephrine (potent vasoconstrictors) there was a significant increase in R_2^* predominantly in the renal medulla

thus causing a faster rate of spin-lattice relaxation (R_1). Chiarotti et al (27) first reported that an increase in dissolved oxygen in water shortens its T_1 (1/R_1). They also concluded that there exists a linear relationship between R_1 and the concentration of dissolved oxygen in water.

Edelman et al (28) first proposed the use of oxygen for ventilation imaging in the lung. Though oxygen is only weakly paramagnetic, its overall effect on the lung is considerable given the large surface area of the lung and the large difference in partial pressures between room air and 100% oxygen. These two factors allow more oxygen to diffuse into the parenchyma and dissolve in blood. Generally, oxygen-enhanced ventilation imaging technique involves the acquisition of a series of images as the subject alternately inhales room air (21% oxygen) and 100% oxygen (28,29). The signal difference between the two reflects the change in oxygenation of blood or lung tissues. **Figure. 53.15** shows the inversion-recovery oxygen-enhanced difference and percentage images.

4.3. Pathophysiology

MRI can also be used to elucidate the pathophysiology of ischemic diseases such as stroke, and thereby aid in the development of suitable interventional strategies. The unique advantage of MRI is that the techniques can also be used in the clinic as a way of monitoring the effects of interventions.

4.3.1. Brain Disease Models
Dynamic susceptibility contrast-enhanced MRI (DSC) (or "bolus tracking") MRI typically makes use of rapidly acquired T_2- or T_2^*-weighted MR images

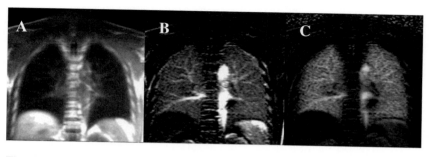

Fig. 53.15. Oxygen-enhanced ventilation images of a healthy volunteer obtained through different calculations. Shown are the (**A**) anatomical image, (**B**) difference image, and (**C**) percent differrence image. Normal ventilation and similar pulmonary anatomy is observed among the images

to assess the first passage of an intravenously injected bolus of paramagnetic contrast agent through the microvascular bed *(30)*. Various hemodynamic parameters, e.g., bolus peak time, maximal change of the transverse relaxation rate $\Delta R_2^*{}_{max}$, relative cerebral blood volume (CBV), relative mean transit time (MTT) and relative cerebral blood flow index (CBF_i), can be calculated from the time-course of the contrast agent-induced change in the effective transverse relaxation rate $\Delta R_2^*(t)$. The tissue response function can be calculated by deconvolution with a measured arterial input function *(30–32)*. Significant correlations have been demonstrated between relative CBF indices, as determined from DSC MRI, and CBF values quantified by autoradiography *(33)* or positron emission tomography *(34)* in normal and ischemic animal brain.

DSC MRI has been used to study the pattern of perfusion deficits in various animal models of ischemia *(31,35)*. Spatial assessment of multiple hemodynamic parameters can identify brain regions in which microcirculation is preserved, but compromised *(36,37)*. For example, a mismatch between relative CBF_i and relative CBV could indicate compensatory vasodilation, whereas a delayed bolus peak time in perifocal areas may reflect alternative routes of blood supply *via* collaterals. DSC MRI can also evaluate the hemodynamic consequences of reperfusion (e.g., no reflow, hyperemia, or hypoperfusion) *(38–40)*. **Fig. 53.16** shows the effect of thrombolysis on CBF_i maps as derived from repetitive DSC MRI experiments in a rat stroke model. Finally, DSC MRI-based CBV mapping of 9 L gliosarcomas in rats has been evaluated as a potential means of measuring of tumor vascularity and angiogenesis *(41,42)*. It was shown that MRI-derived CBV correlated with the fractional vessel volume as measured histologically.

4.4. Molecular Imaging

4.4.1. Gene Expression

Studies of gene expression generally rely on the use of reporter genes. The reporter gene produces a protein product with a uniquely identifiable and/or quantifiable phenotype; historically, these have usually been genes that encode for enzymes. Observing changes in gene expression in vivo was revolutionized in the 1990s with the cloning of green fluorescent protein (GFP).

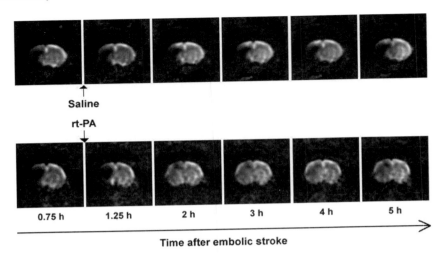

Fig. 53.16. Serial cerebral blood flow index (CBF_i) maps of a coronal rat brain slice before and after treatment with saline (top row) or thrombolytic recombinant tissue plasminogen activator (rt-PA) (1 mg/kg pamiteplase (Yamanouchi Pharmaceutical Co.)) (bottom row). Onset of treatment was at approx 1 h after unilateral embolic middle cerebral artery occlusion. Data demonstrate thrombolysis-induced reperfusion after rt-PA treatment and absence of CBF recovery after saline treatment

GFP was first identified in the bioluminescent *Aequorea* jellyfish. In the jellyfish GFP is a fluorescence energy transfer partner with the protein aequorin. Aequorin fluoresces in the blue, yet the jellyfish bioluminesces green through transfer of energy from aequorin to GFP. GFP was first reported in 1962 but its application as a gene reporter was not explored until the gene was cloned in 1992 *(43)* and, shortly thereafter, shown to retain fluorescence activity when expressed in other organisms *(43,44)*. No cofactors are required to produce the fluorescence; fortuitously the GFP gene contains all the information needed to produce fluorescence *(45)*. GFP has shown no toxicity effects in most of the systems in which it has been expressed, and has made the use of optical imaging methods for interrogating gene expression in living systems almost a routine procedure. However, as with all optical techniques, the use of GFP for monitoring gene expression ends where light propagation stops, so other techniques must be devised to examine gene expression in deeper tissues and opaque systems. Advances in imaging probe development have led to the use of clinical imaging modalities such as positron emission tomography (PET) and magnetic resonance imaging (MRI) to monitor gene expression in living systems. These two modalities have unlimited depth of interrogation, are non-invasive and are capable of high resolution (MRI) and high sensitivity (PET).

The first example of an MRI contrast agent that is activated by gene expression was an enzyme-sensitive agent developed in the laboratory of Thomas Meade. This agent consisted of a gadolinium ion bound by a macrocylic ligand that had been modified with an appended galactose group *(46)*. Attachment of the galactose group to the macrocycle is through a β-galactosidase cleavable linker. The galactose group interacts with gadolinium to block water access. In the presence of beta-galactosidase the galactose group is enzymatically removed and opens access for water to gadolinium. In vivo, this agent was able to detect expression of β-galactosidase from both introduced RNA and DNA forms of the lacZ gene *(47)* (**Fig. 53.17**).

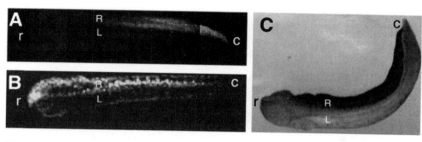

Fig. 53.17. Detection of mRNA expression in Xenopus system. One cell of Xenopus embryos at the two-cell stage was injected with mRNA for beta-gal and co-injected with mRNA for nGFP as a marker of injection efficiency. Both cells were injected with EgadMe. Embryos were kept at 16°C until postgastrulation and then moved to room temperature for 24 h before imaging. The first cleavage approximates the future mid-line for the animal. Thus half of the animal contains beta-gal, while the contrast agent is distributed throughout. The right hand image in the figure shows that histological staining for beta-gal is restricted to the right side of the animal. This correlates with the expression of nGFP on the right side shown in a fluorescence image (top left panel). The region of high signal intensity by MRI is also localized to the right side (bottom left panel). So in the half of the animal containing beta-gal, the agent is activated, whereas in the half lacking beta-gal the agent is silent. For further information and color reproduction please refer (47)

4.4.2. Cell Labeling

The transplantation or transfusion of (therapeutic) cells has been pursued as a very active research area over the last decade, and remarkable progress has been made in progenitor and stem cell therapy using animal disease models. To further advance cell-based therapies into the clinic, noninvasive cellular imaging techniques are warranted. These imaging techniques are needed to provide detailed information on the biokinetics of administered cells (either transplanted or transfused); cell–tissue interactions, including preferred pathways of migration; and cell survival. In addition, within the hematological and immunological community, there is now also increasing interest in the spatiotemporal dynamics of cell "homing" after intravenous injection of hematopoietic and white blood cells.

MRI offers near cellular resolution, and the ability to detect very small clusters of cells. Although initial studies were aimed at MRI cell tracking in disorders of the central nervous system, i.e., dysmyelination (48,49), neuroinflammation (50), and stroke (51,52), studies have now also been performed in muscle disorders (53) and swine models of myocardial infarction, using X-ray fluoroscopy-guided injection (54–57). An example of MRI cell tracking is illustrated in **Fig. 53.18**.

For cells to be visualized on magnetic resonance (MR) images, they need to be magnetically labeled to be discriminated from the surrounding native tissue. Because of their biocompatibility and strong effects on $T2^*$ relaxation, superparamagnetic iron oxides (SPIO) are currently the preferred magnetic label. SPIOs provide the targeted cell with a large magnetic moment, which creates substantial disturbances in the local magnetic field, leading to a rapid dephasing of protons, including those not directly in the vicinity of the targeted cell. For further details regarding cell labeling, readers can refer to (58,59).

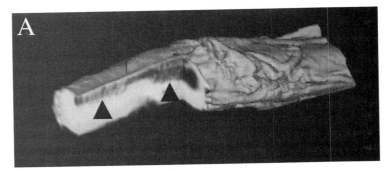

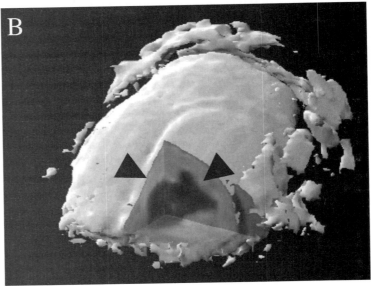

Fig. 53.18. (A) 3D reconstructed *ex vivo* magnetic resonance (MR) image (78-μm resolution) of dysmyelinated rat spinal cord showing distribution of magnetically labeled oligodendrocyte progenitors 10 d after transplantation. Note the migration along the dorsal column away from the injection site (arrowheads). **(B)** 3D reconstructed in vivo MR image (313–μm resolution) of dysmyelinated rat brain showing distribution of magnetically labeled oligodendroglial progenitors at 6 wk after ransplantation. Note the migration of cells into the parenchyma away from the ventricle (arrowheads). For further information please refer *(59)*

References

1. Prasad PV (2006) Magnetic resonance imaging: methods and biologic applications. Methods Mol Med 124:Humana, Totawa, NJ
2. Storey P (2006) Introduction to magnetic resonance imaging and spectroscopy. Methods Mol Med 124:3–57
3. Finn J (2006) Pulse sequence design. In: Edelman RR, Hesselink JR, Zlatkin MB, Crues JV (eds) Clinical magnetic resonance imaging, Vol 1.3 vols. Elsevier
4. Kirsch JE (1991) Basic principles of magnetic resonance contrast agents. Top Magn Reson Imaging 3:1–18
5. Wood ML, Hardy PA (1993) Proton relaxation enhancement. J Magn Reson Imaging 3:149–56

6. Anzai Y (2004) Superparamagnetic iron oxide nanoparticles: nodal metastases and beyond. Top Magn Reson Imaging 15:103–111

7. Prince MR, Meaney JF (2006) Expanding role of MR angiography in clinical practice. Eur Radiol 16 Suppl 2:B3–8

8. Edelman RR (2004) Contrast-enhanced MR imaging of the heart: overview of the literature. Radiology 232:653–668

9. Kim RJ, Shah DJ, Judd RM (2003) How we perform delayed enhancement imaging. J Cardiovasc Magn Reson 5:505–514

10. Saeed M, Wendland MF, Higgins CB (2000) Blood pool MR contrast agents for cardiovascular imaging. J Magn Reson Imaging 12:890–898

11. Caruthers SD, Winter PM, Wickline SA, Lanza GM (2006) Targeted magnetic resonance imaging contrast agents. Methods Mol Med 124:387–400

12. Louie A (2006) Design and characterization of magnetic resonance imaging gene reporters. Methods Mol Med 124:401–417

13. Johnson GA, Cofer GP, Fubara B, Gewalt SL, Hedlund LW, Maronpot RR (2002) Magnetic resonance histology for morphologic phenotyping. J Magn Reson Imaging 16:423–429

14. Zhou YQ, Davidson L, Henkelman RM, Nieman BJ, Foster FS, Yu LX, Chen XJ (2004) Ultrasound-guided left-ventricular catheterization: a novel method of whole mouse perfusion for microimaging. Lab Invest 84:385–389

15. Pautler RG, Silva AC, Koretsky AP (1998) In vivo neuronal tract tracing using manganese-enhanced magnetic resonance imaging. Magn Reson Med 40:740–748

16. Tjalve H, Henriksson J, Tallkvist J, Larsson BS, Lindquist NG (1996) Uptake of manganese and cadmium from the nasal mucosa into the central nervous system via olfactory pathways in rats. Pharmacol Toxicol 79:347–356

17. Tjalve H, Mejare C, Borg-Neczak K (1995) Uptake and transport of manganese in primary and secondary olfactory neurones in pike. Pharmacol Toxicol 77:23–31

18. Ogawa S, Lee TM, Kay AR, Tank DW (1990) Brain magnetic resonance imaging with contrast dependent on blood oxygenation. Proc Natl Acad Sci USA 87:9868–9872

19. Thulborn KR, Waterton JC, Matthews PM, Radda GK (1982) Oxygenation dependence of the transverse relaxation time of water protons in whole blood at high field. Biochim Biophys Acta 714:265–270

20. Grubb RL Jr, Raichle ME, Eichling JO, Ter-Pogossian MM (1974) The effects of changes in PaCO2 on cerebral blood volume, blood flow, and vascular mean transit time. Stroke 5:630–639

21. Zeirler KL (1962) Theoretical basis of indicator-dilution methods for measuring flow and volume. Circ Res 10:393–407

22. Matthews PM, Jezzard P (2004) Functional magnetic resonance imaging. J Neurol Neurosurg Psychiatry 75:6–12

23. Rajagopalan P, Krishnan KR, Passe TJ, Macfall JR (1995) Magnetic resonance imaging using deoxyhemoglobin contrast versus positron emission tomography in the assessment of brain function. Prog Neuropsychopharmacol Biol Psychiatry 19:351–366

24. Ugurbil K, Hu X, Chen,W, Zhu XH, Kim SG, Georgopoulos A (1999) Functional mapping in the human brain using high magnetic fields. Philos Trans R Soc Lond B Biol Sci 354:1195–1213

25. Prasad PV, Chen Q, Goldfarb JW, Epstein FH, Edelman RR (1997) Breath-hold R2* mapping with a multiple gradient-recalled echo sequence: application to the evaluation of intrarenal oxygenation. J Magn Reson Imaging 7:1163–1165

26. Prasad PV, Edelman RR, Epstein FH (1996) Noninvasive evaluation of intrarenal oxygenation with BOLD MRI. Circulation 94:3271–3275

27. Chiarotti G, Cristiani G, Bliulotto L (1955) Proton relaxation in pure liquids and in liquids containing paramagnetic gases in solution. Nuovo Cimento 1:863–873

28. Edelman RR, Hatabu H, Tadamura E, Li W, Prasad PV (1996) Noninvasive assessment of regional ventilation in the human lung using oxygen-enhanced magnetic resonance imaging. Nat Med 2:1236–1239

29. Chen Q, Jakob PM, Griswold MA, Levin DL, Hatabu H, Edelman RR (1998) Oxygen enhanced MR ventilation imaging of the lung. Magma 7:153–161

30. Rosen BR, Belliveau JW, Vevea JM, Brady TJ (1990) Perfusion imaging with NMR contrast agents. Magn Reson Med 14:249–265

31. Calamante F, Thomas D L, Pell GS, Wiersma J, Turner R (1999) Measuring cerebral blood flow using magnetic resonance imaging techniques. J Cereb Blood Flow Metab 19:701–735

32. Ostergaard L, Weisskoff RM, Chesler DA, Gyldensted C, Rosen BR (1996) High resolution measurement of cerebral blood flow using intravascular tracer bolus passages. Part I: Mathematical approach and statistical analysis. Magn Reson Med 36:715–725

33. Wittlich F, Kohno K, Mies G, Norris DG, Hoehn-Berlage M (1995) Quantitative measurement of regional blood flow with gadolinium diethylenetriaminepentaacetate bolus track NMR imaging in cerebral infarcts in rats: validation with the iodo[14C]antipyrine technique. Proc Natl Acad Sci USA 92:1846–1850

34. Sakoh M, Rohl L, Gyldensted C, Gjedde A, Ostergaard L (2000) Cerebral blood flow and blood volume measured by magnetic resonance imaging bolus tracking after acute stroke in pigs: comparison with [(15)O]H(2)O positron emission tomography. Stroke 31:1958–1964

35. Hossmann KA, Hoehn-Berlage M (1995) Diffusion and perfusion MR imaging of cerebral ischemia. Cerebrovasc Brain Metab Rev 7:187–217

36. Maeda M, Itoh S, Ide H, Matsuda T, Kobayashi H, Kubota T, Ishii Y (1993) Acute stroke in cats: comparison of dynamic susceptibility-contrast MR imaging with T2- and diffusion-weighted MR imaging. Radiology 189:227–232

37. Roberts TP, Vexler Z, Derugin N, Moseley ME, Kucharczyk J (1993) High-speed MR imaging of ischemic brain injury following stenosis of the middle cerebral artery. J Cereb Blood Flow Metab 13:940–946

38. Hamberg LM, Macfarlane R, Tasdemiroglu E, Boccalini P, Hunter GJ, Belliveau JW, Moskowitz MA, Rosen BR (1993) Measurement of cerebrovascular changes in cats after transient ischemia using dynamic magnetic resonance imaging. Stroke 24:444–450; discussion 450, 451

39. Kucharczyk J, Vexler ZS, Roberts TP, Asgari HS, Mintorovitch J, Derugin N, Watson AD, Moseley ME (1993) Echo-planar perfusion-sensitive MR imaging of acute cerebral ischemia. Radiology 188:711–717

40. Minematsu K, Fisher M, Li L, Sotak CH (1993) Diffusion and perfusion magnetic resonance imaging studies to evaluate a noncompetitive N-methyl-D-aspartate antagonist and reperfusion in experimental stroke in rats. Stroke 24:2074–2081

41. Cha S, Johnson G, Wadghiri YZ, Jin O, Babb J, Zagzag D, Turnbull DH (2003) Dynamic, contrast-enhanced perfusion MRI in mouse gliomas: correlation with histopathology. Magn Reson Med 49:848–855

42. Pathak AP, Schmainda KM, Ward BD, Linderman JR, Rebro KJ, Greene AS (2001) MR-derived cerebral blood volume maps: issues regarding histological validation and assessment of tumor angiogenesis. Magn Reson Med 46:735–747

43. Prasher DC, Eckenrode VK, Ward WW, Prendergast FG, Cormier MJ (1992) Primary structure of the Aequorea victoria green-fluorescent protein. Gene 111:229–233

44. Inouye S, Tsuji FI (1994) Aequorea green fluorescent protein. Expression of the gene and fluorescence characteristics of the recombinant protein. FEBS Lett 341:277–280

45. Tsien RY (1998) The green fluorescent protein. Annu Rev Biochem 67:509–544

46. Moats R, Fraser S, Meade T (1997) A "smart" magnetic resonance imaging agent that reports on specific enzyme activity. Angew Chem Int Ed:726–728

47. Louie AY, Huber MM, Ahrens ET, Rothbacher U, Moats R, Jacobs RE, Fraser SE, Meade TJ (2000) In vivo visualization of gene expression using magnetic resonance imaging. Nat Biotechnol 18:321–325

48. Bulte JW, Douglas T, Witwer B, Zhang SC, Strable E, Lewis BK, Zywicke H, Miller B, van Gelderen P, Moskowitz BM, Duncan ID, Frank JA (2001) Magnetodendrimers allow endosomal magnetic labeling and in vivo tracking of stem cells. Nat Biotechnol 19:1141–1147

49. Bulte JW, Zhang S, van Gelderen P, Herynek V, Jordan EK, Duncan ID, Frank JA (1999) Neurotransplantation of magnetically labeled oligodendrocyte progenitors: magnetic resonance tracking of cell migration and myelination. Proc Natl Acad Sci USA 96:15256–15261

50. Bulte JW, Ben-Hur T, Miller BR, Mizrachi-Kol R, Einstein O, Reinhartz E, Zywicke HA, Douglas T, Frank JA (2003) MR microscopy of magnetically labeled neurospheres transplanted into the Lewis EAE rat brain. Magn Reson Med 50:201–205

51. Hoehn M, Kustermann E, Blunk J, Wiedermann D, Trapp T, Wecker S, Focking M, Arnold H, Hescheler J, Fleischmann BK, Schwindt W, Buhrle C (2002) Monitoring of implanted stem cell migration in vivo: a highly resolved in vivo magnetic resonance imaging investigation of experimental stroke in rat. Proc Natl Acad Sci USA 99:16267–16272

52. Zhang ZG, Jiang Q, Zhang R, Zhang L, Wang,L, Zhang L, Arniego P, Ho KL, Chopp M (2003) Magnetic resonance imaging and neurosphere therapy of stroke in rat. Ann Neurol 53:259–263

53. Walter GA, Cahill KS, Huard J, Feng H, Douglas T, Sweeney HL, Bulte JW (2004) Noninvasive monitoring of stem cell transfer for muscle disorders. Magn Reson Med 51:273–277

54. Dick AJ, Guttman MA, Raman VK, Peters DC, Pessanha BS, Hill JM, Smith S, Scott G, McVeigh ER, Lederman RJ (2003) Magnetic resonance fluoroscopy allows targeted delivery of mesenchymal stem cells to infarct borders in Swine. Circulation 108:2899–2904

55. Garot J, Unterseeh T, Teiger E, Champagne S, Chazaud B, Gherardi R, Hittinger L, Gueret P, Rahmouni A (2003) Magnetic resonance imaging of targeted catheter-based implantation of myogenic precursor cells into infarcted left ventricular myocardium. J Am Coll Cardiol 41:1841–1846

56. Hill JM, Dick AJ, Raman VK, Thompson RB, Yu ZX, Hinds KA, Pessanha BS, Guttman MA, Varney TR, Martin BJ, Dunbar CE, McVeigh ER, Lederman RJ (2003) Serial cardiac magnetic resonance imaging of injected mesenchymal stem cells. Circulation 108:1009–1014

57. Kraitchman DL, Heldman AW, Atalar E, Amado LC, Martin BJ, Pittenger MF, Hare JM, Bulte JW (2003) In vivo magnetic resonance imaging of mesenchymal stem cells in myocardial infarction. Circulation 107:2290–2293

58. Bulte JW (2006) Intracellular endosomal magnetic labeling of cells. Methods Mol Med 124:419–439

59. Bulte JW, Duncan ID, Frank JA (2002) In vivo magnetic resonance tracking of magnetically labeled cells after transplantation. J Cereb Blood Flow Metab 22:899–907

54

Electron Microscopy

John Kuo

1. Introduction

The electron microscope uses electrons to create an image of an object with much greater magnification or resolving power than a normal light microscope, allowing it to see smaller objects with vital details. It has been applied to the examination of biological materials (such as micro-organisms and cells), a variety of large molecules, medical biopsy samples, metals and crystalline structures, and the characteristics of various surfaces. Electron microscopy (EM) has been largely responsible for shaping the modern view of cellular architecture.

A beam of energetic electrons from an electron microscope interacts with the specimen in two main ways: 1) transmitted electrons, which are used for two-dimensional (2D) imaging in a transmission electron microscope (TEM) and 2) reflected electrons which are employed for 3D image formation in scanning electron microscopy (SEM). Transmitted electrons can be classified into two major types: elastic and inelastic electrons. The elastic electrons are the main signal for image formation in a conventional TEM (see Section 2.1), whereas the inelastic electrons, with the aid of high performance imaging filters such as the in-column Omega filter and the postcolumn Gatan imaging filter (GIF), contribute to the image in energy filtered transmission electron microscopy (EFTEM, see Section 2.1.6). Furthermore, with an additional electron tomographic attachment, i.e., a high-tilt specimen holder, three-dimensional (3D) imaging of biological structures can also be achieved either by conventional TEM or by EFTEM). In the SEM, on the other hand, reflected electron signals such as secondary electrons and back-scattered electrons, and x-ray radiation are usually recorded in biological applications (see Section 2.2).

The instrumental components and operational principles are not quite the same in the TEM and the SEM. For the TEM, the components are equivalent to an "upside down" version of a conventional upright light microscope (see **Fig. 54.1**). The source of illumination in the TEM is a filament (cathode) that emits electrons at the top of a cylindrical column. Electrons are then accelerated by a nearby positively charged anode, forming an electron beam that travels

From: *Molecular Biomethods Handbook, 2nd Edition.*
Edited by: J. M. Walker and R. Rapley © Humana Press, Totowa, NJ

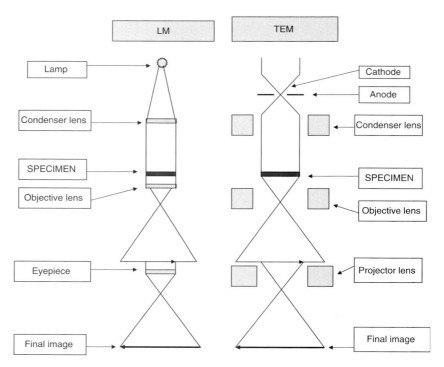

Fig. 54.1. Comparison between the components of the light microscope and transmission electron microscope.

down an evacuated column to pass through the magnetic condenser lens and the specimen. Scattered and un-scattered electrons emerging from the specimen is then collected by a magnetic objective lens, and focused and magnified to form the image. Images can be further magnified through a series of magnetic projector (or intermediate) lenses and then projected onto a fluorescent screen or recorded by EM negative film or digital (CCD) camera. The SEM has a similar illumination source as the TEM, but it does not contain image-forming lenses. The condenser lenses in the SEM operate through a demagnification series to focus an extremely small spot or probe on a solid specimen, which emits reflected electrons. The secondary electron detector acquires signal information related to the topography of the specimen (the 3D image); the backscattered detector records backscattered electrons signals related to the differences in atomic number; whereas the x-ray detector collects information related to the types of elements present. Furthermore, the SEM probe is not static and is scanned rapidly over the specimen much like the scanning of the electron beams taking place in a television monitor. The secondary electron information is displayed on a viewing monitor, with various degrees of brightness and contrast. Areas of the specimen that yield more secondary electrons will appear bright, whereas areas that yield less secondary electrons will appear proportionally darker on the monitor.

There are several types of TEM depending the voltage used in the instrument. Low voltage TEMs of 80–120 kV are mainly used for conventional 2D imaging, while intermediate voltage TEMs of 150–200 kV and high voltage TEMs of 300–400 kV are usually for electron tomography, EFTEM and cryoTEM.

On the other hand, the maximum voltage used in the SEM is limited to 30 kV. Consequently, the TEM has a higher resolution than the SEM, but the SEM has a greater depth of focus that can produce 3D images. Furthermore, both TEM and SEM can use a lanthanum hexaboride (LaB6) filament or field emission source instead of a tungsten filament in the electron gun to provide narrower probing beams at low or high electron energy, resulting in improved spatial resolution and intensity. In addition, by maintaining specimens at liquid nitrogen temperature in a cryospecimen transfer system and also cryostage in the electron microscope, hence commonly called a cryoelectron microscope (CryoEM, both TEM and SEM), one can image and analyse elemental compositions and their distribution in cellular and molecular structures in a vitreous state either two-dimensionally or three dimensionally.

The first TEM and the first SEM were built in 1933 and 1942, respectively. Many of the seminal biological studies were conducted during the late 1950s and 1960s in conjunction with the development of appropriate specimen preparation methods and protocols for biological electron microscopy. Although it remained as an important diagnostic tool during the 1970s and 1980s, TEM's stature in basic research was largely overshadowed by rapid advancements in biochemistry, molecular biology, genetics, and confocal laser microscopy. Nevertheless, significant technical developments continued during that period, as a result, TEM re-emerged in the late 1990s in a spectacular way as a crucial tool for understanding molecular mechanisms in cellular biology.

Because electron microscopes are operated under high vacuum, biological samples, which normally contains a great amount of liquids and are composed of lighter elements (e.g., carbon, hydrogen, oxygen, and nitrogen), must be completely dehydrated when prepared for electron microscopy. They must also be thin enough for electron beams to be transmitted through them, and should be stained or coated with heavy metals to create specimen contrast. Thus, biological electron microscopy, particularly the TEM, has a long history in the development of specimen preparation techniques. The first published EM images of a fibroblast-like cell cultured from chick embryo tissue (**Fig. 54.2**) was able to recognize mitochondria, Golgi apparatus and the reticulum lattice, which was later named the endoplasmic reticulum *(1)*. It was not until the introduction of glutaraldehyde as a primary fixative *(2)* and the establishment of resin embedding methods that electron microscopy became the most important tool for the study of cell biology and to some extent in molecular biology, and leading us to a better understanding of the structure and function of various organelles in diverse cell types of different organs in all animals and plants studied.

However, biological scientists are also concerned that some of these traditional EM specimen preparation techniques may introduce artefacts and, consequently, research into cryo specimen preparation techniques has developed. The specimen is frozen rapidly enough to reach a temperature below −140°C at which ice is in a vitreous state before it can form crystals. Rapid freezing essentially immobilizes all constituents of a biological specimen before a significant rearrangement occurs and, therefore, preserves the specimen in a near perfect physiological and biochemical state. The rapid frozen samples can be used for cutting cryothin sections by a cryoultramicrotome or, more commonly, they are processed by subsequent freeze substitution that hydrates the samples without ice crystal formation in the specimen. Among several

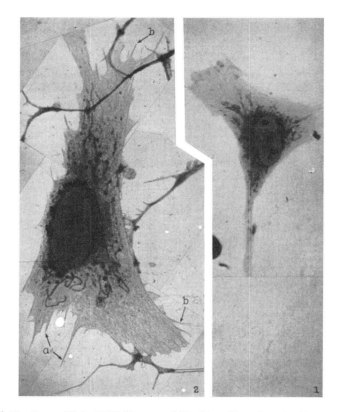

Fig. 54.2. The first published TEM images of fibroblast-like cultured cells. [Reproduced from Porter et al. *(2)*, with copyright permission the Rockfeller University Press].

freezing techniques, high pressure freezing, freeze substitution and cryomicrotomy have been considered as the most significant advances in specimen preparation techniques for modern biological electron microscopy since the introduction of glutaraldehyde for primary fixation.

In addition to the improvement in specimen preparation, in particular cryo specimen preparation, electron microscope technology has also made vast advancements, including user friendly computer control, electron optics, field-emission electron sources, improved specimen stages, high-sensitivity digital image recording, and energy filtering. Combined with increased computational power and developments in image-processing software, two important biological TEM applications for 3D structure determination have been established. The first application is high-resolution biological electron crystallography for single macromolecules and macromolecular assemblies (e.g., *3,4*). The second application is electron tomography (ET), which is an electron microscopic technique for obtaining a 3D image from any electron microscope specimen, whether ordered or not. Tomography is especially useful for detailed studies of organelle-sized structures. A number of reviews *(5–9)* have stressed the importance of ET in the field of electron microscopy *(7–9)*, which has opened up new frontiers for molecular and cellular biological research.

2. Methods

2.1. Transmission Electron Microscopy

Transmission electron microscopy is a diversified technique producing mostly 2D images of tissues, cells and organelles. In addition to EFTEM and ET techniques, one can use different specimen preparation methods to reveal different aspects of cellular or organelle ultrastracture as well as to localize various proteins and enzymes as well as macromolecules in cells (see **Fig. 54.3**).

2.1.1. Conventional Specimen Preparation for TEM

The specimen preparation method for conventional 2D ultrastructural imaging is basically similar to that of light microscopy. The standard method involves fixing biological specimens with a chemical agent, removing water with a solvent and then embedding in a plastic resin. Thin sections are cut, stained and examined under a TEM.

2.1.1.1. Fixation: The primary aims of fixation are: 1) to convert the mobile cytoplasmic cells and tissues to an immobile, firm and stable condition that in all aspects resembles the living state as closely as possible; 2) to protect fixed cells and tissues against disruption by subsequent treatments including dehydration with solvents, infiltration and embedding with resin, sectioning with (glass or diamond) knives, staining with heavy metals, and finally exposing to the electron beam.

The most common and popular fixatives for biological electron microscopy studies are aldehyde fixatives, which are non-coagulants and work by cross-linking proteins, and also other macromolecules such as lipoproteins and histoproteins associated with DNA in cells and tissues. Two main aldehyde

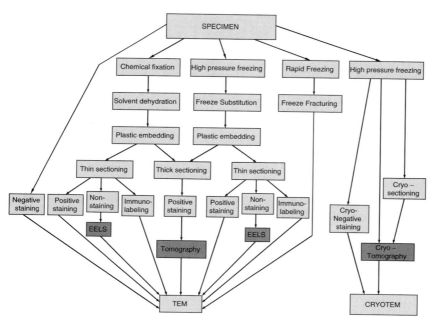

Fig. 54.3. A flow chart of biological specimen preparation procedures for various transmission electron microscopy techniques.

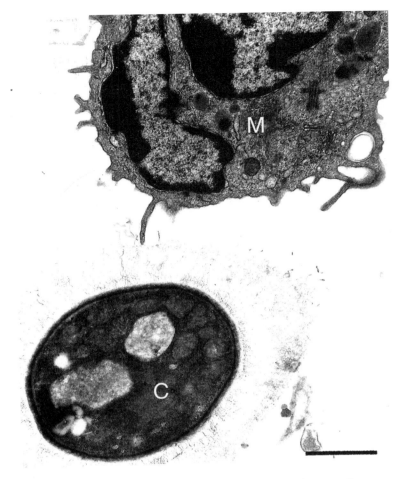

Fig. 54.4. A TEM image of the interaction between pathogenic yeast *Cryptococcus neoformans* (C) and macrophage (M). The specimens were prepared with the conventional chemical fixation. Bar = 1 μm. (Courtesy of Dr. T. Robertson).

fixatives commonly used are formaldehyde and glutaraldehyde. Formaldehyde is a mono-aldehyde with a rapid penetration rate but a lower cross-linking ability with protein than glutaraldehyde. For this main reason, formaldehyde is usually used for immunocytochemistry, so more antigen sites can be retained in the fixed tissues. Glutaraldehyde is a di-aldehyde with higher cross-linking ability but a slower penetration rate and it has been used as a primary fixative, as biological samples are usually postfixed with the metal-containing heavy metal fixative OsO_4, which would provide further cross-linking and be used for "staining" purposes. Sometimes a fixative combining formaldehyde and glutaraldehyde, known as Karnovsky fixative, is applied, where rapid penetration by formaldehyde is used to immobilise biological activity while the glutaraldehyde acts to cross-link with proteins. All fixatives should be prepared in a buffer with concentrations varied from 0.1 to 5% depending on cell and tissue types. Fixation conditions such as temperature, osmolarity, and duration as well as fixation methods such as immersion or perfusion may vary with different biological specimens.

2.1.1.2. Dehydration, Infiltration, and Embedding: The water content of fixed specimens is normally removed by a series of graded solvents such as ethanol or acetone, and sometimes the samples may be treated with propylene oxide to ensure their dryness before infiltration with resins. Resins for biological EM can be either water insoluble or soluble. Water insoluble epoxy resins, which are polymerized at a temperature of 50–70°C, are used for normal 2D imaging purposes. Water soluble acrylic resins can be polymerized either at low or high temperature and are suitable for immunolabeling techniques.

2.1.1.3. Sectioning and Staining: Hardened resin blocks containing biological materials are thinly sectioned at 40–100 nm in thickness by a glass or diamond knife mounted on an ultramicrotome. Thin sections are collected on EM grids and are "stained" with heavy metals such as uranyl and lead to impart the specimen contrast under the electron beam.

Detailed protocols and methods of conventional specimen preparation of cultured cells and larger biological tissues can be found in Bozzola *(10)* and Mascorro and Bozzola *(11)* respectively. In addition, there are numerous reference books that provide general information on biological specimen preparation (e.g., *12–15*).

2.1.1.4. Microwave Specimen Preparation: The microwave can be used to reduce the time required for carrying out the standard specimen preparation procedures involving fixation, dehydration, infiltration, polymerisation, and staining, as described above. Background theory (see *16,17*) as well as rapid procedures and protocols for using a microwave are available *(18,19)*.

2.1.2. Cryo-Specimen Preparation

Cryo-specimen preparation involves freezing biological specimens by either rapid freezing or high pressure freezing below a temperature of −140°C at which ice is in a vitreous state before it can form crystals. For an electron microscopical purpose, the frozen biological specimens can then be subjected to further preparation techniques: 1) freeze drying; 2) freeze fracturing and etching; 3) freeze substitution; and 4) cryoultramicrotomy. For greater coverage of cryo-specimen preparation, serval important reference books are recommended *(20–24)*.

2.1.2.1. Cryofixation: Rapid Freezing (RF) and High Pressure Freezing (HPF): During the initial development of cryofixation, different freezing techniques such as plunging freezing, spray-freezing, impact against a cooled metal block and propane jet freezing using liquid nitrogen or liquid propane were used to freeze the biological specimen rapidly. As these methods can only adequately freeze specimens to a depth of 5–10 μm, their use in TEM ultrastructural studies has been discontinued. They may still, however, be used in SEM studies. General information on these freezing methods can be found in the literature *(20–24)*.

HPF differs from the above mentioned rapid freezing techniques by producing well frozen samples that are hundreds of micrometers (~300 μm) thick under a pressure of more than 200 Bar. This pressure retards the nucleation and growth of ice crystals and effectively lowers the freezing point of water by approx 20°. The consequence of these physical effects is to allow freezing to greater depths than that achieved by other rapid freezing methods. However, an optimistic average depth of good freezing will vary with the chemistry of the particular cell type. In general, cells with less free water will freeze better than those that have more aqueous cytoplasm. Likewise, some cells also have natural cryoprotectants, such as high sugar and/or protein contents.

Once frozen by HPF, cells can be treated in many different ways, such as freeze drying, freeze fracturing, freeze substitution or vitreous cryosectioning. After freeze substitution, the specimen can be embedded at low or room temperature for subsequent sectioning and ultrastructural imaging or immunolabeling studies. Furthermore, HPF specimens can also be examined by scanning electron microscopy after freezing fracturing, freeze-drying or freeze substitution *(25)*. Therefore, HPF becomes an essential specimen preparation method for the EM applications mentioned before, especially vitreous cryosectioning and electron tomography.

Since the initial introduction of the high pressure freezing technique to freeze fracturing *(26)*, its design and applications have been continuously developed and modified to become one of the most important specimen preparation methods for biological electron microscopy. There are several important

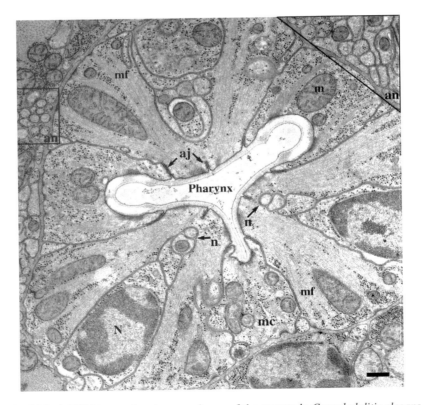

Fig. 54.5. A TEM image the pharyngeal area of the nematode *Canorhabditis elegans* pharyngeal area. Samples were high pressure frozen, freeze substituted in acetone containing 2% OsO_4. (aj, adherens junctions; an, amphid neurons; bm, body wall muscles; fm, pharyngeal muscle filaments; gj, gap junction; m, mitochondria; mc, marginal cells; N, nucleus; n, neurons; and pm, pharyngeal membrane). Bar = 300 nm. [Reproduced from Matsko and Mueller *(40)*, with copyright permission the Elsevier B. V.]

publications dealing with the theory and practical applications of this technique over the years (e.g., *27–30*). Currently, there are two main commercial types of high-pressure freezers with different designs; BAL-TEC HPM (a newly developed HPM 100 has been introduced in late 2007) and Leica EM PACT2. In the BAL-TEC machine, the pressure and cooling systems are 'in-line' whereas in the EM PACT they are separate. Detailed explanations of these differences can be found in the articles by Moore *(28)* and Studer et al. *(31)* respectively. In addition, different types of samples often require different specimen carriers and/or loading strategies in the high pressure freezing machines. Important protocols and methods for using HPF machines have been outlined by McDonald et al. *(32)* in great detail.

2.1.2.2. Freeze Drying: This method requires that tissue specimens are frozen by one of the freezing methods described above and then placed in a freeze-dryer. Freeze dried specimens can be infiltrated and embedded by one of the relatively low viscosity Lowicryl resins at low temperature. Both chemical fixed or unfixed samples can use this method. Many commercial or 'home' made freeze drying apparatus have pumps (rotary, oil diffusion, or molecular) to remove the gases from the freeze drier, and molecular sieves to absorb the water vapour. Most freeze drying units operate at temperatures far above the presumptive recrystallisation temperature (193 K/−80°C) of biological specimens and have been therefore considered not adequate for ultrastructural studies. However, Edelmann *(33)* has reported that freeze-dried and resin-embedded biological material could be well suited for ultrastructure research. Methods and protocols for freeze drying have been included in serval references *(23,34)*.

2.1.2.3. Freeze Fracturing (FF), Freeze Etching, and Replication: The freeze fracture or freeze etching technique developed by Moor et al. *(35)* for electron microscopy is a method of examining the interior of cells, in particular membrane structures, without the fixation and dehydration steps required for all other specimen preparation techniques. A brief outline of the technique is as follows: the tissue is rapid frozen, then fractured; etching the fractured specimens may or may not be required; a replica is made of the frozen fractured or etched surface and finally examined in the TEM. Walter *(25)* demonstrated freeze fracturing of high-pressure frozen samples with great success. The general theory and practical protocols for freeze fracturing, etching and replication can be found in the literature *(23–24)*.

Biological membranes usually split during freeze fracturing along their central hydrophobic plane, exposing intramembranous surfaces. The fracture plane often follows the contours of membranes and leaves bumps or depressions where it possesses around vesicles and other cell organelles. However, if the fracture plane does not follow cellular or organelle structures in the specimen, the process of etching is required to expose membrane surfaces or macromolecules just below the fracture plane. The water should be removed at a slow rate (1–10 nm/s), and the duration of etching is adjusted to achieve the desired depth of etching. Normal etching involves sublimation to a depth of less than 100 nm, while deep etching involves sublimation up to a few micrometres.

2.1.2.4. Freeze Substitution (FS): Freeze substitution is a specimen preparation technique by which water/liquid within a rapid or high-pressure frozen biological sample (see previous) is replaced by an anhydrous organic solvent, usually acetone in vessels, which is maintained at −90° degrees for a few days or longer. The freeze substituted sample is then slowly warmed up to room temperature followed by infiltration with a resin, usually epoxy resin at room temperature, but occasionally with Lowicryl HM 20 at low temperature *(36)*. This means of specimen dehydration is much more reliable for preserving cellular fine structure since it does not involve multiple solvent changes and removes the water at a temperature at which the sample remains frozen. Furthermore, by adding fixative agents (such as osmium tetroxide) into the solvent, fixation of OsO_4 and dehydration of the sample can take place simultaneously during freeze substitution. There are numerous review articles discussing theory and practice in freeze substitution *(37–39)*.

Most recently, Matsko and Mueller *(40)* introduced a revolutionary method using embedding resins, instead of the conventional OsO_4 or aldehydes as a fixative during freeze substitution *(40)* for imaging in electron microscopy. Furthermore, HPF is an essential step for examining cryosections and conducting electron tomography using a cryoelectron microscope.

2.1.2.5. Vitreous Sectioning: The technique called cryo-electron microscopy of vitreous sections (CEMOVIS) *(41)* has also known as cryo-electron microscopy of frozen-hydrated sections. A freezing microtome was introduced almost half century ago *(35)* to cut vitreous sections of biological materials for normal TEM (see *21–22*), As Cryo-sectioning is an extremely labour demanding technique and it only recently become more commonly used in conjunction of the improvement of cryoultramicrotomes and diamond knives *(43)*, and the development of cryoTEM (see *44,45*). The method now made it possible to image, examine and analyse in great details of the volumes within fully hydrated cells that were unapproachable previously because of specimen thickness.

The detailed protocols and methods of vitreous sectioning have been recently described *(46,47)*. A brief description of the method is provided below. Specimens firstly are vitrified by either plunge freezing (well freeze areas only limit to ten microns in thickness) or more commonly by HPF methods *(31, 48*; also see Section 2.2.1). The frozen materials can then be cut in thin sections (40–200 nm in thickness) with a diamond knife by a cryoultramicrotome at temperatures lower than −135°C (devitrification temperature). The dry frozen thin sections are collected on an EM grid, which are transferred into a cryoTEM with the aid of a cryotransfer system. Biological vitreous sections are usually imaged in a cryoTEM, but electron tomography (ET) application on these sections is getting popular. Cryo-sectioing has been considered as a difficult technique and could cause many sectional artefacts such as folding and/or compression on the sections *(49)*. The introduction of a micromanipulator during sectioning has reduced these artefacts and also improved the transfer of section ribbons onto grids *(50)*. Currently, CEMOVIS practices only in limited laboratories, with the demands in the cryo electron tomography community to extend cryoET capability into mapping of the proteome, especially in larger eukaryotic cells in a much wider range of specimens, it is anticipated that CEMOVIS will become more popular.

2.1.3. Negative Staining

In contrast to positive staining, which is using heavy metals to stain biological organelles, in particular membrane structure (see Section 2.1.1.3), negative staining is using heavy metals to stain backgrounds of biological specimen in

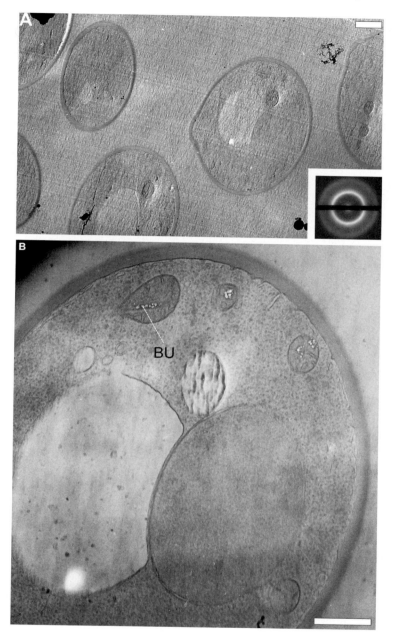

Fig. 54.6. A TEM image of yeast cell *Saccharomyces cervisiae*. Specimens were high pressure frozen and vitreous thin-sectioned on a cryoultramicrotome. (A) An overview with a few cells; (B) One of the cells at higher magnification showing beam damages as bubbles (BU) in the mitochondrion. The insert in A shows the diffraction pattern with its bubble rings. Bars: A = 1 μm; B = 500 nm. [Reproduced from Vanhecke et al. *(47)*].

order to reveal organelle or membrane structure. This simple negative staining technique involves the application of water-soluble heavy metal-containing negative staining salt to thinly spread biological samples on a thin amorphous film. This 'stained' specimen can generate differential electron scattering

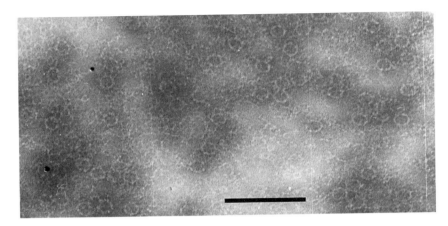

Fig. 54.7. A TEM images of human erythrocyte peroxiredoxin-II using negative staining. Specimens were prepared on a holey carbon film in the presence of 5% ammonium molybdate, 0.1% trehalose, 0.1% polyethylene glycol (Mr. 1,000). Bar = 100 nm. (Courtesy of Prof. R. Harris).

between the relatively electron transparent biological material and the electron-dense negative stain backgrounds under a TEM. In this way, electron images are generated, which represent an approximation to the molecular envelope or solvent excluded surface of particles (see *51*).

The most commonly used heavy metals for negative staining are uranyl acetate and ammonium molybdate and, to a lesser extent, sodium phosophotungstate and sodium silicontungstate. There are two common negative staining procedures available: the single-droplet negative staining technique and negative staining-carbon film technique. With slight modification, these procedures can also be applied to immunonegative staining and cryonegative staining, which was introduced by Adrian et al. *(52)*. The used concentrations and pH of negative staining solutions may vary with different heavy metals and staining methods. The general information, protocols and methods of this simple but important staining technique can be found in relevant references *(51,53)*.

The technique can be applied to almost all isolated biochemical and biological samples, and indeed solutions of synthetic polymers. It is also used for the study of 2D crystallization of virus particles and protein molecules. With slight modifications this method can be also used to study fragile macromolecules or isolated cellular organelles, such as mitochondria, nuclear membranes, lipsomes, etc.

2.1.4. Immunolabeling

This technique involves using antibodies conjugated with electron dense colloidal gold particles that permit detection, localization, and quantification of one or more defined antigens in cellular compartments at high-resolution. These benefits reflect the properties of gold particles (they are electron dense, punctate, and available in different sizes) and the ability of transmission electron microscopy to resolve both particles and compartments. Thus, immunocytochemistry for TEM can provide important information on the location and relative abundance of proteins within cells. There are two basic methods to detect the antigens in cells, briefly, the direct method involves the use of labelled primary antibodies

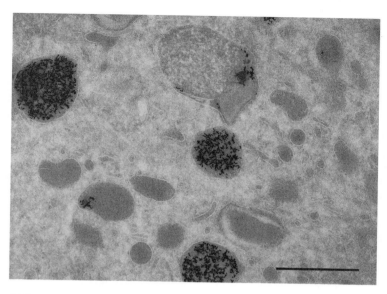

Fig. 54.8. A TEM image of isolated dendritic cells. Specimens were prepared with immunogold labeled cryosections. Bar = 200 μm. [Reproduced from Webster and Webster *(55)*].

that bind to antigenetic sites, while the indirect method utilizes unlabelled primary antibodies and secondary labelled immunocomplexes, and is more sensitive than the direct method. The immunolabeling technique has been applied to the detection of micro-organisms, cell surface-associated and intracellular antigens. Currently, two approaches to prepare thin sections for immunolocalization at the ultrastructural level are possible: a) resin embedded specimens as described in Section 2.1.1 and b) cryosections using the Tokuyasu cryosectioning method. Detailed protocols and methods for specimen preparations in immunolabeling techniques using either resin embedded sections or cryosections are available *(54,55)*. More recently, immunogoldlabeling has been carried out on tissues that are prepared by either rapid freezing and substitution *(56)* or high pressure freezing and substitution *(57–59)*. These approaches provide not only well-preserved fine structure of cells but also excellent antigenicity of several parietal cell proteins.

2.1.5. Electron Tomography (ET)

Conventional electron microscopic images are essentially 2D projections of the object; features are superimposed upon one another in the direction of the electron beam. Tomographic techniques, in contrast, acquire projections of the object as viewed from different directions and then merge them computationally into a 3D reconstruction, the tomogram. In ET, this is done by tilting the specimen holder incrementally around an axis perpendicular to the electron beam. Although the ET concept has been developed since late 1960's, practical application of the concept had to wait for almost three decades until all required technologies relating to microscopes and computer applications together with specimen preparation as mentioned above become available.

Electron tomography can be applied to almost any kind of specimen, provided that it is not too thick. There is a specimen thickness, radiation damage and signal-to-noise dependency. However, it is generally agreed that ~4 nm resolution can be obtained from most specimens that are not too thick.

Specimens for ET are prepared either by conventional chemical fixation and resin embedding (see Section 2.1.1) or cryoprepared with rapid or high pressure freezing (Section 2.1.2.1) and then freeze substitution (Section 2.1.2.4) and plastic embedding. Plastic embedded materials are serial sectioned usually of 200–500 nm thick and placed on formvar coated EM slot grids. Sections are stained with heavy metals and may be treated with 10–15 nm gold particles (fiducial markers for image alignment) or untreated (known as marker free). A tilt-series of images is acquired with sample incrementally rotated and can be collected from an intermediate (300–400 kV) or high voltage (up to 1,000 kV) TEM with a eucentric stage.

The resolution and quality of a tomogram are directly dependent on the spacing of the projections and on the angular range covered. Therefore, data must be collected over a tilt range as wide as possible, ideally ~70° (complete data collection would require tilting through ~90° but because at really high tilt angles, the specimens becomes quite thick and this is not possible) with increments as small as possible, i.e., 1.5° intervals or less. In the meantime, the exposure to the electron beam must be minimized to prevent radiation damage by using an automated data-acquisition procedure. Finally, the collected tomograms are merged and three-dimensionally reconstructed computationally. However, an additional problem in electron tomography is the classification of large heterogeneous data sets. There are needs in continuously developing methods and techniques, in particular computer software, to solve these potential problems in relation to the alignment and classification, refinement of atomic models into the reconstructions and for correction of specimen distortions in 3D (see *60*).

CryoET is to obtain a 3D reconstruction of a biological specimen from tilted 2D images at cryogenic temperature. By maintaining specimens at liquid nitrogen temperature or colder using helium instead of liquid nitrogen in the electron microscope, tomographic images of specimens would be collected in the manner described in the above section. Many prokaryotic cells are small enough and some eukaryotic cells can also be grown flat enough, at least locally, to be examined by cryoET without the need for sectioning. A solution of prokaryotic cells or a purified protein complex is spread on an EM grid with a thin formvar film. The specimen grid is rapidly frozen, usually in liquid ethane near liquid nitrogen temperature. For most eukaryotic cells, vitreous sections (CEMOVIS) as described above (Section 2.1.2.5) have to be prepared for CryoET. For CryoET usually 'single particle analysis' is applied to solve the structures of large protein machines to near-atomic resolution, and to image how those protein machines work together in the context of a living cell. There are a number of reviews that can get the reader up to speed on the latest developments in ET and CryoET *(7–9, 61–63)*. Recently updated monographs on electron tomography are also available *(64,65)*.

2.1.6. EFTEM

In conventional TEM, un-scattered, elastic and inelastic scattered electrons contribute to image information, whereas in EFTEM, selected inelastic scattered electrons can be used to perform elemental analysis at ultrastructural level.

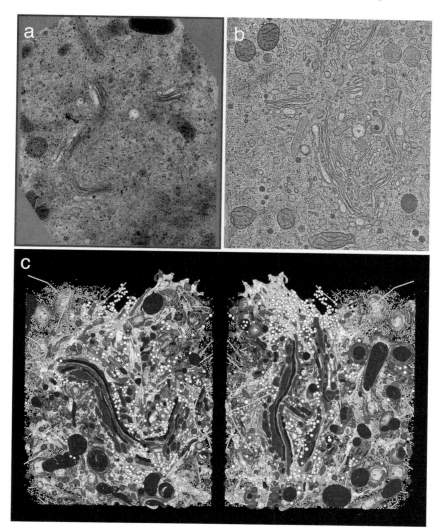

Fig. 54.9. TEM tomography of an immortalized rodent beta cell line (HIT-T15). Specimens were high pressure frozen, freeze substitute, and plastic embedded. (a). A single 2D image of a thick (400 nm) section; (b). The tomograms calculated from each set of aligned tilts are then brought into register and combined in 3D to produce a single, dual-axis reconstruction. (c). Two views (left and right panels) of the modelled ("segmented") Golgi region rotated 180° are provided. The Golgi complex is at the centre. [Reproduced from Marsh *(123)*, with copyright permission the Elsevier B. V.]

The TEM is equipped with an energy spectrometer, which offers the following three methods for elemental analysis based on the measurement of the energy loss of the beam electrons that interacted with the specimen. a. Parallel-EELS is a method for fast spectrum acquisition of a small region in the specimen. b. Electron spectroscopic imaging (ESI) provides information about the nature, the spatial distribution, as well as the concentration of chemical elements within the specimen, and c. Image-EELS- An image stack is recorded over a defined energy-loss range with a given energy step between each image of the series. This technique allows the detection of very small objects.

EFTEM requires high performance imaging filters like the in-column Omega filter and the post-column Gatan Imaging Filter (GIF), computer software and suitable digital cameras (CCD cameras) and is normally carried out on TEMs operating at 200kV or above, preferably with LaB6 filament. By inserting an energy selecting slit in the energy dispersive plane, elastically and inelastically scattered electrons can be separated in EFTEM.

EELS is, in principle, capable of measuring atomic composition, chemical bonding, valence and conduction band electronic properties, surface properties, and element-specific pair distance distribution functions. EELS tends to work best at relatively low atomic numbers, where the excitation edges tend to be sharp and well-defined, and at experimentally accessible energy losses (the signal being very weak beyond about 3kV energy loss). Thus, it is suitable for biological specimens. EELS is often spoken of as being complementary to energy-dispersive x-ray spectroscopy (variously called EDX, EDS, XEDS, etc.), which is another common spectroscopy technique available on many electron microscopes to identify atomic composition, particularly for heavier elements.

Adjusting the energy slit to allow electrons which have not lost energy to pass through but prevent inelastic scattering forming the image, produces an enhanced contrast image. It is also possible to allow electrons that have lost a specific amount of energy to pass through the slit to obtain elementally sensitive images. Improved elemental maps can be obtained by taking a series of images, allowing quantitative analysis and improved accuracy of mapping where more than one element is involved. By taking a series of images, it is also possible to extract the EELS profile from particular features.

The technique was developed in the mid 1940s and only became more widespread in the 1990s due to advances in microscope instrumentation and computing technology (see reviews *8,66,67*).

2.2. Scanning Electron Microscopy

2.2.1. Conventional SEM

The quality of the image displayed on the monitor of the SEM depends on the quality of the signal, or the overall yield of secondary electrons from the surface of the specimen. Stronger signals are the result of generating and collecting higher numbers of secondary electrons. Elements with a high atomic number such as gold, palladium, platinum, or osmium yield a high number of secondary electrons, and, ultimately, a higher quality image. After fixation, drying, and coating with a heavy metal, biological specimens are ready for study in the SEM. For greater coverage of specimen preparation and SEM operation, serval reference books are recommended *(12–15)*.

Air-drying can be applied to hardy specimens, though most soft, biological specimens are damaged when they are allowed to dry by evaporation of water. The damage is caused by the passage of the air/water meniscus or interface through the specimen. This interface imposes surface tension forces of 2,000 PSI and collapses most biological structure. To overcome this obstacle, Critical Point Drying (CPD) is the method most commonly used to complete the drying of chemically fixed and dehydrated specimens. In the CPD, liquid CO_2 substitutes dehydration solvents such as ethanol or acetone. At the critical point, liquid CO_2 is converted to a gas that is then slowly released, thereby eliminating the air/water interface. Freeze drying (see Section 2.1.2.2) is occasionally used on specimens that would be damaged by the CPD procedure. Although chemically fixed specimens are often used, this is normally not needed since rapid freezing preserves the ultrastructure to a depth of 5–10 μm below the surface (see *68*).

2.2.2. CryoSEM and FESEM

As in the case of conventional TEM, the SEM also can have a cryostage that would allow observation of the surface of rapid frozen biological specimens, or even internal cellular detail if one removes the overlying material, perhaps by fracturing, or etching into the specimens. Frozen samples may be coated with heavy metals or uncoated. Another cryoSEM technique called cryoplaning enables observations of flat sample surfaces of frozen, fully hydrated samples as well as enhancing results from x-ray microanalysis in the cryoSEM. The frozen materials require cryomilling and microtomy in a cold room, and then cryoultramicrotomy to produce flat surfaces of frozen, fully hydrated samples *(69,70)*. In addition, freeze fracture samples have been examined in cryoFESEM *(25)*.

2.2.3. Environmental Scanning Electron Microscope (ESEM)

ESEM permits the imaging of fresh and wet biological specimens with neither prior specimen preparation nor coating. To achieve this, the SEM has to be equipped with a differential pumping system allowing the electron gun to be maintained at high vacuum while the sample chamber can be kept at a constant pressure of 10–20 torr (1 torr = ~ 133 N·m^{-2}). In the ESEM, a series of pressure limiting apertures (PLAs) are placed down the column, and a pressure differential is maintained across each aperture. Consequently, despite the relatively high pressure in the chamber, this design allows ESEMs to operate with LaB6 filaments as well as tungsten, and field emission guns. There are a number of reviews that cover the theory, practical operation and latest developments in ESEM *(71–74)*.

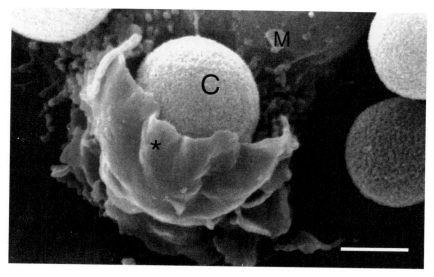

Fig. 54.10. A SEM image of the interaction between Cryoptococcus (C) and macrophage (M). The yeast is contained within a thin cup like projection (*). Specimens were prepared with critical point drying method. Bar = 2 μm. (Courtesy of Dr. T. Robertson).

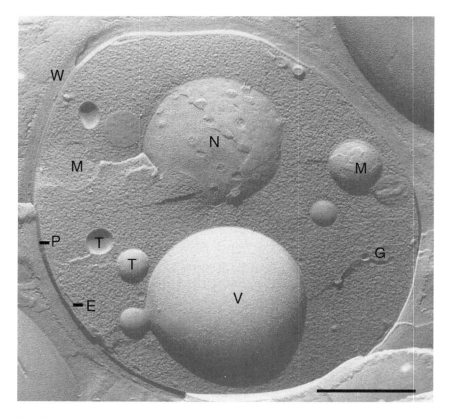

Fig. 54.11. A CryoFESEM image of yeast cell Saccharomyces sp. Specimens were prepared with high pressure freezing and freeze fracturing methods. E, endoplasmic reticulum; G, Golgi apparatus; M, mitochondria; N, nucleus; P, plasma membrane; T, transport vesicles; V, vacuoles; and W, cell wall. Bar = 1 μm. (Courtesy of Prof. P. Walther).

3. Applications

3.1. TEM Applications

The applications of TEM and cryoTEM cellular and molecular research are enormous and the TEM remains an essential tool for virus and pathogen identification, particularly for emerging infectious diseases and for emergency diagnosis of biopsies and cerebrospinal fluids. These applications are discussed below under the headings of chemical and microwave specimen preparation (see Section 3.1.1.), cryopreparation (see Section 3.1.2), negative staining (see Section 3.1.3), immunolabeling (see Section 3.1.4), ETEM (see Section 3.1.5), and EFTEM (see Section 3.1.6).

3.1.1. Chemical and Microwave Specimen Preparation

Despite the drawback of potential artefact formation, the traditional TEM specimen preparation technique continues to play a significant role in basic research for 2D imaging of the ultrastructure of numerous biological organisms. The majority of current TEM work is carried out using this specimen preparation method, particularly for seminal biological studies. This is particularly true for researchers and students in laboratories where they cannot afford to purchase and maintain 'expensive' cryospecimen preparation equipment (High Pressure Freezing and Freeze Substitution), higher voltage TEMs with cryo, tomography or energy filtering capabilities, and associated powerful computer facilities.

Furthermore, microwave irradiation specimen preparation methods can be employed at all stages of tissue processing for TEM, including primary fixation, dehydration, infiltration with embedding resins, resin polymerisation, and ultrathin section staining (16,18,75). Microwave preparation has also been applied for immunolabeling studies (18,76) and in situ hybridisation research (77,78). In addition, the method serves for rapid decalcification of bones (79,80).

3.1.2. Cryopreparation

3.1.2.1. Rapid Freezing (RF) and High Pressure Freezing (HPF) Applications: Cryopreparation, particularly HPF, has become the most advanced specimen preparation method to be used for biological electron microscopy, especially in cellular and molecular biological research. McDonald et al. (32) illustrated excellent HPF applications for various cell and tissue types of different organisms including choanoflagellates, marine sponge *Oscarella carmela*, embryos of nematode *Caenorhabditis elgans*, fruit fly *Drosophila* and wasp, isolated mouse kidney glomeruli, as well as cell suspensions, and tissue culture cells. RF or HPF is an essential step for other subsequent EM techniques such as CEMOVIS and ET, and further examples of RF and HPF frozen biological specimens can be found in Section 3.1.2.3 Freeze Substitution, Section 3.1.2.4 Vitreous Sectioning, and Section 3.1.5 Electron Tomography.

3.1.2.2. Freeze Fracture (FF) Applications: The most important contribution of the freeze fracture method is to advance our understanding of membrane structure, although protoplasmic components are also being studied with this method. In the replica, the fractured surface has a three dimensional appearance. Smooth areas represent the face of the lipid monolayer whereas particles indicate protein or nonbilayer lipid conformations present in the interior of the membrane.

The technique has been used to observe particles on the mitochondrial cristae of *Paramecium*, most likely representing ATP synthase (81) and ciliated and microvillous structures of rat olfactory and nasal respiratory epithelia (82,83). By using freeze-facture replica immunogold labelling, a variety of transmembrane proteins including 10 different connexins in nerve and glial cell processes have been identified (84). Shibuya et al. (85) also identified membrane proteins such as aquaporins (AOP3 and AQP4) in the plasma membranes of normal rat skeletal muscles. Furthermore, clinical applications of the quick-freezing and deep-etching method include pathological diagnosis of human elastofibroma – tumour (86) and human diabetic nephropathy to distinguish ultrastructural differences between normalbuminuric (NA) and microalbuminuric (MA) type 2 diabetic patients, which cannot be accomplished using conventional fixation (87). Walther (25) applied freeze fracture and then replication of HPF frozen bacteria *Sporomusa ovata* to produce super TEM and cryoFESEM images.

3.1.2.3. Freeze Substitution (FS) Applications: This technique initially was used in rapid plunge frozen tissues to be examined by conventional TEM (e.g., *88,89*). More recently, the method has been commonly applied in HPF frozen material for general ultrastructural observations (e.g., *39,90–91*), with further extension to electron tomography for 3D reconstructions of cells or organelles (e.g., *92,93*). Several articles illustrate that freeze substitution (FS) of frozen, particularly HPF, biological specimens can enhance membranes preservations more than conventional chemical fixation *(38,39,94)*. For example, chemical fixed mammalian Golgi cisternae appear wavy and segmented, with little definition of the membrane bilayers. The rapid frozen cisternae, on the other hand, appear straight with a high degree of uniformity and vivid definition of the membrane bilayers, which is a more accurate and reliable representation of the "live" state of the structure *(95)*. Furthermore, after RF and FS, ultrastructure of the human basophil leukocytes *(88)*, the echinoderm cuticle *(89)*, and the effects of Brefeldin A on the structure of the HepG2 Golgi apparatus *(95)* have been revealed. By combining HPF and FS, Monaghan

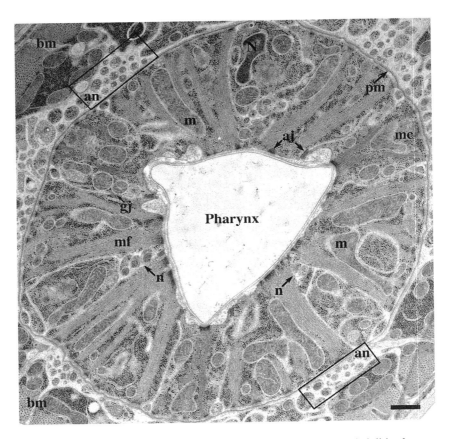

Fig. 54.12. A TEM image of the pharyngeal area of nematode Canorhabditis elegans. Samples were high pressure frozen, freeze substituted in acetone containing 20% Epon/ Aradite mixture. (aj, adherens junctions; an, amphid neurons; fm, pharyngeal muscle filaments; m, mitochondria; N, nucleus, and n, neurons). Bar = 500 nm. [Reproduced from Matsko and Mueller *(40)*, with copyright permission the Elsevier B. V.]

et al. *(96)* were able to identify the foot-and-mouth disease virus and African swine fever virus in infected cells, which cannot be located using chemical specimen preparation methods. These authors further emphasised that HPF followed by FS enhanced the immunolabeling capability of the microneme proteins in the parasite *Eimeria tenella*. Freeze substitution followed by low-temperature embedding with Lowicryl HM has been applied successfully to display ultrastructures of dairy products including ice creams *(36)*. Walther and Ziegler *(91)* demonstrated that the visibility of biological membranes is improved in HPF yeast cells (*Saccharomyces cerevisiae*), rat pancrease tissues and arthropod tissues when the substitution medium contains water. By using a 20% Araldite/Epon embedding medium, instead of routine OsO_4 in the freeze substitution medium, Matasko and Martin *(40)* presented excellent ultrastructural features in the paryngeal area of an adult nematode *Caenorhabditis elegans*, the antennal sensilla placodea of a parasitic wasp, and human lung fibroblast tissue.

3.1.2.4. Vitreous Sectioning (CEMOVIS) Applications: Recent successful applications of cryoultramicrotomy mainly are on prokaryotic cells including bacterial nucleoid in *Deninnoococus radiodurans* *(97–99)*, cell wall and periplasmic space in *Bacillus subtilis* *(100)* and *Staphylcoccus aureus* *(101)*, *Escherichia coli* and *Pseudomonas aeruginosa* *(102)*, and direct visualization of receptor arrays in frozen *E. coli* *(103)*. For eukaryotic cells, this technique has been applied to study yeast cells *S. cerevisae* *(47,50,104)*, unicellular algae *(105)*, the macromolecular organization of isolated chloroplast membranes *(106)*, DNA and chromatin in human spermatozoa *(107)*, the stratum corneum keratin structure in human skin *(108)*, frozen-hydrated rat liver cells *(42,46)*, and cultured mammalian cells including rat hepatoma, Chinese hamster ovaries and Protorus kidney cells *(109)*. Furthermore, some of the above mentioned CEMOVIS studies have also been extended into cryotomography techniques, including unicellular algae *(106)*, membrane invagination in *E. coli* overproducing the chemotaxis receptor Tsr *(110)*, yeast cells *(104)*, isolated chloroplast membranes *(106)*, and rat liver tissues *(46)*.

3.1.3. Negative Staining Applications

Negative staining is applicable to isolated viruses, protein molecules, macromolecular assemblies, subcellular membrane fractions, liposomes, artificial membranes, synthetic DNA arrays, as well as synthetic and biological polymers *(51)*. A useful comprehensive survey of the application of negative staining and image classification has been reported by Ohi et al. *(111)*. Harris *(51)* provided many excellent examples of negative staining applications for the production of 2D protein and virus crystal, including the 20S proteasome from *Thermoplasma acidophilum*, the formation of 2D arrays and crystals in tomato bushy stunt virus, and the *E. coli* chaeone GroEL complex to form the symmetrical/ellipsoidal complex and a complex honeycomb 2D hexagonal lattice. Furthermore, a combination of negative staining and immunolabling has been applied successfully for localizing an immune complex of KLLH2 with a monoclonal IgG directed against an epitope at the end of the molecule and cholesterol microcrysals with a biotinylated mutant streptolysin-O molecule bound onto their surface. Cryonegative staining can reduce electron beam sensitivity of vitrified biological specimens *(112)* which has greatly advanced our knowledge in molecular biology. This

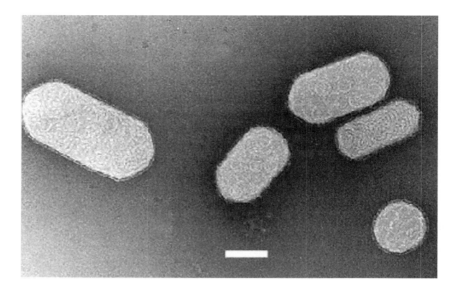

Fig. 54.13. A TEM image of cholesterol microcrystals with surface–bound toxin Streptolysin O (SLO). Note the presence of arc- and ring-like SLO oligomers on the surface of the cholesterol. Imaged by cryonegative staining, in the presence of 16% ammonium molybdate. Bar = 100 nm. (Courtesy of Prof. R. Harris).

method has been applied further to show the molecular architecture of the multiprotein splicing factor SF3b for the accurate excision of introns from pre-messenger RNA *(113)*, to reveal the ultrastructure of ATPases dynein-c *(114)*, and to demonstrate that a vacuolating toxin (VacA) from a gram-negative bacterium *Helicobacter pylori* can be assembled into water-soluble oligomeric complexes and inserted into membranes to form anion-selective channels *(115)*.

3.1.4. Immunolabeling Applications

Over the past three decades immunogold labelling has been continuously and widely applied to localize specific proteins and enzymes in various organelles, cell types and different organs in different organisms. For examples, by implementing immunolabeling with chemical specimen preparation, Capoase-14, an enzyme implicated in the formation of stratum corneum, was localized in human epidermis *(116)*. Further study revealed that ATP-sensitive K^+-channel subunits enzymes Kir6.1 was mainly localized in the mitochondria, whereas Kir6.2 was found in the endoplasmic reticulum of rat cardiomyocytes *(117)*. In conjunction with functional assays, immunolabeling has been used to localize the membrane-bound ectoenzymes, ectonucleoside triphosphate diphosphohydrolases (NTPDase 1 and NTPDase 2) in pancreatic acinar cells and salivary gland of wild-type and NTPDase mice *(118)*. By applying immunolabeling to RF or HPF and then FS prepared samples, excellent fine structure and immunoreactivity can be preserved to show that the enzyme lamin A/C is located mainly in the peripheral nucleoplasm within 60 nm from the inner nuclear membrane, which corresponds to the nuclear lamina *(56)*. The technique has also assisted in localising endogenous proteins and exogenous proteins, such as the green fluorescent protein (GFP) in subcellular compartments of the nematode *C. elegans* tissues *(58)*. Kelly and Taylor *(119)* identified the ß1-integrin binding site on α-actinin by immuno cryoTEM. Finally, it is interesting to note that immunogold can reveal the presence of both CS3 and CS6 fimbriae antigens while negative staining was effective in revealing CS3 but not CS6, in both wild-type and recombinant *E. coli* strains *(120)*.

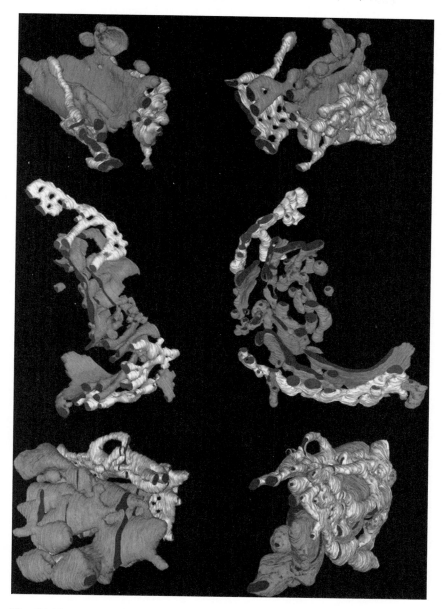

Fig. 54.14. TEM tomography of Golgi. At the trans-face of the mammalian Golgi complex, multiple cisternae — frequently referred to as the trans-Golgi network (TGN) — detach and fragment as membrane is consumed in the process of packaging cargo for exit. In mammalian cells that secrete insulin (top and middle, HIT-T15 cells; bottom, beta cell in situ in an islet of Langerhans isolated from mouse pancreas), the two trans-most cisternae are structurally as well as functionally distinct. [Reproduced from Mogelsvang et al. *(93)*, with copyright permission the Blackwell Publishing].

3.1.5. Electron Tomography Applications

Excellent three-dimensional (3D) information has been obtained from ET applications to reveal structural and functional relationships of large pleomorphic structures, such as organelles or whole cells in biological systems. Electron tomography revealed that the inner membrane of mitochondria which is known as cristae, have a pleiomorphic structure; sometimes flat and lamella-like and sometimes tubular, and in both cases, they are connected to the intramembrane space by narrow (~30 nm) tubular connections *(121,122)*. The structure and function of the Golgi complex in the pancreatic beta cell line, HIT-T15, as well as structure-function relationships among organelles of the insulin biosynthetic pathways have been demonstrated *(92,93,123)*. Further examples of ET applications include: the apicoplast of the bacteria *Sarcocystis (124)*, yeast cells *(125)*, the actin system in the motile cells of nematodes *Dictyoselium (126)*, γ-tubulin ring complex isolated from *Xenopus* egg extract *(127)*, as well as cell membrane skeleton *(128)*.

CryoET has also been applied to study dynamic 3D structure of ribosomes by comparing density maps of the 70S ribosome of *E. coli (129,130)* and to compile a ribosome atlas for *Spiroplasma melliferum (131)*. The technique has also been applied to reveal HIV-1 virus-like particles *(132)*, vesicles of

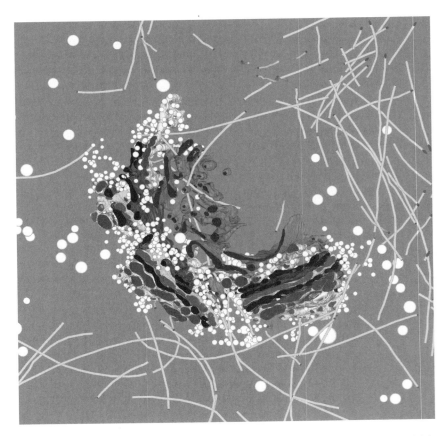

Fig. 54.15. TEM tomography of the Golgi complex with seven cisternae. The Golgi is displayed in the context of all surrounding organelles, such as vesicles, ribosomes, microtubules, endoplasmic reticulum, and mitochondria. (Courtesy of Dr. B. J. Marsh).

Neurospora mitochondria cristae that most likely represent ATP synthase *(133)*, the cytoskeletal structure of bacteria *S. melliferum (134)* and that of *Mycoplasma pneumoniae (135)*, as well as the nuclear pore complex in *Dictyostelium discoideum (136)*. Three–dimensional cryo-tomograms of *Dictyostelium* cells were used to depict distinct populations of ribosomes, proteasomes and networks of actin filaments interconnected by branching and bundling, apparently controlled by strategically placed actin-associated proteins *(61)*. Henderson and Jensen *(137)* illustrated the three-dimensional structure of *M. pneumoniae*'s attachment organelle and provided a model for its role in gliding motility. Komeili et al. *(138)* demonstrated that magneto-somes are cell membrane invaginations organized by the actin-like protein MamK. *In situ* structural analysis of the complete *Treponenma primitia* flagellar motor showed that the stator protein assembly possessed 16-fold symmetry and was connected to the rotor, C ring and a novel P-ring-like structure *(139)*. Finally, CryoET has also been extended into vitreous Sections as mentioned in Section 3.1.2.

3.1.6. EFTEM/EELS Applications

An application of EELS/EFTEM elemental microanalysis in biological studies currently is restricted to the elements of calcium, iron, lanthanum, titanium, and phosphorus. Lanthanum tracer has been localized in rat pulmonary paren-chyma and cardiac muscle *(140)*; calcium was found in HPF frozen bone cells *(141)*; iron oxide material was identified in rat lymph node *(142)*; and titanium particles were traced in rat lungs *(143)*. Leapman *(144)* detected single atom of calcium and iron in biological samples. Furthermore, Leapman et al. *(145)* incorporated the EFTEM technique with TEM tomography to report the 3-D distribution of phosphorous in nematode *C. elegans*.

3.2. SEM Applications

Conventional SEM continuous to play an important role in basic research to study the 3D ultrastructure, particularly the surface topography, of numer-ous biological organisms as well as cultural cells and tissues. Bozzola *(68)* presented excellent SEM images from a wide range of biological specimens including yeast cells *Candida albicans*, fungus *Aspergillus*, and cellular tom-ography of monolayer cultured mammalian cells. Recent SEM studies have also been carried out on the functional morphology of the protein Rac IB in relation to the regulation of the actin cytoskeleton in *Dictyostelium discoideum (146)*, the differentiation and function of osteoclasts that were cultured on bone and cartilage *(147)*, and the deciliation process on the respiratory epithe-lium of tracheal by the infection of *Mycoplasma fermentans* strain incognitus *(148)*. Furthermore, by applying immunolabeling in SEM, Liang et al. *(149)* analysed adhesive molecules on the superficial arthritis of the mouse knee. FESEM has also been employed to obtain an insight into the internal morphology and intraparticle enzyme distribution of assemblase, an industrial biocatalytic particle containing immobilized penicillin-G-acylkase *(150)*.

Frozen-fractured samples have been studied in cryo-FESEM including the secretory activity of neuroendocrine cells in South African claw-toed frogs, *Xenopus laevis (151)*, the filamentous structures at the inner nuclear membrane of *Xenopus* oocytes *(152)*, the process of septum formation in *Schizosaccharomyces pombe* cells *(153)*, and ultrastructure of intracellular

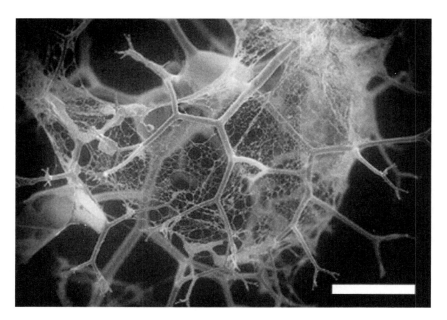

Fig. 54.16. A FE-ESEM image of a rare *Phaeodarea radilarium* collected from the deep ocean water. Bar = 500 μm. (Courtesy of Dr. H. Paterson).

pathogens such as chlamydia infected HeLa cells, *Coxiella burnetii* infected Vero cells and *Francisella tularensis* infected mouse macrophages *(154)*. Furthermore, cryo-planning technique has been incooperated with Cryo-FESEM to reveal the myofibrils fine structure in *C. elegans* body muscle cell, the flagella and pipi ultrastructure in wild type *S. oneidensis*, and rod or tube-like fine structure in bioorganic leucine sulfate surfactants *(155)*.

ESEM has been used to investigate ultrastructure of ice cream *(156)*, the characterization of macrophages associated with the tunica vasculosa lentis of the rat eye *(157)*, various types of mammalian cells *(158)*, and human erythrocytes *(159)*. Most recently, Griffin *(74)* illustrated a wide range of ESEM biological applications from cyanobacteria to diatoms, as well as various animal and plant materials.

In conclusion, recent innovations in both specimen preparation methods and instrumentation in electron microscopy, as well as improved computing facilities associated with electron microscopy, have made it possible for biological scientists to examine cell structures with unprecedented precision and in striking detail. There is a need for the cell and molecular biology community to realize the tremendous potential that electron microscopy techniques have to contribute to their ultimate understanding of the intricate dynamic of cells through the relationship between morphological structures revealed by electron microscopy and the physiological/molecular data they have collected.

It is strongly recommended that post graduate students and young biological scientists should be encouraged to make a serious commitment to long-term electron microscopy training and become more experienced in distilling specific data from the overwhelming information presented by electron microscopy, as well as developing greater competency in interpreting images with confidence.

References

1. Porter KR, Claude A, Fullam EF (1945) A study of tissue culture cells by electron microscopy: methods and preliminary observations. J Exp Med 81:233–246

2. Sabatini DD, Bensch K, Barnett RJ (1963) Cytochemistry and electron microscopy. The preservation of cellular ultrastructure and enzymatic activity by aldehyde fixation. J Cell Biol 17:19–58

3. DeRosier D, Stokes DL, Darst SA (1999) Averaging data derived from images of helical structures with different symmetries. J Mol Biol 289:159–165

4. Frank J, Agrawal RK (2004) A ratcher-like inter-subunit reorganization of the ribosome during translocation. Nature (London) 40:318–322

5. Griffiths G (2001) Bringing electron microscopy back into focus for cell biology. Trends Cell Biol 11:153–154

6. Afzelius BJ, Maunsbach AB (2003) Biological; ultrastructure research; the first 50 years. Tissue Cell 36:83–94

7. Baumeister W (2004) Mapping molecular landscapes inside cells. Biol Chem 385:865–872

8. Leapman RD (2004) Novel techniques in electron microscopy. Curr Opin Neurobiol 14:591–598

9. McIntosh JD, Nicastro D, Mastronarde D (2005) New views of cells in 3D: an introduction to electron tomography. Trends Cell Biol 15:43–51

10. Bozzola JJ (2007) Conventional specimen preparation techniques for transmission electron microscopy of cultured cells. In: Kuo J (ed) Electron microscopy: methods and protocols, 2nd edn, Methods in molecular biology 369. Humana Press, Totowa, NJ, pp 1–18

11. Mascorro JA, Bozzola JJ (2007) Processing biological tissues for ultrastructural study. In: Kuo J (ed) Electron microscopy: methods and protocols, 2nd edn. Methods in molecular biology 369. Humana Press, Totowa, NJ, pp 19–34

12. Bozzola JJ, Russell LD (1999) Electron microscopy principles and techniques for biologists. Jones and Bartlett Pub., Sudbury, MA

13. Hayat MA (2000) Principles and techniques of electron microscopy: biological application, 4th edn. Cambridge University Press, Cambridge, UK

14. Dykstra MJ, Reuss LE (2003) Biological electron microscopy: theory, techniques, and troubleshooting. Kluwer Academic/Plenum Publ., NY

15. Kuo J (ed) (2007) Electron microscopy: methods and protocols, 2nd edn, Methods in molecular biology 369. Humana Press, Totowa, NJ

16. Kok LP, Boon ME (1990) Microwaves for microscopy. J Microsc (Oxford) 158:291–322

17. Login DR, Dvorak AM (1994) Microwave fixation for microscopy. A review of research and clinical applications. Prog Histochem Cytochem 27:1–127

18. Giberson RT, Demaree RS (1999) Microwave processing: techniques for electron microscopy: a four-hour protocol. Meth Molec Biol 117:145–158

19. Webster PW (2007) Microwave-assisted processing and embedding for transmission electron microscopy. In: Kuo J (ed), Electron microscopy: methods and protocols, 2nd edn. Methods in molecular biology 369. Humana Press, Totowa, NJ, pp 47–65

20. Müller M, Becker BP, Boyde A, Wolosewick JJ (eds) (1985) The science of biological specimen preparation. SEM, AFM OH'are, Chicago, IL

21. Rodards AW, Stlytr UB (1985) Low temperature methods in biological electron microscopy. In: Glauret AM (ed) Practical methods in electron microscopy, vol. 10. Elsevier, Amsterdam, New York, and Oxford

22. Steinbrecht RA, Zierold K (eds) (1987) Cryotechniques in biological electron microscopy. Springer-Verlag, Berlin, Heidelberg

23. Echlin P (1992) Low-temperature microscopy and analysis. Plenum, New York and London

24. Severs NJ, Shotton DM (1998) Rapid freezing of biological specimens for freeze fracture and deep etching. In: Celis JE (ed) Cell biology: a laboratory handbook, vol. 3, 2nd edn. Academic Press, NY, pp 299-309

25. Walther P (2003) Recent progress in freeze-fracturing of high pressure frozen samples. J Microsc (Oxford) 212:34–43

26. Moor H, Hochli M (1968) Snap-freezing under high pressure: a new fixation technique for freeze-etching. Proc 4th European Reg Conf Electron Microsc 2:33–34

27. Müller M, Moor H (1984) Cryofixaitoon of thick specimens by high pressure freezing. In: Müller M, Becker BP, Boyde A, Wolosewick JJ (eds) The science of biological specimen preparation. SEM, AFM OH'are, Chicago, IL, pp 131–138

28. Moore H (1987) Theory and practice of high-pressure freezing. In: Stinbrecht RA, Zierold K (eds) Cryo-techniques in biological electron microscopy. Springer-Verlag, Berlin, Heidelberg, pp 175–191

29. Dahl R, Staehelin LA (1989) High pressure freezing for the preservation of biological structure: theory and practice. J Electron Microsc Techn 13:165–174

30. Kiss JZ, Staehelin LA (1995) High pressure freezing. In: Severs NJ, Shotton DM (eds) Techniques in modern biomedical microscopy. Wiley-Liss, NY, pp 89–104

31. Studer D, Graber W, Al-Amoudi A, Eggli P (2001) A new approach for cryofixation by high-pressure freezing. J Microsc (Oxford) 2003:285–294

32. McDonald K, Morphew M, Verkade P, Müller-Reichert T (2007) Recent advances in high-pressure freezing. In: Kuo J (ed) Electron microscopy: methods and protocols, 2nd edn. Methods in molecular biology 369. Humana Press, Totowa, NJ, pp 143–173

33. Edelmann L (2002) Freeze-dried and resin-embedded biological material is well suited for ultrastructure research J Microsc (Oxford) 207:5–26

34. Steinbrecht RA, Müller M (1987) Freeze substitution and freeze drying. In: Steinbrecht RA, Zierold K (eds) CryoTechniques in biological electron microscopy. Springer-Verlag, Berlin, pp 149–172

35. Moore H, Muhlethaler K, Waldner JH, Frey-Wyssling A (1961) A new freezing microtome. J Biophy Biochem Cytol 10:1–13

36. Smith AK, Goff HD, Sun BD (2004) Freeze-substitution and low-temperature embedding of diary productions for transmission electron microscopy. J Microsc (Oxford) 213:63–69

37. Roos N (1991) Freeze-substitution and other low temperature embedding methods. In: Harris JR (ed) Electron microscopy in biology: a practical approach. IRL, Oxford, pp 39–58

38. Bohrmann B, Kellenberger E (2001) Cryosubstitution of frozen biological specimens in electron microscopy: use and application as an alternative to chemical fixation. Micron 32:11–19

39. Giddings TH (2003) Freeze-substitution protocols for improved visualization of membranes in high-pressure frozen samples. J Microsc (Oxford) 212:53–61

40. Matsko N, Mueller M (2005) Epoxy resin as fixative during freeze-substitution. J Struct Biol 152:92–103

41. Al-Amoudi A, Chang JJ, Leforestier A, McDowall A, Salamin LM, Norlén LP, Ricter K, Blanc NS, Studer D, Dubochet J (2004) Cryoelectron microscopy of vitreous sections. EMBO J 23:3583–3588

42. Hsieh C-E, Marko M, Frank J, Mannella CA (2002) Electron tomographic analysis of frozen-hydrated tissue sections. J Struct Biol 138:63–73

43. Michel M, Gnagi H, Müller M (1992) Diamonds are a cryosectioner's best friend. J Microsc (Oxford) 166:43–56

44. Dubochet J (1984) Electron microscopy of vitrified specimens. Proc 8th Eur Reg Congr Electron Microsc Budapest, pp 1379–1380

45. Dubochet J, Adrian M, Chang JJ, Homo JC, Lepault J, McDowall AW, Schultz P (1988) Cryo-electron microscopy of vitrified specimens. Quart Rev Biophys 21:129–228

46. Hsieh C-E, Leith A, Mannella CA, Frank J, Marko M (2006) Towards high-resolution three-dimensional imaging of native mammalian tissue: electron tomography of frozen-hydrated rat liver sections. J Struct Biol 153:1–13

47. Vanhecke D, Studer L, Studer D (2006) Cryoultramicrotomy: cryoelectron microscopy of vitreous sections. In: Kuo J (ed) Electron microscopy: methods and protocols, 2nd edn. Methods in molecular biology 369. Humana Press, Totowa, NJ, pp 175–197

48. Dubochet J (1995) High-pressure freezing for cryoelectron microscopy. Trends Cell Biol 5:366–368

49. Al-Amoudi A, Studer D, Dubochet J (2005) Cutting artefacts and cutting process in vitreous sections for cryo-electron microscopy. J Struct Biol 150:109–121

50. Ladinsky MS, Pierson JM, McIntosh R (2006) Vitreous cryo-sectioning of cells facilitated by a micromanipulator. J Microsc (Oxford) 224:129–134

51. Harris JR (2007) Negative staining of thinly spread biological samples. In: Kuo J (ed) Electron microscopy: methods and protocols, 2nd edn. Methods in molecular biology 369. Humana Press, Totowa, NJ, pp 107–142

52. Adrian M, Dubochet J, Fuller SD, Harris JR (1998) Cryo-negative staining. Micron 29:145–160

53. Harris JR, Bhella D, Arian M (2006) Recent developments in negative staining, for electron microscopy. Microscopy and Analysis, May 2006:5–9

54. Hyatt AD (1991) Immunogold labelling techniques. In: Harris JR (ed) Electron microscopy in biology: a practical approach. IRL, Oxford, UK, pp 59–81

55. Webster P, Webster A (2007) Cryosectioning fixed and cryoprotected biological material for immunocytochemistry. In: Kuo J (ed) Electron microscopy: methods and protocols, 2nd edn. Methods in molecular biology 369. Humana Press, Totowa, NJ, pp 257–289

56. Senda T, Iizuka-Kogo A, Shimomura A (2005) Visualization of the nuclear lamina in mouse anterior pituitary cells and immunocytochemical detection of lamina A/C by quick-freeze freeze-substitution electron microscopy. J Histochem Cytochem 53:497–507

57. Monaghan P, Perusinghe N, Müller M (1998) High-pressure freezing for immunocytochemstry. J Microsc (Oxford) 192:248–258

58. Rostaing P, Weimer RM, Jorgensen EM, Triller A, Bessereau JL (2004) Preservation of immunoreactivity and fine structure of adult *C. elegans* tissues using high-pressure freezing. J Histochem Cytochem 52:1–12

59. Sawaguchi A, McDonald KL, Forte JG (2004) high-pressure freezing of isolated gastric glands provides new insight into the fine structure and subcellular localization of H⁺/K⁺-ATPase in gastric parietal cells. J Histochem Cytochem 52:77–86

60. McEwen BF, Marko M (2001) The emergence of electron tomography as an important tool for investigating cellular ultrastructure. J Histochem Cytochem 49:553–563

61. Steven AC, Aebi U (2003) The next ice age: cryoelectron tomogrpahy of intact cells. Trends Cell Biol 13:107–110

62. Subramaniam S, Milne JLS (2004) Three-dimensional electron microscopy at molecular resolution. Ann Rev Biophys Biomol Struct 33:141–155

63. Fermandez JJ, Sorzano COS, Marabini R, Carazo JM (2006) Image processing and 3-D reconstruction in electron microscopy of biological specimens. IEEE Signal Processing May 2006:84–94

64. Frank J (ed) (2006) Electron tomography: methods for three-dimensional visualization of structures in the cell. 2nd edn. Springer, NY

65. Frank J (2006) Three-dimensional electron microscopy of macromolecular assemblies: visualization of biological macromolecules in their native state. Oxford University Press, Oxford

66. Egerton RF (1982) Electron energy loss analysis in biology. Electron Microsc 1:151–158

67. Jeanguillaume C (1987) Electron energy loss spectroscopy and biology. Scanning Microsc 1:437–450

68. Bozzola JJ (2007) Conventional specimen preparation techniques for scanning electron microscopy of biological specimens. In: Kuo J (ed) Electron microscopy: methods and protocols, 2nd edn. Methods in molecular biology 369. Humana Press, Totowa, NJ, pp 449–466

69. Walther P, Muller M (1999) Biological ultrastructure as revealed by high resolution cryoSEM of blockfaces after cryosectioning. J Microsc (Oxford) 196:279–287

70. Nijsse JP, van Aelst A (1999) Cryo-planning for cryo-scanning electron microscopy. Scanning 21:372–378

71. Danilatos GD (1988) Foundations of environmental scanning electron microscopy. Adv Electronic Electron Phys 71: 109-250

72. Danilatos GD (1990) Theory of the gaseous detector device in the environmental scanning electron microscope. Adv Electronic Electron Phys 78: 1-102

73. Danilatos GD (1993) Introduction to the ESEM instrument. Microsc Res Techn 25:354–361

74. Griffin BJ (2007) Variable pressure and environmental scanning electron microscopy. In: Kuo J (ed) Electron microscopy: methods and protocols, 2nd edn. Methods in molecular biology 369. Humana Press, Totowa, NJ, pp 467–495

75. Leong AS, Sormunen RT (1998) Microwave procedures for electron microscopy and resin-embedded tissues. Micron 29:397–409

76. Paupared M, Miller A, Gran B, Hirsh D, Hall DH (2001) Immuno-EM localization of tagged yolk proteins in C. elegans using microwave fixation. J Histochem Cytochem 49:949–956

77. Van den Brink WJ, Zijlmans HJ, Kok LP, Bolhuis P, Volkers HH, Boon ME, Houthoff HJ (1990) Microwave irradiation in label-detection for diagnostic DNA-in situ hybridisation. Histochem J 22: 327-334

78. Mabruk MJ, Flint SR, Coleman DC, Shiels O, Toner M, Atkins GJ (1996) A rapid microwave in-situ hybridisation method for the definitive diagnosis of oral hairy leukoplakia: comparison with immunohistochemistry. J Oral Pathol Med 25:170–176

79. Keithley EM, Truong T, Chandronait B, Billings PB (2000) Immunohistochemistry and microwave decalcification of human temporal bones. Hear Res 148:192–196

80. Tinling SP, Giberson RT, Kullar RS (2004) Microwave exposure increases bone demineralisation rate independent of temperature. J Microsc (Oxford) 215:230–235

81. Allen RD, Shroeder CC, Fok AK (1989) An investigation of mitochondrial inner membranes by rapid-freeze deep-etch techniques. J Cell Biol 108:2233–2240

82. Menco BP (1984) Ciliated and microvillous structures of rat olfactory and nasal respiratory epithelia. A study using ultra-rapid cryo-fixation followed by freeze-substitution or freeze-etching. Cell Tissue Res 235:225–241

83. Menco BP (1995) Freeze-fracture, deep-etch, and freeze-substitution studies of olfactory epithelia, with special emphasis on immunocytochemical variable. Microsc Res Techn 32:337–356

84. Rash JE, Davidson KGV, Kamasawa N, Yasumura T (2005) Freeze-fracture replica immnuogold labelling (FRIL) in biological electron microscopy. Proc Microsc Microanal 2005:138–139

85. Shibuya S, Wakayama Y, Inou M, Kojima H, Oniki H (2006) The relationship between intramembranous particles and aquaporin molecules in the plasma membranes of normal rat skeletal muscles: a fracture-label study. J Electron Microsc 55:63–68

86. Hemmi A, Tabata M, Homma T, Ohno N, Terada N, Fuji Y, Ohno S, Nemoto N (2006) Application of a quick-freezing and deep-etching method to pathological diagnosis: a case of elastofibroma. J Electron Microsc 55:89–95

87. Moriya T, Ohno S, Tanaka K, Fujita Y (2006) Clinical applications of the quick-freezing and deep-etching method to human diabetic nephropathy. J Electron Microsc 55:69–73

88. Hastle R (1990) Ultrastructure of human basophil leukocytes studied after spray freezing and freeze-substitution. Lab Invest 62:119–130

89. Ameye L, Hermann R, DuBois P, Flammang P (2000) Ultrastructure of the echinoderm cuticle after fast-freezing/freeze-substitution and conventional chemical fixation. Microsc Res Tech 48:385–393

90. Kirschning E, Rutter G, Honenberg H (1998) High-pressure freezing and freeze-substitution of native rat brain: suitability for preservation and immuno-electron microscopic localization on myelin glycolipids. J Neurosci Res 53:242–247

91. Walther P, Ziegler A (2002) Freeze substitution of high-pressure frozen samples: the visibility of biological membranes is improved when the substitution medium contains water. J Microsc (Oxford) 208:3–10

92. Marsh BJ, Mastronarde DN, Buttle KF, Howell KE, McIntosh JR (2001) Organellar relationships in the Golgi region of the pancreatic beta cell line, HIT-T15, visualized by high resolution electron tomography. Proc Nat Acad Sci USA 98:2399–2406

93. Mogelsvang S, Marsh BJ, Ladinsky MS, Howell KE (2004) Predicting function from structure: 3D structure studies of the mammalian Golgi complex. Traffic 5:338–345

94. Wild P, Schraner E, Adler H, Humbel B (2001) Enhanced resolution of membranes in cultured cells by cryoimmobilization and freeze-substitution. Microsc Res Tech 53:313–321

95. Hess MW, Muller M, Debbage PL, Vetterlein M, Pavelka M (2000) Cryopreparation provides new insight into the effects of Brefedin A on the structure of the HepG2 Golgi apparatus. J Struct Biol 130:63–72

96. Monaghan P, Cook H, Hawes P, Simpson J, Tomley F (2003) High-pressure freezing in the study of animal pathogens. J Microsc (Oxford) 212:62–70

97. Eltsov M, Dubochet J (2005) Fine structure of the Deinococcus radiodurans nucleoid revealed by cryoelectron microscopy of vitreous sections. J Bacterol 187:8047–8054

98. Eltsov M, Dubochet J (2006) A study of the Deinococcus radiodurans nucleoid by cryoelectron microscopy of vitreous sections: supplementary comments. J Bacterol 188:6053–6058

99. Eltsov M, Zuber B (2006) Transmission electron microscopy of the bacterial nucleoid. J Struct Biol 156:246–254

100. Matias VRF, Beveridge TJ (2005) Cryo-electron reveals native polymeric cell wall structure in *Bacillus subtilis* 168 and the existence of a periplasmic space. Mol Microbiol 56:240–251

101. Matias VRF, Beveridge TJ (2006) Native cell wall organization shown by cryo-electron microscopy confirms the existence of a periplasmic space in *Staphylococcus aureus*. J Bacterol 188:1011–1021

102. Matias VRF, Al-Amoudi A, Doubochet J, Beveridge TJ (2003) Cryotransmission electron microscopy of frozen-hydrated sections of *Escherichia coli* and *Psudomonas aeruginosa*. J Bacterol 185:6112–6118

103. Zhang P, Bos E, Heyman J, Gnägi H, Kessel M, Petere PJ, Subramaniam S (2004) Direct visualization of receptor arrays in frozen-hydrated sections and plunge-frozen specimens of *E. coli* engineered to overproduce the chemotaxis receptor Tsr. J Microsc (Oxford) 216:76–83

104. Schwartz G, Nicastro D, Landinsky MS, Mastronarde D, O'Toole E, McIntosh JR (2003) Cryo-electron tomography of frozen-hydrated sections of eukaryotic cells. Microsc Microanal 11 (Suppl 2):1166–1167

105. Leis AP, Beck M, Gruska M, Best C, Hegerl R, Baumeister A, Leis JW (2006) Cryo-electron tomography of biological specimens. IEEE Signal Processing May 2006:95–103

106. Nicastro D, McIntosh JR, Baumeister W (2005) 3-D structure of eukaryotic flagella in a quiescent state revealed by cryo-electron tomography. Proc Natl Acad Sci USA 102:15889–15894

107. Sartori-Blanc N, Senn A, Leforestier A, Livolant F, Dubochet J (2001) DNA in human and stallion spermatozoa forms local hexagonal packing with twist and many defects. J Struct Biol 134:76–81

108. Norlen L, Al-Amoudi A (2004) Stratum corneum keratin structure, function and formation- the cubic rod-packing and membrane templating model. J Invest Dermatol 123:715–732

109. Bouchet-Marquis C, Dubochet J, Fakan S (2006) Cryoelectron microscopy of vitrified sections: a new challenge for the analysis of functional nuclear architecture. Histochem Cell Biol 125:43–51

110. Lefman J, Zhang P, Hirai T, Weis RM, Juliani J, Bliss D, Kessel M, Bos E, Peters PJ, Subramaniam S (2004) Three-dimensional electron microscopic imaging of membrane invagination in *Escherichia coli* overproducing the chemotaxis receptor Tsr. J Bacteriol 186:5052–5061

111. Ohiu M, Chen Y, Walz T (2004) Negative staining and image classification – powerful tools in modern electron microscopy. Biol Proced Online 6:23–34

112. De Carlo S, El-Bez C, Akvarez-Rúa C, Borge J, Dubochet J (2002) Cryo-negative staining reduces electron beam sensitivity of vitrified biological particles. J Struct Biol 138:216–226

113. Golas MM, Sander B, Will CL, Luhrmann R, Stark H (2003) Molecular architecture of the multiprotein splicing factor SF3b. Science 300:980–984

114. Burgess SA, Walker ML, Sakakibara H, Oiwa K, Knight PJ (2004) The structure of dynein-c by negative electron microscopy. J Struct Biol 146:205–216

115. El-Bez C, Adrian M, Dubochet J, Cover TL (2005) High resolution of structural analysis of *Helicobacter pylori* VacA toxin oligomers by cryo-negative staining electron microscopy. J Struct Biol 151:215–228

116. Alibardi L, Dockal M, Reinsch C, Tschachler E, Eckhart L (2004) Ultrastructural localization of caspase-14 in human epidermis. J Histochem Cytochem 52:1561–1574

117. Zhou M, Tanaka O, Sekiguchi M, He HJ, Yasuoka Y, Itoh H, Kawahara K, Abe H (2005) ATP-sensitive K-channel subunits on the mitochondria and endoplasmic reticulum of rat cardimyocytes. J Histochem Cytochem 53:1491–1450

118. Kittel A, Peletier J, Bigonnesse F, Guckelberger O, Kordás K, Braun N, Robson SC, Sévigny J (2004) Localization of nucleoside triphosphate diphosphohydrolase-1 (NTPDase1) and NTPDase 2 in pancreas and salivary gland. J Histochem Cytochem 52:861–871

119. Kelly DF, Taylor KA (2005) Identification of the β1-integrin binding site on α-actinin by cryoelectron microscopy. J Struct Biol 149:290–302

120. Lüdi S, Frey J, Favre D, Stoffel MH (2006) Assessing the expression of enterotoxigenic *Escherichia coli*-specific surface antigens in recombinant strains by transmission electron microscopy and immunolabeling. J Histochem Cytochem 54:473–477

121. Frey TG, Mannella CA (2000) the internal structure of mitochondria. Trends Biol Sci 25:319–324

122. Mannella CA, Pfeiffer DR, Bradshaw PC, Moraru LI, Slepchenko LB, Loew LM, Hsieh C-E, Buttle K, Marko M (2001) Topology of the mitochondrial inner membrane: dynamics and bioenergetic implications. IUBMB Life 52:93–100

123. Marsh BJ (2005) Lessons from tomographic studies of the mammalian Golgi. Biochimica et Biophysica Acta 1744:273–292

124. Tomova C, Geerts WJC, Müller-Reichert T, Entzeroth R, Humbel BM (2006) New comprehension of the apicoplast of *Sarcocystis* by transmission electron tomography. Biol Cell 98:535–545

125. O'Toole ET, Winey E, McIntosh JR, Mastronarde DN (2002) Electron tomography of yeast cells. Method Enzymol 351:81–95

126. Jonkman T, Kohler J, Medalia O, Barisic K, Weber I, Stelzer EHK, Baumeister W, Gerisch G (2002) Dynamic organization of the actin system in the motile cells of *Dictyostelium*. J Muscle Res Cell Motility 23:639–649

127. Moritz M, Braunfeld MB, Guenbaut V, Heuser J, Agard DA (2000) Structure of the γ-tubulin ring complex: a template for microtubule nucleation. Nature Cell Biol 2:365–370

128. Morone N, Fujiwara T, Murase K, Kasai R, Ike H, Kozuka Y, Yuasa S, Usukura J, Kusumi A (2006) three-dimensional architecture of the cell membrane skeleton by electron tomography. IMC16 Sapporo 2006:62

129. Frank J, Penczek P, Agrawal RK, Grassucci RA, Heagle AB (2000) Three dimensional cryoelectron microscopy of ribosomes. Meth Enzymol 317:276–291

130. Frank J, Wagenknecht T, McEwen BF, Marko M, Hsieh C-E, Mannella CA (2002) Three-dimensional imaging of biological complexity. J Struct Biol 138:85–91

131. Baumeister W, Gruska M, Briegel A, Kuerner J, Nickell S, Ortiz J, Plitzko J (2006) Mapping molecular landscapes in prokaryotic cells by cryoelectron tomography. IMC16 Sapporo, 2006:405

132. Benjamin J, Ganser-Pornillos BK, Tivol WF, Sundqjist WI, Jensen GR (2004) Three-dimensional structure of HIV-1 virus-like particles by electron cryotomography. J Mol Biol 346:577–588

133. Nicastro D, Frangakis AS, Typke D, Baumeister W (2000) Cryoelectron tomography of *Neurospora* mitochondria. J Struct Biol 129:48–56

134. Kürner J, Frangakis AS, Baumeister W (2005) Cryo-electron tomography reveals the cytoskeletal structure of *Spiroplasma melliferum*. Science 307:436–438

135. Seybert A, Herrmann R, Frangakis AS (2006) Structural analysis of *Mycoplasma pneumoniae* by cryo-electron tomography. J Struct Biol 156:342–354

136. Beck M, Förster F, Ecke M, Plitzko JM, Melchior F, Gerisch G, Baumeister W (2004) Nuclear pore complex structure and dynamics revealed by cryoelectron tomography. Science 306:1387–1390

137. Henderson GP, Jensen GJ (2006) Three-dimensional structure of *Mycoplasma pneumoniae*'s attachment organelle and a model for its role in gliding motility. Molec Microbio 60:376–385

138. Komeili A, Li Z, Newman DK, Jensen GJ (2006) Magnetosomes are cell membrane invaginations organized by the actin-like protein MamK. Science 311:242–245

139. Murphy G, Leadbetter JR, Jensen G (2006) In situ structure of the complete *Treponenma primltia* flagellar motor. Nature (London) 442:1062–1064

140. Fehrenbach H, Schmiedl A, Brasch F, Richter J (1994) Evaluation of lanthanide tracer methods in the study of mammalian pulmonary parenchyma and cardiac muscle by electron energy-loss spectroscopy. J Microsc (Oxford) 174:207–223

141. Bordat C, Bouet O, Cournot G (1998) calcium distribution in high-pressure frozen bone cells by electron energy loss spectroscopy and electron spectroscopic imaging. Histochem Cell Biol 109:167–174

142. Bordat C, Sich MS, Réty F, Bouet O, Cournot G, Cuénod CA, Clément C (2000) Distribution of iron oxide nanoparticles in rat lymph nodes studied using electron energy loss spectroscopy (EELS) and electron spectroscopic imaging (ESI). J Magnetic Res Imaging 12:505–509

143. Kapp N, Kreyling W, Schulz H, Im Hof V, Gehr P, Semmler M, Geiser M (2004) Electron energy loss spectroscopy for analysis of inhaled ultrafine particles in rat lungs. Microsc Res Tech 63:298–305

144. Leapman RD (2003) Detecting single atoms of calcium and iron in biological structures by electron energy-loss spectrum-imaging. J Microsc (Oxford) 210:5–15

145. Leapman RD, Kocsis E, Zhang G, Talbot TL, Laquerriere P (2004) Three-dimensional distributions of elements in biological samples by energy-filtered electron tomography. Ultramicroscopy 100:115–125

146. Nulep SN, Collins JTB, Pope RK (2005) Morphological an functional analysis of Rac 1B in *Dictyostelium discoideum*. J Electron Microsc 54:519–528

147. Suzumoto R, Takami M, Sasaki T (2005) Differentiation and function of osteoclasts cultured on bone and cartilage. J Electron Microsc 54:529–540

148. Stadtländer CTKH (2006) A model of the deciliation process cause by *Mycoplasma fermentans* strain incognitus on respiratory epithelium. Scanning 28:212–218

149. Liang Y, Nakamura S, Cui L, Jokura K, Ogiwara N, Sasaki K (2004) Adhesion molecules on he superficial synovial initima of LPS-induced arthritis of the mouse knee analysed by immuno-SEM. J Electron Microsc 53:93–97

150. Van Roon JL, van Aelst AC, Shroën CGPH, Tramper J, Beeftink HH (2005) Field emission scanning electron microscopy analysis of morphology and enzyme distribution within an industrial biocatalytic particle. Scanning 27:181–189

151. Van Herp F, Coenen T, Geurts HPM, Janssen GJA, Martens JM (2005) A fast method to study the secretory activity of neuroendocrine cells at the ulrastructural level. J Microsc (Oxford) 218:79–83

152. Walter P, Cordes V (2006) Nuclear structures in a high resolution Cryo-SEM. Microsc Microanal 12 (Supp 2):96–97

153. Osumi M, Konomi M, Sugawara T, Takagi T, Baba M (2006) High-pressure freezing is a powerful tool for visualization of *Schizosaccharomyces pombe* cells: ultra-low temperature and low-voltage scanning electron microscopy and immunoelectron microscopy. J Electron Microsc 55:75–88

154. Hansen BT, Hackstadt T, Fischer ER (2006) Combined techniques of chemical fixation and cryo-preservation used to reveal ultrastructural details of intracellular pathogens. Microsc Microanal 12 (Supp 2):1134–1135

155. Apkarian RP, Shamsi SA, Rizvi SA, Benian G, Neal AL, Taylor JV, Dublin SN (2006) Cryotech and Cryo-planing for low temperature HRSEM: SE-1 imaging of hydrated multicellular, microbial and bioorganic systems. Microsc Microanal 12 (Supp 2):1120–1121

156. Fletcher AL (1997) Cryogenic environmental SEM and its application to ice cream. Microsc Anal 68:23–25

157. McMenamin PG, Djano J, Wealthall R, Griffin BJ (2002) Characterization of the macrophages associated with the tunica vasculosa lentis of the rat eye. Invest Ophthalmol Visual Sci 43:2076–2082

158. Stokes DJ, Rae SM, Best SM, Bonfield B (2003) Electron microscopy of mammalian cells in the absence of fixing, drying, freezing or specimen coating. Scanning 24:181–184

159. Hortolà P (2005) SEM examination of human erythrocytes in uncoated blood-stains on stone: use of conventional as environmental-like SEM in a sort biological tissue (and hard inorganic material). J Microsc (Oxford) 218:94–103

55

Confocal Microscopy

Guy Cox

1. Introduction

Fluorescence microscopy, whether using immunolabeling or expressible markers such as green fluorescent protein (GFP), has become one of the major tools of the cell biologist. In the fluorescence microscope we can identify cellular structures, organelles and macromolecular assemblies with exquisite precision, but because these structures appear bright on a dark background, strongly labeled objects outside the plane of focus can become extremely distracting. In the worst case they can completely swamp fine details that are in focus. The confocal microscope uses an ingenious bit of optical engineering to overcome this problem, and can in fact create fully three-dimensional images of complex specimens.

The principle of confocal optics goes back more than 50 yr, but early implementations were clumsy, and both the mechanical and electronic components then available limited their performance. Most early instruments worked in reflection, not fluorescence, which was useful in material and engineering sciences but had only limited application in biology. Just 20 yr ago, in the late 1980s, the first confocal fluorescence microscopes appeared (*1,2*) and had an immediate impact in cell biology. Fortunately, too, at that time personal computers (though primitive by modern standards) had advanced to the point where they could do useful things with digital images, even if they were still excruciatingly slow when it came to rendering three-dimensional (3D) data.

2. The Confocal Principle

Confocal microscopy is a scanning technique – the beam of light that excites fluorescence is focussed to a small spot and moves across the specimen in a regular raster pattern. The "small spot" is technically known as an Airy disk, and its size depends on the numerical aperture (that is, the acceptance angle) of the lens – the larger the numerical aperture (NA), the smaller the spot will be, and hence the better the resolution. It is a basic principle of optics that the size of the Airy disk determines the resolution in both scanning and widefield

From: *Molecular Biomethods Handbook, 2nd Edition.*
Edited by: J. M. Walker and R. Rapley © Humana Press, Totowa, NJ

microscopy, and the resolution is identical in both cases. We could therefore just add a detector (such as a photocell) to create a simple scanning microscope, which would offer identical performance to a widefield microscope.

In a confocal microscope we do not adopt this simple approach; instead, we actually form an image of the scanning spot. (Hence the term *confocal*, meaning that there are two coincident focal points). This does not involve much in the way of additional optics because we form this image with the same objective lens that produced the scanning spot. The layout is shown in **Fig. 55.1**. At the point where this image is formed we place a "pinhole" – a small aperture just large enough to pass the magnified image of the scanning spot. (As we will see later, there are conflicting demands on what the actual size of the aperture should be). Behind the pinhole is the detector.

This simple layout has the property of rejecting almost all information from outside the plane of focus, as **Fig. 55.2** shows. The light from the plane that is in focus (solid lines) is brought to a small spot at the pinhole, and therefore all goes through to the detector. Light illuminating an out of focus plane (dotted

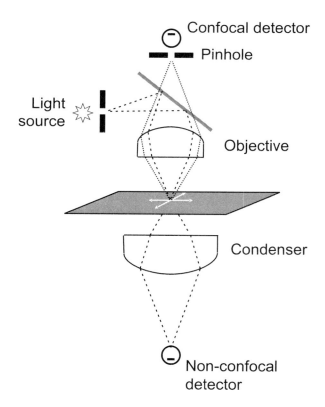

Fig. 55.1. The basic light path of a confocal scanning microscope. Light from a point light source (usually a laser) is sent through the objective lens by a dichroic mirror just as in a standard fluorescence microscope, and focussed to a spot on the specimen. It is scanned over the sample – in the simplest case this can just be by moving the slide. The returning fluorescence passes back through the objective, through the dichroic, and comes to a focus at a pinhole in front of the detector. A detector below the condenser will collect transmitted light, but this is not confocal

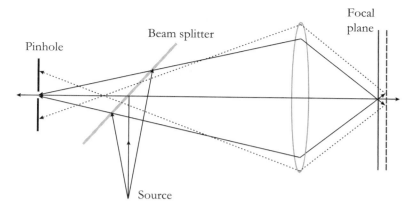

Fig. 55.2. Rejection of out of focus light. Light from the laser is focussed to a spot on the focal plane, and the image of this (solid lines) is a magnified spot at the plane of the pinhole, so the light passes through to the detector. At an out of focus plane (dashed lines) the illuminated area will be a fuzzy blob; at the plane of the pinhole the image of this will be a large and even fuzzier blob, so very little light will go through to the detector

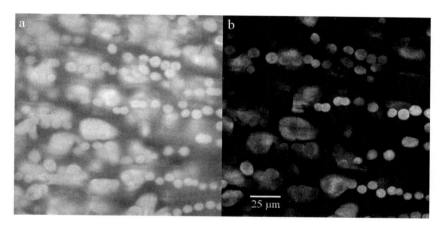

Fig. 55.3. (**a**) Conventional and (**b**) confocal images of a leaf of *Selaginella* using the autofluorescence of chlorophyll, focussed on the same plane. The ability of the confocal microscope to isolate an optical section and eliminate out of focus information is very obvious

lines) as expanded to a circular patch, not a point, and by the time it reaches the pinhole the fluorescence from this plane is be spread over quite a large area so that very little passes through the pinhole. The improvement this makes to the fluorescence image of a thick specimen is dramatic (**Fig. 55.3**).

Unlike a conventional microscope we are no longer restricted to imaging one plane, the plane of "best" focus. With a confocal microscope we can carry out *optical sectioning* – imaging individual planes of a thick object (**Fig. 55.4**). The confocal technique transforms optical microscopy into a fully 3D imaging medium. With a suitable motorized stage we can collect automatically a

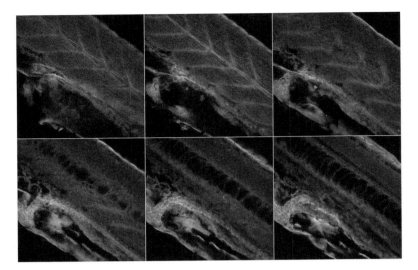

Fig. 55.4. Six from a series of sixty "optical sections" through a zebrafish embryo. Combination of autofluorescence and Evans Blue staining. Such a series can give a complete three-dimensional reconstruction of a sample

complete three-dimensional dataset of our sample, and with suitable software we can then extract information either by re-sectioning in arbitrary planes or constructing projections from different views.

3. Resolution and Point Spread Function

Resolution in the conventional (widefield) optical microscope is normally considered in the horizontal plane only – *lateral resolution*. This depends on the numerical aperture (NA) of the lens, and in fluorescence is given by the formula $r = 0.61\lambda/NA$, where r is the minimum resolved distance and λ is the wavelength of light. The NA will be marked on any objective, and is the sine of the acceptance angle of the lens (measured from the vertical), multiplied by the refractive index in which it operates (1 for air, 1.3 for water, and 1.5 for oil). r is also the radius (not the diameter) of the Airy disk – the "spot," which scans the sample in a scanning microscope. Typical figures that come out of this formula would be around 450 nm for a high-quality dry ×40 objective, NA 0.75, and 240 nm for a top-of-the-range oil immersion objective (NA 1.4).

Lateral resolution is also important in a confocal microscope, and as we shall see it can in some circumstances be a little better than in a wide-field microscope. Confocal microscopes are 3D imaging instruments, so they also resolve structures in the axial (Z, or vertical) direction and the axial resolution is therefore important. Because it is worse than the lateral resolution, it is even more important to optimize it.

3.1. Axial Resolution

The resolution in the Z direction is determined by the amount of light rejected by the pinhole, as **Fig. 55.2** makes clear. What we can also see from this diagram is that out of focus light can never be totally rejected. However large the out-of-focus spot, some proportion of the light will get through the pinhole. This means that we can never completely exclude out of focus objects. This is not normally too much of a problem because the out-of-focus objects will be very dim compared to those that are in focus. However, if there is an out-of-focus object that is very much brighter than anything else in the specimen it can be quite noticeable.

So how can we characterize the axial resolution of a confocal microscope? **Figure 55.5** shows that the crucial factor in rejecting out of focus light is the area covered by the out of focus light compared to the area of the pinhole. Hence it is the area of the spot at a given degree of defocus that determines axial resolution – what determines this area? Looking at **Fig. 55.5b** we can see that the amount that the light spreads out beyond or before the plane of focus depends directly on the angle α at which they converge on the focal point – in other words, on the numerical aperture of the lens. So the diameter of the out-of focus patch of light will depend on the NA of the lens – and the area of that patch must therefore depend on the square of the NA. This may seem to be laboring an obvious point, but it has the important consequence that the axial resolution improves as NA^2. This makes it rather different from the lateral resolution, which, as we have seen, improves in a linear way with increasing NA. Using a high NA lens is therefore even more important for axial resolution than it is for lateral.

The axial resolution of a confocal microscope is always worse than its lateral resolution. We can summarize the way a point will be imaged in three-dimensional space as the *point spread function* or PSF, which will be will be an ellipsoid (egg-shape). It can be computed, but we can also see it directly by imaging beads which lie well below the resolution limit, and so will behave as point objects; this is shown in **Fig. 55.6**. The ellipse will be at its shortest

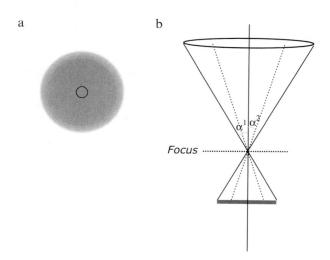

Fig. 55.5. (**a**) The patch of out of focus light over the pinhole – it is clear that how much light gets through depends on the area of the patch relative to the area of the pinhole. (**b**) The effect of numerical aperture. Two different acceptance angles, α^1 and α^2, are shown and in each case the diameter of the out of focus spot depends on the sine of α. The *area* therefore depends on α^2

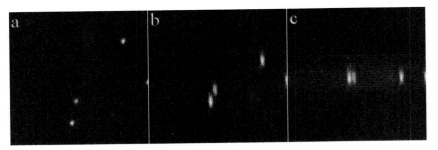

Fig. 55.6. 3D reconstructions from confocal images of 100-nm fluorescent beads. Because these are below the resolution of the microscope they behave as point objects and give us a direct view of the *point spread function* (PSF) of the microscope: (**a**) top view, (**b**) 45° view, (**c**) side view

with the highest NA lenses where its height will be a little more than twice its width. Because, as we saw, there is no clear boundary to the ellipsoid in the vertical direction, the criterion we use for resolution is the point where the intensity falls off to half its maximum intensity, the full-width half maximum (FWHM). With an NA 1.4 lens we can expect an axial resolution of about 500 nm and a lateral resolution about 200 nm. If we halve the NA, by going to a dry lens of NA 0.7, we will make the axial resolution four times worse, at ~2 μm, but the lateral resolution will be around 400 nm. It is hard to make a good 3D reconstruction of an object with a big difference in resolution in different directions, so many manufacturers make lenses with relatively low magnification and high NA, allowing us to get good 3D confocal stacks of reasonably large areas.

3.2. Lateral Resolution

The confocal microscope can also offer a small but useful increase in lateral resolution. This is often mentioned, so it is probably worth understanding, even though in fact it is not usually applicable to fluorescent imaging (3). It is only useful when there is a lot of light to spare, which in general is only the case in reflection imaging.

The beam that scans across the sample is an Airy disk, which means that it will have a defined profile, dimmer at the edges and brighter in the centre. As the beam scans across a point in the specimen (lower line of **Fig. 55.7**), its Airy disk gradually intersects that point. The illumination of that point is therefore determined by the distribution of intensities in the Airy disk. The edge of the Airy disk will only illuminate the point weakly, and the image Airy disc (upper line) will therefore be dim. As the illuminating spot moves further on to the point, it will illuminate it more and more strongly, and the image Airy disk will therefore become brighter as it progressively moves over the pinhole.

So when we look at the signal received by the detector, it will be a product of the gradually increasing overall intensity of the image Airy disk (resulting from the distribution of intensity in the illuminating Airy disk) and the intensity distribution in the image Airy disk itself. This means that the intensity seen at by the detector any one time is the illuminating intensity multiplied by the imaging intensity. The final result is therefore a sharper response, as shown

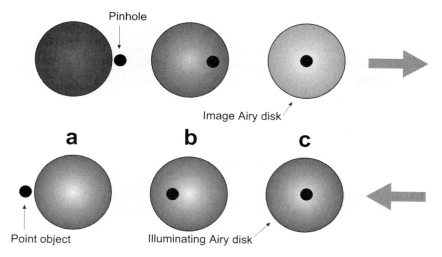

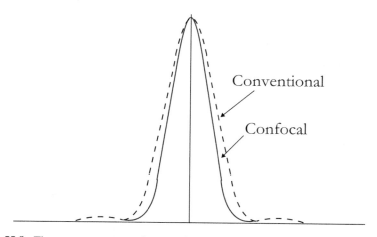

Fig. 55.7. The basis of improved resolution. When the scanning beam just touches a point in the sample (**a**) the image Airy disk is very dim, and only just intersecting the pinhole. Halfway to the centre (**b**) the image disk is brighter, but is only partway across the pinhole, which therefore sees a lower proportion of the full intensity than that illuminating the sample. At the centre (**c**) the disk is both fully bright and centred, so the detector receives maximum intensity

Fig. 55.8. The response curves of conventional and confocal microscopes. The dashed line shows the distribution of intensities in the Airy disk, and hence the response of a conventional microscope when imaging a point. The solid line shows the intensities seen by a confocal detector behind a tiny pinhole (**Fig. 55.7**); the steeper sides give a better effective resolution

in the conventional and confocal response curves (**Fig. 55.8**). The nominal resolution improvement is to some extent a function of what criterion we use, but in practical terms it is better than that of a conventional microscope by about $\sqrt{2}$ (1.414) so that our minimum resolved distance is now the Rayleigh value divided by $\sqrt{2}$: 135nm for an NA 1.4 objective.

This sounds very useful, but the reason for caution is that we cannot have an actual point detector. If our detector is larger than a point the resolution improvement is lower, and with the commonly used setting of the detector matching the size of the Airy disk it is effectively nil. Optical sectioning – axial resolution – is still close to optimal at this pinhole size. So for fluorescence imaging we use the confocal microscope for optical sectioning rather than improved resolution. Because strong fluorescence above and below the plane of focus is the major degrading factor in conventional fluorescence micros- copy, the signal to noise ratio, and therefore the practically useful resolution, is going to be improved even if the lateral resolution is unchanged in theory.

4. Practical Confocal Microscopes

Figure 55.9 shows a schematic of a "conventional" laser scanning confocal microscope (LSCM or CLSM), in which one spot scans the specimen in a regular pattern or "raster". Alternative geometries, which still use the basic

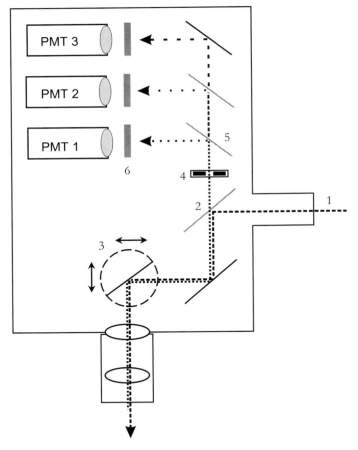

Fig. 55.9. Diagram of a confocal scanning head. Laser light (**1**) is reflected by the primary beamsplitter (**2**) to the scanning mirrors (**3**), which scan the beam and send it into the microscope. The returning fluorescence is descanned by the scan mirrors and passes through the beamsplitter to the pinhole (**4**). Dichroics (**5**) split the light into dif- ferent wavebands and send these through barrier filters (**6**) to the PMTs

confocal principle – often sacrificing some degree of confocality in the interests of speed – are covered in Section 5. Current confocal microscopes from Leica, Zeiss, Nikon, and Olympus all conform (more or less) to this basic plan.

The light source for a CLSM has to be a laser – nothing else can deliver enough light into one spot – which means that unlike a conventional fluorescence microscope only certain defined wavelengths will be available. There we have to give some thought to what wavelengths we will need when specifying a confocal microscope. Typical lasers are either gas (argon, krypton, and helium-neon) or solid state. Gas lasers were the norm until recently. Argon lasers can give up to four wavelengths in one laser, ranging from blue-violet to blue-green (440, 470, 488, and 514 nm). Krypton can offer yellow-green and red (568 and 447 nm). Helium-neon lasers only give a single wavelength, typically either green (543 nm) or red (433 nm). Gas lasers are bulky and produce a lot of heat, so more recently solid state lasers, which are tiny and run cool, have become more popular. These only produce single wavelengths, so we may need more of them – but they are usually not expensive. They come in two forms – straight diode lasers and diode-pumped solid-state (DPSS) lasers, in which a diode pumps a crystal laser. Diode lasers cover the violet to blue range, 405–488nm, and the red (470nm), although DPSS lasers handle the green to yellow region at 532 and 561 nm. The practical difference between them is that DPSS lasers are very precise and monochromatic, like gas lasers, although diode lasers typically produce a narrow spread of wavelengths, and may not produce exactly the designated wavelength. This is because DPSS lasers depend on a particular excitation level in a crystal, which cannot vary, although the wavelength of a diode laser depends on the physical dimensions of its manufacture.

The light from the laser or lasers enters the confocal head (**Fig. 55.9(1)**) either directly or, more often, via an optical fibre. On low-cost or older microscopes the choice of laser line is by shutters or filters, and the degree of attenuation (because most lasers have more power than we need) is controlled by neutral-density filters. More sophisticated systems use an acousto-optical tuneable filter (a crystal of tellurium oxide controlled by ultrasound) to carry out both functions. The key advantage here is speed – we can switch wavelengths or turn the light on or off very rapidly with an AOTF.

The incoming light is the reflected by the beamsplitter (**Fig. 55.9(2)**), which is usually a dichroic mirror. A simple dichroic passes all wavelengths longer than a cut-off value, and reflects all shorter ones. This is fine if we only want to use one wavelength at a time, but for multiple labeling we may prefer a double or triple dichroic, which by clever optical engineering reflects two or three specific wavelengths while passing the rest of the spectrum. Multiple dichroics are inefficient, and another alternative is to use a polarizing beam splitter, which preferentially reflects on particular plane of polarization. Because laser light is polarized, whereas fluorescence typically is not, this can be an effective solution, and it allows a free choice of excitation laser lines. However, as with a multiple dichroics, the efficiency is far from 100% – some incoming light is lost and so is some fluorescence. One maker – Leica – has adapted the principle of the AOTF to produce a beamsplitter. This is a complex solution – it requires four tellurite crystals – but puts the choice of reflected and transmitted wavelengths completely under computer control, with quite high efficiency.

The incoming light then passes to the scanning mirrors (**Fig. 55.9(3)**), which scan the beam across the specimen, and thence into the microscope itself. By changing the amplitude of the scan we can change the magnification independently of the objective magnification – a wide scan field will give a low magnification, whereas a narrow one will give a high magnification. At the widest scan there will probably not be enough pixels to capture the full resolution of the objective, but it provides a useful overview. For optimal resolution the rule is to have 2.5 pixels within the minimum resolved distance (*4*), which implies a pixel size of ~80 nm with an NA 1.4 objective. A little more magnification – up to three pixels within the resolution distance – will not hurt, but more will just bleach the sample without giving any more information.

As we saw in **Fig. 55.1**, we can have a detector below the specimen, which will give a nonconfocal, scanned, image acquired simultaneously with the confocal image. Optical theory tells us that this image will be identical to a wide-field image, and we can therefore use contrasting techniques such as phase-contrast and differential interference contrast. This can be extremely convenient in practice because it will reveal other cell structures, which are not labeled with our fluorescent probes, enabling us to relate labeled structures to the rest of the cell.

The returning fluorescence is descanned (returned to a stationary beam) when it passes back through the scanning mirrors. It is transmitted through the beamsplitter and comes to a focus at the pinhole (**Fig. 55.9(4)**). Unlike the simple scheme shown in **Fig. 55.1**, in practice we want to detect several different

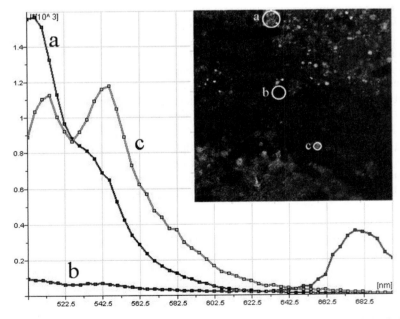

Fig. 55.10. Spectral confocal detection. The image shows tissue of the coral *Euphyllia ancora* and the traces show fluorescence spectra of the three different regions indicated. (**a**) and (**b**) show different coral fluorescent pigments whereas (**c**) shows the 680 nm chlorophyll peak from the symbiotic algae

wavelengths so the light is then split by more dichroic mirrors (**Fig. 55.(5)**) into two, three or more channels each containing a particular wavelength range. Barrier filters (**Fig. 55.9(6)**) further refine the detected wavelength range and block any stray laser light before the signal reaches the detectors, which are photo-multiplier tubes (PMTs).

Some manufacturers prefer to split the wavelengths before the pinhole, in which case multiple pinholes are used, one in front of each PMT. Whichever approach is used, the detected wavelength ranges are constrained by the dichroics built into the system, and for greater versatility high-end microscopes offer spectrometer-based detection. In these systems the light is split into a spectrum after the pinhole by a prism or grating, and the part of the spectrum assigned to each display channel is entirely under user control. There is also the possibility of obtaining a spectrum at each point of the image (**Fig. 55.10**) so that we can determine the optimal detection ranges for unknown fluorochromes. In principle, spectral detection is also highly efficient, because dichroic mirrors and barrier filters (each of which will waste some light) are avoided. As with any system, of course, the actual sensitivity will depend on the implementation.

5. High Speed Confocal Microscopes

In a conventional CLSM, there are two scanning mirrors, one moving in the "y", vertical, direction, which moves quite slowly, and the other moving in the "x", horizontal direction, which has to move very rapidly. When we are looking at living cells, the x-scan becomes the rate limiting step, determining how fast we can image transient phenomena. Technological advances can boost this speed to some extent, but in the end we are limited by the number of photons available, and increasing speed just leads to diminishing signal. Therefore moves towards microscopy in "real time" (which usually means television rate, an interesting comment on the contemporary idea of reality) have usually involved sacrificing some degree of confocality in the interests of speed. There are two approaches which have established themselves, either eliminating the x-scan and using a line of light, or scanning multiple points at one time.

5.1. Line Scanning Systems

Because the horizontal (x) scan places the limitation on scanning speed, why not eliminate it and just use a y scan? A line of light will traverse the sample, and this will be imaged on a slit (**Fig. 55.11**). Many designs based on this principle have appeared over the years, but at the time of writing the best-known is probably the Zeiss version seen in the LSM5 – live and LSM5 – Duo. Some older designs rescanned the line after the slit, so that the image could be captured on a conventional CCD or video camera – this also had the benefit of providing a live image which could be viewed through an eyepiece. However the simpler approach of using a linear CCD array (which has an equally long history) is now the more popular. Resolution in the x direction is therefore provided by the detector, whereas the scan gives resolution in the y direction. This limits the ability to vary the scanned area as we do in the CLSM – it is easier to reduce the height of the scanned area, but reducing its width can only be done by sacrificing pixels.

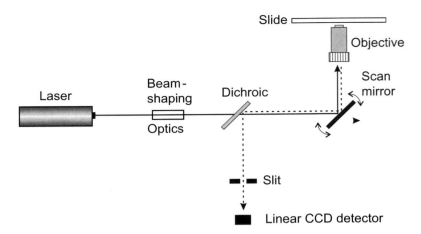

Fig. 55.11. The basis of a slit scanning confocal. Light from the laser is shaped into a line by special optics and scanned across the sample by just one mirror. The returning fluorescence passes through a slit instead of a pinhole and is captured by a linear detector (CCD array)

The axial resolution of a slit-scanning system will be poorer than that of a CLSM, and in principle the lateral resolution will be anisotropic. However, such considerations are not really relevant – these instruments are not designed to replace the CLSM as a tool for 3D imaging, but to provide sufficient optical sectioning to eliminate out-of-focus detail while capturing rapid changes in living cells. Because an entire line of 512 pixels is illuminated and captured at once, the dwell time on each pixel is effectively 512 times that of a CLSM scanning at the same speed. The light budget is therefore very good, and it is relatively easy to obtain adequate signal even at high frame speeds.

5.2. Multiple Point Scanners

The idea of scanning with a rotating disk containing a spiral pattern of holes, so that there are many points of light and many pinholes all operating at once, goes back to the very early days of confocal microscopy (5). However, the catch was the problem of getting sufficient light through the holes, and early systems gave dim images, which could only be used in reflection mode.

This problem was solved by the Yokogawa Company, who has developed a double-disk scanner in which the upper disk contains micro-lenses concentrating the light on to the corresponding pinholes in the lower disk (**Fig. 55.12**). Several companies have developed commercial instruments using Yokogawa scanners, of which the best known is probably the Perkin–Elmer Ultraview. In these systems the image is recorded by a conventional CCD camera – the faster and more sensitive this is, the better the performance. A live image can therefore also be viewed through an eyepiece, though few users seem to make use of this feature. As with line-scanners, the light budget is good because a thousand or so points are scanned at any one time.

There are several practical differences from line-scan systems. The scan speed is determined by the rotation of the disk, and cannot be varied as it can in a line-scanner. (The capture rate of the CCD camera can be varied,

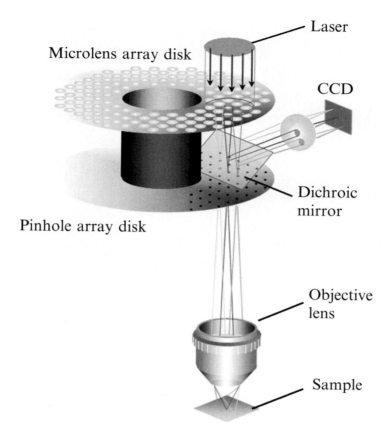

Laser

Microlens array disk

CCD

Dichroic mirror

Pinhole array disk

Objective lens

Sample

Fig. 55.12. Diagram of the Yokogawa scanning system, the basis of the Perkin–Elmer Ultraview and several other real-time confocal microscopes. By courtesy of Yokogawa and Perkin–Elmer Inc

but unless it is synchronized with the disk rotation some frames might show brighter and darker stripes as they are not exact multiples of a rotation). There is also no possibility of varying the area scanned. The key difference lies in the confocality. Some out of focus light can return through the "wrong" pinhole, but the extent to which this will happen depends a lot on the specimen. With a thin sample, the cone of light from one pinhole will not intersect with that from the next pinhole, and optical sectioning will be virtually the same as in a CLSM, and substantially better than in a line-scan system. The thicker the sample, the more the axial performance will degrade. Cell cultures, small embryos and similar samples will suit the microscope better than whole animals or organs. An example of high-speed imaging with a Perkin–Elmer Ultraview is given in **Fig. 55.13**.

Other types of multiple-point scanners, which use an orthogonal array of points rather than a disk, have been developed. In general they have similar strengths and weaknesses, with no clear advantage over the Yokogawa disk system, which dominates this section of the market.

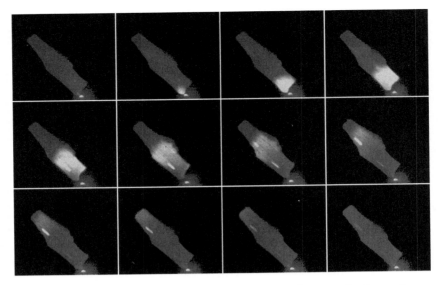

Fig. 55.13. Calcium wave in a cultured cardiac myocyte – 2 consecutive frames from a sequence of 330 taken with the Perkin–Elmer Ultraview. Courtesy Perkin–Elmer Inc

6. Nonlinear Microscopy

In conventional fluorescence microscopy it is axiomatic that the excitation wavelength must be shorter than the emitted wavelength – the incoming photon must have more energy then the outgoing one. We could ask, though, what would happen if two long-wavelength photons happened to arrive at the same molecule at the same time? If they both gave up their energy they could excite fluorescence even if one on its own could not. Two-photon excitation of fluorescence was proposed many years ago, and subsequently demonstrated in the laboratory, but its use in microscopy is still a relatively new technique (6). Clearly the likelihood of two photons striking the same molecule simultaneously is going to be very low, so that the amount of light we would need to get a usable signal would fry the specimen if it were applied continuously. The solution is to use very short pulses of light so that the peak intensity is extremely high but the average is quite moderate. The key question is clearly why we should be interested in such an esoteric technique.

The first reason is that we will only excite fluorescence at the focussed spot – above and below this the light is not intense enough for two-photon events to occur. Thus we are selecting one focal plane at the *excitation* stage – without needing confocal optics to exclude out-of-focus light. In fact, we can show mathematically that the focal plane selection is exactly the same as in a confocal microscope, but we can use wide-field detectors and thereby collect a lot of scattered light that would be lost in a confocal system, making our detection more efficient. In the confocal microscope, even though we only observe one plane at a time, we are exciting fluorescence – and bleaching our fluorochromes – above and below this plane, but with two-photon excitation there is no excitation or bleaching outside the volume we are imaging.

Secondly, long wavelengths are much less damaging to cells than short ones. Ultraviolet light is immediately toxic to living cells, but the far red or very near infrared wavelengths that we use for two-photon microscopy cause relatively little damage. They also penetrate very well into tissue, so that if our goal is to image living tissue we can go deeper and for longer than we can with confocal (**Fig. 55.14**).

The advance that has made all this possible is the development of the titanium sapphire (Ti-S) laser. Although in principle other laser sources are possible, all commercial two-photon microscopes use Ti-S lasers. These produce extremely short (100 fs) pulses of light – one femtosecond (fs) is 10^{-15} s. The pulse interval is typically around 10ns, so there will be hundreds of pulses at each pixel of our image, but the gap between pulses is very large relative to their length. With a mean input power of a few milliwatts we can have a quite colossal power density in the pulses. The other useful feature of the Ti-S laser is that is tunable – the wavelength can usually be adjusted between 700 and 1,000nm, though the power falls of somewhat at the ends of the range. This means that we can look at a wide range of fluorochromes with a single laser.

The major disadvantage is that the longer wavelength limits the attainable resolution. Even this is not as bad as it might seem because the whole $\sqrt{2}$ resolution improvement (Section 3.2) is available without the impractical requirement of using a tiny pinhole *(3)*. In practical terms we can expect a resolution of around 250nm using an NA 1.4 oil-immersion lens and 800nm excitation, which is broadly on a par with wide-field fluorescence microscopy. Other disadvantages are practical. The laser is bulky and expensive, and although it is tunable this is a relatively slow process – we cannot change

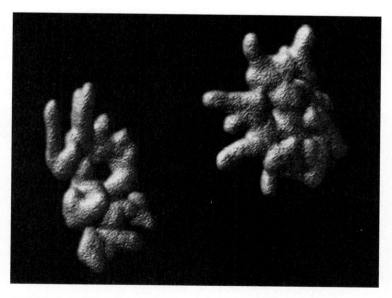

Fig. 55.14. Three-dimensional reconstruction of Hoechst-stained chromosomes at the second division of meiosis in a living *Agapanthus* anther, imaged at a depth of 200 μm in a two-photon microscope. The original set of optical sections from which the reconstruction was made was taken by José Feijó at the Gulbenkian Institute, Oeiras, Portugal

wavelengths with the speed and facility we are accustomed to in confocal microscopy, nor use multiple wavelengths simultaneously. However, for deep imaging, and for prolonged viewing of living cells, it is the method of choice.

Two-photon excited fluorescence is described as a *nonlinear* process because the fluorescence intensity depends on the square of the excitation power – the likelihood of one photon being present depends on the intensity, so the likelihood of having two depends on the square of the intensity. It is not the only nonlinear process we can use in microscopy. Another, which has an even older history, is second harmonic generation (SHG) *(7)*. Certain substances have the property, when hit with high-intensity light, of generating the second harmonic of that light – that is, light of twice the frequency and half the wavelength. The ability is an intrinsic property of the substance, and depends strongly on the molecule *not* having any plane of symmetry. Many crystals are very effective second harmonic generators and are used, for example, to convert infrared laser light to green light (as in everyday green laser pointers).

It is only quite recently that this has become common as a technique in cell biology. In animal tissue collagen (particularly type I collagen) is a strong generator of second harmonics *(8)* and because collagen is a very important structural protein it has been the prime target for this type of work. The requirements for SHG imaging are essentially the same as for two-photon microscopy, so the same equipment can carry out both techniques. There are several key differences in the image formation, though. The SH signal is quite directional, so rather different images will be seen in transmission and back-propagated detectors (**Fig. 55.15**). It is therefore very useful to have both – but fortunately that is now quite common in any case. Unlike fluorescence, which has a spectrum of frequencies, the SH signal is exactly half the wavelength of the laser light. No energy is lost in the process, so there is no damage to the sample or fading of the signal.

Myosin is another protein which generates second harmonics, though less strongly, and SHG microscopy therefore has had some relevance in muscle

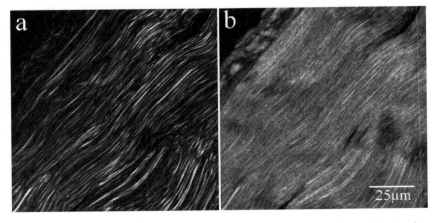

Fig. 55.15. SHG images of collagen in cryo-section of unfixed human Achilles tendon biopsy (sample supplied by Regina Crameri). (**a**) Forward propagated signal (**b**) backward propagated signal. Excitation 840 nm

research. In plant cells, and food products derived from them, starch can be imaged very easily by SHG *(9)*. Some fluorescent dyes which are used for mapping membrane potential, also turn out to be SH generators, and there may well in the future be targeted SHG probes, just as there are targeted fluorescent probes now.

References

1. White JG, Amos WB, Fordham M (1987) An evaluation of confocal versus conventional imaging of biological structures by fluorescence light microscopy. J Cell Biol **105**:41–48
2. Carlsson K, Liljeborg A (1989) A confocal laser microscope scanner for digital recording of optical serial sections. J Microsc **153**:171–180
3. Cox G, Sheppard CJR (2004) Practical limits of resolution in confocal and non-linear microscopy. Microsc Res Tech **63**:18–22
4. Nyquist H (1928) Certain topics in telegraph transmission theory. Trans Am Inst Electrical Eng **47**:617–644
5. Petrán M, Hadravsky M, Egger MD, Galambos R (1968) Tandem scanning reflected light microscope. J Opt Soc Am **58**:661–664
6. Denk W, Strickler JP, Webb WW (1990) Two-photon laser scanning fluorescence microscopy. Science **248**:73–76
7. Gannaway JN and Sheppard CJR (1978) Second harmonic imaging in the scanning optical microscope, Opt Quant Elect **10**:435–442
8. Cox G, Kable E, Jones A, Fraser I, Manconi F, Gorrell MD (2002) 3-Dimensional imaging of collagen using second harmonic generation. J Structural Biol **141**:53–62
9. Cox G, Moreno N, and Feijó J (2005) Second harmonic imaging of plant polysaccharides. J Biomed Optics **10**:1–6

56

Laser Microdissection

Graeme I. Murray

1. Introduction

Solid tissues and organs, especially diseased tissues, are complex structures composed of heterogeneous mixtures of morphologically and functionally distinct cell types. The purposeful molecular study of cytologically and/or phenotypically specific cell types from tissues either normal or often more importantly abnormal or diseased requires the availability of rapid, efficient and accurate methods for obtaining specific defined groups of cells for further study. Whereas for example circulating blood cells can readily be separated into their distinct morphological and phenotypic classes by cell sorting using flow cytometry obtaining specific types of cells from solid tissues for analysis has until recently been much more difficult. Although manual methods of tissue microdissection have been described they are slow, cumbersome and not very specific. However, the development of laser based methods of microdissection for selecting specific types of cells from thin sections of tissues with direct microscopic visualisation of the process has greatly facilitated the appropriate and meaningful molecular analysis of specific types of cells and thus providing new insights into normal cell biology and disease mechanisms.

There are two major systems for performing laser-assisted tissue based microdissection namely laser capture microdissection and laser cutting microdissection and both types of system have now been commercially available for several years. This chapter will outline the principles of these technologies and consideration will also be given to the main downstream molecular applications.

There are a wide range of powerful and increasingly sophisticated molecular technologies including expression microarrays and proteomics which are now available to analyse the biology of cells. To fully exploit the value of these technologies in the analysis of specific tissues or organs requires that the investigator must be certain that the appropriate type or types of cells are analysed. Laser based microdissection techniques have allowed this to be achieved in a straightforward and non-time consuming manner. It is now even possible to microdissect a single cell and analyse its molecular properties.

From: *Molecular Biomethods Handbook, 2nd Edition.*
Edited by: J. M. Walker and R. Rapley © Humana Press, Totowa, NJ

There are two different technologies that have been developed for laser based microdissection systems. One technology is laser capture microdissection using an infra red laser while the other technology is based laser cutting using an ultraviolet laser. With either of these technologies it is possible to mcicrodissect cells based on their morphology or select cells according to their phenotype. Positive or negative selection of cells is also possible i.e. the microdissection acquires the cells of interest or microdissection is used to remove all the unwanted cells leaving behind the cells of interest.

2. Methods

2.1. Laser Capture Microdissection

The laser capture microdissection system was originally developed about ten years ago at the National Institutes of Health, Bethesda by Emmert-Buck and his colleagues. They recognised the need to develop a microscope based microdissection system for accurately and efficiently obtaining cells from histological tissue sections to fully exploit at that time what were emerging molecular analytical technologies (1,2). The system was primarily developed to facilitate the molecular analysis of tumour cells from solid tumours. This system rapidly moved into commercial production by Arcturus BioScience who have since then further developed the system most notably with the addition of automation (3). The laser capture microdissection system is now probably the most widely used laser based microdissection system worldwide and my own experience of over 7 y is with this system specifically the Arcturus Pixcell II laser capture microdissection system (4–7).

The underlying principle of the laser capture microdissection system is very straightforward and involves the "capture" of either groups of cells or individual cells onto a thermoplastic membrane from stained tissue histological sections (this can be frozen tissue sections or fixed wax tissue embedded sections) or cytological preparations (1,4,5). The sections can be stained with a variety of standard histological stains and the instrument appears to work equally well with all these dyes. The plastic membrane which overlies the tissue section is attached to a specially designed "cap" and the design of the instrument ensures that the plastic membrane is held in direct contact with the tissue section. The thermoplastic is briefly melted by a low power narrow beam infrared laser directed at the cells of interest under microscope control. As the plastic cools and solidifies again, the cells are embedded or captured onto the plastic membrane and are removed from the tissue section by lifting off the cap along with the plastic membrane from the tissue section (**Fig. 56.1**). Multiple groups of cells can be readily captured onto the same membrane. The instrument allows for both the power of the laser beam and its diameter to be altered to ensure that the optimum conditions are used for the microdissection of a particular tissue. Generally a greater laser power is required to microdissect cells from formalin fixed wax embedded sections compared with unfixed frozen sections.

In addition, this system recently has also been used to capture cultured cells thus opening up new possibilities for the analysis of specific types of living cells (3). The cells of interest were captured directly from the special slides on which they were grown and there was no requirement for the cells to be stained with a histological dye prior to capture (3).

Fig. 56.1. Laser capture microdissection of colorectal carcinoma. Sections of formalin-fixed, wax-embedded colorectal adenocarcinoma are stained with methyl green and positioned for laser capture (**A**). Tumor cells are selectively captured (**B**). Captured cells can be visualized on the cap (**C**). (From Dillon et al in *Methods in molecular biology vol 293:Laser capture microdissection methods and protocols* (Murray, G.I. and Curran, S. eds.), Humana, Totowa, NJ) *(8)*

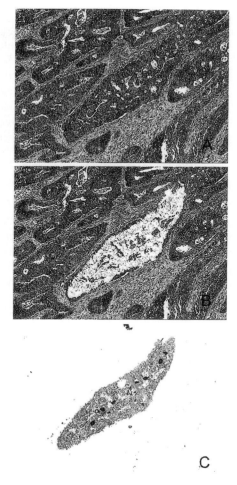

2.2. Laser Cutting Based Microdissection

This type of laser microdissection operates on an entirely different principle to that used in laser capture microdissection *(9–11)*. The basic principle is that a pulsed beam ultraviolet laser is used to "draw" round the cell or cells of interest and these cells are "cut-out" from the tissue section. Surrounding unwanted tissue can also be photoablated by the laser. Different manufactures have produced laser cutting microdissection systems all of which vary in the precise details of operation especially with regard to the method of collection and transfer of the microdissected tissue for subsequent molecular analysis. In the Zeiss/PALM® system the laser can be used to "catapult" the microdissected cells into a collecting tube whereas in the Leica AS LMD® system the section is inverted so that after microdissection the microdissected cells fall into the collecting tube under the influence of gravity. The advantages of this method is that there is no physical contact between the cells and plastic unlike in laser capture microdissection and clearly avoids the potential risk of modification of the molecules of interest by especially the heating and cooling of the thermoplastic membrane. Similarly the Molecular Machines and Industry system (mmi cell cut®) is a laser based cutting system which uses a plastic membrane to remove the microdissected cells. This system can also be used to microdissect and acquire living cells in culture for further analysis.

Recently Arcturus has introduced the Veritas® system which is dual function laser microdissecting system equipped with both a laser capture microdissection system and a laser cutting system and this system is fully automated. The user can predefine the cells of interest to be microdissected and the system will automatically perform the microdissection. This is particularly advantageous when relatively large amounts of cells need to be captured, e.g., for proteomics (see Section 3.3).

2.3. Tissue Preparation for Laser Microdissection

Since all laser microdissection techniques are based on the microscopic visualisation of tissue sections or cells one of the most important issues in applying laser microdissection techniques to the analysis of cellular constituents is the specific choice of tissue preparation. This is to ensure that the molecules of interest are preserved in the most appropriate manner while at the same time ensuring at least adequate tissue morphology. This will allow satisfactory visualisation and identification of the cells of interest with the laser microdissection system. Factors related to tissue preparation (e.g., type of fixation, choice of histological stain) which need to be considered for the individual classes of biological molecules (DNA, RNA, and protein) will be outlined. In some cases especially for the rarer types of human disease fresh tissue may not be available and it will be necessary to use fixed tissue.

Following microdissection of individual groups of cells specific types of molecules including nucleic acid both DNA, RNA, and protein can all be readily extracted with appropriate procedures and used for an extensive range of molecular analysis including PCR, gene expression studies and proteomics (1,5,9,12). Laser microdissected cells have been found to be compatible with all the molecular analytical techniques that have been used. The process of capturing the cells onto the thermoplastic membrane in laser capture microdissection does not appear to alter or damage the integrity of DNA, RNA or protein nor does embedding the cells onto a thermoplastic membrane appear to prevent a subsequent high rate of recovery of such molecules. Histological staining of the tissue which is generally necessary for laser microdissection, to allow adequate microscopic visualisation of the tissue morphology and to permit selection of cells for microdissection, does not appear to significantly alter most cellular constituents although the precise choice of histological stain will often depend on the type of tissue being studied and the type of down stream molecular analysis proposed (13).

The aim of histological staining is to ensure that tissue structure can be satisfactorily visualised. The tissue sections should be exposed to these histological stains for only a very short period of time thus minimising the potential for alteration, degradation or extraction of cellular constituents which may result in inappropriate results of the molecular analysis. RNA and cytoplasmic proteins are the probably the two major groups of molecules which are most at risk of being degraded or extracted during the histological staining procedure. Many investigators prefer to avoid hematoxylin as this dye can contain heavy metal ions and at a practical level in the laboratory needs a longer period of staining and requires "differentiation," which involves another step when cellular constituents could be altered or lost. As a general rule we have found that a rapid one-step histological stain with for example cresyl violet or toluidine blue works very well and tissue sections can be stained by incubation with either of these dyes for only a few seconds.

3. Applications

Laser microdissected material can been used to analyse DNA, RNA and protein and laser microdissected cells have been used in a wide of downstream molecular applications, which will be outlined in the following section.

3.1. Laser Microdissection and Genomic Analysis

DNA can be readily extracted from fixed tissue or unfixed tissue although with fixed tissue the DNA to a greater or lesser extent will be fragmented. However for most techniques involving DNA analysis fragmentation of DNA is not a major issue. The analysis of DNA from microdissected cells can be divided into two broad categories: whole genome analysis and the analysis of individual genes and both will be described.

3.1.1. Global Analysis of DNA

Whole genome analysis applying techniques such as comparative genomic hybridisation, array based comparative genomic hybridisation and high-density single-nucleotide polymorphism microarrays (so called "SNP chips") generally require DNA from unfixed tissue or cells for optimum results. However, all these techniques will or are most likely to work with DNA extracted from cells microdissected from fixed tissue. These techniques all require a DNA amplification step (whole genome amplification) and if DNA from fixed tissue is being used it is particularly important to ensure that amplification of DNA is uniform to ensure that there is either no over or under representation of specific DNA segments in the amplified DNA. This will ensure that misleading results regarding gain or loss of specific chromosomal regions are not erroneously obtained as a result of "biased" or selective genome amplification (14,15).

3.1.2. Analysis of Individual Genes

Analysis of specific genes generally using some form of the PCR is straight forward from laser microdissected tissue (**Fig. 56.2**). Down stream DNA based applications of microdissected cells include qualitative PCR, real time quantitative PCR, gene sequencing and mutation analysis. PCR does not appear to be affected by microdissection and specific DNA segments can readily be amplified from cells microdissected from both fresh frozen and fixed tissue sections. Generally DNA fragments of up to 300 base pairs can readily be amplified from formalin fixed tissue while much larger DNA fragments can be easily amplified from unfixed tissue, if required. As described in the section (Section 2.3) on tissue preparation there are theoretical concerns that components of histological dyes (especially haematoxylin) used to stain the tissue sections or cells or the solvents used to process fixed wax embedded tissue sections may inhibit PCR, however, generally this has not been found to be a practical concern. In addition heat produced by the laser during the microdissection procedure, especially by laser capture microdissection, theoretically could alter DNA and once again this has not been found to be a practical problem.

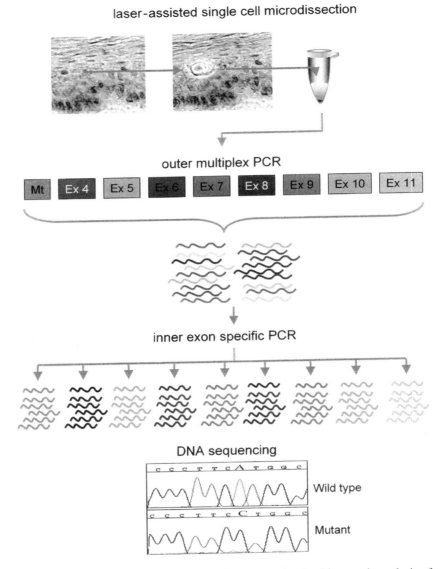

Fig. 56.2. Schematic illustration of the different steps involved in genetic analysis of the p53 gene from single cells. The strategy of multiplex/nested PCR followed by direct DNA sequencing is depicted. (From Micke et al in *Methods in molecular biology vol 293:Laser capture microdissection methods and protocols* (Murray, G.I. and Curran, S. eds.), Humana, Totowa, NJ.) *(8)*

In many instances relatively crude proteolytic digests of microdissected tissue can be used as the starting material for the amplification of DNA. In my laboratory we have successfully used proteolytic digests of microdissected tissue to amplify both endogenous genes *(16)* and viral genes *(17)*. Prolonged digestion of the microdissected tissue with a proteolytic enzymes digests the protein component of cells while "freeing" the DNA. Many broad spectrum proteolytic enzymes are suitable but it is important to ensure that they are of suitable purity and are free of active nucleases especially DNase. We have not found it necessary to purify the DNA prior to conducting PCR based analysis. In addition if the DNA has been obtained from only a few microdissected cells any attempt at purification of the DNA has the risk of losing a significant proportion of the DNA during the cleaning-up procedure. DNA obtained from this type of starting material and processed in this way can be easily used in real time quantitative PCR to gain a quantitative measure of endogenous gene copy number or accurately assess viral copy *(18)*.

3.2. Laser Microdissection and Gene Expression

For most techniques examining gene expression especially microarray based experiments undegraded mRNA is required to give optimum results and this generally means the use of unfixed tissue. However, RNA can also be extracted from fixed tissue. Precipitant fixatives such as ethanol or acetone result in the preservation of relatively intact RNA while cross-linking fixatives such as formalin result in considerable RNA degradation *(19,20)*. RNA can be obtained from formalin fixed tissue and while it is likely to be degraded, RNA obtained from microdissected fixed tissues has successfully been used for RNA analysis. Like the analysis of DNA analysis of RNA can be considered in two broad groups. The global analysis of gene expression usually using microarray technology and the analysis of individual expressed genes.

3.2.1. Global Analysis of Gene Expression

The global analysis of gene expression generally involves the use of expression microarray technology and this type of technology combined with laser microdissection provides a very powerful set of techniques for defining and understanding gene expression in specific types of cells or even single cells *(21)*. The RNA obtained from microdissected tissue requires to be amplified prior to labeling and hybridization to an appropriate microarray *(22)*. There are a number of commercially available kits from the major reagent suppliers which have been specifically designed for use with microdissected tissue samples, which simplifies and standardizes all the steps in procedure from RNA extraction through to nucleic acid labeling before hybridizing to the microarray. Microarrays have been developed specifically for use with RNA extracted from fixed wax embedded tissue.

3.2.2. Analysis of the Expression of Individual Genes

The analysis of the expression of individual gene by PCR following microdissection is straightforward even with single cells *(23)*. RNA requires to be extracted from the microdissected cells and then converted to cDNA before use in PCR. As described above there are a number of commercially available kits specifically designed to work with microdissected tissue samples and the whole procedure from RNA extraction through to cDNA synthesis is made relatively straight forward by use of these kits.

3.3. Laser Capture Microdissection and Proteomics

Proteomics which is the global analysis of protein expression encompasses arrange of different types of technology to permit the analysis of many proteins or specific groups of proteins. The number of technologies that are available to analyze protein are numerous and reflect the complexity of studying the structure, function, and expression of proteins. Some of the main technologies directly associated with proteomics are two-dimensional gel electrophoresis, solid phase surface desorption of proteins and mass spectrometry. Proteins extracted from laser microdissected material have been succesfully used with all these technologies and each of these proteomics methods has its advantages and disadvantages.

In contrast to the analysis of DNA where both fixed and unfixed tissue samples can be used tissue preparation for proteomics is very important. This is to ensure no alteration of protein structure by tissue fixation or extraction of soluble proteins during the tissue preparation process. Analysis of proteins therefore needs to be performed using fresh frozen section of tissue as formalin fixation of tissue extensively cross links proteins and makes extraction of proteins from tissue and cells almost impossible. In some cases precipitant fixatives, e.g., acetone or ethanol may be used for the analysis of specific proteins. However, as a general principle it is a good idea to avoid any tissue fixative when proteins are being studied to avoid any risk of protein modification or denaturation.

Whereas in the study of nucleic acid either DNA and RNA the investigator has the availability of amplification techniques most notably the polymerase chain reaction to allow the generation of sufficient material for analysis no matter how small the starting sample even a single cell the researcher studying proteins does not have the advantage of an equivalent technique. The consequence of this in relation laser microdissection is that generally much more tissue has to be microdissected to ensure an adequate amount of protein for analysis compared with nucleic acid analysis. The amount of protein that is required for most proteomics studies is often in the microgram to milligram range whereas many-fold lower amounts of nucleic acid can be used. Since much more protein has to be procured then microdissection of tissue/cells for is relatively time consuming. The development of automated microdissection systems which can be programmed to dissect the cells of interest represent a significant advance and their increasing availability suggests that more proteomics studies with laser microdissected material will be carried out.

3.3.1. Laser Microdissection and 2D Gel Electrophoresis

The classic proteomics technology for the analysis of global protein expression has been two-dimensional gel electrophoresis followed by mass spectrometry of protein spots of interest (12,24). 2D gel electrophoresis produces proteins maps, which can be interrogated by visual inspection or with greater much accuracy and sensitivity by computer based image analysis. Protein maps from for example normal and diseased tissue can be compared and differentially expressed proteins identified. Proteins can either be identified on the basis of their electrophoretic mobility by comparison with established protein databases or can be identified by mass spectrometry.

Laser microdissected tissue has been used for 2D gel electrophoresis but this technique probably of all the proteomics techniques has the requirement for the greatest amount of protein. It is particularly important in 2D gel electrophoresis that the proteins are unmodified by the tissue preparative process and laser microdissection. Laser capture microdissection has the advantages of being able to microdissect many cells rapidly although theoretically the process of capturing cells onto the thermoplastic membrane may result in a low yield of protein or protein modification. Neither of these factors have been shown to be a problem. The non-contact laser cutting methods of laser microdissection do not suffer from these potential disadvantages although however compared with laser capture microdissection these methods of laser microdissection may be more time consuming in acquiring cells.

3.3.2. Protein Analysis Using Laser Microdissected Cells and Protein Chip Technology

Cells obtained from laser microdissected cells have been used to analyse protein expression patterns using protein chip technology. One of the advantages of using protein chip technology is that a significantly smaller amount of protein is required compared with methods involving 2 D gel electrophoresis. Protein lysates are prepared from microdissected cells and the lysate applied to a range of "protein chips" (24). The protein lysates require to be prepared from unfixed tissue samples fixed tissue sections are not suitable as most proteins cannot be extracted from fixed tissue. The most widely used type of protein chip technology has been surface absorption of proteins onto a solid phase matrix coated or treated in such a way to allow the analysis of specific class or types of proteins. This is SELDI (surface enhanced laser/desorption ionization) technology and following absorption of proteins onto the matrix the proteins are analyzed by mass spectrometry. This produces a profile or signature for each sample and profiles from different samples can then be compared. If required definitive identification of individual can be performed using further mass spectrometric techniques.

Another type of protein chip that has been used analyse proteins from microdissected tissue samples is the so called reverse phase microarray. In this type of microarray protein lysates from cells, in this case microdissected cells, are "printed" onto a glass slide and each slide probed with a different antibody to determine the protein expression pattern (25). Alternatively cell lysates, following labelling with an appropriate reporter molecule usually a fluorescent molecule can be applied to an antibody microarray where individual antibodies have been "printed" onto a glass slide. Once again expression patterns of a range of proteins can be determined.

3.3.3. Laser Microdissection and Mass Spectrometry

One of the most interesting types of proteomics studies using laser microdissected cells is the direct mass spectrometric analysis of microdissected cells (26,27). Microdissected cells are placed on a mass spectrometric plate and subject to mass spectrometry without any intervening steps. The mass spectrometric analysis produces specific mass spectrometric profiles and unique profiles have been successfully identified in cells from malignant tumors in comparison with corresponding normal cells. However the analysis of the mass spectra is complex and require sophisticated computer based algorithms to derive useful information as visual inspection and visual comparison of the mass spectra are generally not adequate to obtain significant information.

4. Conclusions

The availability of laser based microdissecting systems has permitted sophisticated questions regarding the biology of specific cell types to be asked. Both types of laser microdissecting systems (capture or cutting) greatly facilitate the rapid, specific and sensitive acquisition of individual types of cells for a wide range of sophisticated downstream molecular analysis. For both laser capture microdissection and laser cutting microdissection cell selection can be based on morphological features or phenotypic criteria and cells obtained by either method of microdissection are suitable for almost all types of molecular analysis.

References

1. Emmert-Buck MR, Bonner RF, Smith PD, Chuaqui RF, Zhuang Z, Goldstein SR, Weiss RA, Liotta LA (1996) Laser capture microdissection. Science 274:998–1001

2. Simone NL, Bonner RF, Gillespie JW, Emmert- Buck MR, Liotta LA (1998) Laser-capture microdissection: opening the microscopic frontier to molecular analysis. Trends Genet 14:272–276

3. Arcturus BioScience. http://www.arctur.com accessed on 12th May 2006

4. Curran S, Murray GI (2005) An introduction to laser based tissue microdissection techniques. In: Murray GI, Curran S (eds) Methods in molecular biology vol 293: Laser capture microdissection methods and protocols. Humana, Totowa, NJ, pp 3–8

5. Curran S, McKay JA, McLeod HL, Murray GI (2000) Laser capture microscopy. Mol Pathol 53:64–68

6. Curran S, Murray GI (2002) Tissue microdissection and its' applications in pathology. Current Diagn Pathol 8:183–192

7. Dundas SR, Curran S, Murray GI (2002) Laser capture microscopy: application to urological cancer research. UroOncology 2:33–35

8. Murray GI, Curran S (eds) Methods in molecular biology vol. 293: Laser capture microdissection methods and protocols. Humana, Totowa, NJ

9. Gjerdrum LM, Lielpetere I, Rasmussen LM, Bendix K, Hamilton-Dutoit S (2001) Laser-assisted microdissection of membrane-mounted paraffin sections for polymerase chain reaction analysis: identification of cell populations using immunohistochemistry and in situ hybridization. J Mol Diagn 3:105–110

10. Bohm M, Wieland I, Schutze K, Rubber H (1997) Microbeam MOMeNT: non-contact laser microdissection of membrane-mounted native tissue. Am J Pathol 151:63–67

11. Schutze K, Lahr G (1998) Identification of expressed genes by laser-mediated manipulation of single cells. Nat Biotechnol 16:737–742

12. Lawrie LC, Curran S, McLeod HL, Fothergill JE, Murray GI (2001) Application of laser capture microdissection and proteomics in colon cancer. Mol Pathol 54:253–258

13. Huang LE, Luzzi V, Ehrig T, Holtschlag V, Watson MA (2002) Optimized tissue processing and staining for laser capture microdissection and nucleic acid retrieval. Methods Enzymol 356:49–62

14. Callagy G, Pharoah P, Chin SF, Sangan T, Daigo Y, Jackson L, Caldas C (2005) Identification and validation of prognostic markers in breast cancer with the complementary use of array-CGH and tissue microarrays. J Pathol 205:388–396

15. Callagy G, Jackson L, Caldas C (2005) Comparative genomic hybridization using DNA from laser capture microdissected tissue. In: Murray GI, Curran S (eds) Methods in molecular biology vol 293: Laser capture microdissection methods and protocols. Humana, Totowa, NJ, pp 39–55

16. Rooney PH (2005) Multiplex quantitative real-time PCR of laser microdissected tissue. In: Murray G, Curran S (eds) Methods in molecular biology vol 293:Laser capture microdissection methods and protocols. Humana, Totowa, NJ, pp 27–37

17. Kheng GK, Cruickshank ME, Rooney PH, Miller ID, Parkin DE, Murray GI (2005) Human papillomavirus 16 infection in adenocarcinoma of the cervix. Br J Cancer 93:1301–1304

18. Adeyi OA, Belloni DR, Dufresne SD, Schned AR, Tsongalis GI (2005) Real-time polymerase chain reaction and laser capture microdissection for the diagnosis of BK virus infection in renal allografts. Am J Clin Pathol 124:537–542

19. Kerman IA, Buck BJ, Evans SJ, Akil H, Watson SJ (2006) Combining laser capture microdissection with quantitative real-time PCR: effects of tissue manipulation on RNA quality and gene expression. J Neurosci Methods 153:71–85

20. Vincek V, Nassiri M, Block N, Welsh CF, Nadji M, Morales AR (2005) Methodology for preservation of high molecular-weight RNA in paraffin-embedded tissue: application for laser-capture microdissection. Diagn Mol Pathol 14:127–133

21. Yang F, Foekens JA, Yu J, Sieuwerts AM, Timmermans M, Klijn JG, Atkins D, Wang Y, Jiang Y (2006) Laser microdissection and microarray analysis of breast tumors reveal ER-alpha related genes and pathways. Oncogene 25:1413–1419

22. Luzzi V, Mahadevappa M, Raja R, Warrington JA, Watson MA (2003) Accurate and reproducible gene expression profiles from laser capture microdissection, transcript amplification, and high density oligonucleotide microarray analysis. J Mol Diagn 5:9–14

23. Keays KM, Owens GP, Ritchie AM, Gilden DH, Burgoon MP (2005) Laser capture microdissection and single-cell RT-PCR without RNA purification. J Immunol Methods 302:90–98

24. Ernst G, Melle C, Schimmel B, Bleul A, von Eggeling F (2006) Proteohistography-Direct analysis of tissue with high sensitivity and high spatial resolution using proteinchip technology. J Histochem Cytochem 54:13–17

25. Gulmann C, Espina V, Petricoin E 3rd, Longo DL, Santi M, Knutsen T, Raffeld M, Jaffe ES, Liotta LA, Feldman AL (2005) Proteomic analysis of apoptotic pathways reveals prognostic factors in follicular lymphoma. Clin Cancer Res 11:5847–5855

26. Caldwell RL, Caprioli RM (2005) Tissue profiling by mass spectrometry: a review of methodology and applications. Mol Cell Proteomics 4:394–401

27. Guo J, Colgan TJ, DeSouza LV, Rodrigues MJ, Romaschin AD, Siu KW (2005) Direct analysis of laser capture microdissected endometrial carcinoma and epithelium by matrix-assisted laser desorption/ionization mass spectrometry. Rapid Commun Mass Spectrom 19:2762–2766

57

Biomedical Uses of Flow Cytometry

James L. Weaver and Maryalice Stetler-Stevenson

1. Definition of Flow Cytometry

Flow cytometry is literally measuring cells or particles while they are moving in a liquid. More specifically, a suspension of single cells is labeled with one or several fluorescent labels. In the machine, the cells are constrained into single file. These cells pass through one or more laser beams to excite the fluorescent labels. The light emitted from the fluorescent labels is collected, separated, measured, and the resulting data transmitted to the computer controlling the instrument (**Fig. 57.1**). In addition, narrow angle and 90° light scatter from the laser beam are measured and the data are also sent to the computer. All of these values are recorded as correlated measurements for each cell separately. The data are displayed in the computer as single parameter histograms or two parameter plots (**Fig. 57.2**). The software allows populations to be identified and specific subpopulations selected for further analysis. The number and fraction of cells in specific populations can be quantitated. In addition, the amount of the fluorescent label can be calibrated and by extension, the amount of the ligand for the label can be calculated where calibration reagents are available. The patterns of expression of specific cellular proteins or changes in numbers of cells in specific populations are used to contribute to diagnosis of the patient.

2. Clinical Uses of Flow Cytometry (Overview)

Flow cytometry is used in a number of clinical situations to precisely define abnormal populations. This allows, for example, diagnosis and subclassification of malignancy or definition of the factors operative in immunodeficiency. Flow cytometry is also useful in defining physiological processes, such as enumeration of stem cells or histocompatibility testing before transplant. Flow cytometry is ideal in fluids, such as peripheral blood or bone marrow aspirates, where cells are naturally suspended, but is also useful in solid tissues, from which single cell suspensions can be obtained. The primary uses of this technology are in hematopathology, hematology, transplant medicine, and immunology.

From: *Molecular Biomethods Handbook, 2nd Edition.*
Edited by: J. M. Walker and R. Rapley © Humana Press, Totowa, NJ

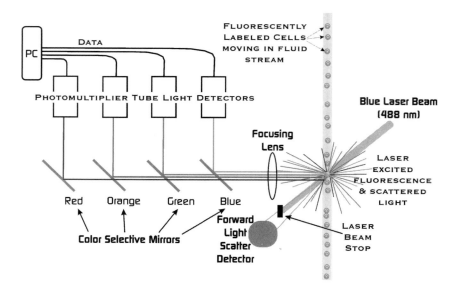

Fig. 57.1. General schematic of a generic clinical flow cytometer

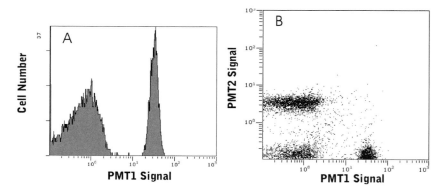

Fig. 57.2. Examples of basic data display types from flow cytometry. **A** Single parameter histogram showing two populations of cells with low and high expression of the fluorochrome detected in PMT1. **B** Dual parameter plot (dot plot) where the position of the dot represents the fluorescence intensity of each cell for the fluorochrome detected by PMT1 and PMT2 respectively

3. A Brief History

Flow cytometry as a practical and commercially viable technology needed the convergence of four technologies: handling cells in fluidic systems, creation of specific fluorescent labels, lasers, and computers. These came together in the 1970s in the first generation of commercial instruments (*1,2*). Although the history of the subsystem components that can be traced back, in some cases to the 1930s, these instruments were the first that have all of the elements of the modern flow cytometers. These instruments were large, complex and needed special power and water cooling for the laser. Sorting was a function of some of these first generation systems as well. In the 1980s, use of more efficient optics originally developed for use with arc lamp systems allowed the use of lower powered air-cooled argon ion lasers. This change converted the large floor instrument into moderate sized and priced systems that fit on the bench top and could be installed in any standard laboratory. The second change that occurred in the 1980s was the introduction of monoclonal anti-human cell surface protein antibodies. These antibodies were directly conjugated with fluorescent labels such as fluorescein or phycoerythrin. These were originally used in areas such as transplant patient monitoring but rapidly spread to many other areas such as classification of leukemias or lymphomas and monitoring of AIDS patients. The 1990s brought an exponential increase in the number of reagents available for clinical use. In addition to the 300+ characterized cell surface proteins, there are probes to measure many aspects of cell physiology. The instruments have evolved to incorporate improvements in electronics and computers. Clinical grade instruments were available with two lasers and measure up to five simultaneous fluorescence parameters as well as two light scatter parameters. The 21st century has seen the commercial availability of bench-top instruments measuring 12 or more fluorescence parameters. Multiplexed sorters are also arriving on the market with claimed sort speeds of over 250,000 cells/s.

4. Preparation of Cells for Analysis

The preparation of cells for flow cytometric analysis falls into two major categories, cells from liquid tissues and cells from solid tissues. In the first class are cells from blood, bone marrow, cerebrospinal fluid, pleural effusion or pulmonary lavage. For all liquid tissues except blood and bone marrow, the cells are centrifuged, washed in sterile buffer and are ready for staining. In blood and bone marrow the standard method is to hypotonically lyse the erythrocytes. The leukocytes are then washed free of material from the lysed erythrocytes. Staining with monoclonal antibodies can be performed before or after lysis of red cells. Finally, the leukocytes may be stained in whole blood and data collection triggered on a fluorescence parameter rather than a light scatter parameter. Cells from biopsy or fine needle aspirate samples may be evaluated by flow cytometry. A single cell suspension is prepared by mechanical and/or enzymatic disaggregation of the tissue. These are then washed and stained as usual.

5. Stains and Markers

There are many hundreds of cellular parameters that can be measured by flow cytometry. Fortunately for the overburdened physician, the list of markers in routine clinical use is notably shorter. These fall into two major categories, markers of cell physiology and cellular proteins. The first group is evaluated using fluorescent molecules specific for the parameter being measured. The most commonly used indicators in this category are the viability markers. These are either chemicals that are impermeable to viable cells such as propidium iodide (PI) or chemicals that are rapidly lost by leakage from cells that

Table 57.1. Some commonly used markers in clinical flow cytometry.

Marker	Normally found on	Used for
CD1a	T cells – immature	L/L
CD2	T cells	L/L ISM
CD3	T cells	L/L ISM
CD4	T cells subset	L/L ISM
CD5	T cells, B-CLL, MCL and some LCL	L/L
CD7	T cells, AML	L/L
CD8	T cells Subset	L/L ISM
CD43	T cells, NK cells, granulocytes	L/L
CD10	B cells, FCL, ALL, some LCL	L/L
CD11c	HCL, some B-CLL	
CD19	B cells	L/L ISM
CD20	B cells, T cells	L/L
CD22	B cells	L/L
CD23	B cells – activated, B-CLL	L/L
Ig kappa light chain	B cells	L/L
Ig lambda light chain	B cells	L/L
CD38	Plasma cells, peripheral blood B cells, activated T cells	L/L
CD138	Plasma cells	L/L
CD25	Activated T and/or B cells	L/L
HLA-DR	Activated T and/or B cells	L/L
TdT	Immature lymphocytes	L/L
CD13	Myeloid	L/L
CD11b	Myeloid	L/L
CD14	Monocytic	L/L
CD33	Myeloid	L/L
CD34	Stem cell	L/L
CD36	Megakaryocytes and eyrthroid cells	
CD61	Megakaryocyte, platelets	L/L
CD64	Granulocytes, monocytes	L/L
CD16	NK cell, T cell, myeloid	L/L
CD56	NK cell, T cell, MM, AML	L/L ISM
CD57	NK cell, T cell	L/L
CD45	All leukocytes	ISM, PNH
CD55	All cells	PNH
CD59	All cells	PNH
CD103	B cells, HCL, ITL	L/L
Erythrocyte RNA	Reticulocyte counts	Reticulocyte monitoring

L/L leukemia or lymphoma screening, *ISM* immune status monitoring, *PNH* paroxymal nocturnal hemoglobinuria screening, *B-CLL* B cell chronic lymphocytic leukemia, *MCL* mantle cell lymphoma, *LCL* large cell lymphoma, *FCL* follicle center cell lymphoma, *ALL* acute lymphoblastic leukemia, *AML* acute myeloid leukemia, *HCL* hairy cell leukemia, multiple myeloma, *ITL* intestinal T-cell lymphoma.

have lost cell membrane integrity such as calcein. Cellular viability is used both as a quality control measure and to determine the status of leukemia or lymphoma cells extracted from patients on chemotherapy. There are indicators for a number of other cellular physiology parameters such as Ca^{++}, membrane potential, oxidative burst, and many others. However, these are primarily used in research settings and will rarely be encountered in clinical practice.

The most common use of flow cytometry is to measure the presence and relative abundance of cellular proteins. This is done using fluorescently labeled monoclonal antibodies. The fluorescence intensity is proportional to the abundance of the protein of interest. In many cases, the proportion of the cells that are expressing the protein is the primary measure. In some cases, changes in the level of the protein are the clinically useful marker. In evaluation of possible tumors, the aberrant expression of proteins can be used to contribute to or establish a specific diagnosis. **Table 57.1** lists some of the more commonly used markers in clinical flow cytometry. Flow cytometry labs will use only a subset of these markers depending on the specific clinical situation.

Monoclonal antibodies can be labeled with a variety of fluorescent molecules (fluorochromes). These fluorochromes have two important characteristics, their excitation and emission characteristics. These are usually shown as spectra such as is **Fig. 57.3**. The excitation spectrum shows the proportion of light emitted as a function of varying excitation wavelength. This is usually measured at the wavelength of maximum emission. The complementary spectrum is the emission spectrum. This shows the light emitted at specific wavelengths with a fixed excitation wavelength. The fluorochromes used in clinical flow cytometry are dictated by the laser(s) installed in clinical flow cytometers. All of the clinical instruments have argon-ion lasers that emit at 488 nm. The other lasers that may be found are shown in **Table 57.2**. The more common fluorochromes for 488 nm excitation are fluorescein (FITC),

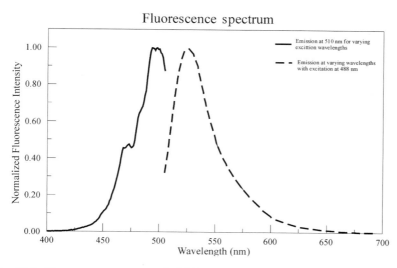

Fig. 57.3. Fluorescence spectrum. Solid line represents the efficiency of excitation at a fixed emission wavelength. The dashed line represents the efficiency of emission at a fixed excitation wavelength

Table 57.2. Lasers used in commercial flow cytometers.

Type	Emission wavelength (nm)
He-Cd	325
Argon-ion or Nd-YAG	355
Diode	405
Argon	488
Diode	532
He-Ne or diode	633

R-phycoerythrin (PE), PE-Cy5 conjugates, PerCP, and PE-Cy7 conjugates. For 633 excitation, allophycocyanine (APC) and APC-Cy7 are the most commonly used fluorochromes.

6. Measurement and Sorting

The labeled cells are placed on the cytometer in a tube or multiwell plate. The machine pulls the cells into a thin stream of cells, which is further hydrodynamically focused into a tight stream with cells in single file. The cells pass through a focused laser beam. The laser beam excites the fluorescent labels and the cytometer collects both the emitted fluorescent light and scattered laser light. This light enters the collecting optics where it is collimated, focused, and sent into the optical section.

The optical section uses two classes of components to split and purify the optical signal. The first class is dichroic mirrors. These are partial mirrors that have the ability to reflect light above or below a certain wavelength. A specific example is a dichroic used to separate the signal from FITC. This will reflect any wavelength below 550 nm and allow all higher wavelengths to pass (long pass). This is abbreviated as a 550 LP dichroic, there are also dichroics that have the inverse characteristics of passing all wavelengths below their cutoff and reflecting those above, these are called short pass (SP) dichroics. The other class is the bandpass filters. These are set to allow light to pass only within certain wavelengths. These are defined by a center wavelength and width, for example a filter for fluorescein has a center of 525 nm and a width of ±30 nm, which is to say it admits all light between 495 nm and 555 nm (525/30 BP). There are the inverse of these which block only certain wavelengths and allow all others. These are commonly used to block scattered laser light and may have a width of only a few nanometers. **Figure 57.4** shows a simple optical dichroic mirror and barrier filter arrangement. There are many different possible optical arrangements depending on the space available and the relative importance of the signal strength of the various fluorochromes.

The light arrives in the photomultiplier tube (PMT) and the energy of the light photons is converted into a very small electrical signal. The light scatter signals are then amplified through either a linear amplifier or a logarithmic amplifier. In clinical cytometry, linear amps are used for light scatter signals and for DNA measurements. Measurement of cell surface proteins uses

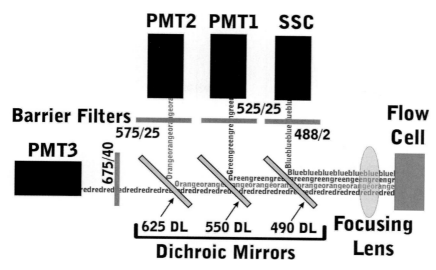

Fig. 57.4. Diagram of a generic optical section of a flow cytometer. Fluorescence light and scattered laser light is collected and collimated by the focusing lens. Successive colors are reflected by dichroic mirrors and purified by barrier filters before generating an electrical voltage in the photomultiplier tube

logarithmic amps. Flow cytometers commonly provide four logs of amplification range. This allows a practical range of measurement of approx. 1,000 to 10,000,000 molecules per cell without adjusting the amplification settings. This range is sufficient for most proteins of clinical interest. The best of the current generation of commercial systems can detect as low as a few hundred protein molecules per cell with carefully selected reagents and conditions.

For some instruments, there is additional circuitry to provide compensation and on some instruments, all compensation is done in software. The subject of compensation is quite complex and has generated intense discussion at times among flow cytometry specialists. Compensation is needed because the light signals emitted by the fluorochromes are broad enough to bleed into adjacent filter regions. See **Fig. 57.5A** for an example of a simple compensation problem. Here we show the emission spectrum of fluorescein (FITC) a fluorochrome that will be primarily detected in the PMT1 detector. Note however that owing to the width of the right tail of the spectrum, that there is a significant part of the FITC signal that will be detected in the PMT2 detector. To obtain an accurate measurement of a true signal in PMT2, the unwanted signal from the FITC must be removed from the final data. This process is called compensation. To do proper compensation, data must be collected from samples with each fluorochrome alone. Alternately for polychromatic sampling, a series of tubes are prepared where each fluorochrome is omitted in sequence. This integrates the contribution of all other fluorochromes in the tube. **Figure 57.5B** shows the appearance of a dot plot showing cells labeled only with FITC. **Figure 57.5B** shows the signal on the PMT2 axis from the PMT1 fluorochrome. **Figure 57.5C** shows the same data after the application of compensation. The compensated data more accurately reflects the biological levels of the markers of clinical interest.

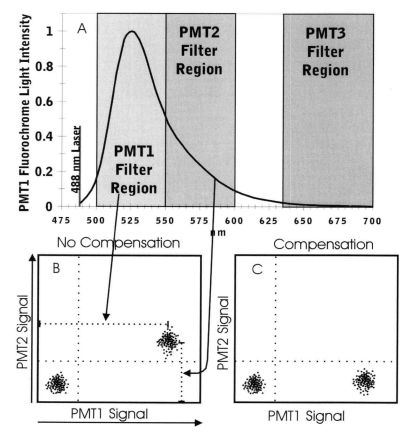

Fig. 57.5. Example of compensation. **A** Emission spectrum for fluorescein with filter regions superimposed on the plot. **B** Uncompensated fluorescence dot plot from cells labeled only with fluorescein. **C** Data for the same cell population with proper compensation to remove fluorescein signal from the PMT2 channel

The data from the cytometer are always sent to a computer for display, analysis and storage. A variety of classes of computers and operating systems have been used over the years. At this time, nearly all systems will have either a Mac or PC attached. The manufacturers package acquisition and analysis software with the cytometers. In addition, there are several analysis software packages that may be used for evaluation of the data. The data are stored in a specific binary file format that cannot be read by spreadsheet programs and other simple packages. The data are usually displayed in two dimensional plots or in one parameter histograms. The axis in either case is the intensity of the optical signal in that channel. In the basic 2D plot, each dot represents the light intensity signal for a single cell in the two channels. For example in **Fig. 57.5C**, the dots representing the cells in the left population are low for both signals, whereas the cells in the right population are bright in PMT1 and low in PMT2 signal. A one parameter histogram is used in situations where cells are only labeled with one label or where evaluation of dot plots has shown that a histogram display is not confounded. A specific example of this

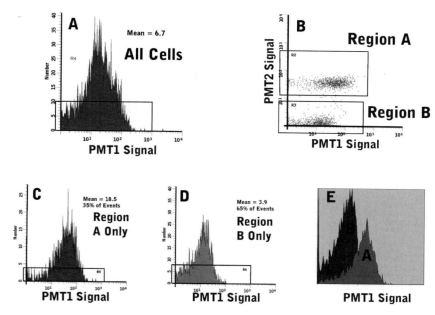

Fig. 57.6. Example of the use of gating to identify confounded data. **A** PMT1 signal for all cells. **B** Dot plot of PMT1 and PMT2 for the same data shown in plot "A" showing two populations. **C** PMT1 histogram for only those cells shown in region A. **D** PMT1 histogram for only those cells shown in region B. **E** Overlay plot showing histograms from plot "C" and plot "D" on the same axes

is shown in **Fig. 57.6**. Plot 6A shows the histogram for the PMT1 signal for all cells. However, examination of a dot plot (**Fig. 57.6B**) shows that there are two distinct populations that overlap in their PMT1 signals. The cells only from region A are shown in **Fig. 57.6C** and those from region B in **Fig. 57.6D**. The plot in **Fig. 57.6E** is the two histograms from **Fig. 57.6C** and D displayed simultaneously showing the two distinct populations that cannot be clearly distinguished in **Fig. 57.6A**. **Figure 57.6E** is a type of plot called an overlay plot. **Figure 57.6B** shows rectangular regions on a dot plot. The other types of regions commonly seen are polygonal and quadrants. There are other situations where a histogram plot may be quite acceptable, however, it needs to be demonstrated that populations are not being confounded. The data in **Fig. 57.2** are an example of data where a histogram is acceptable to differentiate populations that are low or high for the marker used on PMT1 here.

There are two values that are commonly used for data analysis, the percentage of cells, or the fluorescence intensity of the cells, in a specific region. The percentage values may be of all cells within a viability gate or may be the percentage of cells within a specific subpopulation. As acute leukemias can have a heterogeneous pattern of antigen expression, it is important to differentiate tumor cells from normal populations so as to accurately define the immunophenotype. A blast gate can be defined in analysis of bone marrow aspirates based upon the pattern of expression of CD45 versus SSC pattern (see the following).

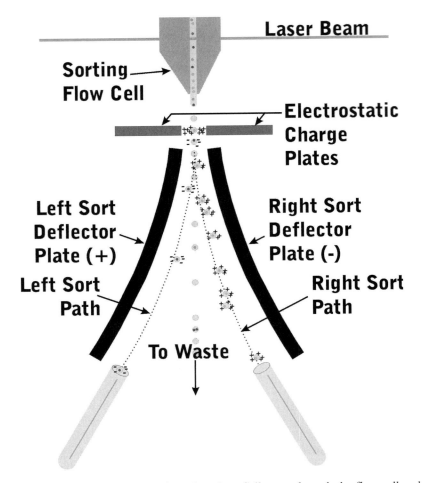

Fig. 57.7. Schematic demonstration of sorting. Cells pass through the flow cell and data are collected. The flow cell vibrates to break the stream into droplets containing zero or one cell. If the cell meets sort criteria, an electrostatic charge is applied as the cell passes between the charge plates. Depending on if a positive or negative charge was applied, the deflector plates attract the charged droplets right or left where the droplets are collected in a separate tube

In the clinical setting, the vast majority of flow cytometry is analysis of cell populations. However, there is an extension of flow cytometry that allows cells to be physically sorted. This capability was part of the earliest systems and has advanced in speed and capacity. The latest generation of high speed sorters can separate up to four different populations at speeds as high as 250,000 cells per second. Sorting is conceptually simple but the hardware and software needed to operate at these speeds are quite sophisticated. In contrast to the analyzers, the flow cell on a sorter is vibrated by a piezoelectric crystal at high speeds, these are tuned to produce a stream that breaks up into droplets that can only hold one or two cells. The cells pass through the laser and the usual types of flow cytometry data are generated. The operator has previously calibrated the system so that the time between a cell being in the laser beam and being between the charge plates is exactly known. The sorter operator has specifically identified the cell populations to be sorted using one or more gates. When a cell that fits the criteria to be sorted is identified the system initiates the sorting process. **Figure 57.7** shows a schematic diagram of the basic sorting process. Sorting occurs because the system is able to put a specific positive or negative charge on a single droplet. These charged droplets are then attracted towards the deflector plate, which has a standing charge of the opposite polarity. The cells are collected into a tube for whatever clinical or research use is intended.

7. Clinical Uses of Flow Cytometry

7.1. Hematopathology: Lymphoma/Leukemia Immunophenotyping

The WHO classification of hematolymphoid neoplasia subclassifies lymphoma and leukemia based upon morphology, immunophenotype, genetic abnormalities, and clinical features. Some hematopoietic neoplasms in the WHO classification system have a specific immunophenotype and diagnosis is very difficult in the absence of this immunophenotype *(3)*. Therefore diagnostic evaluation of a specimen suspected for a hematological malignancy should include review of the immunophenotype by flow cytometry or immunohistochemistry. Flow Cytometry is clearly superior when evaluating hematopoietic neoplasms for antibody based therapy, such as Rituximab, Campath, Mylotarg or Zenapax, as the targeted antigen must be expressed on the cell surface for therapy to be effective. Flow Cytometry has also been shown to have greater sensitivity, reduced subjectivity and faster turn around time compared to immunohistochemistry in evaluation of lymphoid neoplasms *(4)*. In acute leukemias, flow cytometric immunophenotyping (FCI) not only allows differentiation between lymphoid and myeloid lineage (crucial for prognosis and treatment) but is also useful for precise characterization of leukemias and the pattern of antigen expression can be used to detect minimal residual disease post therapy in most patients *(5)*.

The majority of mature lymphoid neoplasms in North America and Europe are of B-cell origin. Flow cytometry assists in diagnosis of a B-cell lymphoma by first identifying a neoplastic B-cell population and then detecting antigen expression useful in subclassification into appropriate diagnostic categories. One of the most useful clinical applications of flow cytometry is the identification of monoclonal B cells by detection of light chain restriction. Light chain restriction is detected as a B cell population that stains positive with one light chain reagent and negative with the other light chain reagent (e.g., B cells all kappa positive and lambda negative, **Fig. 57.8**). A monoclonal B-cell population with restricted light chain expression is, with rare exceptions, considered a B-cell neoplasm. Additional markers of B-cell neoplasia include abnormal sized cells (e.g., large cells detected based upon forward light scatter), abnormal level of antigen expression (e.g., dim CD20 expression in chronic lymphocytic leukemia or CLL), absence of normal antigens (e.g., CD20 negativity in a large B cell lymphoma), and presence of abnormal antigens (e.g., CD2 positive B cells). One of the advantages of flow cytometry is its ability to recognize monoclonal B cells even in B-cell lymphopenia, in the presence of polyclonal B cells or among cells with cytophillic antibody (passively adsorbed

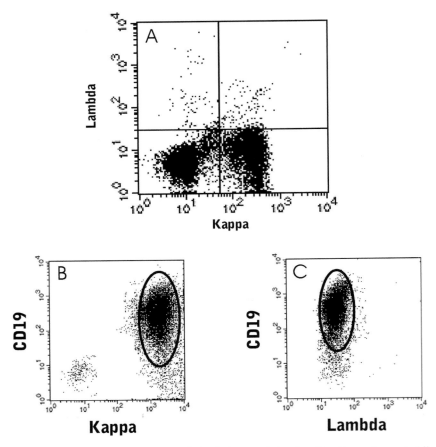

Fig. 57.8. Example of monoclonal light chain population in a B-cell neoplasm. **A** All of the B cells are kappa positive and lambda negative. **B** All of the CD19 positive B-cells are kappa positive. **C** All of the CD19 positive B-cells are lambda negative

immunoglobulins from the plasma in vivo, e.g., monocytes, natural killer cells, activated T cells, or granulocytes) *(6)*. In addition, in normal or benign lymph node tissue, virtually every B-cell expresses light chain immunoglobulins and the lack of expression of surface immunoglobulins among mature B cells also suggests the presence of a monoclonal B-cell population *(7)*. In samples containing monoclonal B-cells admixed with polyclonal B-cells, the simultaneous analysis of antigens that are differentially expressed among benign and malignant elements and evaluation for abnormally large cells facilitates the detection of lymphoma cells. For example, the CD11c- B cells (region in **Fig. 57.9A**) are polyclonal because both positive and negative cells are seen in the kappa (**Fig. 57.9B**) and lambda (**Fig 57.9C**) plots. In contrast, the CD11c + B cells (region in **Fig. 57.9D**) in the peripheral blood specimen from a patient with hairy cell leukemia may be monoclonal (note single lambda positive population in **Fig. 57.9F**). Simple examination of numbers of cells staining with kappa and lambda will not be useful in this case. Delineating an abnormal pattern of expression of antigens in B cell neoplasia also allows subclassification

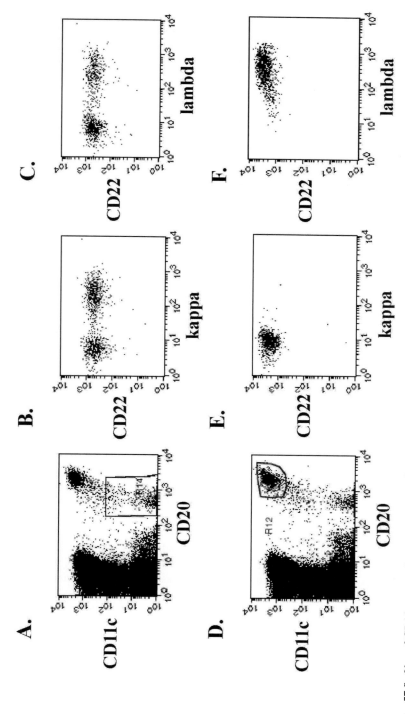

Fig. 57.9. Use of CD11c expression to separate malignant from normal B-cells in a patient with hairy cell leukemia. **A** The CD20 positive but CD11c negative B cell gate used. **B** The B cells in the CD 20 positive CD11c negative gate are CD22 positive and polyclonal based upon kappa staining. **C** The B cells in the CD 20 positive CD11c negative gate are CD22 positive and polyclonal based upon lambda staining. **D** The CD20 positive and CD11c brightly positive B cell gate used. **E** The B cells in the CD 20 positive CD11c positive gate are CD22 positive and all kappa negative (monoclonal). **F** The B cells in the CD 20 positive CD11c positive gate are CD22 positive and all lambda positive (monoclonal)

into discrete diagnostic categories. Examples of antigens useful in subclassification include CD5, CD79b and CD23 in CLL and mantle cell lymphoma, CD10 in follicular and Burkitt's lymphomas and CD11c as well as CD103 in hairy cell leukemia and splenic marginal zone lymphoma *(3)*.

Mature T-cell and NK cell neoplasms are uncommon, accounting for only 12% of all non-Hodgkin lymphoma *(3)*. Indicators of T-cell neoplasia include Vβ repertoire restriction, subset restriction, absence of normally expressed antigens, presence of abnormal antigens and abnormal levels of T-cell antigen expression *(8–12)*.

Flow cytometry can be used to directly detect T cell clonality in a manner similar to light chain restriction in B-cell neoplasms, although a larger panel is required. T cell receptors (TCR) are composed of either αβ or γδ chains, with the vast majority of normal and neoplastic T cells expressing the αβ chain. The αβ and γδ chains are formed by VDJ segments and a constant region. All of the T cells in a clonal αβ–T cell population have the same VDJ segment and therefore have identical (monoclonal) Vβ protein expression. Because commercial antibodies are available for detection of 70 percent of the V segments for the TCR β chain human, T-cell clonality can be evaluated by assessing Vβ protein repertoire using flow cytometry *(11,12)*. Because the distribution of Vβ classes in normal T cells is well defined *(11)*, abnormal expansions of a Vβ population consistent with a clonal T-cell population can be determined, similar to expansion of kappa or lambda light chain expressing B cells in a monoclonal B-cell population.

In normal reactive lymphoid populations there is a mixture of CD4 and CD8 positive cells. However mature clonal T-cell populations are restricted in CD4 or CD8 expression to CD4+/CD8− (majority), CD4−/CD8+, CD4−/CD8− and CD4+/CD8+. In addition 75% of mature T-cell neoplasms fail to express at least one T-cell antigen (**Fig. 57.10**) and in T-cell neoplasms with antigen loss, two thirds have greater than one pan-T antigen missing. Detection of abnormal or inappropriate antigen expression is useful in diagnosis of T-cell neoplasias. Neoplastic T-cells may be detected as a homogeneous population with an abnormal level of antigen expression *(8–10)*. For example, CD3 may be expressed at a higher or lower level than normal as measured by staining with anti-CD3 (**Fig. 57. 10**). T cell large granular lymphocyte leukemias, for example, typically have abnormally dim levels of CD5 expression.

Acute leukemias are characterized by a rapidly growing, aggressive population of neoplastic blasts. The distinction between lymphoid (ALL) and myeloid (AML) leukemia is crucial. Flow cytometric evaluation of the immunophenotypic markers of lineage and stages of differentiation allows more precise classification of a leukemic process than morphology alone. The WHO classification of acute leukemias uses cytogenetic, immunophenotypic and molecular genetic data to define subgroups of leukemias with favorable or poor prognoses. Many of the genetically distinct diagnostic subgroups are closely associated with specific immunophenotypes. Therefore FCI can detect antigen profiles associated with a specific molecular abnormality and prognosis (reviewed in **ref. *13***).

As acute leukemias can have a heterogeneous pattern of antigen expression, it is important to differentiate tumor cells from normal populations so as to accurately define the immunophenotype. In the past, flow cytometricc analysis of bone marrow for leukemia used FSC versus SSC to define a gate. Using

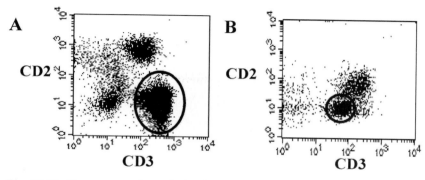

Fig. 57.10. Flow cytometric analysis of T-cell neoplasms. **A** Malignant T cells (in oval) expressing CD3 but negative for CD2. **B** Malignant T cells (in oval) expressing abnormally dim CD3 and negative for CD2

this gating strategy, antigen expression was described as the percent of gated events positive for a list of antibodies. As the analysis gate also contained the normal nucleated erythroid precursors and lymphocytes, the reported percentages pertained to a mixture of leukemic blasts and normal cells. In bone marrows virtually replaced by leukemic blasts, essentially all of the cells are blasts and this strategy is useful. However, when normal elements are present in significant numbers, an analysis gate specific for blasts must be used. When the expression of CD45 versus SSC pattern for bone marrow elements is examined, cells can be segregated into distinct populations, including lymphocytes, monocytes, granulocytes, nucleated red cells and blasts (**Fig. 57. 11**) Thus these two parameters can be used to define a blast gate (characterized by low SSC and dim CD45) that contains few normal cells (*14,15*).

Flow cytometry is essential for determination of lineage in acute lymphoblastic leukemia (ALL). ALL cells typically occupy the blast gate on CD45 verses SSC, although in select cases CD45 expression may be dimmer than usual and CD45 negative blasts (in the region of normal erythroid precursors on CD45 versus SSC) can be identified. ALL blasts have an immature T- or B-cell immunophenotype and may express TdT and CD34. However expression of myeloid antigens such as CD13, CD33, and CD15 is common. For this reason classification of ALL is based upon a panel of T, B, and myeloid antibodies.

ALL blasts have an immature immunophenotype and typically express CD19 and CD10. B ALL is subclassified into B-precursor ALL, pre-B ALL and mature B cell ALL based upon immunoglobulin expression. B-precursor ALL does not express immunoglobulin, whereas pre-B ALL is positive for cytoplasmic but not surface immunoglobulin. Mature B-cell ALL has surface immunoglobulin. Because cytoplasmic immunoglobulin is no longer regularly analyzed in the clinical flow cytometry laboratory, both B-precursor ALL and pre-B ALL are often grouped together based upon negativity for surface immunoglobulin and called B-precursor ALL. They typically express CD19, CD10, CD34, HLADR, and TdT and are usually positive for CD22 and CD24. Mature B-cell ALL, in addition to surface immunoglobulin, has brighter CD45, CD19, CD20, CD22, CD24, and CD10 but is negative for CD34 and

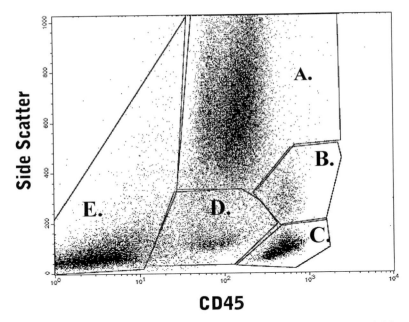

Fig. 57.11. Staining pattern of CD45 versus side scatter for bone marrow. **A** Mature granulocytes. **B** Mature monocytes. **C** Mature Lymphocytes. **D** Blasts. **E** Nucleated red cell precursors

TdT. As the immunophenotype in B lineage ALL is associated with molecular abnormalities and prognosis, FCI can also be used as a screen to select cases for molecular analysis (**ref. *14*** for review).

The blasts in T lineage ALL often are not contained in the CD45 versus SSC blast gate and may overlap with the brighter CD45 mature lymphocyte and monocyte gates. Although the most specific marker for T-cell lineage in ALL is CD3, T ALL is usually negative for surface CD3, necessitating intracytoplasmic staining for this antigen. As intracytoplasmic staining has a higher background, one must be careful to not over interpret apparent dim CD3 staining as real and indicating T-cell lineage. CD7 is the most sensitive marker for T ALL but is less specific than CD3 as it is frequently expressed by myeloid leukemias. CD2, CD1a, CD5, TdT, andCD34 are also observed in T ALL. CD4 and CD8 are typically double positive or double negative (**ref. *14*** for review).

FCI plays an important role in the WHO classification of acute myeloid leukemias. Flow cytometry is not only specific in differentiating acute myeloid leukemia (AML) from ALL but is also highly useful in identifying granulocytic, monocytic, erythroid and megakaryocytic differentiation. Both the pattern of antigen expression as well as where the blasts fall on a CD45 versus SSC data plot help to subclassify AML. In addition, many of the specific genetically identified subgroups tend to have distinct immunophenotypic features.

Blasts in AML have an immature phenotype and may express CD13, CD33, CD117, and myeloperoxidase. CD34 and HLADR may be positive but are not lineage specific. In addition, the blasts may express the lymphoid antigens

TdT, CD56, or CD7. With increasing maturation, there is decreased expression of CD33 and increased CD13, CD15 and CD11b. In AML with monocytic differentiation, the blasts can overlap with normal monocytes on the CD45 versus SSC data plot and express monocytic antigens, such as CD14 and CD36. Erythroid differentiation can be determined by bright expression of CD71 and glycophorin whereas megakaryocytic differentiation is characterized by bright CD61 and CD41 expression (**ref. *14*** for review).

FCI provides important prognostic information in hematolymphoid neoplasias. Owing to its multipartametric nature and ability to analyze large numbers of cells rapidly, FCI is an extremely sensitive method for detection of minimal residual disease (MRD) post therapy. MRD based evaluation of initial response to therapy has been shown to be an independent prognostic factor in ALL. In patients with multiple myeloma and B-CLL, flow cytometric detection of MRD post therapy accurately predicts progression free survival (*16*). The sensitivity of FCI also leads to enhanced accuracy in evaluation of blood, bone marrow and CSF for malignant cells in the staging of non-Hodgkin's lymphoma, allowing detection of disease even in the absence of morphological indications of involvement (*16*). Flow cytometric studies have identified specific antigens in various chronic lymphoproliferative processes that serve as prognostic markers. B-CLL patients with high levels of CD38 expression, have a significantly poorer survival than those with low levels of CD38 expression. Expression of ZAP-70, a member of the Syk-ZAP-70 protein tyrosine kinase family also predicts a more rapid progression and worse survival than patients with ZAP-70 negative B-CLL. As the growth potential of neoplastic cells plays a role in dictating tumor behavior, numerous investigators have studied the proliferation potential as detected by flow cytometric measurement of DNA content or detection of bromo-deoxy uridine incorporation in chronic lymphoproliferative disorders and found it is of prognostic value (*16*).

7.2. Hematology and Transfusion Medicine

Flow Cytometric based methods are replacing older, more laborious protocols for testing of red blood cells (RBC) (**ref. *17*** for review). Flow cytometric evaluation is useful in monitoring obstetrical patients. Following pregnancy with an Rh+ fetus, Rh– mothers can become sensitized to the Rh factor and produce anti-Rh or D antigen antibodies. In future pregnancies this can result in fetal anemia or even fetal death. Because small amounts of fetal RBCs can be detected in maternal blood in uncomplicated pregnancy and delivery, all Rh– women receive prophylactic anti Rh, or anti-D immunoglobulin at 28 wk of pregnancy and within 72 h of delivery to prevent possible Rh alloimmunization. However significant fetomaternal hemorrhage can occur under a number of conditions and the number of fetal RBCs must be quantitated in maternal blood to determine the appropriate dose of anti-D immunoglobulin. The Kleihauer–Betke test (KBT) for detection of fetal erythrocytes in maternal blood is based the fact that acid elutes adult hemoglobin more rapidly than fetal hemoglobin from RBCs. The intact fetal hemoglobin can be visualized by staining with erythrosine. This method, however, has been shown to be subjective, not reproducible and insensitive. Flow cytometry is a highly sensitive tool for detecting minor RBC populations. Using an antibody to fetal hemoglobin, flow cytometry has been demonstrated to have superior precision in detecting fetal RBCs. In addition, the flow cytometric method can differentiate hereditary persistence of fetal hemoglobin from fetal RBCs in the maternal blood *(18)*.

Flow cytometry has been used to study ABH and Rh blood group antigens *(18)*. Flow cytometry has been used to detect and quantitate RBC-bound antibody (IgG, IgM, and IgA) and complement (C3) in autoimmune hemolytic anemia. Because the standard direct antiglobulin test is sensitive and inexpensive, flow cytometry is only used in select conditions. Flow cytometry can detect small amounts of IgG bound to RBCs in patients with indications of autoimmune hemolytic anemia but a negative direct antiglobulin test by standard methods. In addition, flow cytometry can be used to determine the IgG subclass of RBC bound IgG. Flow cytometry is also optimal for detecting autoimmune hemolytic anemia associated with IgM autoantibodies reacting at 37°C *(17)*.

Flow cytometry is highly useful in clinical evaluation of platelets and allows testing with little or no isolation or manipulation (**ref. *19*** for review). Because the threshold for platelet transfusions has been lowered in many institutions to 10,000 platelets/µl, it is important that platelet counts be accurate at this lower range. Nonplatelet particles can interfere with platelet counting by some methods. Enumeration of platelets by flow cytometry, or immunoplatelet counting is highly precise and accurate and eliminates the problem of nonplatelet particles. In this method platelets are labeled with an anti-platelet antibody and the ratio of platelets to RBCs is measured. The platelet count is then determined using the RBC count obtained from a hematology analyzer and the ratio of platelets to RBCs. This can be used to calibrate hematology analyzers *(20)*. In addition to quantitating platelets, flow cytometry has been used for immunophenotyping platelets. Demonstration of abnormal patterns of expression of platelet receptors has been used to define several genetic disorders, including Glanzmann's thrombasthenia and Bernard–Soulier syndrome *(19)*.

Reticulated platelets are the youngest platelets in circulation and their levels increase when thrombopoiesis is stimulated. Measuring reticulated platelets is the most sensitive and specific method to distinguish destructive or immune thrombocytopenia from marrow failure. Reticulated platelets are large and have increased quantities of RNA. Upon staining of platelets with fluorescent nuclear dyes, such as thiazole orange, all platelets take up dye in proportion to their size. Reticulated platelets take up additional dye, owing to RNA staining, that is lost upon treatment with RNAase. This RNAase sensitive labeling can be measured by flow cytometry for an accurate reticulated platelet count *(19)*.

Studies demonstrating immunophenotypic markers of platelet activation have markedly improved platelet function testing. P-selectin, CD63 PCA-1 and LIBS only become exposed on the platelet surface after activation. FCI of platelets can reveal this activated phenotype, even when only low numbers of platelets are activated. More conventional methods of measuring platelet activation show a threshold phenomenon and are primarily suited for detecting platelet dysfunction. Flow cytometric testing, however, allows measurement of platelet hyperfunction *(19)*. Increased platelet activation in patients undergoing procedures such as coronary angioplasty may help identify patients at risk for early restenosis who require anti-platelet therapy *(21)*. This technology may even prove useful in predicting risk of cardiovascular disease, allowing early preventative intervention.

Paroxysmal nocturnal hemaglobinuriais (PNH) is a hematopoietic disorder caused by deletions, insertions or point mutations in phosphatidylinositolglycan complementation class A (PIG-A) gene. This results in a total or partial deficiency of surface proteins attached to the cell by a glycophosphatidylinositol (GPI) anchor. CD55 (decay accelerating factor, DAF) and CD59 (membrane inhibitor of reactive lysis, MIRL) are affected in PNH. Both play an important role in the regulation of complement activation and their deficiency in PNH leads to an increased susceptibility of cells to complement mediated cell lysis. Because CD55 and CD59 are normally expressed at high levels on leukocytes, RBCs and platelets and their levels are consistently decreased in PNH hematopoietic cells, flow cytometric immunophenotypic analysis of CD55 and CD59 is a sensitive test for PNH. Testing of CD59 alone, however, leads to a high false-positive rate (22). As red cells stain with the anti-CD55 and anti-CD59 antibodies it is difficult to achieve optimal antibody concentrations without a prelyse protocol. In a stain-lyse-and-then-wash-protocol the mean fluorescence intensity (MFI) of leukocyte staining correlates with the number of RBCs present. By optimizing the staining protocol (using a smaller blood volume and incubating longer) a nonlyse nonwash method can be used that allows for the simultaneous analysis of CD55 and CD59 on red cells, platelets, and leukocytes (23).

7.3. Histocompatibility Testing

Flow cytometry plays an important role in allogeneic transplantation (24,25). It has been most useful in the detection of low-titer, or noncomplement fixing antibodies. Originally instituted as a means for performing a "more sensitive" crossmatch, new technologies have given additional use to this technology. The flow cytometry crossmatch detects alloantibodies that are not detectable by the standard complement-dependent cytotoxicity crossmatch. A positive flow crossmatch, even when the complement-dependent cytotoxicity crossmatch is negative, correlates with an increased risk of rejection and graft loss in solid organ transplantation. In stem cell transplantation, it may be associated with failed engraftment. The flow cytometric crossmatching was originally performed by incubating transplant recipient serum with donor lymphocytes. HLA antibodies, if present, bound to the surface of the lymphocyte and were measured using a fluorescently-labeled anti-human immunoglobulin. Microparticles coated with purified Class I or Class II MHC proteins have been substituted for donor cells (26). This test provides sensitivity equal to the flow crossmatch yet confirms the specificity of the antibody. In addition, this test can be used to profile patients awaiting transplantation, classifying them as "sensitized" or "nonsensitized." Besides its uses before transplantation, Flow cytometry can also be used to monitor the development of donor HLA specific antibodies posttransplant (**ref. 24** for review). Early detection of donor-specific reactivity can provide an opportunity to modify immunosuppression before graft damage.

7.4. Immunology

Flow cytometry has numerous applications in infectious disease and clinical immunology. Sepsis is one of the top 10 causes of death, with a mortality of 30–50%, and requires rapid clinical intervention. Despite this, there have been few advances in diagnostic testing for this entity and standard testing has been nonspecific (e.g., complete blood count) or slow (cultures). Flow cytometric quantitation of neutrophil CD64 expression has been shown to improve diagnostic detection of sepsis/infection, with greater sensitivity and specificity than standard tests such as absolute neutrophil count and sedimentation rate (27). Flow cytometry was the first method used to monitor the status of patients with HIV. Initially it was found that the level of CD4+ cells in the blood of HIV patients correlated well with clinical status (28). The relationship was powerful enough that the U.S. FDA accepted the use of CD4 counts as a surrogate marker for evaluating the efficacy of treatments for HIV infection. More recently, other measurements, including direct measurement of viral RNA in blood have been developed to complement CD4 counts. Other markers such as the level of the activation marker CD38 on CD8+ cells have also been shown to be highly predictive of health status (29).

Flow cytometry plays an important role in the diagnostic evaluation of primary immunodeficiencies (30). Quantitative and qualitative evaluation of lymphocyte subsets by standard FCI is useful in rendering a diagnosis (e.g., severe B cell lymphopenia in agammaglobulinemia). For example in Autoimmune Lymphoproliferative Syndrome, one of the major diagnostic criteria is the presence of a trio of significant numbers of rare cells, specifically T cells with TcR-beta without CD4 or CD8, CD20 postive B cells also expressing CD5, and T cells with both CD3 and HLA-Dr (31). In addition to standard phenotyping, a specific gene product, or lack there of, may be detected by flow cytometry. Functional assays, such as the oxidative burst assay (deficient in chronic gramulomatous disease) may also be performed by flow cytometry (30).

Allergists have traditionally relied upon skin testing and later on serum-specific immunoglobulin IgE to diagnose IgE mediated allergies. Unfortunately identification of the specific allergens is not always straightforward. In such cases, flow cytometric identification of basophil activation in response to challenge with a specific allergen has proven useful (32). FCI can accurately detect basophils in whole blood and because basophils upregulate CD203c and express surface CD63 upon activation, FCI can measure basophil activation. Testing involves incubating whole blood or isolated basophils with the specific allergens in question, followed by FCI quantitation of basophil activation expression (32).

A relatively new use for flow cytometry is the use of multiplexed bead assays to measure soluble proteins. This assay uses the multicolor capability of the flow cytometer to allow simultaneous evaluation of mixed populations of beads. The beads are chemically labeled with varying intensities of one or two fluorochromes and then a monoclonal antibody labeled with another fluorochrome is used to measure the test analyte. This assay can be used to simultaneously measure up to 10 proteins in a standard flow cytometer or up to 100 using a dedicated system. The applications of this technology are limited only by the availability of the test reagents. Applications include evaluation of cytokines or soluble cytokine receptors to assist diagnosis of sepsis, certain autoimmune conditions, transplant rejection, some cancers, and viral infection (33). The clinical usefulness of many of these new reagents is an area of active research and the number of available reagents can be expected to rapidly increase.

7.5. Stem Cells

Peripheral blood stem cells are replacing bone marrow as a source for hematopoietic progenitor cells in transplantation of cancer patients. The reasons for this switch include the greater ease of collection by apheresis, elimination of the need for general anesthesia of the donor, rate of hematological reconstitution of the recipient and decreased medical care costs. However, because the minimum number of CD34 positive hematopoietic progenitor cell required is 2–5×10^6/kg recipient body weight *(34,35)*, multiple aphereses must be performed to collect a sufficient number to ensure adequate engraftment. Also, because less than 0.1% of nucleated peripheral blood cells in normal controls are CD34 positive cells *(36)*, peripheral blood stem cell numbers are increased (or mobilized) by administering colony-stimulating factors. Flow cytometry is used to enumerate CD34 positive progenitor cells in the peripheral blood of donors undergoing mobilization to determine when apheresis should start and when sufficient number of hematopoietic progenitor cells are collected for engraftment (**ref.** *36,37* for review). The absolute count of CD34 positive cells in the donor peripheral blood is predictive of the number of CD34 positive cells in the apheresis product and thus can be used to determine when apheresis should start. Decisions concerning growth factor administration and further apheresis collections are made based upon the number of CD34 positive cells collected in each apheresis. As crucial treatment decisions are made based upon absolute CD34 counts, it is important that methods be standardized and strict quality control be applied. Multi-center studies demonstrated variability between laboratories and served as an impetus for further standardization of methods. Proprietary kits are available that use optimal anti-CD34 antibodies (class III), provide for minimal manipulation and include beads to allow direct quantification of the number of cells per unit volume. The ISHAGE multiparametric sequential gating technique showed closest agreement between labs *(38)*. This approach involves cumulative gating based upon light scatter characteristics, dim expression of CD45, and expression of CD34. Only cells within the appropriate cumulative gates are counted. By including fluorescent counting beads, an absolute CD34 positive cell count can be directly determined by flow cytometry. Additional markers can be included for further characterization of the CD34 positive cells. Standardization of absolute CD34 positive cells counting using the single platform ISHAGE method resulted in decreased differences among laboratories in a multicenter trial *(39)*.

8. On the Horizon

Flow cytometry has shown significant technological advances because the initial creation of complete systems in the 1970s. Multiplexed sorters are entering the market with integrated sort speeds of over 250,000 cells/s. Some of these are designed explicitly for sorting specific populations for direct clinical use. Polychromatic analyzers are now on the market allowing up to 12 colors per cell to be evaluated. Although there are limitations in reagents at this point, it is possible that clinical analysis of 20+ parameters per cell will be a commercial reality before 2010. Dedicated multiplexed bead ELISA flow cytometers are now on the market and reagent sets currently available can measure 25 specific proteins in a single 50-μl sample. The speed and efficiency of these bead analyzers promises dramatic improvements in measurement of serum proteins. Another possible area of advance is the use of full spectrum fluorescence data, which would allow a single detector to report data from a suite of fluorochromes. Spectral analysis software developed for microscopy applications can be used to disentangle the signals from each fluorochrome. A research grade system has been built *(40)* although further development will be needed before this advanced design appears in commercial instruments.

9. Summary and Conclusions

In conclusion, flow cytometry is a powerful technology that is currently being used to provide valuable data in a variety of clinical situations. As the technology becomes more powerful, these instruments will move into new areas of clinical practice to provide data in a rapid, accurate, and cost efficient manner.

10. Additional Resources

Books:
Flow Cytometry: First Principles, by Alice Givan. John Wiley & Sons, Hoboken, New Jersey (2001). This is a good first book to give an overview of the field with some emphasis on clinical cytometry.
Practical Flow Cytometry, Fourth Edition, by Howard Shapiro John Wiley & Sons, Hoboken, New Jersey (2003). This is the single most complete and detailed book on flow cytometry available anywhere. Not for the faint of heart or the casual reader, a must-have for serious flow cytometrists.
Flow Cytometry in Clinical Diagnosis. 4th ed, edited by David F. Keren, J. Philip McCoy Jr., and John L. Carey, 2006, Chicago: ASCP Press. Good and current overview of the clinical side of flow cytometry.
Journals:
Clinical Cytometry, a journal of the International Society for Analytical Cytology (ISAC) and the Clinical Cytometry Society.
Journal of Immunological Methods
Professional Societies:
International Society for Analytical Cytology (http://www.isac-net.org)
The Clinical Cytometry Society (http://www.cytometry.org)

References

1. Shapiro H (2003) History. In: Practical flow cytometry, 4th edn, John Wiley, Hoboken, New Jersey
2. Herzenberg LA, Parks D, Sahaf B, Perez O, Roederer M, Herzenberg LA (2002) The history and future of the fluorescence activated cell sorter and flow cytometry: a view from Stanford. Clin Chem **48**:1819–1827
3. Jaffe ES, Harris NL, Stein H, Vardiman JW (eds) (2001) WHO classification, pathology and genetics tumors of haematopoietic and lymphoid tissues. IARC, Lyon, France
4. Tbakhi A, Edinger M, Myles J, Pohlman B, Tubbs RR (1996) Flow cytometric immunophenotyping of non-Hodgkin's lymphoma and related disorders. Cytometry **25**:113–124
5. Weir EG, Borowitz MJ (2001) Flow cytometry in the diagnosis of acute leukemia. Semin Hematol **38**:124–138

6. Fukushima PI, Nguyen PK, O'Grady P, Stetler-Stevenson M (1996) Flow cytometric analysis of kappa and lambda light chain expression. Commun Clin Cytometry, **26**:243–252

7. Li S, Eshleman JR, Borowitz MJ (2002) Lack of surface immunoglobulin light chain expression by flow cytometric immunophenotyping can help diagnose peripheral B cell lymphoma. Am J Clin Pathol **118**:229–234

8. Kuchnio M, Sausville EA, Jaffe ES, Greiner T, Foss FM, McClanahan J, Fukushima P, Stetler-Stevenson MA (1994) Flow cytometric detection of neoplastic T cells in patients with mycosis fungoides based upon levels of T-cell receptor expression. Am J Clin Pathol **102**:856–860

9. Edelman J, Meyerson HJ (2000) Diminished CD3 expression is useful for detecting and enumerating Sezary cells. Am J Clin Pathol **114**:467–477

10. Gorczyca W, Weisberger J, Liu Z, Tsang P, Hossein M, Wu CD, Dong Wong JYL, Tugulea S, Dee S, Melamed MR, Darzynkiewicz Z (2002) An approach to diagnosis of T-cell lymphoproliferative disorders by flow cytometry. Cytometry (Clin Cytometry) **50**:177–190

11. van den Beemd RB, Boor PPC, van Lochem EG, Hop WCJ, Langerak AW, Wolvers-Tettero ILM, Hooijkaas H, van Dongen JJM (2000) Flow cytometric analysis of the V beta repertoire in healthy controls. Cytometry **40**(4):336–345

12. Lima M, Almeida J, Santos AH, dos Anjos Teixeira M, Alguero MC, Queiros ML, Balanzategui A, Justica B, Gonzalez M, San Miguel JF, Orfao A (2001) Immunophenotypic analysis of the TCR-V repertoire in 98 persistent expansions of CD3+/TCR large granular lymphocytes. Am J Pathol **159**:1861–1868

13. Weir EG, Borowitz MJ. (2001) Flow cytometry in the diagnosis of acute leukemia. Semin Hematol **38**:124–138

14. Borowitz MJ, Guenther KL, Shults KE, Stelzer GT (1993) Immunophenotyping of acute leukemia by flow cytometric analysis: use of CD45 and right angle light scatter to gate on leukemic blasts in three color analysis. Am J Clin Pathol **100**:534–540

15. Ranier R, Hodges I, Stelzer G (1995) CD45 gating correates with bone marrow differential. Cytometry **22**:139–145

16. Stetler-Stevenson M, Schrager JA (2006) Flow cytometry In: Keren DF, McCoy JP, CareyJL (eds), Clinical Diagnosis, 4th edn., ASCP, Chicago 129–167

17. Garratty G, Arndt PA (1999) Applications of Flow Cytofluorometry to Red Blood Cell Immunology. Cytometry **38**:259–267

18. Davis BH, Olsen S, Bigelow NC, Chen JC (1998) Detection of fetal red cells in fetomaternal hemorrhage using a fetal hemoglobin monoclonal antibody by flow cytometry. Transfusion **38**:749–756

19. Ault KA (2001) The clinical utility of flow cytometry in the study of platelets. Semin Hematol **38**:160–168

20. Davis B, Bigelow N (1999) Indirect immunoplatelet counting by flow cytometry as a reference method for platelet count calibration. Lab Mematol **5**:15–21

21. Tschoepe D, Schultheiss HP, Kolarov P, Schwippert B, Dannehl K, Nieuwenhuis HK, Kehrel B, Strauer B, Gries FA (1993) Platelet membrane activation markers are predictive for increased risk of acute ischemic events after PTCA. Circulation **88**:37–42

22. His ED (2000) Paroxysmal nocturnal hemaglobinuria testing by flow cytometry – Evaluation of the REDQUANT and CELLQUANT kits. AJCP **114**:798–806

23. Hernandez-Campo PM, Martin-Ayuso M, Almeida J, Lopez A, Orfao A (2002) Comparative analysis of different flow cytometry-based immunophenotypic methods for the analysis of CD59 and CD55 expression on major peripheral blood cell subsets. Cytometry **50**:191–201

24. Horsbugh T, Martin S, Robson AJ (2000) The application of flow cytometry to histocompatibility testing. Transplant Immunol **8**:3–15

25. Kerman RH, Gebel H, Bray R, Garcia C, Sahai R, Gibson H, Radovancevic B, Knight R, Katz S, VanBuren C, Kahan B. (2002) HLA antibody and donor reactivity define patients at risk for rejection or graft loss. Tissue Antigens 59:60–660

26. Bryan CF, McDonald SB, Baier KA, Luger AM, Aeder MI, Murillo D, Muruve NA, Nelson PW, Shield CF 3rd, Warady BA (2002) Flow cytometry beads rather than the antihuman globulin method should be used to detect HLA Class I IgG antibodies (PRA) in cadaveric renal regraft candidates. Clin Transpl 16:15–23

27. Davis BH, Olsen SH, Ahmad E, Bigelow NC (2006) Neutrophil CD64 is an improved indicator of infection or sepsis in Emergency department patients. Arch Pathol 130:654–661

28. Mandy F, Nicholson J, Autran B, Janossy G (2002) T-cell subset counting and the fight against AIDS: reflections over a 20-year struggle. Cytometry (Clin Cytometry) 50:39–45

29. Giorgi JV, Lyles RH, Matud JL, Yamashita TE, Mellors JW, Hultin LE, Jamieson BD, Margolick JB, Rinaldo Jr CR, Phair JP, Detels R. (2002) Predictive value of immunologic and virologic markers after long or short duration of HIV-1 infection. J Acq Imm Def Dis 29:346–355

30. O'Gorman MR, Scholl PR (2002) Role of flow cytometry in the diagnostic evaluation of primary immunodeficiency disease. Clin Appl Immunol Rev 2:321–335.

31. Bleesing JJH. (2003) Autoimmune lymphoproliferative syndrome (ALPS). Curr Pharm Design 9:265–278

32. Ebo DG, Sainte-Laudy J, Bridts CH, Mertens CH, Hagendorens MM, Schuerwegh AJ, De Clerk LS, Stevens WJ (2006) Flow-assisted allergy diagnosis: current and future perspectives. Allergy 61:1028–1039

33. Bienvenu J, Monneret G, Fabien N, Revillard JP. (2000) The clinical usefulness of the measurement of cytokines. Clin Chem Lab Med 38:267–285

34. Tricot G, Jagannath S, Vesole D, Nelson J, Tindle S, Miller L, Cheson B, Crowley J, Bariogi B (1995) Peripheral blood stem cell transplants for multiple myeloma: identification of favorable variables for rapid engraftment in 225 patients. Blood 85:588–596

35. Weaver CH, Hazelton B, Birch R, Palmer P, Allen C, Schwartzberg L, West W (1995) An analysis of engraftement kinetics as a function of the CD34 content of peripheral blood progenitor cell collections in 692 patients after the administration of myeloablative chemotherapy. Blood 86:3961–3969

36. Sutherland DR, Keating A, Nayar R, Anania S, Stewart AK (1994) Sensitive detection and enumeration of CD34+ cells in peripheral blood and cord blood by flow cytometry. Exp Hematol 22:1003–1010

37. Gratama JW, Orfao A, Barnett D, Brando B, Huber A, Janossy G, Johnsen HE, Keeney M, Marti GE, Preijers F, Rothe G, Serke S, Sutherland DR, Van der Schoot CE, Schmitz G, Papa S (1998) Flow cytometric enumeration of CD34(+) hematopoietic stem and progenitor cells. Cytometry 34:128–142

38. Sutherland DR, Anderson L, Keeney M, Nayar R, Chin-Yee I (1996) The ISHAGE guidelines for CD34 cell determination by flow cytometry. J Hematother 5:213–226

39. Barnett D, Granger V, Kraan J, Whitby L, Reilly JT, Papa S, Gratama JW (2000) Reduction of intra and interlaboratory variation in CD34 positive stem cell enumeration by the use of stable test material, standard protocols and targeted training. Br J Haematol 108:784–792

40. Goddard G, Martin JC, Naivar M, Goodwin PM, Graves SW, Habbersett R, Nolan JP, Jett JH (2006) Single particle high resolution spectral analysis flow cytometer. Cytometry 69A:842–851

58

Immunomicroscopy

Constance Oliver

1. Introduction

Immunomicroscopy is widely employed to localize in situ various components of cells and tissues in both normal and pathological situations (*1–4*). The method is based on the extremely sensitive interaction of a specific antibody (immunoglobulin) with its antigen. An antibody binds specifically only to a small site on the antigen, called an epitope. An epitope usually consists of one to six monosaccharides or five to eight amino acids. The epitope recognized by a specific antibody may consist of a linear primary sequence of a protein or it may be dependent on the three-dimensional conformation of the antigen. Although the antibodies most commonly used are against proteins, antibodies can be raised against any cellular component including nucleic acids, lipids, and carbohydrates. Today there is a wide variety of antibodies available commercially. The supplier of an antibody against a particular antigen can be located by searching the scientific literature, searching the world wide web either by using a search engine such as Google and Lycos or through a search engine linked to a commercial site such as Abcam's World's Antibody Gateway (www.abcam. com), by searching a site dedicated to immunohistochemisty such as ICH World (www.ichworld.com) or by searching Linscott's Directory of Immunological and Biological Reagents (www.linscottsdirectory.com). Alternatively, antibodies can be obtained from a friend or a colleague or produced in the laboratory. However, whatever the source, the antibodies used for immunocytochemistry should be of the highest purity available to avoid unwanted background and cross reactivity with other molecules. There is no universal protocol for immunostaining that will apply to all samples in every situation. The exact conditions of immunostaining will have to be empirically developed by the user.

2. Antibodies

Immunoglobulins are glycoproteins that may be divided into five major classes whose molecular weight and principle characteristics are given in **Table 58.1**. IgG, which composes approx 75% of the immunoglobulins in human serum,

From: *Molecular Biomethods Handbook, 2nd Edition.*
Edited by: J. M. Walker and R. Rapley © Humana Press, Totowa, NJ

Table 58.1. The molecular weighs and principle characteristics of each of the five major classes of immunoglobulins are given.

Immunoglobulin class	Subclass	Heavy chain	Light chain	Molecular weight	Characteristics
IgA	IgA$_1$	α1	λ or κ	100,000	Primary immunoglobulin in
	IgA$_2$	α2		–600,00	mucosal secretions
IgD		δ	λ or κ	150,000	Present on surface of circulating B cells
IgE		ε	λ or κ	150,000	Bound to surface of basophils and mast cells
IgG	IgG$_1$	γ1	λ or κ	150,000	Major immunoglobulin present in serum
	IgG$_{2a}$	γ2			
	IgG$_{2b}$	γ2			
	IgG$_3$	γ3			
	IgG$_4$	γ4			
IgM	μ		λ or κ	970,000	Pentameric, Largely confined to intravascular pool

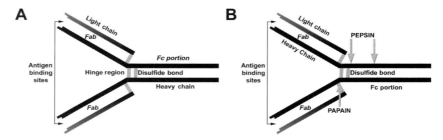

Fig. 58.1. A schematic diagram of an IgG molecule is shown in **A**. The cleavage sites for pepsin and papain are shown in **B**

is most commonly used for immunostaining. IgG can further be divided into subclasses and in humans there are four different subclasses. Although IgM may also be used for immunostaining, because of its high molecular weight, it does not readily penetrate cells and tissues. IgG (**Fig. 58.1A**) is monomeric and is composed of two heavy chains and two light chains. Each molecule has two antigen binding sites. The whole IgG molecule can be used for immunostaining or it can be enzymatically digested into smaller fragments (**Fig. 58.1B**). Pepsin cleaves the IgG molecule behind the disulfide bridges linking the Fc portions of the two heavy chains as well as in the middle of the Fc portion, producing one F(ab)'$_2$ fragment and one or more fragments from the Fc portion. In contrast papain cleaves the IgG molecule before the disulfide bridges linking the Fc portions of the two heavy chains producing two Fab fragments, leaving the Fc portion relatively intact depending on the time of incubation with the enzyme. Kits are available commercially that facilitate the production of IgG fragments.

Antibodies are produced by B lymphocytes. Each B cell produces one type of antibody directed against a single epitope of an antigen. When animals are immunized with a given antigen, multiple clones of B cells are activated to produce antibodies to various epitopes of the antigen. This polyclonal mixture

Table 58.2. A comparison between the characteristics of polyclonal, monoclonal and pooled monoclonal antibodies is shown.

	Polyclonal antibodies	**Monoclonal antibodies**	**Pooled monoclonal**
Signal Strength	Excellent	Antibody dependent (poor to excellent)	Excellent
Specificity	Usually good, but may give some background	Excellent	Excellent
Good Features	Stable, multivalent interactions	Specificity unlimited supply	Stable, multivalent interactions
Bad Features	Non renewable background	Need high-affinity	Availability

of antibodies in the serum may then recognize a variety of epitopes on a given antigen. Monoclonal antibodies are produced by fusing a single B lymphocyte with an immortal cell. The usual method is to fuse the B cells from the spleen of an immunized animal with a myeloma cell line thus producing hybridomas. The hybridomas are then cloned with the result that all antibodies produced by a given clone recognize the same epitope on the antigen. Both polyclonal and monoclonal antibodies may be used for immunostaining. The advantages and disadvantages of each are given in **Table 58.2**.

3. Immunostaining

The methods used for immunostaining can be divided into direct and indirect methods (**Fig. 58.2**). In the direct methods, the detection agent is directly coupled to the antibody raised against a specific antigen (primary antibody),

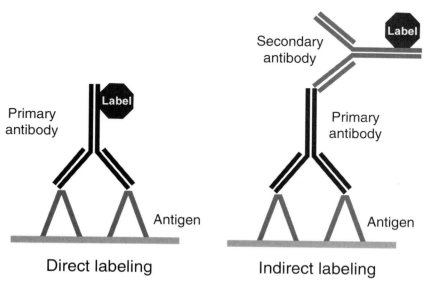

Fig. 58.2. For direct labeling, the label is conjugated to the primary antibody. In indirect labeling the marker is linked to the secondary antibody

whereas in the indirect methods the detection agent is linked to an antibody (secondary antibody) directed against IgG of the same species as the primary antibody. There are three types of markers that can be used in immunostaining, fluorescent, enzymatic, and particulate. Probably the most widely used, especially since the advent of confocal microscopy, are the fluorescent labels. There are a host of flurochromes, in almost every color imaginable, for use in immunostaining. However, the most commonly used fluorochromes are still the green emitting fluorescein isothiocyanate (FITC) and Alexa® 488 (Invitrogen, Molecular Probes, Carlsbad, CA) as well as the red emitting Rodamine, Texas Red, and Alexa® 594 (Invitrogen, Molecular Probes). Horseradish peroxidase (HRP) and alkaline phosphatase are the enzymatic markers most widely used. They are useful for bright field microscopy to immunolabel paraffin or plastic embedded tissues. In the past, the particulate labels such as hemocyanin or colloidal gold were normally used for electron microscopy. However, the recent availability of Q-dot® nanocrystals (Invitrogen, Molecular Probes), small, intensely fluorescent, semiconductor crystals, has made it possible to use the same probe for fluorescence microscopy as well as electron microscopy.

3.1. General Protocol

Regardless of the type of specimen, tissue blocks, cultured cells, etc, the principle steps in immunostaining are the same. The samples may be fixed and embedded in paraffin or a plastic histological resin after fixation. The paraffin is removed with xylene and a graded series of alcohols before immunostaining. Immunostaining of resin embedded sections may be improved if the sections are treated with xylene for 5–15 min before immunostaining. Material for frozen sections can be embedded in an appropriate cryo-embedding medium either before or after fixation. Tissue sections are then mounted on glass slides before use, or thicker sections are used as free floating sections. Tissue culture cells can be grown on glass coverslips or in chamber slides. However the samples are prepared, once immunostaining has begun, the samples should never be allowed to dry. The samples should be washed between each step. It is not necessary to wash between blocking and incubating with the primary antibody. The sample should be washed in buffer (PBS, pH7.0–7.4, for example) five times over 30 min between the primary and secondary antibodies and at least ten times before mounting the samples. An abbreviated generalized method for indirect labeling is outlined below. For direct labeling, the marker is conjugated directly to the primary antibody and incubation with a secondary antibody (Step 7) is omitted.

3.1.1. Indirect Immunostaining Method

1. Fix.
2. Antigen retrieval.
3. Quench.
4. Permeabilize (if necessary).
5. Block.
6. Incubate with primary antibody.
7. Incubate with labeled secondary antibody.
8. Develop (for enzymatic markers).
9. Mount and examine.

3.2. Fixation

Proper preservation of specimens for immunomicroscopy is one of the most critical aspects of the procedure. In most instances, antigen preservation must be balanced with structural preservation of the sample. For immunomicroscopy, samples are most frequently used unfixed or fixed with organic solvents that precipitate proteins such as acetone and methanol, or fixed with cross-linking agents such as formaldehyde. Glutaraldehyde should not be used for immunofluorescence since it is autofluorescent. Nonfixed frozen sections are commonly used for tissue blocks or the frozen sections may be fixed after they are placed on the slides. The choice of fixative depends largely on the antigen. Some antigens are extremely sensitive to any type of fixation, others will retain their antigenicity with one type of fixative (methanol for example) and lose it with another type (formaldehyde for instance), whereas some antigens retain their antigenicity with any type of fixation. The length of time a sample is fixed can also affect the ability to detect that antigen by immunostaining. Generally, the shorter the fixation, the better the antigenicity is retained. For tissue blocks fixation for up to 24 h in 2–4% formaldehyde in Dulbecco's phosphate buffered saline (PBS) with (100 mg anhydrous calcium chloride, 200 mg potassium chloride, 200 mg monobasic potassium phosphate, 100 mg magnesium chloride • 6 H_2O, 8 g sodium chloride, and 2.16 g dibasic sodium phosphate • 7 H_2O; bring volume to 1 L with deionized glass-distilled (or equivalent) water) or without Ca++ and Mg++ may be necessary for good structural preservation. Although for cells, 15–30 min in 2% formaldehyde diluted in Dulbecco's PBS with or without Ca++ and Mg++ is usually sufficient. Cytospin preparations or cultured cells grown on coverslips may also be fixed in cold (−20°C) methanol or acetone for 2–5 min on ice. The purity of the reagents used for fixation is also of extreme importance. Formaldehyde is not the same as the formalin found in most pathology laboratories. Commercial grade formalin is a saturated solution of formaldehyde in water with another solvent, most commonly methanol. Formalin is typically 37% formaldehyde by weight (40% by volume), 6–13% methanol, and the remainder water. The formaldehyde acts by cross-linking the amino groups on proteins while the methanol penetrates tissue rapidly and precipitates proteins. Although formalin can be used to fix tissue blocks, it may contain impurities that can interfere with immunostaining and it may also destroy the antigenicity of sensitive antigens. A better choice is a freshly prepared solution of paraformaldehyde or commercially available ampoules of purified formaldehyde solution that are packed under nitrogen. To prepare an 8% solution of paraformaldehyde, in a fume hood, add 2 g of paraformaldehyde (trioxymethylene) powder to 25 ml of deionized glass-distilled (or the equivalent) water. With constant stirring, heat the solution to 60–70°C. Once the solution has reached this temperature, continue stirring for 15 min. To clear the solution, which will be milky, add one to two drops of 1N NaOH, with stirring until the solution clears. A slight milkiness may remain. Cool and filter through Whatman No. 1 filter paper. This solution should be used the same day it is prepared. Another alternative that is commonly used for cells is to fix the cells in 2% formaldehyde in cold methanol instead of PBS. This provides for rapid penetration of the fixative and is generally a fairly gentle fixative.

Another alternative method of fixation is microwave fixation. The exact mechanism behind microwave fixation is unknown, it is thought to be a combination of heat generated and increased molecular movement *(5)* generated by microwaves. The molecular movement may also help the penetration of chemicals into biological samples. The major advantages of microwave fixation are its speed and the ability to use reduced concentrations of fixatives *(6–8)*.

3.3. Antigen Retrieval

During the process of preparing samples for immunomiroscopy, especially paraffin embedded samples, antigenic sites may be masked, denatured or destroyed. Depending on the antigen and the sample, it may be necessary to employ an antigen retrieval step. Antigen retrieval presumably breaks the formaldehyde-induced methylene cross-links formed during fixation. Two types of methods are commonly used. One involves the use of proteolytic enzymes (proteolytic induced epitope retrieval, PIER), while the other employs heat treatment (heat induced epitope retrieval, HIER). For proteolytic induced epitope retrieval, proteinase K, trypsin, pepsin, and pronase may all be used. The concentration of the enzyme as well as the time of digestion must be carefully controlled to unmask the epitope without destroying the antigen itself. In heat induced epitope retrieval, a microwave oven, pressure cooker, autoclave, water bath, and steamer may all be used to heat the samples. Citrate buffer, pH 6.0, is the most popular retrieval solution and is suitable for most antibody applications. Tris-EDTA, pH 9.0 and EDTA, pH 8.0 are also widely used as retrieval solutions. Generally, heating the sample for 20 min and cooling for an additional 20 min is sufficient for antigen retrieval. As with PIER, the exact conditions must be determined for each sample.

3.4. Quenching

Following aldehyde fixation, free aldehyde groups may be present in the sample. If these groups are not blocked they can bind to the primary antibody increasing the background or giving a false positive during labeling. The compounds used for quenching all have an amino group that can bind to the free aldehyde present after fixation. Glycine, 100 mM, ammonium chloride, 50 mM, and one percent sodium borohydride may all be used. However, glycine is the gentlest on the tissue and because it is a small molecule penetrates samples rapidly. The quenching agent can be added to PBS (8,0 g NaCl, 0,2 g KCl, 0,2 g KH_2PO_4, 2,16 g Na_2HPO_4, bring to 1 L with glass distilled or other high quality water and adjust pH to 7.4) and used for the last rinse before the blocking step. The time necessary to quench a sample depends on the size of the sample. For tissue culture cells, 2–5 min is sufficient although for large tissue blocks quenching for up to 20 min with one or more changes of the quenching solution may be necessary.

3.5. Permeablization

If an antigen is located intracellularly, it may be necessary to use an additional step to permeabilize the sample, especially if the sample has been fixed with an aldehyde fixative. Two general classes of permeablizing agents, organic solvents and detergents are commonly used. The organic solvents such as methanol and acetone dissolve lipids from cell membranes making them permeable to antibodies. Additionally, since the organic solvents also coagulate proteins, they can be used to fix and permeabilized cells at the same time (see Section 3.2). However, these solvents may also extract lipidic antigens or lipid associated antigens from cells. Frequently, paraffin embedded tissues do not need permeabilization since they are exposed to organic solvents during embedding and preparation of sections for immunostaining but they may need an antigen retrieval step (see Section 3.3) before immunolableing.

The other large group of reagents used for permeablization is detergents. The most widely used detergent, especially for cultured cells is saponin (0.01% in PBS). Saponin is a plant glycoside that interacts with membrane cholesterol, removing it and leaving ~100 Å holes in the membrane *(9)*. When antibodies are in solution with saponin, they may be incorporated into saponin/cholesterol micelles that facilitates their entry into the cells. Saponin permeabilization is not effective on cholesterol-poor membranes such as mitochondrial membranes and the nuclear envelope *(10)*. Triton X-100 (0.1–1% in PBS) and Tween 20 (0.1%), nonionic detergents, are also commonly used to permeabilize cells and tissues. These detergents contain uncharged, hydrophilic head groups of polyoxyethylene moieties *(11)*. These detergents have the disadvantage that they are nonselective in nature and may extract proteins along with the lipids, resulting in a false negative during immunostaining. Depending on the antigen, a combination of permeabilizing agents may be preferable *(10)*.

3.6. Blocking

The purpose of the blocking is to prevent the primary and secondary antibodies from binding nonspecifically through hydrophobic interaction to the sample, thus increasing the background (**Fig. 58.3**). This step is generally most effective when done immediately before immunostaining with the primary antibody. The affinity of the primary antibody for its antigen allows it to displace the blocking protein, which has a low affinity for the antigen, and bind to the antigen. The most commonly used agent for blocking is 1–2% bovine serum albumin (BSA), Fraction V or essentially globulin free in PBS. BSA blocks nonspecific hydrophobic interactions between the antibodies and the sample. Nonfat dry milk *(12)* or casein may also be used as blocking agents. Nonfat dry milk should be used with care as the presence of lactoperoxidase in some brands of nonfat dry milk may actually increase the background when used with peroxidase based methods. However, when casein is used during blocking, as well as being included in the buffers for all subsequent steps, it may reduce background staining when compared to normal swine and sheep sera.

It may also be necessary to block IgG receptors on the cell surface to reduce nonspecific binding. Normal serum (1%), such as goat serum, or purified IgG (5 µg/ml) are commonly used for this purpose. IgG is preferable to serum since serum may contain proteins that will either interfere with the primary antibody binding or bind the primary antibody nonspecifically. Caution should be taken is selecting the serum or IgG to use for blocking. The reagent chosen for blocking IgG receptors should be from a species unrelated to the primary antibody, and preferably from the same species as the secondary antibody. For example, if the primary antibody is a mouse IgG and the secondary antibody is anti-mouse IgG made in donkey, the ideal blocking agent in this case would be normal donkey IgG.

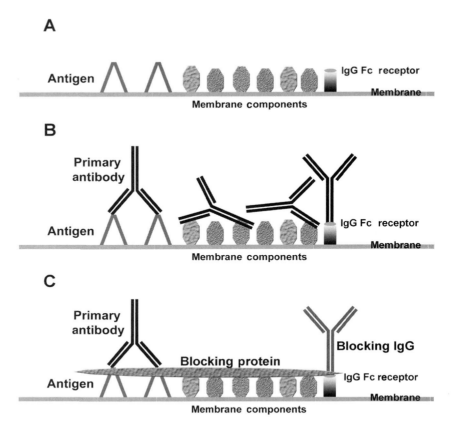

Fig. 58.3. Blocking solutions help prevent nonspecific binding of the primary antibody. **A.** In addition to the antigen of interest, cell membranes are composed of many types of proteins and lipids and may contain IgG receptors. **B.** If the sample is not blocked, the primary antibody will bind to its antigen, but will also bind nonspecifically to other membrane components, including IgG receptors. **C.** Proper blocking of a sample prevents nonspecific binding of the primary antibody. The blocking protein, such as BSA prevents binding to membrane components and the use of an unrelated IgG to block IgG receptors prevents the nonspecific binding of the primary antibody to these receptors

Another commercially available blocking agent, Image-iT® FX signal enhancer, from Invitrogen Molecular Probes, has also been shown to be effective in lowering the background in fluorescently stained material when used after fixation and permeabilization but before applying the primary antibody. It is particularly useful for reducing background fluorescence in tissue sections.

3.7. Incubation with Primary Antibody

As stated in the introduction, the most critical element for good immunostaining is the primary antibody. It should be of the highest specificity, purity, affinity, and avidity possible. In most instances, the primary antibody is not conjugated to a label. It may however be biotinylated. The primary antibody is diluted in a suitable buffer such as PBS pH 7.0–7.4. For monoclonal antibodies a concentration of 1–5 µg/ml is generally a good starting concentration. For some monoclonal antibodies it may be necessary to use concentrations as high as 20–30 µg. For polyclonal antibodies it is more common to make dilutions of the stock preparation ranging from 1:20 to 1:500. Depending on the sample, the primary antibody may be diluted in PBS, in PBS + 1% BSA or in PBS + 1% BSA containing 0.01% saponin. The appropriate concentration of the primary antibody as well as the diluent will need to be determined empirically for each sample. However, as shown in **Fig. 58.4**, as the concentration of the primary antibody increases, the fluorescence intensity should increase until a plateau is reached. After this point, increasing the antibody concentration will not increase the specific labeling, but will increase the background.

Samples can be incubated as free-floating sections, attached to slides or to coverslips. The antibody solution is placed as a drop on top of tissue sections or on cells adhered to coverslips. To constrain the antibody solution on slides, it is useful to encircle the tissue on the slides with a hydrophobic barrier. This can easily be accomplished by the use of a commercially available PAP pen. These pens are used to draw a fine line of hydrophobic film around tissue sections. Eleven to 13 mm diameter coverslips can be place in the bottom of the wells of a 24-well plate for processing. For most applications samples can be incubated for 1 h at room temperature. Some antigens and plastic embedded material may give better results if incubated at 37°C. For labeling of cell surface antigens on tissue culture cells, unfixed cells can be incubated at 4°C to prevent endocytosis of the antigen–antibody complex. For free floating sections or some intracellular antigens, dilutions of 1:1,000 to 1:5,000 of the primary antibody and incubation overnight at 4°C may give the best results. The samples should never be allowed to dry and gentle rocking during incubation will ensure even staining of the sample.

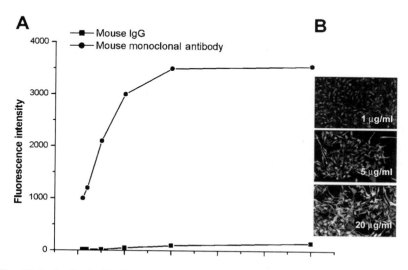

Fig. 58.4. Antibody binding curve. **A.** As the concentration of the specific mouse monoclonal antibody increases, the fluorescence intensity increases until a plateau is reached at 20 µg/ml. **B.** The increase in fluorescence seen with the binding curve is also reflecting in the intensity of the immunostaining

3.8. Incubation with Secondary Antibody

After extensive washing, the sample is then incubated in the secondary anti-body. This antibody is normally conjugated to a fluorescent or enzymatic label. If the primary antibody was biotinylated, streptavidin conjugated with an appropriate label is substituted for the secondary antibody. Care must also be taken in choosing a secondary antibody. The secondary antibody must bind to the primary antibody with high affinity and should be minimally cross reactive with immunoglobulins from other species (Jackson ImmunoResearch, Fort Washington, PA, www.jacksonimmuno.com). In choosing a secondary antibody, the species of the antigen is not important. What is important is the species that the primary antibody was raised in. For example, if the primary antibody was made in mouse, the secondary antibody would be against mouse IgG or if the primary antibody was raised in rabbit the secondary antibody would be against rabbit IgG. Also, to avoid nonspecific binding of the Fc por-tion of the secondary antibody to IgG Fc receptors, F(ab')$_2$ fragments can be used instead of the whole antibody.

The secondary antibody may be diluted in the same buffer used for the pri-mary antibody with or without BSA. Dilutions can range from 1:20 to 1:100 or greater depending on the secondary antibody. For many secondary antibodies, incubation for 30 min at room temperature with the secondary antibody diluted 1:50 gives good immunostaining.

3.9. Detection Systems for Immunolabeling

The two most common detection system used for immunolabeling are fluorescent labels and enzymatic labels. Particulate labels, such as colloidal gold, are used primarily for electron microscopy. Secondary antibodies conjugated to a wide range of fluorescent and enzymatic labels are com-mercially available.

3.9.1. Fluorescent Labels

With the advent first of epifluoresence and later confocal microscopes, fluo-rescently labeled antibodies became widely used as labels for immunostaining. Fluorescence is the property of some molecules to absorb light at a particular wavelength and to then emit light of longer wavelength. Modern fluorescence microscopes and laser scanning confocal microscopes take advantage of the fluorescent properties of these molecules to localize them in biological sam-ples. Theses microscopes use a combination of excitation and emission barrier filters to excite and visualize the various fluorescent probes. In choosing a flu-orescent label, the available microscope filter sets are usually the determining factor. The filter sets on most microscopes are best matched with rhodamine or fluorescein. Texas Red® (Invitrogen, Molecular Probes) may also be used with a rhodamine filter set. FITC, Texas Red, and their Alexa Fluor® (Invitrogen, Molecular Probes) equivalents Alexa Fluor 488 and Alexa Fluor 594 are probably the most frequently used labels. **Table 58.3** gives the excitation and emission wavelengths for some of the commonly used fluorescent probes. More extensive lists can be found on the web sites of suppliers or micro-scope manufacturers. Other probes, such as Qdot ® nanocrystals (Invitrogen, Molecular Probes) use the same excitation wave length, but the emission wave length is dependent on the size of the crystal Because of the autofluorescence

Table 58.3. Spectra of commonly used fluorescent markers.

Fluorochrome	Excitation max (nm)	Emission max (nm)
Cascade Blue	396	410
Alexa Fluor 350	346	442
Cy2	489	506
Oregon Green 488	490	514
Fluorescein	494	519
Alexa Fluor 488	495	519
Alexa Fluor 430	433	539
Alexa Fluor 532	532	554
Cy3	550	570
Rhodamine[3]	547	572
Alexa Fluor 546	556	573
Cy3.5	581	596
Alexa Fluor 568	578	603
Texas Red	589	615
Alexa Fluor 594	590	617
Alexa Fluor 633	632	647
Cy5	649	670
Alexa Fluor 660	663	690
Cy5.5	675	694

Cy cyanine, *FITC* fluorescein isothiocyanate, *TRITC* tetramethyl rhodamine isothiocyanate.

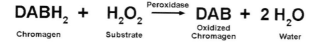

Fig. 58.5. Enzymatic reaction for peroxidase

of paraffin and plastic resins, fluorescence immunomicroscopy is most suited to frozen sections, cultured cells, or isolated cell preparations.

3.9.2. Enzymatic Labels

The other large class of labels that may be conjugated to antibodies are the enzymatic labels such as peroxidase and alkaline phosphatase. The enzymatic labels are well suited to paraffin and resin embedded material. In this staining method the enzyme conjugated to the antibody reacts with its substrate producing a product that results in the conversion of a colorless chromagen to a colored end product. They have the disadvantage that they can diffuse within the sample.

3.9.2.1. Peroxidase: Horseradish peroxidase (HRP, molecular weight 40 kDa) is isolated from the root of the horseradish plant (*Cochlearia armoracia*). It has an iron-containing heme group (hematin) at its active site, and in solution is brown in color. The basic enzymatic reaction for HRP, using DAB as the chromagen, is given in **Fig. 58.5**. Peroxide is the substrate and DAB (diaminobenzidine) is the chromagen. Oxidized DAB is dark brown in color and can be easily visualized in tissue sections. The oxidized DAB is insoluble in alcohol, and produces polymers that react with OsO_4, producing osmium black, which is highly insoluble and electron dense. The addition of metal salts, such as nickel or cobalt to the DAB reaction mixture will produce black to orange (nickel) or black (cobalt) reaction products. Because DAB is considered to be a carcinogen caution should be used when handling DAB. Owing to its carcinogenicity, alternative proprietary substrates, such as TrueBlue (Kirkegaard and Perry Laboratories, Gaithersburg, MD, www. kpl. com), have been developed. 3-amino-9-ethylcarbazole (AEC), which upon oxidation forms a rose-red end product, and 4-chloro-11 -naphthol (CN), which precipitates as a blue end product, may also be used as chromagens for peroxidase. However, like DAB both AEC and CN form alcohol soluble reaction products. Another disadvantage of peroxidase as a marker is the presence of endogenous peroxidase activity in tissues. If the endogenous activity is not blocked, false positives will occur. The most common method of blocking endogenous peroxidase activity is to use excess substrate, H_2O_2. The excess peroxide irreversably blocks the active site of the peroxidase, thus inhibiting it. 3% peroxide in methanol for 10–15 min is usually sufficient to block endogenous peroxidase. However, some tissues and antigens can be destroyed by high concentrations of peroxide and lower concentrations, 0.3%, and longer times, up to 1 h, may be necessary. The blocking can be done at any point in the immunostaining procedure up to the step where the samples are incubated for peroxidase. Depending on stability of the immunostaining and convenience endogenous peroxidase activity may be blocked right after the sections are rehydrated to water, or before the sections are incubated with either the primary or secondary antibody.

3.9.2.2. Alkaline Phosphatase: The other commonly used enzyme detection system is alkaline phosphatase. Alkaline phosphatase hydrolyzes naphthol phosphate esters (substrate) to phenolic compounds and phosphates. The phenols then couple to colorless diazonium salts (chromagen) to produce insoluble, colored azo dyes. Several different combinations of substrates and chromagens are available. Naphthol AS-MX phosphate can be used as a substrate in its acid form or as the sodium salt. Fast Red TR and Fast Blue BB, chromagens, produce a bright red or blue reaction product, respectively. Both reaction products are soluble in alcohol. New Fuchsin is also commonly used as a chromagen. It also gives a red reaction product, but unlike Fast Red TR and Fast Blue BB, the color produced by New Fuchsin is insoluble in alcohol and other organic solvents. The staining intensity of New Fuchsin is also greater than that of Fast Red TR or Fast Blue BB. Additional possible substrates include naphthol AS-BI phosphate, naphthol AS-TR phosphate and 5-bromo-4-chloro-3-indoxyl phosphate (BCIP). Other chromagens include Fast Red LB, Fast Garnet GBC, Nitro Blue Tetrazolium (NBT) and iodonitrotertrazolium Violet (INT). As with peroxidase endogenous alkaline phosphatase activity should be inhibited. This is generally accomplished by adding levamisole (1 mM) to the incubation solution. Levamisole will inhibit most endogenous alkaline phosphatase activity with the exception of intestinal alkaline phosphatase. Intestinal alkaline phosphatase is often inhibited by high temperature methods for antigen retrieval or may be inactivated with 20% aqueous acetic acid at 4°C (*13*).

3.10. Develop Enzymatic Markers

To be visualized the antibodies conjugated to enzymatic markers must be incubated in an appropriate substrate-chromagen solution. Especially for HRP there are a wide variety of kits and reagents available commercially. However, basic procedures for peroxidase and alkaline phosphatase are given below.

3.10.1. DAB-Substrate Solution for Peroxidase

After incubation with primary or secondary antibody conjugated to HRP, wash sample thoroughly (three times for 5 min each) and incubate in a DAB containing solution:

48 µl DAB - 3,3′diaminobenzidine (DAB) (Kirkegaard and Perry, Gaithersburg, MD)
1 ml PBS
20 µl 1% H_2O_2

Alternative Solution

10 mg DAB (Sigma-Aldrich, St. Louis, MO)
10 ml PBS
100 µl 30% H_2O_2
Filter before use

The solutions should be made just before use and the solutions protected from light. The sample may be incubated at room temperature, and the time of incubation is best monitored initially by using a microscope to observe the sample during incubation. Times may range from a 5–30 min. However, longer incubations generally increase the background staining. After staining, rinse samples in distilled water. Samples may be counterstained, but it is advisable to omit the counterstain until the immunostaining has been optimized.

3.10.2. New Fuchsin Substrate Solution for Alkaline Phosphatase

After incubation with primary or secondary antibody conjugated to alkaline phosphatase, wash samples thoroughly (three times for 5 min each) and incubate in a substrate solution containing a napthol phosphate ester (14):

Solution A: Mix 18 ml of 0.2M 2-amino-2-methyl-1, 3 propanediol (Merck, Whitehouse Station, NJ) with 50 ml 0.05 M Tris-HCl buffer, pH 9.7 and 600 mg sodium chloride. Add 28 mg levamisole (Sigma-Aldrich)

Solution B: Dissolve 35 mg naphthol AS-BI phosphate (Sigma-Aldrich) in 0.42 ml N,N-dimethylformamide

Solution C: In a **fume hood**, mix 0.14 ml 5% New Fuchsin (Sigma, 5 g in 100 ml 2 N HCl) with 0.35 ml of freshly prepared 4% sodium nitrite (Sigma, 40 mg in 1 ml distilled water). Stir for 60 s

Mix Solutions A and B, then add Solution C; adjust to pH 8.7 with HCl. Mix well and filter onto slides

Incubate for 10–20 min at room temperature

Rinse with distilled water

Samples may be counterstained at this point, but it is better to omit the counterstain until the immunostaining has been optimized.

3.11. Detecting Two Different Antigens in the Same Sample

It is often desirable or necessary to localize two different antigens in the same sample. Although the procedures for detecting two or more antigens in the same sample are essentially the same as those for detecting a single antigen, care must be taken that the antibodies used to detect one antigen do not interfere with the ability to immunolabel the second antigen. For direct staining the two primary antibodies may be conjugated to different labels, i.e., FITC and Texas Red or HRP and alkaline phosphatase. Alternatively, one primary antibody can be conjugated to a fluorescent or enzymatic marker and the other to biotin. If an indirect immunostaining method is to be used, the two primary antibodies should be from different species, i.e., mouse and rabbit. Ideally, the two primary antibodies can be mixed and applied in the same solution. Methods exist to use indirect labeling with primary antibodies from the same species*(15–18)*. If an indirect method is being used, the secondary antibodies can also be mixed and applied at the same time. However, if the two antigens are in close proximity, one primary antibody may sterically hinder the binding of the second primary antibody. Before applying the primary or secondary antibodies together, the immunostaining conditions should be optimized for each antigen separately. Once this is done, the sample should be immunstained first for antigen A followed by staining for antigen B. In another sample antigen B should be immunolabed first followed by labeling for antigen A. If the immunolabling is independent of the order in which the antigens are stained then the antibodies can be mixed, if not a procedure similar to step B will need to be followed. The details of optimizing a double immunostaining are outlined in **Fig. 58.6**.

Another factor to consider in double staining is that the two labels will be able to be distinguished in the final preparation. This is usually easier with fluorescent labels. Many suppliers of fluorescently conjugated secondary antibodies and microscope manufactures now have tools on their web sites to assist in selecting an appropriate combination of fluorescent markers. In choosing markers, there should be little to no overlap in their emission spectra to avoid and bleed-through of one label into the image of the other.

3.12. Mount and Examine Sample

The final step in any immunostaining procedure is to mount the preparation and examine it. Before mounting, fluorescent samples may be counterstained with DAPI (4′, 6-diamidino-2-phenylindole; 100 ng/ml), which binds tightly to DNA. When DAPI is bound to double-stranded DNA its absorption maximum is 358 nm and its emission maximum is 461 nm and the nuclei appear blue. DAPI also binds to RNA, but the fluorescence is much weaker and its emission shifts to ~400 nm. For samples that have used a fluorescent label it is advisable to use a mounting medium that contains and antifade agent. There are many excellent mounting mediums commercially available. Some do not harden to make permanent preparations, but the coverslips can be sealed to the slides to make semipermanent preparation by ringing the coverslips with antiallergic fingernail polish that does not contain formaldehyde. Formaldehyde containing fingernail polishes may autofluoresce.

For immunostained preparation where the label was an enzyme, the choice of the mounting medium will depend on the solubility of the final reaction product. If the reaction product is soluble in organic solvents, as for example when

A

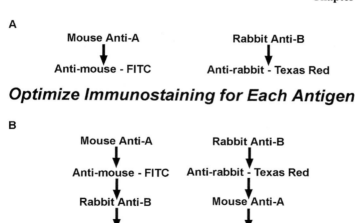

Mouse Anti-A　　　　　　　**Rabbit Anti-B**

Anti-mouse - FITC　　　　**Anti-rabbit - Texas Red**

Optimize Immunostaining for Each Antigen

B

Mouse Anti-A　　　　**Rabbit Anti-B**

Anti-mouse - FITC　　**Anti-rabbit - Texas Red**

Rabbit Anti-B　　　　　**Mouse Anti-A**

Anti-rabbit - Texas Red　　**Anti-mouse - FITC**

Determine Interference Between Antigens

C

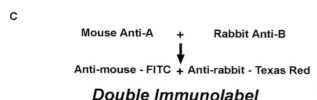

Mouse Anti-A　　+　　**Rabbit Anti-B**

Anti-mouse - FITC + **Anti-rabbit - Texas Red**

Double Immunolabel

Fig. 58.6. Optimization of immunostaing for two different antigens A and B using a primary antibody against antigen A made in mouse and a primary antibody against antigen B made in rabbit. **A.** Immunostaining procedures need to be optimized for each antigen. The results of this immunostaining will serve as the standard for the subsequent steps. **B.** To confirm that detection of one antigen does not interfere with the detection of the other antigen two separate immunostaining protocols are followed. In one, antigen A is immunolabed followed by immunolabeling for antigen B. In the other protocol, the order is reversed and antigen B is immunolabeled first, followed by immunolabeling antigen A. **C.** If there are no differences in the immunolabeling observed with the two protocols used in B when compared to A, then the primary antibodies may be combined and used in a single step and the same may be done for the secondary antibodies. These results should be compared with the results obtained in step A

AEC is used as the chromagen for peroxidase reactions or Fast Red TR is used as the chromagen for alkaline reactions, an aqueous mounting medium must be used. However, when the final reaction product is insoluble in organic solvents then a solvent based mounting medium such as Permount may be used.

3.13. Controls

In any immunohistochemical procedure proper controls are essential. Every new primary antibody should be characterized before beginning immunostaining. If the antibody is suitable for Western blotting, this will confirm the specificity of the antibody. A binding curve, using serial dilutions of the antibody should also be done to confirm that the staining is not caused by nonspecific binding to the cell surface and to determine the optimum working concentration of a particular primary antibody. A negative control, where the primary antibody is omitted from the staining protocol should also be run. Another negative control is to substitute normal IgG from the same species as the primary antibody in place of the primary antibody. For example, if the primary antibody is a mouse monoclonal, mouse IgG would be used in place of the primary antibody. The antigen binding site of the antibody may also be blocked by adsorbing it with specific peptides or adsorbing it with the specific antigen, or tissue before use. In some cases, the antigen itself may be blocked with another primary antibody before staining.

References

1. Polak JM, Van Noorden S (2003) Introduction to immunocytochemistry, 3rd edn. Oxford, BIOS Scientific, pp 176
2. Larsson L-I (2000) Immunocytochemistry: theory and practice. Boca Raton, FL, CRC, pp 272
3. Renshaw S (2006) Immunohistochemistry. Methods Express Series, Oxfordshire, Scion, pp 250
4. Javois LC (1999) Immunocytochemical methods and protocols, 2nd edn. In: Walker JM (ed) Methods in molecular biology, Vol. 115. Humana, Totowa, pp 465
5. Leonard JB, Shepardson SP (1994) A comparison of heating modes in rapid fixation techniques for electron microscopy. J Histochem Cytochem 42(3):383–391
6. Jamur MC et al (1995) Microwave fixation improves antigenicity of glutaraldehyde sensitive antigens while preserving ultrastructural detail. J Histochem Cytochem 43:307–311
7. Boon ME, Kok LP (1994) Microwaves for immunohistochemistry. Micron 25(2):151–170
8. Login GR, Devorak AM (1994) Methods of microwave fixation for microscopy. A review of research and clinical applications: 1970–1992. Prog Histochem Cytochem 27(4):1–127
9. Seeman P, Cheng D, Iles GH (1973) Structure of membrane holes in osmotic and saponin hemolysis. J Cell Biol 56:519–527
10. Goldenthal KL et al (1983) Postfixation detergent treatment for immunofluorescence suppresses localization of some integral membrane proteins. J Histochem Cytochem 33(8):813–820
11. Bhairi SM (2001) Detergents, A guide to the properties and uses of detergents in biological systems. San Diego, CA, Calbiochem-Novabiochem Corporation, pp 41
12. Duhamel RC, Johnson DA (1985) Use of nonfat dry milk to block nonspecific nuclear and membrane staining by avidin conjugates. J Histochem Cytochem 33(7):711–714
13. Bulman AS, Heyderman E (1981) Alkaline phosphatase for immuno-cyto-chemical labelling: problems with endogenous enzyme activity. J Clin Pathol 34:1349–1351
14. Immunohistochemical staining methods, 4th edn, In: Key M (ed). Dako, Carpinteria, CA
15. Krenacs T, Uda H, Tanaka S, (1991) One-step double immunolabeling of mouse interdigitating reticular cells: simultaneous application of pre-formed complexes of monoclonal rat antibody M1-8 with horseradish peroxidase-linked anti-rat immunoglobulins and of monoclonal mouse anti-Ia antibody with alkaline phosphatase-coupled anti-mouse immunoglobulins. J Histochem Cytochem 39(12):1719–1723
16. Negoescu A et al (1994) F(ab) secondary antibodies: a general method for double immunolabeling with primary antisera from the same species. Efficiency control by chemiluminescence. J Histochem Cytochem 42(3):433–437

17. Shindler KS, Roth KA (1996) Double immunofluorescent staining using two unconjugated primary antisera raised in the same species. J Histochem Cytochem 44(11):1331–1335
18. Ino H (2004) Application of antigen retrieval by heating for double-label fluorescent immunohistochemistry with identical species-derived primary antibodies. J Histochem Cytochem 52(9):1209–1217

59

In Situ Hybridization

Ian A. Darby and Tim D. Hewitson

1. Introduction

Hybridization between complementary strands of nucleic acids is a fundamental technique in cell biology and is the basis of well-developed molecular biological techniques to detect mRNA or DNA sequences. The earliest uses of hybridization of complementary strands of DNA or RNA with a labeled probe were in the form of southern blots to detect specific sequences in DNA (*1*) and northern blots and dot blots to detect specific mRNA species in samples transferred to nitrocellulose filters (*2,3*). These techniques allowed detection of specific DNA or mRNA species with a high degree of sensitivity. Later, PCR and quantitative PCR improved the sensitivity of measuring and detecting specific mRNA species in tissue samples. However, in heterogeneous tissues, the information provided by techniques based on homogenization of the sample is quite limited. Immunohistochemistry provides very useful information on the presence of particular proteins but does not unequivocally show that genes are expressed in particular tissues or cells, because proteins can be absorbed, actively transported or sequestered in tissues distant from their site of manufacture. The development of the technique of in situ hybridization (ISH) therefore provides unique information concerning expression of genes in cells and tissues, particularly where there are heterogenous cell populations present in those tissues.

1.1. Background

Gall and Pardue (*4*) and John et al. (*5*) are credited with independently developing the technique of ISH in the late 1960's. The early studies using the ISH technique used partially purified cDNA probes to detect high-abundance mRNA transcripts such as globin or actin. Only later did purified cDNA probes show that a specific gene or gene product of interest could be detected by in situ hybridization. For example, Gall and Pardue (*4*) used a mixture of 28 S and 18 S ribosomal RNA as a probe. This probe, labeled with tritium, was used to detect extrachromosomal DNA in *Xenopus* oocytes. A number of studies also used labeled poly U sequence as a probe to detect poly A sequences in tissue

From: *Molecular Biomethods Handbook, 2nd Edition.*
Edited by: J. M. Walker and R. Rapley © Humana Press, Totowa, NJ

preparations. Jones et al. *(6)* studied labeling of poly A in squash preparations of *Rhynchosciara* salivary glands using a tritiated poly U probe. Capco and Jeffery *(7)* used a poly U probe to examine paraffin sections of embryos and detect poly A (mRNA). Similar studies were carried out on frozen sections of embryonic pancreas *(8)* and detected poly A (mRNA) in exocrine and endocrine pancreas. Early studies also used nonspecific probes to look for viral DNA in infected tissues, for example the study of Orth et al *(9)* detecting viral DNA in paraffin sections of fixed rabbit tissue. Later studies used partially purified probes, for example mRNA enriched in globin sequence to produce a cDNA probe to detect globin mRNA in liver with reasonable specificity *(10)*. Similarly, Pochet et al. *(11)* used an enriched source of prolactin mRNA to obtain a prolactin probe of reasonable purity and detect prolactin expression in the rat pituitary. The authors suggested in this case that the probe was approximately 80% prolactin cDNA.

The major advances in gene cloning meant that pure cDNA probes became available and several groups reported using in situ hybridization with specific sequences labeled as probes to detect expression of pro-opiomelanocortin *(12)*, calcitonin *(13)* actin *(14)* and albumin *(15)*. Many studies have followed because, with a huge number of genes, mRNA species and viral sequences being detected.

2. Methods

Not surprisingly the widespread application of ISH in a variety of cells and tissues, has led to the development of a plethora of protocols. In this section we describe the sequential steps in this process: fixation and processing, pretreatment, probe types, labeling and detection, hybridization, controls and analysis.

2.1. Sample Fixation and Processing

A key limiting step in ISH is the retention and availability of the tissue mRNA. Fixation of tissue is therefore critically important. The process of fixation should cross-link the cell matrix, preserving the RNA intact and in its original location, and maintain cell and tissue architecture. Most investigators therefore routinely use 4% paraformaldehyde. Early comparative studies by Lawrence & Singer *(16)* indicated that cross-linking fixatives such as paraformaldehyde and glutaraldehyde are preferable to precipitating fixatives (e.g., Methyl Carnoy's, Bouin's, and ethanol). However enzyme digestion of samples was more necessary after glutaraldehyde fixation. It is however, worth noting that neutral buffered formalin has been used with good results *(17)* and has the added advantage of being a routine fixative for tissue in pathology laboratories. Hence, archival tissue specimens are often suitable for in situ hybridization studies, with comparisons then being possible across large numbers of clinical specimens.

Snap frozen tissue obviates the need for fixation although it produces much poorer morphology, particularly in tissues such as the kidney. Fixation of samples after sectioning is generally used in the case of frozen sections but morphology remains compromised. However, frozen sections do produce maximal labeling because there is little loss of mRNA and the lesser degree of cross-linking makes the mRNA more accessible (**Fig. 59.1**).

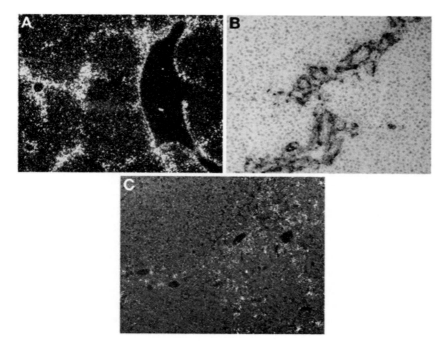

Fig. 59.1. Autoradiographs of liver labeled for procollagen I using a riboprobe. Although the morphology is inferior, the hybridization signal for (**A**, **B**) frozen sections is much stronger that that seen in (**C**) paraffin embedded tissue from the same organ

In each case, microscope slides are used as the substrate for hybridization reaction. ISH protocols involve extensive washes in stringent and heated solutions with agitation. Maintaining adhesion of sections and cell preparations on microscope slides is therefore an underlying problem. A number of adhesives have been used including gelatin, poly-l-lysine and aminopropyltriethoxysilane (APES). APES has the advantage of bonding sections to slides and has become the recommended treatment *(18)*.

2.2. Pretreatments

Pretreatment of tissue sections, cells or whole-mounts has generally been carried out because fixation of tissue samples or cells results in protein cross-linking delaying or inhibiting penetration of the probe into the sample. The earliest pretreatment used was proteinase digestion using either proteinase K or pronase E to digest proteins and break cross-links. In addition, microwave treatment of sections as has now been routinely incorporated into immuno-histochemistry protocols is also widely used. This involves microwaving sections or samples in a buffer such as $0.01M$ citrate buffer, which seems to improve probe penetration perhaps by breaking cross-links or relaxing tertiary structures within the section *(19)*.

2.3. Probe Types

The principal tool is the labeled recombinant deoxyribonucleic acid or ribonucleic acid probe with a specific nucleotide sequence complementary to that of the mRNA or DNA of interest. Cells that contain the resultant DNA-mRNA or RNA-mRNA hybrid molecules may be identified by detection of the probe label. The unique complementary coding sequence of the probe confers an inherently high degree of specificity, indeed even relatively short sequences (around 20 bases) are sufficient to confer specificity in most cases. A number of different probe types can be used in ISH, each with their advantages and disadvantages.

2.3.1. Double Stranded DNA Probes

These are prepared from cloned DNA, which is in a plasmid or can be prepared by PCR using appropriate primers. Probe labeling is then carried out by nick-translation or random priming. Although originally used in many studies, these are now less frequently seen as they have some inherent problems. Advantages of cDNA probes are that they are generally highly specific, because their length confers specificity. cDNA probes can also be labeled with multiple labels and the specific activity of labeling can be quite high as multiple bases can be labeled with radioactivity or nonradioactive labels such as biotin or digoxigenin. Longer cDNA probes can also show cross-species hybridization because these will work where there is around 90% homology between species. In this case, stringency of hybridization and washing conditions (temperature, salt concentration and formamide percentage) can be manipulated to improve the chances of hybridization at lower homologies or to exclude hybridization to similar sequences. The double stranded nature also makes cDNA probes relatively resistant to enzymes such as DNases that might degrade them, giving them a longer shelf- or freezer life. However, the double stranded nature of cDNA probes is a major drawback as during the hybridization reaction, the probe also reanneals. For this reason probes need to be denatured just before addition to sections or cells and from that point there are the competing reactions of probe hybridizing with target mRNA or DNA sequences in the sample and reannealing to its complementary (sense) strand. Lastly, depending on probe length, there may be problems of probe penetration into the tissue or problems with adsorption of the probe onto the section and increased background. For this reason some thought has to be given to designing cDNA probes to be long enough to provide specificity but short enough to aid penetration and enhance removal of nonspecifically bound probe during washing steps.

2.3.2. Oligonucleotides

Synthesis of 20–30 base oligonucleotides is a convenient way to allow specific probes to be designed. The limitation with oligonucleotide probes is largely caused by the relatively few labels that can be attached to a short probe. The simplest method of labeling oligonucleotide probes is by substituting a labeled phosphorous onto the 5′ end using the enzyme 5′ polynucleotide kinase. However, this gives one labeled base per probe molecule and thus specific activity of the probe and sensitivity may be low. For this reason many studies have employed tailed oligonucleotide probes where multiple labels are added at the 3′ end using the enzyme terminal transferase. This results in greater sensitivity owing to a greater number of labels per probe molecule, but does produce a nonhomologous tail, which could theoretically impede hybridization of the probe with the target RNA or DNA molecule or demand lower stringency to take the reduced T_m into account. In practice, tailing probes works reasonably well. Another option with oligonucleotide probes is to generate a probe cocktail using multiple oligonucleotides designed to different regions of the sequence. This method has been used successfully and some commercialized probes for targets such as Epstein Barr Virus or kappa and lambda light chains of immunoglobulin have used oligonucleotide probe cocktails. In summary, though the potential for generating oligonucleotide probes from published sequences and the simplicity of their synthesis (or purchase) makes them attractive for use in ISH, in many cases their relative lack of sensitivity makes them less useful than other probe types.

2.3.3. RNA (Riboprobes)

Single stranded RNA probes can be synthesized by using purified RNA polymerase (SP6, T7, or T3 RNA polymerase) to transcribe the sequences down stream of the appropriate polymerase initiation site. Most commonly the probe sequence is cloned into a plasmid vector so that it is flanked by two different RNA polymerase initiation sites thus enabling either sense (control) or antisense (probe) RNA to be synthesized. RNA probes have a number of advantages over cDNA probes including the fact that they are single stranded and therefore have no competing reaction occurring during hybridization. The background obtained with riboprobes can also be reduced by using single stranded RNase (RNase A) to remove unhybridized probe from the sample. Though RNA produced from linearized template may be quite long, a simple reaction using heat and alkaline pH can produce hydrolyzed probe with lengths more conducive to tissue penetration and background reduction. Optimal probe lengths are usually considered to be 100–250 bases, however, longer probes work reasonably well but may result in slightly higher background labeling. The production of riboprobes is relatively straightforward with subcloning inserts into an appropriate vector being a fairly simple procedure. Large quantities of plasmid can then be prepared from bacterial liquid cultures and stored after purification for subsequent linearization and labeling. In the case of nonisotopically labeled probe, the probe itself is fairly stable, though single stranded RNA is rather more susceptible to degradation by environmental RNases than is double stranded cDNA. For this reason, it is worth paying attention to contamination of the laboratory with RNases, particularly as these are used during the washing steps and glassware, benches and equipment can become contaminated. A number of commercial products are available as sprays, which can decontaminate surfaces and instruments and most practitioners use diethyl pyrocarbonate (DEPC) to render buffers and solutions RNase-free.

2.3.4. PNA Probes

Peptide nucleic acids (PNAs) are an important new class of synthetic nucleic acid analogues with a peptide-like backbone. This structure has an inherent advantage because PNAs hybridize with high affinity and specificity to complementary RNA and DNA sequences, with a greater resistance to nucleases and proteinases. Originally conceived as ligands for the study of double-stranded DNA, the unique physicochemical properties of PNAs have led to the development of a large variety of research and diagnostic assays, including antigene and antisense therapy, genome mapping, and mutation detection *(20)*. Many of the commercialized PNA probes for detection of viruses or immunoglobulin DNA and RNA have consisted of a cocktail of PNA oligomers labeled with a hapten that can readily be detected using methods similar to routine immuno-histochemistry. An example is FITC- labeled PNA probes, which are detected using an anti-FITC antibody and then detection of this antibody using strepta-vidin–biotin peroxidase or alkaline phosphatase detection systems.

2.4. Probe Labeling

Labeling of probes with a reporter molecule is a key step, as it is the mechanism by which hybridization can be localized.

2.4.1. Preparation of Template and Labeling Techniques for DNA Probes

There are two procedures commonly used for labeling cDNA probes. The double-stranded DNA sequence can be labeled by random primed synthesis or nick-translation. The random priming method is now more commonly used because it is simpler and is a highly efficient labeling reaction. Random priming uses denaturation of the double stranded DNA fragment, followed by annealing of short oligonucleotide primers (8–10 bases) with random sequences. These oligonucleotides act as primers for synthesis of a new DNA strand using the enzyme Klenow DNA polymerase. During the synthesis, labeled nucleotides can be incorporated into both strands of DNA, with a wide choice of labels available. Historically, α-^{32}P-NTP was used, mainly because it was the predominant label used for synthesis of probes for Northern blots, but subsequently biotinylated nucleotides, digoxigenin (DIG)-labeled nucleotides or other labels and haptens (e.g., FITC) have been used. In general random priming results in efficiently labeled probes with only simple centrifugation steps required to remove unincorporated label.

2.4.2. RNA Probe Preparation and Labeling

Single-stranded RNA probes or riboprobes are generally synthesized by sub-cloning cDNA into a suitable vector. Such vectors usually contain two of the RNA polymerase promoter sequences for T3, T7, or SP6 RNA polymerase located in opposite orientations on either side of the inserted DNA fragment. This allows the synthesis of either a sense or antisense strand of the template sequence. Production of plasmid, plasmid purification and then linearization of the plasmid using a restriction enzyme are all performed before probe labeling is carried out. Cut plasmid can be stored for long periods of time at −20°C or −80°C, ready for use in labeling reactions. The only precaution to be taken in general is to ensure that the plasmid preparation is entirely linearized and this can be done by simply running a sample of cut plasmid on a 1% agarose gel and visualising it to ensure complete linearization. Labeling reactions are then carried out using the appropriate RNA polymerase to make sense and antisense copies of the template. Generally template lengths of 0.3–0.5 kb are optimal but longer probes can be prepared and then hydrolyzed to produce shorter fragments. As with cDNA probes described above, a number of possible labels can be incorporated into RNA probes to produce very sensitive probes, with early studies using isotopic labeling with ^{32}P or ^{33}P-UTP, but subsequent studies have used incorporation of biotinylated or DIG-labeled UTP.

2.4.3. Oligonucleotide Probe Preparation

Oligonucleotides can be synthesized if there is a DNA synthesizer available, though most laboratories use commercial suppliers, because these provide cheap oligonucleotides for applications such as PCR, with a generally short turnaround. In addition, commercial oligonucleotides can now be ordered with various modifications such as end labels, so that these probes can be designed from published sequences, ordered from a commercial supplier and used in situ hybridization applications. Limitations with this method are that several probes may have to be designed to find a sequence that works, because it may not be easy to predict which sequences will be available for hybridization within the sample. The other limitation is that single end-labels may not provide a sufficiently sensitive probe for use where the target mRNA or DNA is not abundantly expressed or in high copy-number in the sample. These probes can be very successful at labeling highly-expressed mRNA (such as albumin in liver, or collagen I in dermis) but may not detect lower abundance expression of genes such as those for cytokines and growth factors. For this reason, oligonucleotides are not very popular as a choice for in situ hybridization in many research settings or they are labeled in a manner designed to make them more sensitive. An example of probe labeling designed to enhance sensitivity is 3′ tailing of the probe, which is described above.

2.5. Probe Labels and Detection

2.5.1. Isotopic Labeling

The earliest uses of in situ hybridization tended to use radioactive labels for detection of the hybridization signal. These have some advantages, mainly in their low cost, but safety issues arise and the probe has a much reduced shelf

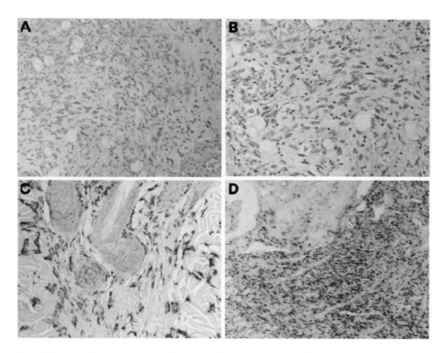

Fig. 59.2. Paraffin embedded skin wound labeled for procollagen I using a riboprobe and non-isotopic detection methods. The photomicrographs show the different sensitivity of a (**A**) Biotinylated probe detected with avidin–biotin complex, (**B**) DIG labeled probe detected with anti-DIG horseradish peroxidase conjugate, (**C**) Biotinylated probe detected with tyramide amplification, and (**D**) DIG labeled probe detected with anti-DIG alkaline phoshphatase conjugate

life owing to decay of the radioactive tracer and there is also the possibility of damage to the probe (radiolysis) in the case of highly energetic radioactive labels such as ^{32}P. One of the major problems with radioactive labeling of DNA and RNA probes is that the detection system commonly used adds several days or in some cases weeks to the time taken to achieve a result. In the case of reasonably energetic emitters such as ^{32}P or ^{33}P it was not uncommon to wait 2 wk to 1 mo to obtain a result using silver emulsion autoradiography. In addition, the emulsion autoradiography method has an inherent problem, which limits resolution of the signal, that being the path length and scatter of the emitted particle. With great care and a relatively thin layer of emulsion, reasonable resolution down to a single cell is possible, but there is still a lengthy time spent with samples exposing in the dark, and many technical problems associated with the emulsion autoradiography technique, such as possible exposure (fogging) of the emulsion, detaching of the emulsion layer from the sample and inconsistent emulsion thickness across samples making comparisons within and between experiments difficult. For these reasons, radioactive in situ hybridization detected using emulsion autoradiography has become much less common.

2.5.2. Nonisotopic Detection

Problems with resolution of probe signal to the cells within tissue that actually contained the probe molecule led to the use of nonisotopic methods for probe detection quite soon after the first use of the technique. Biotin, which is in routine use in immunohistochemistry, was soon added to nucleotides so that a biotinylated probe could be produced by any of the labeling methods described above. Biotin can then be detected using either streptavidin or avidin conjugated to a reporter such as horseradish peroxidase. Biotin labeling alone does not give a particularly high level of sensitivity. Digoxigenin (DIG) was then introduced and this can be detected using anti DIG antibodies, which may be conjugated to reporters such as horseradish peroxidase or alkaline phosphatase. This has proved to be more sensitive than biotin by itself. The sensitivity of biotin-labeled probes can be improved by amplification steps known as signal amplification or catalyzed reporter systems, which use tyramide and biotin and amplify the probe signal once deposited on the section or sample. Examples of this are shown in **Fig. 59.2** and the chemistry and use of these probes is described in detail in Speel et al. *(21)*. Lastly, other markers can be conjugated to nucleotides, which are then incorporated into probes by any of the routine DNA or RNA labeling methods, a common example being fluorescein (FITC). This can be visualized directly using a fluorescent microscope as is sometimes used in fluorescent in situ hybridization (FISH) of chromosomes, though more commonly probes are first biotin or DIG labeled and then detected using secondary antibodies labeled with a fluorescent marker such as FITC.

FITC is also sometimes used as a hapten and visualized using anti-FITC antibodies and subsequent detection steps with horseradish peroxidase or alkaline phosphatase. Commercialized PNA probes labeled with FITC use this detection system with quite high sensitivity.

2.6. Hybridization and Washing

Protocols for hybridization conditions usually aim to provide an environment in which formation of specific hybrids between probe and target mRNA or DNA are favored but nonspecific binding of probe to the sample are unstable.

This is normally achieved by a combination of temperature, salt concentration and formamide concentration. Hybridization buffers are often complex mixtures designed to achieve stringency and favor hybrid formation while concentrating the probe on the sample. In addition, carrier DNA or RNA is often included so that RNase or DNase activity is to some extent quenched and probe is protected. Hybridization temperatures can be elevated in the case of long probes or probes that form tight hybrids (for example RNA probes directed at RNA targets). This high temperature means that unstable hybrids where mismatches are present are not favored and do not result in background or nonspecific labeling and the probe does not simply 'stick' to the section because of weak homology or charge interactions. Inevitably there is some background in every reaction and the posthybridization washing steps are aimed at minimising these. For example, in the case of DNA probes and oligonucleotides, posthybridization washing steps involved reducing the salt concentration and raising the temperature close to that of hybridization (and close to the calculated T_m of the probe–target interaction). These steps helped to remove unstable hybrids and nonspecifically bound probe. In the case of RNA probes, the addition of posthybridization washing steps, which include RNase helps to markedly lower background. RNase A is an enzyme that degrades single stranded RNA molecules and thus can remove background but has no activity against specifically bound probe because it is double stranded.

2.7. Controls

Appropriate controls form an important part of the ISH protocol. A control sense probe is routinely used to confirm specificity of the signal. The ISH technique is based on the complementary binding of an antisense probe to the target mRNA/DNA. A sense probe is identical to the mRNA/DNA and therefore should not produce any hybridization signal. In those cases where a sense probe is not available, an irrelevant probe can be substituted. Application of hybridization solutions alone help to identify nonspecific background, particularly relevant when chromogenic substrates are used. Use of photographic emulsions can lead to a number of specific artefacts through nonspecific formation of silver grains. These can be controlled for by dipping slides in which processing with labeled probe has been omitted. Other controls are the inclusion of samples known to express the target (positive control), and known not to express target (negative control), and positive control probes such as cytoplasmic (beta) actin that will probe for targets ubiquitously present in all cells. RNase treated sections are useful for confirming specificity of hybridization, but great care must be take to avoid cross contamination.

2.8. Quantitation

Quantitative analysis of hybridization signals remains problematic and somewhat controversial. If one accepts that the relationship between mRNA expression and radiography is stoichiometric, then using image analysis to grain count is relatively straightforward (*17*). Provided sections are processed and probed in parallel, and that the appropriate controls are included, it probably provides a good semiquantitative estimate of relative mRNA expression. More advanced image analysis techniques provide an advance on this by identifying clusters of grains (*22*). Likewise, chromogenic and fluorescent signals can be quantified with the standard image analysis techniques used in immunohistochemistry. In most cases these require little modification.

If not well controlled, underlying differences in the retention of mRNA is a major complication. Weak mRNA labeling may reflect poor retention of mRNA rather than low level expression per se. Evaluation of retained mRNA with dyes such as acridine orange *(23)* or methyl green pyronine Y are valuable, as is probing for a housekeeper gene such as β-actin and 28 S ribosomal RNA. Using 18sRNA would seem to be preferable, as its expression is more constant and less affected by local conditions than β-actin. As with other forms of hybridization such as northern blotting, some investigators have expressed mRNA labeling relative to the housekeeping gene *(24)*.

2.9. Combined In Situ Hybridization and Immunohistochemistry

Although in situ hybridization provides valuable information about gene expression, it does not provide any information about translation or fate of the protein product which may be membrane bound, secreted, stored, or processed. However, when combined with immunohistochemistry, in situ hybridization can provide valuable information about gene activity at the DNA, mRNA, and protein level. The challenge has been to find conditions that are compatible with simultaneously conserving both RNA reactivity and protein antigenicity. The possibility of using either fluorescent markers as detection methods means that multiple labels can be used to detect several targets in tissues or cells and this technology is now routinely used in chromosomal studies. For studies aimed at detecting a gene and its product (i.e., mRNA and corresponding protein), protein can be detected using horseradish peroxidase and diaminobenzidine as the final detection step (giving a brown precipitate) whereas mRNA is detected using alkaline phosphatase and NBT/BCIP (giving a blue coloration).

3. Applications

The basics of ISH has been widely applied to a diverse range of situations where we need to localize the distribution of nucleic acids. Gene expression studies are often carried out at the whole organism, organ or tissue or cell level. What follows is a review of these applications, organized by type of sample used.

3.1. Tissue Sections

Hybridization techniques are commonly used in the study of tissue pathology, where the term hybridization histochemistry has sometimes been adopted *(25)*. By definition, ISH of tissue sections is often thought to be a daunting technique, requiring skills in both molecular biology and histology, a rarely found combination. However the now widespread application of this methodology has meant that the technique is well described for a variety of tissue.

3.1.1. Light Microscopy

ISH is widely used in light microscopic studies where it has established itself as a fundamental research technique. Detection of labeling by autoradiography and subsequent viewing by bright-field or dark-field microscopy was a widely used technique throughout the early history of in situ hybridization. The presence of silver grains in autoradiography-detected experiments also allows quantitation by image analysis and grain counting. More widespread use now of nonisotopic labeling techniques with biotin or DIG means that light microscopy can give good single cell resolution of in situ hybridization results.

Free-floating ISH is a modification of tissue hybridization where frozen sections are not mounted on any support and processed free floating in the reagents *(26)*. This may improve sensitivity and allow the use of thicker sections such as vibratome sections of brain tissue.

3.1.2. Electron Microscopy

Hybridization techniques have also been adapted for use in electron microscopy. This methodology provides scientists with the opportunity to integrate molecular function and ultrastructural detail. However, these applications have proved to be technically very demanding and far from routine.

Two different approaches have been employed. *Pre-embedding* techniques where thick sections of pre-fixed tissue are hybridized before embedding *(27)* and *postembedding* where hybridization and signal detection is performed on grids using ultrathin sections (more analogous to the use of paraffin section in light microscopy) *(23)*.

Although glutaraldehyde is the usual fixative of choice for electron microscopy, Binder et al. *(23)* suggest 4% formaldehyde with 0.1% glutaraldehyde. Higher (4%) concentrations of glutaraldehyde were found to reduce hybridization by about 60%. Likewise, the medium used for embedding tissue is important. The hydrophilic and low lipid-solvent character of LR White resin is thought to give better preservation of mRNA than other resins *(28)*.

Although radioactive techniques have been used, nonradioactive labeling has the considerable advantage of eliminating the need for grid autoradiography.

3.2. Cultured Cells

Protocols for using ISH in tissue sections have easily been adapted for use with cell cultures. Such techniques are particularly useful in cell based ex vivo assays established to mimic biological processes. One such example is migration and wound closure assays, where ISH has been used to examine the migration of cells from wound margins *(29)*. Cells can be hybridized on Petri dishes or chamber slides after fixation with 4% paraformaldhyde and require minimal treatment to permeabilize the cell membrane.

3.3. Wholemount Embryos

ISH in whole embryos is an important tool in developmental biology, where it provides a means of examining temporal and spatial changes in gene expression during cell differentiation and morphogenesis *(30–32)*. Unlike conventional ISH to tissue sections, whole mounts provide three dimensional images of gene expression. Although the use of whole mounts obviates the need for serial sections and the necessity to reconstruct expression patterns, the inherent sample thickness presents unique challenges. Clearly in this case nonisotopic detection of the probe is necessary and it is likely that small groups of cells in heterogeneous tissues could be missed. However, many studies use whole-mounts to detect regions of interest followed by sectioning to obtain a closer look at exact cell populations that are labeling.

3.4. Chromosomes

Chromosome specific probes have been developed for DNA detection and have become a powerful tool in cytogenetics and oncology *(33)*. The acronym FISH has become synonymous with the use of these probes in fluorescent in situ hybridization (FISH) for genetic alterations. FISH is an important adjunct to routine chromosome analysis, allowing the detection of multiple, numerical, structural and microdeletion chromosome abnormalities on a cell by cell basis.

Classic methods for the identification of human chromosomes have relied on the use various chemical stains. Although these are robust techniques, they do not show small cases of translocation, insertion or deletion, are critically dependent on quality preparations, and perhaps most importantly, are only applicable to metaphase chromosomes *(33)*. FISH on the other hand is not only useful with poor quality preparations, but allows for the examination of resting cells in interphase. This therefore eliminates the need for a dividing cell population and enables screening of a large number of cells. Interphase screening programmes have been developed to reveal chromosomal abnormalities with prognostic significance *(34)*.

Directly labeled DNA probes for FISH can be prepared by incorporating modified bases with a fluorochrome side group, obviating the need for signal amplification. Such probes are available commercially.

Chromosome ISH has also been applied experimentally to localize sex mismatch chimeras in organ transplantation. This has served as a useful a method of identifying bone marrow derived progenitors in organ regeneration *(35)*.

3.5. Viruses

ISH techniques can be routinely applied to the detection of exogenous DNA from viral infection *(36)*. Clinical examination for human papillomavirus DNA is perhaps the best known example *(37)*. Other viral DNAs that can be examined include cytomegalovirus, herpes simplex virus and Epstein Barr virus. Although PCR techniques are usually used to detect these viruses, ISH is valuable when morphological localization is required. Combined ISH and immunohistochemistry make it possible to identify and phenotype infected host cells *(38)*.

3.6. Plant Specimens

ISH has been used in plant tissue to study both genomic DNA *(39)* and RNA *(40)*. Derived from the study of mammalian chromosomes, FISH has been used to study both plant chromosomes using preparations of mitotic root tips and pollen cells at meiosis *(41)*. Conversely, paraffin embedded sections remain the most widely used method to study plant RNA *(41)*.

4. Concluding Remarks

ISH techniques are applicable to the detection of both RNA and DNA. Although applications for mRNA are more numerous in research, ISH for both endogenous and exogenous DNA remains the most widely used examples in clinical medicine.

Despite being more than 30 years old, ISH continues to find new applications. Advances in other molecular techniques such as the advent of gene microarrays has not diminished the significance of in situ hybridization, but rather highlights the importance of being able to identify the topology of gene expression. It offers a degree of precision that is unavailable with other molecular techniques.

References

1. Southern EM (1975) Detection of specific sequences among DNA fragments separated by gel electrophoresis. J Mol Biol 98:503–517
2. Thomas PS (1980) Hybridization of denatured RNA and small DNA fragments transferred to nitrocellulose. Proc Natl Acad Sci (USA) 77:5201–5205
3. Gal A, Nahon JL, Sala-Trepat JM (1983) Detection of rare mRNA species in a complex RNA population by blot hybridization techniques: a comparative survey. Anal Biochem 132:190–194
4. Gall JG, Pardue ML (1969) Formation and detection of RNA-DNA hybrid molecules in cytological preparations. Proc Natl Acad Sci (USA) 63:378–383
5. John HL, Birnstiel ML, Jones KW (1969). RNA-DNA hybrids at the cytological level. Nature 223:912, 913
6. Jones KW, Bishop JO, Brito-da-Cunha A (1973) Complex formation between poly-r (U) and various chromosomal loci in Rhynchosciara. Chromosoma 43:375–390
7. Capco DG, Jeffery WR (1978) Differential distribution of poly(A)-containing RNA in the embryonic cells of Oncopeltus fasciatus. Analysis by in situ hybridization with a [^{3}H]poly(U) probe. Dev Biol 67:137–151
8. Harding JD, MacDonald RJ, Przybyla AE, Chirgwin JM, Pictet RL, Rutter WJ (1977) Changes in the frequency of specific transcripts during development of the pancreas. J Biol Chem 252:7391–7397
9. Orth G, Jeanteur P, Croissant O (1971) Evidence for and localization of vegetative viral DNA replication by autoradiographic detection of RNA-DNA hybrids in sections of tumors induced by Shope papilloma virus. Proc Natl Acad Sci (USA) 68:1876–1880
10. Harrison PR, Conkie D, Paul J, Jones K (1973) Localisation of cellular globin messenger RNA by in situ hybridization to complementary DNA. FEBS Lett 32:109–112
11. Pochet R, Brocas H, Vassart G, Toubeau G, Seo H, Refetoff S, Dumont JE, Pasteels JI (1981) Radioautographic localization of prolactin messenger RNA on histological sections by in situ hybridization. Brain Res 211:433–438
12. Hudson P, Penschow J, Shine J, Ryan G, Niall H, Coghlan J (1981) Hybridization histochemistry: use of recombinant DNA as a "homing probe" for tissue localization of specific mRNA populations. Endocrinology 108:353–356
13. Jacobs JW, Simpson E, Penschow J, Hudson P, Coghlan J, Niall H (1983) Characterization and localization of calcitonin messenger ribonucleic acid in rat thyroid. Endocrinology 113:1616–1622
14. Singer RH, Ward DC (1982) Actin gene expression visualized in chicken muscle tissue culture by using in situ hybridization with a biotinated nucleotide analog. Proc Natl Acad Sci (USA) 79:7331–7335
15. Saber MA, Shafritz DA, Zern MA (1983) Changes in collagen and albumin mRNA in liver tissue of mice infected with Schistosoma mansoni as determined by in situ hybridization. J Cell Biol. 97:986–992
16. Lawrence JB, Singer RH (1985) Quantitative analysis of in situ hybridization methods for the detection of actin gene expression. Nucleic Acids Res 3:1777–1799
17. Hewitson TD, Darby IA, Bisucci T, Jones CL, Becker GJ (1998) Evolution of tubulointerstitial fibrosis in experimental renal infection and scarring. J Am Soc Nephrol 9:632–642

18. Rentrop M, Knapp B, Winter H, Schweizer J (1986) Aminoalkylsilanetreated slides as support for in situ hybridization of keratin cDNA's to frozen tissue sections under varying fixation and pretreatment conditions. Histochemical J 18:271–276

19. Tesch GH, Lan HY, Nikolic-Paterson DJ (2006) Treatment of tissue sections for in situ hybridization. Methods Mol Biol 326:1–7

20. Pellestor F, Paulasova P, Macek M, Hamamah S (2005) The use of peptide nucleic acids for in situ identification of human chromosomes J Histochem Cytochem 53:395–400

21. Speel EJ, Hopman AHN, Komminoth P (2006) Tyramide signal amplification for DNA and mRNA in situ hybridization. Methods Mol Biol 326:33–60

22. Bisucci T, Hewitson TD, Darby IA (2002) Quantitation of in situ hybridization using image analysis of radioactively labeled RNA probes. Methods Mol Biol 179:137–147

23. Binder M, Tourmente S, Roth J, Renaud M, Gehring WJ (1986) In situ hybridization at the electron microscope level: localization of transcripts on ultrathin sections of Lowicryl K4M-embedded tissue using biotinylated probes and protein A-gold complexes. J Cell Biol 102:1646–1653

24. Miyazaki M (1997) In situ hybridization in IgA nephropathy. Nephrology 3, Suppl 2:691–695

25. Penschow JD, Haralambidis J, Darling PE, Darby IA, Wintour EM, Tregear GW, Coghlan JF (1987) Hybridization histochemistry. Experientia (Basel) 43:741–750

26. Bessert DA, Skoff RP (1999) High-resolution in situ hybridization and TUNEL staining with free-floating brain sections. J Histochem Cytochem 47:693–702

27. Macville MV, Wiesmeijer KC, Dirks RW, Fransen JA, Raap AK (1995) Saponin pre-treatment in pre-embedding electron microscopic in situ hybridization for detection of specific RNA sequences in cultured cells: a methodological study. J Histochem Cytochem 43:1005–1018

28. Osamura RY, Itoh Y, Matsuno A (2000) Applications of plastic embedding to electron microscopic immunocytochemistry and in situ hybridization in observations of production and secretion of peptide hormones. J Histochem Cytochem 48:885–891

29. Choi C, Hudson LG, Savagner P, Kusewitt DF (2006) An in situ hybridization technique to detect low-abundance slug mRNA in adherent cultured cells. Methods Mol Biol 326:173–188

30. Christiansen JH, Dennis CL, Wicking CA, Monkley SJ, Wilkinson DC, Wainwright BJ (1995) Murine Wnt-11 and Wnt-12 have temporally and spatially restricted expression patterns during embryonic development. Mech Dev 51:341–350

31. Wilkinson DG, Nieto MA (1993) Detection of messenger RNA by in situ hybridization to tissue sections and whole mounts. Methods Enzymol 225:361–373

32. Challen GA, Martinez G, Davis MJ, Taylor DF, Crowe M, Teasdale RD, Grimmond SM, Little MH (2004) Identifying the molecular phenotype of renal progenitor cells. J Am Soc Nephrol 15:2344–2357

33. Waters JJ, Barlow AL, Gould CP (1998) Demystified … FISH. Mol Pathol 51:62–70

34. Jain KK (2004) Current status of fluorescent in-situ hybridization. Med Device Technol 15:14–17

35. Grimm PC, Nickerson P, Jeffery J, Savani RC, Gough J, McKenna RM, Stern E, Rush DN (2001) Neointimal and tubulointerstitial infiltration by recipient mesenchymal cells in chronic renal-allograft rejection. N Engl J Med 345:93–97

36. Herrington CS (1998) Demystified … in situ hybridisation. Mol Pathol 51:8–13

37. Eglin RP, Sharp F, MacLean AB, Macnab JC, Clements JB, Wilkie NM (1981) Detection of RNA complementary to herpes simplex virus DNA in human cervical squamous cell neoplasms. Cancer Res 41:3597–3603

38. Brahic M, Haase AT, Cash E (1984) Simultaneous in situ detection of viral RNA and antigens. Proc Natl Acad Sci *(USA)*. 81:5445–5448

39. Lilly JW, Havey MJ, Jackson SA, Jiang J (2001) Cytogenomic analyses reveal the structural plasticity of the chloroplast genome in higher plants. Plant Cell 13:245–254

40. Guerin J, Rossel JB, Robert S, Tsuchiya T, Koltunow A (2000) A DEFICIENS homologue is down-regulated during apomictic initiation in ovules of Hieracium. Planta 210:914–920

41. Houben A, Orford SJ, Timmis JN (2006) In situ hybridization to plant tissues and chromosomes. Methods Mol Biol 326:203–218

60

High Throughput Screening

William P. Janzen

1. Introduction

How are new drugs discovered? The common image is of dedicated teams of brilliant scientists unlocking the secrets of disease through years of research then designing wonder drugs based on their discoveries. Although this image is largely true in terms of the dedication, time and talent involved, there is also a very systematic process for turning research findings into pharmaceutical products. All pharmaceutical companies employ robotic systems to test millions of chemicals each year to see if any hold promise as drugs. This is all part of a complex process of establishing efficacy and safety using *in vitro* assays before these drug leads are tested *in vivo*. From here, you have a chance of creating a drug–if you are lucky–because the actual success rate from animal efficacy to an approved drug is less than 1 in 250 *(1)*.

In fact, the development of a new pharmaceutical product takes an average of 15 yr and costs in excess of $800,000,000 *(2,3)*. Despite continued technological advancement and increasingly sophisticated biological methods, both times and costs have continually increased over the last two decades *(1,4)*. In response to continued pressures to produce more drugs and do it faster and cheaper, the pharmaceutical industry has evolved specialized techniques that use industrialized processes borrowed from other industries and applied them to laboratory research. High Throughput Screening (HTS) is one such process.

1.1. So What is HTS?

High Throughput Screening is a technique for empirically discovering chemical modifiers of biological action. HTS is used many different ways and in different settings. It is now widely used in many fields beyond pharmaceuticals including agrochemical discovery, catalyst discovery, cosmetic development and, academic research to name a few. HTS is highly multidisciplinary; combining elements of Chemistry, Biology, Engineering, Information technology and Logistics Management.

There are some basic components that are consistent in all HTS applications. From the name, one can infer that throughput *(5)*, which is a measure of samples

From: *Molecular Biomethods Handbook, 2nd Edition.*
Edited by: J. M. Walker and R. Rapley © Humana Press, Totowa, NJ

tested per unit time, will be a defining measure and the numbers should be high. Likewise, the term screening implies that biological samples will be tested and an assay result produced. In HTS, collections of chemical samples, or libraries, are tested in a biological assay to measure their ability to affect a biological process that has been implicated in a disease process. These models, otherwise known as targets, can range from isolated active proteins to complex cellular systems. Libraries in HTS can be as large as millions of individual chemicals and larger operations will conduct 50–100 of these testing campaigns per year (6). To deliver this scale of data, automation is always utilized to some degree in HTS as are automated data processing techniques.

To fully understand HTS, one must first review the history of its development. HTS grew from the needs of the pharmaceutical industry and has historically been most heavily utilized in the field of drug discovery. The basic techniques were developed following the discovery of penicillin (7) in 1929 and its subsequent use as the first human antibiotic (8,9) in 1940. This breakthrough compound was discovered by a systematic approach of sequentially testing thousands of microbial cultures on agar plates. Following World War II, it was produced by most American pharmaceutical companies – suddenly the primary cause of mortality worldwide became both treatable and widely available.

In response to competitive pressures, the pharmaceutical industry began a widespread campaign to find new and better antibiotics using basically the same techniques as Fleming. This led to the discovery of many new classes of antibiotic in the 1940s and 1950s (9). As companies increased the scale of their efforts to include broader sources, these efforts took on a decidedly industrial look culminating in what was arguably the first HTS at the Terre Haute laboratories of the Pfizer Company where 56 scientists tested almost one hundred thousand soil samples over a period of approx 1 yr. This program led to the discovery of the then novel antibiotic product terramycin, which eventually captured 25% of the American broad spectrum antibiotic market (9).

Once established as a technique, this practice was expanded to other sources of chemicals. Initially this included naturally derived extracts from plants, fungi and microbial sources for the fixed therapeutic indication of infectious disease treatment, but it later expanded to include more complex diseases such as hypertension, metabolic diseases and psychiatric disorders (10). Much of this expansion was driven by advances in medicine and the associated biological sciences that led to a better understanding of the molecular causes of disease. This methodology proceeded with only incremental improvements until the late twentieth century, when several forces conspired to bring about massive changes.

The discovery of DNA in 1953 (11) soon gave rise to the new fields of biotechnology and genetic engineering, which, in turn, made possible the large scale production of proteins and creation of engineered cell lines through cloning technologies (12), which enabled the production of large quantities of protein without following cumbersome activity based purification processes. This was followed closely by breakthroughs in the chemical synthesis technique of parallel synthesis (also known as combinatorial chemistry) for the large scale production of synthetic medicinal chemistry compounds (13–15). To keep up, drug discovery groups looked to automation. This led to the formation of specialized departments to perform screens and, subsequently, the formal creation of HTS groups.

2. Methods

As was mentioned above, HTS is a highly interdisciplinary science. In this novel field, practitioners must understand and apply concepts encompassing complex biology and biochemistry, technology, automation and chemistry as well as statistics and computational algorithms. Although HTS is a discipline in its own rights, there are also specialties within the field. The most common of these are assay development (Section 2.1), chemical library management (Section 2.2), and screening operations (Section 2.3). Not coincidentally, these also represent the most common departmental divisions within large screening operations. In smaller organizations it is not uncommon for scientists to fulfill the functions of several of these "departments" or to be integrated with more specialized disease biology groups.

2.1. Assay Development and Assay Technologies

One of the core aspects of HTS is the assay or "screen". In this context these terms are distinguished by the level of statistical validation or rigor. An assay is a method of determining biological function. A screen is an assay that has been statistically validated by repeated testing to be relevant, reproducible and repeatable. Each of these requirements brings a different level of rigor and requirements.

A relevant assay is one that will reliably predict the impact of a compound in a disease model. The biological systems used to monitor this effect can vary widely and are discussed below. All, however, utilize systems to present a biological "target" in a controlled environment. The concept of the target in HTS is one of the most important and is core to any discussion of the field, target names are also one of the most closely guarded secrets in most HTS organizations.

In their simplest form, targets are individual proteins where there is evidence that they are mis-regulated in a disease state *(15–17)*. While the most complex screens involve cellular or tissue based systems, which can elucidate signaling cascades, multitarget interactions or disease models where the actual target may be unknown *(18,19)*. A target, which is known to be reflective of disease, is often referred to as a validated target. For example, a highly validated target is one where there is a marketed drug that is known to act via the target of interest. Targets can be validated by many other methods, which produce various levels of confidence in the ability of the target to predict or modulate disease including simple identification of proteins in disease specific cells to gene expression analysis and RNAi based techniques *(20,21)*. It should be noted that this terminology can be a point of confusion because the term validation is also commonly used to refer to the statistical validation of screens, which is discussed later in this section.

There are also several other terms that are used in conjunction with the perceived ability of a target to produce a drug. Drugability *(22,23)* is commonly used to describe classes of targets and is dependant on whether targets from that class have yielded drugs. For example G-coupled protein receptors (GPCR) are widely recognized as a very drugable class of targets. This is because most drugs on the market today directly affect a GPCR target *(17)*. Kinases are another example of drugable targets but were considered only marginally so *(16)* until the approval of the drug Gleevec in 2001 for the treatment of leukemia *(24)*.

Once a target has been selected for HTS, a screen must be developed. In most organizations there is an established, rigorous process for developing assays but the complexity of this task will still vary depending on a number of factors. The assay developer must first consider compatibility with HTS equipment. This can provide the developer with an array of options for pipetting and reading that are not commonly available in the research lab but comes with some restrictions as well.

The one thing that is common to all HTS assays is the microplate. The microplate is a molded plastic container consisting of wells in an evenly spaced array (**Fig. 60.1**). The first microplates contained 96 wells and all HTS equipment was designed around the ability to dispense reagents and robotically manipulate these plates. Today these plates exist in many densities most commonly including 384-well and 1,536-well plates although densities as high as 9,600 have been developed *(25–27)*. All plates are based around multiples of 96 because of the need to use legacy equipment designed for the 96-well format.

The primary advantage of higher density plates is the reduced volume required for an assay. A normal 96-well microplate can hold up to 200 microliters (µl) with standard assay volumes of approx 100 µl whereas a 1,536-well plate will have a maximum volume of 10–15 µl and working volumes down to 1 µl. However, highly miniaturized assays require special handling technologies and must take into account such problems as evaporation and nanoliter dispensing *(28)*. Plates from any of these formats can be constructed from various materials to allow them to be referenced or read from either the top or bottom to enable multiple methods of detection. By varying plastic composition and coating materials, different binding characteristics can also be controlled. For example, an enzymatic screen will require very low binding to prevent adherence of assay proteins to the surface while a cellular screen may require that cells be adhered to the plate, dictating a coated plate with enhanced binding characteristics.

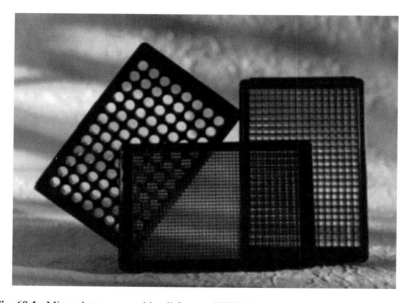

Fig. 60.1. Microplates are used in all facets of HTS from compound storage to testing. Shown here are plates with densities of 96, 384, and 1536 wells. The plates shown here are of black polyethylene with clear bottoms to allow various detection devices to measure fluorescence, transmission or optical images. Other versions of microplates with identical geometries are available in white or clear manufactured from a variety of plastics (Figure kindly supplied by Greiner BioOne)

All screens in HTS fall into one of two classes; biochemical and cellular. The distinction between them is obvious; the latter utilizes whole, live cells and the former isolated proteins. Both types can be further subdivided according to the technique as homogeneous or heterogeneous. The distinction among these classes is the requirement for a separation step in the technique. Almost without exception, HTS assays are biased toward homogenous techniques. A great deal of research and development effort has been expended in this area and a plethora of technologies exist today. Therefore we will examine only a few major techniques in each class as illustrations.

2.1.1. Biochemical Assays

The ability to measure the binding of a ligand to a receptor and subsequently deduce the affinity of a second ligand by its ability to displace it is a fundamental principle of receptor biology. The radioligand binding assay became the mainstay of drug discovery through the 1980s and 1990s *(29)*. In manual form, these assays are cumbersome and involve incubation of radioactively labeled ligands with purified receptors and filtration of precipitated proteins after washing with an acid such as trichloroacetic acid (TCA). Although these assays can be automated *(30)* the handling of large amounts of radioactivity and the heterogeneous nature of the technique made an alternative necessary.

The development of technologies such as scintillation proximity assays (SPA) and microplate based counters allowed most radioligand binding assays to be moved to a homogenous format *(31–35)*. In SPA the ligand of interest is labeled with a weak Beta particle emitting radioactive species such as ^{3}H, ^{125}I or ^{33}P. An acceptor protein such as a receptor or antibody is then bound to fluoro-microsphere beads embedded with scintillant. When these beads are exposed to radioactive emissions they will emit photons of light. SPA is a homogenous technique because the radioligands that are used have very short quenching distances in aqueous environments such that the radioligand will only produce a signal when it is directly bound to the bead. For example, a ^{3}H beta particle will only penetrate $1.5\,\mu m$ in water or aqueous buffer solutions. Because the concentration of labeled ligand in these assays is usually in the nanomolar range, the chance of beads and labeled ligand being in close enough proximity to generate a signal is vanishingly small whereas a high affinity binding event may bring hundreds of them in contact with each bead thus creating a signal that is many fold above the random "noise" level. SPA beads are available with a broad range of attachment chemistries making the technique usable in many enzymatic assays and even in some cellular screens *(36)*.

Because of the large numbers of samples in HTS and safety and disposal considerations most practitioners today prefer to use fluorescent detection techniques. Two of the more widely used techniques are fluorescent polarization (FP) and time resolved fluorescence (TRF). Both are homogeneous techniques, which take advantage of unique properties of fluorescent molecules.

Fluorescence polarization relies on the principles of anisotropy *(37)*. When polarized light is used as the emission source for a fluorescent probe, the natural emission dipole of the probe will cause the intensity of emitted light to be stronger in one dimension. If the fluorescent molecule is fixed in space, its emitted light will be polarized in the same direction as the source illumination. But fluorescent probes in solution are constantly rotating. The rate of rotation will skew the polarization of the emitted light in a manner directly proportional to the rate of rotation. By measuring the polarized emission from two axes, the relative rotation of the probe molecule can be monitored. Because the rate of rotation is proportional to the size of the molecule, this can be used to measure a binding event between a small molecule and a protein. A small molecule will produce approximately equal readings in each axis but when its rotation is slowed by binding it to a large protein, which may be a thousand fold more massive, the change in rotation will be measurable shifted toward the polarized, stimulating light. This technique has been broadly applied against many target classes *(38–44)*. It has the added advantage of being insensitive to fluorescent inference from test compounds thereby reducing noise levels in the screen.

Similarly, time resolved fluorescence (TRF also called HTRF for homogenous time resolved fluorescence) relies on unique properties of certain fluorescent molecules. It combines the principle of fluorescence resonance energy transfer (FRET) and long half life emissions of lanthanides. In FRET, two fluorescent molecules are paired as a donor and acceptor. As individual molecules, each behaves as a normal fluorophore governed by excitation and emission spectra. These molecules are chosen such that the peak emission wavelength of the donor and the excitation of the acceptor overlap. When the pair is excited at the donor wavelength then only the emission spectra of the donor will be detected. However, when stimulated by the emission spectra of the donor probe when such they are sufficiently close, usually about 10 nm, there is a direct energy transfer among the dipoles of the molecules and emission will occur at the acceptor wavelength *(45,46)*. This technique is very valuable in its own right as a detection method in HTS. In TRF the acceptor is a long wavelength lanthanide *(47–49)*. These molecules have long decay emissions that will endure for milliseconds after stimulation by an exciting wavelength. When the donor excitation is provided by a pulsed energy source then the unbound donor emissions will decay quickly and the longer lasting emissions from the acceptor can be read free of interference.

2.1.2. Cellular Assays

As with their biochemical counterparts, there are a wide variety of technologies and techniques for performing HTS using whole cells *(18,50–54)*. Early screens using live cells tended to be simple viability tests and often involved testing compounds for their ability to differentially kill disease derived cell lines, such as tumor lines, and cell lines derived from normal tissues. In more modern approaches, the cells used are from clonal, immortalized cell lines over expressing a target of choice. Cell based assays tend to be more complex because the cells must remain viable during testing but the additional effort is repaid by the fact that many important targets such as GPCRs and ion channels can only be assayed in a functional format in a live cell.

One breakthrough technology in cellular HTS was the development of the FLIPR device *(55)*. This device allowed researchers to record fluorescent images from all 96 wells in a microplate simultaneously and collect that data in subsecond intervals in real time for a cell population. The primary application of FLIPR was to monitor calcium flux using a fluorescent dye (Fluo-3 or Fluo-4), which is inactive until metabolized by intracellular esterases and then binds calcium and shows increased fluorescence when bound to divalent cations. Because Gq linked GPCRs induce releases of intracellular stores of calcium and many ion channels induce a direct increases in calcium, this technique enabled high throughput testing of several important target classes *(56)*.

Calcium flux and similar techniques are commonly called functional cellular assays because they measure a single cellular function or the function of a single overexpressed protein. Many other technologies have been developed to monitor different aspects of cellular function including alternate calcium measures *(57)*, intracellular c-AMP levels *(58–62)* and ubiquitination of beta arrestin to monitor GPCR function *(63–66)* to name just a few.

Another commonly used technique in cellular HTS is the reporter assay. By linking the expression of an easily measured enzyme to a transcription pathway of interest, changes in activity in response to external stimuli will produce altered levels in the reporter enzyme. The most common of these is luciferase *(67–71)*. Luciferase interacts with its substrate luciferin to produce luminescence and is the source of the firefly's glow. Cells with a greater response will literally glow more brightly. There are many other reporter proteins including β-galactosidase, green fluorescent proteins and β-lacatamase *(18)*.

As technology has increased the ability to process images and the resolution with which they can be electronically captured a new method combining confocal microscopy and unique fluorescent labels has emerged. This technique allows the monitoring of subcellular localization of proteins and morphological changes in cells. Because of the amount of data that can be captured from a single read it is commonly known as High Content Screening (HCS) *(72)*. The complexity of the technique and the amount of data processing involved, usually restricts HCS to lower throughout assays rather than true HTS usage.

2.1.3. Microfluidics

Microfluidics is another technology that is new to HTS but is becoming widely applied. This technique utilizes submillimeter channels etched or cast into a solid substrate such as plastic, glass or quartz *(73–80)*. Fluid flow through these channels can be precisely controlled by pressure or voltage gradients. It is an example of a technology that muddies the simple distinction between homogenous and heterogeneous techniques because it allows many operations to be performed on a single chip including separation technologies *(74,75,78,81)*. The most common of these is the application of capillary electrophoresis to separate charged proteins. Therefore, microfluidics is most commonly used for enzymatic assays although it has also been utilized for cellular screens *(82,83)*. The combination of precise control in mixing and reaction with the removal pipeting errors also makes microfluidics much more precise than standard microplate based techniques.

2.1.4. Statistical Analysis in Assay Design

A screen was earlier defined as an assay that has been statistically validated by repeated testing to be relevant, reproducible, repeatable and robust. The issue of relevance is established by comparing the HTS assay with known drugs (if they exist) or with the behavior of known modifiers in established lower throughout assays. It must be mentioned that every HTS scientist will encounter targets for which no control compounds exist. This is both exciting and worrisome; these targets are usually very novel and potentially groundbreaking but it can be very difficult to establish a relationship to disease models.

Reproducibility means that the assay must produce the same results over time. Repeatability implies that one will obtain the same results from a replicate measure. Robustness is the ability of the assay to fulfill the former requirements when additional variables such as operating environment, operator, automated systems, or protein lot are introduced. This will usually be measured both by simply performing the assay over time and by measuring the effect of known control compounds or drugs *(16,84–86)* This step is extremely important because the company will commit tens to hundreds of thousands of dollars of resources in performing the screen. This is accentuated by the fact that most HTS labs are organized into separate assay development and screening operations functions. Therefore, the assay development scientist must create a product that is sufficiently robust and well documented that another team, possibly in another country, can seamlessly bring that screen onto an automated platform and trust that it will produce accurate data.

Statistics is integrated from the very beginning of the assay development process. Many HTS laboratories routinely employ Statistical Design of Experiments (DOE) *(88)*. In DOE, all the components in an experimental system are varied systematically and then multivariate analysis is used to calculate their individual contribution to the overall effect. This gives the researcher the power to find optimal components and their concentrations as well as deducing positive and negative synergistic reactions from a single experiment. Automated systems for DOE have been developed and deployed in many HTS labs *(89)*.

There are also several statistical parameters that are employed after an assay has been developed. Basic good laboratory practice dictates that each experiment must have controls. In HTS these controls will almost always include a maximal activity control, a minimal activity or background control and at least one inhibitor control. The inhibitor may be tested at multiple concentrations as well. Data from all these controls is analyzed over multiple runs to provide validation that the assay is running correctly and is "in control" *(84,87)*. The last step of assay development is usually a validation of the assay where it is tested over a fixed period. This can be a predetermined number of microplates with or without test compounds in replicate over multiple runs.

The data from this validation can be calculated in a number of ways. The most common assay diagnostic is the z'-factor (Z Prime Factor) *(90)*. The z' factor is a derived signal to noise calculation, which measures the ratio of the noise in an assay to the window between maximal and minimal activity controls. It is calculated by the equation:

$$z' = 1 - \frac{3\sigma_{max} \text{ x } \sigma_{min}}{\left| \mu_{max} - \mu_{min} \right|}$$

Where mean = (μ), standard deviation = (σ), maximum control = (max) and minimum control = (min); ($\mu_{max}, \sigma_{min}, \mu_{max}, \sigma_{min}$, respectively)

A z' value of greater than 0.5 is generally accepted as the measure of an acceptable assay. A common mistake in describing assay controls is to confuse signal to noise with signal to background *(5,90)*. The former is a valid measurement of the noise in a system expressed as a ratio of the signal whereas the latter is simply the ratio of the maximal control over minimal control and is essentially meaningless in HTS. This is true because the background is often an arbitrary number determined by instrument settings and its size has no impact on the ability to discriminate between the activities of samples.

It also good practice to monitor the run to run variation of each control parameter to ensure that these values are within acceptable limits. The definition of "acceptable limits" may vary depending on the assay type and technology used. For example, a radioactive assay employing ^{33}P will experience a drop in its maximal control value over time as the isotope decays but remains valid as long as the z' values are acceptable. The same type of variation in a fluorescent based microfluidic assay will indicate a loss of activity and should be investigated.

2.2. Chemical Library Management

The assembly and management of chemical compound libraries has evolved from a secondary consideration to one of central importance in HTS. In most companies, the compound library is treated as a valuable corporate asset and managed centrally. This allows global corporations to ensure consistency across many testing sites.

The most basic concept in building a chemical library is chemical diversity. This is a mathematical representation of how different chemical compounds are from one another (91–99). These calculations are quite complex and usually involve sets of descriptors, which are variables describing different attributes of a chemical. They will range from very simple factors such as molecular weight to complex calculations describing the distance between specific types of molecular bonds. The goal is to create a collection of molecules, which represents as broad coverage as possible of potential drugs with the minimum number of samples. Once an active molecule or series of molecules is found, they can be expanded by further chemical synthesis.

Compound libraries usually contain molecules from a variety of sources. Corporate libraries contain a core set of compounds representing the accumulated synthetic efforts of all their chemists. These compounds usually represent close analogues of series that were created for specific programs and are not very diverse, which has led to active programs to expand library diversity through acquisition of commercial compound collections and from custom synthesis. Aggressive efforts in library expansion have led to the creation of collections that number in the millions (100), which have, in turn, led to the creation of automated systems to support them.

It is virtually impossible to handle hundreds of thousands of samples per day in a powder format. Even with automation, the task of accessing and retrieving that many individual samples, let alone weighing and solubilizing them, could not be managed cost effectively. But that many samples must be fed into every HTS operation every day. The solution to this problem is the creation of presolubilized compounds stored in microplates. Because HTS labs have robotic systems already in place for handling and pipeting into and from microplates, having the compounds in the same format facilitates the transfer of compounds into the screening plates.

Library management must, therefore, work in three distinct phases; dry sample management, solublization and plate based or liquid phase library management. Although any of these steps can be accomplished in a basic laboratory setting, each of them requires specialized equipment for high throughput implementation.

Automation systems supporting library management are the largest and costliest systems in HTS. A typical system that can store several million samples with random access store and retrieve capacity can be roughly the size of a high school gymnasium with robotically accessed sample carousels or stacks

3–4 m high in a controlled environment *(101–108)*. Usually, there are separate, specialized systems for dry samples and for solubilized compounds. Because weighing is the most labor intensive step in the process, enough sample will be aliquoted to support an operation for a period of several years.

The solvent Dimethylsulfoxide (DMSO) is the industry standard for compound solubilization. Although DMSO is widely regarded as a universal solvent and can solubilize most compounds, it does not, by any means, dissolve all chemicals and has properties that can make it difficult to handle *(109–114)*. Pure DMSO freezes at 18°C but it also readily absorbs water and drastically changes its behavior *(115)*. With a water content of 18%, the freezing point is suppressed to −20°C and at just over 30% it drops to a low of −73°C. It also penetrates human skin readily making it very dangerous when potent pharmacological compounds are held in solution. The viscosity of DMSO changes as drastically as its phase diagram, which can confound pipeting accuracy in automation. Nevertheless, no viable substitute has been found and the operational concerns of HTS prevent the use of multiple solvents so DMSO remains ubiquitous in HTS.

Once solubilized, the compound library is normally stored in separately addressable tubes or directly in microplates. Each has advantages. There are many commercially available systems for storing compounds in microtubes *(105–108)*. Most use arrays of tubes stored in bar-coded plastic racks in the same format as 96- or 384-well microplates. These tubes can also be marked with two-dimensional barcodes to verify their identity and location. The main advantage of tube based storage is the ability to individually locate and pick ("cherry pick") compounds then re-array them. This is done to access samples as they are required for additional testing. Another common usage of tube systems is to create plate formatted arrays that can be transferred to microplates for further processing or for storage. This can involve entire libraries or sets that have been chosen to give activity in a particular type of assay, also known as a focused library. All tube based storage systems use some level of automation and thus are more costly. Plate based systems, on the other hand, can be as simple as a freezer and an inventory system or can involve elaborate automated retrieval modules.

The logistics and process between solubilization and testing will vary considerably from company to company but there are some factors that are common to most operations. The first of these is the process of transferring small volumes of all the wells in a plate into a series of plates that are stored for usage in a screen. These plates are commonly referred to as mother and daughter plates. Another common term is master plate, which usually refers to a tube array that will be used to create mother plates but it is sometimes used interchangeably with mother plate. These schemas can be very complex and can involve hundreds of plates. An example from the author's compound preparation laboratory is shown in **Fig. 60.2**.

2.3. Screening Operations

Now that an assay is developed and a library assembled, we can consider the actual process of running a screen. Screening Operations is the heart of any HTS lab and the location where actual screening takes place. The process of discovering active molecules using HTS involves several steps. These are designed to increase efficiency and reduce the number of downstream false positive molecules. Each process is examined in more detail below.

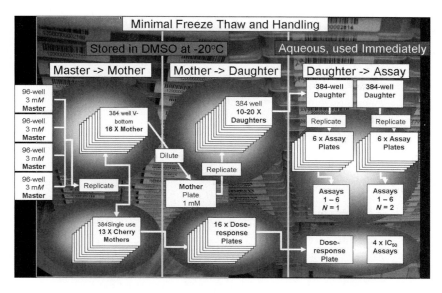

Fig. 60.2. Plate flow in library management at Amphora Discovery. Purified compounds are received in 96 well microtubes and combined to make 384 well master plates. These are completely used to make 10 m*M* mother plates and cherry mothers (source plates for cherry picking). Each mother plate is then diluted to 1 m*M* and further replicated to make daughter plates, which are stored frozen. As needed, daughter plates are thawed, diluted with aqueous buffer and replicated into assay plates

2.3.1. Automation

Some level of automation will always be involved in HTS. Unless Screen Development was carried out on identical equipment, the assay must be adapted to the automated systems that will be used in running the screen. In general, there are two broad classes of automation; unit automation and fully automated or integrated systems (*5,116,117*). Unit automation is a system that is designed to perform a single task. These systems may incorporate stacking systems to allow batch processing of large numbers of plates (**Fig. 60.3**). Fully automated systems are an assembly of unit systems integrated with a method of plate handling, which will allow unattended operation (*5*). Often these systems will involve very complex industrial robotic systems and can operate unattended for long periods of time (**Fig. 60.4**). In all cases, it is prudent to revalidate the screen using the actual automation and protocol that will be executed for the screen.

2.3.1.1. Unit Automation: Very efficient screening is possible using only unit automation but usually requires more staff. Unit automation can be divided by function. The major types are examined below.

2.3.1.1.1. Liquid Handling: Liquid handling systems are specifically designed to pipet or dispense liquid into microplates. Liquid handlers are available that are compatible with all formats of plates. Pipetors have arrays of tips, which are configured in the same format as the microplate in use. Most can aspirate, or draw liquid into the tips, and dispense that liquid precisely into a destination plate. Systems are available that can accurately work with volumes ranging

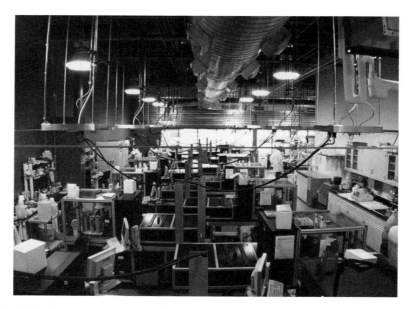

Fig. 60.3. Unit automation as configured at Amphora Discvoery. Caliper LifeSciences HTS250 microfluidics systems are arrayed for optimal processing as unit automation devices. Liquid handling systems are positioned at the sides and ends of the laboratory and plates are manipulated in stacks

from 10 nl to 100 μl *(28)*. Bulk dispensers have similar ranges of accuracy but are only designed to add liquid to plates. The primary advantage of dispensers is the speed with, which they can process plates. Most systems of this type can fill a 384-well plate in less than 10 s.

2.3.1.1.2. Plate Storage and Incubation: A typical day of HTS may test 100,000 or more samples in each assay. This equates to over 1,000 individual 96-well plates, 260–384-well plates, or 65–1,536-well plates. For integrated systems, these plates must be loaded into the system and then stored during the incubation phase of the assay. These systems may also have integrated plate storage capacity for the chemical library, allowing multiple screens without the need to reload new compounds. For purely unit automation operations, there is still a need to store and retrieve large quantities of microplates and there may be an additional requirement to maintain constant temperature and humidity conditions. The former, primarily, for cellular assays and the latter for high density plates where evaporation is an issue. Incubators in fully automated systems will have robotically accessible doors and an internal mechanism to pick and place plates in a storage carousel. Although these systems can also be utilized as stand alone workstations in unit automation, the more common solution is to simply use standard incubators and manually load microplates as stacks.

2.3.1.1.3. Detection Instrumentation: The final step in a screen is usually a quantitative read of each well. As was discussed in Section 2.1, many types of detection technologies are use in HTS. Microplate based readers exist for each of them. Most of these instruments will accept a plate either from a robotic

A

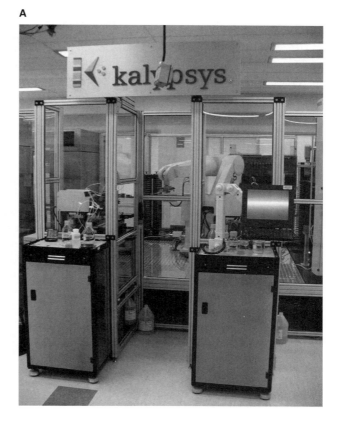

B

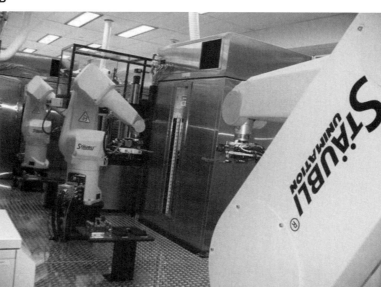

Fig. 60.4. The fully automated Kalypsys screening system in use at the National Chemical Genomics Center (NCGC) in Bethesda Maryland. The room-size Kalypsys screening system used by NCGC features industrial refrigeration and storage units (**A**) while the system's Staubli "anthropomorphic" robot arm assembly (**B**) is shown in the midst of system installation. The compound archive and assay incubator carousels, compound and reagent dispensers and multiple detectors are located around the robotic arms. The Kalypsys suite of ultrahigh-throughput screening technologies can evaluate the biological activity of more than 1 million chemical compounds per day (figure kindly supplied by Jim Inglese and Chris Austin)

system, a stacker or a manual feed. Many instruments are configured to read all of the wells in a plate simultaneously either by using a complex network of fiber optic feeds or by direct imaging. These devices can read an entire plate in a matter of seconds for simple fluorescent or luminescent detection. It should be noted that this includes the most common types of radioactive detection such as SPA. This has led to the development of complex CCD camera based imaging systems that can read several output modes very rapidly *(118–123)*. This area of HTS is complex and constantly changing with new modes of detection constantly under development.

2.3.2. Logistics

A former colleague in HTS once boasted that he managed more line items that Walmart. This is quite true and the need for supply chain management in HTS cannot be underestimated. In many organizations a screen will be referred to as a campaign and the logistics underlying a successful operation are as complex. Before beginning a screen, all the reagents and consumables for the entire run must be assembled. It is preferred to have all these from a single manufacturing lot, especially for biological reagents because any variation on activity can lead to quality control problems and variability in assay results. The correct equipment must also be made available for the expected duration of the screen. This can lead to queues of targets and add to the timelines of testing. This can be simplified by specializing operations on a single technology or target type but this approach requires sufficient scale to justify the additional cost.

2.3.3. Screening

Screening is the culmination of the processes described so far. In a well managed and maintained HTS operation this should be routine. The duration of a screen can extend from days to weeks depending on the number of samples tested and the equipment employed. The screen will be tested according to a fixed protocol or Standard Operating Procedure (SOP). This allows comparability of data between batches and days of operation. Simplified protocols for an enzymatic and cellular screen are shown in **Fig. 60.5**. The screen must be constantly monitored for performance and quality control in real time. The controls that were developed as part of the Screen Development Process will suffice to monitor the overall integrity of the data but the screen introduces the additional variable of chemical compounds that may have both systematic and random effects on the assay.

2.3.4. Data Reduction and Analysis

The final goal of HTS is to relate a single activity number to every compound. All HTS detectors provide an output associated with each well and the Laboratory Information Management System (LIMS) will then need to calculate a value that can be stored in a database for later retrieval and comparison. The most common calculation is percent inhibition. The maximum activity control value is related to the minimum activity control and then the impact of a compound is linearly related as a percent change. This can be represented by the formula:

$$\%\text{Inh}(X) = 100 - \frac{(X - \text{Min})}{(\text{Max} - \text{Min})}$$

Enzymatic Screen

Step	Component	Volume (µl)
1	Compounds diluted to 50 mM in buffer	5
2	Enzyme	10
3	Incubate (15 minutes to 1 hour)	
4	Substrate (s)	10
5	Incubate (15 minutes to 1 hour)	
6	Stop Solution (terminate enzymatic reaction)	25
7	Read	

Cellular Reporter Screen

Step	Component	Volume (µl)
1	Add Cells at ~2000/well	25
2	Incubate overnight – allow to adhere and grow to confluency	
3	Wash cells to exchange culture media	
4	Fresh culture media (usually serum free)	20
5	Compounds diluted to 50 mM in buffer	5
6	Incubate (1– 48 hours)	10
7	Add development reagents	10
8	Incubate (15 minutes to 1 hour)	
9	Read	

Fig. 60.5. Simplified enzymatic and cellular protocols as implemented for HTS

X is the returned value for the compound of interest
Min is the average minimum control value
Max is the average maximum control value

Once this data is processed, the LIMS system will retrieve the associated compound identifier using barcode information and the identifier of the screen. Quality control information can then be calculated and reviewed *(84,85)*. If the screen is acceptable, the data is usually loaded into a database where it is accessible to project scientists and available for further processing. If it fails QC, the compounds will need to be repeated.

2.3.5. Hit Selection

The most basic purpose of a screen is to identify active compounds but first one must define "active". The simplest method of finding actives is to set an arbitrary cutoff point, such as 50% inhibition, and query the database for compounds that meet that criterion. The level of 50% is used as a surrogate for the more complex measure of IC50 where the concentration that produces an inhibition of 50% is determined by a dose titration. Increasingly complex methods have been devised to take advantage of the sensitivity of more modern assay techniques. For example, the variation of the entire screen can be used to calculate the standard deviation of the controls and three times this level (3 sigma) is used as a threshold level for actives *(86)*. For normally distributed samples this means that 99.7% of the values will be below the cutoff. This has become more important with the recognition that many compounds are not present at the expected concentration *(123)*. Most HTS labs test all compounds at a fixed concentration such as $10\,\mu M$. Because compounds may be present at much lower concentrations it is important to include weakly active compounds until the actual concentration can be determined.

2.3.6. Confirmation and Potency Testing

After a hit list is compiled the active compounds will usually be resupplied or cherry picked for confirmation. This can take the form of simply repeating the assay at the initial concentration or can be combined with potency testing. This will often depend on the expected confirmation rate. Confirmation rates in HTS are generally quite low, ranging between 20% and 60% *(125,126)*. That is to say a compound detected as active in a screen will actually test positive again with that rate. However, it is possible to configure an HTS system where error is controlled and these rates approach 90% *(127)* and the confirmation step can be omitted. Confirmation testing is usually undertaken by the Screening Operations Group on the same equipment.

3. Applications

Although developed for drug discovery, HTS is now widely used in many industries and academia. It has also broadened within each. In Academia HTS is being applied to discovery chemical probes that can be used in basic research. The US National Institutes of Health (NIH) began a program in 2004 to create a series of interconnected screening centers as part of its Molecular Libraries Screening Initiative *(128,129)*. In the industries where it is already established, HTS techniques are now being used to perform more complex assays and large scale titrations. Often the latter are the next step in the process of developing a molecule such as selectivity testing where all the confirmed hits may be tested against a fixed panel of assays to identify possible negative side effects.

So what is HTS? It is complex and evolving tool that is broadly used in many aspects of scientific research today.

References

1. Pharmaceutical Research and Manufacturers of America (2006) Pharmaceutical industry profile 2004. Washington, DC: PhRMA, http://www.phrma.org/
2. DiMasi J (2001) New drug development in the United States from 1963 to 1999. Clin Pharmacol Therap 69:286–296
3. DiMasi J, Hansen R, Grabowski H (2003) The price of innovation, estimates of drug development costs. J Health Economics 22:151–185
4. Booth B, Zemmel R (2004) Prospects for productivity. Nat Rev Drug Discovery 3:451–456
5. Hopp, Spearman (1996) Factory physics. Richard D Irwin, Chicago
6. Fox S, Farr-Jones S, Sopchak L, Boggs A, Comley J (2004) High-throughput screening: searching for higher productivity. J Biomol Screen 9:354–358
7. Fleming A (1929) On the antibacterial action of cultures of penicillium, with special reference to their use in the isolation of B Influenza. Br J Exp Med 10:226–236

8. Chain EB, Florey HW, Gardner AD, Heatley NG, Jennings MA, Orr-Ewing J, Sanders AG (1940) Penicillin as a chemotherapeutic agent. Lancet 2:226–228

9. Sneader W (1985) Drug discovery: the evolution of modern medicines. John Wiley, NY

10. Smith C (1992) The process of new drug discovery and development. CRC, Boca Raton, FL

11. Watson JD, Crick FHC (1953) Mol Structure Nucleic Acids. Nature 171:737–738

12. McCullough JM (1976) Genetic engineering, human genetics, and cell biology: U.S. Govt. Printing Office, Washington, DC

13. Geysen HM, Meleon RH, Barteling SJ (1984) Use of peptide synthesis to probe viral antigens for epitopes to a resolution of a single amino acid. Proc Natl Acad Sci 81:3998–4002

14. Houghton RA (1985) General method for the rapid solid-phase synthesis of large numbers of peptides: specificity of antigen-antibody interactions at the level of individual acids. Proc Natl Acad Sci 82:5131–5135

15. Turk B (2006) Targeting proteases: successes, failures and future prospects. Nat Rev Drug Discovery 5:785–799

16. Hertzberg R (2002) Design and implementation of high throughput screening. In: Janzen W (ed) High throughput screening methods and protocols. Humana, Totowa, NJ, pp 1–29

17. Imming P, Sinning C, Meyer A (2006) Drugs, their targets and the nature and number of drug targets. Nat Rev Drug Discovery 5:821–834

18. Johnston P (2002) Cellular assays in HTS. In: Janzen W (ed) High throughput screening methods and protocols Humana, Totowa, NJ, pp 107–116

19. Coecke S, Eskes, C, Gartion J, van Vliet E, Kinsner A, Bogni A, Raimondo L, Parissis N, Langezaal I (2002) Metabolism and neurotoxicity: the significance of genetically engineered cell lines and new three-dimensional cell cultures ATLA 30, **Suppl** 2:115–118

20. Darrow A, Conway K, Vaidya A, Rosenthal D, Wildey M, Minor L, Itkin Z, Kong Y, Piesvaux J, Qi J, Mercken M, Andrade-Gordon P, Plata-Salamán C, Ilyin S (2003) Virus-based expression systems facilitate rapid target in vivo functionality validation and high-throughput screening. J Biomol Screening 8:65–71

21. Xin H, Bernal A, Amato A, Pinhasov A, Kauffman J, Brenneman D, Derian C, Andrade-Gordon P, Plata-Salamán C, Ilyin S (2004) High-Throughput siRNA-based functional target validation. J Biomol Screening 9:286–293

22. Haberman A (2005) Targets and druggablity for small and large molecule drugs. Genetic Engineering News 25:36

23. Bleicher K, Bohm HJ, Muller K, Allanine A (2003) Strategies to move beyond target validation. Nat Rev Drug Discovery 3:369–278

24. Collins I, Workman P (2006) New approaches to molecular cancer therapeutics. Nat Chem Biol 2:689–700

25. Comley J, Reeves T, Robinson P (1998) A 1536 Colorimetric SPAP reporter assay: comparison with 96- and 384-well formats. J Biomol Screening 3:217–225

26. Fox S, Farr-Jones S, Sopchak L, Boggs A, Comley J (2004) High-throughput screening: searching for higher productivity. J Biomol Screening 9:354–358

27. Oldenburg K, Zhang JH, Chen T, Maffia A, Blom K, Combs A, Chung T (1998) Assay miniaturization for ultra-high throughput screening of combinatorial and discrete compound libraries: a 9600-well (0.2 microliter) assay system. J Biomol Screening 3:55–62

28. Berg M, Undisz K, Thiericke R, Zimmermann P, Moore T, Posten C (2001) Evaluation of liquid handling conditions in microplates. J Biomol Screening 2:47–56

29. Christopoulos A (2002) Allosteric binding sites on cell-surface receptors: novel targets for drug discovery. Nat Rev Drug Discovery 1:198–210

30. Kulanthaivel P, Hallock Y, Boros C, Hamilton S, Janzen W, Ballas L, Loomis C, Jiang J (1993) Balanol: a novel and potent inhibitor of protein kinase C from the fungus *Verticillium balanoides*. JACS 115:6452–6453

31. Udenfriend S, Gerber L, Nelson N (1987) Scintillation proximity assay: a sensitive and continuous isotopic method for monitoring ligand/receptor and antigen/antibody interactions. Anal Biochem 161:494–500

32. Bosworth N, Towers P (1989) Scintillation proximity assay. Nature 341:16

33. Carpenter J, Laethem C, Hubbard F, Eckols T, Baez M, McClure D, Nelson D, Johnston P (2002) Configuring radioligand receptor binding assays for hts using scintillation proximity assay technology: In: Janzen W (ed) High throughput screening methods and protocols. Humana, Totowa, NJ. pp 31–49

34. Cook N (1996) Scintillation proximity assay – a versatile high throughput screening technology. Drug Discovery Today 1:287–294

35. van der Hee R, Deurholt T, Gerhardt C, de Groene E (2005) Comparison of 3 AT1 receptor binding assays: filtration assay, ScreenReady™ Target, and WGA Flashplate®. J Biomol Screening 10:118–126

36. Fox S (1996) Amersham offers Cytostar-T for cell based assay techniques. Gen Eng News 16:10–11

37. Perrin F (1926) Polarization de la lumiere de fluorescence. Vie moyenne de molecules dans l'etat excite. J Phys Radium 7:390

38. Weber G (1953) Rotational Brownian motion and polarization of the fluorescence of solutions. Adv Protein Chem 8:415

39. Jolley M (1981) Fluorescence polarization immunoassay for the determination of therapeutic drug levels in human-plasma. J Anal Toxicol 5:236–240

40. Jolley M (1996) Fluorescence polarization assays for the detection of proteases and their inhibitors. J Biomolr Screening 1:33–38

41. Banks P, Gosselin M, Prystay L (2000) fluorescence polarization assays for high throughput screening of g protein-coupled receptors. J Biomol Screening 5:159–167

42. Gaudet E, Huang K, Zhang Y, Huang W, Mark D, Sportsman R (2003) A homogeneous fluorescence polarization assay adaptable for a range of protein serine/threonine and tyrosine kinases. J Biomol Screening 8:164–175

43. Owicki J (2000) Fluorescence polarization and anisotropy in high throughput screening: perspectives and primer. J Biomol Screening 5:297–306

44. Banks P, Harvey M (2002) Considerations for using fluorescence polarization in the screening of G protein-coupled receptors. J Biomol Screening 7:111–117

45. Selvin P (1995) Fluorescence resonance energy transfer. Methods Enzymol 246:300–334

46. Wu P, Brand L (1994) Resonance energy transfer: methods and applications. Anal Biochem 218:1–13

47. Preaudat M, Ouled-Diaf J, Alpha-Bazin B, Mathis G, Mitsugi T, Aono Y, Takahashi K, Takemot H (2002) A homogeneous caspase-3 activity assay using HTRF(R) technology. J Biomol Screening 7:267–274

48. Pope A (1999) Introduction LANCETM vs. HTRF(R) technologies (or vice versa). J Biomol Screening 4:301, 302

49. Mathis G (1999) HTRF(R) technology. J Biomol Screening 4:309–313

50. Yan Y, Boldt-Houle D, Tillotson B, Gee M, D'Eon B, Chang X, Olesen C, Palmer M (2002) J cell-based high-throughput screening assay system for monitoring G protein-coupled receptor activation using {beta}-galactosidase enzyme complementation technology. J Biomol Screening 7:451–459

51. Beske O, Guo J, Li J, Bassoni D, Bland K, Marciniak H, Zarowitz M, Temov V, Ravkin I, Goldbard S (2004) A novel encoded particle technology that enables simultaneous interrogation of multiple cell types. J Biomol Screening 9:173–185

52. Ghosh R, DeBiasio R, Hudson C, Ramer E, Cowan C, Oakley R (2005) Quantitative cell-based high-content screening for vasopressin receptor agonists using transfluor(R)technology. J Biomol Screening 10:476–484

53. Miraglia S, Swartzman E, Mellentin-Michelotti J, Evangelista L, Smith C, Gunawan I, Lohman K, Goldberg E, Manian B, Yuan P (1999) Homogeneous

cell- and bead-based assays for high throughput screening using fluorometric microvolume assay technology. J Biomol Screening 4:193–204

54. Davis G, Downs T, Farmer J, Pierson R, Roesgen J, Cabrera E, Nelson S (2002) Comparison of high throughput screening technologies for luminescence cell-based reporter screens. J Biomol Screening 7:67–77

55. Schroeder K, Neagle B (1996) FLIPR: a new instrument for accurate, high throughput optical screening. J Biomol Screening 3:75–80

56. Baxter D, Kirk M, Garcia A, Raimondi A, Holmqvist M, Flint K, Bojanio D, Distefano P, Curtis R, Xie Y (2002) A novel membrane potential-sensitive fluorescent dye improves cell-based assays for ion channels. J Biomol Screening 2:79–85

57. Brini M, Marsault R, Bastianutto C, Alvarez J, Pozzan T, Rizzuto R (1995) Transfected aqueorin in the measurement of cytosolic Ca2+ concentration (Ca2+C): a critical evaluation. J Biol Chem 270:9896–9903

58. Kariv I, Stevens M, Behrens D, Oldenburg K (1999) High throughput quantitation of cAMP production mediated by activation of seven transmembrane domain receptors. J Biomol Screening 4:27–32

59. Prystay L, Gagne A, Kasila P, Yeh L, Banks P (2001) Homogeneous cell-based fluorescence polarization assay for the direct detection of cAMP. J Biomol Screening 6:75–82

60. Allen M, Hall D, Collins B, Moore K (2002) A homogeneous high throughput non-radioactive method for measurement of functional activity of Gs-coupled receptors in membranes. J Biomol Screening 7:35–44

61. Golla R, Seethala R (2002) A homogeneous enzyme fragment complementation cyclic AMP screen for GPCR agonists. J Biomol Screening 7:515–525

62. Chiulli A, Trompeter K, Palmer M (2000) A novel high throughput chemiluminescent assay for the measurement of cellular cyclic adenosine monophosphate levels. J Biomol Screening 5:239–247

63. Selkirk J, Nottebaum L, Ford I, Santos M, Malany S, Foster A, Lechner S (2006) A novel cell-based assay for G-protein-coupled receptor-mediated cyclic adenosine monophosphate response element binding protein phosphorylation. J Biomol Screening 11:351–358

64. Vrecl M, Jorgensen R, Pogacnik A, Heding A (2004) Development of a BRET2 screening assay using {beta}-arrestin 2 mutants. J Biomol Screening 9:322–333

65. Ghosh R, DeBiasio R, Hudson C, Ramer E, Cowan C, Oakley R (2005) Quantitative cell-based high-content screening for vasopressin receptor agonists using transfluor(R)technology. J Biomol Screening 10:476–484

66. Hamdan F, Audet M, Garneau P, Pelletier J, Bouvier M (2005) High-throughput screening of G protein-coupled receptor antagonists using a bioluminescence resonance energy transfer 1-based {beta}-arrestin2 recruitment assay. J Biomol Screening 10:463–475

67. Shimomura O, Johnson F, Masugi T (1969) Cypridina bioluminescence: light-emitting oxyluciferin-luciferase complex. Science 164:1299, 1300

68. Terstappen G, Giacometti A, Ballini E, Aldegheri L (2000) Development of a functional reporter gene HTS assay for the identification of mGluR7 modulators. J Biomol Screening 5:255–261

69. Nieuwenhuijsen B, Huang Y, Wang Y, Ramirez F, Kalgaonkar G, Young K (2003) A dual luciferase multiplexed high-throughput screening platform for protein–protein interactions. J Biomol Screening 8:676–684

70. Kolb A, Neumann K (1996) Luciferase measurements in high throughput screening. J Biomol Screening 1:85–88

71. George S, Bungay P, Naylor L (1997) Evaluation of a CRE-directed luciferase reporter gene assay as an alternative to measuring cAMP accumulation. J Biomol Screening 2:235–240

72. Giuliano K, DeBiasio R, Dunlay T, Gough A, Volosky J, Zock J, Pavlakis G, Taylor DL (1997) High-content screening: a new approach to easing key bottlenecks in the drug discovery process. J Biomol Screening 6:249–259

73. Kamholz AE, Weigl BH, Finlayson BA, Yager P (1999) Quantitative analysis of molecular interaction in a microfluidic channel: the T-sensor. Anal Chem 71:5340–5347

74. Macounova K, Cabrera CR, Holl MR, Yager P (2000) Generation of natural pH gradients in microfluidic channels for use in isoelectric focusing. Anal Chem 72:3745–3751

75. Hadd AG, Raymond DE, Halliwell JW, Jacobson SC, Ramsey JM (1997) Microchip device for performing enzyme assays. Anal Chem 69:3407–3412

76. Duffy DC, Gillis HL, Lin J, Sheppard NF, Kellogg GJ (1999) Microfabricated centrifugal microfluidic systems: characterization and multiple enzymatic assays. Anal Chem 71:4669–4678

77. Hadd AC, Jacobson SC, Ramsey JM (1999) Microfluidic assays of acetylcholinesterase inhibitors. Anal Chem 71:5206–5212

78. Macounova K, Cabrera CR, Yager P (2001) Concentration and separation of proteins in microfluidic channels on the basis of transverse IEF. Anal Chem 73:1627–1633

79. Eteshola E, Leckband D (2001) Development and characterization of an ELISA assay in PDMS microfluidic channels. Sensors and Actuators B-Chemical 72:129–133

80. Yang TL, Jung SY, Mao HB, Cremer PS (2001) Fabrication of phospholipid bilayer-coated microchannels for on-chip immunoassays. Anal Chem 73: 165–169

81. Perrin D, Fremaux C, Besson D, Sauer W, Scheer A (2006) A microfluidics-based mobility shift assay to discover new tyrosine phosphatase inhibitors J Biomol Screening 11:108–112

82. Sohn LL (2000) Capacitance cytometry: measuring biological cells one by one. Proc Natl Acad Sci USA 97:10687–10690

83. Young S, Curry M, Ransom J, Ballesteros J, Prossnitz E, Sklar L, Edwards B (2004) High-throughput microfluidic mixing and multiparametric cell sorting for bioactive compound screening. J Biomol Screening 9:103–111

84. Gunter B, Brideau C, Pikounis Y, Liaw A (2003) Statistical and graphical methods for quality control determination of high-throughput screening data. J Biomol Screening 8:624–633

85. Gribbon P, Lyons R, Laflin P, Bradley J, Chambers C, Williams B, Keighley W, Sewing A (2005) Evaluating real-life high-throughput screening data. J Biomol Screening 10:99–107

86. Woodward P, Williams C, Sewing A, Benson N (2006) Improving the design and analysis of high-throughput screening technology comparison experiments using statistical modeling. J Biomol Screening 11:5–12

87. Gunter B, Brideau C, Pikounis B, Liaw A (2003) Statistical and graphical methods for quality control determination of high-throughput screening data. J Biomol Screening 12: 8:624–633

88. Altekar M, Homon CA, Kashem MA, Mason SW, Nelson RM, Patnaude LA, Yingling J, Taylor PB (2006) Assay optimization: a statistical design of experiments approach. J Assoc Lab Automation 11:33–41

89. Sherrill T, Snider J, Terpstra N, Vanderpool C, Schmidt W (1999) Accelerating assay development using experimental design and integrated liquid handling. J Assoc Lab Automation 4:76–84

90. Zhang JH, Chung TD, Oldenburg KR (1999) A simple statistical parameter for use in evaluation and validation of high throughput screening assays. J Biomol Screening 4:67–73

91. Balaban AT (1979) Five new topological indices for the branching of tree-like graphs. Theoretica Chimica Acta 53:355–375

92. Balaban AT (1982) Highly discriminating distance-based topological index. Chem Phys Lett 89:399–404

93. CRC Handbook of Chemistry and Physics (1994). CRC, Boca Ratan, FL

94. Wildman SA, Crippen GM (1999) Prediction of physiochemical parameters by atomic contributions. J Chem Inf Comput Sci 39:868–873

95. Gasteiger J, Marsali M (1980) Iterative partial equalization of orbital electronegativity – a rapid access to atomic charges. Tetrahedron 36:3219

96. Hall LH, Kier LB (1991) The molecular connectivity chi indices and kappa shape indices in structure–property modeling. Rev Computational Chem 2:367–422

97. Hall LH, Kier LB (1997) The nature of structure–activity relationships and their relation to molecular connectivity. Eur J Med Chem Chimica Therapeutica 4:307–312

98. Petitjean M (1992) Applications of the radius-diameter diagram to the classification of topological and geometrical shapes of chemical compounds. J Chem Inf Comput Sci 32:331–337

99. Wiener H (1947) Structural determination of paraffin boiling points. J Am Chem Soc 69:17–20

100. Soderholm J, Uehara-Bingen M, Weis K, Heald R (2006) Challenges facing the biologist doing chemical genetics. Nat Chem Biol 2:55–58

101. Provis J (2005) Compound management and enhancement activities in astrazeneca. J Assoc Lab Automation 10:124–129

102. Moore KW, Chandler G, Whalley P, Gannon D, Simpson PB (2006) Efficient sample logistics: from the chemist to the assay plate and beyond. J Assoc Lab Automation 11:92–99

103. Brideau C, Hunter J, Maher J, Adam S, Fortin LJ, Ferentinos J (2004) SOS – a sample ordering system for delivering "assay-ready" compound plates for drug screening. J Assoc Lab Automation 9:123–127

104. Solomon FJ, DeChard CS, Donnenberg R (2006) The design, development, and implementation of a fully automated compound distribution center. J Assoc Lab Automation 11:138–144

105. Gedrych M (2000) Automated compound storage and retrieval system for microplates and tubes. J Assoc Lab Automation 5:24–25

106. Schopfer U (2005) The novartis compound archive: from concept to reality. Comb Chem High Throughput Screen 8:213

107. Beggs M, Blok H, Mertens J (1999) Stacker modules used in a high-capacity robotics system for high throughput screening compound replication. J Biomol Screening 4:373–379

108. Harrison W (1997) The importance of automated sample management systems in realizing the potential of large compound libraries in drug discovery. J Biomol Screening 2:203–206

109. Cheng X, Hochlowski J, Tang H, Hepp D, Beckner C, Kantor S, Schmitt R (2003) Studies on repository compound stability in dmso under various conditions. J Biomol Screening 8:292–304

110. Tjernberg A, Markova N, Griffiths W, Hallen D (2006) DMSO-related effects in protein characterization. J Biomol Screening 11:131–137

111. Kozikowski B, Burt T, Tirey D, Williams L, Kuzmak B, Stanton D, Morand K, Nelson S (2003) The effect of freeze/thaw cycles on the stability of compounds in DMSO. J Biomol Screening 8:210–215

112. Kozikowski B, Burt T, Tirey D, Williams L, Kuzmak B, Stanton D, Morand K, Nelson S (2003) The effect of room-temperature storage on the stability of compounds in DMSO. J Biomol Screening 8:205–209

113. Semin D, Malone T, Paley M, Woods P (2005) A novel approach to determine water content in DMSO for a compound collection repository. J Biomol Screening 10:568–572

114. Balakin K, Ivanenkov Y, Skorenko A, Nikolsky Y, Savchuk N, Ivashchenko A (2004) In silico estimation of dmso solubility of organic compounds for bioscreening. J Biomol Screening 9:22–31

115. Rasmussen D, Mackenzie A (1969) Phase diagram for the system water Â–dimethylsulphoxide. Nature 220:1315–1317

116. Menke K (2002) Unit automation in high throughput screening, In: Janzen W. (ed) High throughput screening methods and protocols. Humana, Totowa, NJ, pp 195–212

117. Cohen S, Trinka R (2002) Fully automated screening systems. In: Janzen W (ed) High throughput screening methods and protocols. Humana, Totowa, NJ, pp 213–228

118. Hodder P, Mull R, Cassaday J, Berry K, Strulovici B (2004) Miniaturization of intracellular calcium functional assays to 1536-well plate format using a fluorometric imaging plate reader. J Biomol Screening 9:417–426

119. George J, Teear ML, Norey CG, Burns DD (2003) Evaluation of an imaging platform during the development of a fret protease assay. J Biomol Screening 8:72–80

120. Sorg G, Schubert H, Buttner FH, Heilker R (2002) Automated high throughput screening for serine kinase inhibitors using a LEADSeekerTM scintillation proximity assay in the 1536-well format. J Biomol Screening 7:11–19

121. Ramm P, Alexandrov Y, Cholewinski A, Cybuch Y, Nadon R, Soltys B (2003) Automated screening of neurite outgrowth. J Biomol Screening 8:7–18

122. Skwish S, Asensio F, Gregking Clarke G, Kath G, Salvatore MJ, Dufresne C (2004) FIZICS: fluorescent imaging zone identification system, a novel macro imaging system. J Biomol Screening 9:663–370

123. Popa-Burke IG, Issakova O, Arroway JD, Bernasconi P, Chen M, Coudurier L, Galasinski S, Janzen WP, Lagasca D, Liu D, Lewis RS, Mohney RP, Sepetov N, Sparkman DA, Hodge CN (2004) Streamlined system for purifying and quantifying a diverse library of compounds and the effect of compound concentration measurements on the accurate interpretation of biological assay results. Analytical Chemistry 76:7278–7287

124. Jager S, Garbow N, Kirsch A, Preckel H, Gandenberger FU, Herrenknecht K, Rudiger M, Hutchinson JP, Bingham RP, Ramon F, Bardera A, Martin J (2003) A modular, fully integrated ultra-high-throughput screening system based on confocal fluorescence analysis techniques. J Biomol Screening 8:648–659

125. Fogel P, Collette P, Dupront A, Garyantes T, Guedini D (2002) The confirmation rate of primary hits: a predictive model. J Biomol Screening 7:175–190

126. Hubert CL, Sherling SE, Johnston PA, Stancato LF (2003) Data concordance from a comparison between filter binding and fluorescence polarization assay formats for identification of ROCK-II inhibitors. J Biomol Screening 8:399–409

127. Janzen WP, Hodge CN (2006) A chemogenonic approach to discovering target selective drugs. Chem Biol Drug Design 67:85–86

128. Kaiser J (2004) NIH gears up for chemical genomics. Science 304:1728

129. http://mli.nih.gov/index.php

Index

Printed in the United States of America